P9-CQB-879

ANESTHESIA EQUIPMENT: PRINCIPLES AND APPLICATIONS

ANESTHESIA EQUIPMENT: PRINCIPLES AND APPLICATIONS

Second Edition

Jan Ehrenwerth, MD
Professor of Anesthesiology
Yale University School of Medicine
New Haven, Connecticut

James B. Eisenkraft, MD
Professor of Anesthesiology
Icahn School of Medicine at Mount Sinai
New York, New York

James M. Berry, MD
Professor of Anesthesiology
Vanderbilt University Medical Center
Nashville, Tennessee

ELSEVIER
SAUNDERS

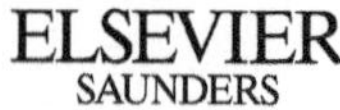

SAUNDERS

1600 John F. Kennedy Blvd.
Ste 1800
Philadelphia, PA 19103-2899

ANESTHESIA EQUIPMENT: PRINCIPLES AND APPLICATIONS, SECOND EDITION ISBN 978-0-323-11237-6

Notices

Knowledge and best practice in this field are constantly changing. As new research and experience broaden our understanding, changes in research methods, professional practices, or medical treatment may become necessary.

Practitioners and researchers must always rely on their own experience and knowledge in evaluating and using any information, methods, compounds, or experiments described herein. In using such information or methods they should be mindful of their own safety and the safety of others, including parties for whom they have a professional responsibility.

With respect to any drug or pharmaceutical products identified, readers are advised to check the most current information provided (i) on procedures featured or (ii) by the manufacturer of each product to be administered, to verify the recommended dose or formula, the method and duration of administration, and contraindications. It is the responsibility of practitioners, relying on their own experience and knowledge of their patients, to make diagnoses, to determine dosages and the best treatment for each individual patient, and to take all appropriate safety precautions.

To the fullest extent of the law, neither the Publisher nor the authors, contributors, or editors, assume any liability for any injury and/or damage to persons or property as a matter of products liability, negligence or otherwise, or from any use or operation of any methods, products, instructions, or ideas contained in the material herein.

ISBN 978-0-323-11237-6

Executive Content Strategist: William Schmidt
Content Specialist: Joanie Milnes
Publishing Services Manager: Patricia Tannian
Project Manager: Carrie Stetz
Design Direction: Louis Forgione

Printed in the United States of America

Last digit is the print number: 9 8 7 6 5 4 3 2

To my wonderful wife, Mary Ann, without whose love and encouragement this book would not have been possible

Jan Ehrenwerth

To Gail, Michelle, and Jonathan, my loving family

James B. Eisenkraft

To my collaborator of 35 years, Dr. Elizabeth Heitman, who has always been my role model as an editor

James M. Berry

Contributors

Michael A. Acquaviva, MD
Assistant Professor of Clinical Anesthesia, Riley Hospital for Children, Indianapolis, IN
Breathing Circuits

Brenton Alexander, BS
University of California Irvine School of Medicine, Irvine, CA
Blood Pressure Monitoring

Steven J. Barker, MD, PhD
Professor and Head, Department of Anesthesiology, Professor of Aerospace Engineering, University of Arizona, Tucson, AZ
Pulse Oximetry

Richard Beers, MD
Associate Chief of Anesthesia, Veterans Administration Medical Center; Professor of Anesthesiology, SUNY Upstate Medical University, Syracuse, NY
Infection Prevention: Recommendations for Practice

James M. Berry, MD
Professor of Anesthesiology, Vanderbilt University Medical Center, Nashville, TN
Monitoring Ventilation; Perioperative Informatics; Vigilance, Alarms, and Integrated Monitoring Systems; Ergonomics of the Anesthesia Workspace

Gerardo Bosco, MD, PhD
Assistant Professor, Department of Biomedical Sciences, University of Padova, Italy
Anesthesia at High Altitude

Sorin J. Brull, MD
Professor of Anesthesiology, Mayo Clinic College of Medicine, Jacksonville, FL
Monitoring Neuromuscular Blockade

Enrico Camporesi, MD
Professor of Anesthesiology, University of South Florida, Tampa, FL
Anesthesia at High Altitude; Anesthesia in Difficult Locations and in Developing Countries

Maxime Cannesson, MD
Associate Professor of Clinical Anesthesiology, Department of Anesthesiology and Perioperative Care, University of California Irvine School of Medicine, Irvine, CA
Blood Pressure Monitoring

Jeffrey B. Cooper, PhD
Professor of Anesthesia, Harvard Medical School; Department of Anesthesia, Critical Care & Pain Medicine, Massachusetts General Hospital; Executive Director, Center for Medical Simulation, Boston, MA
Risk Management and Medicolegal Aspects of Anesthesia Equipment

Stephen F. Dierdorf, MD
Professor and Vice Chair, Department of Anesthesia, Indiana University School of Medicine, Indianapolis, IN
Pediatric Anesthesia Systems and Equipment

Jan Ehrenwerth, MD
Professor of Anesthesiology, Yale University School of Medicine, New Haven, CT
Medical Gases: Storage and Supply; Electrical and Fire Safety

John H. Eichhorn, MD
Professor of Anesthesiology, College of Medicine, Provost's Distinguished Service Professor, University of Kentucky, Lexington, KY
Machine Checkout and Quality Assurance

James B. Eisenkraft, MD
Professor of Anesthesiology, Icahn School of Medicine at Mount Sinai, New York, NY
The Anesthesia Machine and Workstation; Anesthesia Vaporizers; Waste Anesthetic Gases and Scavenging Systems; Respiratory Gas Monitoring; Monitoring Ventilation; Hazards of the Anesthesia Delivery System

Roger Eltringham, MB
Consultant Anesthesiologist, Gloucestershire Royal Infirmary, Gloucester, United Kingdom
Anesthesia in Difficult Locations and in Developing Countries

Chris R. Giordano, MD
Assistant Professor of Anesthesiology, Department of Anesthesiology, University of Florida College of Medicine, Gainesville, FL
Capnography

Nikolaus Gravenstein, MD
The Jerome H. Modell, MD, Professor of Anesthesiology, Professor of Neurosurgery and Periodontology, Department of Anesthesiology, University of Florida College of Medicine, Gainesville, FL
Capnography

Simon C. Hillier, MB ChB
Professor of Anesthesiology and Pediatrics, Dartmouth Medical School, Dartmouth Hitchcock Medical Center, Lebanon, NH
Pediatric Anesthesia Systems and Equipment

Robert S. Holzman, MD
Senior Associate in Perioperative Anaesthesia, Children's Hospital Boston; Professor of Anaesthesia, Harvard Medical School, Boston, MA
Anesthesia Delivery in the MRI Environment

Nicole Horn, MD
Assistant Professor of Clinical Anesthesia, Riley Hospital for Children, Indianapolis, IN
Breathing Circuits

Michael B. Jaffe, PhD
Advanced Technology, Philips Respironics, LLC, Wallingford, CT
Respiratory Gas Monitoring; Standards and Regulatory Considerations

Ken B. Johnson, MD
Professor and Director, Center for Patient Simulation, Carter M. Ballinger Presidential Chair in Anesthesiology, Department of Anesthesiology, University of Utah, Salt Lake City, UT
Simulation Equipment, Techniques, and Applications

Wilton C. Levine, MD
Assistant Professor, Department of Anesthesia, Critical Care & Pain Medicine; Associate Medical Director of the Operating Rooms, Perioperative Services, Massachusetts General Hospital, Boston, MA
Infusion Pumps

Robert G. Loeb, MD
Associate Professor of Anesthesiology, University of Arizona, Tucson, AZ
Ergonomics of the Anesthesia Workspace

S. Nini Malayaman, MD
Assistant Professor of Anesthesiology, Drexel University College of Medicine, Philadelphia, PA
Medical Gases: Storage and Supply

Keira P. Mason, MD
Senior Associate in Perioperative Anesthesia, Director of Radiology Anesthesia and Sedation, Children's Hospital Boston; Associate Professor of Anaesthesia, Harvard Medical School, Boston, MA
Anesthesia Delivery in the MRI Environment

Diana G. McGregor, MB BS
Clinical Professor, Department of Anesthesiology, Stanford University School of Medicine, Stanford, CA
Waste Anesthetic Gases and Scavenging Systems

William L. McNiece, MD
Associate Professor, Division of Pediatric Anesthesia, Department of Anesthesia, Indiana University School of Medicine, Indianapolis, IN
Pediatric Anesthesia Systems and Equipment

Raj K. Modak, MD
Assistant Professor of Anesthesiology, Assistant Director of Cardiac Anesthesia-TEE, Director, PACU, Yale University School of Medicine, New Haven, CT
Anesthesia Ventilators

George Mychaskiw II, DO
Chair, Department of Anesthesiology, Nemours Children's Hospital, Orlando, FL
Medical Gases: Storage and Supply

Mohamed Naguib, MD
Professor of Anesthesiology, Department of General Anesthesiology, Anesthesiology Institute, Cleveland Clinic, Cleveland, OH
Monitoring Neuromuscular Blockade

Jolie Narang, MD
Director of Neurointerventional Anesthesia, Department of Anesthesiology, Montefiore Medical Center, Bronx, NY
Electrocardiographic Monitoring

Michael A. Olympio, MD
Professor of Neuroanesthesiology, Wake Forest Baptist Medical Center, Winston-Salem, NC
Anesthesia Ventilators

David G. Osborn, ME(E)
International Standards Manager, Philips Healthcare, Andover, MA
Standards and Regulatory Considerations

Bijal R. Parikh, MD
Attending Anesthesiologist and Clinical Instructor, Department of Anesthesia and Perioperative Medicine, Saint Barnabas Medical Center, Livingston, NJ
Temperature Monitoring

James H. Philip, ME(E), MD, CCE
Anesthesiologist and Director of Bioengineering, Department of Anesthesiology, Perioperative and Pain Medicine, Brigham and Women's Hospital; Professor of Anaesthesia, Harvard Medical School, Boston, MA
Closed-Circuit Anesthesia

Timothy J. Quill, MD
Professor of Anesthesiology, Dartmouth-Hitchcock Medical Center, Lebanon, NH
Blood Pressure Monitoring

Henry Rosenberg, MD
Director, Department of Medical Education and Clinical Research, Saint Barnabas Medical Center, Livingston, NJ; President, Malignant Hyperthermia Association of the United States
Temperature Monitoring

William H. Rosenblatt, MD
Professor of Anesthesiology, Yale University School of Medicine, New Haven, CT
Airway Equipment

Brian S. Rothman, MD
Assistant Professor of Anesthesiology, Vanderbilt University Medical Center, Nashville, TN
Monitoring Ventilation

Keith J. Ruskin, MD
Professor of Anesthesiology and Neurosurgery, Yale University School of Medicine, New Haven, CT
Computing and the Internet in Clinical Practice

Harry A. Seifert, MD, MSCE
Adjunct Assistant Professor of Clinical Anesthesiology, The Children's Hospital of Philadelphia, Philadelphia, Pennsylvania
Electrical and Fire Safety

Maire Shelly, MB
Consultant in Intensive Care Medicine, Acute Intensive Care Unit, University Hospital of South Manchester, Manchester, United Kingdom
Humidification and Filtration

George Sheplock, MD
Associate Professor of Clinical Anesthesia, Riley Hospital for Children, Indianapolis, IN
Breathing Circuits

David G. Silverman, MD
Professor of Anesthesiology, Director of Departmental Clinical Research, Yale University School of Medicine, New Haven, CT
Monitoring Neuromuscular Blockade

Theodore Craig Smith, MD
Professor of Anesthesiology (retired), University of Pennsylvania, Philadelphia, PA
Breathing Circuits

Craig Spencer
Consultant in Anaesthesia & Critical Care, Lancashire Teaching Hospitals, Preston, United Kingdom
Humidification and Filtration

Collin Sprenker
Research Coordinator, Florida Gulf-to-Bay Anesthesiology, Tampa, FL
Anesthesia in Difficult Locations and in Developing Countries

Paul St. Jacques, MD
Associate Professor, Quality and Patient Safety Director, Department of Anesthesiology, Vanderbilt University Medical Center, Nashville, TN
Perioperative Informatics

Tracey Straker, MD, MPH
Associate Professor of Clinical Anesthesiology, Albert Einstein College of Medicine; Director of Advanced Airway Rotation, Montefiore Medical Center, New York, NY
Airway Equipment

John T. Sullivan, MD, MBA
Associate Chief Medical Officer, Northwestern Memorial Hospital, Residency Program Director, Associate Professor of Anesthesiology, Northwestern University Feinberg School of Medicine, Chicago, IL
Risk Management and Medicolegal Aspects of Anesthesia Equipment

Elizabeth M. Thackeray, MD, MPH
Assistant Professor, Department of Anesthesiology, University of Utah, Salt Lake City, UT
Simulation Equipment, Techniques, and Applications

Daniel M. Thys, MD
Professor Emeritus, Department of Anesthesiology; Chairman Emeritus, Department of Anesthesiology, St. Luke's-Roosevelt Hospital Center, College of Physicians & Surgeons, Columbia University, New York, NY
Electrocardiographic Monitoring

Steven G. Venticinque, MD
Professor of Clinical Anesthesiology and Surgery, University of Texas Health Science Center at San Antonio, San Antonio, TX
Machine Checkout and Quality Assurance

Kyle A. Vernest
Senior Clinical Engineer, Department of Anesthesia, Critical Care, and Pain Medicine, Massachusetts General Hospital, Boston, MA
Infusion Pumps

Scott G. Walker, MD
Director of Pediatric Anesthesia, Associate Professor of Clinical Anesthesia, Riley Hospital for Children, Indianapolis, IN
Breathing Circuits

Matthew B. Weinger, MD
Professor of Anesthesiology, Biomedical Information, and Medical Education; Director, Center for Research & Innovation in Systems Safety; Vanderbilt University School of Medicine and the VA Tennessee Valley Healthcare System, Nashville, TN
Vigilance, Alarms, and Integrated Monitoring Systems; Ergonomics of the Anesthesia Workspace

Ross H. Zoll, MD, PhD
Partner, Atlantic Anesthesia, Virginia Beach, VA
Noninvasive Temporary Pacemakers and Defibrillators

FOREWORD

It is paradoxical that in the late twentieth century, when anesthesia machines and equipment were much simpler, reading *Anesthesia Equipment: Principles and Applications* edited by Drs. Jan Ehrenwerth and James Eisenkraft was mandatory. At that time in most health care facilities, the absence of on-site–trained technicians made each anesthesia caregiver his or her own biomedical technician. Analogous to early aviators, anesthesia caregivers were required to understand the mechanics of their equipment as well as make minor repairs. Today, anesthesia workstations and equipment are complex and computer based. Now there is an information explosion from multiple e-media sources. Does this absolve health care providers from possessing an intimate knowledge of the basics of their equipment? The answer is a resounding no! If anything, the second edition of *Anesthesia Equipment: Principles and Applications* becomes even more important, as the clinician is continually bombarded with data on the well-being of his or her equipment. Deciphering early clues from a potential equipment failure and addressing them in a timely fashion can mean the difference between an uneventful anesthetic procedure and one with a significant complication or adverse outcome.

For this edition, Jan Ehrenwerth and James Eisenkraft are joined by James Berry. All are acknowledged leaders in this field. Incorporating vital material from the first edition, they have completely redesigned this seminal publication. Keeping an easy-to-read and understandable style, they have spent a huge amount of time revising the graphics and tables. The figures are clear and crisp, with the associated educational message easy to understand. Indeed, the editors are so compulsive that even the colors in graphs explaining vaporizer operation are color coded (sevoflurane = yellow, desflurane = blue, and isoflurane = purple). The tables are clear and not so overloaded with data that they become unreadable. The chapters, written by experts in specific areas, follow a template, which enhances their ability to deliver a message clearly and rapidly and augments their educational value. Parenthetically, two of the chapters written by the editors are so outstanding that I recommend them to candidates preparing for their oral board examinations and now the recertification examination. Chapter 3, "Anesthesia Vaporizers," dissects the inner workings of the modern vaporizer and, perhaps more important, adroitly deals with the nuances of vaporizer malfunction in a clinical setting. Chapter 31, "Electrical and Fire Safety," makes these topics so understandable that readers may think they could be an electrical engineer or fire marshal!

The real strength of the second edition of *Anesthesia Equipment: Principles and Applications* lies in the breadth of topics covered. This is not an anesthesia workstation book. Rather, it addresses areas that the clinician is likely to encounter on an everyday basis. The last part of the book, *Safety, Standards, and Quality*, brings all the chapter themes together under the larger topic of patient safety, a core value of our specialty. It addresses such provocative topics as risk management and the development and impact of regulations and standards.

The editors have taken a very complex group of topics, and by use of their skills as clinicians and educators, have made the material meaningful to the novice as well as seasoned attending clinicians. In looking at the value of the book, perhaps Albert Einstein said it best: "Everything should be made as simple as possible, but not simpler."

Paul Barash, MD
Professor of Anesthesiology
Yale University School of Medicine
New Haven, CT

PREFACE

Anesthesia equipment and technologies have evolved significantly since publication of the first edition of *Anesthesia Equipment: Principles and Applications* 20 years ago. In many areas the function of the equipment (e.g., anesthesia workstation) remains the same, but the process has changed to make the systems more accurate, more reliable, and compatible with electronic medical record-keeping and data handling systems. There are many potential benefits to be gained from these largely computer-based advances, such as better ergonomics, intelligent alarm systems, and unlimited potential for data mining to help improve outcomes. This evolution has necessitated an increasing appreciation of the more sophisticated equipment that we use on a daily basis. In 2003, the journal *Anesthesia and Analgesia* added a section on Technology, Computing, and Simulation, with Steven J. Barker, MD, PhD, serving as the first section editor. In an accompanying editorial entitled "Too much technology," Barker[1] cautioned against "black box complacency" and concluded that "Today's problem is not simply too much reliance on technology. Our problem is not enough education in the basis of technology, its limitations, its relationship with physiology, and its integrated use in patient care." His challenge to the reader was to improve "technoeducation" for the benefit of future anesthesiologists and the safety of our patients. This book is intended to meet that challenge.

As in the first edition, the approach taken to describe equipment is first to define the principles of operation, including, where applicable, the physics and technologic aspects. Once the principles of operation are understood, the applications and limitations should be a logical continuation. Clinical relevance and safety aspects have been emphasized throughout.

This volume is organized into seven parts. Part I, *Gases and Ventilation*, covers this topic as used in contemporary anesthesia delivery systems for inhaled anesthetics. Although we focus on systems used in the United States, the principles should be applicable to other systems used elsewhere. Obsolete systems have been omitted except where they may be useful to illustrate important principles. This particularly applies in the case of measured flow vaporizing systems, such as the Copper Kettle and Verni-Trol.

Part II, *System Monitors*, discusses the basic monitors of the anesthesia delivery system that ensure correct functioning.

Part III, *Patient Monitors*, describes the additional equipment used for basic anesthetic monitoring as defined by the standards most recently published by the American Society of Anesthesiologists.

Part IV describes *Other Equipment* that is not logically categorized in other groups.

Part V covers *Computers, Alarms, and Ergonomics*. These features are the basis of the distinction between contemporary systems and their predecessors.

Part VI describes *Special Conditions* in which anesthesia delivery systems may be used, as well as the principles of closed circuit anesthesia techniques.

Part VII includes chapters related to *Safety, Standards, and Quality*. Studies of critical incidents and adverse outcomes involving anesthesia equipment continue to show that pure failure of equipment is uncommon, whereas use error and failure to recognize spurious data are the leading culprits.

There is extensive coverage of most anesthesia equipment; omitted are ultrasound and echocardiography equipment, as well as rapid infusion systems. There is also no discussion of cardiopulmonary bypass or extracorporeal oxygenation hardware and techniques. These devices are omitted because they are somewhat specialized, not exclusive to anesthesiology practice, and are extensively covered in other texts. There is a significant allocation of space to safety, standards, and regulatory issues, along with quality assurance topics.

The editors wish to acknowledge the hard work of all those who have made this second edition possible, especially the contributors, without whose expertise this book would not exist. We would also like to thank the many equipment manufacturers for supplying technical information and outstanding illustrations.

We would also like to acknowledge all of those who have taught and mentored us throughout the years. Finally, we are grateful to the outstanding staff at Elsevier, especially Joanie Milnes, Carrie Stetz, and William Schmitt, who greatly facilitated the production and publication of this text.

Jan Ehrenwerth, MD
New Haven, CT

James B. Eisenkraft, MD
New York, NY

James M. Berry, MD
Nashville, TN

1. Barker SJ. Too much technology? *Anesth Analg* 97:938–939, 2003.

CONTENTS

PART VI
SPECIAL CONDITIONS

PART VII
SAFETY, STANDARDS, AND QUALITY

PART I

GASES AND VENTILATION

CHAPTER 1

MEDICAL GASES: STORAGE AND SUPPLY*

S. Nini Malayaman • George Mychaskiw II • Jan Ehrenwerth

CHAPTER OUTLINE

OVERVIEW

Anesthesia providers were once expected to know a great deal about the storage and supply of medical gases. In both large and small institutions, anesthesiologists often had to rely on their own knowledge and skill in this area to manage the many aspects of medical gases, from purchasing to troubleshooting.

Changes in technology and institutional organization have relieved the anesthesiologist of the majority of these responsibilities. However, this should not excuse anesthesia providers from understanding the basic facts and safety principles associated with the use of medical gases for anesthesia. Invariably, other health care providers and administrators have little knowledge regarding these systems and look to anesthesia professionals for guidance in the use and handling of these gases in the hospital or clinic setting.

With few exceptions, the only medical gases encountered by practicing anesthesiologists today are oxygen, nitrous oxide, and medical air. For safety reasons, flammable agents are rarely, if ever, used in operating rooms (ORs) today. Nitrogen is used almost exclusively to power gas-driven equipment. Helium, carbon dioxide, and premixed combinations of oxygen and helium or carbon dioxide are generally no longer used. In certain uncommon clinical situations, other gases may be used. Helium is occasionally used as an adjunct in the ventilation of patients undergoing laryngeal surgery because of its low density and flow-enhancing characteristics. Carbon dioxide is infrequently used in the management of anesthesia for repair of selected congenital heart defects. Finally, nitric oxide is currently available for use as a pulmonary vasodilator. Anesthesiologists who use these gases must be fully versed in their characteristics and safe handling. For detailed information and numerous references relating to the handling and use of these and other unusual medical gases, along with a wealth of general information about medical gas cylinders, the reader is directed to publications from the Compressed Gas Association.[1,2]

*Portions of this chapter are reproduced by permission from Eisenkraft JB: The anesthesia delivery system, part I, vol 3. In *Progress in Anesthesiology*, San Antonio, TX, 1989, Cannemiller Memorial Education Foundation.

Medical gas manufacturers are subject to more stringent government and industry regulations and inspections than they have been in the past. This has helped markedly reduce the number of accidents related to medical gases. For these reasons, anesthesia training programs may not emphasize instruction in the various aspects of storing and using medical gases.

In addition, the recent increased concern regarding the safety of anesthetized patients has helped reduce the number of gas-related injuries. Inspired oxygen monitors with lower limit alarms provide the anesthesia practitioner with an early warning when the oxygen supply becomes inadequate or is contaminated with another gas. Mixed-gas monitoring and analysis is also becoming more common and provides the practitioner with an important way to quickly detect contaminants or unusual gas mixtures before the patient is injured. If the oxygen monitor fails, pulse oximetry can alert the anesthesiologist to problems with patient oxygenation related to inadequate oxygen supply.

MEDICAL GAS CYLINDERS AND THEIR USE

Medical gases are stored either in metal cylinders or in the reservoirs of bulk gas storage and supply systems. The cylinders are almost always attached to the anesthesia gas machine. Bulk supply systems use pipelines and connections to transport medical gases from bulk storage to the anesthesia machine.

Virtually all facilities in which anesthesia is administered are equipped with central gas supply systems. Anesthesia practice is currently undergoing change in this regard, and many anesthetics are administered outside the OR, and even outside the hospital, where a central gas supply system may be unavailable. The current emphasis on providing care away from the hospital—such as in dental clinics, mobile lithotripsy units, and mobile magnetic resonance imaging facilities—will only increase the demands on the anesthesia provider to ensure a safe and continuous gas supply. E-cylinders are sometimes the only source of medical gas for anesthesia machines in these settings. If an anesthetic is being administered using only E-cylinders, then *both* the anesthesiologist and related support personnel must first ensure that an adequate supply of reserve cylinders is available. In addition, the amount of gas in the cylinders being used must be continually monitored, and the cylinders must be replaced before they are completely emptied. The importance of this cannot be overemphasized. Many anesthesia practitioners today have not been confronted with the possibility of running out of oxygen and having to change a tank while administering an anesthetic—but the evolving nature of anesthesia practice away from traditional facilities is likely to make this a more common occurrence. If an anesthesiologist anticipates this situation, it is imperative that the anesthesia machine be equipped with two oxygen cylinder yokes so that oxygen delivery can continue when the empty tank is changed.

Anesthesia practitioners should be familiar with two sizes of gas cylinders. The cylinder most often used by anesthesia providers is the E-cylinder, which is approximately 2 feet long and 4 inches in diameter. E-cylinders are also routinely used as portable oxygen sources, such as when a patient is transported between the OR and an intensive care unit (ICU). H-cylinders are larger, approximately 4 feet long and 9 inches in diameter, and are generally used as a source of gas for small or infrequently used pipeline systems. They may be used as an intermediate or long-term source of gas at the patient's bedside. Almost all hospitals store H-cylinders of oxygen in bulk as a back-up source in case the pipeline oxygen fails or is depleted. H-cylinders of nitrogen are often used to power gas-driven medical equipment. H-cylinders that contain oxygen, nitrous oxide, or air have occasionally been used in ORs and are connected to the anesthesia machine via special reducing valves and hoses. Such uncommon configurations are not only potentially hazardous, they also defeat certain safeguards. Any practitioner who uses such a system must become thoroughly familiar with it and must be certain it complies with applicable regulations and guidelines.[1-5]

Oxygen Tanks

Oxygen (O_2) has a molecular weight of 32 and a boiling point of −183° C at an atmospheric pressure of 760 mm Hg (14.7 pounds per square inch in absolute pressure [psia]). The boiling point of a gas—that is, the temperature at which it changes from liquid to gas—is related to ambient pressure in such a way that as pressure increases, so does the boiling point. However, a certain *critical temperature* is reached, above which it boils into its gaseous form no matter how much pressure is applied in the liquid phase. The critical temperature for oxygen is −118° C, and the *critical pressure*, which must be applied at this temperature to keep oxygen liquid, is 737 psia. Because room temperature is usually 20° C and therefore in excess of the critical temperature, oxygen can exist only as a gas at room temperature.

E-cylinders of oxygen are filled to approximately 1900 pounds per square inch gauge pressure (psig) at room temperature: 1 atmosphere (atm) is 760 mm Hg, which equals 0 psig or 14.7 psia. At high pressures, psig and psia are virtually the same. When full, the cylinders contain a fixed number of gas molecules, the so-called *fixed mass* of that gas. These gas molecules obey Boyle's law, which states that pressure times volume equals a constant ($P_1V_1 = P_2V_2$), provided temperature does not change. A full E-cylinder of oxygen with an internal volume of 5 L (V_1) and a pressure of 1900 psia (P_1) will therefore evolve approximately 660 L (V_2) of gaseous oxygen at atmospheric pressure (P_2, or 14.7 psia). Thus Boyle's law gives the approximate value:

$$V_2 = (P_1 \times V_1) / P_2 = (1900 \times 5) / 14.7 = 660 \text{ L}$$

If the oxygen tank's pressure gauge reads 1000 psig, the tank is approximately 50% full (1000 ÷ 1900) and will evolve only 330 L (660 × 50%) of oxygen (Fig. 1-1). If such a tank were to be used at an oxygen flow rate of 6 L/min, it would empty in just under an hour (330 ÷ 6 = 55 minutes). Likewise, a full (2200 psig) H-cylinder will evolve 6900 L of oxygen at atmospheric pressure. It is important to understand these principles when oxygen tanks are being used to supply the machine or a ventilator or to transport a patient. Because oxygen exists only as a gas at room temperature, the tank's pressure gauge can be

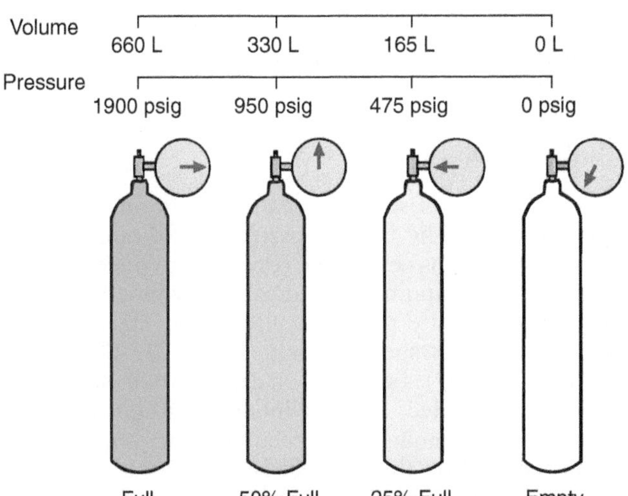

FIGURE 1-1 ■ Oxygen remains a gas under high pressure. The pressure falls linearly as the gas flows from the cylinder; thus, in contrast to nitrous oxide, the pressure remaining always reflects the amount of gas remaining in the cylinder. (Modified from Bowie E, Huffman LM: *The anesthesia machine: essentials for understanding,* 1985. With permission from Datex-Ohmeda, Madison, WI.)

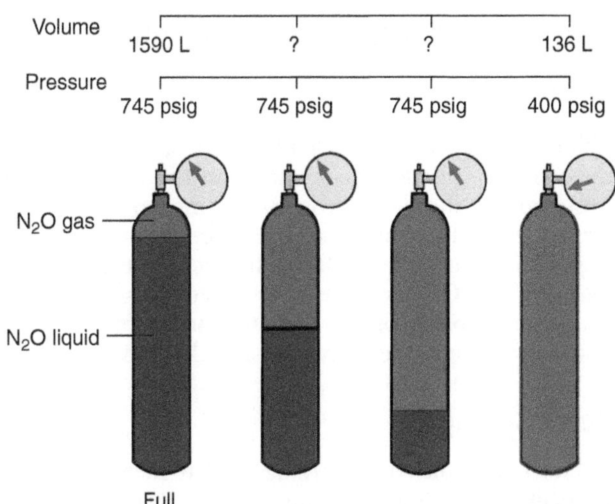

FIGURE 1-2 ■ At ambient temperature (20° C), nitrous oxide liquefies under high pressure, and the pressure of the gas above the liquid remains constant *independent* of how much liquid remains in the cylinder. Only when all the liquid has evaporated does the pressure start to fall, and then it does so rapidly as the residual gas flows from the cylinder. (From Bowie E, Huffman LM: *The anesthesia machine: essentials for understanding,* 1985. With permission from Datex-Ohmeda, Madison, WI.)

used to determine how much gas remains in the cylinder. Clearly, if a machine is equipped with two E-cylinders of oxygen, only one should ever be open at any time to ensure that both tanks are not emptied simultaneously.

Nitrous Oxide Tanks

Nitrous oxide (N_2O) has a molecular weight of 44 and a boiling point of −88° C at 760 mm Hg. Because it has a critical temperature of 36.5° C and critical pressure of 1054 psig, nitrous oxide can exist as a liquid at room temperature (20° C). E-cylinders of nitrous oxide are filled to 90% to 95% of their capacity with liquid nitrous oxide. Above the liquid in the tank is nitrous oxide vapor, that is, gaseous nitrous oxide. Because the liquid nitrous oxide is in equilibrium with its vapor phase, the pressure exerted by the nitrous oxide vapor is its saturated vapor pressure (SVP) at the ambient temperature.

A full E-cylinder of nitrous oxide will evolve approximately 1590 L of gaseous nitrous oxide at 1 atm (14.7 psia). As long as some liquid nitrous oxide remains in the tank and temperature remains constant (20° C), the pressure in the tank will be 745 psig, or the SVP of nitrous oxide at 20° C (Fig. 1-2). It should be clear that, unlike oxygen, the content of a tank of nitrous oxide cannot be determined from the pressure gauge. It can, however, be determined by removing the tank, weighing it, and subtracting the empty weight stamped on each tank (tare weight); the difference is the weight of the contained nitrous oxide. Avogadro's formula for volume states that 1 g of molecular weight of any gas or vapor occupies 22.4 L at standard temperature and pressure. Thus, 44 g of nitrous oxide occupies 22.4 L at 0° C and 760 mm Hg pressure. At 20° C this volume increases to 24 L (22.4 × 293 ÷ 273); thus each gram of nitrous oxide is equivalent to 0.55 L of gas at 20° C.

Only when all the liquid nitrous oxide in the tank has been used up and the tank contains only gaseous nitrous oxide, can Boyle's law be applied. In this instance, when the tank pressure (P_1) is 745 psig from gas only and the internal volume (V_1) of the E-cylinder is approximately 5 L, the volume (V_2) of nitrous oxide gas that will be evolved at atmospheric pressure (P_2) is represented by the following equation:

$$V_2 = (P_1 \times V_1) / P_2$$

$$(745 \times 5) / 14.7 = 253.4\ \text{L}$$

At this point the tank is 16% full (253 ÷ 1590). A tank showing a pressure of 400 psig at 20° C will evolve 136 L [(400 ÷ 745) × 253] of nitrous oxide gas.

While anesthesia is being administered, it is not practical to remove the nitrous oxide cylinder from the anesthesia machine and weigh it accurately enough to determine how much nitrous oxide is left. When the nitrous oxide is being used rapidly, the latent heat of vaporization causes the cylinder itself to become cold. If humidity is sufficient in the surrounding atmosphere, some moisture (or even frost) may collect on the outside surface of the cylinder over the portion that is filled with liquid nitrous oxide. The moisture line, or frost line, which may drop as the gas is used, can provide an indication of when the nitrous oxide will run out. A number of tapes and devices are available to mark the cylinders for this purpose, but their reliability has not been tested. If nitrous oxide is to be used as an anesthetic, it is best to begin with a full cylinder because the length of time the cylinder will last can be calculated. For example, a full E-cylinder of nitrous oxide used at a flow rate of 3 L/min will last about 9 hours (3 × 60 × 9 = 1620 L). When the pressure in the cylinder begins to fall, approximately 250 L are left to be evolved, and the tank will soon need to be replaced.

CHARACTERISTICS OF GAS CYLINDERS

Size

Table 1-1 gives a list of the sizes, weights, and volumes of the common cylinders that contain various medical gases. As noted, the anesthesia provider will most often encounter oxygen and nitrous oxide in E-cylinders and a variety of gases in H-cylinders. Although other gas cylinders are found in the OR—such as those used for gas-powered equipment, laparoscopy equipment, and lasers—these are not likely to be in the domain of anesthesia personnel.

Color Coding

Table 1-2 lists the color markings used to identify medical gas cylinders. Although the internationally accepted color for oxygen is white, green is used in the United States, primarily for reasons of tradition; in addition, yellow is used to identify compressed air, which represents another exception to international standards. Anesthesiologists working in countries other than the United States should be aware of these differences. Because nitric oxide (NO) cylinders are not standardized in color and are frequently supplied as bare aluminum, it is important to check the label and not solely rely on color coding to identify a compressed gas.

Cylinder Markings

Certain codes are stamped near the neck on all medical gas cylinders. The U.S. Department of Transportation (DOT), which has extensive regulations concerning the marking and shipping of medical gas cylinders, requires a code to indicate that the cylinder was manufactured according to its specifications (Fig. 1-3). The service pressure (in psig) is stamped on each cylinder and should never be exceeded. Each cylinder is also given its own serial number and commercial designation; the final code stamped on the cylinder is usually the date of the last inspection and the inspector's mark. Medical gas cylinders must be inspected at least once every 10 years, at which time they should also be tested for structural integrity; this is done by filling the cylinder to 1.66 times the normal service pressure. The date of this inspection is often circled with a black marker to indicate that the cylinder has been checked by the supplier (Fig. 1-4).

TABLE 1-1 **Typical Volume and Weight of Available Contents of Medical Gas Cylinders***

Cylinder Style and Dimensions	Nominal Volume (in³/L)	Unit of Measure	Air	CO_2	Cyclopropane	He	N_2	N_2O	O_2	*Mixtures of Oxygen* He	*Mixtures of Oxygen* CO_2
B	87/1.43	psig		838	75				1900		
3.5 x 13 in		L	370		375				200		
8.89 x 33 cm		lb-oz	1-8	1-7.25					—		
		kg		0.68	0.66				—		
D	176/2.88	psig	1900	838	75	1600	1900	745	1900	†	†
4.25 x 17 in		L	375	940	870	300	370	940	400	300	400
10.8 x 43 cm		lb-oz	—	3-13	3-5.5	—	—	3-13	—	†	†
		kg		1.73	1.51	—	—	1.73	—	†	†
E	293/4.80	psig	1900	838		1600	1900	745	1900	†	†
4.25 x 26 in		L	625	1590		500	610	1590	660	500	660
10.8 x 66 cm		lb-oz	—	6-7		—	—	6-7	—	†	†
		kg		2.92		—	—	2.92	—	†	†
M	1337/21.9	psig	1900	838		1600	2200	7.45	2200	†	†
7 x 43 in		L	2850	7570		2260	3200	7570	3450	2260	3000
17.8 x 109 cm		lb-oz	—	30-10		—	—	30-10	122 cu ft	†	†
		kg		13.9		—	—	13.9	—	†	†
G	2370/38.8	psig	1900	838		1600		745		†	†
8.5 x 51 in		L	5050	12300		4000		13800		4000	5330
17.8 x 109 cm		lb-oz	—	50-0		—		56-0		†	†
		kg		22.7		—	—	25.4		†	†
H or K	2660/43.6	psig	2200			2200	2200	745	2200‡		
		L	6550			6000	6400	15800	6900		
		lb-oz	—			—	—	64	244 cu ft		
		kg	—			—	—	29.1	—		

*Computed contents are based on normal cylinder volumes at 70° F (21.1° C), rounded to no greater than 1% variance.

†The pressure and weight of mixed gases vary according to the composition of the mixture.

‡275 cu ft/7800 L cylinders at 2490 psig are available on request.

Modified from Compressed Gas Association: *Characteristics and safe handling of medical gases, publication P-2*, ed 7. Arlington, VA, 1989, Compressed Gas Association.

All medical gas cylinders should come from the supplier accompanied by a tag with three perforated sections, each designating a different stage of use: *empty*, *in use*, and *full*. The portion of the tag marked "full" should be removed when a cylinder is put into service. This is not usually critical, however, because it is generally obvious when a cylinder is in use; making use of the tag marker becomes important when an empty cylinder is removed from the machine. If the tag is not used correctly at the outset, the problem is compounded with each successive stage of the cylinder's use, and the final result is storage of an empty cylinder as a full one. Although a discrepancy in weight may alert a user to an incorrectly labeled cylinder, this error may be easily overlooked in an emergency situation.

TABLE 1-2 Color Marking of Compressed Gas Containers Intended for Medical Use

Gas	U.S. Color	Canadian Color
Oxygen	Green	White*
Carbon dioxide	Gray	Gray
Nitrous oxide	Blue	Blue
Cyclopropane	Orange	Orange
Helium	Brown	Brown
Nitrogen	Black	Black
Air	Yellow*	Black and white
Mixture other than oxygen and nitrogen	A combination of colors corresponding to each component gas	
Mixture of Oxygen and Nitrogen		
Oxygen 19.5%-23.5%	Yellow*	Black and white
All other oxygen concentrations	Black and green	Pink

*Historically, vacuum systems have been identified by white in the United States and yellow in Canada. Therefore it is recommended that white *not* be used in the United States and yellow *not* be used in Canada as markings to identify containers for use with any medical gas.

Modified from Compressed Gas Association: *Standard color marking of compressed gas containers intended for medical use, publication C-9*, ed 3. Arlington, VA, 1988, Compressed Gas Association.

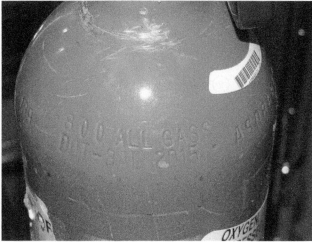

FIGURE 1-3 ▪ Some of the cylinder markings on an E-cylinder. *DOT* indicates that the cylinder was manufactured according to the specifications of the United States Department of Transportation (DOT); *3AL* indicates the tank is aluminum. *2015* indicates the maximum filling pressure of the cylinder in pounds per square inch gauge pressure (psig), the number to the right is the cylinder serial number, and *ALL GASS* is the tank owner's name.

Pressure Relief Valves

All medical gas cylinders must incorporate a mechanism to vent the cylinder's contents before explosion from excessive pressure.[6] Explosion can result from exposure to extreme heat, such as in the event of a fire, or from accidental overfilling. These mechanisms are of three basic types—the fusible plug, frangible disk assembly, and safety relief valve—and are incorporated into the cylinder; as such, they cannot be inspected by the user. The *fusible plug*, made of a metal alloy with a low melting point, will melt in a fire and allow the gas to escape. With certain gases, such as oxygen or nitrous oxide, this can aggravate the fire because oxygen and nitrous oxide are both strong oxidizers. The *frangible disk assembly* contains a metal disk designed to break when a certain pressure is exceeded and thereby allow the gas to escape through a discharge vent. Finally, the *safety relief valve* is a spring-loaded mechanism that closes a discharge vent. If the pressure increases, the valve opens and remains open until the pressure decreases below the valve's opening threshold. Some cylinders have combination devices that incorporate a fusible metal plug with one of the other two mechanisms.

Connectors

Figure 1-5 illustrates the tops of typical valves for both small (E) and large (H) cylinders. As previously mentioned, large cylinders have valve outlets that are coded and are unique to the gas content of the cylinder. The coding is based on the threads and diameter of the outlet port orifice.[4] Regulators to reduce and control the pressure of the gas, also specific for each type of gas, are attached to these threaded valve ports. It is highly

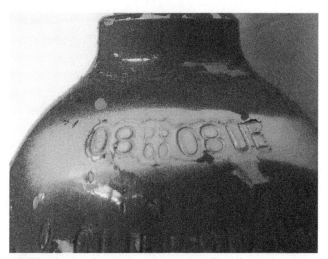

FIGURE 1-4 ▪ An E-cylinder of oxygen. The inspection date, August 2008, has been painted white to indicate the cylinder was checked at the time it was delivered to the facility. All cylinders must be checked for leaks and structural integrity with an overpressure test at least once every 10 years.

unsafe to use a regulator for one type of gas on a valve port of a cylinder of another type of gas.

Small cylinders have cylindrical ports or holes in their valves to receive the yoke, either on an anesthesia machine or free standing, from which the gas will flow. A washer, usually made of Teflon, is necessary to make this connection gas tight. Care must be taken to ensure that the retaining screw that holds the cylinder in the yoke is not placed into the safety relief device instead of in its intended location in the conical depression opposite the valve port (Fig. 1-5, *A*). The connection between cylinder valve and yoke is made gas specific by the pin index safety system for small cylinder connections.

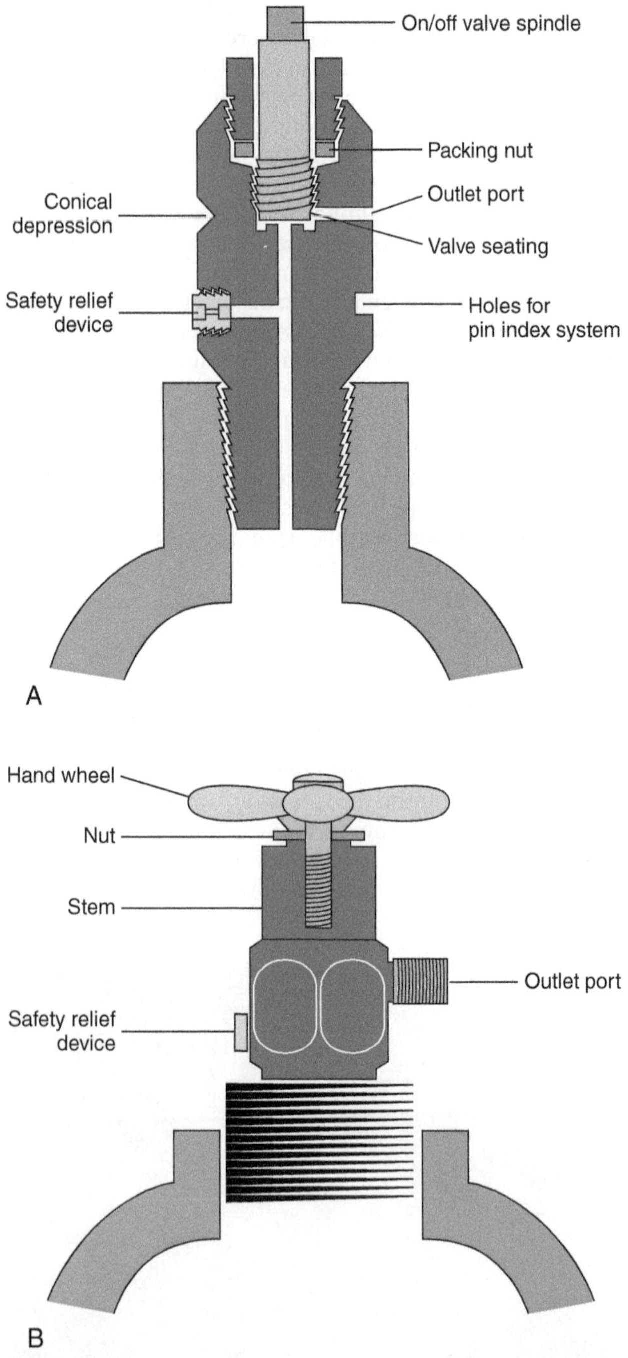

GAS CYLINDER SAFETY ISSUES

Prevention of Incorrect Gas Cylinder Connections

In the past, cylinders containing the wrong gas—for example, nitrous oxide instead of oxygen—were sometimes connected to anesthesia gas delivery systems, with disastrous results. This led to the development of systems designed to help ensure use of the correct cylinder. Most of the gas tanks used for anesthesia are E-cylinders or other small cylinders, for which the pin index safety system was developed in 1952. The pin index system[4] relies on two 5-mm stainless steel pins on the cylinder yoke connector just below the fitting for the valve outlet port. Seven different pin positions are possible depending on the type of gas in the cylinder (Fig. 1-6). The yoke connector for an oxygen cylinder, for

FIGURE 1-5 ■ Typical cylinder valves. **A,** A small cylinder packed valve, such as would be found on an E-cylinder. Note that the female-type port is not unique to the gas type. **B,** A large cylinder packed valve, such as would be seen on an H-cylinder. Note that the male type of outlet port has a unique diameter and threads as a safety feature intended to help ensure correct connections. (Modified from Davis PD, Parbrook EO, Parbrook GD: *Basic physics and measurement in anesthesia*, ed 3. Oxford, UK, 1984, Butterworth-Heinemann.)

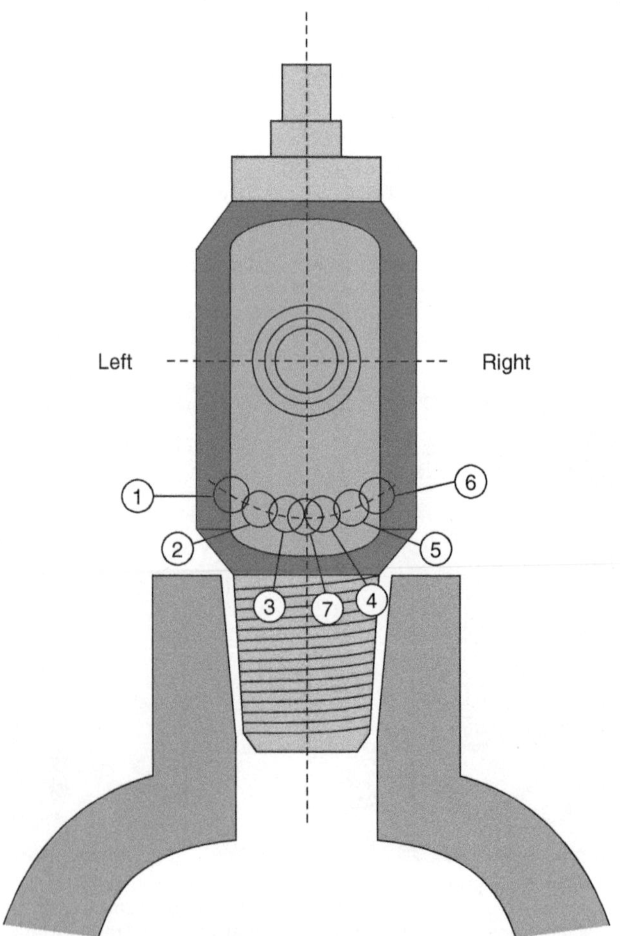

FIGURE 1-6 ■ Pin index safety system pin location is shown, looking at the placement of holes in the tank. Pins are placed precisely complementary in the tank yoke. Two pins are used to identify each type of gas. Pin configurations are listed in Table 1-3.

example, has pins at positions 2 and 5 (Fig. 1-7). Pin positions for the various gases are listed in Table 1-3. These pins fit exactly into the corresponding holes in the cylinder valve (Fig. 1-8). This system provides an additional safety feature and, along with color coding, is designed to ensure that the correct gas is connected to its corresponding cylinder yoke. Obviously, connectors with either damaged or missing index pins are unsafe and should not be used under any circumstances. Because a pin can easily be lost or damaged when a cylinder is handled roughly, the person changing the cylinder must make certain that both pins are intact.

Securing Cylinders Against Breakage

Gas cylinders should always be secured when placed in an upright position. If left freestanding, a cylinder can easily fall over in such a way that it would fracture at the neck (Fig. 1-9). The cylinder's highly pressurized gas would be suddenly released, and the cylinder would become an unguided missile of tremendous force; in fact, the cylinder could generate enough force to penetrate a cinder-block wall several feet thick. The potential danger of such an occurrence is obvious. *Therefore, all gas cylinders must be secured when they are upright.* If that is not possible, the cylinder can be laid on its side. Individual E-cylinders can be placed in a broad-based wheeled carriage for support when in use.

Transfilling

Anesthesia personnel should never attempt to refill small cylinders from larger ones. Even if gas-tight connections were possible, the risk of explosion from the heat of compression in the small cylinder would still be serious. In addition, there is always the possibility that the wrong gas would be placed in the cylinder. The practice of transfilling is also forbidden. Medical gases must be obtained *only* from a reputable commercial supplier.

Cylinder Hazards

A study of 14,500 medical gas cylinders consecutively delivered from supposedly reputable suppliers found 120 (0.83%) with potentially dangerous irregularities.[7] Forty cylinders were delivered either empty or partially filled, 3 were found to be dangerously overfilled to near-bursting pressures, and 6 cylinders of compressed air were found to be contaminated with volatile hydrocarbons. Thirty cylinders were unlabeled, and the labels of many others were illegible, having been painted over. Another 4 cylinders were incorrectly color coded, 5 large cylinders were fitted with incorrect valve outlet ports (which is especially dangerous because an oxygen valve on an air cylinder enables air to be fed into an oxygen outlet), 14 valve assemblies were found to be loose, and 4 valve assemblies were inoperable. On a large number of cylinders, the current inspection date was either absent or had been painted over so as to be illegible. Numerous examples were cited of cylinders being improperly stored or secured. The results of this study serve to remind anesthesia practitioners of the danger of assuming that gas supplies are perfectly safe. All facilities should have an established system to ensure that each cylinder of medical gas is inspected and tested upon delivery to the facility.

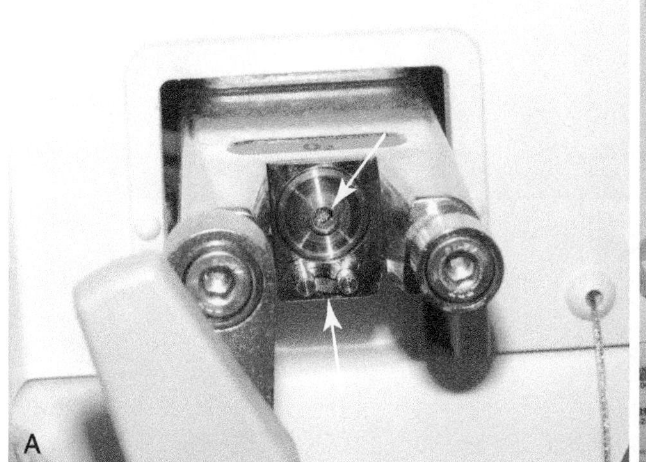

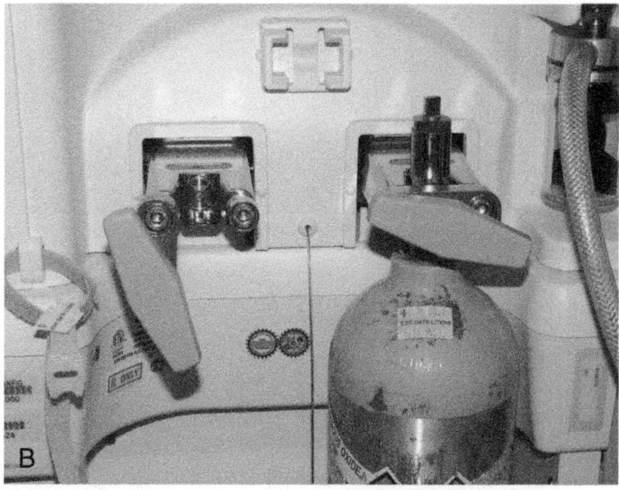

FIGURE 1-7 **A,** Cylinder yoke on the anesthesia machine. Note the two pins for the pin index system at the bottom of the yoke (*bottom arrow*) and the hole (*top arrow;* not gas specific) that aligns with the outlet port of the tank. **B,** Oxygen yoke with the tank removed and the N_2O tank in place.

TABLE 1-3 **Pin Index Safety System**

						Mixtures of Oxygen	
	Air	Cyclopropane	N_2	N_2O	O_2	He	CO_2
Pin positions	1-5	3-6	1-4	3-5	2-5	2-4	1-6

The pin index system relies on two 5-mm stainless steel pins on the cylinder yoke connector just below the fitting for the valve outlet port. Seven different pin positions are possible depending on the type of gas in the cylinder (the seventh pin position is for a gas not used in the United States). See Figures 1-6 and 1-7 for pin locations.

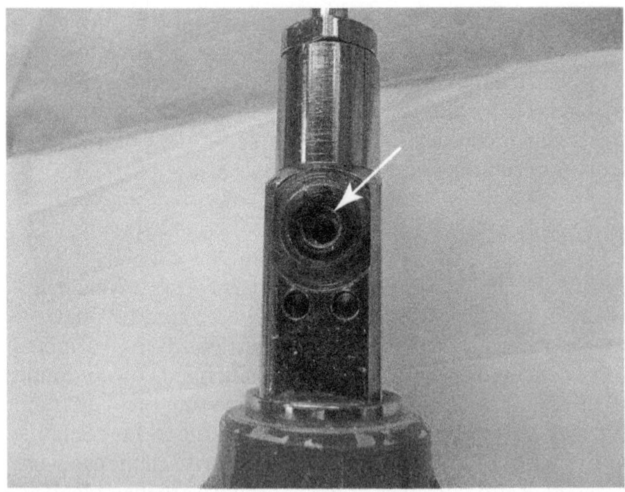

FIGURE 1-8 ■ Cylinder valve at the top of an E-cylinder shows the two holes for the pin index system and the outlet port with an attached washer (*arrow*).

GUIDELINES FOR USE OF MEDICAL GAS CYLINDERS

Numerous rules govern the safe handling of cylinders that contain medical gases.[1,2] Summarized below are practical points that anesthesia practitioners must consider on a routine basis.

Supply

As noted, medical gases should be purchased only from a reputable commercial supplier. Outside metropolitan areas, the only supplier of any type of compressed gas may be the local welding company. Purchasing medical gases from such a source can be appropriate once it has been established that this supplier meets all safety requirements and standards for the manufacture and supply of medical gases. Such verification should be incorporated into the system to promote maximum safety.

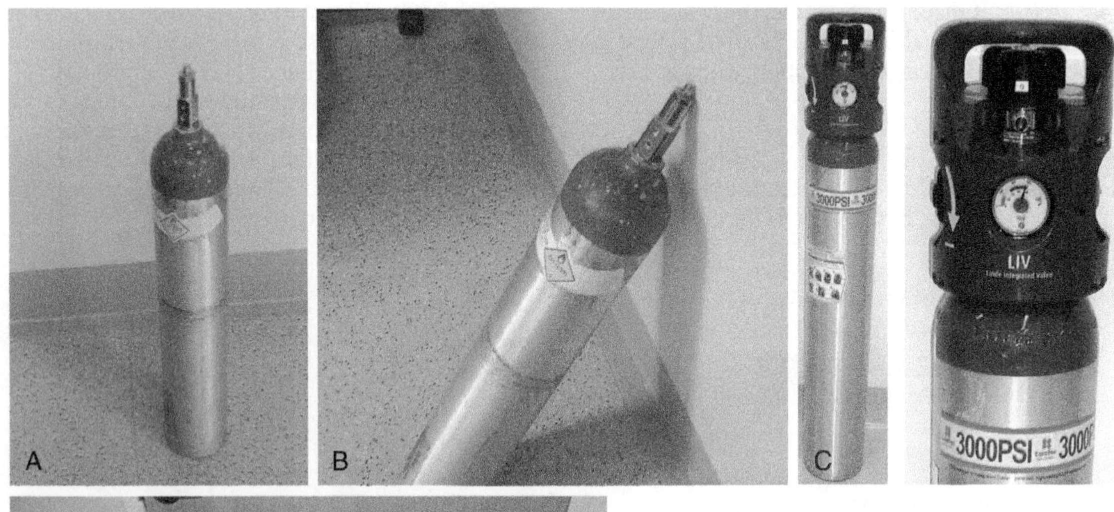

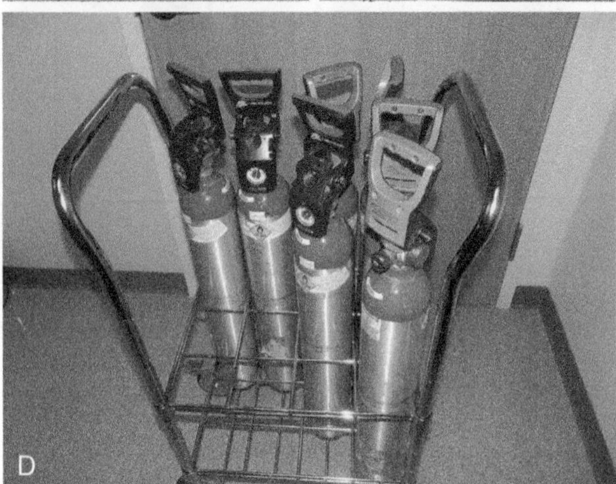

FIGURE 1-9 ■ **A,** Gas cylinders must never be left standing upright and unsecured. They are vulnerable to being knocked over easily, such as by opening a door. Cylinders that fall directly to the floor, and especially cylinders that fall so that the top hits a wall (**B**), are at great risk for breaking at the cylinder neck. This creates a dangerous "unguided missile," in which the high-pressure gas escapes out the narrow neck and rockets the cylinder forward with enough force to penetrate a brick wall. **C,** Oxygen cylinders are now available with a maximum pressure of 300 psi and a capacity of 1000 L of oxygen. These would present an even greater hazard if ruptured. **D,** If upright, individual cylinders should be secured in some type of holder, such as a rolling stand for E-sized cylinders.

Storage

Specific regulations and standards govern the storage of medical gas cylinders.[2,3] For example, full cylinders and empty cylinders must be stored separately, each in its own "tank room" if possible. Small cylinders should be placed in nonflammable racks, and large cylinders should be chained to a wall. At least one anesthesiologist in each facility should be aware of these requirements and how they are being implemented. Anesthesia caregivers should also assume responsibility for all aspects of medical gas supplies.

Transport and Installation

Medical gas cylinders must be handled with care. As previously mentioned, a broken cylinder can have serious consequences, as can valve assemblies damaged by rough handling. Cylinders should undergo a final inspection just before they are used. If questions arise concerning the safety or content of a cylinder, it should not be used; instead, an investigation should be undertaken before returning the cylinder to the supplier. Before a small E-cylinder is installed in the hanger yoke, the plastic wrapping surrounding the cylinder valve outlet must be completely removed. If this is not done, the plastic wrapper will prevent the gas from entering the inlet in the hanger yoke. All cylinders should be opened slightly, or "cracked," immediately before installation to clean any residual oil, grease, or debris from the valve outlet port that would otherwise be released into the anesthetizing apparatus. Furthermore, cylinders should always be opened *slowly* to prevent dramatic heating of the suddenly pressurized piping. If an abnormal odor is detected when the cylinder is opened, gas should be collected from the tank and analyzed by gas chromatography to detect hydrocarbon contamination.[8] Once a problem is confirmed, the cylinder in question should be sequestered, not returned to the supplier, and the appropriate local and federal authorities contacted.

Connections between gas cylinders and anesthesia machines must be tight. Figure 1-10 illustrates the proper method for balancing the tank when securing it to or removing it from the yoke. Washers are necessary for small cylinder yokes and occasionally need replacement; the old washer must be removed before placing a new washer. Having two washers in place simultaneously will create a leak and may defeat the pin index system. If a hissing noise is heard when a cylinder is opened, a leak is present. Tightness can always be checked by dripping soapy water onto the connection and inspecting it for bubbles. A connection should never be overtightened in an attempt to compensate for a leak; doing so may damage or even crack the cylinder valve. As in all aspects of anesthesia practice, brute force is almost never appropriate.

Once a new cylinder is in place, the pressure must be checked on the applicable gauge. Correct pressures for full cylinders are listed in Table 1-1. Overpressurized cylinders are dangerous and must be removed at once and reported to the supplier.

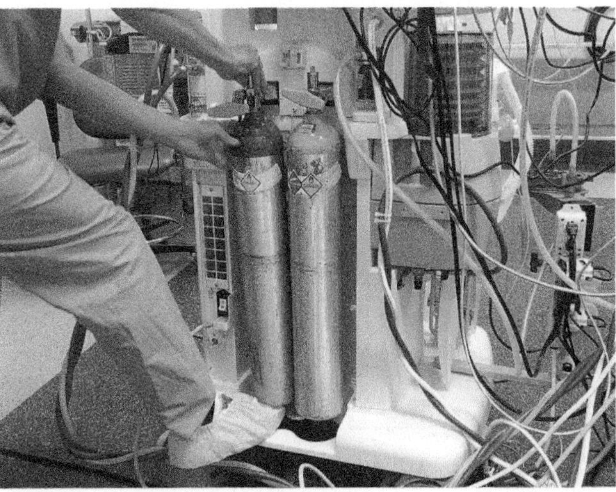

FIGURE 1-10 ■ Proper method for attaching an E-cylinder to the yoke of an anesthesia machine. The tank is first supported on the anesthesiologist's foot while the holes on the tank are aligned with the pins in the yoke. The tank is then slid into place on the yoke, and the T-handle is tightened to make a gas-tight seal.

MEDICAL GAS PIPELINE SYSTEMS

Medical gas pipeline systems consist of three main components: 1) a central supply of gas, 2) pipelines to transport gases to points of use, and 3) connectors at these points that connect to the equipment that delivers the medical gas. Anesthesia caregivers are primarily concerned with piped oxygen and nitrous oxide; however, ORs may have two other medical gas supply pipelines: one for compressed air and another for nitrogen to power gas-driven equipment.

Detailed standards and guidelines exist for the use of medical gas delivery systems. In North America, these are published by the American National Standards Institute (ANSI), the American Society of Mechanical Engineers (ASME), the Compressed Gas Association (CGA), the National Fire Protection Association (NFPA), the Canadian Standards Association (CSA), and the American Hospital Association (AHA).[9] In the United States, a hospital must meet the NFPA standards to be accredited by The Joint Commission (TJC) and often to obtain insurance coverage. The construction of a medical facility is governed by standards, and the procedures required for operating a medical gas system must be followed by the plant engineering and maintenance departments. Problems in the construction of gas pipelines have led to anesthesia deaths; anesthesia providers should therefore be aware of these standards and the gas delivery system at their facility.[10]

MEDICAL GAS CENTRAL SUPPLY SYSTEMS

The central supply (bulk storage) system is the source of medical gases distributed throughout the pipeline system. For oxygen, the central supply can be a series of standard cylinders connected by a manifold system or, for larger

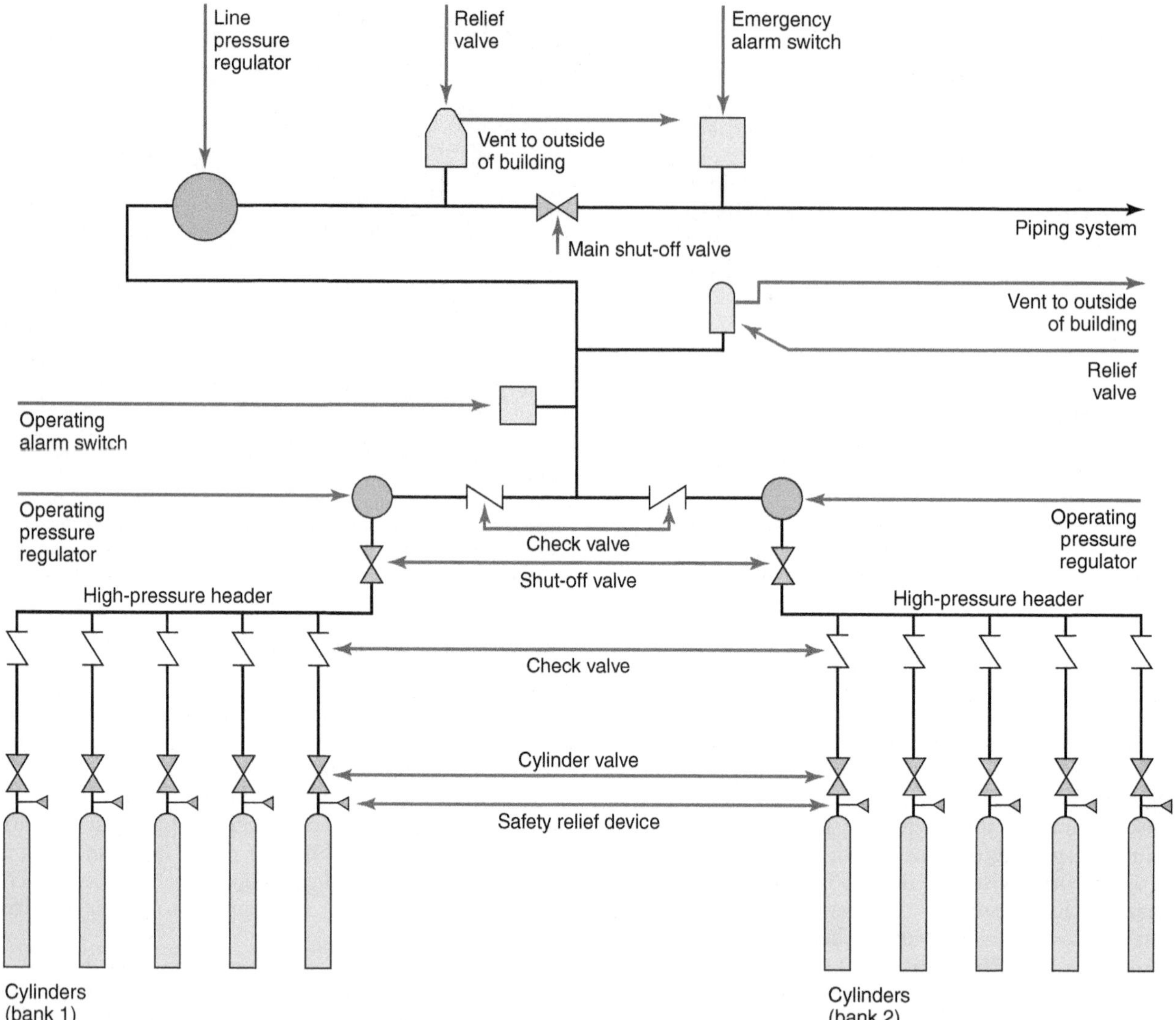

FIGURE 1-11 Typical cylinder (H size) supply system, as would be seen in a small hospital or a freestanding facility. There is no reserve supply. (From CSA Standard Z305.1-1975, *Nonflammable medical-gas piping systems.* Toronto, 1975, Canadian Standards Association.)

installations, pressure vessels of liquid oxygen with accompanying vaporizers. For medical air, the supply can be cylinders of compressed air, cylinders of oxygen and nitrogen with the gases mixed by a regulator, or air compressors. In general, for nitrous oxide or nitrogen, a series of cylinders, or liquid Dewar tanks, with a manifold system is used.

Oxygen

Central supply systems that carry oxygen are both the most common and the most important supply systems; as such, they have received considerable attention. Standards for bulk systems that involve the storage of oxygen as a liquid are contained in NFPA Publication 55.[11] Oxygen systems are extensively covered in NFPA Publication 99[12] and in the CSA Standard Z305.1.[13]

Very small systems have a total storage capacity of less than 2000 cubic feet (cu ft) of gas (a single H-cylinder of oxygen contains 244 cu ft, or 6900 L) and have additional standards when based in nonhospital facilities. Systems in very small hospitals may store oxygen in a series of standard H-cylinders connected by a manifold or high-pressure header system. These systems typically do not have reserve supplies. In Figures 1-11 and 1-12, note that there are two banks of cylinders; all central supply systems for medical gases must be present in duplicate, with two identical sources able to provide the needed medical gas interchangeably. These are often referred to as the *primary* and *secondary* supplies (not to be confused with the entirely separate *reserve system*).

The larger the oxygen demand of the facility, the more complex the supply system. Most hospitals store their bulk oxygen in liquid form (Fig. 1-13), which enables the hospital to maintain a large reservoir of oxygen in a relatively small space. One cubic foot of oxygen stored at a temperature of −297° F (−183° C) expands to 860 cu ft of oxygen at 70° F (21° C).[14] Because 1 cu ft is equal to 28.3 L, this amount of liquid oxygen provides 24,338 L at room temperature and pressure, the equivalent of 3.5 H-cylinders of oxygen.

Liquid oxygen is stored in a special container and kept under pressure. This container has an inner and outer

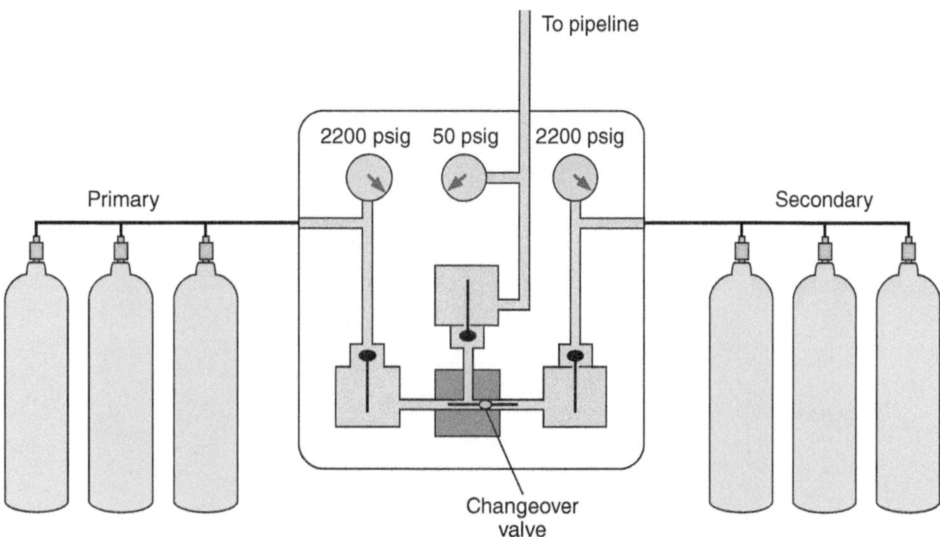

FIGURE 1-12 ■ A simplified version of Figure 1-11. The oxygen is supplied in H-cylinders from both a primary and a secondary supply. The tanks are connected by a manifold; when the tanks are full, the pressure is 2200 psig. A changeover valve automatically switches to the secondary supply once the primary supply has been exhausted. A reducing valve decreases the pressure to 50 psig before the oxygen enters the hospital pipeline. (Modified from Davis PD, Parbrook EO, Parbrook GD: *Basic physics and measurement in anesthesia,* ed 3. Oxford, UK, 1984, Butterworth Heinemann.)

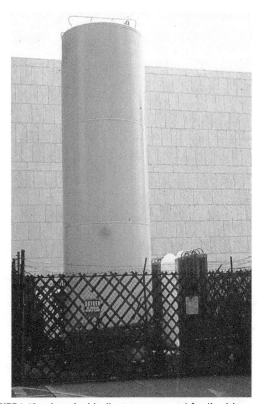

FIGURE 1-13 ■ A typical bulk-storage vessel for liquid oxygen.

layer separated by layers of insulation and a near vacuum. This construction is similar to that of a thermos bottle and keeps the liquid oxygen cold by inhibiting the entry of external heat (Fig. 1-14).

Liquid oxygen systems must be in constant use to be cost effective. If the system goes unused for a period of time, the pressure increases as some of the liquid oxygen boils. The oxygen is then vented to the atmosphere. The liquid oxygen system contains vaporizers that heat the liquid and convert it to a gas before it is piped into the hospital. Environmental and mechanical heat sources can be used to aid in vaporization.

Liquid oxygen can be extremely hazardous, and fires are an ever-present danger. In addition, personnel can receive severe burns if they come in contact with liquid oxygen or an uninsulated pipe carrying liquid oxygen.

Small hospitals typically require central supply systems that store oxygen in replaceable liquid oxygen cylinders and a reserve of oxygen stored in high-pressure H-cylinders. The reserve system is automatically activated when the main supply, with its component primary and secondary storage, fails or is depleted (Fig. 1-15). Hospitals of average size may store liquid oxygen in bulk pressure vessels rather than in liquid oxygen cylinders. The storage vessel is filled from a liquid oxygen supply truck through a cryogenic hose designed to function at extremely low temperatures. In such a system, the size of the reserve system depends on the rate of oxygen use because the reserve must constitute at least an average supply for 1 day, but preferably 2 to 3 days. This supply may be stored in a series of high-pressure H-cylinders. However, large hospitals are required to have a second liquid oxygen storage vessel as the reserve system because of the impracticality of storing and connecting enough cylinders to provide an average day's reserve supply of oxygen (Fig. 1-16).

Built into all these central supply systems for oxygen are a variety of mandatory safety devices. Pressure relief valves are designed to open if pressure in the system exceeds the normal level by 50%. This prevents the rupture of vessels or pipes from the excessive pressure generated by a frozen valve or a malfunctioning pressure regulator. Alarm systems indicate when the supply in the main storage vessel is low and when the reserve supply has been accessed. An oxygen alarm should activate a rehearsed protocol within the hospital that results in contact with the oxygen supplier and subsequent verification that an oxygen delivery is on the way.[15] Pressure alarms built into the

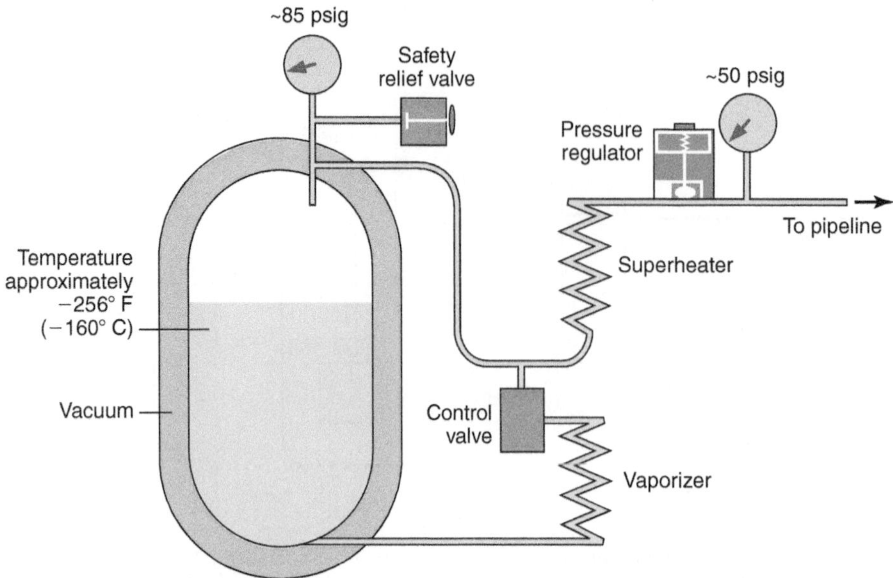

FIGURE 1-14 ■ Diagram of a liquid oxygen supply system. The vessel resembles a giant vacuum bottle. The liquid oxygen is at approximately −256° F (−160° C). Pressure inside the vessel is maintained at approximately 85 psig. When oxygen is used from the top of the vessel, it first passes through a superheater and then through the pressure regulator to keep the pipeline pressure at 50 psig. During times of rapid use, the temperature in the tank may fall, along with the vapor pressure. The control valve causes liquid oxygen to pass through the vaporizer, which adds heat and thus maintains the pressure in the tank. (Modified from Davis PD, Parbrook EO, Parbrook GD: *Basic physics and measurement in anesthesia*, ed 3. Oxford, UK, 1984, Butterworth-Heinemann.)

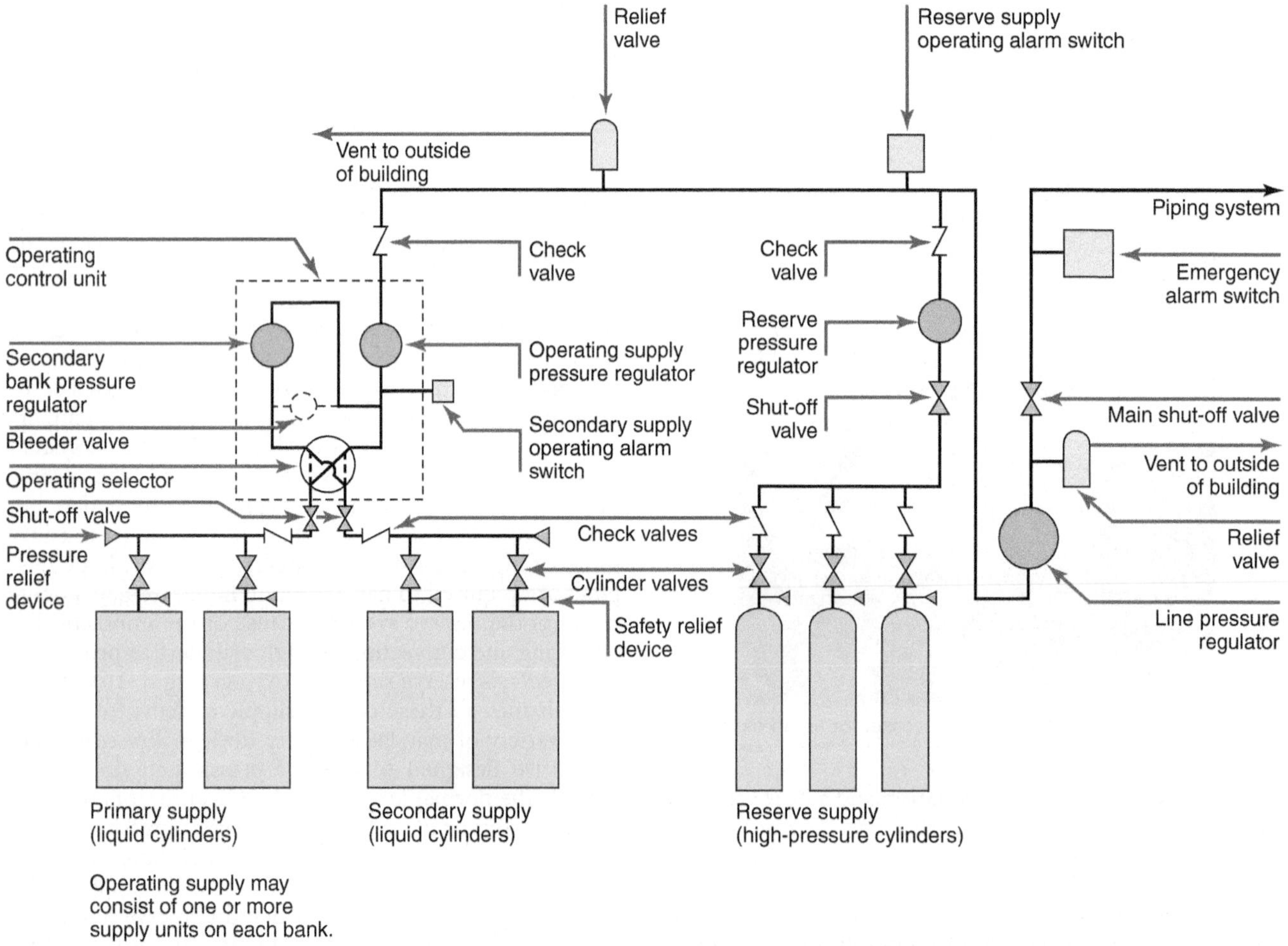

Relief valve
Reserve supply operating alarm switch
Vent to outside of building
Piping system
Operating control unit
Check valve
Check valve
Emergency alarm switch
Reserve pressure regulator
Secondary bank pressure regulator
Operating supply pressure regulator
Shut-off valve
Main shut-off valve
Bleeder valve
Secondary supply operating alarm switch
Vent to outside of building
Operating selector
Shut-off valve
Check valves
Relief valve
Pressure relief device
Cylinder valves
Safety relief device
Line pressure regulator
Primary supply (liquid cylinders)
Secondary supply (liquid cylinders)
Reserve supply (high-pressure cylinders)
Operating supply may consist of one or more supply units on each bank.

FIGURE 1-15 ■ Typical cryogenic cylinder supply system for liquid oxygen with a high-pressure cylinder reserve supply, as would be seen in a small hospital. The redundant primary and secondary liquid cylinders are intended to be the continuous oxygen source; there is an automatic switchover to the other bank when one is depleted and ready for replacement. The reserve supply is automatically activated when both banks of cylinders are depleted or fail. (From CSA Standard Z305.1–92, *Nonflammable medical gas piping systems*. Toronto, 1992, Canadian Standards Association.)

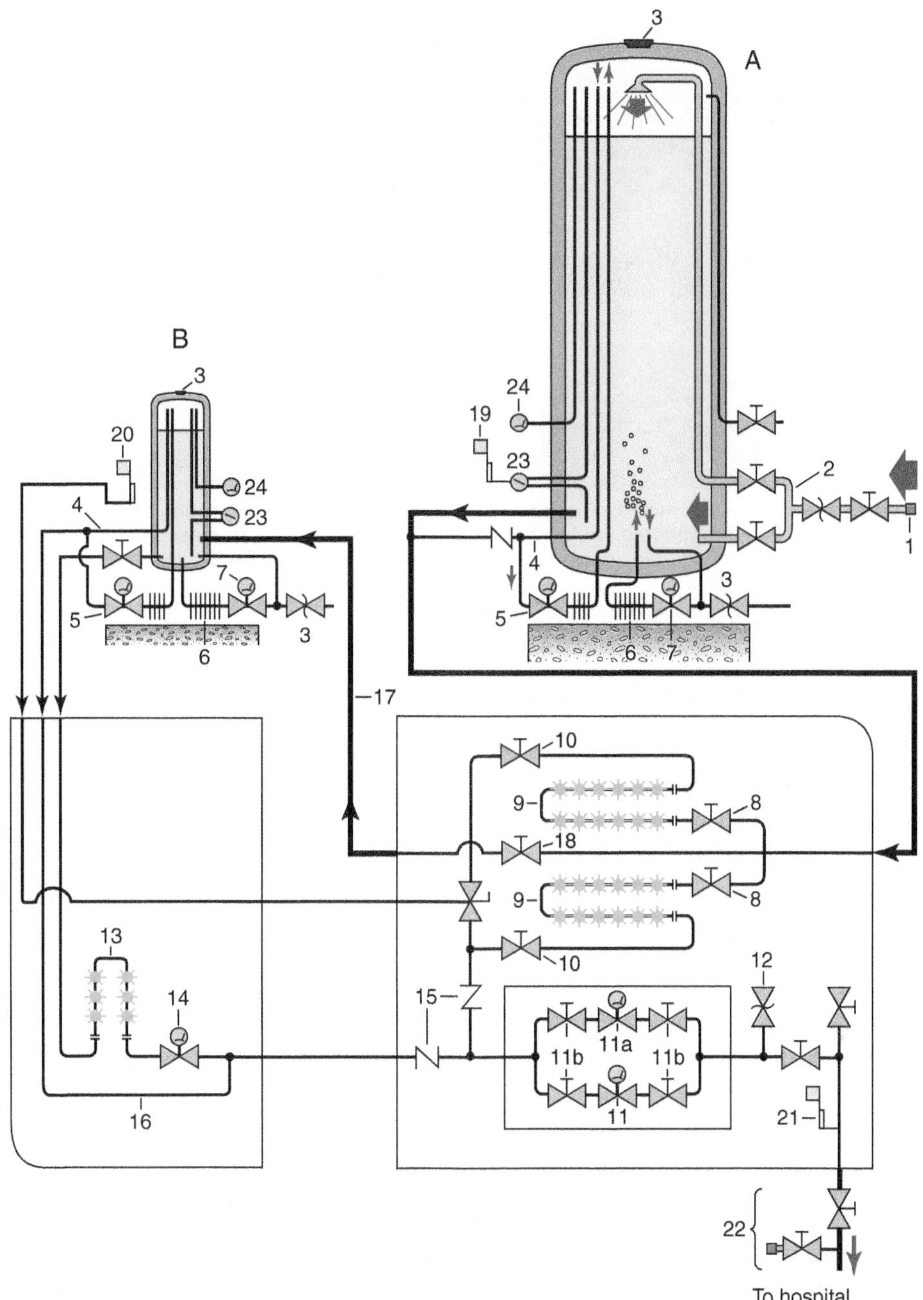

FIGURE 1-16 ■ Typical bulk supply system for oxygen, as would be seen in a large hospital. Very large hospitals may require more than one system of this magnitude. **A,** Main liquid oxygen reservoir. **B,** Reserve liquid oxygen reservoir. *1,* Connection to supply vehicle; *2,* top and bottom fill lines; *3,* reservoir pressure relief valves; *4,* "economizer" circuit; *5,* gas regulator in pressure-building circuit; *6,* pressure-building vaporizer; *7,* liquid regulator in pressure-building circuit; *8,* cryogenic liquid-control valves; *9,* liquid vaporizers; *10,* downstream valves for isolation of vaporizers; *11,* primary line pressure regulator; *11a,* secondary line pressure regulator; *11b,* valves to isolate regulators for repair; *12,* pressure relief valve for main pipeline; *13,* reserve system liquid vaporizer; *14,* reserve system line pressure regulator; *15,* gas flow check valves; *16,* reserve system "economizer" line; *17,* reserve system fill line; *18,* valve controlling flow to reserve system from main cylinder; *19,* low liquid level alarm; *20,* reserve in use alarm; *21,* main line pressure alarm; *22,* main shut-off valve and T-fitting; *23,* liquid level indicators; *24,* vapor or "head" pressure gauges. In normal operation, liquid oxygen flows from the lower left of the main vessel (**A**) via a cryogenic pipe through valves (*8*) and to the vaporizer (*9*), where the liquid becomes gaseous oxygen. It then flows through pressure regulators (*11*) and hence into the supply pipeline to the hospital. (From Bancroft ML, du Moulin GC, Hedley-Whyte J: Hazards of bulk oxygen delivery systems. *Anesthesiology* 1980;52:504-510.)

main supply line sound when the line pressure varies by 20% in either direction from the normal operating pressure of approximately 55 psig. Pressure alarms should also be located in various areas in the pipeline to detect oxygen supply problems beyond the main connection (Fig. 1-17).

All these alarm systems must sound in two different locations: the hospital maintenance or plant engineering department and an area occupied 24 hours a day, such as the telephone switchboard. These alarms should be periodically tested as part of a regular maintenance program

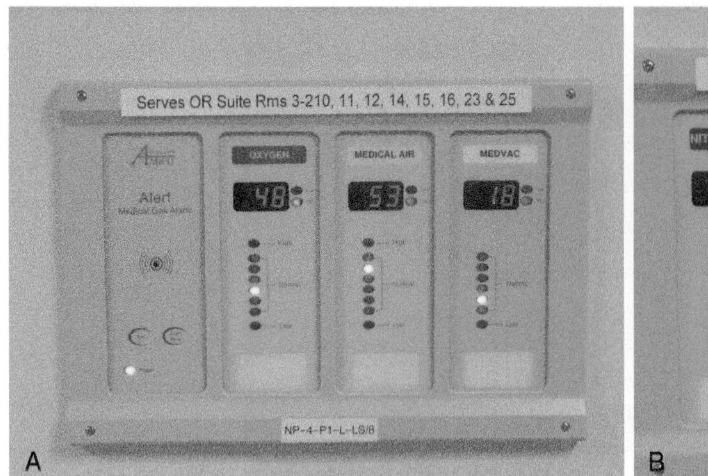

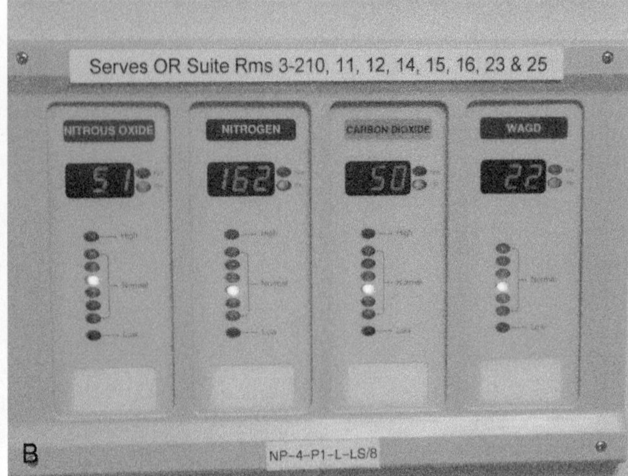

FIGURE 1-17 ■ **A,** Bank of pressure gauges that monitor the gases in one zone of the operating room. These gauges are for oxygen, air, and vacuum. Note that the rooms being monitored are identified on the top of the panel. **B,** A second gas monitoring panel for N_2O, nitrogen, CO_2, and waste gases. Note that colored lights indicate whether the line pressures are in the normal range; alarms are triggered for high or low pressures.

because failure of such alarms has led to crisis situations. Testing the various alarms can be difficult but is possible if the system is properly designed.

Another critical safety feature is the T-fitting located at the point where the central supply system joins the hospital piping system. This fitting allows delivery of an emergency supply of oxygen from a mobile source in the event of extended failure, extensive repair, or modification of the hospital's central supply.

The location and housing of oxygen central supply systems are governed by strict standards.[11] A bulk oxygen storage unit should be located away from public areas and flammable materials.

Oxygen Concentrators

The use of oxygen concentrators to deliver oxygen to the anesthesia circuit has gained attention recently. Oxygen is generated by the selective adsorption of the components of air with molecular sieve technology. These sieves consist of rigid structures of silica and aluminum, with additional calcium or sodium as cations.[16] Air is forced through the sieves under pressure, and oxygen and nitrogen are generated. The oxygen is then used clinically, and the nitrogen is vented to the atmosphere. The maximum oxygen concentration produced by concentrators is approximately 90% to 96%, with the balance made up mostly of argon.[17,18]

Oxygen concentrators are commonly used in remote locations and developing countries, but in some cases they have been configured to supplement a hospital's existing liquid oxygen system as a reserve or a secondary supply.[17] Oxygen concentration may vary with gas flow, and concentrators are most effective at delivering oxygen at flows of less than 4 L/min to anesthesia machines.[18] Accumulation of argon may occur, however, in low-flow conditions, so the use of an oxygen monitor is essential.[19] As the current emphasis on cost cutting in medical care continues, along with cost increases of supplied liquid and gaseous oxygen, oxygen concentrators are likely to come into wider use.

Medical Air

The central supply of medical air can come from three sources: 1) cylinders of compressed air that have been cleaned to medical quality by filtration distillation; 2) a proportioning system (relatively uncommon) that receives oxygen and nitrogen from central sources, mixes them in a proportion of 21% oxygen to 79% nitrogen, and delivers this mixture to the medical air pipeline (these systems usually have compressed air cylinders or an air compressor as a reserve system); and 3) air compressors (Fig. 1-18), the most common source of medical air in hospitals. The compressor works by compressing ambient air and then delivering the pressurized air to a reservoir or holding tank.[14] The medical air is then fed to the pressure regulator and travels from there to the hospital piping system.

Air compressor systems are subject to rigorous standards.[12,13] As with other systems (i.e., vacuum or electrical generators), redundancy is important. Duplicate compressors are necessary, each with the capacity to meet the entire hospital's medical air needs if the other fails. The system must be used only for the medical air pipeline and not for the purpose of powering equipment. If air is to be used for powering equipment, a separate *instrument air system* must be installed. (The requirements for this system are specified in NFPA-99.) The compression pumps must not add contaminants to the gas, and the air intake must be located away from any street or other exhaust. It is particularly important that the pumps be located away from the hospital's vacuum system exhaust. The air must first be thoroughly dried to remove water vapor and then filtered to remove dirt, oil, and other contaminants. The condensed water is then properly disposed of to eliminate potential breeding grounds for bacteria, such as those that cause Legionnaire's disease. Valves, pressure regulators, and alarms analogous to those in oxygen supply systems are needed. In addition, the piping should not be exposed to subfreezing temperatures.

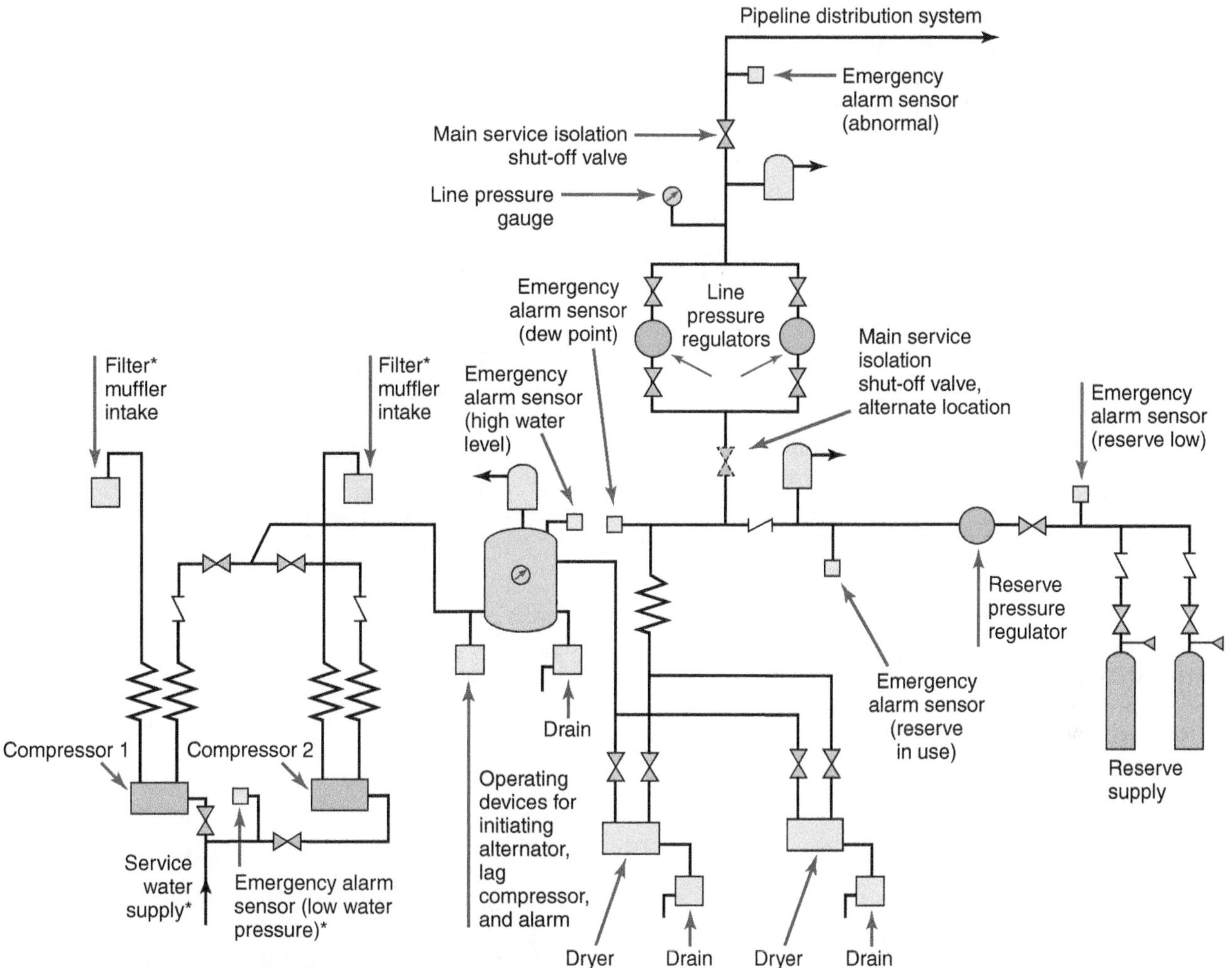

FIGURE 1-18 ■ A typical duplex medical air compressor system. Compressors (*lower left*) draw in ambient air and send high-pressure air to a holding tank. It is critical that these air intakes not be located near any source of air pollution, such as a garage or the exhaust from the facility's vacuum system. The air from the holding tank is dried and filtered on its way to pressure regulators, which deliver gas at about 55 psig into the pipeline system. *Where required. (From *Standard Z305.1–92, Nonflammable medical gas piping systems.* Toronto, 1992, Canadian Standards Association.)

Nitrous Oxide

Specific standards exist for nitrous oxide systems, and certain portions of the more general standards of the NFPA and CSA are applicable as well.[20] A nitrous oxide central supply system may be warranted, depending on the expected daily use of the gas. If demand is sufficient, such a system could be cost effective compared with attaching small cylinders to each anesthesia machine. Even though anesthesiologists are the only people who use the nitrous oxide system, they must delegate the responsibility for the operation and maintenance of the central nitrous oxide system to other hospital personnel.

Nitrous oxide central supply systems are usually of the cylinder-manifold type, as shown in Figure 1-11. Again, it is necessary to have two separate banks of cylinders with an automatic crossover; however, large institutions may need a bulk liquid storage system similar to the one used for oxygen, shown in Figure 1-16. In this case, the storage of liquid nitrous oxide requires an insulated container similar to that used for liquid oxygen.

Helium

Helium is commonly supplied in an E-size cylinder with a flowmeter that delivers it into the fresh-gas flow, but H-size cylinders are also used. Anesthesia machines are available that incorporate a helium flowmeter on the manifold, usually in place of medical air (see Fig. 1-18, *A*). Although this design incorporates some of the anesthesia machine's safety features, care must be taken to avoid delivering hypoxic gas mixtures. On new machines, helium tanks are supplied premixed with oxygen as a 3:1 He/O_2 mixture. This prevents the risk of hypoxia that occurs when 100% helium tanks are used on the machine.

Nitric Oxide

Inhaled nitric oxide is approved and regulated by the U.S. Food and Drug Administration as a pharmaceutical product, not as a medical gas. It is provided as 800 ppm nitric oxide diluted in nitrogen and available in D cylinders (353 L at 2000 psig) or the larger 88 cylinders (1963 L at 2000 psig). The selected concentration of inhaled nitric oxide is delivered into the inspiratory limb of the breathing system. A monitoring device to measure the concentrations of oxygen, nitric oxide, and nitrogen dioxide (a toxic byproduct) is placed downstream of the nitric oxide inlet. Ikaria, Inc. (Hampton, NJ) produces the INOmax DS delivery system, which electronically controls the amount of nitric oxide injected into the circuit, monitors delivered concentrations, and adjusts nitric oxide to maintain a constant concentration despite variations in fresh gas flow (Fig. 1-19).

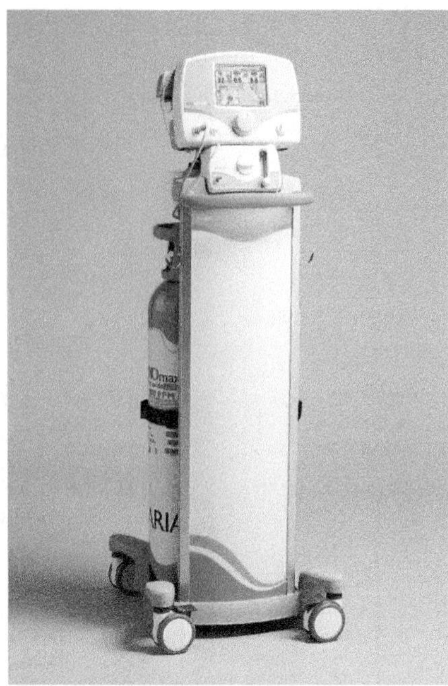

FIGURE 1-19 ■ Ikaria INOmax DS delivery system delivers a constant, operator-determined concentration of nitric oxide with sensors to detect oxygen, nitric oxide, and nitrogen dioxide. (Courtesy Ikaria, Hampton, NJ.)

Nitrogen

Even though a nitrogen central supply system is designed to supply gas only for powering OR equipment, it is still subject to the same standards outlined above. Nitrogen supply systems are frequently smaller than those for nitrous oxide but are of essentially the same design, in which a series of H-cylinders are connected by a manifold (pressure header) system that feeds a pressure regulator. A typical nitrogen control panel is illustrated in Figure 1-20. Again, because this system services the OR, it is important to delegate responsibility for maintenance. Although relatively uncommon, some systems are designed to mix central nitrogen with oxygen to create medical air. It is also possible to store nitrogen as a liquid for a centrally supplied system.

Central Vacuum Systems

Although not a source of medical gas, the central vacuum system is no less important and demands the same attention to detail as a medical gas system. Inadequate or failed suction can be disastrous in the face of a surgical or anesthetic crisis.

Certain standards exist for the central vacuum source and vacuum piping system; the Canadian standards are considered the most complete and current.[13] Larger ORs must have enough suction to remove 99 L/min of air. Factors such as normal wall suction (−7 psig), total flow of the system, and the length of the longest run of pipe must be considered to maintain adequate suction. Two independent vacuum pumps must be present, each one capable of handling the peak load alone. An automatic switching device distributes the load under normal conditions and automatically shifts if one unit fails. Emergency power connections are essential, and the pumps must be located away from oxygen and nitrous oxide storage. There must be traps to collect and safely dispose of any solid or liquid contaminants introduced into the system, and the system piping must not be exposed to low temperatures to prevent condensation. The type and location of the vacuum system exhaust is specified and must not be near the intake for the medical air compressor.

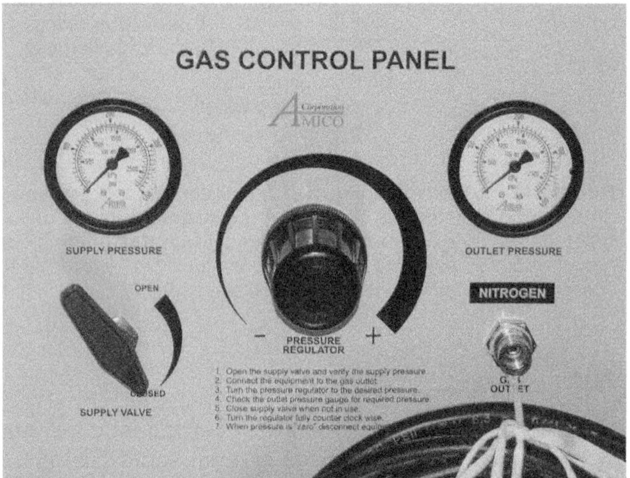

FIGURE 1-20 ■ An operating room control panel for nitrogen. The outlet pressure of nitrogen can be controlled by the variable pressure regulator. In this manner, the exact pressure can be set to meet the demands of the piece of equipment being powered.

MEDICAL GAS PIPELINES

Medical gas must travel through a pipeline to reach its designated point of use. The potential for serious injury to a patient from a medical gas pipeline mishap has led to the development of detailed standards.[12,13]

Planning

In any new construction, physicians must provide architects and engineers with the number and desired locations of any gas outlets. Anesthesiologists need to decide whether they want one or two sets of outlets for anesthesia gases in each OR and whether they want wall and/or ceiling-mounted distribution of the gases. Representatives from all the departments that will use the system should be involved in planning the location of the outlets. A basic layout for a portion of a piping system is illustrated in Figure 1-21. Extensive planning is necessary for

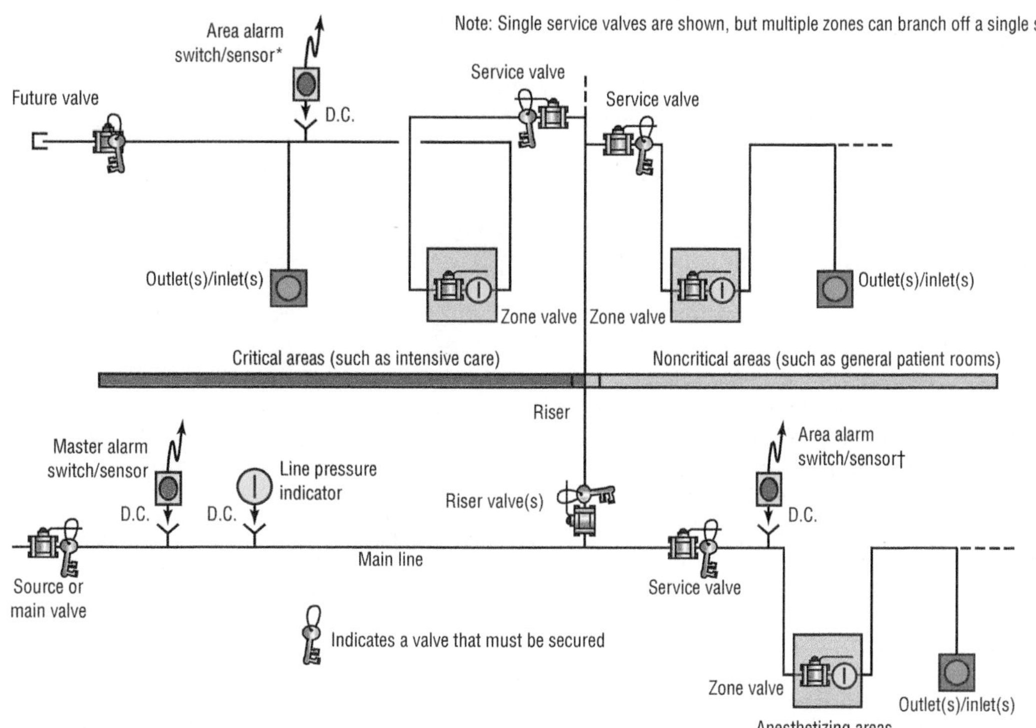

FIGURE 1-21 ■ A representative portion of the pipeline system for oxygen in a hospital. Note that separate similar designs are needed for the other medical gases. The schematic is representational, demonstrating a possible arrangement of required components. It is not intended to imply a method, materials of construction, or more than one of many possible and equally compliant arrangements. Alternative arrangements are permitted. *Area alarms are required in critical care locations (e.g., intensive care units, coronary care units, angiography laboratories, cardiac catheterization laboratories, postanesthesia recovery rooms, and emergency rooms) and anesthetizing locations (e.g., operating rooms and delivery rooms). †Locations for switches/sensors are not affected by the presence of service or inline valves. (From *NFPA 99-2012. Health care facilities.* Copyright 2011, National Fire Protection Association. Quincy, MA, 02269.)

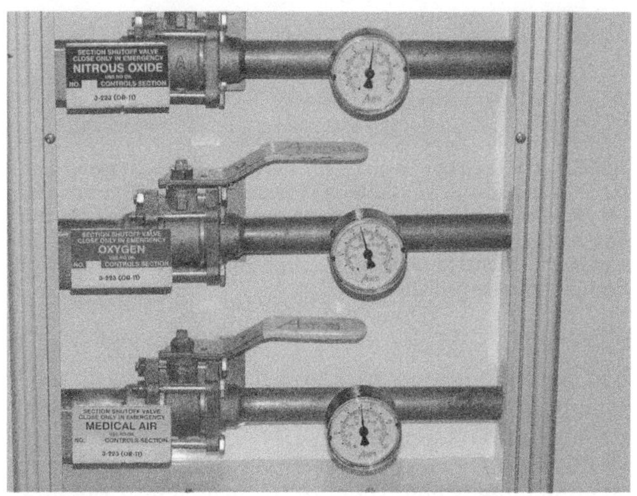

FIGURE 1-22 ■ Typical shut-off valves for the gases supplied in operating rooms (ORs). Each gas must have its own shut-off valve, and a separate set of valves must be present for each OR.

each separate medical gas pipeline, and anesthesiologists must be aware of all appropriate requirements. For example, each anesthetizing location must have a separate shut-off valve (Fig. 1-22), and other areas such as the postanesthesia care unit (PACU) require zone shut-off valves.

Detailed standards must be followed with respect to the specific type of pipe used, typically seamless copper tubing, as well as the cleaning, soldering, and supporting of the pipe within the walls.[8,12,13] In addition, pipelines must be protected, such as by enclosure in conduits, especially when they run underground. Pipes located inside risers and walls must be labeled in a specific way and at given intervals.

Once drafted, the plans must be examined to verify that all standards have been met. Given the fact that the construction of medical gas pipelines is relatively uncommon, it is possible that a given engineering, architectural, or building firm has never constructed one before. Any changes made in the plans should be recorded in the as-built drawings to enable hospital personnel to discern the exact location of the pipes if problems arise.

Additions to Existing Systems

Even more difficult than planning a new medical gas pipeline system is adding to an existing system. In addition to all the planning outlined above, the interaction between the old facility and the new one must be considered. The central supply system may need to be expanded to include new pipeline systems, which may necessitate the difficult task of shutting down the existing pipeline system. Extreme precision is required for such an operation, and procedural standards exist both for modifying or adding to existing systems.[13]

Installation and Testing

Installation of a pipeline should be overseen by a representative from the medical facility, and the testing should actively involve several individuals who will use the system. Prior to installation, the copper tubing used for the medical gas pipeline must be clean and free of contamination. The lengths of pipe must be stored with both ends sealed with rubber or plastic caps to prevent contamination. After the pipelines have been installed, but before the outlet valves are installed at each gas outlet location, high-pressure gas must be used to blow the pipeline free of any particulate matter.

The pipeline system involves pressure regulators that function to maintain normal outlet pressure (e.g., 55 psig for oxygen). Also, there must be pressure relief devices that automatically vent the gas if the pressure increases by 50% above the normal operating pressure. High- and low-pressure alarms and shut-off valves are required at various locations throughout the system. The locations of all these should be marked on a map of the institution.

The pipeline terminates at various locations within the hospital. A connector is installed at these termination points to allow the interface of various pieces of medical equipment, such as the anesthesia machine or ventilator. The connectors installed at each outlet of the pipeline are subject to detailed requirements.[12,13] Two basic types of connectors are used: one is the quick coupler, which is made by several manufacturers and allows rapid connection and disconnection of fittings and hoses (Figs. 1-23 and 1-24). The other is a noninterchangeable thread system called the *diameter index safety system* (Fig. 1-25).[5] Both systems have gas-specific fittings to prevent incorrect connections. Improper use of a gas outlet or use of an incorrect fitting essentially defeats the purpose of the built-in safeguards of the system. Accordingly, the station outlets must have back-up automatic shut-off valves in case the quick coupler is damaged or removed. All outlets, hoses, and quick couplers should be properly labeled and color coded.

Gas outlets in the OR may be located in either the wall or the ceiling. If the gas hoses are run along the floor, they must be made of noncompressible materials to prevent obstruction in case the hose is run over by a piece of heavy equipment. Outlets may be suspended from the ceiling in columns or as freestanding hose drops (Fig. 1-26), or they may be integrated into a multiservice gas boom (Fig. 1-27). These gas booms can be configured with all the anesthetic gases as well as vacuum systems, electrical outlets, monitor connections, and even data and telephone lines. They can be rotated to several different positions and can be raised or lowered as necessary.

Testing of the pipeline begins after the couplers have been installed. Before the walls are closed, the pipeline is subjected to 150 psig, and each joint is examined for leaks. The system then undergoes a 24-hour standing pressure test, in which the system is filled with gas to at least 150 psig, disconnected from the gas source, and closed. If the pressure is the same after 24 hours, no leaks are present. Cross-connection testing involves pressurizing each pipeline system separately with test gas and verifying that only the outlets of that particular system—for example, compressed air—are pressurized. This is particularly important when additions or modifications are made to existing pipeline systems.

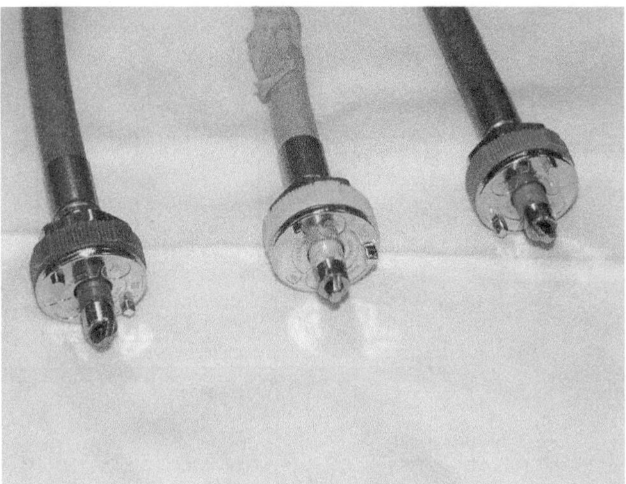

FIGURE 1-23 Common types of quick couplers used in hospitals. Note that each has a specific pin configuration for the individual gas. The quick coupler and the attached hose should be color coded for the specific gas.

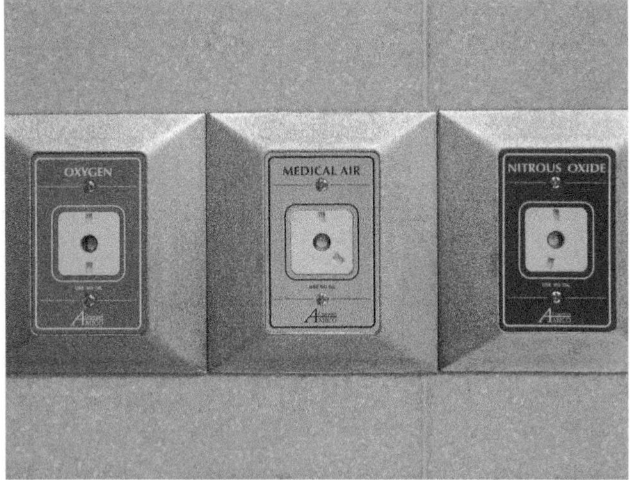

FIGURE 1-24 Wall connections for oxygen, air, and nitrous oxide in a safety-keyed quick-connect system. The GE Healthcare (Waukesha, WI) quick-connect system is shown, in which each gas is assigned two specific pins with corresponding inlet holes within the circumference of the circle. In this manner, the connection is made gas specific.

After the correct connections have been verified, each pipeline is connected to its own central supply of gas, and the pipelines are purged with their own gases. The content of gas from every station outlet must then be analyzed. An oxygen analyzer can be used for the oxygen (100%) and medical air (21%) outlets. The concentrations of nitrous oxide and nitrogen must be 100% according to chromatography or other appropriate analysis.

All the gas systems must be properly verified. According to NFPA-99, "testing shall be conducted by a party technically competent and experienced in the field of medical gas and vacuum pipeline testing and meeting the

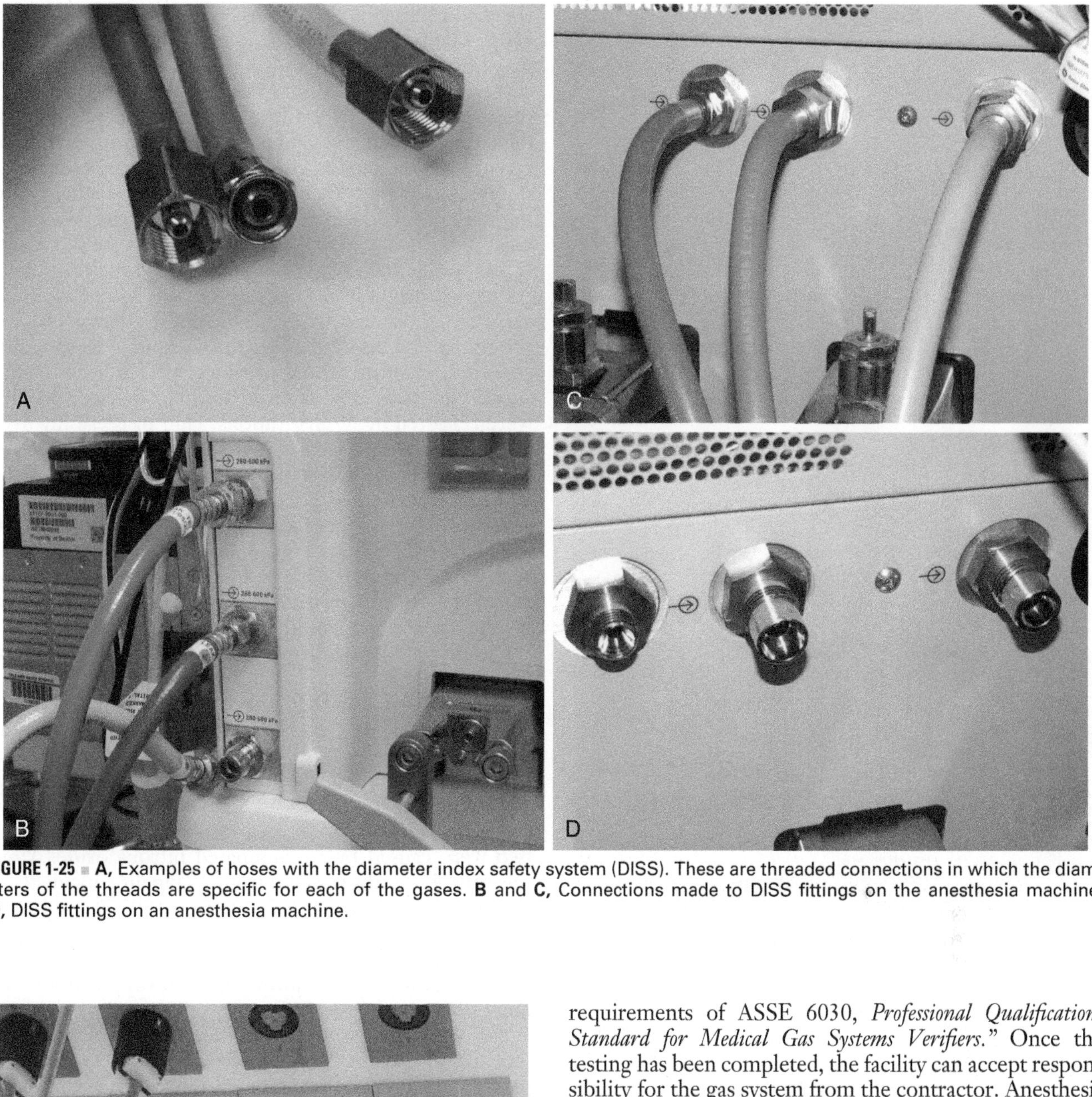

FIGURE 1-25 ■ **A,** Examples of hoses with the diameter index safety system (DISS). These are threaded connections in which the diameters of the threads are specific for each of the gases. **B** and **C,** Connections made to DISS fittings on the anesthesia machine. **D,** DISS fittings on an anesthesia machine.

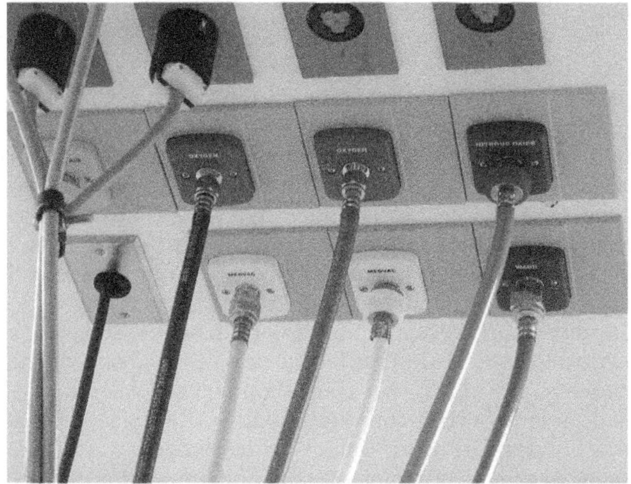

FIGURE 1-26 ■ Freestanding ceiling hose drops in an operating room. Note the proximal ends of the hoses (nearest to the ceiling) have diameter index safety system connections. The distal ends (nearest to the anesthesia machine) have quick-coupler connections (see Fig. 1-23).

requirements of ASSE 6030, *Professional Qualifications Standard for Medical Gas Systems Verifiers.*" Once the testing has been completed, the facility can accept responsibility for the gas system from the contractor. Anesthesiologists should certainly be involved in verifying the correctness of the gas supplies. Major problems with new systems have been identified by anesthesiologists after the system was "certified" safe for use.[21] Australia has a rigorous "permit to work" system modeled after a similar system in the United Kingdom, with specific steps that must be followed before gas supplies can be used.[22,23]

Contamination of medical gas pipelines has become a concern,[8] and rigorous standards have been developed to prevent contamination. Gas samples should be taken at the same time from both the source of the system and the most distant station outlet. If analysis by gas chromatography demonstrates contaminants present above the maximum allowable level, the system should be purged and retested. If purging the system fails to solve the problem, extensive troubleshooting may be necessary. Detailed records of all testing must be maintained and should be available for inspection by TJC. Once the testing has been satisfactorily completed, the system is ready for use.

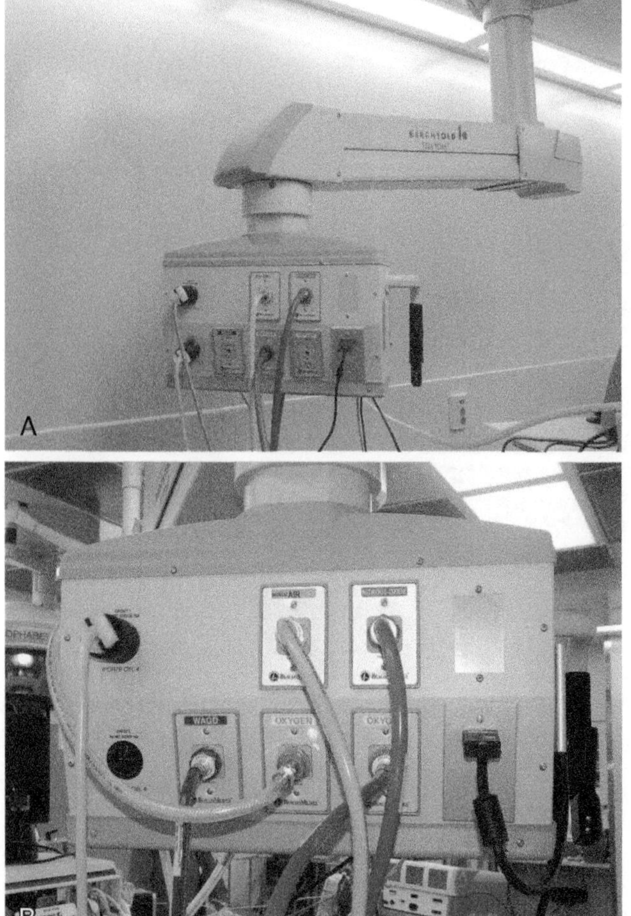

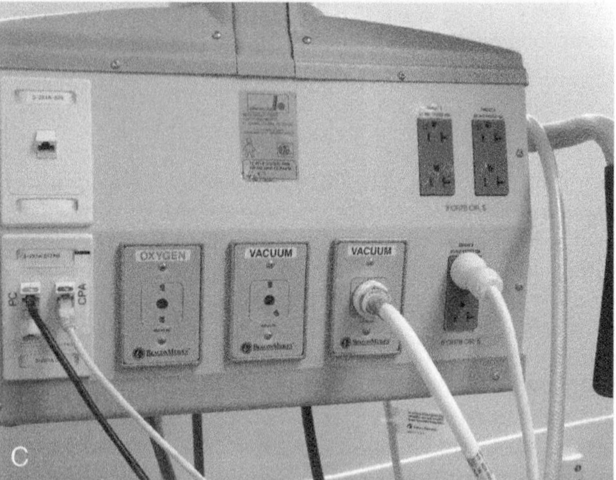

FIGURE 1-27 ■ **A** to **C**, The distribution head for an articulating multiservice gas boom. Compressed gases, vacuum, waste anesthesia gas, computer/Internet, and electrical connections can all be integrated at one location. The articulated arm can be raised, lowered, or rotated in a wide arc.

HAZARDS OF MEDICAL GAS DELIVERY SYSTEMS

A number of deaths have occurred as a result of incorrect installation or malfunction of medical gas delivery systems. The exact number is not known, however, because the medical literature contains few publications on medical gas delivery systems. Physicians and administrators may be reluctant to discuss or publish details of accidents that occur at their facilities. Often, only personnel within the medical facility are aware of an accident. If the accident is either serious or results in litigation, it may be reported in the media. However, it is likely that many, if not most, accidents that involve medical gas delivery systems are not reported, which may prevent the dissemination of valuable information that could help prevent future accidents. One attempt was made to learn about problems with bulk gas delivery systems by conducting a survey of hospitals with anesthesia residency training programs.[24] One third of the hospitals responding reported problems, three of which were deaths. In this survey, 76 malfunctions in medical gas delivery systems were reported by 59 institutions. Half of these involved insufficient oxygen pressure, crossed pipelines, depletion of central supply gas, failure of alarms, pipeline leaks, and freezing of gas regulators. Insufficient oxygen pressure was most frequently reported from pipelines damaged during unrelated hospital construction projects, such as resurfacing a parking lot above a buried pipeline. Another frequent problem was debris or other material in pipelines, which could be eliminated by adhering to the prescribed procedures for testing newly installed gas piping systems.

Between 1964 and 1973 in the United Kingdom, 29 deaths or permanent complications were reported to the Medical Defense Union, a malpractice insurance company. These resulted from problems in the gas supply or anesthetic apparatus.[25] Three cases were the result of either an error or failure in piped oxygen supplies, and two were caused by contaminated nitrous oxide. More recently, 45 deaths resulted from 26 pipeline incidents in the United States from 1972 through 1993.[26] A substantially higher number of "near misses" also occurred during this period, and patient death was prevented by prompt discovery of improper oxygen supply and treatment of exposed patients.[26]

Errors on the part of commercial suppliers when filling liquid oxygen bulk reservoirs have endangered patients and, in at least one instance, have harmed a patient. A supplier succeeded in filling a liquid oxygen reservoir with liquid nitrogen by bypassing the indexed, noninterchangeable safety valve connection designed to prevent such an occurrence.[27] A hypoxic gas mixture was thus delivered to anesthetized patients. Fortunately, however, the ensuing problems were quickly recognized and catastrophe averted by a switch to tank oxygen supply. In another more recent episode, two patients received a hypoxic gas mixture that led to the death of one of the patients.[28] In this case a 100-L container of "liquid oxygen" was delivered and connected to the hospital's gas pipeline approximately 1 hour before patients were anesthetized. This container actually contained almost pure nitrogen. It is interesting to note that no inspired oxygen analyzer was in use at the time of the accident.

Several other problems with bulk oxygen delivery systems have been reported. In one case, the delivery of a large volume of liquid oxygen caused a sudden drop in the temperature of the system, which resulted in a regulator freezing in a low-pressure mode.[29] Insufficient oxygen pressure resulted, and attempts to correct the problem quickly revealed that a low-pressure alarm had been disconnected during a recent modification of the system. In an attempt to restore regulator function, several maneuvers were performed that worsened the situation by allowing excessive pressure (100 psig) into the hospital pipeline. This caused reducing valves on anesthesia machines to rupture. In this case, injury to patients was avoided by the quick thinking of the anesthesiologists in the OR. A more tragic incident involved a child who sustained cardiac arrest and subsequent brain damage when an oxygen pipeline valve was simply turned off.[30] Another case of a hypoxic mixture coming from oxygen outlets involved a problem with the regulator in the oxygen pipeline; the regulator failed, causing a decreased oxygen pressure that allowed high-pressure compressed air to enter the oxygen system through an air-oxygen blender connected to both outlets in the neonatal intensive care unit.[31]

Accidental cross-connecting of pipelines represents a clearly recognized threat to patients.[32-34] Exposure of patients to incorrect gases proves the inadequacy of the testing of that pipeline. An additional source of error may arise when the pipeline is connected to the anesthesia machine. According to one report, several deaths were caused by the connection of a nitrous oxide pipeline to the oxygen inlet on the anesthesia machine with the corresponding connection of the oxygen pipeline to the nitrous oxide inlet.[35] In other instances, repair of the hoses that run from the outlet to the machine led to the interchange of the oxygen and nitrous oxide quick coupler female adapters. As a result, the nitrous oxide pipeline was connected to the oxygen inlet, causing the death of one patient, among other catastrophes.[36,37]

One published report of contamination of gas pipeline systems involved a newly constructed hospital building.[8] During cross-connection testing of the gas pipelines, a distinct "organic chemical" odor was detected. Gas chromatography revealed the presence of a volatile hydrocarbon at a concentration of 10 ppm. Four days of purging reduced this contaminant to 0.1 ppm in the oxygen pipeline and 0.4 ppm in the medical air pipelines. The original outlet tests also showed a fine, black powder being expelled from gas outlets. Subsequent investigation revealed that during installation, the ends of the pipe segment were color coded with spray paint. Later, when the pipe ends were being prepared for soldering, they were sanded down, and the paint particles settled inside the pipeline. This particulate contamination was eliminated by the purging process.

Contamination of a hospital oxygen pipeline system by other chemicals was also reported when the solution used to clean the oxygen supply tubing between the supply tank and the hospital pipeline had not been flushed out.[38] In this case, all the hospital outlets had to be shut down, and patients were switched to tank supplies while the problem was identified and the pipeline system flushed with fresh oxygen.

A commercial firm that conducts tests of new hospital gas pipelines conducted a study of 10 hospitals in which a total of 1668 gas outlets were examined. At seven hospitals, all outlets failed the gas purity tests. Of the 1668 outlets, 331 (20%) failed for a variety of reasons, such as unacceptably high moisture, volatile hydrocarbons, halogenated hydrocarbon solvents, unidentified odors, and particulate matter such as solder flux. Contamination of new medical gas pipelines appears to be a common problem that merits close attention. A report in the 2012 fall newsletter of the Anesthesia Patient Safety Foundation further emphasizes this problem. During a construction project, a new oxygen line was built and was leak tested with nitrogen. Subsequently, the nitrogen was not fully purged from the line and entered the main hospital oxygen supply. The inspired oxygen concentration decreased to 2% to 3% in 8 to 9 operating rooms.[39]

Another frequently reported cause of mishaps in oxygen supply is a problem with oxygen blending devices, such as those found on ventilators to decrease the inspired oxygen percentage.[40,41] These devices are subjected to heavy use and are exposed to multiple mechanical stresses as ventilators are moved about. Again, the importance of monitoring the delivered oxygen concentration cannot be overemphasized.

Although the potential hazards of using medical gas delivery systems are many, such mishaps are largely preventable with close attention to the applicable standards.

PROCEDURES

When a new medical gas delivery system is constructed, both the medical staff and the plant engineering department must be involved in all stages of the process to prevent building inadequacies or inconveniences into the system that might otherwise limit its value or even create a hazard. The medical facility must clearly designate the lines of responsibility for the medical gas delivery system among the hospital staff members. One suggestion is for institutions to have four departments—plant engineering, maintenance, anesthesia, and respiratory therapy—delegate responsibility for the gas delivery systems to one or more members of each department. Each member of the group should possess a thorough understanding of the institution's systems, and each person must be able to manage any problem that might occur. Consideration should be given to use of an outside contractor who specializes in the construction of new and refurbished medical pipeline systems.

Excellent communication must be established with the company that supplies the bulk gas. The gas supplier should supply the hospital with a list of emergency contacts and should notify the institution whenever a bulk gas delivery is scheduled. In this way, the delivery can be overseen by the appropriate committee member. Had this been done in certain situations, several of the problems cited above could have been avoided.

Communication between the supplier and the hospital's representatives is important when the gas delivery system undergoes any work. In addition, representatives from both the institution and the supplier should be aware of any construction that might affect the gas system. In one case, such precautions could have prevented crushing of the underground pipes of an oxygen bulk supply system during the resurfacing of a hospital parking lot.[24] Hospitals need to develop protocols and designate a responsible person to respond to medical gas alarms, including a complete failure of the oxygen system. The necessity of such plans is illustrated by a situation in which a tornado destroyed a hospital's central bulk oxygen supply.[42]

Interdepartmental communication is also critical. All affected departments must be notified when the gas supply system is to be shut off for repair or periodic maintenance. A near-crisis situation arose when an engineering department shut down piped oxygen supplies during the operating schedule without notifying anyone else in the hospital.[24] Although this incident occurred many years ago, such incidents still occur but often go unreported, especially if no patients are injured. After repair or maintenance, a qualified person should inspect the system before it is put back into service. The patient death that resulted from the interchanged quick couplers could have been prevented had this procedure been followed.

Anesthesia providers are often complacent about their gas supply until either a problem or a catastrophe occurs. Almost all injuries to patients and problems related to medical gases are preventable, even those caused by natural disasters. Building and maintaining a safe medical gas system requires a great deal of effort on the part of many individuals but is vital to the integrity of health care facilities.

REFERENCES

1. *Safe handling of compressed gas in containers*: Publication P–1, ed 11, Arlington, VA, 2008, Compressed Gas Association.
2. *Characteristics and safe handling of medical gases*:Publication P–2, ed 9, Arlington, VA, 2006, Compressed Gas Association.
3. Dorsch JA, Dorsch SE: Medical gas cylinders and containers. In *Understanding anesthesia equipment*, ed 5, Baltimore, 2008, Lippincott Williams & Wilkins, pp 12–15.
4. *American National, Canadian, and Compressed Gas Association standard for compressed gas cylinder valve outlet and inlet connections*:Publication V–1 ed 12, Arlington, VA, 2005, Compressed Gas Association.
5. *Diameter index safety system*:Publication V–5, ed 6, Arlington, VA, 2008, Compressed Gas Association.
6. *Pressure relief device standards: Part 1. Cylinders for compressed gases*: Publication S–1.1, ed 13, Arlington, VA, 2007, Compressed Gas Association.
7. Feeley TW, Bancroft ML, Brooks RA, et al: Potential hazards of compressed gas cylinders: a review, *Anesthesiology* 48:72–74, 1978.
8. Eichhorn JH, Bancroft ML, Laasberg H, et al: Contamination of medical gas and water pipelines in a new hospital building, *Anesthesiology* 46:286–289, 1977.
9. Slack GD: *Medical gas and vacuum systems*, Chicago, 1989, American Hospital Association.
10. Eichhorn JH: Medical gas delivery systems, *Int Anesthesiol Clin* 19(2):1–26, 1981.
11. *Compressed gases and cryogenic fluids code, NFPA 55*, Quincy, MA, 2010, National Fire Protection Association.
12. Gas and vacuum systems. In *Health care facilities code, NFPA-99*. Quincy, MA, 2012, National Fire Protection Association, pp 25-73.
13. *Nonflammable medical gas pipeline systems, Z305.1-92*, Toronto, 1992, Canadian Standards Association.
14. Dorsch JA, Dorsch SE: Medical gas piping systems. In *Understanding anesthesia equipment*, ed 2, Baltimore, 1984, Williams & Wilkins, pp 16–37.
15. Bancroft ML, duMoulin GC, Hedley-Whyte J: Hazards of hospital bulk oxygen delivery systems, *Anesthesiology* 52:504–510, 1980.
16. Penny M: Physical and chemical properties of molecular sieves: the pressure absorption cycle, *Health Service Estate (HSE)* 61:44–49, 1987.
17. Friesen RM: Oxygen concentrators and the practice of anesthesia, *Can J Anaesth* 39:R80–R84, 1992.
18. Rathgeber J, Zuchner K, Kietzmann D, Kraus E: Efficiency of a mobile oxygen concentrator for mechanical ventilation in anesthesia: studies with a metabolic lung model and early clinical results, *Anaesthesist* 44:643–650, 1995.
19. Wilson IH, vanHeerden PV: Domiciliary oxygen concentrators in anaesthesia: preoxygenation techniques and inspired oxygen concentrations, *Br J Anaesth* 65:342–345, 1990.
20. *Standard for nitrous oxide systems at consumer sites*: Publication G-8.1, ed 4, Arlington, VA, 2007, Compressed Gas Association.
21. Krenis LJ, Berkowitz DA: Errors in installation of a new gas delivery system found after certification, *Anesthesiology* 62:677–678, 1985.
22. Seed RF: The permit to work system, *Anaesth Intensive Care* 10:353–358, 1982.
23. Howell RSC: Piped medical gas and vacuum systems, *Anaesthesia* 35:679–698, 1980.
24. Feeley TW, Hedley-Whyte J: Bulk oxygen and nitrous oxide delivery systems: design and dangers, *Anesthesiology* 44:301–305, 1976.
25. Wylie WD: There, but for the grace of God, *Ann R Coll Surg Engl* 56:171–180, 1975.
26. Petty WC: Medical gases, hospital pipelines, and medical gas cylinders: how safe are they? *AANA Journal* 63:307–324, 1995.
27. Sprague DH, Archer GW: Intraoperative hypoxia from an erroneously filled liquid oxygen reservoir, *Anesthesiology* 42:360–362, 1975.
28. Holland R: "Wrong gas" disaster in Hong Kong, *Anesthesia Patient Safety Foundation Newsletter* 4(3):26, 1989.
29. Feeley TW, McClelland KJ, Malhotra IV: The hazards of bulk oxygen delivery systems, *Lancet* 1:1416–1418, 1975.
30. Epstein RM, Rackow H, Lee AA, et al: Prevention of accidental breathing of anoxic gas mixtures during anesthesia, *Anesthesiology* 23:1–4, 1962.
31. Carley RH, Houghton IT, Park GR: A near disaster from piped gases, *Anaesthesia* 39:891–893, 1984.
32. N_2O asphyxia [editorial], *Lancet* 1:848, 1974.
33. The Westminster inquiry [editorial], *Lancet* 2:175–176, 1977.
34. Macintosh R: Wrongly connected gas pipelines, *Lancet* 2:307, 1977.
35. McCormick JM: National fire protection codes—1968, *Anesth Analg* 47:538–545, 1968.
36. Mazze RI: Therapeutic misadventures with oxygen delivery systems: the need for continuous in-line oxygen monitors, *Anesth Analg* 51:787–792, 1972.
37. Robinson JS: A continuing saga of piped medical gas supply, *Anaesthesia* 34:66–70, 1979.
38. Gilmour IJ, McComb C, Palahniuk RJ: Contamination of a hospital oxygen supply, *Anesth Analg* 71:302–304, 1990.
39. It could happen to you! Construction contaminates oxygen pipeline. *APSF Newsletter* 27(2):35, 2012.
40. Otteni JC, Ancellin J, Cazalaa JB: Defective gas mixers, a cause of retro-pollution of medical gas distribution pipelines, *Ann Fr Anesth Reanim* 16:68–72, 1997.
41. Lye A, Patrick R: Oxygen contamination of the nitrous oxide pipeline supply, *Anaesth Intensive Care* 26:207–209, 1998.
42. Johnson DL: Central oxygen supply versus mother nature, *Respir Care* 20:1043, 1975.

CHAPTER 2

THE ANESTHESIA MACHINE AND WORKSTATION

James B. Eisenkraft

CHAPTER OUTLINE

ANESTHESIA GAS DELIVERY SYSTEM

The modern anesthesia gas delivery system is composed of the anesthesia machine, anesthesia vaporizer(s), ventilator, breathing circuit, and waste gas scavenging system. The basic arrangement of these elements is the same in all contemporary anesthesia gas delivery systems (Fig. 2-1). The anesthesia machine receives gases under pressure from their sources of storage (see Chapter 1), creates a gas mixture of known composition and flow rate, and delivers it to a concentration-calibrated vaporizer, which adds a controlled concentration of potent, inhaled, volatile anesthetic agent. The resulting mixture of oxygen—with or without a second gas such as nitrous oxide, air, or helium (heliox)—is delivered to the machine's common gas outlet (CGO). This gas mixture flows continuously from the CGO into the patient breathing circuit. The breathing circuit represents a microenvironment in which the patient's lungs effect gas exchange, so that by controlling the fresh gas mixure's composition, flow rate, and ventilatory parameters, the patient's arterial partial pressures of oxygen, nitrous oxide, anesthetic agent, and carbon dioxide can be controlled. Fresh gas flows continuously into the breathing system, most commonly a circle breathing system. Gas must therefore be able to leave the circuit, otherwise the pressure would increase and possibly lead to barotrauma—unless a completely closed system is used. If ventilation is spontaneous or assisted, excess gas leaves the circuit via the adjustable pressure-limiting (APL) valve. If the lungs are mechanically ventilated, the ventilator bellows or piston acts as a counterlung, exchanging its volume with the patient's lungs via the breathing circuit. In this case, excess gas exits the breathing circuit at end expiration via the ventilator pressure relief valve. The gas that exits the circuit is waste gas that enters the waste gas scavenging system to

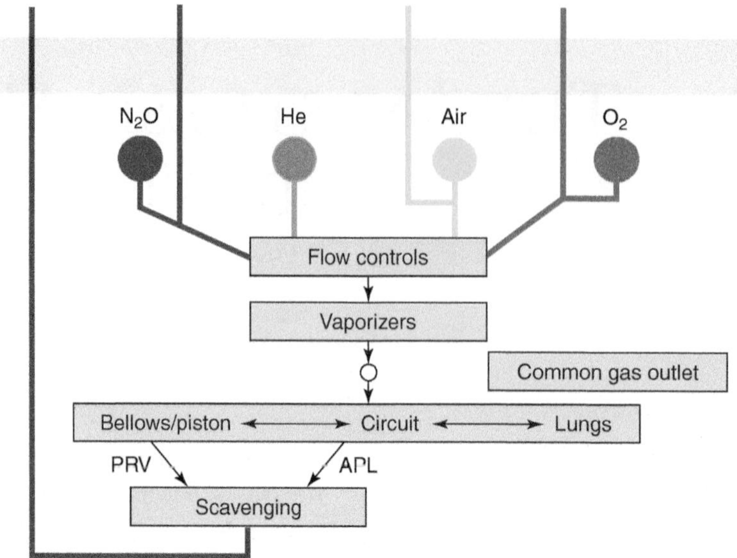

FIGURE 2-1 Organization of the anesthesia delivery system. APL, adjustable pressure-limiting; PRV, pressure relief valve.

be discharged outside the facility. An understanding of the structure and function of the gas delivery system is essential to the safe practice of anesthesia.

Anesthesia Machine and Workstation

Gas delivery systems continue to evolve as advances in technology and safety are incorporated into current designs. The recent evolution can be traced through the voluntary consensus standards that have been developed with input from manufacturers, users, and other interested agencies. The current voluntary consensus standard that describes the features of a contemporary system is published by the American Society for Testing and Materials (ASTM).[1] This document, standard F1850-00, published in March 2000 and reapproved in 2005, is entitled *Standard Specification for Particular Requirements for Anesthesia Workstations and Their Components*. It introduces the term "workstation" in distinction to "anesthesia (or gas) machine." The *anesthesia workstation* is defined as a system for the administration of anesthesia to patients consistsing of the anesthesia gas supply device (i.e., the machine), ventilator, and monitoring and protection devices. This standard supersedes anesthesia machine standard F1161-88, published in 1989 by the ASTM.[2] Standard F1161-88 had superseded the original anesthesia machine standard (Z79.8-1979) published in 1979 by the American National Standards Institute (ANSI).[3] Like its predecessors, ASTM standard F1850-00 has been voluntarily adopted by anesthesia machine manufacturers. The standard is not mandated, but it is highly unlikely that a new manufacturer would build, or would a purchaser be likely to purchase, a workstation that did not comply with the current standards.

The evolution of the anesthesia workstation and advances in technology have led to many changes in design. Although basic operations remain the same, the components are more technologically advanced. For example, in many new models—such as the Dräger Apollo (Fig. 2-2) and the GE Aisys (Fig. 2-3)—the

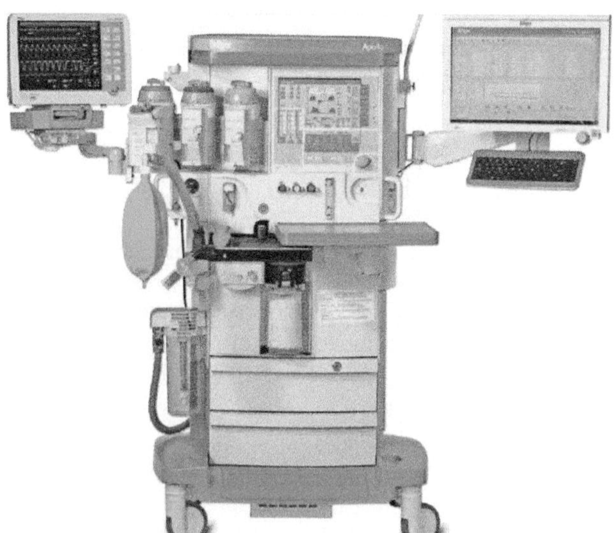

FIGURE 2-2 Apollo anesthesia workstation. (Courtesy Dräger Medical, Telford, PA.)

familiar rotameter tubes are replaced by virtual flowmeters displayed on a computer screen. The gas flow-control needle valves may be replaced by electronically controlled gas-mixing devices. This chapter describes the basic components and functions of a traditional anesthesia machine (i.e., the gas delivery device described in standard F1850-00) to enable the reader to appreciate some of the changes that have been made in the most recent models.

In the United States, the two largest manufacturers of gas delivery systems—machines, ventilators, vaporizers, and scavenging systems—are Draeger Medical Inc. (Telford, PA) and GE Healthcare (Waukesha, WI). This chapter reviews the features of a basic anesthesia delivery system, making reference to Dräger and GE (Datex-Ohmeda brand) products when appropriate. The flow of compressed gases from the point of entry into the machine, through the various components, and to the exit at the

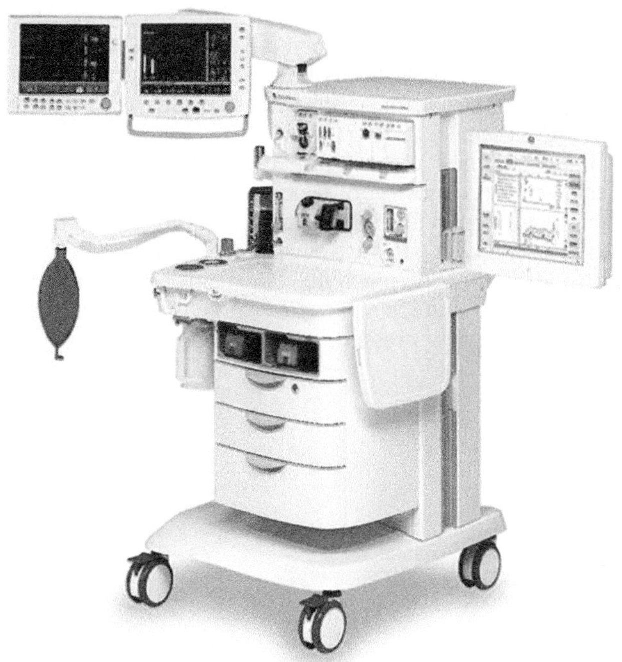

FIGURE 2-3 ■ Datex-Ohmeda Aisys Carestation. (Courtesy GE Healthcare, Waukesha, WI.)

CGO is described. The function of each component is discussed so that the effects of failure of that component, as well as the rationale for the various machine checkout procedures, can be appreciated. This approach provides a framework from which to diagnose problems that arise with the machine. Of note, the individual machine or workstation manufacturer's operator and service manuals represent the most comprehensive reference for any specific model of machine, and the reader is strongly encouraged to review the relevant manuals. The manufacturers also produce excellent educational materials,[4-6] and a number of simulations are also available on the Internet.[7-9]

Basic Anesthesia Machine

Although older anesthesia machines were completely pneumatic and required only a supply of gas under pressure, contemporary machines are electronic *and* pneumatic and therefore must be connected to an electrical outlet for normal, uninterrupted operation. When the main ON/OFF switch is turned on, both the pneumatic and the electronic functions are enabled.

In the OFF position, most of the electronic functions of the workstation are disabled, with the exception of the battery charger that charges the backup battery and the convenience electrical outlets on the back of the workstation, which are used to supply power to additional monitors (e.g., bispectral index) or a heated, pressurized desflurane vaporizer. The pneumatic functions maintained are the oxygen supply to the oxygen flush system and, in most machines, the auxiliary oxygen flowmeter.

When the ON/OFF switch is turned to ON, the workstation electronics go through a powering-up protocol that may include an automated checkout procedure that lasts several minutes. In case of an emergency, the automated checkout can be bypassed, but a record of this is maintained in the workstation's computer. In the ON position, the pneumatic functions permit delivery of an anesthetic gas mixture from the flowmeters and the concentration-calibrated vaporizer.

Pneumatic Systems

The gas flow arrangements of a basic two-gas anesthesia machine are shown in Figure 2-4. The machine receives each of the two basic gases, oxygen (O_2) and nitrous oxide (N_2O), from two supply sources: a tank or cylinder source and a pipeline source. The storage and supply of these gases to the operating room (OR) is described in Chapter 1.

The basic functions of any anesthesia machine are to receive compressed gases from their supplies and to create a gas mixture of known composition and flow rate at the CGO. The relation between pressure and flow is stated in Ohm's law:

$$\text{Flow} = \frac{\text{Pressure}}{\text{Resistance}}$$

Controlling the flow of gases from high-pressure sources through the machine to exit the CGO at pressures approximating atmospheric pressure requires changes in pressure and/or resistance. Modern anesthesia machines also incorporate certain safety features designed to prevent the delivery of a hypoxic mixture to the patient circuit. These features include the oxygen supply pressure failure alarm, pressure sensor shut-off ("fail-safe") system, and gas flow proportioning systems.

The anesthesia machine gas pathways have been conveniently divided by some authors into three systems[10]:

1. A high-pressure system that includes parts upstream of the first-stage regulator, where oxygen pressures are between 45 and 2200 psig
2. An intermediate pressure system that includes parts between the pipeline gas inlet/downstream outlet of the first-stage pressure regulator and the gas flow control valves, where oxygen pressures are between 55 and 16 psig
3. A low-pressure system that includes all parts downstream of the gas flow control valves, where pressures are normally slightly greater than atmospheric pressure

Other authors consider the high-pressure system to be simply all parts upstream of the gas flow control valves and the *low-pressure system* to be all parts downstream of the gas flow control valves. Indeed, this is in agreement with the system descriptions in the U.S. Food and Drug Administration 1993 preuse checkout recommendations.[11] Either way, the most important definition is that of the low-pressure system, the one to which most preuse checkouts refer.

Oxygen Supply Sources: Pipelines and Cylinders

Pipeline oxygen is supplied to the wall outlets in the OR at a pressure of 50 to 55 psig. *Gauge pressure* is pressure above ambient atmospheric pressure. Ambient atmospheric pressure at sea level is usually considered to be equivalent to 760 mm Hg, or 14.7 psia. The wall outlet connectors are gas specific, but only within each manufacturer's connector system. Thus an Ohmeda oxygen hose connector will not fit into an Ohmeda nitrous oxide wall outlet, but neither will it fit into an oxygen wall outlet in a Chemtron system. Thus the medical gas wall outlets and connectors are not interchangeable among the various gases or with the vacuum (Fig. 2-5). A color-coded hose conducts the pipeline oxygen from the wall outlet to the anesthesia machine's oxygen inlet. At the machine end of the hose, the connectors are gas specific by a national standard (Fig. 2-6) known as the *diameter index safety system* (DISS) that ensures that the correct gas enters the correct part of the anesthesia machine.[12] To standardize connections, many institutions are replacing the manufacturer's gas-specific wall outlets with DISS connectors (Fig. 2-7).

The machine's oxygen pipeline inlet incorporates a check valve that prevents leakage of oxygen from the machine if the pipeline is not connected and oxygen tanks are in use (Fig. 2-8). Failure of this valve would cause oxygen to leak from the machine. Upstream of the pipeline inlet in the machine is a pressure gauge that displays the pipeline gas supply pressure (see Fig. 2-4).

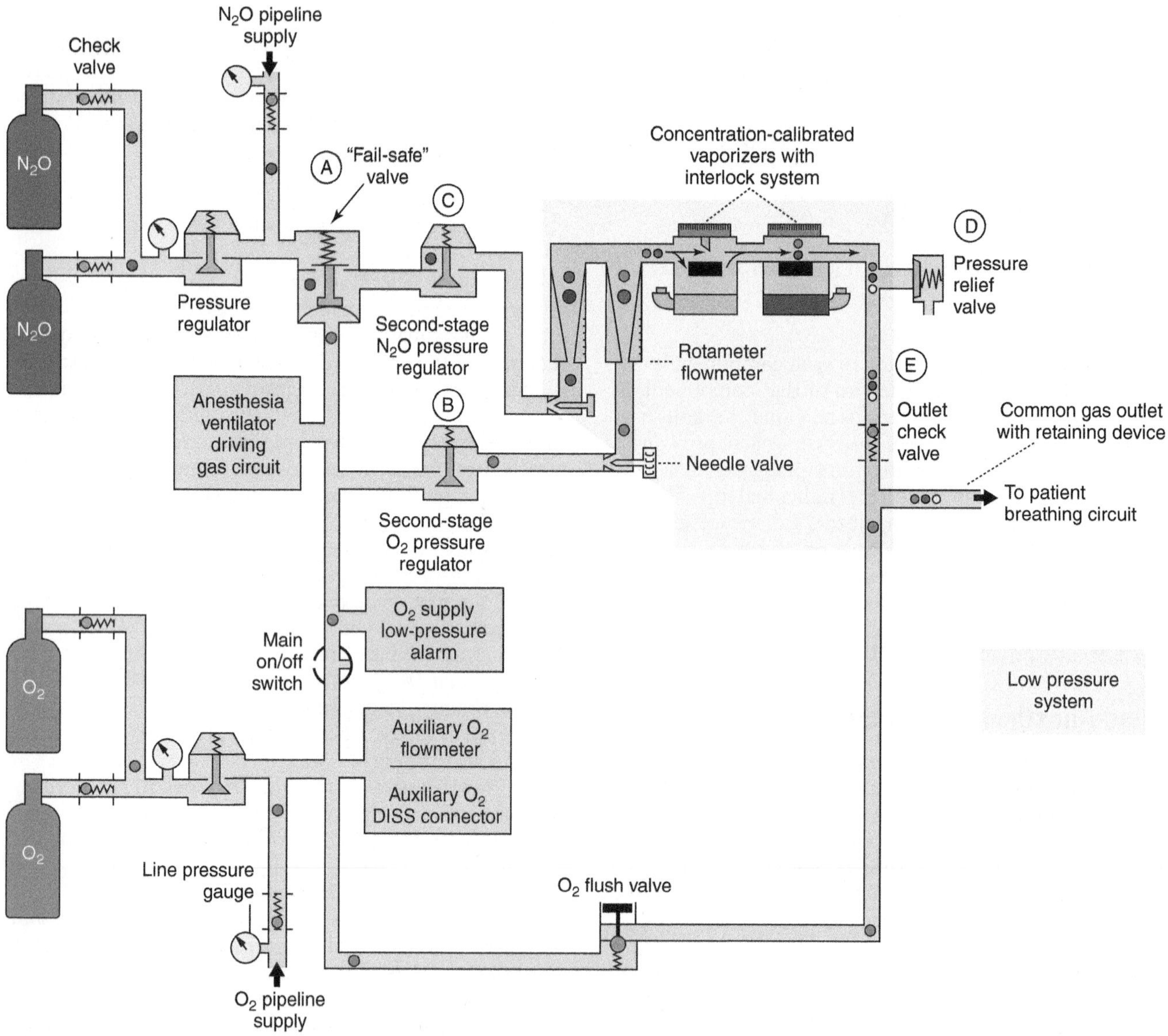

FIGURE 2-4 Schematic of flow arrangements of a generic contemporary anesthesia machine. *A,* The fail-safe valve in older GE Healthcare Datex-Ohmeda machines is termed a *pressure-sensor shut-off valve*; in more recent models, this valve has been replaced by a balance regulator. In Draeger Medical Inc., machines, the fail-safe valve is the oxygen failure protection device (OFPD). *B,* A second-stage oxygen pressure regulator is used in Datex-Ohmeda machines but not in Draeger Narkomed models. *C,* A second-stage nitrous oxide pressure regulator is used in Datex-Ohmeda Modulus machines that have the Link-25 Proportion Limiting System but not in Draeger machines. *D,* A pressure relief valve used in certain Datex-Ohmeda machines but not in Draeger machines. *E,* The outlet check valve used in Datex-Ohmeda machines, except Modulus II Plus and Modulus CD models, is not used in Draeger machines. The oxygen connection for the anesthesia ventilator driving gas circuit is *downstream* of the main ON/OFF switch in Draeger machines, as shown here. In Datex-Ohmeda machines, the takeoff is *upstream* of the main ON/OFF switch. DISS, diameter index safety system. (Modified from *Checkout: a guide for preoperative inspection of an anesthesia machine.* Park Ridge, IL, 1987, American Society of Anesthesiologists. Reproduced by permission of the American Society of Anesthesiologists, 520 N. Northwest Highway, Park Ridge, IL.)

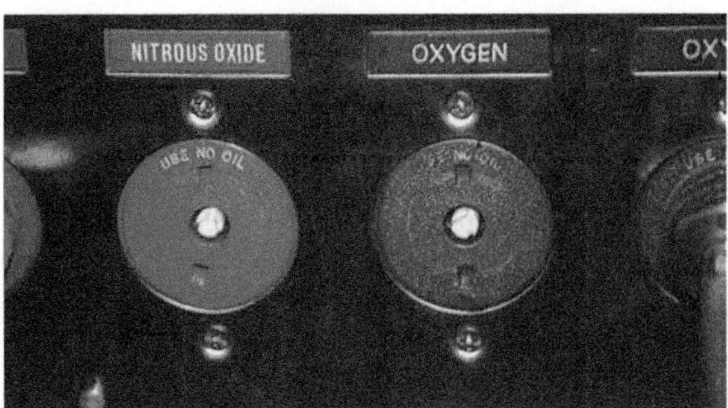

FIGURE 2-5 ■ Medical gas–specific wall outlet connectors. (Courtesy GE Healthcare, Waukesha, WI.)

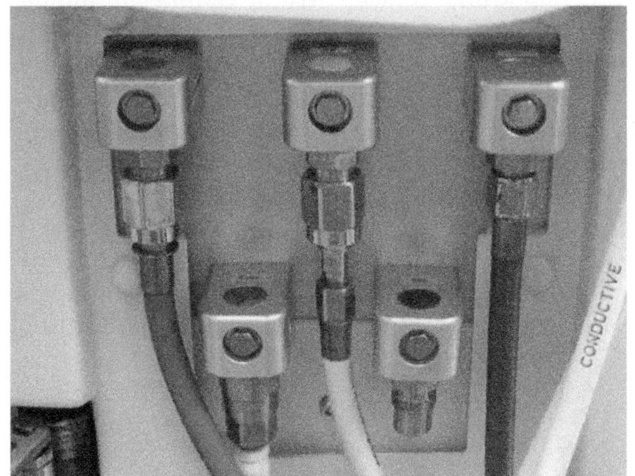

FIGURE 2-6 ■ Diameter index safety system hose connections to workstation pipeline supply connections.

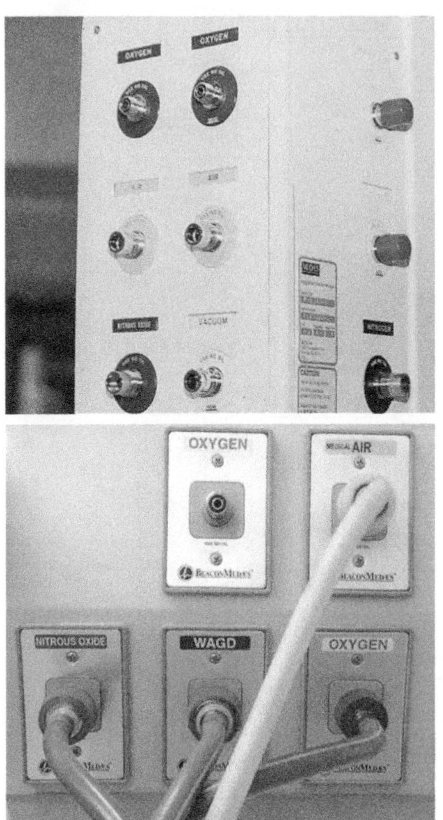

FIGURE 2-7 ■ Diameter index safety system wall connectors. Blue is nitrous oxide, green is oxygen, yellow is room air, white is the hospital vacuum, and purple is the waste gas scavenging vacuum.

Tank oxygen is supplied to the machine from the back-up E-cylinders attached via the oxygen hanger yokes (Fig. 2-9). The medical gas *pin index safety system* ensures that only an oxygen tank fits correctly into an oxygen hanger yoke (see Chapter 1).[13] Although manipulation is possible, a medical gas cylinder should never be forced to fit into a hanger yoke.

The pressure in a full oxygen tank is normally between 1900 and 2200 psig. Oxygen enters the hanger yoke at this pressure and then passes through a strainer nipple (Fig. 2-10) designed to prevent dirt or other particles from entering the machine. The oxygen then flows past a hanger yoke ("floating") check valve to enter the anesthesia machine at high pressure.

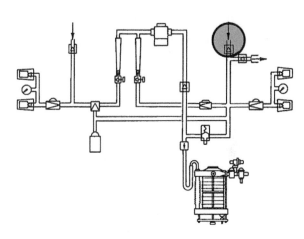

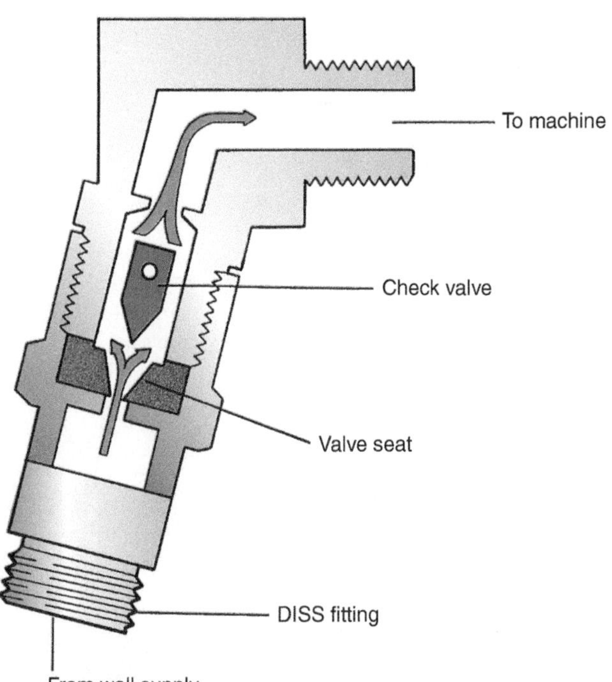

FIGURE 2-8 ■ Machine pipeline inlet check valve. The flow of oxygen from the wall supply opens the pipeline inlet valve. If the wall supply hose were disconnected with the tank oxygen in use, the pressure of oxygen in the machine would force the check valve to its seated position, preventing loss of oxygen via this connector. DISS, diameter index safety system. (From Bowie E, Huffman LM: *The anesthesia machine: essentials for understanding.* Madison, WI, 1985, GE Datex-Ohmeda.)

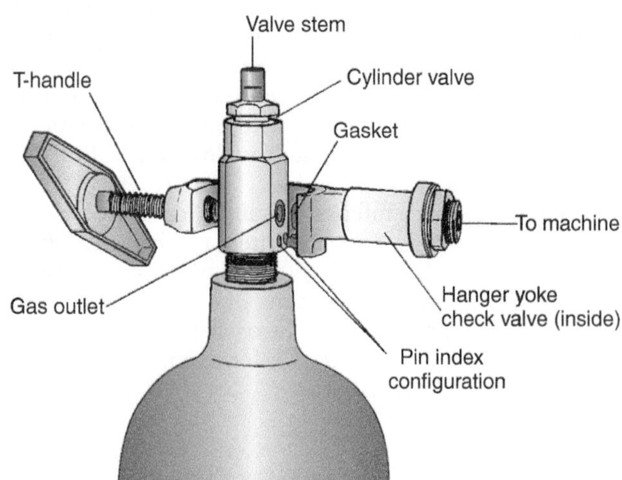

FIGURE 2-9 ■ **Hanger yoke for an oxygen tank showing the pin-indexed safety system.** (From Bowie E, Huffman LM: *The anesthesia machine: essentials for understanding.* Madison, WI, 1985, GE Datex-Ohmeda.)

Several considerations apply before a tank is hung in a yoke. First, the plastic wrapper that surrounds the tank valve must be removed. Then the valve is opened slowly, or "cracked," to allow gas to exit the tank and blow out any particles of dirt that may be lodged in the outlet. The tank is then hung in the yoke. The gas outlet hole is aligned with the strainer nipple, and the two yoke pins are aligned with the corresponding holes in the tank. The tank should never be turned through 180 degrees and then hung in the yoke because a tightened T-handle screw might damage the tank valve-stem pressure relief mechanism (see Chapter 1). Although changing the oxygen tank on an anesthesia machine may seem straightforward, one study showed that a significant number of senior residents in a simulator could not perform this task satisfactorily, possibly because it is generally performed by technical staff.[14] Checking to see that a backup tank contains sufficient oxygen is an important part of the preuse checkout and also ensures that a tank wrench is available for opening and closing the tank valve.[15]

Oxygen is also available in freestanding E-size tanks pressurized to 3000 psig (1000 L gaseous oxygen) that incorporate a regulator that delivers oxygen at 50 psig to a DISS connector. Thus, if the pipeline fails, the machine's

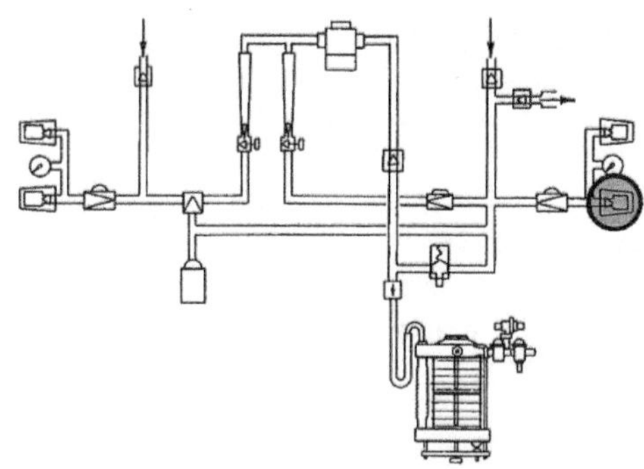

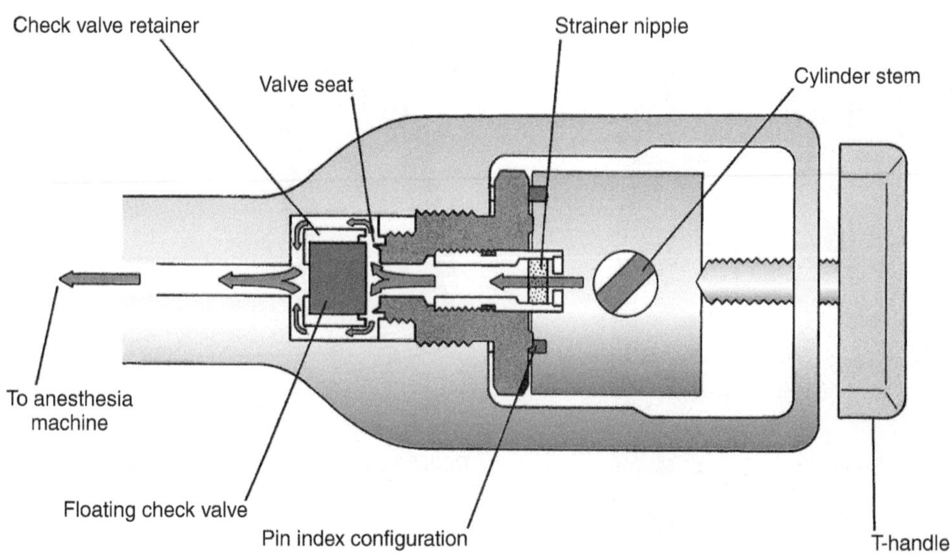

FIGURE 2-10 ■ **Cross-section of hanger yoke showing flow of oxygen from the tank through the strainer nipple into the machine.** (From Bowie E, Huffman LM: *The anesthesia machine: essentials for understanding.* Madison, WI, 1985, GE Datex-Ohmeda.)

oxygen hose could be connected to this tank outlet if the wall end of the hose has a DISS fitting (Figs. 2-11 and 2-12).

Some anesthesia machines have two hanger yokes for oxygen. Once oxygen has passed through the check valve, the two hanger yokes are connected by high-pressure tubing, to which an oxygen pressure gauge is also connected (see Fig. 2-16). This gauge measures the pressure of the oxygen cylinder supply connected via hanger yokes. On many machines, both yokes may share one pressure gauge. In this case, to measure the tank pressure, the pipeline supply is first disconnected from the machine and both tanks are turned off. Next, the oxygen flush button is depressed to drain all oxygen from the machine, and the tank and pipeline gauge readings should both fall to zero. One tank is then turned on, and its pressure is noted on the gauge. The tank is then turned off, the oxygen flush button is again depressed, and the tank gauge pressure falls to zero. The second tank is then opened and its pressure noted. The second tank is then closed, and the oxygen flush button is depressed. The pipeline connector is then reattached to the wall oxygen outlet.

As previously noted, a check valve in each oxygen hanger yoke is designed to prevent oxygen from flowing out of the machine through the strainer nipple. This valve prevents loss of gas via the hanger yoke when no oxygen tank is hanging in one yoke, but an oxygen tank in the other yoke is being used to supply the machine (see Fig. 2-16). These valves also prevent transfilling of one oxygen tank to the other, if two tanks are hanging on the machine and both are on. In other words, without a check valve, oxygen would tend to flow from the full tank to the empty one if both were open. If the check valve were not present, the transfilling and sudden compression of oxygen into the empty cylinder could cause a rapid temperature rise in the pipes, gauge, and tank with an associated risk of fire. This is known as an *adiabatic change*, in which the state of a gas is altered without the gas being permitted to exchange heat energy with its surroundings.[5]

If there are two hanger yokes for oxygen but only one tank is hanging, a yoke plug should be inserted and tightened in the empty yoke. Thus, if an oxygen check valve leaks, loss of oxygen from the empty hanger yoke is prevented by the yoke plug (Fig. 2-13).

The pressure gauges used in the traditional machine to measure pipeline supply pressure or tank supply pressure (Fig. 2-14) are of the Bourdon tube design. In principle, the Bourdon tube is a coiled metal tube sealed at its inner end and open to the gas pressure at its outer end (see Chapter 9). As gas pressure rises, the coiled tube tends to straighten. A pointer attached to the inner-sealed end thereby moves across a scale calibrated in units of pressure. If the Bourdon tube were to burst, the inside of the gauge could be exposed to high pressure. The gauge is therefore constructed with a special heavy glass window and a mechanism designed to act as a pressure fuse so that gas is released from the back of the casing if the pressure suddenly rises. The cylinder and pipeline pressure gauges for the gases supplied to the machine are generally situated in a panel on the front of the anesthesia machine (see Fig. 2-14). In some workstations, pressure is sensed by a pressure transducer and is displayed on a screen (Fig. 2-15).

Cylinder Pressure Regulator

A *pressure regulator* is a device that converts a variable, high-input gas pressure to a constant, lower output pressure. As previously mentioned, tank oxygen enters the machine at pressures of up to 2200 psig depending on how full the tank is. These variable, high-input pressures are reduced to a constant, lower output pressure of 45

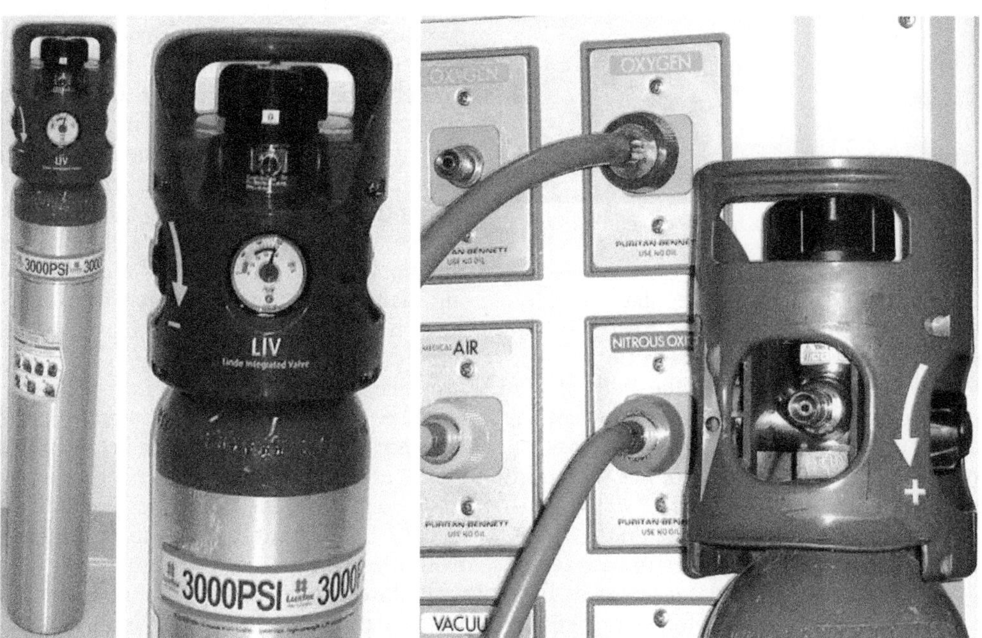

FIGURE 2-11 ■ *Left,* Oxygen tank pressurized to 3000 psig when filled. *Right,* The tank valve incorporates a regulator with a diameter index safety system (DISS) oxygen connector that supplies oxygen at 50 psig. The anesthesia machine oxygen hose is shown connected to a DISS wall outlet for oxygen.

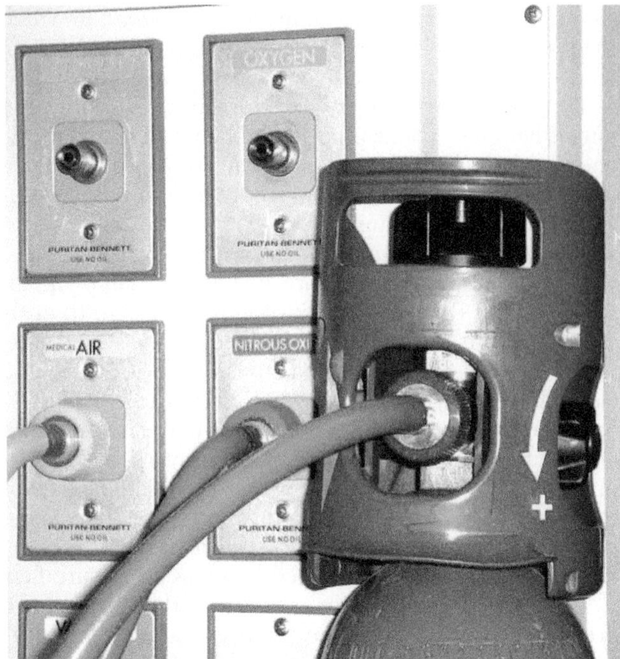

FIGURE 2-12 ■ If the wall oxygen supply fails, the machine's oxygen hose can be disconnected from the wall and reconnected to the 50 psig diameter index safety system connector on the oxygen tank shown in Figure 2-11.

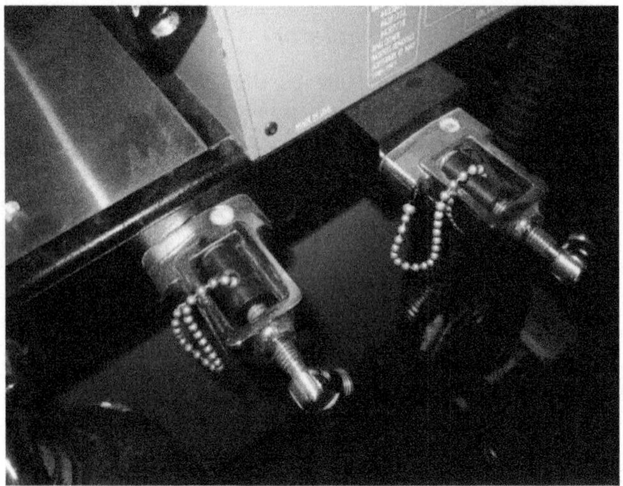

FIGURE 2-13 ■ Yoke plugs in unused tank hanger yokes.

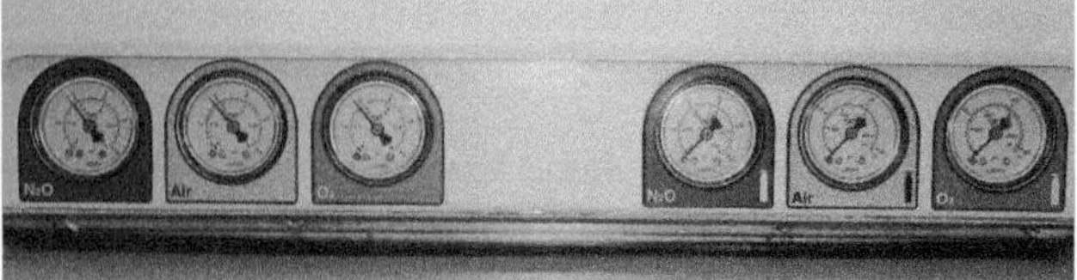

FIGURE 2-14 ■ Gas supply pressure gauges on the front panel of an anesthesia workstation. The three on the left display pipeline supply pressures; those on the right display cylinder supply pressures (note cylinder symbols).

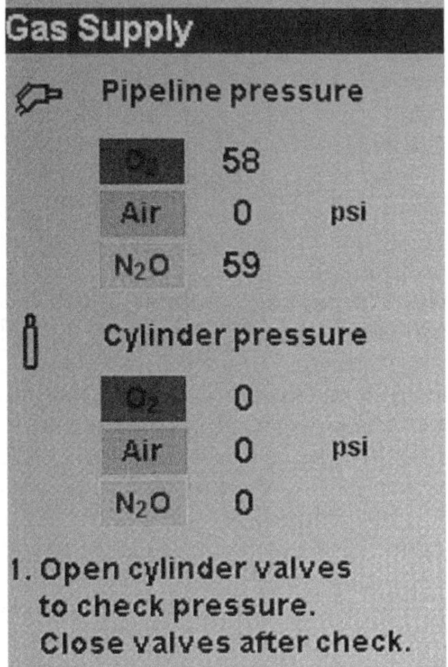

FIGURE 2-15 ■ Pipeline and cylinder gas supply pressures in this workstation are measured by pressure transducers and are displayed digitally on the workstation screen during checkout.

psig by the oxygen cylinder pressure regulator, sometimes termed the *first-stage regulator* (see Fig. 2-4). As noted in Figure 2-16, the tank oxygen from both yokes flows to a common pathway leading to the inlet of the regulator. One regulator serves the two oxygen hanger yokes and is located under the machine's work surface.

The principles of action of the regulator are shown in Figure 2-17.[16,17] This is described as a *direct-acting regulator* because the high-pressure gas tends to open the valve. In an *indirect-acting regulator*, the high-pressure gas tends to close the valve. In essence, the regulator works by balancing the force of a spring against the forces that result from gas pressures acting on a diaphragm. Oxygen at tank pressure enters the high-pressure inlet and is applied over a small area to the valve seat (see Fig. 2-17), and the valve opening is opposed by a return spring. The valve seat is connected by a thrust pin to a diaphragm in the low-pressure chamber of the regulator. Upward movement of the diaphragm is opposed by a spring that exerts a pressure of 45 psig on the diaphragm. The adjustment of this spring is such that oxygen may flow from the high-pressure inlet across the valve seat and into the low-pressure chamber. If pressure in the low-pressure chamber exceeds 45 psig, the diaphragm moves upward and closes the valve opening, halting the flow of oxygen from high- to low-pressure chambers, until the gas pressure exerted on the diaphragm falls below 45 psig. The pressure in the low-pressure chamber and the low-pressure piping of the machine when supplied by the tanks is thereby kept at a constant 45 psig. A cessation of flow from the low-pressure chamber, such as would occur if the oxygen flow control valve meter were closed, causes pressure to build up here, closing the regulator valve and halting the flow of gas from the cylinder into the regulator.

Failure of the pressure reduction function of a regulator can transmit excessively high pressure (up to 2200 psig) to the machine's low-pressure system (see Fig. 2-17). To protect against such occurrences, the regulator incorporates a pressure relief valve in the low-pressure

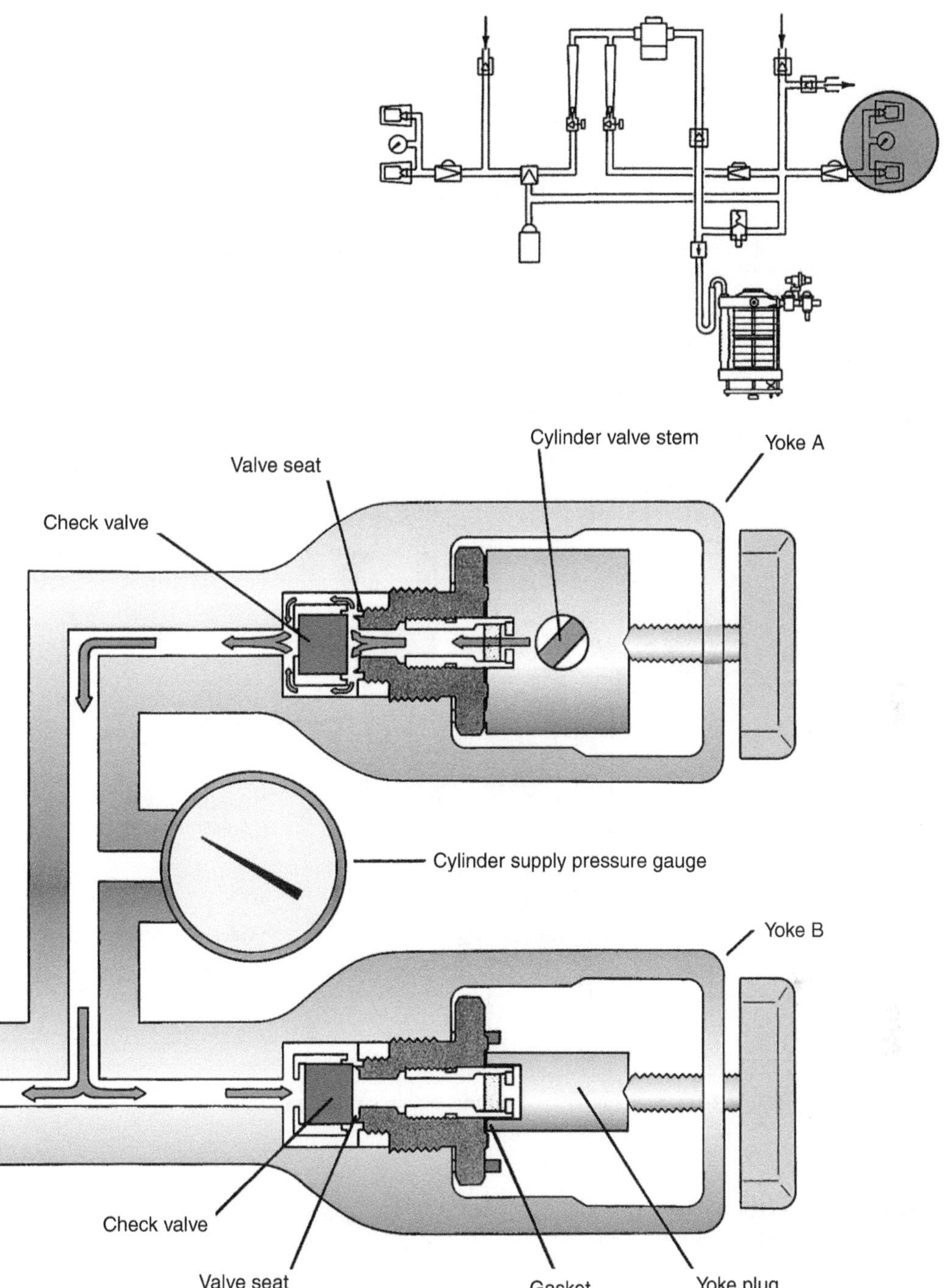

FIGURE 2-16 ■ Double-hanger yoke assembly with oxygen tank hanging in yoke A. Gas flows into the machine via the floating check valve. Gas cannot escape via yoke B because the oxygen pressure closes the check valve. If gas should leak past the check valve, its flow is prevented by the yoke plug, which has been tightened into yoke B, occluding the yoke nipple. (From Bowie E, Huffman LM: *The anesthesia machine: essentials for understanding.* Madison, WI, 1985, GE Datex-Ohmeda.)

chamber in which excess pressures are vented to the atmosphere. If the diaphragm were to rupture or develop a hole, the regulator would fail and gas would escape around the adjustment screw and spring. The high flow of escaping oxygen makes a loud sound, alerting the anesthesiologist to the possibility of a regulator failure. Such a hole represents a significant leak in the high-pressure system or intermediate-pressure system through which oxygen would be lost. Figure 2-4 shows that even if the tanks were turned off and the pipeline supply were in use, a ruptured diaphragm in the regulator would cause loss of oxygen from the machine's high-pressure system or intermediate-pressure system and a possible failure of oxygen supply to the flowmeters. Such a machine should be withdrawn from service until the problem has been corrected by an authorized service technician. Meanwhile, oxygen may be supplied to the patient by a self-inflating (Ambu) bag connected to a portable supply of oxygen, such as a transport oxygen cylinder with its own pressure-reducing valve and flowmeter.

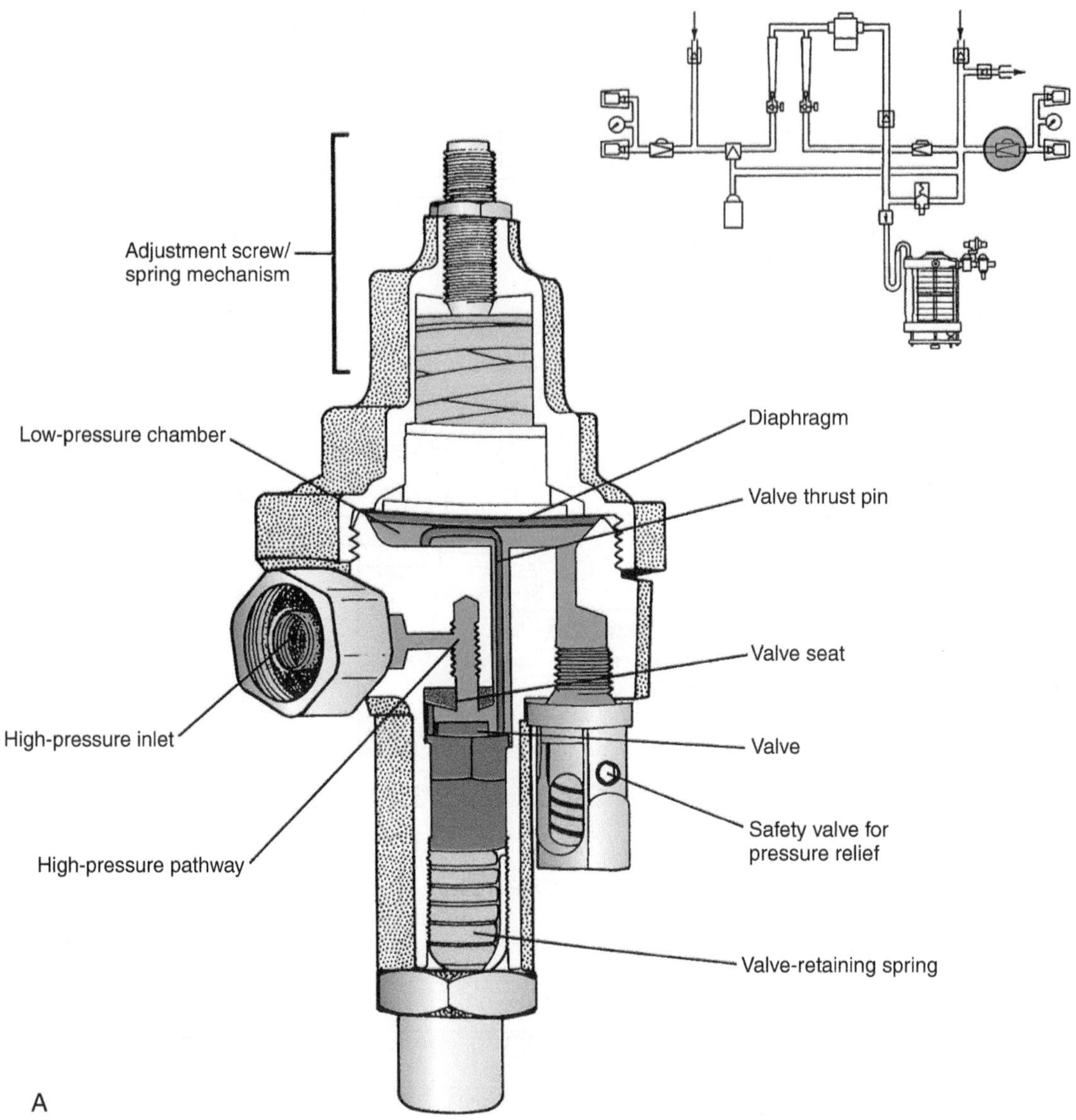

FIGURE 2-17 ■ **A,** Schematic of a direct-acting oxygen pressure regulator.

OXYGEN SUPPLY TO THE INTERMEDIATE-PRESSURE SYSTEM

Oxygen is typically supplied to the machine's pipeline connector inlet at pressures of 50 to 55 psig, whereas the tank oxygen supply is regulated to enter at 40 to 45 psig. This difference in supply pressures is deliberate; if the pipeline is connected and the oxygen tanks are open, oxygen is preferentially drawn from the pipeline supply. This is because the higher pressure (50 to 55 psig) from the pipeline supply closes the valve in the first-stage oxygen regulator, thereby preventing the flow of oxygen from the tank. However, at times, such as during heavy oxygen use, the pipeline pressure may fall below 45 psig. In this case, oxygen would be drawn from the tanks if they were open. Thus, once the tank supply has been checked, it should be turned off to prevent loss of the backup oxygen supply. Also, if the tank is left open, oxygen might leak around the plastic washer between the tank and the yoke.

An awareness of the differential in supply pressures of oxygen to the machine is essential.[14] If a pipeline crossover is suspected, such as when a hypoxic gas is flowing through the oxygen pipeline to the piping in the machine, the machine *must be disconnected* from the pipeline supply if the backup oxygen supply is to be used. For example, if a hypoxic gas (e.g., nitrous oxide) is accidentally used to supply the oxygen pipeline at a supply pressure of greater than 45 psig, the anesthesiologist cannot deliver the true oxygen from the backup tanks because the pressure from the wall supply is greater than that from the first-stage oxygen regulator.

FLOW PATHWAYS FOR OXYGEN IN THE INTERMEDIATE-PRESSURE SYSTEM

Having entered the machine intermediate-pressure system at 50 to 55 psig (pipeline) or 40 to 45 psig (tank

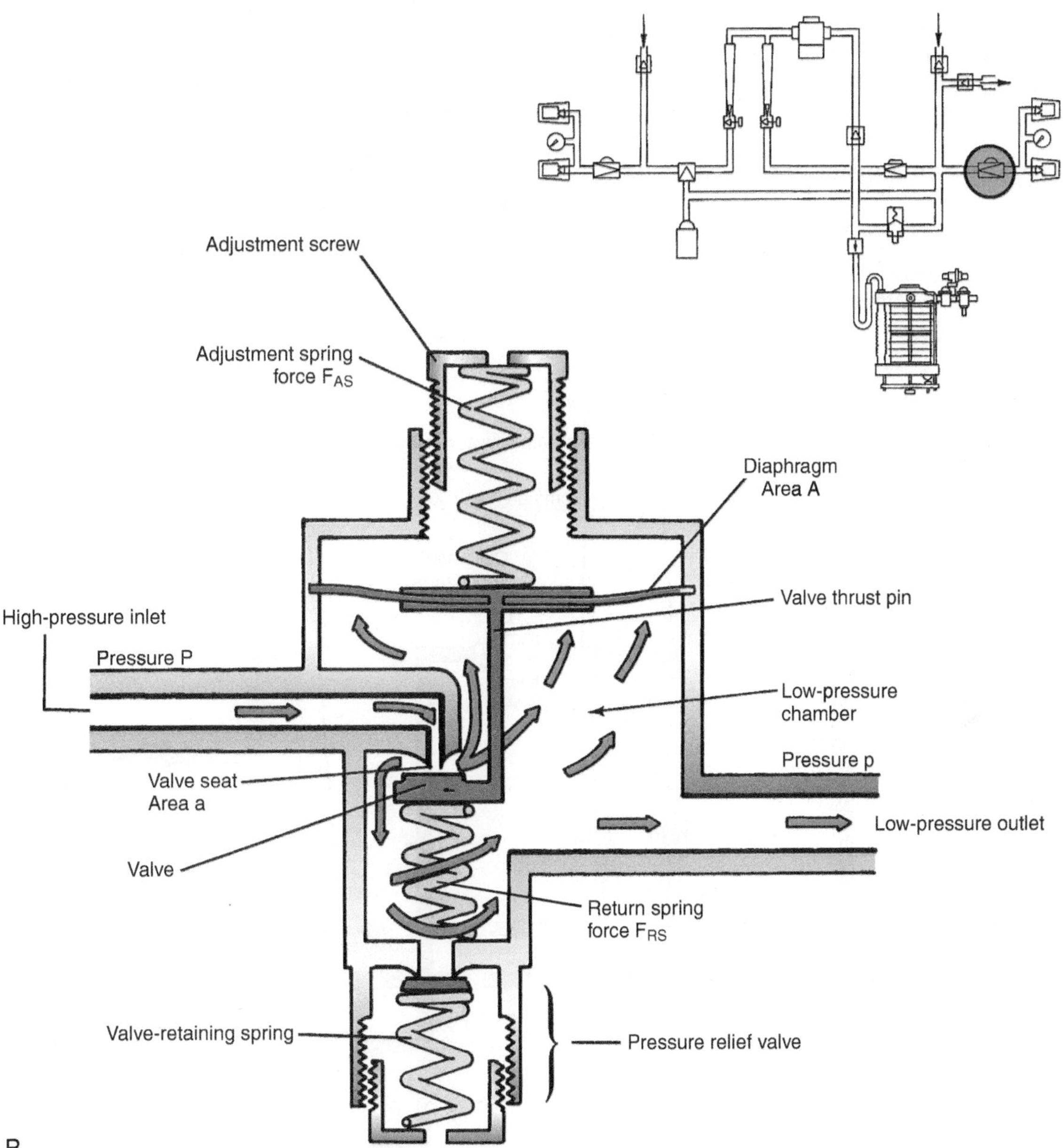

FIGURE 2-17, cont'd ■ **B,** An inside look at the regulator as oxygen pressure is reduced. In principle, the regulator functions by balancing forces acting on the diaphragm. Gas under high pressure (*P*) enters the regulator and is applied to the valve over the area of the seat (*a*). Because Force = Pressure × Area, the force resulting from high-pressure gas is $P \times a$. Valve opening is initially opposed by the force of the return spring, F_{RS}. Because of the small area of the valve orifice, gas flowing through it enters the next chamber at a lower pressure (*p*). This lower pressure is applied over the large area of the diaphragm (*A*) at a force of $p \times A$. Upward movement of the diaphragm is opposed by the force of the adjustment spring, F_{AS}. The valve and diaphragm are connected by a thrust pin and move as one unit according to the forces applied in either direction. In equilibrium, the forces acting on the diaphragm are equal: $(P \times a) + F_{AS} = (p \times A) + F_{RS}$. The reduced pressure $p = [(F_{AS} - F_{RS}) + (P \times a)]/A$. The regulator is designed such that *p* is fairly constant despite changes in *P*. (From Bowie E, Huffman LM: *The anesthesia machine: essentials for understanding.* Madison, WI, 1985, GE Datex-Ohmeda.)

first-stage regulator), oxygen can flow or pressurize in several directions.

Oxygen Flush

As soon as any oxygen supply is connected to the machine, pressing the oxygen flush button results in a flow of oxygen to the machine CGO at 35 to 75 L/min.[1] Figure 2-18 shows that this pathway bypasses the main pneumatic and electronic ON/OFF switches and that the pressure at the CGO could increase the supply pressure to the machine unless some pressure relief mechanism is present. To avoid barotrauma in a patient, extreme caution is therefore necessary when oxygen flush is used. Contemporary machines incorporate a pressure-limiting device to prevent such potentially harmful pressures, particularly if the flush is activated during the inspiratory phase of positive-pressure ventilation (see Chapter 6).

The workstation standard requires that the oxygen flush valve be self-closing and designed to minimize unintended operation by equipment or personnel.[1] A modern design for an oxygen flush button is shown in Figure 2-19; note that the button is recessed in a housing to prevent accidental depression and that the valve is self-closing.

Auxiliary Oxygen Flowmeter

Most contemporary machines incorporate an auxiliary oxygen flowmeter that delivers oxygen, usually via a pressure-reducing regulator, to an accessible nipple at flows typically up to 10 L/min (Fig. 2-20). This is the source used to connect devices that deliver supplemental oxygen to a nasal cannula, face mask, or self-inflating reservoir bag, such as an Ambu bag. Similar to the oxygen flush, this flowmeter is active when the machine's main ON/OFF switch is off.

Auxiliary Diameter Index Safety System Oxygen Source

Many workstations provide an auxiliary source of oxygen at pipeline pressure (50 to 55 psig) via a DISS connector while the machine is connected to a pipeline supply. An available DISS connector can be beneficial if the

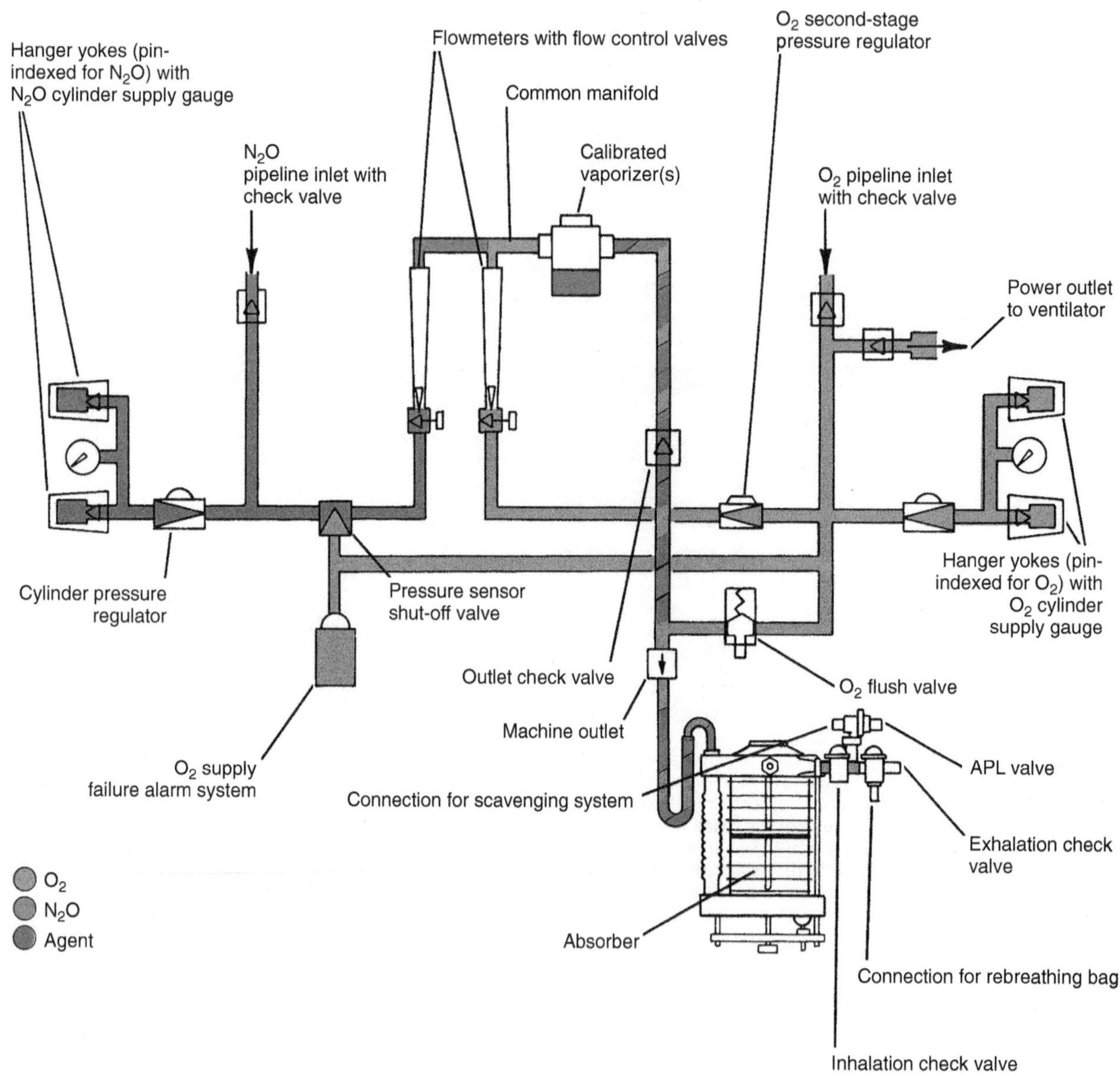

FIGURE 2-18 Schematic showing principal pathways for oxygen flow or pressurization in a basic GE Healthcare Datex-Ohmeda machine. APL, adjustable pressure-limiting valve. (From Bowie E, Huffman LM: *The anesthesia machine: essentials for understanding.* Madison, WI, 1985, GE Datex-Ohmeda.)

machine's oxygen hose and the wall oxygen outlets have quick-connect fittings (Figs. 2-20 and 2-21). The outlet can be used to drive a Sanders-type jet ventilator,[18] a Venturi-based suctioning device, or other device that requires pipeline oxygen pressure.

Unless otherwise stated, oxygen flows to, or pressurizes, the components that follow it only when the main ON/OFF switch is in the ON position (see Fig. 2-4).

Oxygen Supply Failure Alarm System

Oxygen pressurizes an oxygen supply failure alarm system such that if the supply pressure falls, usually below 30 psig, an alarm is triggered (see Figs. 2-4 and 2-18). Some older machine models use a canister pressurized with oxygen that emits an audible alarm for at least 7 seconds when the pressure falls below the threshold. Contemporary machines use a pressure-operated electrical switch that ensures a continuous audible alarm when the oxygen supply pressure falls below the threshold setting.

The workstation standard requires that whenever oxygen supply pressure falls below the manufacturer-specified threshold, a medium-priority alarm is activated within 5 seconds. After the alarm has been activated, it may be released by the user for a period of up to 120 seconds but is automatically reset after restoration of oxygen supply pressure to a level above the alarm threshold.[1]

Pneumatically Powered Anesthesia Ventilator

Oxygen at a pressure of 50 to 55 psig (pipeline) or 45 psig (tanks) is used as the power source for pneumatically driven anesthesia ventilators, such as the GE Datex-Ohmeda 7000, 7800, and 7900 series and the Dräger AV-E. In Datex-Ohmeda machines, when the ventilator connection is made, the valve opens to permit compressed oxygen to flow to the ventilator (Fig. 2-22). In Dräger Narkomed 2, 3, and 4 machines, the oxygen takeoff to drive the ventilator is *downstream* of the machine main ON/OFF switch, so the ventilator cannot be operated if the machine is turned off (see Fig. 2-4). In older model Ohmeda machines, the oxygen takeoff to the ventilator circuit is *upstream* of the main ON/OFF switch.

During operation, pneumatically powered ventilators consume large quantities of oxygen. If the machine is being supplied by a backup E-cylinder, that cylinder's contents are rapidly exhausted because it is also supplying oxygen to the patient circuit.[19-21] In ventilators that use 100% oxygen as the driving gas—such as the Datex-Ohmeda 7000, 7800, and 7900 series—the ventilator oxygen consumption is in excess of the minute ventilation set on the ventilator (i.e., Rate × Bellows tidal volume). The Dräger AV-E is more economical in terms of oxygen because it uses oxygen to drive a Venturi that entrains air. The air-oxygen mixture is then used as the final driving gas mixture that enters the ventilator bellows housing (see Chapter 6).

In some workstations, if the pressurized supply of oxygen is lost but air is not, the ventilator may switch to being powered by compressed air (Fig. 2-23). Of course, this is not an issue in workstations that use a piston ventilator powered by an electric motor.

Pressure Sensor Shut-off (Fail-Safe) Valves

When the main ON/OFF switch is in the ON position, oxygen pressurizes and holds open a pressure-sensor shut-off valve. These valves reduce or interrupt the supply of nitrous oxide and other hypoxic gases (e.g., carbon dioxide and helium), but not air, to their flowmeters if the oxygen supply pressure falls below the threshold setting. This valve, in relation to control of the nitrous oxide supply, is the fail-safe system designed to prevent the unintentional delivery of a hypoxic mixture from the flowmeters.

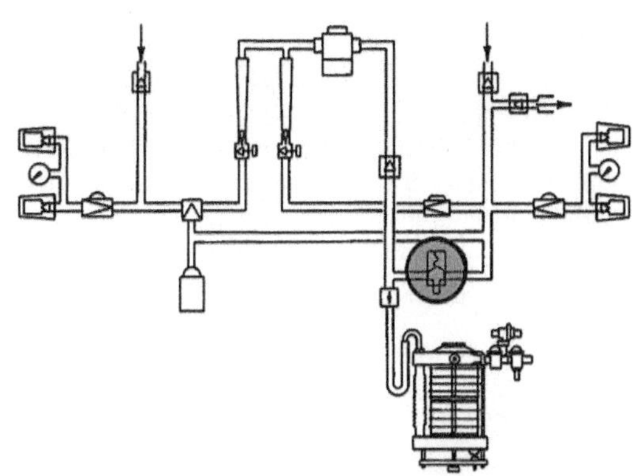

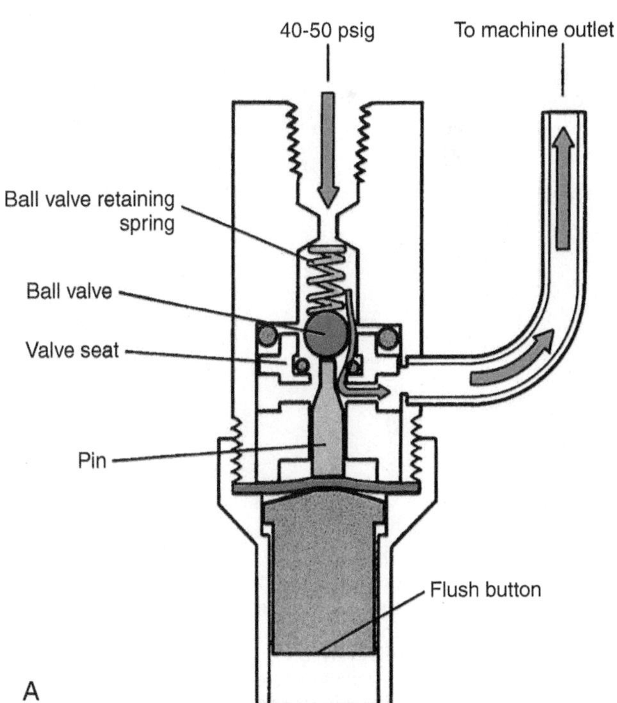

FIGURE 2-19 ▪ **A,** Schematic of oxygen flush valve in closed position. Note that it is recessed to prevent accidental activation. When depressed, oxygen flows from the common gas outlet at a rate of 35 to 75 L/min. Depending on the pressure relief arrangements, the oxygen may be delivered at pipeline supply pressure. (From Bowie E, Huffman LM: *The anesthesia machine: essentials for understanding.* Madison, WI, 1985, GE Datex-Ohmeda.)

Continued

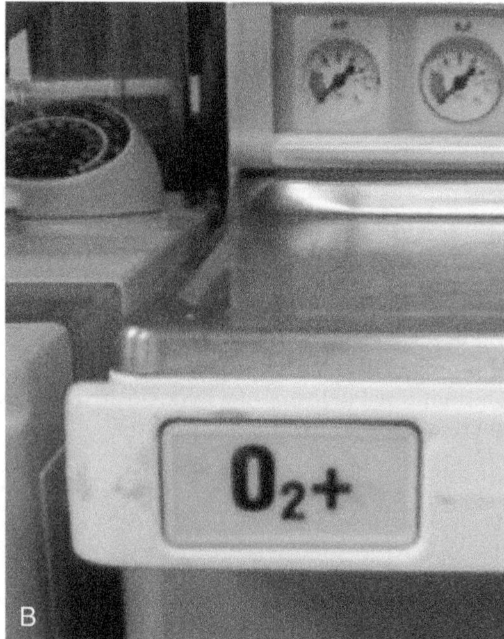

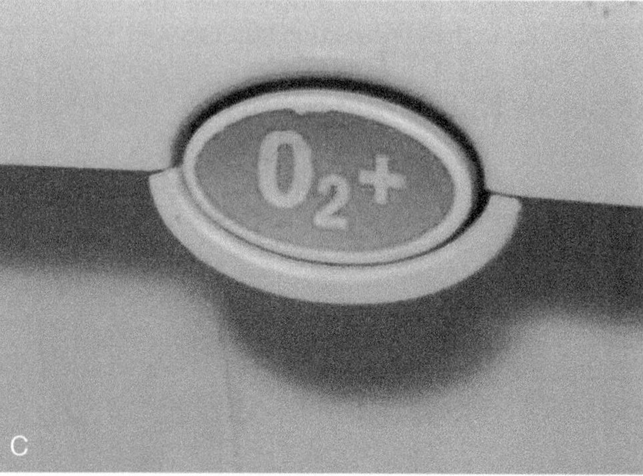

FIGURE 2-19, cont'd ■ **B** and **C,** Examples of oxygen flush valve buttons. Note that they are flush with the front of the workstation to avoid accidental activation.

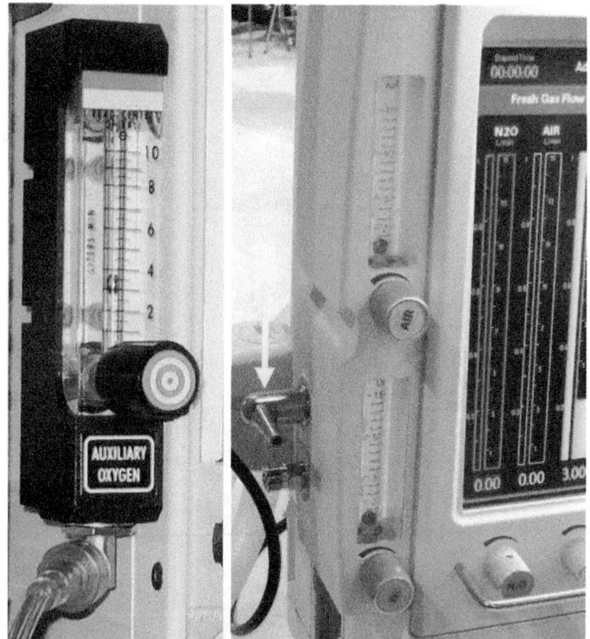

FIGURE 2-20 ■ *Left,* Auxiliary oxygen flowmeter and delivery nipple. Flow can be adjusted up to 10 L/min. Pressure available varies according to the setting of the pressure regulator. Note that if a hypoxic gas enters the oxygen inlet of the machine, the same gas will be delivered to the auxiliary oxygen flowmeter. There is no oxygen analyzer to confirm that the gas flowing from this outlet is, in fact, oxygen. *Right,* A machine with both auxiliary oxygen and auxiliary air flowmeters supplies gas at flows of up to 15 L/min to the auxiliary nipple (*yellow arrow*). The auxiliary air-oxygen mixture is used when a lower fraction of inspired oxygen is needed for delivery by nasal cannula, such as when a fire hazard is present. The *green arrow* indicates a diameter index safety system 55-psig oxygen connector.

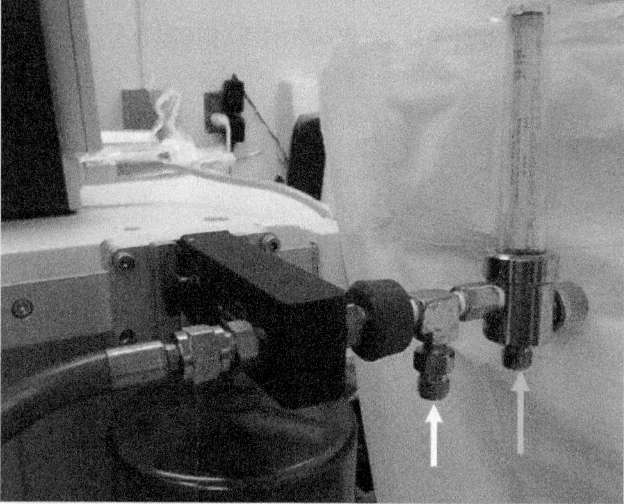

FIGURE 2-21 ■ An auxiliary diameter index safety system 55-psig oxygen outlet (*white arrow*) supplied from the machine's intermediate-pressure system for oxygen can be used to drive a Sanders-type jet ventilating system via an inline pressure-reducing valve and toggle switch. The auxiliary oxygen flowmeter is combined in this assembly. An integral pressure regulator reduces pressure to the auxiliary oxygen flowmeter so that oxygen is delivered at much lower pressures at the outlet of the flowmeter (*green arrow*).

The action of turning the machine's main ON/OFF switch to the OFF position allows the oxygen pressure in parts of the machine downstream of the switch (normally 45 to 55 psig) to be vented to the atmosphere. The resulting decrease in oxygen pressure causes the fail-safe valves to interrupt the supply of all other gases, usually with the exception of air, to their flow-control valves. The design of the fail-safe system differs between the Dräger and Datex-Ohmeda machines.

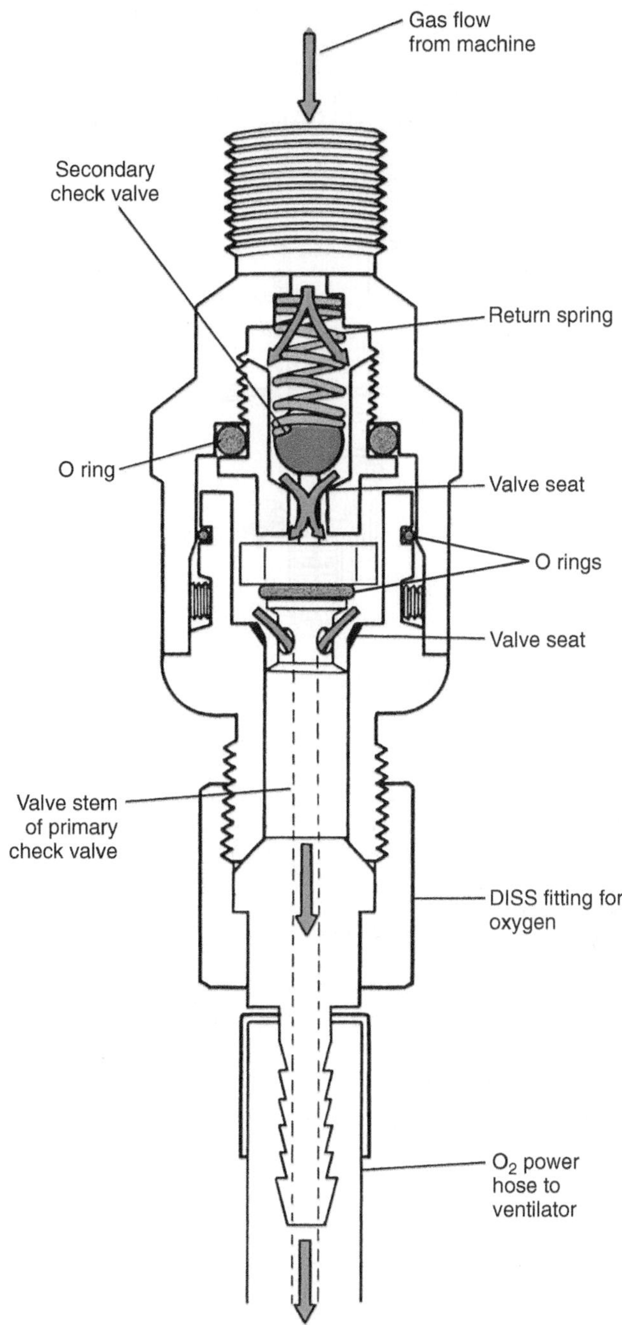

FIGURE 2-22 Oxygen power outlet to a ventilator. While the diameter-indexed safety system (*DISS*) fitting on the ventilator's oxygen supply hose is screwed on to the connector, the valve is lifted from its seat, permitting oxygen to flow to the ventilator's power hose. (From Bowie E, Huffman LM: *The anesthesia machine: essentials for understanding.* Madison, WI, 1985, GE Datex-Ohmeda.)

In older model Datex-Ohmeda machines, when the oxygen supply pressure in the intermediate-pressure system falls below 20 to 25 psig, the flow of nitrous oxide to its flowmeters is completely interrupted. The pressure sensor shut-off valve used by the older model Datex-Ohmeda machines is an all-or-nothing threshold arrangement—open at oxygen pressures greater than 20 to 25 psig and closed at pressures below 20 psig (Fig. 2-24).[22,23]

In the Datex-Ohmeda Aestiva/5 workstation, a more recent model, the fail-safe valve is not an all-or-nothing design; it is a variable valve in a balance regulator, in which the secondary regulator for oxygen reduces the pressure to approximately 30 psig in the intermediate-pressure system (see Fig. 2-4). The oxygen pressure is then piloted to the balance regulator, where it is applied to the oxygen side of the regulated diaphragm. If the pressure of oxygen is sufficient, the diaphragm pushes against a mechanism that opens the flow pathway for nitrous oxide. If the oxygen piloting pressure decreases, the mechanism begins to close off the pathway for nitrous oxide in proportion to the decrease in piloted oxygen pressure. The balance regulator for nitrous oxide completely closes when the pressure of oxygen falls to 0.5 psig. Balance regulators for heliox and carbon dioxide interrupt the flow of these gases when the piloted oxygen pressure falls below 10 psig.[4]

The fail-safe valve in Narkomed 2, 3, and 4 machines is called an *oxygen failure protection device* (OFPD) and, as in the Datex-Ohmeda systems, there is one for each of the gases supplied to the machine (Fig. 2-25). As the oxygen supply pressure falls and the flow of oxygen from the machine's flowmeter decreases, the OFPDs proportionately reduce the supply pressure of other gases to their flowmeters. The supply of nitrous oxide and other gases is thereby completely interrupted when the oxygen supply pressure falls to below 12 ± 4 psig.[24] Therefore, the OFPD functions similarly to the balance regulator in the Datex-Ohmeda Aestiva/5.

Both fail-safe valve designs ensure that at low- or zero-oxygen supply pressures, only oxygen may be delivered to the machine's CGO. However, as long as the oxygen supply *pressure* is adequate, other gases may flow to their flowmeters. The fail-safe system does not ensure oxygen *flow* at its flowmeter, only a supply *pressure* to the oxygen

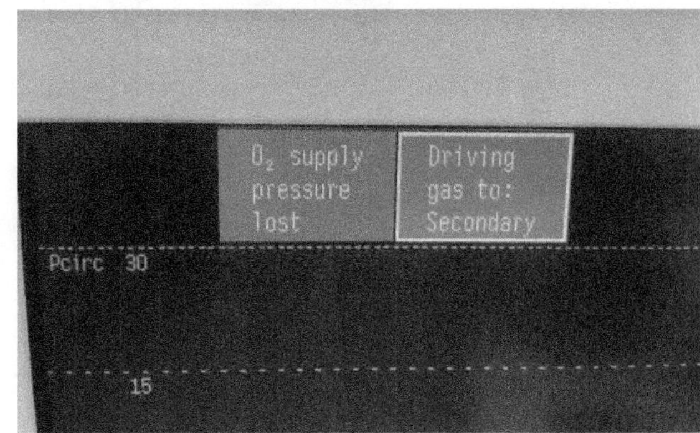

FIGURE 2-23 If the oxygen supply to the workstation fails but the air supply is maintained, the workstation can switch to the secondary gas (air) to drive the bellows ventilator. An alert is displayed on the workstation screen. Air can be delivered at the common gas outlet as set on the air flowmeter.

flowmeter. Thus a normally functioning fail-safe system would permit flow of 100% nitrous oxide, provided the machine has an adequate oxygen supply *pressure*. The term "fail-safe" therefore represents something of a misnomer because it does not ensure oxygen *flow* (Fig. 2-26).

Flowmeters

Oxygen flows to the oxygen flow control valve and flowmeter(s), traditionally rotameters. Supply pressure to the oxygen flowmeters differs in Datex-Ohmeda and Dräger machines. In contemporary Datex-Ohmeda machines, the oxygen supply pressure to the flowmeters is regulated to a constant, lower pressure—14 to 30 psig, depending upon the model—by a second-stage regulator. This regulator (see Figs. 2-4 and 2-18) ensures a constant supply pressure to the Datex-Ohmeda oxygen flowmeter. Thus, even if the oxygen supply pressure to the machine decreases below 45 to 50 psig, as long as it exceeds the set second-stage regulated downstream pressure, the flow setting on the oxygen flowmeter is maintained. Without this second-stage regulator, if the oxygen supply pressure were to fall, the oxygen flow at the flowmeter would decrease. If another gas (e.g., nitrous oxide) was also being used, a hypoxic gas mixture could result at the flowmeter manifold.

The second-stage oxygen regulator used in Datex-Ohmeda machines is similar in terms of principle of operation to that of the first-stage regulator (see Fig. 2-17). However, because it normally handles lower pressures than the first-stage regulator, it neither requires nor incorporates a pressure relief valve.

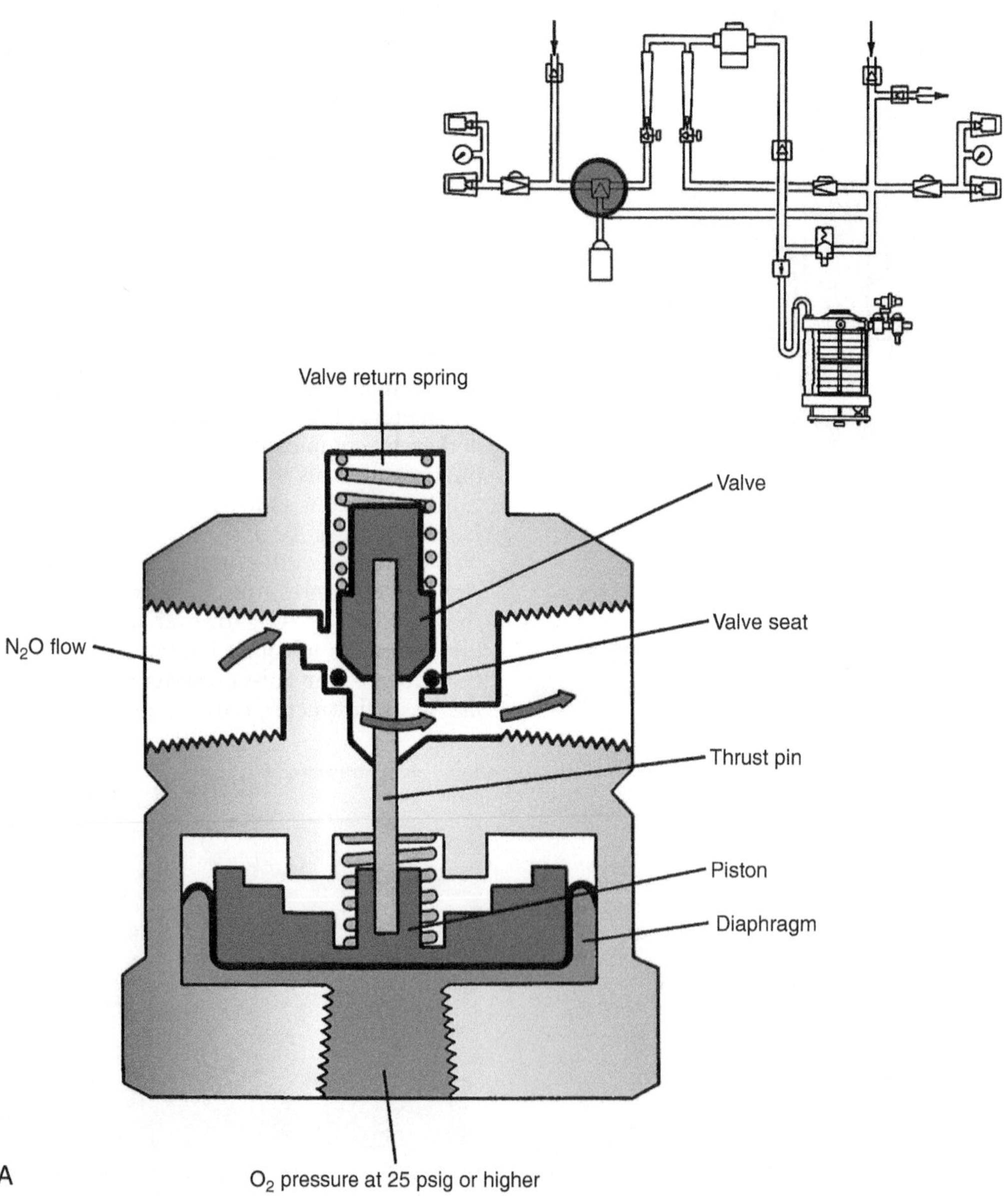

FIGURE 2-24 ■ **A,** GE Healthcare Datex-Ohmeda pressure sensor shut-off ("fail-safe") valve in a traditional machine. If oxygen supply pressure on the diaphragm exceeds the threshold, in this case 25 psig, the valve is lifted from its seat and nitrous oxide can flow to its flowmeter.

Continued

Narkomed anesthesia machines do not use a second-stage oxygen pressure-regulator valve (see Fig. 2-4). These machines have OFPDs that interface the supply pressure of oxygen with that of nitrous oxide and the other gases supplied to the machine.[6] The OFPD consists of a seat-nozzle assembly connected to a spring-loaded piston (see Fig. 2-25). When deactivated, the spring is expanded, forcing the nozzle against the seat so that no gas can flow through the device to the flowmeter. As oxygen pressure increases, it is applied to the piston, which in turn forces the nozzle away from its seat so that gas can flow through the OFPD. The OFPD responds to oxygen pressure changes such that as pressure falls, the other gas flows will fall in proportion. When the oxygen supply pressure is less than 12 ± 4 psig, the OFPD is completely closed.[24] A decrease in oxygen supply pressure causes a proportionate decrease in the supply pressures of each of the other gases to their flowmeters. As the oxygen supply pressure and flow decrease, all other gas flows are decreased in proportion to prevent the creation of a hypoxic gas mixture at the flowmeter level (see the preceding section). The operation of the OFPD can be demonstrated. With the Narkomed machine supplied from pipeline oxygen (55 psig), set 6 L/min flows of both nitrous oxide and oxygen; if the pipeline oxygen is disconnected and the tank oxygen supply is opened (45 psig), flow of both oxygen and nitrous oxide will be observed to have decreased at the rotameters.

The use (GE Datex-Ohmeda) or nonuse (Dräger) of a second-stage oxygen regulator affects the total gas flow emerging from the CGO of the machine if the oxygen

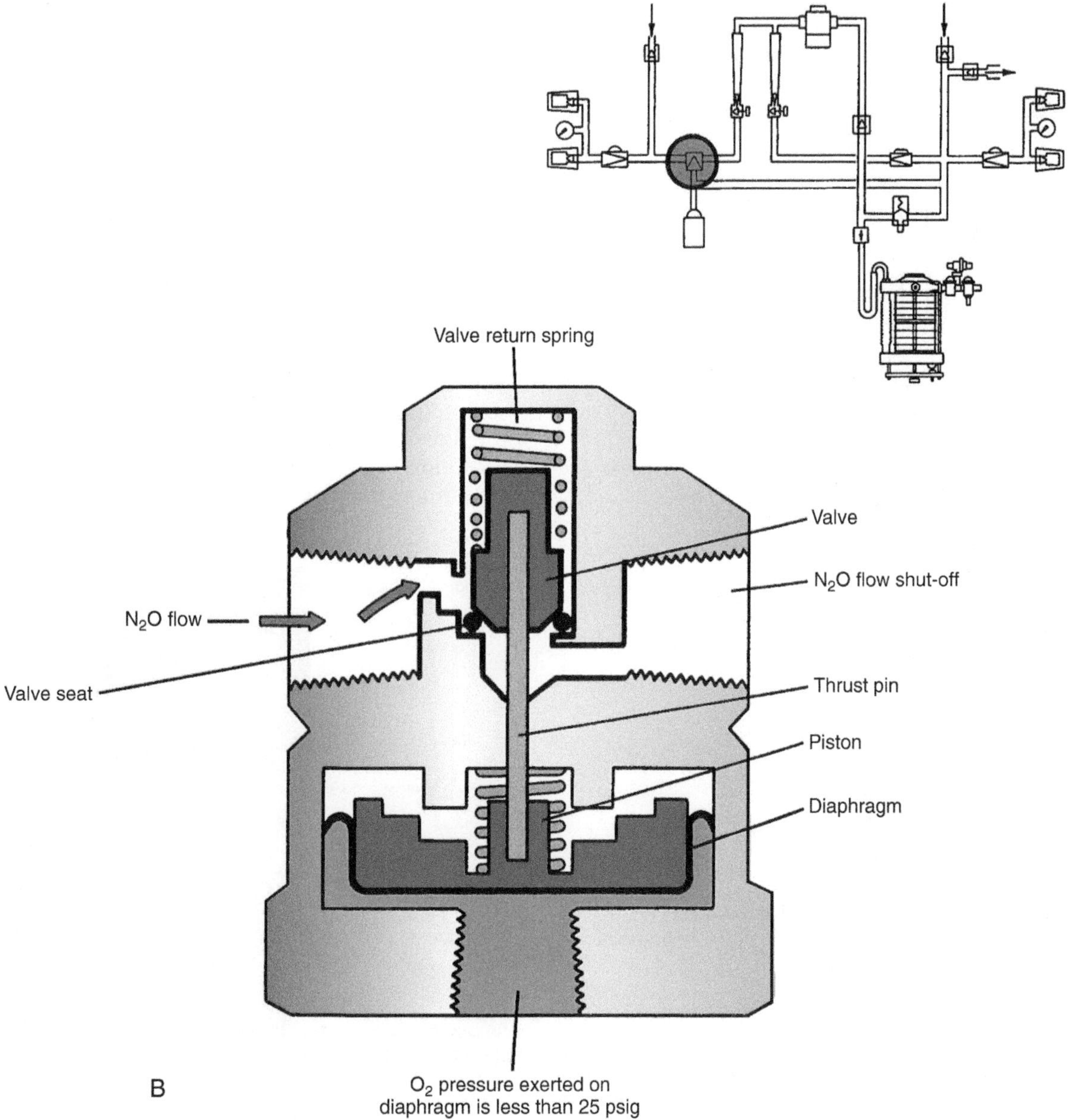

FIGURE 2-24, cont'd ■ **B,** If the oxygen supply pressure falls below the threshold setting for the valve return spring pressure, the valve is no longer held off its seat and interrupts the flow of nitrous oxide to its flowmeter. A pressure sensor shut-off valve is present for each gas (but not oxygen) supplied to the machine. In the GE Healthcare Aestiva/5 machine, a balancing valve replaces the pressure sensor shut-off valve. This is a variable valve, rather than an open or shut valve. (From Bowie E, Huffman LM: *The anesthesia machine: essentials for understanding.* Madison, WI, 1985, GE-Datex-Ohmeda.)

supply pressure falls. In an older model Datex-Ohmeda machine, as long as the oxygen supply pressure exceeds the set threshold of the second-stage regulator, all gas flows are maintained at the original flowmeter settings. In a Narkomed machine, if the oxygen supply pressure falls from normal (45 to 55 psig), all gas flows decrease in proportion via the OFPDs. A decrease in total gas flow from the machine's CGO might result in rebreathing, depending on the breathing circuit in use.

NITROUS OXIDE

Like oxygen, N_2O may be supplied to the machine either from the pipeline system at 50 to 55 psig or from the backup E-cylinder supply on the machine itself. Nitrous oxide from the tank supply enters the nitrous oxide–specific yokes at pressures of up to 745 psig (at 20° C); it then passes through a first-stage regulator similar to that for oxygen, which reduces this pressure to 40 to 45 psig (see Fig. 2-4). The pin index safety system is designed to ensure that only a nitrous oxide tank can hang in a nitrous oxide hanger yoke. As with oxygen, a check valve in each yoke prevents the backflow of nitrous oxide if no tank is hung in the yoke (see Fig. 2-8).

The nitrous oxide pipeline is supplied from liquid nitrous oxide or from banks of large tanks of nitrous oxide, usually H-cylinders (see Chapter 1). The pressure in the pipeline is regulated to 50 to 55 psig to supply the outlets in the OR. Once it enters the anesthesia machine, nitrous oxide must flow past the pressure-sensor shut-off (fail-safe) valve to reach its flow control valve and flowmeter.

In Datex-Ohmeda anesthesia machines that have the Link-25 proportion limiting system, a second-stage nitrous oxide regulator further reduces gas pressure so that nitrous oxide is supplied to its flowmeter at a nominal 26 psig (Fig. 2-4).[22] The actual downstream pressure of this second-stage nitrous oxide regulator is adjusted at the factory or by an authorized field service representative to ensure correct functioning of the proportioning system.

OTHER MEDICAL GASES

Some anesthesia machines are designed to deliver other gases such as air, helium, heliox, and even carbon dioxide (Figs. 2-27 and 2-28). If another medical gas is supplied to the machine, the arrangements are similar to those for the nitrous oxide supply. Thus, there is a DISS gas-specific connector for a pipeline supply and a pin-indexed gas-specific hanger yoke for the tank supply. Supply pressure gauges are provided for the supply source (pipeline or tank), and a fail-safe valve controls the flow of each gas to its flowmeter, with the possible exception of air, according to the oxygen supply pressure in the machine.

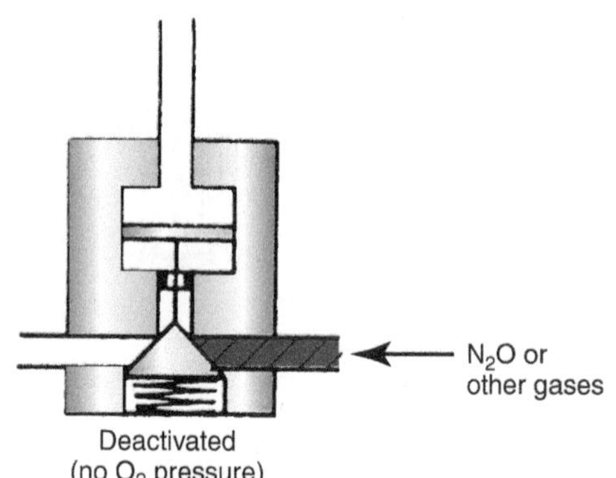

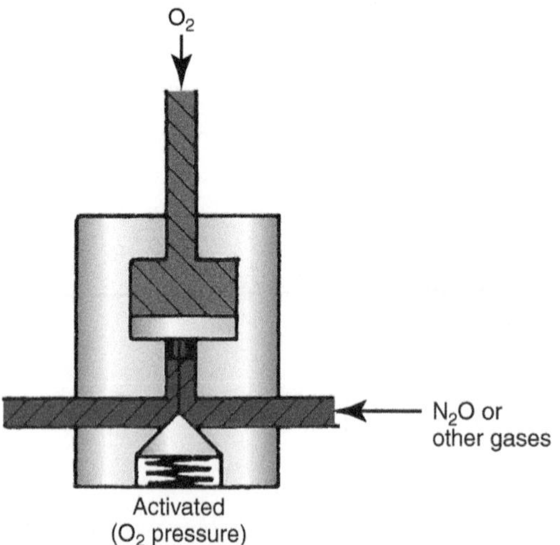

FIGURE 2-25 Draeger Medical Inc. oxygen failure protection device (OFPD). As the supply pressure of oxygen decreases from the normal value of 55 psig, the OFPD proportionately decreases the nitrous oxide supply pressure to the nitrous oxide flowmeter; the flow is interrupted completely when oxygen supply pressure is 12 ± 4 psig. There is an OFPD for each gas (but not oxygen) supplied to the machine; thus a four-gas machine would have three OFPDs. This is a variable fail-safe valve. (Courtesy Dräger Medical, Telford, PA.)

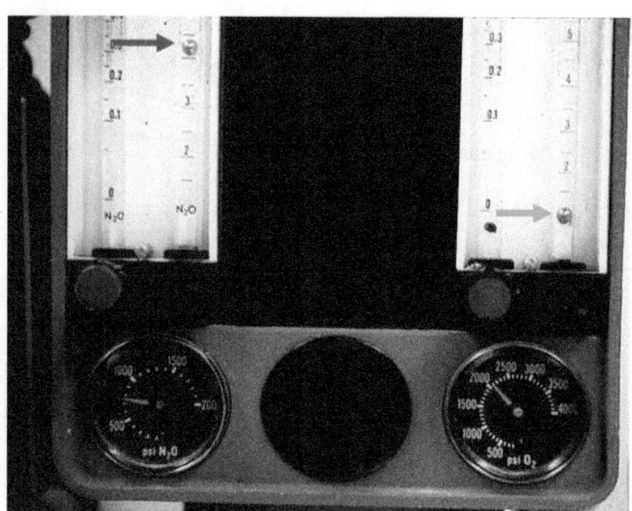

FIGURE 2-26 Limitation of the fail-safe system. In this machine, because the supply pressure of oxygen is adequate (2000 psig from the tank and therefore 45 psig in the machine), nitrous oxide may flow to its flowmeter and beyond (4 L/min; *blue arrow*) even though the oxygen flow control valve is turned off and no oxygen is flowing (*green arrow*). The term *fail-safe* is therefore somewhat of a misnomer; the system cannot prevent delivery of a hypoxic gas mixture because the valve is pressure sensitive rather than flow sensitive.

ANESTHESIA MACHINE GAS PIPING SYSTEM

Within the anesthesia machine, piping conducts compressed gases from point of entry, through the various components, and to the CGO. The workstation standard requires that this piping be capable of withstanding four times the intended service pressure without rupturing.[1] It further specifies that between the cylinders or the pipeline inlet and the flow control valves, the maximum leakage of each gas cannot exceed 10 mL/min at normal working pressure (30 mL/min at a pressure of 30 cm H_2O with the vaporizers in both the ON and OFF positions).[1] The standard requires that gas piping connectors be noninterchangeable or that the content of each pipe be identifiable by a marking at each junction.[1] Such a system is designed to prevent crossover of gases within the machine.

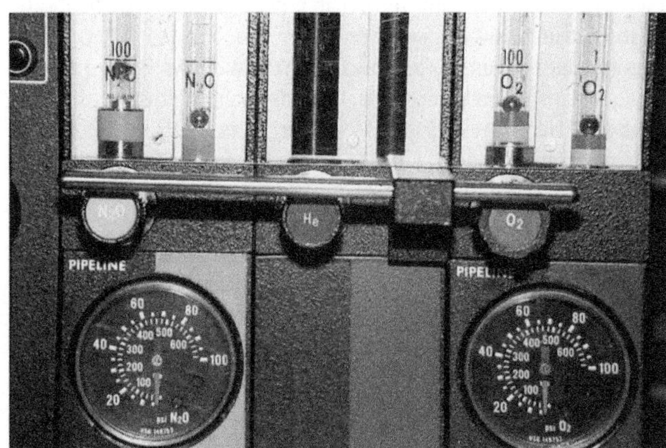

FIGURE 2-27 ■ Potential for a hyperoxic mixture. This machine is designed to deliver oxygen, nitrous oxide, and helium. If it were set to deliver a mixture of oxygen at 1 L/min and helium at 3 L/min (i.e., 25% O_2/75% He) for laser surgery of the airway and the helium tank became empty, the machine would deliver 100% oxygen and create a potential fire hazard. In this case, an oxygen analyzer with a high-concentration alarm is essential. Newer machines are designed to deliver a mixture of helium and oxygen (heliox).

Control of Gas Flows

Two separate components deliver the intended gas flow: a variable resistor device controls the flow, and another device measures the flow.

Mechanical Rotameter Flowmeters

In a basic anesthesia machine, the proportions of oxygen and nitrous oxide and other medical gases controlled by the machine, as well as total gas flows delivered to the CGO, are adjusted by flow control needle valves and vertical glass tube rotameter flowmeters. There may be one rotameter or two rotameters in series (see Figs. 2-27 and 2-28) for each gas.[1] If two are present for any gas, the first permits accurate measurement of low flows (usually up to 1 L/min), and the second permits measurement of higher flows (of up to 10 or 12 L/min). Each flowmeter is calibrated for discharge through the CGO into a standard atmosphere (760 mm Hg) at 20° C.[1] In North America, the oxygen flowmeter is normally positioned on the right side of a rotameter bank downstream of the other flowmeters and closest to the CGO (see Figs. 2-4 and 2-28). If a leak occurs in one of the other flowmeter tubes, this position is the least likely to result in a hypoxic mixture.[25] Where oxygen and other gases are delivered

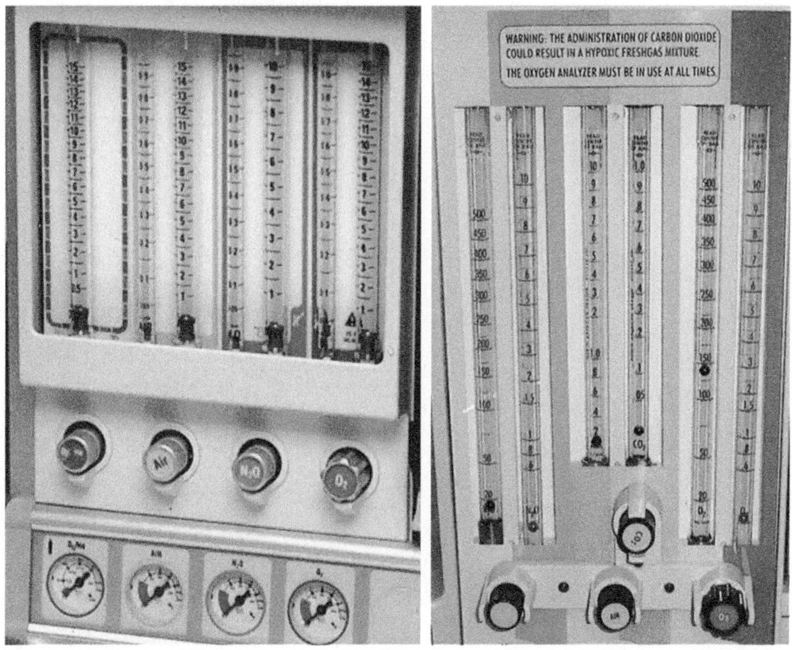

FIGURE 2-28 ■ Flowmeter banks on a four-gas Datex-Ohmeda (GE Healthcare, Waukesha, WI) anesthesia machine (*left*) and a four-gas Dräger Medical (Telford, PA) machine *(right)*. Flowmeters for each gas are arranged in series. The oxygen flows first through a rotameter, where low flows (<1 L/min) are measured, and then through a rotameter, where high flows (<10 L/min) are measured. In the United States, the oxygen flowmeters are on the right side of the flowmeter bank when viewed from the front. One gas flow control knob is present for each gas, even if there are two (low and high) flowmeter tubes for that gas.

by their flowmeters into a common manifold, the oxygen is delivered downstream of all other gases.[1]

The vertical rotameter is an example of a constant-pressure, variable-orifice flowmeter. Its operation is based on the principle of the Thorpe tube (see Figs. 2-27 and 2-29).[17] Each rotameter consists of a tapered glass tube that has a smaller diameter at the bottom, increasing to a larger diameter at the top and contains a ball or bobbin. The area between the outside of the bobbin and the inside of the glass tube represents the variable orifice, and a certain pressure difference across the bobbin is required to float the bobbin. As the orifice widens, greater and greater flows are required to create the same pressure difference across the bobbin, which floats higher in the tapered glass tube.

At low flow rates, gas flow is essentially laminar, and Poiseuille's law applies.[17] Thus,

$$\text{Flow} = (\pi \times P \times r^4)/(8 \times \eta \times L)$$

where π is the constant 3.142, P is the pressure difference across the bobbin, r is the radius of the tube, η is the viscosity of the gas, and L is the length of the bobbin or float. When flows are greater and the orifice is larger, turbulent flow occurs, in which case:

$$\text{Flow} \propto P \propto r^2 \propto \text{Length}^{-1} \propto 1/\sqrt{\text{Density}}$$

Flowmeters use a physical property of the gas to measure flow. In the case of low flows, when flow is laminar, the property used is the viscosity of the gas. At high flows, when flow is turbulent or orificial, gas density is used to measure flow.

Rotameters are precision instruments. Flow tubes are manufactured for specific gases, calibrated with a unique float, and are meant to be used within a certain range of temperatures and pressures. Whether the flow indicator float is a ball or a bobbin, flow on the calibrated scale should be read at the highest and widest portion of the float. Flowmeters are not interchangeable among gases. If a gas is passed through a rotameter for which it has not been calibrated, the flows shown are likely inaccurate. Theoretical exceptions to this are as follows. At low flows, flow rates of gases with similar viscosities, such as oxygen and helium, are read identically at 202 and 194 micropoise (μP), respectively; at high flows, gases of similar density—such as nitrous oxide and carbon dioxide, both of which have an atomic mass of 44—are read identically. Again, flowmeters are *not* interchangeable among medical gases, and modern machines are manufactured so that they cannot be interchanged.

The gas flow to the rotameter tube is controlled by a touch- and color-coded knob, which is linked to a needle valve (see Fig. 2-29). In the United States, the oxygen control knob is green, as is everything related to oxygen;

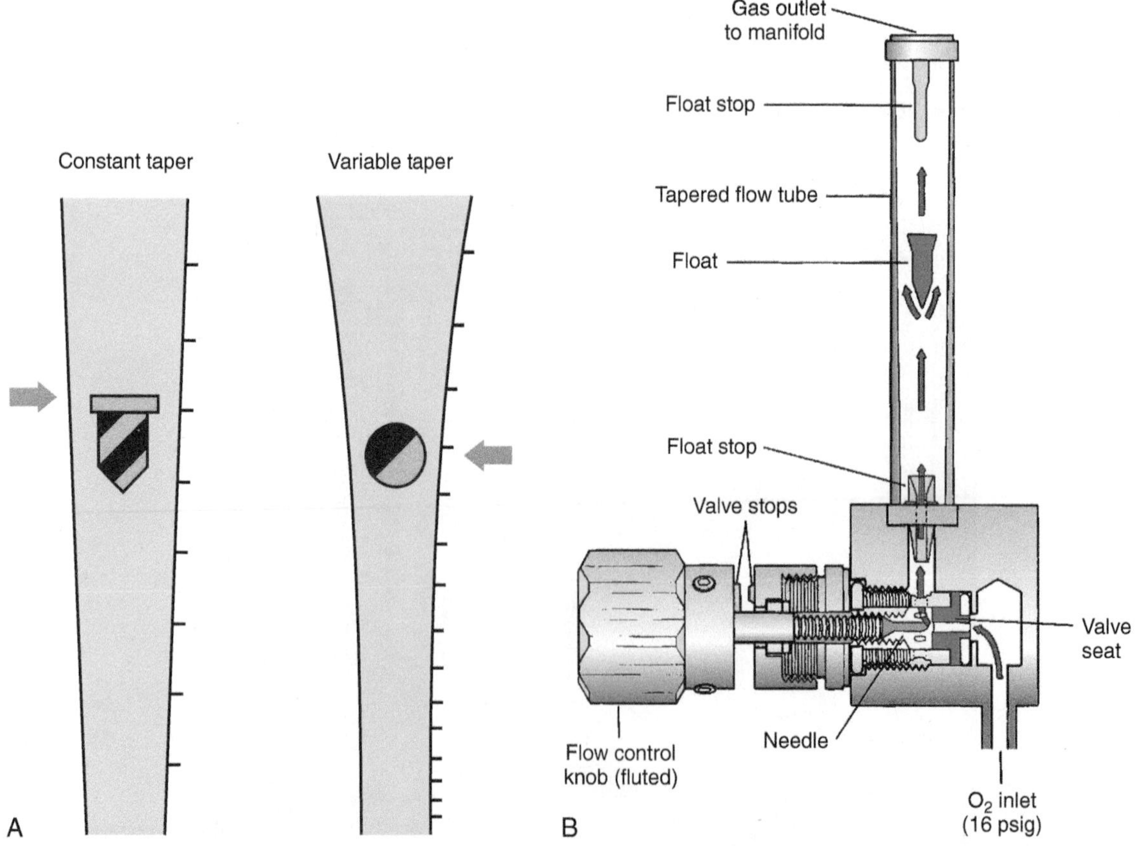

FIGURE 2-29 **A,** Constant- and variable-taper design tube flowmeters. **B,** Schematic section of an oxygen flowmeter and flow control valve. Designs may use a ball or an elongated float, as shown. Note that the flow control knob for oxygen is fluted (touch coded) to distinguish it from the other knobs, which are knurled. Minimum oxygen flow is achieved by valve stops in this GE Healthcare Datex-Ohmeda flow control system. (B, From Bowie E, Huffman LM: *The anesthesia machine: essentials for understanding.* Madison, WI, 1985, GE Datex-Ohmeda.)

it is also fluted and larger in diameter than the other gas flow control knobs.[1] The nitrous oxide control knob is smaller, blue, and ridged or knurled, but not fluted like the oxygen knob (Fig. 2-30).

Anesthesia machine manufacturers offer the option of oxygen flow that cannot be completely discontinued when the machine's main ON/OFF switch is turned on—that is, when the machine is capable of delivering an anesthetic. This is because either a mechanical valve stop ensures a minimum oxygen flow of 200 to 300 mL/min past the partially open needle valve (see Fig. 2-29, *right*), or a gas flow resistor permits a similar flow of 200 to 300 mL/min to bypass a completely closed oxygen flow control needle valve.

The workstation standard requires that each flowmeter assembly be clearly and permanently marked with the appropriate color, unit of measure, and the name or chemical symbol of the gas it measures. The manufacturer should ensure that the flowmeters and tubes are not interchangeable among the different gases or between the low-flow (0 to 1 L/min) and high-flow (1 to 10 L/min) rotameter tubes for each gas. Flowmeters may also be pin indexed to eliminate the possibility of installing a flowmeter intended for a different gas.

Flowmeter tubes are fragile and are therefore protected on the machine by a plastic window. Individual flow control knobs may also be surrounded by a shield to prevent accidental alterations of the settings (Fig. 2-31). To obtain a true reading of flow, the rotameter tubes must be kept vertical to prevent the ball or bobbin from touching the sides of the glass tube. The flow should be read at the middle of the ball or at the top of the bobbin (see Fig. 2-29). The ball or bobbin is more likely to stick at low flows and where the tube is narrowest. Electrostatic charges and dirt may also interfere with the bobbin's free movement; in this respect, a ball is superior to a bobbin because a ball is less likely to stick.

Flowmeters are individually calibrated by the manufacturer against a master flowmeter for each gas. In clinical practice, flowmeter calibration is most easily checked by setting gas flows to produce desired nitrous oxide–oxygen concentrations and using a gas analyzer to check the composition of the gas mixture emerging from the machine's CGO.

The positioning of the oxygen flowmeter in the bank of several gas flowmeters is important. The anesthesia workstation standard requires that the oxygen flowmeter be placed on the right side of the flowmeter group when the workstation is viewed from the front. It is also the most downstream flowmeter, closest to the CGO, to make hypoxia less likely in the event of a leak in one of the other flowmeters. Thus, if the oxygen flowmeter is placed upstream of a leaking nitrous oxide flow tube, oxygen would be lost through the leak and an excess of nitrous oxide would flow to the CGO.[25] Although these considerations were important in the past,[26] they may be less so now because the use of an oxygen analyzer in the inspiratory limb of the breathing system has become the standard of care.

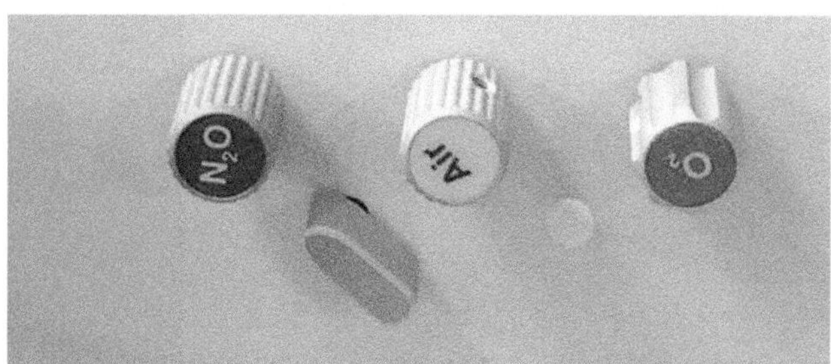

FIGURE 2-30 Gas flow control knobs. Oxygen is on the right and is fluted (touch coded). The second gas in this machine, air or nitrous oxide, must be selected by the switch. Note the absence of any guard device to prevent unintended changes in knob position. The flow control knobs for nitrous oxide and air are smaller than those for oxygen and are knurled.

OXYGEN RATIO MONITORING AND PROPORTIONING SYSTEMS

A major consideration in the design of contemporary anesthesia machines is the prevention of delivery of a hypoxic gas mixture to the patient. The fail-safe system described above only interrupts, or proportionately reduces and ultimately interrupts, the supply of nitrous oxide and other gases to their flowmeters if the oxygen supply *pressure* to the machine decreases. It does not prevent delivery of a hypoxic mixture to the CGO.

In contemporary anesthesia machines, oxygen and nitrous oxide flow controls are physically interlinked either mechanically (Datex-Ohmeda machines) or mechanically and pneumatically (Dräger machines) so that a fresh gas mixture containing at least 25% oxygen is created at the level of the rotameters when nitrous oxide and oxygen are being delivered.[4,6] In other contemporary workstations, proportioning is achieved by electronically controlled valves.

Datex-Ohmeda anesthesia machines use the Link-25 proportion-limiting control system to ensure an adequate percentage of oxygen in the gas mixture. In this system, the sizes of the openings of the oxygen and nitrous oxide

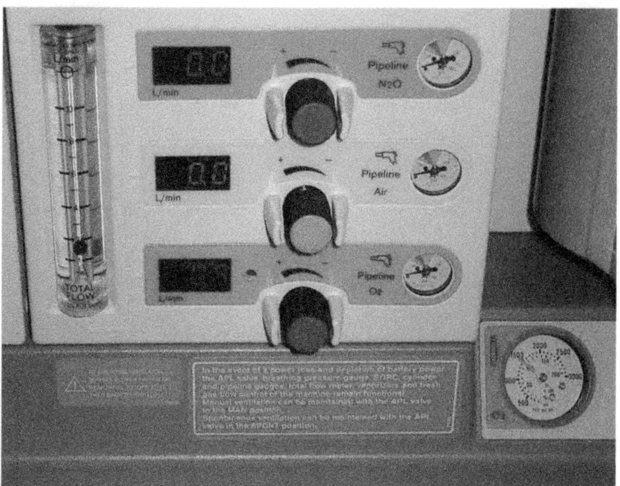

FIGURE 2-31 Front view of a Dräger Fabius GS workstation (Dräger Medical, Telford, PA) showing a vertical arrangement of the flow control knobs. The knobs are less susceptible to accidental changes in flow by the protective half-sleeves on either side of each knob (compare with Fig. 2-30).

flow control needle valves are proportioned and the supply pressures of these gases to their flow control valves are precisely regulated by second-stage (low-pressure) regulators. In addition, a gear (sprocket) with 14 teeth is integral with the nitrous oxide flow control spindle, and a sprocket with 29 teeth can rotate on a threaded oxygen flow control valve spindle, like a nut on a bolt (Fig. 2-32). The two sprockets are connected by a precision stainless-steel linked chain. Because of the 14:29 ratio of gear teeth, for every 2.07 revolutions of the nitrous oxide flow control spindle, an oxygen flow control, set to the lowest oxygen flow, rotates once. Because the sprocket on the oxygen flow control spindle is thread mounted so that it can rotate on the oxygen control valve spindle, oxygen flow can be increased independently of the flow of nitrous oxide. However, regardless of the oxygen flow set, if the flow of nitrous oxide is sufficiently increased, the chain will cause the oxygen sprocket to rotate and move outward toward the oxygen flow control knob. Eventually, a tab on the oxygen sprocket engages with a tab on the oxygen flow control knob, causing it to rotate in a counterclockwise manner, opening the oxygen needle valve and thereby causing the oxygen flow to increase. If nitrous oxide flow is decreased, the oxygen flow remains at the increased setting unless it is manually decreased. The proportioning of nitrous oxide to oxygen (75% to 25%) is completed because the nitrous oxide flow control valve is supplied from a second-stage gas regulator that reduces nitrous oxide pressure to a nominal 26 psig, adjusted as previously described, before it reaches the flow control valve. The oxygen flow control valve is supplied at a pressure of 14 psig from a second-stage oxygen regulator (Figs. 2-4 and 2-33). The Link-25 system permits the nitrous oxide and oxygen flow control valves to be set independently of one another, but when a setting of nitrous oxide concentration more than 75% is attempted, the oxygen flow is automatically increased to maintain at least 25% oxygen in the resulting mixture. This system thus increases the minimum flow of oxygen

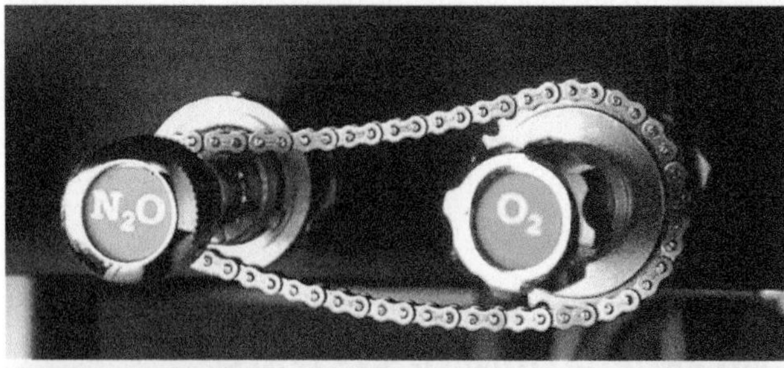

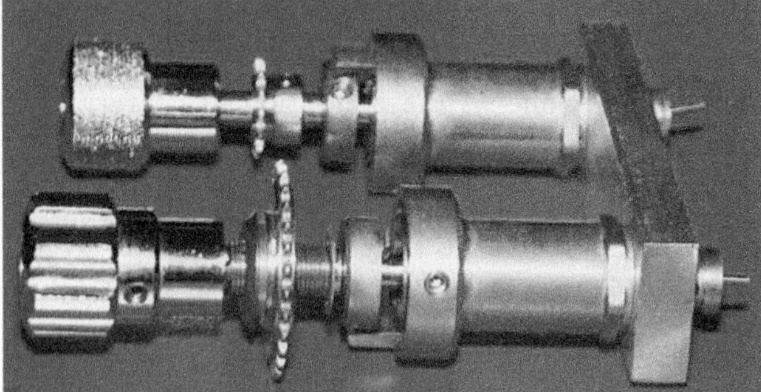

FIGURE 2-32 ■ Datex-Ohmeda Link-25 Proportion Limiting System (GE Healthcare, Waukesha, WI). *Top:* Front view of flow control knobs, sprockets (N_2O, 14 teeth; O_2, 29 teeth), and stainless-steel link chain. *Bottom:* Side view shows N_2O sprocket fixed on the spindle, whereas the O_2 sprocket can move on the threaded O_2 spindle, like a nut turning on a bolt.

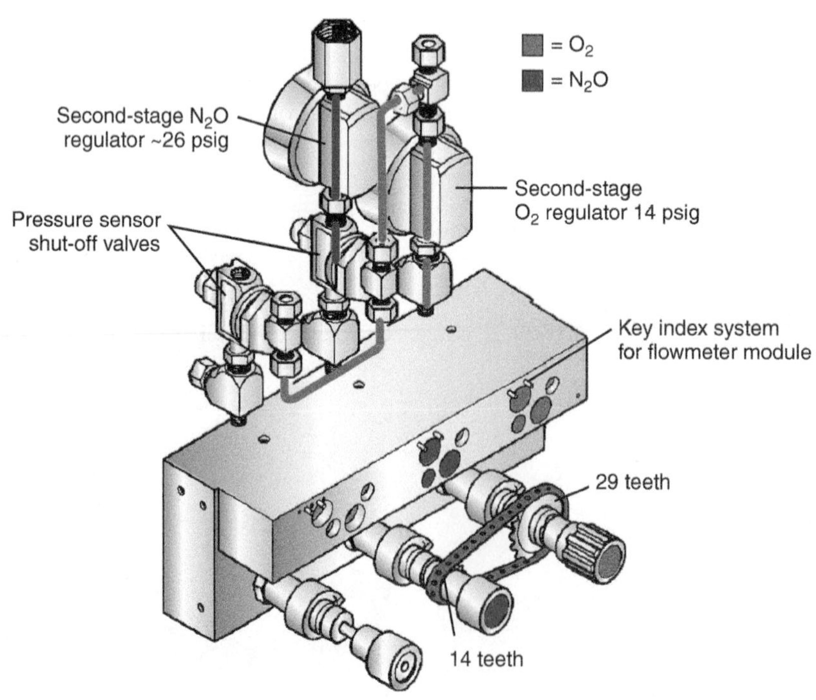

FIGURE 2-33 ■ Schematic of Datex-Ohmeda Link-25 Proportion Limiting System (GE Healthcare, Waukesha, WI). A second-stage regulator for both O_2 and N_2O ensures that their flow control needle valves have a constant input pressure. Because Flow = Pressure/Resistance, in this system pressure is constant and resistance is adjusted via the needle valve orifices to maintain flow proportionality.

according to the nitrous oxide flow setting by further opening the oxygen needle control valve.[4]

The Link-25 system interconnects only the nitrous oxide and oxygen flow control valves. If the anesthesia machine has flow controls for other gases, such as pure helium or air (see Figs. 2-27 and 2-28), a gas mixture containing less than 25% oxygen could be set at the level of the flowmeters. This potential hazard is addressed on more modern machines by supplying helium in tanks that contain a mixture of helium and oxygen (heliox) in a 75:25 ratio.

Older models of Narkomed machines use the *oxygen ratio monitor controller* (ORMC; Fig. 2-34) to limit the flow of nitrous oxide according to the oxygen *flow*, which creates a mixture of at least 25% oxygen at the flowmeter level when these two gases are being used.[6,27] Newer models use the *sensitive oxygen ratio controller* (S-ORC) proportioning system. In principle, both ORMC and S-ORC work similarly. At oxygen flow rates of less than 1 L/min, concentrations of oxygen greater than 25% are delivered.

The ORMC and S-ORC function much the same: as oxygen flows past the flow control needle valve and up the rotameter tube, it encounters a resistor that creates a backpressure, which is applied to the oxygen diaphragm (see Fig. 2-34); as nitrous oxide flows past its flow control valve and up into the rotameter tube, it also encounters a resistor that causes a backpressure on the nitrous oxide diaphragm. The two diaphragms are linked by a connecting shaft, whose ultimate position depends on the relative backpressures, and therefore flows, of nitrous oxide and oxygen. One end of the connecting shaft controls the orifice of a slave valve, which in turn controls the supply pressure of nitrous oxide to its flow control valve. When the oxygen flow is high, the shaft moves to the left and opens the slave control valve. Conversely, if the flow of nitrous oxide is increased excessively, the shaft moves to the right, closing the slave valve orifice and limiting the

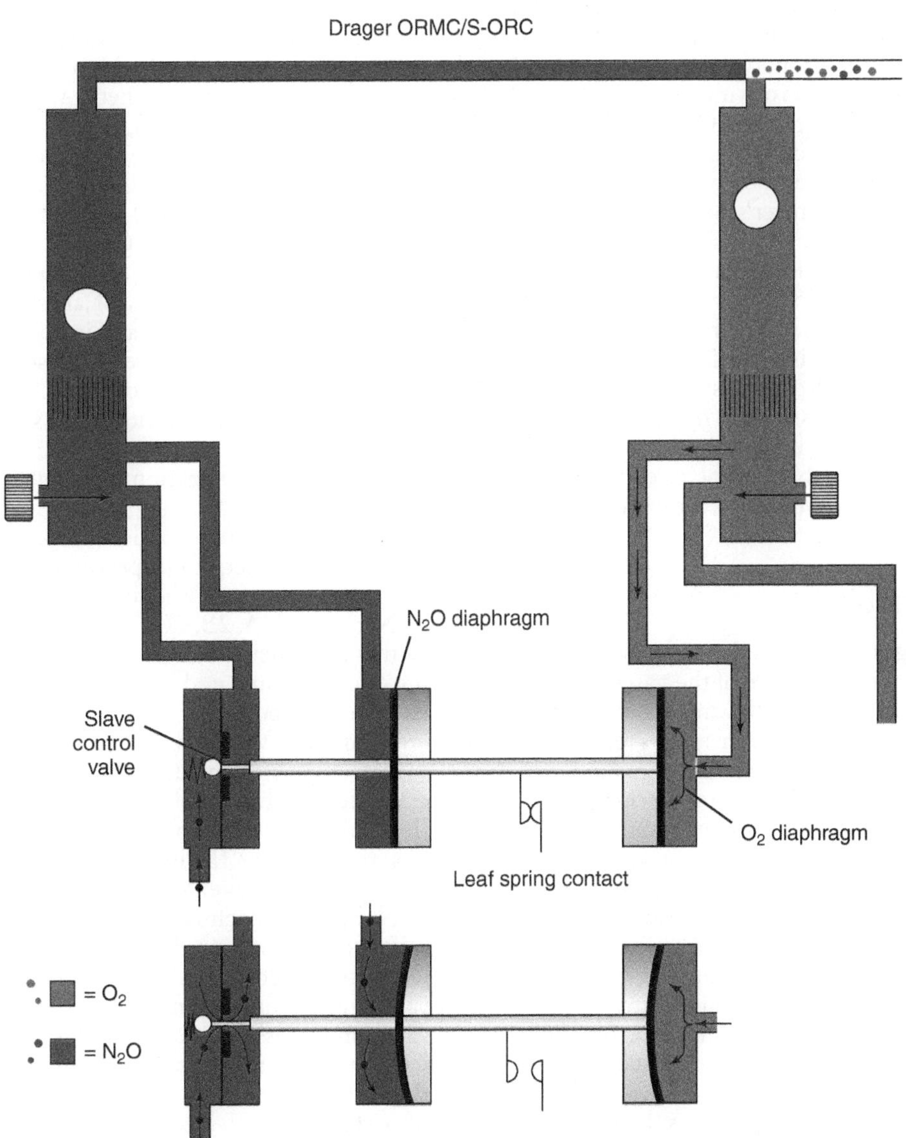

FIGURE 2-34 ■ Dräger Medical oxygen ratio monitor controller (*ORMC*) and sensitive oxygen ratio controller (*S-ORC*) principles. In this system, resistance is kept constant by fixed resistors just downstream of each needle valve, and flow of N_2O is kept proportioned by controlling pressure upstream of the N_2O needle valve. (From Schreiber PJ: *Anesthesia systems.* Telford, PA, 1985, North American Dräger.)

supply pressure, and thereby the flow, of nitrous oxide to its flow control valve.[6]

The Dräger ORMC and S-ORC differ from the Datex-Ohmeda Link-25 Proportioning Limiting System in a number of ways. First, the ORMC and S-ORC do not use second-stage oxygen and nitrous oxide regulators. Second, the ORMC and S-ORC limit the flow of nitrous oxide according to the flow of oxygen, whereas the Link-25 system increases the flow of oxygen as the nitrous oxide flow is increased. In the Link-25 system, once the oxygen flow has been increased via the link chain and gears, the oxygen flow remains at the increased setting even if the nitrous oxide flow is deliberately decreased. With the ORMC and S-ORC systems, if the system is acting to decrease the flow of nitrous oxide because the user has decreased the oxygen flow, when the flow of oxygen is increased again, the nitrous oxide flow will increase to its original setting. Third, like the Link-25 system, the ORMC and S-ORC function only between nitrous oxide and oxygen and there is no interlinking of oxygen with other gases, such as air or helium, that might be delivered by the machine. Thus, when a third or fourth gas is in use, the proportioning systems afford no protection against a hypoxic mixture at the CGO. Although of elegant design, the ORMC, S-ORC, and Link-25 systems are subject to mechanical and/or pneumatic failure (see Chapter 30) and should be tested according to the manufacturer's instructions during the preuse machine checkout.[28] Fourth, even if the systems are functioning correctly, they ensure delivery of no less than 25% oxygen at the flowmeter level. An oxygen leak downstream of the flowmeters, or the addition of high concentrations of a potent volatile inhaled anesthetic (e.g., 18% desflurane) also downstream of the proportioning systems, could result in a hypoxic mixture (i.e., <21% oxygen) being delivered from the machine CGO. An oxygen analyzer in the patient circuit is therefore essential if a potentially hypoxic mixture is to be detected and thereby prevented.

Vaporizer Manifolds

After individual gas flows have been measured by their respective rotameters, a mixture of the gases is created in a manifold downstream of the flowmeters. From here the gas mixture flows to the vaporizer manifold, where concentration-calibrated vaporizers are mounted on the machine. In older model Narkomed machines, the Dräger Vapor 19.1 vaporizers are permanently mounted and are not intended to be removed by the user. These vaporizers are mounted in series; that is, fresh gas flows through each vaporizer, albeit via a bypass channel, on its way to the CGO. An interlock device ensures that only one vaporizer can be turned on at any one time.

Contemporary anesthesia machines are designed so that the vaporizers are easily removable by the user. These vaporizer manifolds are designed such that no gas from the flowmeters enters any part of a vaporizer that is turned off, not even the vaporizer's bypass channel. When a vaporizer is turned on, fresh gas enters only that vaporizer. This is important to understand when it comes to checking the machine's low-pressure system. To check a vaporizer for leaks, it must be turned on to become connected to the low-pressure system of the machine. (Vaporizer manifolds are discussed in more detail in Chapter 3.)

Some departments maintain an anesthesia machine on which no vaporizers have been mounted; this makes an available "clean machine" for use with patients susceptible to malignant hyperthermia. In this case the gas mixture created at the flowmeter manifold is conducted directly to the CGO.

Common Gas Outlets and Outlet Check Valves

The fresh gas mixture produced by the settings of the flowmeters for oxygen, nitrous oxide, and/or other gases and vapor from one concentration-calibrated vaporizer exit the machine via the CGO. Some Datex-Ohmeda machines—such as the Modulus I, Modulus II, and Excel models—have an outlet check valve situated between the vaporizers and the CGO (Fig. 2-35) and a pressure relief valve (see Fig. 2-4). The pressure relief valve, as its name suggests, prevents the buildup of excessive pressures upstream of the outlet check valve. In some Datex-Ohmeda machines (Excel, Modulus I with Selectatec switch), the pressure relief valve is located downstream of the outlet check valve. In all machines, these components are located upstream from where the oxygen flush flow would join to pass to the CGO.

The use or nonuse of an outlet check valve varies among the various models of anesthesia machine. The pressure relief mechanism and its location with respect to an outlet check valve, if present, also vary. The reader is encouraged to review the schematic of machines in use to understand the configuration of its system.

The purpose of the outlet check valve is to prevent reverse gas flow, a situation that could permit fresh gas to reenter the vaporizer ("pumping effect") if the vaporizer did not have its own outlet check valve or specialized design. This effect, if not prevented, can cause increased concentrations of anesthetic agent output (see Chapter 3).

Narkomed 2A, 2B, 2C, 3, and 4 machines are designed so that an outlet check valve is not required. The pumping effect is eliminated by the special design of the vaporizers. The Modulus II Plus and Modulus CD machines are equipped with Datex-Ohmeda TEC 4 or TEC 5 vaporizers, which incorporate a baffle system and a specially designed manifold to prevent the pumping effect; this makes an outlet check valve unnecessary. Nevertheless, the Modulus II Plus and Modulus CD machines do have a pressure relief valve upstream of the CGO.[29]

Narkomed machines do not have a separate pressure relief valve. If required, pressure relief occurs when the pressure exceeds 18 psig through the specially designed vaporizers. The presence or absence of an outlet check valve and pressure-relief valve is of some significance when it comes to leak testing the low-pressure system of the anesthesia machine; it also affects the performance of a transtracheal jet ventilating system connected to the CGO.

Transtracheal jet ventilation systems are sometimes needed by anesthesiologists for use in an emergency.

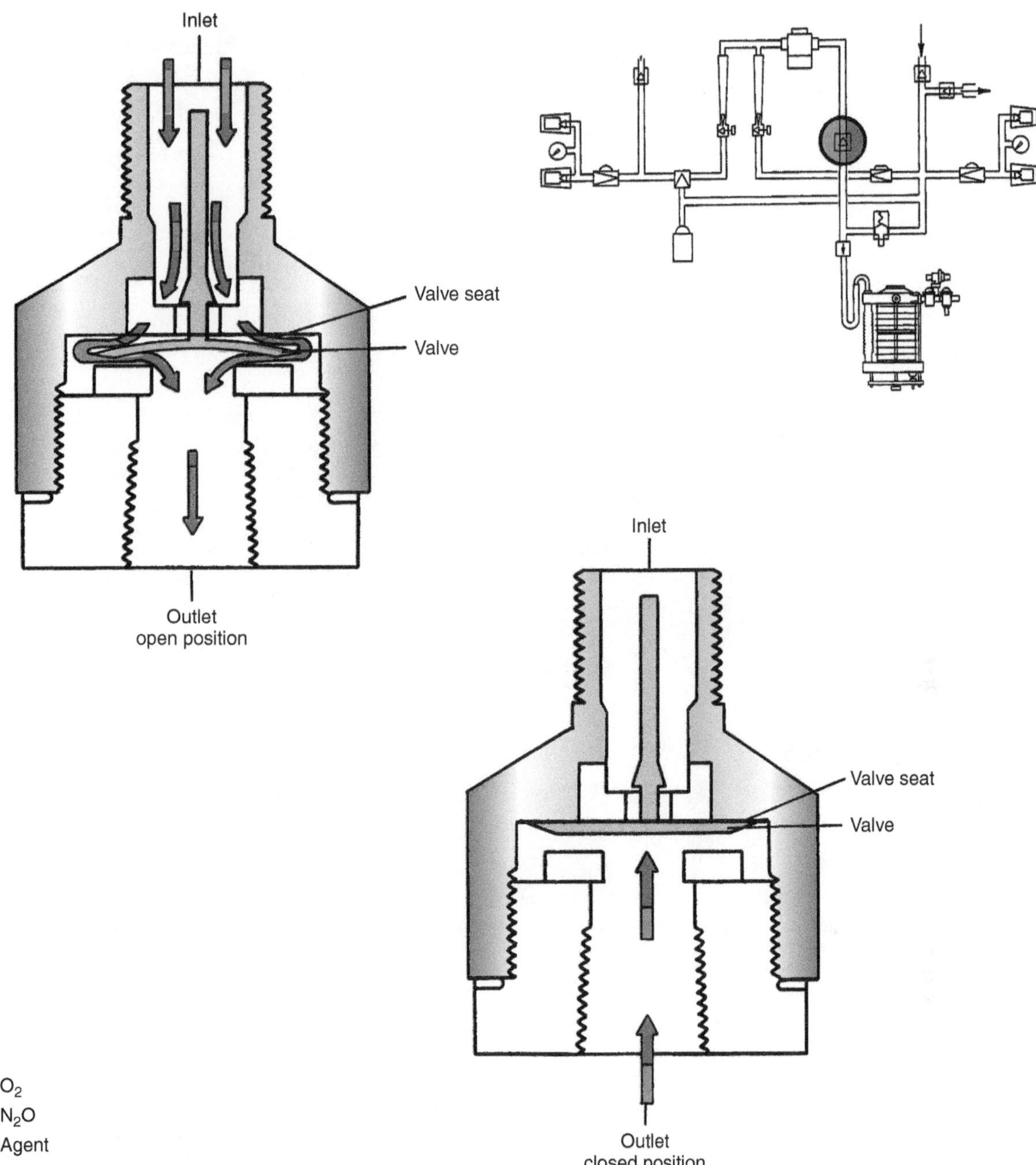

FIGURE 2-35 ▪ Machine outlet check valve located between the vaporizer and the common gas outlet. This valve is present on Datex-Ohmeda Modulus I, Modulus II, and Excel machines but not on Modulus II Plus or Modulus CD or on Dräger Medical Narkomed (Telford, PA) machines. The valve is designed to permit gas flow from the vaporizers to the common gas outlet and to prevent reverse gas flow, which might cause a pumping effect on the vaporizer. Increased pressure at the common gas outlet causes the valve to close. (From Bowie E, Huffman LM: *The anesthesia machine: essentials for understanding.* Madison, WI, 1985, GE Datex-Ohmeda.)

Ideally, a purpose-designed Sanders-type transtracheal jet ventilation system is available in every anesthetizing location and certainly in the difficult airway cart. This system is connected via a pressure-reducing valve and toggle switch to a separate 50-psig oxygen source.[18] However, some anesthesia care providers have described "homemade" systems designed to be connected to the machine CGO via a 15-mm connector, and ventilation is achieved by intermittent depression of the oxygen flush button.[30-32] The driving pressure of such systems is limited by the threshold-opening pressure of the pressure-relief mechanism, if present (see Fig. 2-4). In the case of Modulus II Plus or Modulus CD machines, the pressure relief valve opens at 2.2 to 2.9 psig. In the case of Narkomed machines equipped with vaporizers, it opens at 18 psig. In the case of Modulus I and Modulus II machines (outlet check valve present) and Narkomed machines without vaporizers (no pressure relief system), the driving pressure available at the CGO is 45 to 55 psig, depending on whether the tank or pipeline oxygen supply to the machine is in use (see Fig. 2-4). The "cracking" pressure of the relief mechanisms—that is,

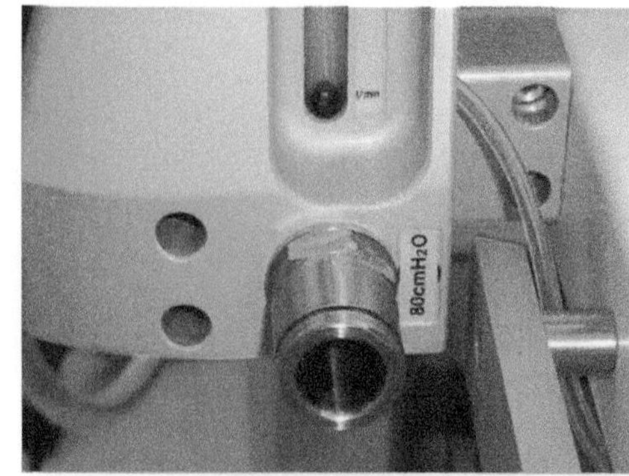

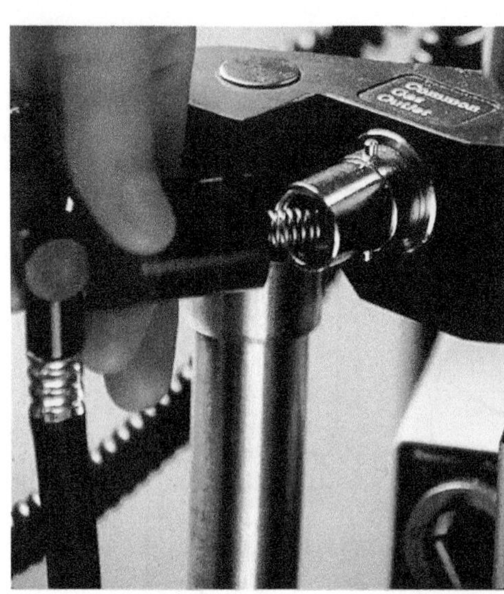

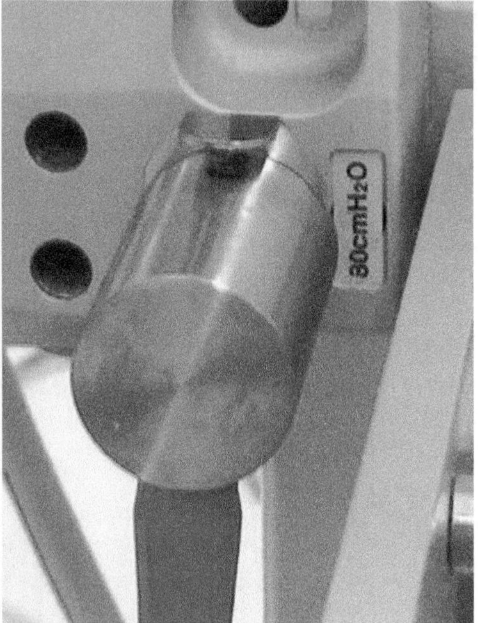

FIGURE 2-36 ■ *Left,* Spring-loaded bayonet fitting retaining device at the common gas outlet (CGO) of a Datex-Ohmeda (GE Healthcare, Waukesha, WI) anesthesia machine. *Right,* CGO (*top*) and retaining device (*bottom*) on a GE ADU workstation. These devices are designed to prevent accidental disconnection of the hose that connects the CGO to the patient breathing circuit.

the pressure at which the relief valve first begins to open—provides some guide to the potential driving pressure available for the transtracheal ventilating system. In practice, pressures a little higher than the cracking pressure are generated because of both the flow restriction offered by the relief valve and that offered by the ventilating system. It should be noted, however, that anesthesia machine oxygen flush systems were not designed or intended by the manufacturers to be used for transtracheal jet ventilation. For these reasons anesthesia machine oxygen flush systems should not be used for this purpose.

The anesthesia workstation standard requires anesthesia machines to have only one CGO. When that CGO is connected to the breathing system by a fresh gas supply hose, the usual arrangement in most ORs, the CGO must be provided with a manufacturer-specific retaining device.[1] The purpose of the retaining device is to help prevent disconnection or misconnections between the machine's CGO and the patient circuit. Thus a disconnection here would result in failure to deliver the intended gas mixture, with possible entrainment of room air if a hanging bellows design of ventilator or a piston ventilator were used; this could result in a hypoxic mixture in the circuit in addition to patient awareness as a result of failure of delivery of inhaled anesthetic. The machine manufacturers use their own proprietary retaining devices (Fig. 2-36). The workstation standard requires that the CGO have a 15-mm female fitting or a coaxial fitting with a 15-mm internal diameter and 22-mm external diameter. It must not incorporate a 19-, 23-, or 30-mm conical fitting because these are specific for other parts of the delivery system, specifically the patient circuit and the waste gas scavenging system (see Chapter 16).

Concerns about disconnections at the CGO have led to some machine and workstation designs in which the outlet is not accessible to the user. Examples include the Datex-Ohmeda Aestiva/5; the Datex-Ohmeda Aespire, Avance, and Aisys Carestations that use the Advanced Breathing System; and the Dräger Apollo workstation.

The Aestiva/5 machine has an *auxiliary* CGO that, when selected, diverts the fresh gas flow to this outlet, switching out the circle system (Fig. 2-37). This allows use of a rebreathing system. The auxiliary CGO must be selected to perform the machine's low-pressure system leak check. Once the leak check is complete, the user

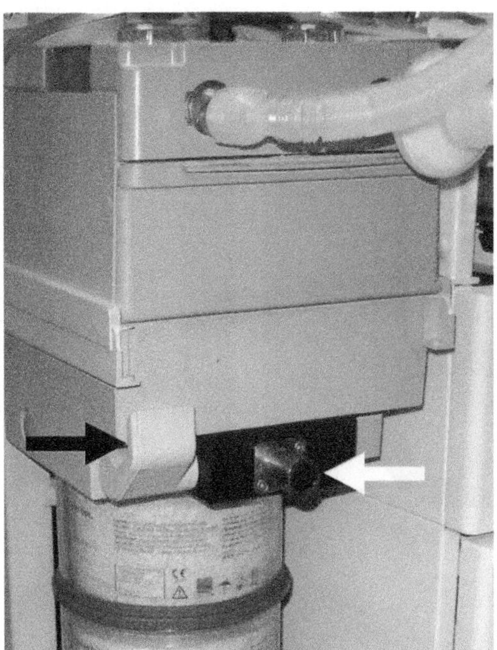

FIGURE 2-37 ■ Auxiliary common gas outlet (*white arrow*) on a Datex-Ohmeda Aestiva/5 machine (GE Healthcare, Waukesha, WI). This outlet is enabled and the connection to the circle system is disabled by pressing down the lever (*black arrow*) to the left of the outlet. This outlet is used to perform the low-pressure system leak check or to connect a noncircle system.

must remember to switch out the auxiliary CGO to use the circle system.

An auxiliary CGO similar to that of the Aestiva/5 is an option on GE machines that use the Advanced Breathing System. In one case report, a massive leak developed in an Aisys Carestation during a neurosurgical procedure. Being unable to correct the situation, the authors reported completing the anesthetic by switching to a Bain circuit connected to the alternate CGO.[33]

The Datex-Ohmeda ADU and the Dräger Fabius GS have accessible CGOs, whereas the Dräger Apollo workstation does not and therefore can be used only with a circle breathing system.

ANESTHESIA MACHINE LOW-PRESSURE SYSTEM CHECKOUTS

The anesthesia delivery system should be checked each day before the first procedure and when any change has been made to the system. Such changes include replacement of the ventilator bellows or anesthesia circuit and movement of the anesthesia machine in the operating room; moving the machine may cause kinking or compression of the tubing, which in turn may produce interference with gas delivery, ventilator function, or waste gas scavenging. Thus, in addition to a complete check at the start of each day, a shortened check of the delivery system should precede each procedure.

In August 1986, the U.S. Food and Drug Administration (FDA) published its Anesthesia Apparatus Checkout Recommendations, which included 24 steps.[34] A study subsequently reported that anesthesia practitioners did not appropriately apply this checkout protocol.[34] In 1993, the FDA published a revised checkout that had only 14 steps (see Table 32-1 in Chapter 32).[11] One of the most important steps in these checks is that of checking the machine's low-pressure system for leaks.

Testing for Leaks in the Anesthesia Machine and Breathing System

Many traditional anesthesia machines, for which the FDA 1986 and 1993 checks were designed, remain in service around the world. The following discussion of checking the low-pressure system for leaks is therefore still relevant. In particular, an appreciation of the principles of the low-pressure system check and its relation to the presence or absence of an outlet check valve is essential. Application of the incorrect check could result in a large leak being missed.

Item 16 in the FDA 1986 checklist described what should be done before each patient procedure. This check evaluates the components of the delivery system downstream of the flowmeters (i.e., the low-pressure system) and should detect gross leaks that may be due to cracked rotameter tubes, leaking gaskets and vaporizers, and leaks in the anesthesia circuit. In this generic test, the APL valve, or "pop-off valve," is closed, and the patient circuit is occluded at the patient end. The system is then filled via the oxygen flush until the reservoir bag is just full but with negligible pressure in the system. Oxygen flow is set to 5 L/min and then slowly decreased until pressure no longer rises above approximately 20 cm H_2O (Fig. 2-38). This set flow is said to approximate the total rate of gas leak, which should be no greater than a few hundred milliliters per minute. The reservoir bag should then be squeezed to a pressure of about 50 cm H_2O to verify that the system is gas tight. If the leak is large enough, the circuit pressure may fall to zero (Fig. 2-39).

The advantages of this test routine are that it can be performed quickly and that it checks the patient circuit as well as the low-pressure components of the machine in models that *do not* have an outlet check valve. Disadvantages of this process are that it is relatively insensitive to small leaks, and in machines that have an outlet check valve—such as the Modulus I, Modulus II, and Excel models—only the patient circuit downstream of the outlet check valve is tested for leaks.

The generic check is insensitive because it depends on volume. Thus, in this test, a large volume of gas—in effect, that contained in the circuit tubing, absorber, and reservoir bag—is compressed. The circuit pressure gauge is then observed for any changes. The term *compliance* expresses the relationship between volume and pressure and is defined as change in volume per unit change in pressure. Because of the large volume of gas compressed and the high compliance of the distensible reservoir bag, relatively large changes in volume (i.e., leaks) may exist with minimal changes in pressure. The anesthesiologist performing the check is looking for a pressure decrease as an indicator of gas leakage; however, relatively large leaks may go undetected by this test.

The second limitation of the FDA 1986 generic check is related to the presence or absence of an outlet check

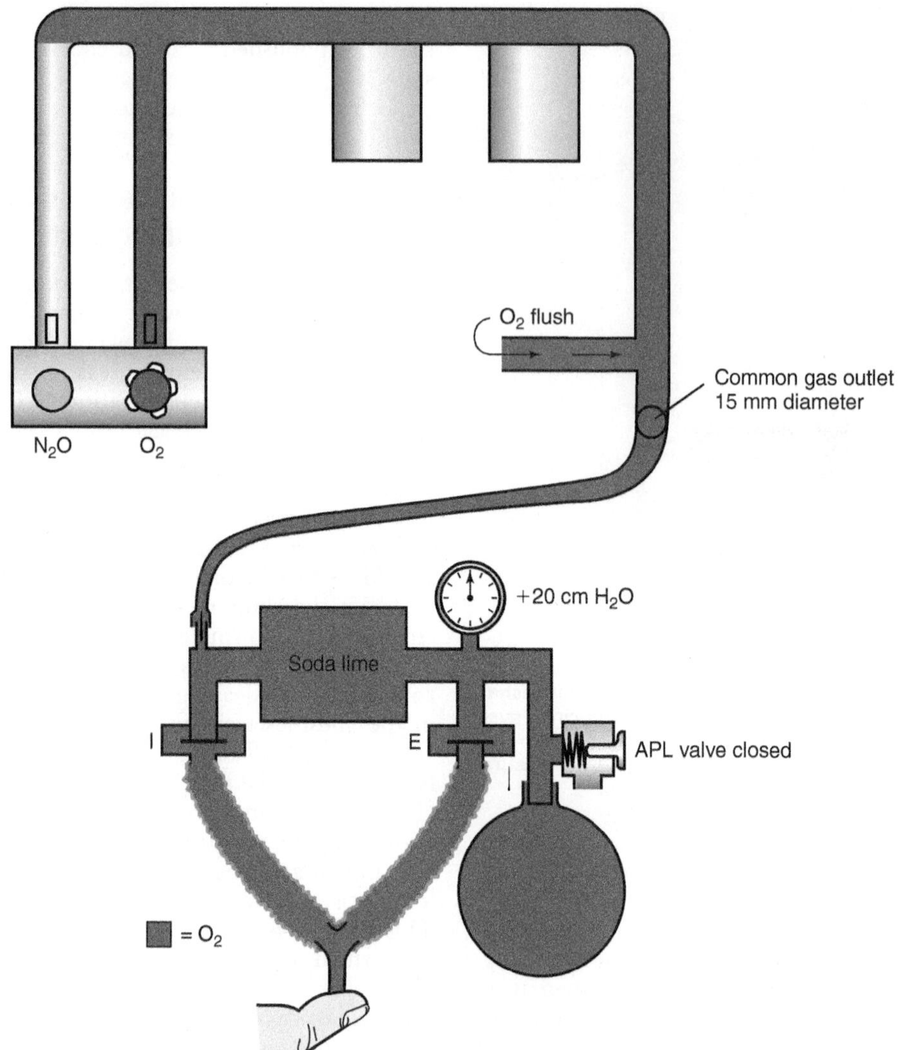

FIGURE 2-38 The U.S. Food and Drug Administration 1986 generic leak check procedure of low-pressure system in a machine with no outlet check valve. In the absence of a leak, pressure is maintained at 20 cm H_2O. APL, adjustable pressure limiting. (From Eisenkraft JB: The anesthesia delivery system, part II. In Eisenkraft JB, editor: *Progress in anesthesiology, vol 3.* San Antonio, TX, 1989, Dannemiller Memorial Educational Foundation. Reproduced by permission.)

valve. Application of the generic leak check in this situation tests only for leaks in components downstream of the outlet check valve (Fig. 2-40).

The limitations of the FDA 1986 generic leak checkout make it obvious that specialized leak checks of the low-pressure system must be used, and the operator's manual for each machine should be consulted for details. Tests described for the Narkomed and Datex-Ohmeda machines are briefly reviewed in the following sections to illustrate the differences in system design, function, and check.

Narkomed Machines: No Outlet Check Valve

Dräger Medical recommends the following test procedure for checking the anesthesia breathing system and fresh gas delivery system.[35] In this test, all gas flow control (flowmeter) valves are closed, and the machine system main power switch is turned to STANDBY or OFF. In this position, no gas should flow to the flowmeters or from the CGO, and all vaporizer concentration dials are set to ZERO concentration. The inspiratory and expiratory valves are short circuited with 22-mm diameter circuit hose (Fig. 2-41). The shortest possible length of hose should be used to minimize contained gas volume. The MANUAL/AUTOMATIC selector valve is set to the MANUAL (bag) position. The APL (pop-off) valve is closed by turning it fully clockwise. The reservoir bag is removed, and the test terminal is attached to the bag mount (see Fig. 2-41). A sphygmomanometer squeeze bulb is connected to the hose barb on the test terminal. It should now be apparent that the total volume of the circuit components has been drastically reduced by the removal of the circle system tubing: a circle with each limb 152 cm (5 feet) in length has a volume of about 1200 mL, and the reservoir bag has a volume of 3 L. The sphygmomanometer bulb is squeezed by hand until the pressure shown at the breathing system pressure gauge indicates a pressure higher than 50 cm H_2O. The gauge is then observed for a decrease in pressure. Per manufacturer specifications, the pressure should not decrease to less than 30 cm H_2O over a 30-second observation period.[14] Because the volume of gas being compressed in this test is minimal (i.e., circuit compliance

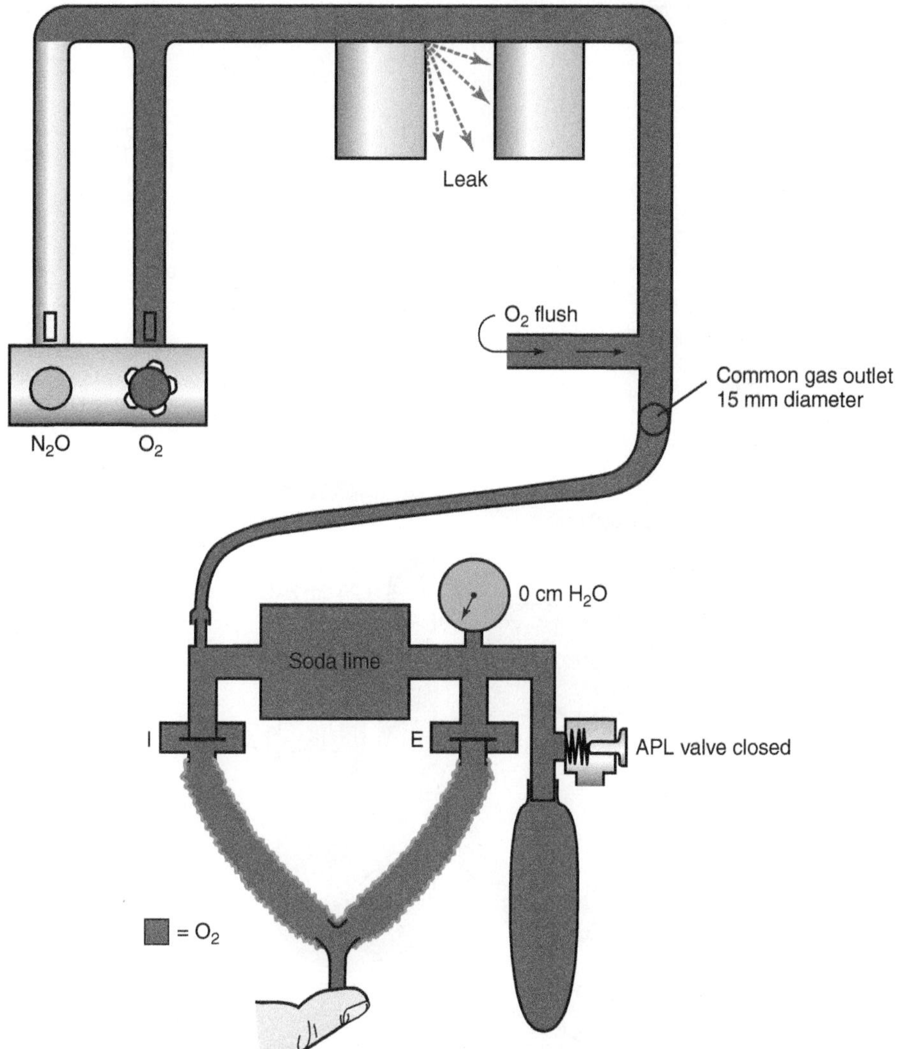

FIGURE 2-39 ■ **The U.S. Food and Drug Administration 1986 generic leak check procedure in a machine with no outlet check valve. A leak at the vaporizer mount results in failure of the system to hold pressure, which in this case has fallen to zero. Such a leak would not be detectable if an outlet check valve were present because pressure applied at the common gas outlet would not be transmitted into the vaporizer manifold. APL, adjustable pressure limiting.** (From Eisenkraft JB: The anesthesia delivery system, part II. In Eisenkraft JB, editor: *Progress in anesthesiology, vol 3.* San Antonio, TX, 1989, Dannemiller Memorial Educational Foundation. Reproduced by permission.)

has been significantly decreased), small gas leaks will result in a decrease in pressure that is observable on the circuit pressure gauge.

The positive-pressure leak check should be repeated sequentially with each vaporizer turned on and set at any concentration greater than 0.4%. This checks for leaks in individual vaporizers (e.g., filler caps, selector switches, and vaporizer mounts).

The test specifications given in this section apply to an anesthesia breathing system without accessories, such as the volumeter, sidestream gas analyzer, and other adapters. Test limits will be exceeded if accessory items are included in the test. The specific suppliers of the accessory items should be contacted for leak specifications of their devices.

Leaks in the patient circuit components can be distinguished from leaks in the low-pressure part of the Narkomed machine. If a leak has been identified with the combined circuit machine positive-pressure leak check, as described above, the sphygmomanometer bulb can be connected to the machine's CGO with a 15-mm (tracheal tube) connector and to a pressure gauge with a three-way stopcock. With this arrangement, only the anesthesia machine, as opposed to machine and circuit in the previous test, is pressurized to 50 cm H_2O. A decrease in pressure indicates a leak within the machine upstream of the CGO.

Datex-Ohmeda Machines with an Outlet Check Valve

In some Datex-Ohmeda machines, the presence of an outlet check valve complicates positive-pressure testing of the machine's low-pressure system (see Fig. 2-40). Application of positive pressure downstream of the valve causes it to close, so only components downstream of the CGO are checked for leaks. Positive-pressure ventilation and opening of the oxygen flush valve cause the check valve to close (see Figs. 2-4 and 2-41). For this reason, GE Healthcare developed a *negative pressure leak test* to be performed with a special suction bulb

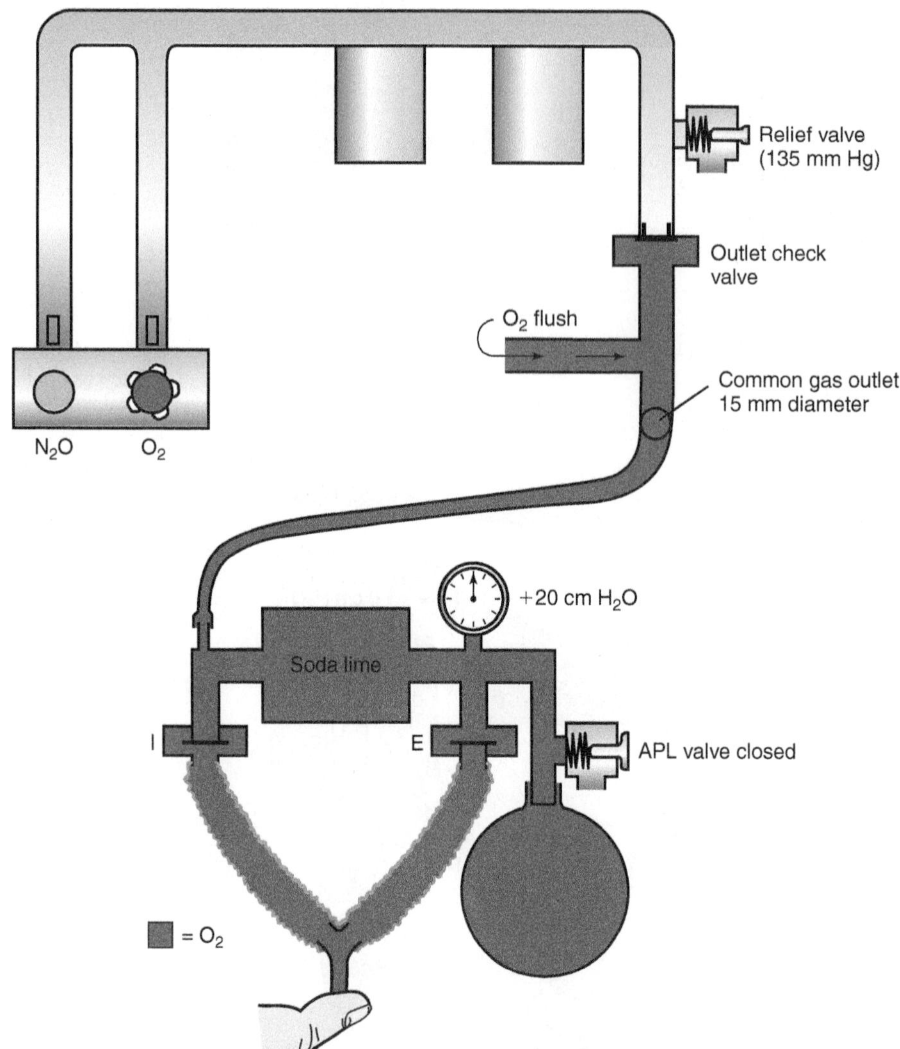

FIGURE 2-40 ■ Application of the U.S. Food and Drug Administration 1986 generic leak check procedure to a system with an outlet check valve. In this case, application of a positive backpressure of 20 cm of water causes the check valve to close so that only those components downstream of the outlet check valve are leak tested. APL, adjustable pressure limiting. (From Eisenkraft JB: The anesthesia delivery system, part II. In Eisenkraft JB, editor: *Progress in anesthesiology, vol 3.* San Antonio, TX, 1989, Dannemiller Memorial Educational Foundation. Reproduced by permission.)

device that is supplied with machines having this valve (Fig. 2-42).

First, the adequacy of the leak testing device should be checked by sealing the inlet connector of the bulb and squeezing the bulb until it is collapsed. The bulb is then released, and the time taken to reinflate it is observed. If reinflation occurs in less than 60 seconds, the device should be replaced.[29] The device is checked periodically, at times of machine servicing, to ensure that the vacuum produced by the evacuated bulb is at least -65 mm Hg.

The device is then used to check the machine.[23] First, the anesthesia machine's system master switch and all vaporizers are turned off so that no gases are flowing in the low-pressure parts of the machine. Each gas supply is then opened by turning on the backup cylinder valves or by connecting the pipeline supply. The flow control valves (rotameters) are turned fully to the OPEN position. Thus with the master switch turned off and the flowmeters open, no gas is flowing, but the entire system is accessible for testing. The testing bulb is attached to the machine's CGO via a 15-mm connector and is repeatedly squeezed and released until it remains collapsed. If the bulb reinflates within 30 seconds (Fig. 2-43), a leak of as little as 30 mL/min is present. The test procedure is repeated with each vaporizer turned to the ON position to look for leaks in the individual vaporizers. If the source is not easily correctable, the machine should be withdrawn from service. When the leak tests are complete, the negative-pressure bulb is removed from the CGO. Because the leak check described is conducted with all the flow-control valves open, components up to and including the machine's main ON/OFF control switch are also tested for leaks.

The negative pressure leak check described for Datex-Ohmeda machines results in the outlet check valve being held open by the -65 mm Hg vacuum (see Figs. 2-42 and 2-43) and air or gas being sucked into the system through any leaks. If such leaks were present while the machine

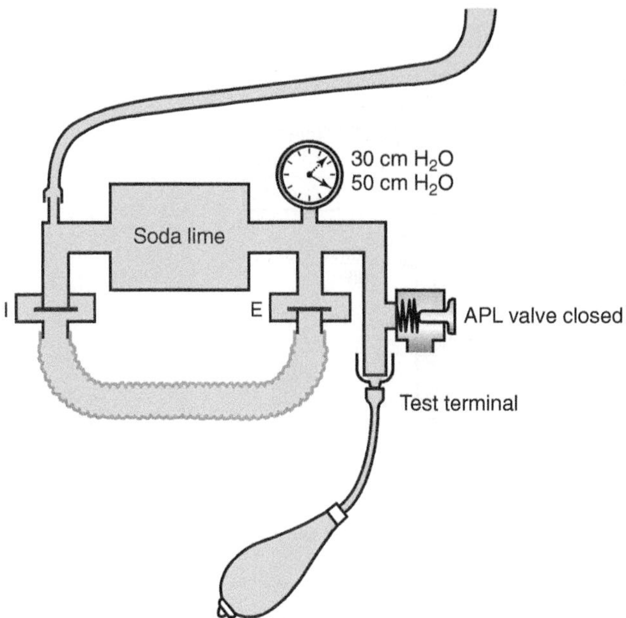

FIGURE 2-41 Narkomed positive-pressure leak check (Dräger Medical, Telford, PA). The system is pressurized to 50 cm H_2O and the pressure gauge observed for 30 seconds. To pass this leak check, the pressure must not fall below 30 cm H_2O within 30 seconds. APL, adjustable pressure limiting. (From Eisenkraft JB: The anesthesia delivery system, part II. In *Progress in anesthesiology, vol 3.* San Antonio, TX, 1989, Dannemiller Memorial Educational Foundation. Reproduced by permission.)

was in service, anesthesia gases would escape from the system. If the anesthesia machine is found to have a leak, it should be withdrawn from use until an authorized agent has repaired the leak, rechecked the system, and certified that the machine is fit to be put back into clinical service.

Datex-Ohmeda Machines Without an Outlet Check Valve

GE Healthcare recommends the negative leak test procedure described above to check for leaks in Modulus II Plus and Modulus CD machines, which have no outlet check valves.[36] Although the bulb could, in principle, be used to check for leaks in a Narkomed machine, Draeger Medical does not provide specifications for the application of such a leak check device on their products. Item 5 of the FDA's 1993 Anesthesia Apparatus Checkout Recommendations describes the use of a negative-pressure suction bulb to check a machine's low-pressure system for leaks. They require that the bulb stay fully collapsed for at least 10 seconds. A study comparing tests for leak testing the low-pressure system reported that only the negative-pressure leak test detected all leaks and concluded that "adoption of the negative-pressure test as a universal [low-pressure system] leak test may prevent the risks associated with using the wrong test for the particular anesthesia machine."[37]

These descriptions of the pneumatic system apply in principle to all anesthesia machines and workstations, but, as previously stated, many of the traditional mechanical components are being replaced by more modern devices, such as those described in the following paragraphs.

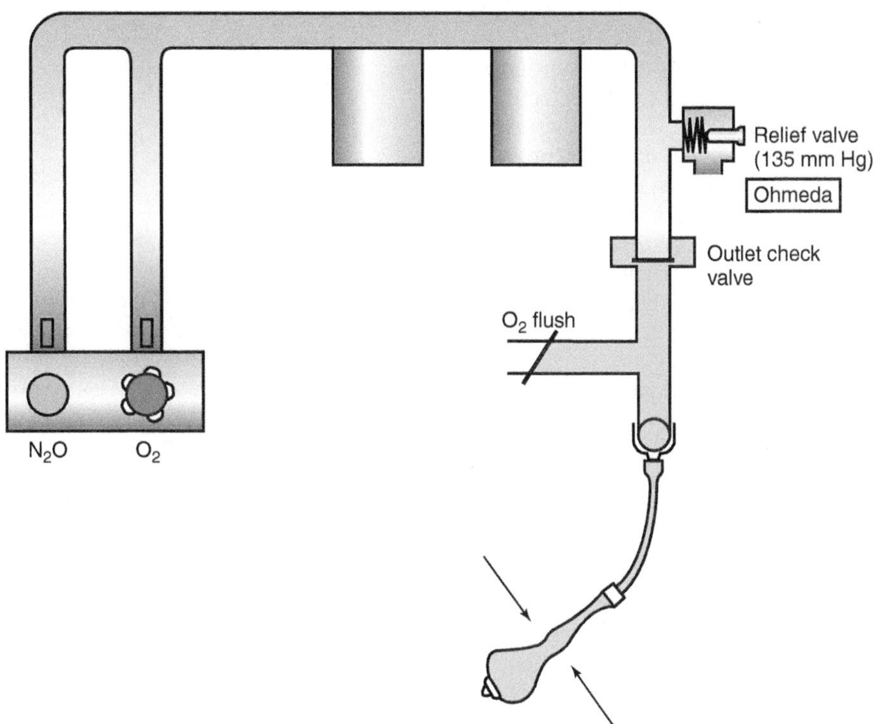

FIGURE 2-42 Datex-Ohmeda (GE Healthcare, Waukesha, WI) negative-pressure leak check procedure in a machine with an outlet check valve. (From Eisenkraft JB: The anesthesia delivery system, part II. In *Progress in anesthesiology, vol 3.* San Antonio, TX, 1989, Dannemiller Memorial Educational Foundation. Reproduced by permission.)

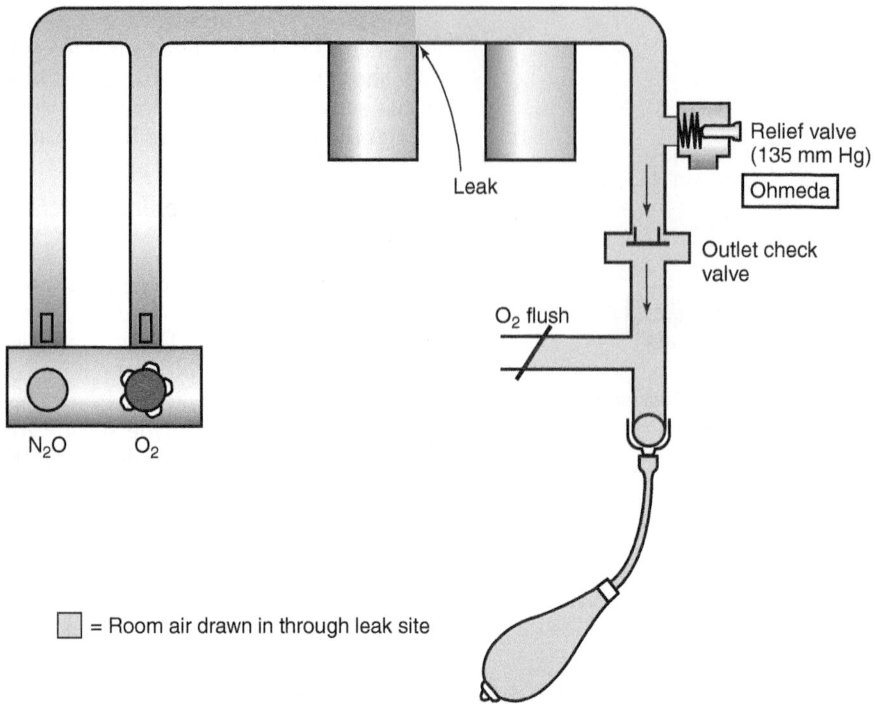

FIGURE 2-43 Datex-Ohmeda (GE Healthcare, Waukesha, WI) negative-pressure leak check procedure. When there is a leak in the machine, the evacuated bulb reinflates. (From Eisenkraft JB: The anesthesia delivery system, part II. In *Progress in anesthesiology, vol 3.* San Antonio, TX, 1989, Dannemiller Memorial Educational Foundation. Reproduced by permission.)

Datex-Ohmeda Aestiva/5. The Aestiva/5 is an example of a modern basic anesthesia machine (Fig. 2-44). Gauges on the front panel display the gas supply pressures, and a main ON/OFF switch enables electronic and pneumatic functions. Gas flows are controlled with the traditional needle valves and glass rotameter tubes. The majority of the vaporizers are mechanical Tec-type vaporizers. The CGO is not accessible to the user because the fresh gas flow is conducted directly into the absorber–ventilator–circle system unit. An auxiliary CGO can be selected to divert all fresh gas flow to this outlet. This allows use of noncircle breathing systems (e.g., Bain) and provides access to the machine's low-pressure system for application of the negative-pressure leak check. With the exception of the ventilator controls, the system is essentially mechanical and pneumatic so that an anesthetic can be delivered in the absence of electrical power, although the unit does have a backup battery.

Datex-Ohmeda S5/ADU Workstation. The S5/ADU workstation represents the next step toward an all-electronic workstation (Fig. 2-45). Gas pressures are measured by conventional gauges, and gas flow is controlled by knobs and traditional needle valves. Gas flows, however, are measured electronically and are displayed on a color screen as virtual rotameters and as digital values. The workstation has an electronically controlled anesthetic vaporizer that uses agent-specific cartridges (see Chapter 3). Electronic measurement has several benefits:

1. Accuracy is enhanced because there is no confusion over where to read the flow on a traditional rotameter float and the system is sensitive to very low flows.

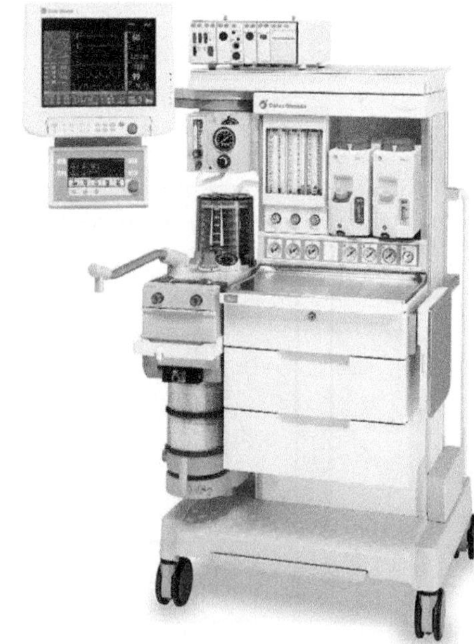

FIGURE 2-44 GE Healthcare (Waukesha, WI) Aestiva/5, a basic anesthesia machine with traditional components: needle valves, glass tube rotameters, and mechanical vaporizers.

2. Proportioning of N_2O and O_2 is performed by computer-controlled solenoid valves that ensure a minimum of 25% oxygen when nitrous oxide is used. Because the vaporizing system is also electronic (see below), it can decrease the flow of nitrous oxide to maintain 25% oxygen when high concentrations of desflurane are used (Fig. 2-46).

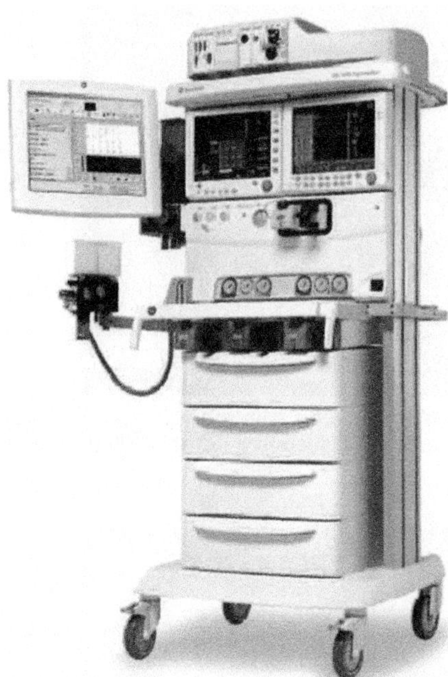

FIGURE 2-45 ■ GE Healthcare (Waukesha, WI) ADU workstation. The next step in evolution: electronic flow sensing, virtual flowmeters, and an electronically controlled vaporizing system.

3. During volume ventilation, the flow measurements are used to ensure that changes in fresh gas flow, respiratory rate, and the inspiration/expiration ratio do not change the tidal volume from that set to be delivered. Thus, if fresh gas flow is increased, the computer immediately decreases the volume delivered from the ventilator bellows.
4. The electronic flow data and anesthesia vaporizer concentration data permit continuous monitoring of volatile anesthetic agent use. The data can also be downloaded to an anesthesia information management system.
5. The electronic display can be easily modified by software changes. This eliminates the need to manufacture different machines for different countries, such as to follow local convention for gas colors.
6. Troubleshooting a computerized system may be easier for service personnel. Repairs may require simple replacement of a module.
7. A partially automated and manually menu-driven check procedure is standard. During checkout the compliance of the breathing system is measured, and this information is used by the ventilator software so that the tidal volume set is delivered to the patient.

Disadvantages. Gas flow cannot be measured when electrical power is lost, but flows can still be controlled by flow control knobs and needle valve assemblies. For this reason, a rotameter flowmeter is available for installation at the CGO to measure the total fresh gas flow, albeit without the normal accuracy. To deliver 40% oxygen with nitrous oxide using the common gas flowmeter in the event of power loss, starting with all gas flows off, it is possible to dial up 2 L/min of oxygen and then nitrous oxide until the total flow is 5 L/min (Fig. 2-47). Loss of electrical power to the ADU workstation would result in failure of the gas analyzer, and therefore in oxygen monitoring, as well as an inability to deliver a potent inhaled anesthetic agent because of the electronic vaporizer. Therefore, if all electrical power were to be lost, the ADU workstation could still deliver N_2O and O_2 to the breathing circuit; ventilation would have to be spontaneous or manual, and intravenous agents would be required to replace the potent inhaled anesthetic.

Other Features. The potent agent vaporizer concentration control dial is electronic, but contrary to electronic convention, an increase in concentration requires counterclockwise rotation of the dial; the dialed-in concentration is displayed on the screen. The CGO is accessible, and the workstation has a backup battery that will energize the anesthesia machine parts of the workstation, but not the physiologic monitors, for 45 to 90 minutes. An indicator on the screen shows the state of the battery charge when it is in use.

Contemporary Anesthesia Workstations

Aisys Carestation. The Aisys Carestation is an example of a fully computerized electronic workstation. When turned on, the workstation goes through an automated check that requires some menu-driven actions by the user. Gas supply pressures are measured electronically by pressure transducers and are displayed digitally on a screen. The supplied gases—O_2, N_2O, and air—pass to an electronically controlled gas mixer, where the desired flows and concentrations are created. The flow of each gas is determined by pressing a key to select the gas flow and then confirming by pressing the ComWheel. Alternatively, the concentration of oxygen in N_2O or air and the total gas flow can be set (Fig. 2-48). The concentrations and individual gas flows are displayed as virtual flowmeters on a computer screen. The gas mixture then passes to an electronic vaporizer, where the electronically set agent concentration is added. Because no CGO is accessible on the basic model, the resulting fresh gas mixture is conducted to the circle breathing system.

The Aisys offers two types of CGO, the *auxiliary common gas outlet* (ACGO) or a *switched common gas outlet* (SCGO). The ACGO is a port on the front of the machine through which fresh gas exits when the ACGO is selected by an adjacent switch. This is similar to the ACGO on the Aestiva/5 described above (see Figs. 2-37 and 2-44). The ACGO allows use of a noncircle system and also provides a place for attaching a negative-pressure bulb for leak testing the low-pressure system, as described above. When selected from the Aisys start-up menu screen, the SCGO mode functionally converts the inspiratory port for the circle into a CGO. It does this by diverting fresh gas so that it bypasses the inspiratory unidirectional valve and emerges through the inspiratory flow sensor.

There are obvious major differences between the Aisys Carestation and the ADU. For example, gas flows are under full electronic control. Having pressed the key for the gas to be controlled, flow is adjusted by turning the com wheel to the desired concentration and then confirming. Adjustment is therefore a two-step process that is implemented only after being actively confirmed. Because this is an electronic control, by convention an

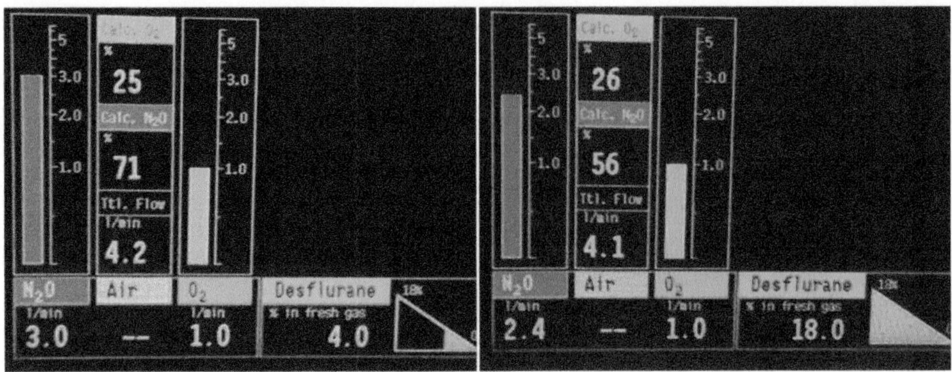

FIGURE 2-46 ■ Electronic proportioning system in the GE Healthcare (Waukesha, WI) ADU. *Left,* Minimum 25% O_2 with N_2O and low concentration of desflurane. *Right,* When desflurane is increased to 18%, the proportioning system automatically decreases N_2O flow to maintain minimum O_2 concentration.

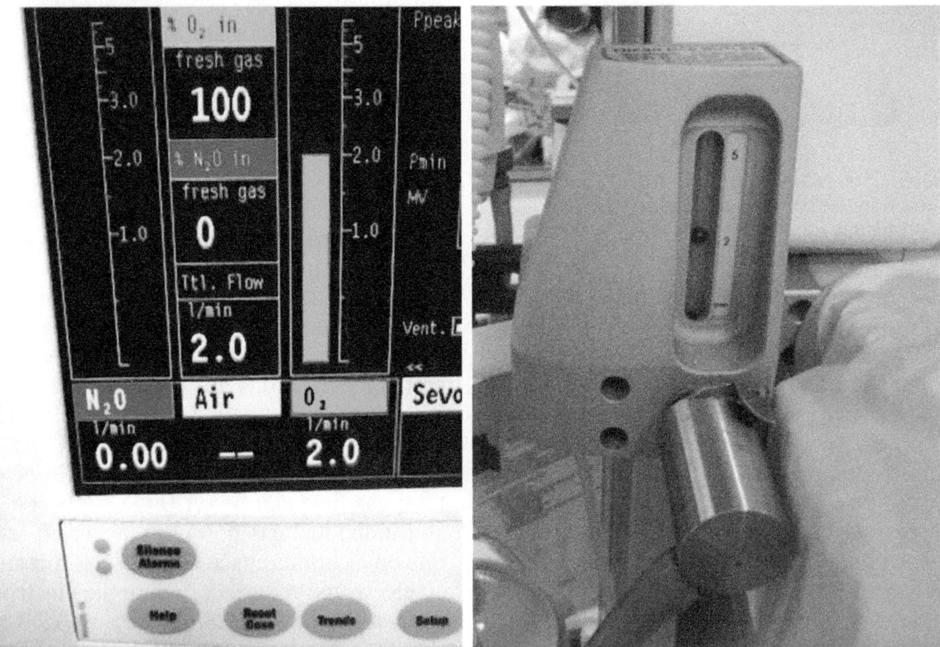

FIGURE 2-47 ■ Virtual flowmeter on a GE Healthcare (Waukesha, WI) ADU workstation screen shows O_2 flow of 2 L/min. If the electrical power fails, gas flow can be approximated from the total gas flow rotameter reading at the common gas outlet.

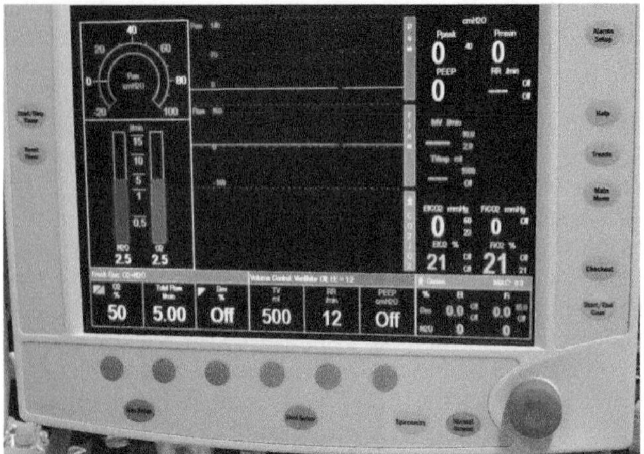

FIGURE 2-48 ■ GE Healthcare (Waukesha, WI) Aisys Carestation showing virtual flowmeter display of N_2O at 2.5 L/min and O_2 at 2.5 L/min. This was achieved by setting a total flow of 5 L/min followed by the desired O_2 concentration of 50%. Gas flows can also be controlled individually by selecting a different screen setup option.

increase in flow and agent concentration is by clockwise rotation of the com wheel. With the traditional needle valve flow control, flow is increased by counterclockwise rotation of the flow control knob. Similarly, with conventional vaporizer dials, concentration is increased by counterclockwise rotation of the dial.

Disadvantages. Power supply failure to the Aisys would result in the electronic gas mixer and vaporizer shutting down. To deal with this possibility, the machine has an alternate oxygen flowmeter (not to be confused with the *auxiliary* oxygen flowmeter) that is a basic mechanical needle valve and rotameter tube (Fig. 2-49). In the event of power loss, the workstation switches to the mechanical, alternate oxygen flow control system so that oxygen can continue to be delivered to the patient breathing system; the same would happen if the gas mixer were to fail. If the gas mixer fails but the electronic vaporizing system is working, potent inhaled agent can be added to the alternate oxygen flow. An ON/OFF switch for the

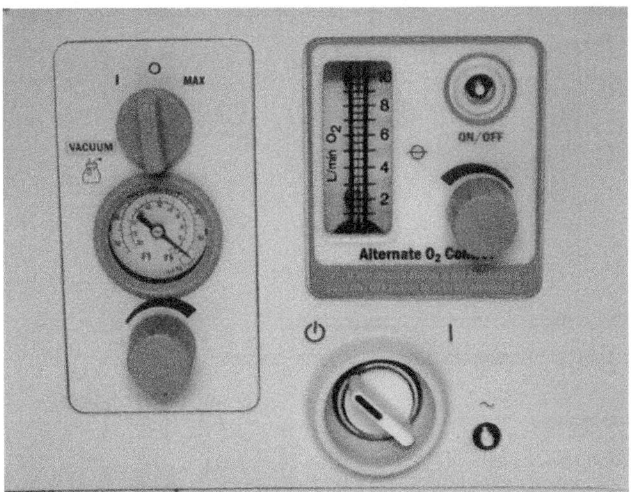

FIGURE 2-49 ■ Alternate O_2 control and rotameter flowmeter on the GE Healthcare (Waukesha, WI) Aisys Carestation for use in the event of electrical power supply failure, failure of the anesthesia screen display, or failure of the O_2-N_2O-air gas mixer module.

alternate oxygen flowmeter can be used and tested if necessary.

During startup, the Aisys goes through a 5-minute automated check that also requires some procedures to be performed by the user, although they can be bypassed in an emergency. The Aisys backup battery is specified to power the anesthesia machine components (vs. the physiologic monitors) for 40 minutes.

As previously mentioned, all anesthesia delivery systems are the same in principle, but the functions of some components have been affected by modern technology. This is illustrated in Figure 2-50, which shows the gas flow arrangements of the Aisys Carestation.

Dräger Fabius GS Premium. The Fabius GS Premium workstation is currently the basic model from Dräger Medical (Fig. 2-51). Conventional pressure gauges on the front of the workstation display the cylinder and pipeline gas supply pressures. Gas flow control is by conventional flow control knobs and needle valves that are arranged vertically rather than horizontally. Gas flow measurement is by flow sensors, rather than by traditional rotameters, and flows are displayed digitally to the left of the flow control knobs and as virtual flowmeter displays on the color screen. A rotameter located to the left of the digital flow readings (see Fig. 2-51) continuously measures the total fresh gas flow with an accuracy specified as ±15%. The majority of vaporizers are of the traditional, mechanical, variable-bypass design. With this workstation, in the event of electrical power loss, an inhaled anesthetic can be delivered because of the total gas flow rotameter and mechanical vaporizers. The fresh gas flow exits the machine via an accessible CGO to be conducted to the breathing system.

An auxiliary oxygen flowmeter is provided. Unlike the GE workstations, which have gas-driven bellows ventilators, the anesthesia ventilator in the Fabius GS is piston driven by an electric motor. The preuse check is not automated, and Dräger states that the checkout procedure pages in the operator's instruction manual be "removed and copied to establish a daily record of machine checks." The company also states that each function should be marked after successful completion of the machine checks.[38] It is essential to perform all the steps of the manufacturer's recommended check procedure because omission of any steps or failure to perform the check properly may result in a large internal gas leak going undetected.[39]

Apollo Workstation. The Dräger Medical Apollo workstation (Fig. 2-52) has an advanced design that incorporates many more electronic features than the Fabius GS. Before use, the workstation requires a manual, menu-driven check followed by an automated check (Figs. 2-53 and 2-54). Gas supply pressures are measured by pressure transducers and are displayed on the color screen. Individual gas flows are controlled by mechanical needle valves and conventional flow control knobs arranged horizontally. As in the Fabius GS Premium described above, gas flows are measured by flow sensors and are displayed digitally and as virtual flowmeters on the screen. A traditional rotameter displays the total fresh gas flow. The majority of the vaporizers are of the traditional, mechanical, variable-bypass design. In the event of electrical power loss with this workstation, an inhaled anesthetic can be delivered because of the total gas flow rotameter and mechanical vaporizers. The anesthesia ventilator uses a piston driven by an electric motor, and the CGO is not accessible to the user; fresh gas flows directly into the autoclavable compact breathing system.

ANESTHESIA MACHINE ELECTRICAL SYSTEMS

Although basically pneumatic, all contemporary anesthesia machines also incorporate electrical systems and require connection to an electrical power supply. Turning the main switch clockwise to ON (Fig. 2-55) energizes the electrical systems of the machine and mechanically opens the flow of gases to the flowmeters, provided gas supply pressure is adequate, so that the machine is capable of delivering an anesthetic. The electrical system powers the alarms and monitors on the machine and also powers the ventilator control system. If the machine's electrical system completely failed, the flow of gases to the flowmeters would continue uninterrupted as long as the machine's main switch is ON. In the event that the AC power supply to the machine fails, a 12-volt battery serves as a backup system to provide power to the workstation's monitors, alarms, ventilator controls, and motor, if so designed. When fully charged, the battery supply provides power for 30 to 45 minutes in most machines. However, a fully charged battery requires that the machine's AC power cord be plugged into an energized electrical receptacle. A battery test indicator is provided on the machine to check for the status of the reserve power battery (see Fig. 2-54). The amount of time a workstation can function when the AC power fails can be extended by connecting the workstation and other

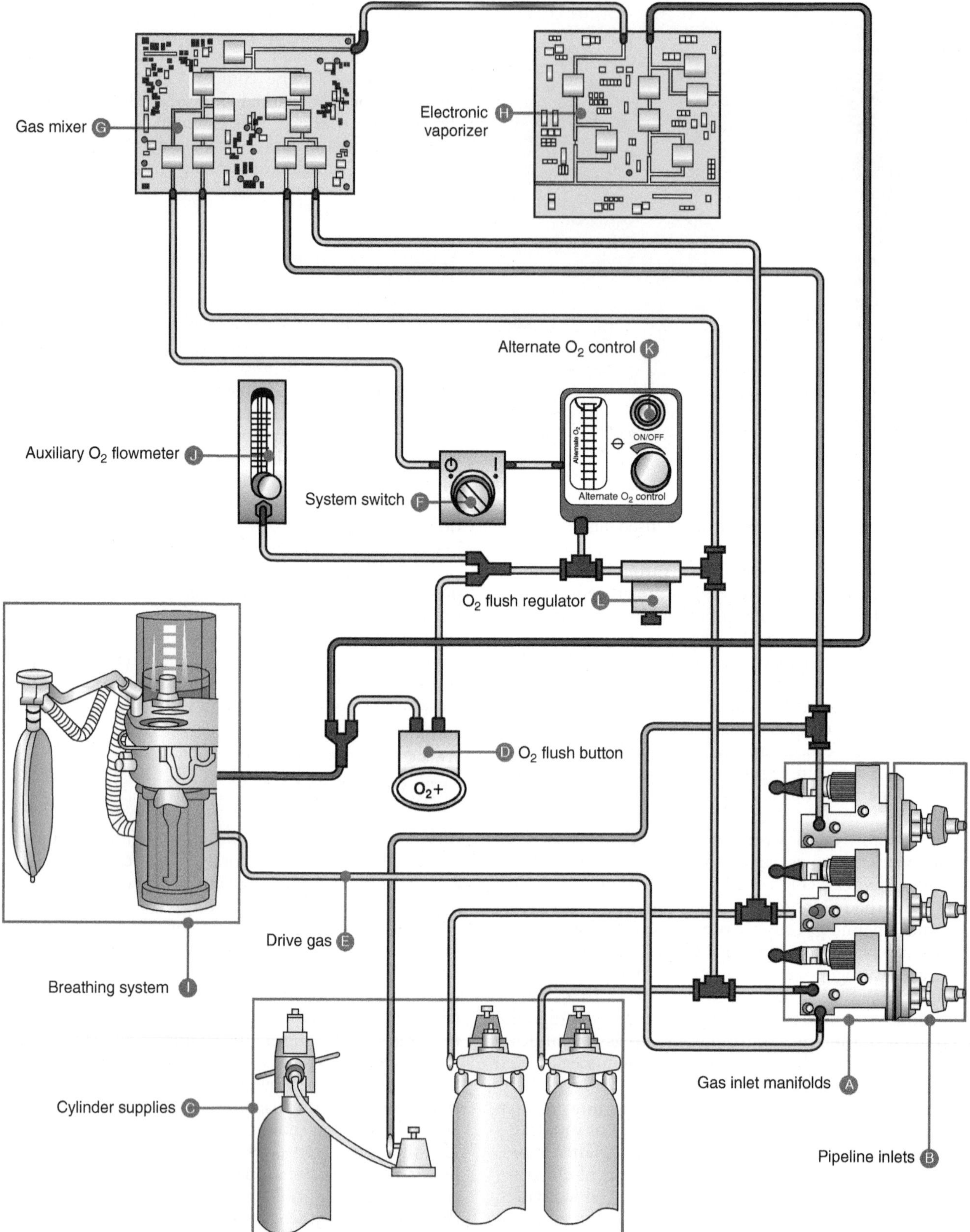

FIGURE 2-50 ■ Gas flow schematic of Aisys Carestation (GE Healthcare, Waukesha, WI). It is essentially the same as the basic machine schematic in Figure 2-4. Electronic components have replaced many of the traditional ones. (From *Explore the anesthesia machine: Aisys*. Madison, WI, 2005, GE Healthcare.)

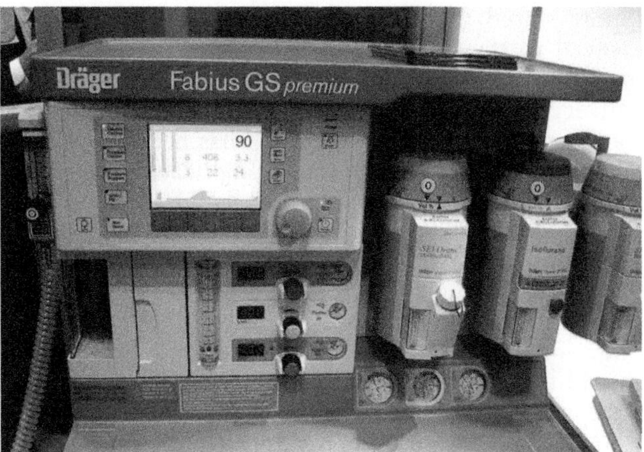

FIGURE 2-51 ■ The Fabius GS Premium workstation (Dräger Medical, Telford, PA). Note needle valve gas flow controls arranged vertically and the electronic display of virtual flowmeters. A total fresh gas rotameter flowmeter permits flow measurement in the event the electronic flow display fails.

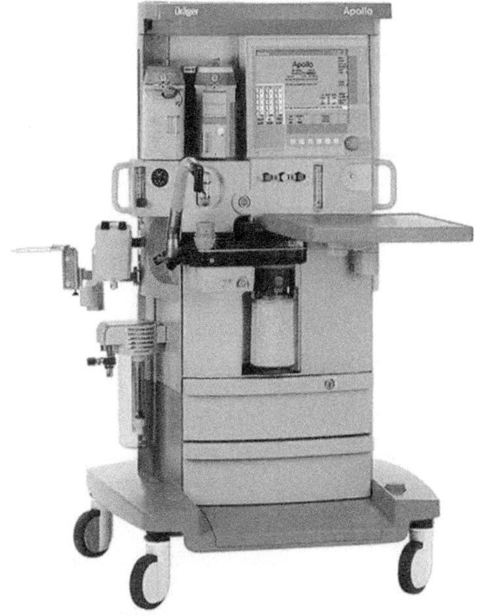

FIGURE 2-52 ■ The Apollo anesthesia workstation (Dräger Medical, Telford, PA).

essential devices, such as the computerized record-keeping system, into an uninterruptible power supply connected to a wall outlet so that its charge is maintained (Fig. 2-56). An uninterruptible power supply source is especially important in computerized workstations; if power is interrupted, the workstation computer may shut down and require a restart, which may take several minutes. This is also a consideration in the design of the workstation's main ON/OFF switch because unintentionally turning off the workstation commits the user to a repeat start-up protocol. In an emergency, the workstation permits the user to bypass the automated check, but that action is logged into the memory.

Contemporary anesthesia machines are commonly equipped with a number of convenience receptacles or outlets to provide AC power to other monitors, such as

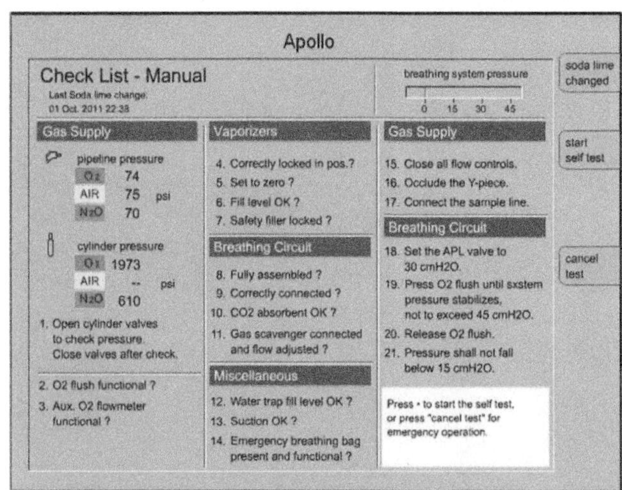

FIGURE 2-53 ■ Screen for manual checklist on the Apollo workstation (Dräger Medical, Telford, PA).

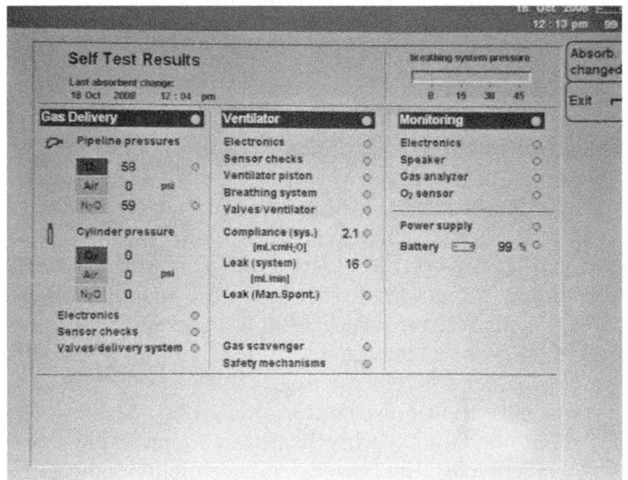

FIGURE 2-54 ■ Screen showing the results of the automated self-test during preuse checkout of the Apollo workstation (Dräger Medical, Telford, PA).

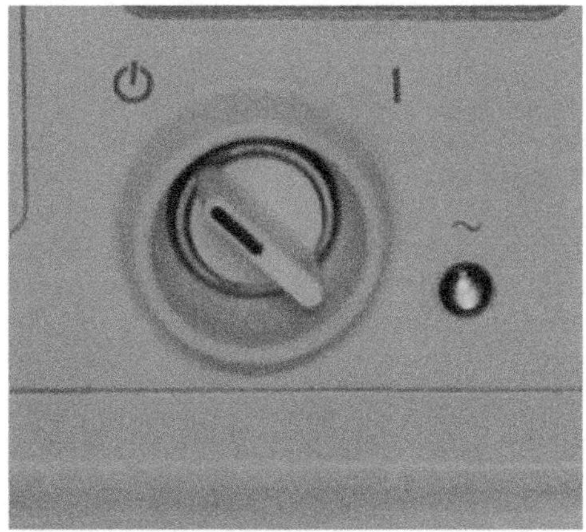

FIGURE 2-55 ■ Main ON/OFF switch. Care must be taken to not accidentally shut down the workstation.

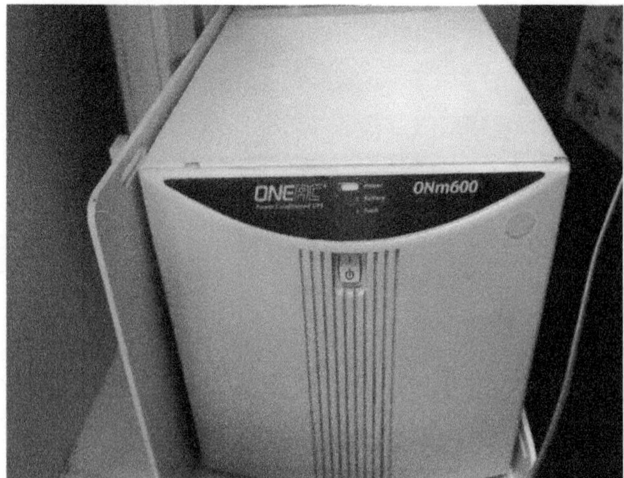

FIGURE 2-56 Uninterruptible power supply unit supplements the workstation backup battery by energizing monitors and automated anesthesia record-keeping systems.

the blood pressure monitor and pulse oximeter. These receptacles are energized via the machine's main AC power cord and are protected by circuit breakers.

The presence of several electrical systems on the machine necessitates that each circuit be protected from overload. This is achieved by using circuit breakers, which vary in number according to the number of circuits present. In principle, however, one circuit breaker protects the machine's main AC power supply, one or more protect the convenience receptacles, and one or more protect the low-voltage (12-volt) DC circuits. It is not uncommon for circuit breakers on the machine to be tripped, usually from overloading a convenience receptacle, such as by connecting an OR table power cord In this case, other convenience receptacles on the same circuit will have their power interrupted. The anesthesiologist should be familiar with the power supply capabilities of the receptacles, the power demands of any equipment connected to them, and the location (which is not always obvious) and function of the circuit breakers on the machine. The manufacturer's manual should be consulted for details on specific models.

ANESTHESIA MACHINE OBSOLESCENCE AND PREUSE CHECKS

With the evolution of the anesthesia machine to the workstations of today, many safety features have been added. As a result, many older models of machine still in use may be considered outdated or even obsolete. The American Society of Anesthesiologists (ASA) Committee on Equipment and Facilities has developed guidelines for determining whether a machine is obsolete (see Chapter 30).[40]

The 1993 FDA checklist is not applicable to many newer workstations. Recognizing this, a subcommittee of the ASA Committee on Equipment and Facilities reviewed the 1993 recommendations in relation to newer workstations and published their findings in 2008 (summarized in Table 32-1 in Chapter 32).[15] The report stated that "anesthesia delivery systems have evolved to the point that one preanesthesia checkout procedure (PAC) is not applicable to all the anesthesia delivery systems currently on the market. For these reasons, a new approach to the PAC has been developed. The goal was to apply guidelines applicable to all anesthesia delivery systems so that individual departments can develop a PAC that can be performed consistently and expeditiously." The 2008 guidelines are intended to provide a template for developing check procedures appropriate for every machine design and practice setting. They discuss which systems and components should be checked, the check interval (e.g., before the first procedure of the day vs. before each patient), and who may be responsible for performing each procedure—the anesthesiologist or the technician. Regardless of who performs the check, the anesthesiologist bears the ultimate responsibility. The reader should refer to the ASA website for the full document and for sample, system-specific preuse checklists that have been developed from the recommendations (www.asahq.org/For-Members/Clinical-Information/2008-ASA-Recommendations-for-PreAnesthesia-Checkout/Sample-Procedures.aspx).

The most important, yet frequently overlooked,[41] step in the preanesthesia check procedure is to ensure the immediate availability of a manual means by which the lungs can be ventilated, such as a functioning (tested) self-inflating resuscitation bag and an auxiliary, and preferably full, tank of oxygen.

REFERENCES

1. American Society for Testing and Materials: *Standard specification for particular requirements for anesthesia workstations and their components. ASTM F-1850-00*, West Conshohocken, PA, 2000, American Society for Testing and Materials.
2. American Society for Testing and Materials: *Standard specification for minimum performance and safety requirements for components and systems of anesthesia gas machines. F1161-88*, Philadelphia, 1989, American Society for Testing and Materials.
3. American National Standards Institute: *Standard specification for minimum performance and safety requirements for components and systems of continuous flow anesthesia machines for human use. ANSI Z79.8-1979*, New York, 1979, American National Standards Institute.
4. *Explore the anesthesia system: Aestiva/5*, Madison, WI, 2003, GE Healthcare.
5. *Explore the anesthesia machine: Aisys*, Madison, WI, 2005, GE Healthcare.
6. Cicman JH, Gotzon J, Himmelwright C, et al: *Operating principles of Narkomed anesthesia systems*, ed 2, Telford, PA, 1998, Draeger Medical.
7. Virtual anesthesia machine simulation, University of Florida. Available online at http://vam.anest.ufl.edu/simulations/vam.php.
8. Modulus II simulation, University of Florida. Available online at http://vam.anest.ufl.edu/simulations/modulusiisimulation.php.
9. Aestiva simulation, University of Florida. Available online at http://vam.anest.ufl.edu/simulations/aestivasimulation.php.
10. Dorsch JA, Dorsch SE: *Understanding anesthesia equipment*, ed 5, Philadelphia, 2008, Lippincott Williams & Wilkins, p 88.
11. U.S. Food and Drug Administration: *Anesthesia apparatus checkout recommendations*, 1993. Available online at http://www.osha.gov/dts/osta/anestheticgases/index.html#Appendix2. Accessed Sept 18, 2011.
12. *Diameter index safety system, CGA V-5*, New York, 1978, Compressed Gas Association.
13. *Compressed gas cylinder valve outlet and inlet connections, pamphlet V-1*, New York, 1977, Compressed Gas Association.

14. Mudumbai SC, Fanning R, Howard SK, et al: Use of medical simulation to explore equipment failures and human-machine interactions in anesthesia machine pipeline supply crossover, *Anesth Analg* 110:1292–1296, 2010.
15. American Society of Anesthesiologists: *Recommendations for preanesthesia checkout procedures.* Available at http://www.asahq.org/for-members/clinical-information/~/media/For%20Members/Standards%20and%20Guidelines/FINALCheckoutDesignguidelines.ashx. Accessed October 13, 2012.
16. Bowie E, Huffman LM: *The anesthesia machine: essentials for understanding*, Madison, WI, 1985, BOC Health Care.
17. Parbrook GD, Davis PD, Parbrook EO: *Basic physics and measurement in anesthesia*, ed 2, Norwalk, CT, 1986, Appleton Century Crofts.
18. Fassl J, Jenny U, Nikiforov S, et al: Pressures available for transtracheal jet ventilation from anesthesia machines and wall-mounted oxygen flowmeters, *Anesth Analg* 110:94–100, 2010.
19. Klemenzson GK, Perouansky M: Contemporary anesthesia ventilators incur a significant "oxygen cost." *Can J Anesth* 51:616–620, 2004.
20. Taenzer AH, Kovatsis PG, Raessler KL: E-cylinder-powered mechanical ventilation may adversely impact anesthetic management and efficiency, *Anesth Analg* 95:148–150, 2002.
21. Szpisjak DF, Javernick EN, Kyle RR, Austin PN: Oxygen consumption of a pneumatically controlled ventilator in a field anesthesia machine, *Anesth Analg* 107:1907–1911, 2008.
22. *Modulus II Plus anesthesia machine: preoperative checklists, operation and maintenance manual*, Madison, WI, 1988, GE Healthcare.
23. *Modulus II anesthesia system: operation and maintenance manual*, Madison, WI, 1987, GE Healthcare.
24. *Narkomed 3 anesthesia system technical service manual*, Telford, PA, 1988, North American Dräger.
25. Eger EI 2nd, Hylton RR, Irwin RH, et al: Anesthetic flow meter sequence: a cause for hypoxia, *Anesthesiology* 24:396, 1963.
26. Hay H: Delivery of an hypoxic gas mixture due to a defective rubber seal of a flowmeter control tube, *Eur J Anaesthesiol* 17:456–458, 2000.
27. *Narkomed 3 anesthesia system: operator's instruction manual*, Telford, PA, 1986, North American Dräger.
28. Gordon PC, James MFM, Lapham H, Carboni M: Failure of the proportioning system to prevent hypoxic mixture on a Modulus II Plus anesthesia machine, *Anesthesiology* 82:598–599, 1995.
29. *Modulus II system service manual*, Madison, WI, 1985, GE Healthcare.
30. Benumof JL, Scheller MS: The importance of transtracheal jet ventilation in the management of the difficult airway, *Anesthesiology* 71:769–778, 1989.
31. Delaney WA, Kaiser R: Percutaneous transtracheal jet ventilation made easy, *Anesthesiology* 74:952, 1991.
32. Gaughan SD, Benumof JL, Ozaki GT: Can the anesthesia machine flush valve provide for effective jet ventilation? *Anesth Analg* 76:800–808, 1993.
33. Kummar P, Korula G, Kumar S, Saravanan PA: Unusual cause of leak in Datex Aisys, *Anesth Analg* 109:1350–1351, 2009.
34. March MG, Crowley JJ: An evaluation of anesthesiologists' present checkout methods and the validity of the FDA checklist, *Anesthesiology* 75:724–729, 1991.
35. *Narkomed 3 anesthesia system: operator's instruction manual*, Telford, PA, 1986, North American Dräger.
36. *Modulus CD anesthesia system: operation and maintenance manual*, Madison, WI, 1991, GE Healthcare.
37. Myers JA, Good ML, Andrews JJ: Comparison of tests for detecting leaks in the low-pressure system of anesthesia gas machines, *Anesth Analg* 84:179–184, 1997.
38. Appendix. *Operator's instruction manual: Fabius GS Software version 4117102-005*, Telford, PA, 2003, Draeger Medical.
39. Eng TS, Durieux ME: Automated machine checkout leaves an internal gas leak undetected: the need for complete checkout procedures, *Anesth Analg* 114:144–146, 2012.
40. Guidelines for determining anesthesia machine obsolescence, *ASA Newsletter* Sept 2004.
41. Demaria S Jr, Blasius K, Neustein SM: Missed steps in the preanesthesia setup, *Anesth Analg* 113:84–88, 2011.

CHAPTER 3

ANESTHESIA VAPORIZERS

James B. Eisenkraft

CHAPTER OUTLINE

GENERAL PRINCIPLES

The term *vapor* describes the gaseous phase of a substance at a temperature at which the substance can exist in either a liquid or solid state below a critical temperature for that substance. If the vapor is in contact with a liquid phase, the two phases will be in a state of equilibrium, and the gas pressure will equal the equilibrium vapor pressure of the liquid. The potent inhaled volatile anesthetic agents—halothane, enflurane, isoflurane, sevoflurane, and desflurane—are mostly in the liquid state at normal room temperature (20° C) and atmospheric pressure (760 mm Hg).[1] Anesthesia vaporizers are devices that facilitate the change of a liquid anesthetic into its vapor phase and add a controlled amount of this vapor to the flow of gases entering the patient's breathing circuit.

The anesthesia care provider should be familiar with the principles of vaporization of the potent inhaled anesthetic agents and their application in both the construction and use of anesthesia vaporizers designed to be placed in the low-pressure system of the anesthesia machine—that is, the fresh gas flow circuit downstream of the gas flow control valves. The 1989 voluntary consensus standard for anesthesia machines (American Society for Testing and Materials [ASTM] F1161-88) required that all vaporizers located within the fresh gas circuit be concentration calibrated and that control of the vapor concentration be provided by calibrated knobs or dials.[2] The most recent standard, ASTM 1850-00, maintains these requirements.[3]

Measured flow systems are not mentioned in the 1989 and subsequent ASTM standards[3] and are therefore considered obsolete as defined in the American Society of Anesthesiologists (ASA) 2004 statement on determining anesthesia machine obsolescence. Despite their obsolescent status, the principles of measured flow vaporizing systems are briefly discussed in this chapter because they provide a basis for understanding the contemporary concentration-calibrated, variable bypass vaporizers used to deliver isoflurane, enflurane, halothane, and sevoflurane.

Desflurane has certain physical properties that preclude its delivery by a conventional variable bypass vaporizer and is therefore discussed in a separate section. The most recently introduced Aladin vaporizing system (GE Healthcare, Waukesha, WI) is a hybrid of the measured flow and variable bypass designs. The Aladin system can accurately deliver desflurane and the other less volatile potent anesthetic agents.

VAPOR, EVAPORATION, AND VAPOR PRESSURE

When placed in a closed container at normal atmospheric pressure and room temperature (given above), a potent inhaled anesthetic is in liquid form. Some anesthetic molecules escape from the surface of the liquid to enter the space above as a gas or vapor. At constant temperature, an equilibrium is established between the molecules in the vapor phase and those in the liquid phase. The molecules in the vapor phase are in constant motion, bombarding the walls of the container to exert *vapor pressure.* An increase in temperature causes more anesthetic molecules to enter the vapor phase—that is, to evaporate; this results in an increase in vapor pressure. The gas phase above the liquid is said to be *saturated* when it contains all the anesthetic vapor it can hold at a given temperature, at which time the pressure exerted by the vapor is referred to as its *saturated vapor pressure* (SVP) at that temperature.

Measurement of Vapor Pressure and Saturated Vapor Pressure

The following description is intended to provide an understanding of how, in principle, the SVP of a potent inhaled volatile anesthetic agent could be measured in a simple laboratory experiment and demonstrate the pressure that a vapor can exert. Figure 3-1, *A,* shows a simple (Fortin) barometer, which is essentially a long, glass mercury-filled test tube inverted to stand with its mouth immersed in a trough of mercury. When the barometer tube is first made vertical, the mercury column in the tube falls to a certain level, leaving a so-called *Torricellian vacuum* above the mercury meniscus. In this system, the pressure at the surface of the mercury in the trough is due to the atmosphere. In a communicating system of liquids, the pressures at any given depth are equal; therefore the pressure at the surface of the mercury in the trough is equal to the pressure exerted by the column of mercury in the vertical tube. In this example, atmospheric pressure is said to be equivalent to 760 mm Hg, because this is the height of the column of mercury in the barometer tube.

In Figure 3-1, *B,* sevoflurane liquid is introduced at the bottom of the mercury column. Being less dense than mercury, it rises to the top and evaporates into the space created by the Torricellian vacuum. The sevoflurane vapor exerts pressure and causes an equivalent decrease in the height of the mercury column. If liquid sevoflurane is added until a small amount remains unevaporated on the top of the mercury meniscus (Fig. 3-1, *C*), the space above the column must be fully saturated with vapor; the pressure now exerted by the vapor is the SVP of sevoflurane at that temperature, and adding more liquid sevoflurane will not affect the vapor pressure. If this experiment is repeated at different temperatures, a graph can be constructed that plots SVP against temperature. Such curves for some of the potent inhaled volatile anesthetic agents are shown in Figure 3-2. Contemporary technologies for measuring the partial pressures or SVPs of gases and vapors are described in Chapter 8.

Boiling Point

The SVP exerted by the vapor phase of a potent inhaled volatile agent is a physical property of that agent and depends only on the agent and the ambient temperature. The temperature at which SVP becomes equal to ambient (atmospheric) pressure and that at which all the liquid agent changes to the vapor phase (i.e., evaporates) is the boiling point of that liquid. Water boils at 100° C at 1 atm because at 100° C, the SVP of water is 760 mm Hg. The most volatile of the agents are those with the highest SVPs at room temperature. At any given temperature, these agents also have the lowest boiling points: desflurane and diethyl ether boil at 22.9° C and 35° C, respectively, at an ambient pressure of 760 mm Hg. Boiling point decreases with decreasing ambient barometric pressure, such as occurs at increasing altitude.

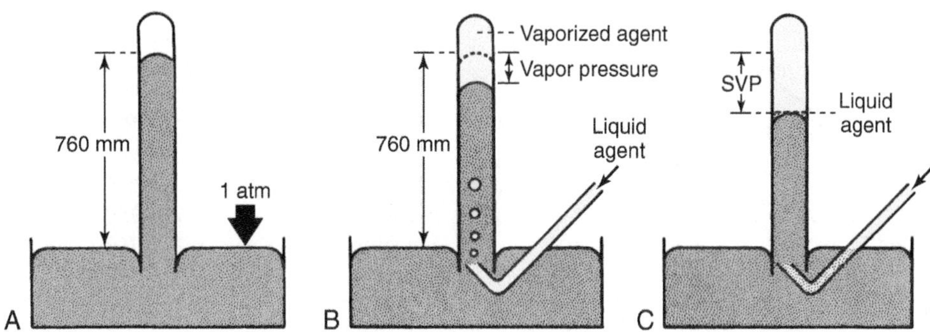

FIGURE 3-1 ■ Measurement of vapor pressures using a simple Fortin barometer. SVP, saturated vapor pressure. (From Eisenkraft JB: Vaporizers and vaporization of volatile anesthetics. In *Progress in anesthesiology,* vol 2. San Antonio, 1989, Dannemiller Memorial Educational Foundation.)

Units of Vapor Concentration

The presence of anesthetic vapor may be quantified either as an absolute pressure, expressed in millimeters of mercury (mm Hg) (or, less commonly, kilopascals [kPa]) or in *volumes percent* (vol%) of the total atmosphere (i.e., volumes of vapor per 100 volumes of total gas). From Dalton's law of partial pressures, the volumes percent can be calculated as the fractional partial pressure of the agent:

$$\text{vol}\,\% = \frac{\text{Partial pressure from vapor}}{\text{Total ambient pressure}} \times 100\,\%$$

Dalton's Law of Partial Pressures

Dalton's law states that the pressure exerted by a mixture of gases, or gases and vapors, enclosed in a given space such as a container is equal to the sum of the pressures that each gas or vapor would exert if it alone occupied that given space or container.[4] A gas or vapor exerts its pressure independently of the pressure of the other gases present. For example, in a container of dry air at 1 atm (760 mm Hg), with oxygen representing 21% of all gases present, the pressure exerted by the oxygen—its partial pressure—is 159.6 mm Hg (21% × 760). Consider the same air at a pressure of 760 mm Hg but fully saturated with water vapor at 37° C (normal body temperature). Because vapor pressure depends on temperature, the SVP for water at 37° C is 47 mm Hg. The pressure from oxygen is therefore now 21% of 713 (i.e., 760 – 47) mm Hg. The partial pressure of oxygen is therefore 149.7 mm Hg.

Note that volumes percent expresses the relative ratio or proportion (%) of gas molecules in a mixture, whereas partial pressure (mm Hg) represents an absolute value. Anesthetic uptake and potency are directly related to partial pressure and only indirectly to volumes percent. This distinction become more apparent when hyperbaric and hypobaric conditions are considered.

Minimum Alveolar Concentration

The *minimum alveolar concentration* (MAC) of a potent inhaled anesthetic agent is the concentration that produces immobility in 50% of patients who undergo a standard surgical stimulus. Used as a measure of anesthetic potency or depth, MAC is commonly expressed as volumes percent of alveolar (end-tidal) gas at 1 atm pressure at sea level (i.e., 760 mm Hg). Table 3-1 shows how MAC expressed in familiar volumes percent can be expressed as a partial pressure in millimeters of mercury. Anesthesiologists should learn to think of MAC in terms of partial pressure rather than in terms of volumes percent because the partial pressure (tension) of the anesthetic in the central nervous system is responsible for the depth of anesthesia. This concept has been advocated by Fink,[5] who proposed the term *minimum alveolar pressure* (MAP), and by James and White,[6] who suggested *minimum alveolar partial pressure* (MAPP). In this text, the term P_{MAC1} (see Table 3-1) is used to express the partial pressure of a potent inhaled agent at a concentration of 1 MAC; thus 1 MAC of isoflurane is equivalent to a P_{MAC1} of 8.7 mm Hg.

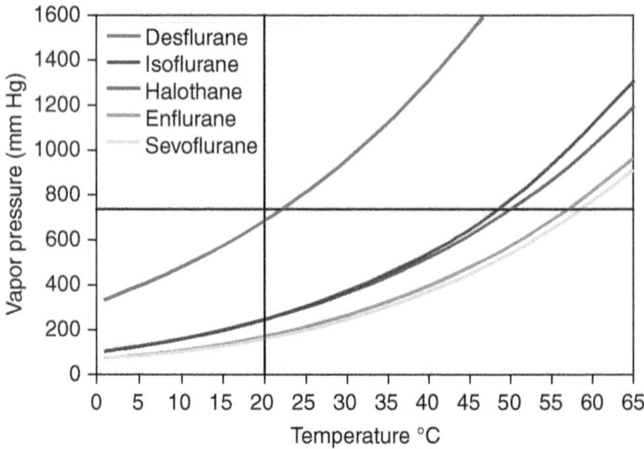

FIGURE 3-2 Vapor pressure curves for desflurane, isoflurane, halothane, enflurane, and sevoflurane.

Latent Heat of Vaporization

Vaporization requires energy to transform molecules from the liquid phase to the vapor phase. This energy is called the *latent heat of vaporization* and is defined as the amount of heat (calories) required to convert a unit mass (grams) of liquid into vapor. For example, at 20° C the latent heat of vaporization of isoflurane is 41 cal/g. The heat of vaporization is inversely related to ambient temperature in such a way that at lower temperatures, more heat is required for vaporization. The heat required to vaporize an anesthetic agent is drawn from the remaining liquid agent and from the surroundings. As vapor is generated and heat energy is lost, the temperatures of the vaporizer and the liquid agent fall. This causes the vapor pressure of the anesthetic to decrease. If no compensatory mechanism is provided, this will result in decreased output of vapor.

Specific Heat

Specific heat is the quantity of heat (calories) required to raise the temperature of a unit mass (grams) of a substance by 1° C. Heat must be supplied to the liquid anesthetic in the vaporizer to maintain the liquid's temperature during the evaporation process, when heat is being lost.

TABLE 3-1 Expression of MAC as a Partial Pressure

Agent	MAC (vol%)	P_{MAC1} (mm Hg)
Halothane	0.75 × 760	5.7
Enflurane	1.68 × 760	12.8
Isoflurane	1.15 × 760	8.7
Methoxyflurane	0.16 × 760	1.2
Sevoflurane	2.10 × 760	16
Desflurane	7.25 × 760	55

Assumes an ambient pressure of 760 mm Hg.

MAC, minimum alveolar concentration; P_{MAC1}, partial pressure of a potent inhaled agent at a concentration of 1 MAC.

Specific heat is also important when it comes to vaporizer construction material. For the same amount of heat lost through vaporization, temperature changes are more gradual for materials with a high specific heat than for those with a low specific heat. *Thermal capacity*, defined as the product of specific heat and mass, represents the quantity of heat stored in the vaporizer body.

Also of importance is the construction material's ability to conduct heat from the environment to the liquid anesthetic. This property is called *thermal conductivity*, defined as the rate at which heat is transmitted through a substance. For the liquid anesthetic to remain at a relatively constant temperature, the vaporizer is constructed from materials that have a high specific heat and high thermal conductivity. In this respect, copper comes close to the ideal; however, bronze and stainless steel have been used more recently in vaporizer construction.

Regulating Vaporizer Output: Variable Bypass Versus Measured Flow

The SVPs of halothane, sevoflurane, and isoflurane at room temperature are 243, 160, and 241 mm Hg, respectively. Dividing the SVP by ambient pressure (760 mm Hg) gives the saturated vapor concentration (SVC) as a fraction (or percentage) of 1 atm. This is an application of Dalton's law, as discussed earlier. The SVCs of halothane, sevoflurane, and isoflurane are therefore 32%, 21%, and 31%, respectively. These concentrations are far in excess of those required clinically (Table 3-2). Therefore the vaporizer first creates a saturated vapor in equilibrium with the liquid agent; second, the saturated vapor is diluted by a bypass gas flow. This results in clinically safe and useful concentrations flowing to the patient's breathing circuit. Without this dilution of saturated vapor, the agent would be delivered in a lethal concentration to the anesthesia circuit.

Contemporary anesthesia vaporizers are concentration calibrated, and most are of the variable bypass design. In a variable bypass vaporizer, such as those made by GE Healthcare (Tec series) and the Dräger Vapor 2000 (Dräger Medical, Telford, PA), the total fresh gas flow from the anesthesia machine flowmeters passes to the vaporizer (Fig. 3-3). The vaporizer splits the incoming gas flow between two pathways: the smaller flow enters the vaporizing chamber, or sump, of the vaporizer and leaves it with the anesthetic agent at its SVC. The larger bypass flow is eventually mixed with the outflow from the vaporizing chamber to create the desired, or "dialed in," concentration (see Fig. 3-3).

In the now-obsolete measured flow, non-concentration-calibrated vaporizers such as the Copper Kettle (Puritan-Bennett; Covidien, Mansfield, MA) or Verni-Trol (Ohio Medical Products, Gurnee, IL), a measured flow of oxygen is set on a separate flowmeter to pass to the vaporizer, from which vapor emerges at its SVP (Fig. 3-4). This flow is then diluted by an additional measured flow of gases (oxygen, nitrous oxide, air, etc.) from the main flowmeters on the anesthesia machine. With this type of arrangement, calculations are necessary to determine the anesthetic vapor concentration in the emerging gas mixture.

With both types of vaporizing systems, there must be an efficient method to create a saturated vapor in the vaporizing chamber. This is achieved by having a large surface area for evaporation. Flow-over vaporizers (Dräger Vapor 2000 series, GE Tec series) increase the surface area using wicks and baffles. In measured flow, bubble-through vaporizers, oxygen is bubbled through the liquid agent. To increase the surface area, tiny bubbles are created by passing the oxygen through a sintered bronze disk in the Copper Kettle, for example, which created large areas of liquid/gas interface, over which evaporation of the liquid agent could quickly occur.

TABLE 3-2 **Physical Properties of Potent Inhaled Volatile Agents**

Agents	Halothane	Enflurane	Isoflurane	Methoxyflurane	Sevoflurane	Desflurane
Structure	$CHBrClCF_3$	$CHFClCF_2OCHF_2$	$CF_2HOCHClCF_3$	$CHCl_2CF_2OCH_3$	$CH_2FOCH(CF_3)_2$	$CF_2HOCFHCF_3$
Molecular weight (AMU)	197.4	184.5	184.5	165.0	200	168
Boiling point at 760 mm Hg (° C)	50.2	56.5	48.5	104.7	58.5	22.8
SVP at 20° C (mm Hg)	243	175	238	20.3	160	664
SV conc. at 20° C and 1 ATA* (vol%)	32	23	31	2.7	21	87
MAC at 1 ATA* (vol%)	0.75	1.68	1.15	0.16	2.10	6-7.25†
P_{MAC1} (mm Hg)	5.7	12.8	8.7	1.22	16	46-55†
Specific gravity of liquid at 20° C	1.86	1.52	1.50	1.41	1.51	1.45
mL vapor per gram liquid at 20° C	123	130	130	145	120	143
mL vapor per mL liquid at 20° C	226	196	195	204	182	207

*1 ATA = one atmosphere absolute pressure (760 mm Hg).
†Age related.
AMU, atomic mass units; conc., concentration; MAC, minimum alveolar concentration; P_{MAC1}, partial pressure of a potent inhaled agent at a concentration of 1 MAC; SVC, saturated vapor concentration; SVP, saturated vapor pressure.

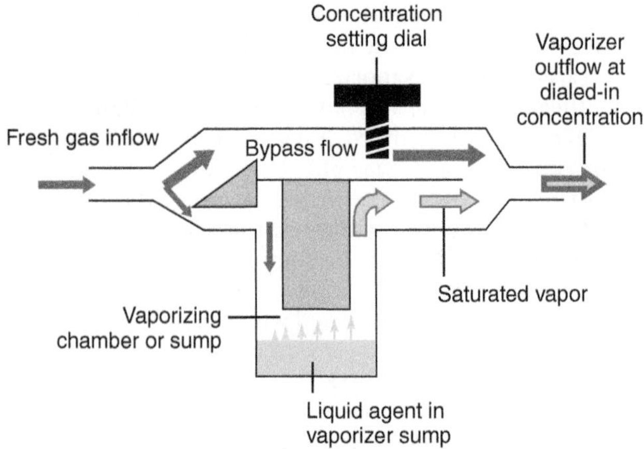

FIGURE 3-3 Schematic of a concentration-calibrated variable bypass vaporizer. Fresh gas enters the vaporizer, where its flow is split between a larger bypass flow and a smaller flow to the vaporizing chamber or sump. In the sump is the agent at its saturated vapor concentration. Saturated vapor mixes with the bypass flow, which dilutes it to the concentration dial setting.

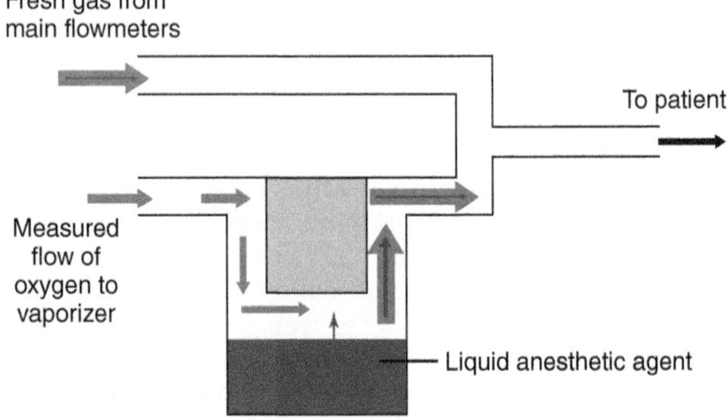

FIGURE 3-4 Schematic of a measured flow vaporizing arrangement. These are commonly known as "bubble-through" vaporizers.

Calculation of Vaporizer Output

At a constant room temperature of 20° C, the SVPs of two commonly used potent inhaled agents are 160 mm Hg for sevoflurane and 238 mm Hg for isoflurane. If ambient pressure is 760 mm Hg, these SVPs represent 21% sevoflurane (160/760) and 31% isoflurane (239/760), each in terms of volumes percent of 1 atm (760 mm Hg).

A concept fundamental to understanding vaporizer function is that under steady-state conditions, if a certain volume of *carrier gas* flows into a vaporizing chamber over a certain period, that same volume of carrier gas exits the chamber over the same period. However, because of the addition of vaporized anesthetic agent, the total volume exiting the chamber is greater than that entering it. In the vaporizing chamber, anesthetic vapor at its SVP constitutes a mandatory fractional volume of the atmosphere (i.e., 21% in a sevoflurane vaporizer at 20° C and 760 mm Hg). Therefore the volume of carrier gas will constitute the difference between 100% of the atmosphere in the vaporizing chamber and that resulting from the anesthetic vapor. In the case of sevoflurane, the carrier gas represents 79% of the atmosphere in the vaporizing chamber at any time. Thus if 100 mL/min of carrier gas flows through a vaporizing chamber containing sevoflurane, the carrier gas represents 79% (100% – 21%) of the atmosphere and the remaining 21% is sevoflurane vapor. By simple proportions, the volume of sevoflurane vapor exiting the chamber can be calculated to be 27 mL ([100/79] × 21) when rounded to the nearest whole number.

In other words, if 100 mL/min of carrier gas flows into the vaporizing chamber, the same 100 mL of carrier gas will emerge together with 27 mL/min of sevoflurane vapor. Another way of expressing this is shown below:

$$\frac{\text{SVP agent (mm Hg)}}{\text{Total pressure (mm Hg)}}$$

$$= \frac{\text{Agent vapor } (x \text{ mL})}{\text{Carrier gas } (y \text{ mL}) + \text{Agent vapor } (x \text{ mL})}$$

$$= \frac{\text{Volume of agent vapor}}{\text{Total volume leaving vaporizer}}$$

Continuing the above example for sevoflurane, y is 100 mL/min, and $160/760 = x/(100 + x)$, from which x can be calculated as 27 mL (rounded to the nearest whole number). Conversely, if x is known, the carrier gas flow y can be calculated. At steady state, the total volume of gas leaving the vaporizing chamber is greater than the total volume that entered, the additional volume being anesthetic vapor at its SVC.

VAPORIZER FUNCTION

Measured Flow Vaporizers

Although measured flow vaporizers are not mentioned in the ASTM anesthesia machine standards published after 1988, it is helpful to review the function of one example, the Copper Kettle. If 1% (vol/vol) isoflurane must be delivered to the patient circuit at a total fresh gas flow rate of 5 L/min (Fig. 3-5), the vaporizer must evolve 50 mL/min of sevoflurane vapor (1% × 5000 mL) to be diluted in a total volume of 5000 mL.

In the Copper Kettle, isoflurane represents 31% of the atmosphere, assuming a constant temperature of 20° C and a constant SVP of 238 mm Hg. If 50 mL of isoflurane vapor represents 31%, the carrier gas flow (x mL) of, oxygen flow x must represent the other 69% (100% – 31%). Thus

$$\frac{50}{31} = \frac{x}{69}$$

$$31x = 50 \times 69$$

$$x = \frac{(50 \times 69)}{31} = 111 \text{ mL}$$

Therefore, if 111 mL/min of oxygen is bubbled through liquid isoflurane in a Copper Kettle vaporizer, 161 mL/min of gas emerges, of which 50 mL is isoflurane vapor and 111 mL is the oxygen that flowed into the vaporizer. This vaporizer output of 161 mL/min must be diluted by an additional fresh gas flow of 4839 mL/min (5000 mL – 161 mL) to create an isoflurane mixture of *exactly* 1% because 50 mL of isoflurane vapor diluted in a total volume of 5000 mL gives 1% isoflurane by volume.

Although this situation is highly unlikely to occur in contemporary practice because of the obsolescence of measured flow vaporizers, if a measured flow system had to be used to deliver isoflurane, the anesthesia provider would likely set flows of 100 mL/min oxygen to the Copper Kettle and 5 L/min of fresh gas on the main flowmeters, which would result in only slightly less than 1% isoflurane (44.9/5044.9 = 0.89%). Multiples of either of the vaporizer oxygen flow and main gas flowmeter flows would be used to create other concentrations of isoflurane from the Copper Kettle. Thus a 200 mL/min oxygen flow to the vaporizer and 5000 mL/min on the main flowmeters would create approximately 1.8% isoflurane. It is important to realize that if there is oxygen flow only to the Copper Kettle vaporizer and no bypass gas flow is set on the main machine flowmeters, lethal concentrations approaching 31% isoflurane would be delivered to the anesthesia circuit, albeit at low flow rates.

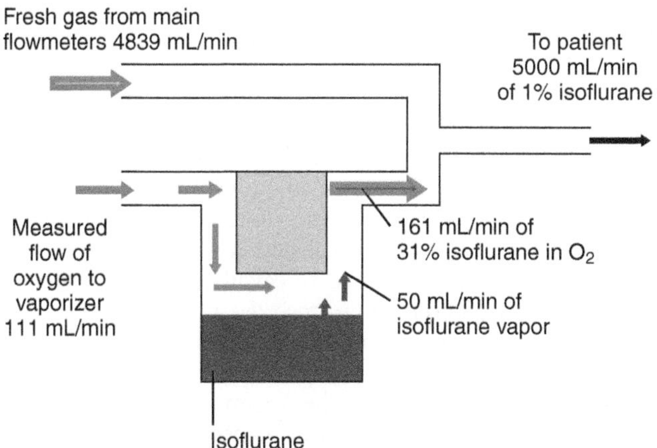

FIGURE 3-5 Preparation of 1% isoflurane by volume using a measured flow vaporizing system. 1% isoflurane in a 5L/min flow requires 50 mL/min isoflurane vapor, diluted in a total volume of 4950 mL fresh gas plus 50 mL isoflurane vapor. Isoflurane saturated vapor concentration is 31%. If 31% = 50 mL, then 69% = 111 mL, the required oxygen inflow per minute; 4839 mL/min (4950 – 111) is the required bypass flow, and final dilution is 1% (50/[50 + 4839 + 111]).

Because halothane and isoflurane have similar SVPs at 20° C, the Copper Kettle flows to be set for halothane would be essentially the same as those for isoflurane when a 1% concentration of isoflurane is to be created with a Copper Kettle. A Copper Kettle arrangement on an older model anesthesia machine is shown in Figure 3-6.

Because enflurane and sevoflurane have similar vapor pressures at 20° C (175 mm Hg and 160 mm Hg, respectively), similar flow settings could be used to create approximately the same agent concentrations with a measured flow system. In the case of sevoflurane, the measured flow vaporizer contains 21% sevoflurane vapor (160/760 = 21%). The oxygen flow therefore represents the remaining 79% of the atmosphere in the Copper Kettle. If precisely 1% sevoflurane is required at a 5 L/min total rate of flow, 50 mL/min of sevoflurane vapor must be generated. If 50 mL represents 21% of the atmosphere in the vaporizer, the carrier gas flow required is 188 mL/min ([50/21] × 79).

If 188 mL/min of oxygen are bubbled through liquid sevoflurane contained in a measured flow vaporizer, 238 mL/min of gas will emerge, 50 mL/min of which is sevoflurane vapor. This must be diluted by a fresh gas flow of 4762 mL/min (5000 – 238) to achieve exactly 1% sevoflurane.

Alternatively, using the formula given previously:

$$\frac{160}{760} = \frac{50}{50 + y}$$

$$y = 188 \text{ mL/min}$$

where y is the oxygen flow to the measured flow vaporizer.

Setting an oxygen flow of 200 mL/min to the vaporizer and 5 L/min on the main flowmeters would result in a sevoflurane concentration of 1.01%, or ([200/79] × 21)/5253.2.

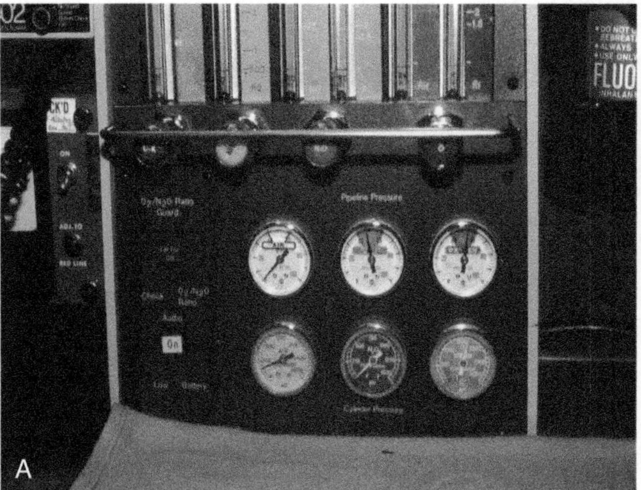

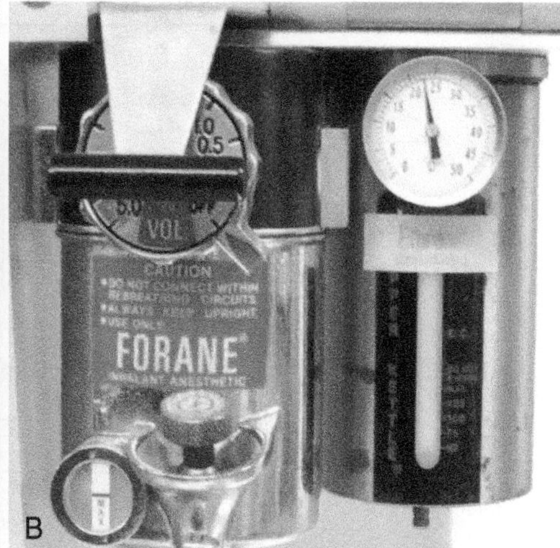

FIGURE 3-6 Copper Kettle vaporizing system (Puritan-Bennett; Covidien, Mansfield, MA). **A,** The oxygen flowmeter knob on the extreme left is marked "C-K" to indicate that it controls oxygen flow to the Copper Kettle. **B,** Close-up of the Copper Kettle.

In the preceding examples, calculations of both the oxygen flow to the measured flow vaporizer and the total bypass gas flow needed to produce the desired output concentrations of vapor were required. This is not only inconvenient, it also predisposes to clinical errors that could result in serious overdose (Fig. 3-7) or underdose of anesthetic. Because of the obvious potential for error with a measured flow vaporizing system, the concurrent continuous use of an anesthetic agent analyzer with high- and low-concentration alarms would be essential for patient safety.[7]

Variable Bypass Vaporizers

In the concentration-calibrated variable bypass vaporizer, the total flow of gas arriving from the anesthesia machine flowmeters is split between a variable bypass and the vaporizing chamber containing the anesthetic agent (see Fig. 3-3). The ratio of these two flows, known as the *splitting ratio*, depends on the anesthetic agent, temperature, and chosen vapor concentration set to be delivered to the patient circuit.

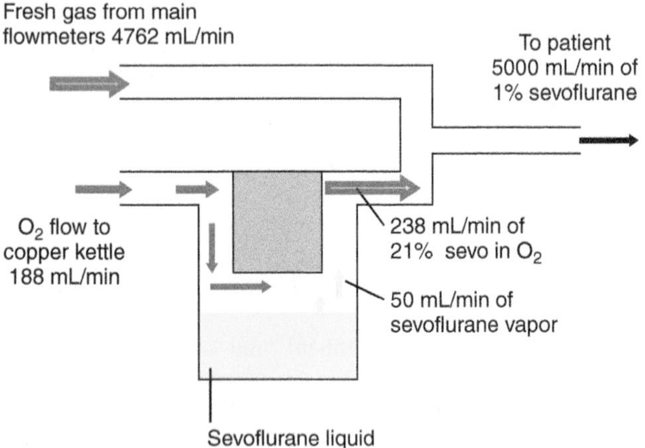

FIGURE 3-7 Preparation of 1% sevoflurane by volume using a measured flow vaporizing system.

As previously discussed, to deliver 1% sevoflurane accurately, a total incoming gas flow of 4950 mL/min must be split so that 188 mL/min flows through the vaporizing chamber and 4762 mL/min flows through the bypass. This results in a splitting ratio of 25:1 (4762/188) between the bypass flow and the vaporizing chamber flow at a temperature of 20° C. A variable bypass vaporizer set to deliver 1% sevoflurane is therefore effectively set to create a splitting ratio of 25:1 for the inflowing gas (Fig. 3-8).

Consider a concentration-calibrated, variable bypass, isoflurane-specific vaporizer set to deliver 1% isoflurane. What splitting ratio for incoming gases must this vaporizer achieve? The SVP of isoflurane at 20° C is 238 mm Hg; therefore the concentration of isoflurane vapor in the vaporizing chamber is 31% (238/760). If carrier gas flows through the vaporizing chamber at a rate of 69 mL/min, isoflurane vapor emerges at 31 mL/min and must be diluted in 3100 mL/min of total gas flow to achieve a 1% concentration because 31/3100 equals 1%. Thus, if carrier gas enters the vaporizer from the flowmeters at 3069 mL/min and is split—such that 3000 mL/min flows through the bypass and 69 mL/min flows through the vaporizing chamber—when the two flows merge, 1% isoflurane is the result. The splitting ratio is therefore 44:1 (3000/69) (Fig. 3-9).

Table 3-3 shows the splitting ratios for variable bypass vaporizers used at 20° C. To ensure complete understanding, the reader is encouraged to calculate these ratios and apply them to different total fresh gas flows arriving from the main flowmeters to the inlet of a concentration-calibrated variable bypass vaporizer. An equation for the calculation of splitting ratios is provided in the Appendix to this chapter.

The concentration-calibrated vaporizer is agent specific and must be used only with the agent for which the unit is designed and calibrated. To produce a 1% vapor concentration, an isoflurane vaporizer makes a flow split of 44:1, whereas a sevoflurane vaporizer makes a flow split of 25:1 (see Table 3-3). If an empty sevoflurane vaporizer set to deliver a 1% concentration were to be filled with

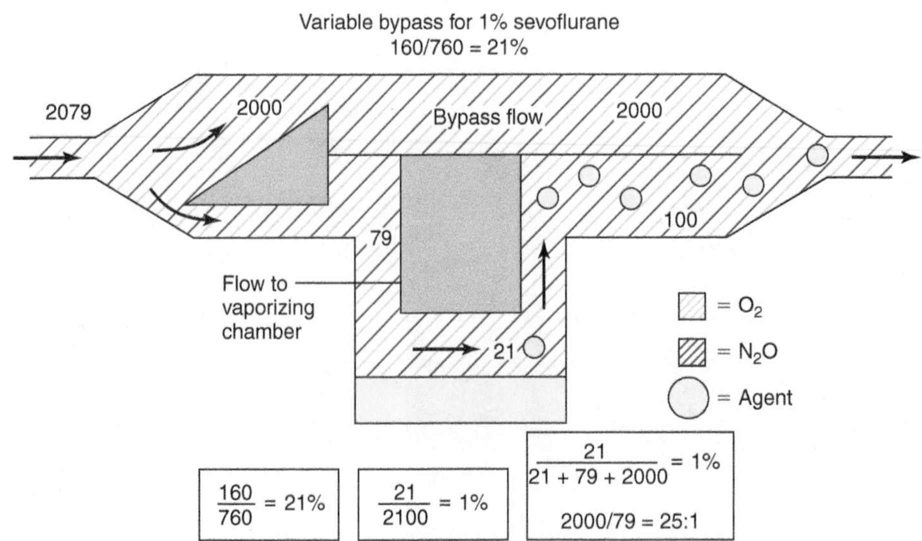

FIGURE 3-8 Preparation of 1% (vol/vol) sevoflurane in a variable bypass vaporizer. To achieve this, a split ratio of 25:1 (bypass flow/vaporizing chamber flow) is created for incoming gas.

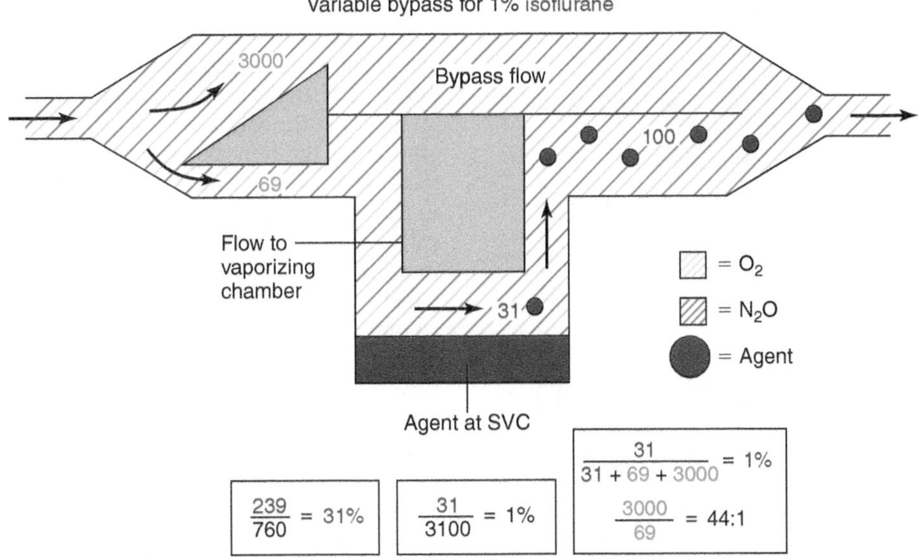

FIGURE 3-9 ■ Preparation of 1% (vol/vol) isoflurane by a variable bypass vaporizer. To achieve this, a split ratio of 44:1 (bypass flow/vaporizing chamber flow) is created for incoming gas.

TABLE 3-3 **Gas Flow Splitting Ratios at 20° C**

	Halothane	Enflurane	Isoflurane	Methoxyflurane	Sevoflurane
1%	46:1	29:1	44:1	1.7:1	25:1
2%	22:1	14:1	21:1	0.36:1	12:1
3%	14:1	9:1	14:1	*	7:1

*Maximum possible is 2.7% at 20° C (see Table 3-2).

isoflurane, the concentration of the isoflurane vapor emerging would be in excess of 1%. Understanding splitting ratios enables prediction of the concentration output of an empty, agent-specific, variable bypass vaporizer that has been erroneously filled with an agent for which it was not designed. The change in concentration output when one agent-specific vaporizer is filled with a different agent can be calculated as the concentration set on the vaporizer dial multiplied by the ratio of the splitting ratios at 20° C (and not as the ratio of the SVPs of the two agents). In the case of the sevoflurane vaporizer set to deliver 1% sevoflurane but filled with isoflurane, the resulting isoflurane concentration will be 1.76% isoflurane (44/25).

Control of Splitting Ratio

In a variable bypass vaporizer, the bypass flow and the vaporizing chamber flow may be thought of as two resistances in parallel. The concentration control dial is used to adjust the ratio of the two resistances to achieve the dialed-in concentration by adjusting the size of a variable orifice. That orifice may be located at the inlet of the vaporizing chamber or at the outlet. In older model vaporizers the variable orifice was located at the inlet to the vaporizing chamber (see Fig. 8-11 in Chapter 8 for an example). In contemporary vaporizers (e.g., GE Healthcare Tec 5; Dräger Medical Vapor 19.n series) the orifice is located at the outlet of the chamber (see Fig. 3-19). The splitting ratios discussed in the previous section describe the *effective flow split* for the fresh gas entering the vaporizer but not where the split is achieved (i.e., whether by the inlet or the outlet of the vaporizing chamber). If the split is achieved at the outlet of the vaporizing chamber, a flow of saturated vapor is metered into the bypass flow and an "exit" splitting ratio can be calculated. In Figure 3-8, to create 1% sevoflurane a controlled flow of 100 mL/min of 21% sevoflurane is mixed with the bypass flow of 2000 mL/min. The ratio of flows is 2000/100 = 20:1. Compare this with the effective flow split of 25:1 for the fresh gas entering the vaporizer from the machine flowmeters.

Similarly, in Figure 3-9, to create 1% isoflurane a controlled flow of 100 mL/min of 31% isoflurane vapor is mixed with the bypass flow of 3000 mL/min; the "exit" splitting ratio is 3000/100 = 30:1. Compare this with the effective flow split of 44:1 for the fresh gas entering the vaporizer.

The location of the variable orifice is of little importance at 1 atm pressure but may have an effect when the vaporizer is used at ambient pressures that are higher or lower than 1 atm. (see later section on Effects of Changes in Barometric Pressure).

Efficiency and Temperature Compensation

Agent-specific concentration-calibrated vaporizers must be located in the fresh gas path between the flowmeter manifold outlet and the common gas outlet on the anesthesia workstation.[3] The vaporizers must be capable of

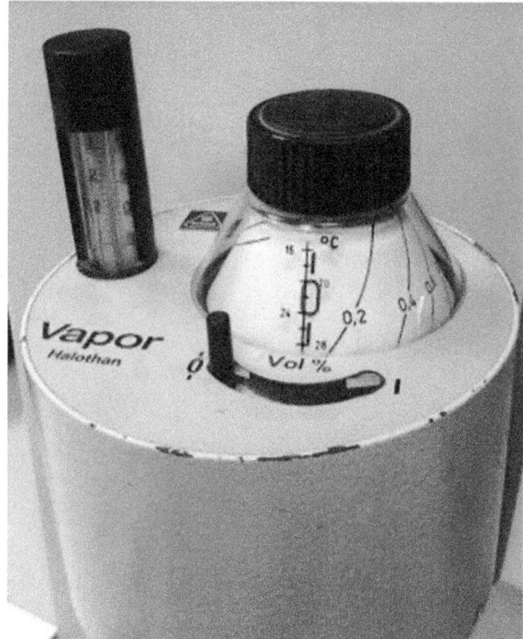

FIGURE 3-10 ■ In the Dräger Vapor vaporizer (Dräger Medical, Telford, PA), temperature compensation is achieved by reading the temperature from the thermometer and using the control dial to align the desired output concentration (slanting) line with the marking for ambient temperature.

accepting a total gas flow of 15 L/min from the machine flowmeters and be able to deliver a predictable concentration of vapor.[3] However, as the agent is vaporized and the temperature falls, SVP also falls. In the case of a measured flow vaporizer or an uncompensated variable bypass vaporizer, this results in delivery of less anesthetic vapor to the patient circuit. For this reason, all vaporizing systems must be temperature compensated, either manually or, as in contemporary vaporizers, automatically.

Measured flow vaporizers incorporate a thermometer that measures the temperature of the liquid agent in the vaporizing chamber. A higher temperature translates to a higher SVP in this chamber. Reference to the vapor pressure curves (see Fig. 3-2) enables a resetting of either oxygen flow to the vaporizer, bypass gas flow, or both to ensure correct output at the prevailing temperature. Although tedious, such an arrangement does ensure the most accurate and rapid temperature compensation. The original Dräger Vapor vaporizer (Fig. 3-10), to be distinguished from the more recent Vapor 19.n and 2000 models fitted to contemporary Dräger workstations, is a variable bypass vaporizer that incorporates a thermometer and a grid of lines on the vaporizer control dial for temperature compensation by which the desired output concentration is matched to the temperature of the liquid agent; turning the control dial changes the size of an orifice in the bypass flow.

Most of the contemporary variable bypass vaporizers, such as the Tec series and the Dräger Vapor 19.n and 2000, achieve automatic temperature compensation via a temperature-sensitive valve in the bypass gas flow. When temperature increases, the valve in the bypass opens wider to create a higher splitting ratio so that more gas flows through the bypass and less gas enters the vaporizing chamber. A smaller volume of a higher concentration of vapor emerges from the vaporizing chamber; this vapor, when mixed with an increased bypass gas flow, maintains the vaporizer's output at reasonable constancy when temperature changes are not extreme.

Temperature-sensitive valves have evolved in design among the different types of vaporizers. Some older vaporizers, such as the Ohio Medical Calibrated Vaporizer, had in the vaporizing chamber, a gas-filled bellows linked to a valve in the bypass gas flow (Fig. 3-11).[8] As the temperature increased, the bellows expanded, causing the valve to open wider. Contemporary vaporizers, such as the Tec series, use a bimetallic strip for temperature compensation.[9] This strip is incorporated into a flap valve in the bypass gas flow. The valve is composed of two metals with different *coefficients of expansion*, or change in length per unit length per unit change in temperature. Nickel and brass have been used in bimetallic strip valves because brass has a greater coefficient of expansion than nickel. As the temperature rises, one surface of the flap expands more than the other, causing the flap to bend in a manner that opens the valve orifice wider, increasing the bypass flow. The principle of differential expansion of metals is applied similarly in the Dräger Vapor 19.n and 2000 series vaporizers, in which an expansion element increases bypass flow and reduces gas flow in the vaporizing chamber as temperature increases.[10] When temperature decreases, the reverse occurs.

The vapor pressures of the volatile anesthetics vary as a function of temperature in a nonlinear manner (see Fig. 3-2). The result is that the vapor output concentration at any given vaporizer dial setting remains constant only within a certain range of temperatures. For example, the Dräger Vapor 2000 vaporizers are specified as accurate to ±0.20 vol% or ±20% of the concentration set when they are used within the temperature range of 15° C to 35° C at 1 atm.[11] The boiling point of the volatile anesthetic agent must never be reached in the current variable bypass vaporizers designed for halothane, enflurane, isoflurane, and sevoflurane; otherwise, the vapor output concentration would be impossible to control and could be lethal.

Temperature Compensation Times

The temperature-compensating mechanisms of contemporary vaporizers do not produce instantaneous correction of output concentration. For example, the Dräger 19.n vaporizer requires a temperature compensation time of 6 min/° C.[12]

Incorrect Filling of Vaporizers

Contemporary concentration-calibrated variable bypass anesthesia vaporizers are agent specific. If an empty vaporizer designed for one agent is filled with an agent for which it was not intended, the vaporizer's output will likely be erroneous. Because the vaporizing characteristics of halothane and isoflurane (SVP of 243 and 238 mm Hg, respectively) and enflurane and sevoflurane (SVP of 175 and 160 mm Hg, respectively) are almost identical at room temperature, this problem mainly applies when halothane or isoflurane is interchanged with enflurane or sevoflurane.

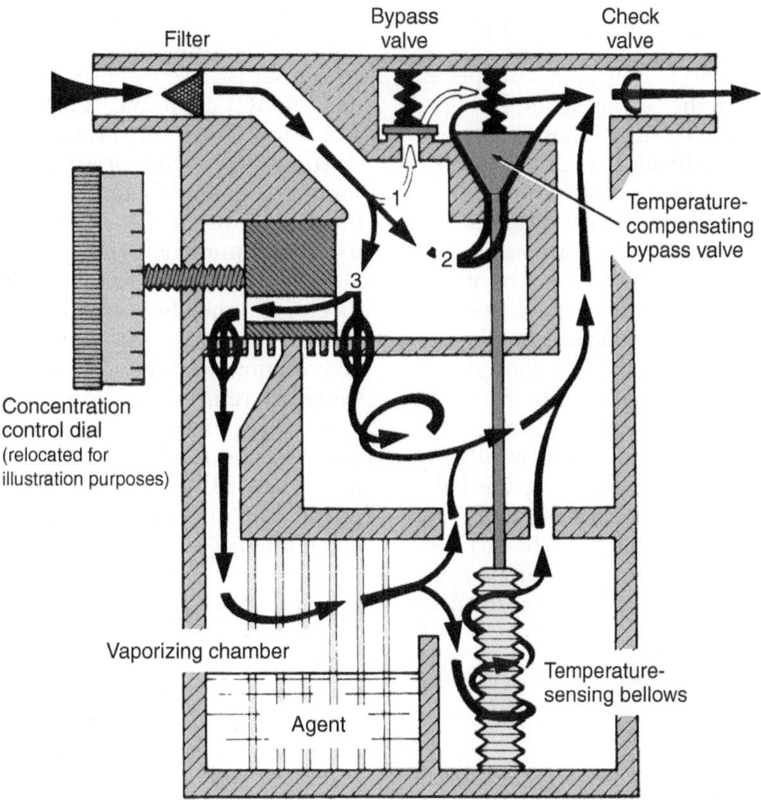

FIGURE 3-11 Schematic of a calibrated vaporizer. Temperature compensation is achieved by a gas-filled temperature-sensing bellows that controls the size of a temperature-compensating bypass valve. Note also the check valve in the vaporizer outlet designed to protect against the pumping effect. (Courtesy GE Healthcare, Waukesha, WI.)

TABLE 3-4 **Output in Volumes Percent and Minimum Alveolar Concentration (MAC in Oxygen) of Erroneously Filled Vaporizers at 22° C**

Vaporizers	Liquid	Setting (%)	Output (%)	Output MAC
Halothane	Halothane	1.0	1.00	1.25
	Enflurane	1.0	0.62	0.37
	Isoflurane	1.0	0.96	0.84
Enflurane	Enflurane	2.0	2.00	1.19
	Isoflurane	2.0	3.09	2.69
	Halothane	2.0	3.21	4.01
Isoflurane	Isoflurane	1.5	1.50	1.30
	Haloflurane	1.5	1.56	1.95
	Enflurane	1.5	0.97	0.57

MAC, minimum alveolar concentration.
From Bruce DL, Linde HW: Vaporization of mixed anesthetic liquids. *Anesthesiology* 60:342-346, 1984.

Bruce and Linde[13] reported on the output of erroneously filled vaporizers (Table 3-4). Erroneous filling affects the output concentration and, consequently, the *potency* output of the vaporizer. In their study, an enflurane vaporizer set to 2% (1.19 MAC) but filled with halothane delivered 3.21% (4.01 MAC) halothane. This is 3.3 times the anticipated anesthetic potency output.

To summarize, if a vaporizer specific for an agent with a low SVP, such as enflurane or sevoflurane, is misfilled with an agent that has a high SVP, such as halothane or isoflurane, the output concentration of the agent will be greater than that indicated on the concentration dial. Conversely, if a vaporizer specific for an agent with a high SVP is misfilled with an agent that has a low SVP, the output concentration of the agent will be less than that indicated on the concentration dial.

In addition, the potency of the agent concentration must be considered in a misfilling situation. A sevoflurane vaporizer set to deliver 2% sevoflurane (1 MAC) misfilled with isoflurane would produce an isoflurane concentration of 3.5% (~3 MAC).

Erroneous filling of vaporizers may be prevented if careful attention is paid to the specific agent and the vaporizer during filling. A number of agent-specific filling mechanisms analogous to the pin index safety system for medical gases are used on modern vaporizers. Liquid anesthetic agents are packaged in bottles that have agent-specific and color-coded collars (Fig. 3-12). One end of an agent-specific filling device fits the collar on the agent bottle, and the other end fits only the vaporizer designed for that liquid agent. Although well designed, these filling devices cannot entirely prevent misfilling.

A number of different filling systems are available (e.g., Quik-Fil [Abbott Laboratories, Abbott Park, IL], Key-Fill [Harvard Apparatus, Holliston, MA]). The agent-specific filling device for desflurane, SAF-T-FILL (Zeneca Pharma, Inc., Mississauga, Canada), is particularly important because a non-desflurane vaporizer must *never* be filled with desflurane.

Vaporization of Mixed Anesthetic Liquids

Perhaps a more likely scenario is that an agent-specific vaporizer, partially filled with the correct agent, is topped off with an incorrect agent. This situation is more complex because it is much more difficult to predict vaporizer output, and significant errors in concentration of delivered vapor can occur. Korman and Ritchie reported that halothane, enflurane, and isoflurane do not react chemically when mixed, but they do influence the extent of each other's ease of vaporization. Halothane facilitates the vaporization of both enflurane and isoflurane and is itself more likely to vaporize in the process.[14] The clinical consequences depend on the potencies of each of the mixed agents and on the delivered vapor concentrations.

If a halothane vaporizer that is 25% full is filled to 100% with isoflurane and set to deliver 1%, the halothane output is 0.41% (0.51 MAC) and the isoflurane output is 0.9% (0.78 MAC; see Table 3-5). In this case, the output potency of 1.29 MAC is not far from the anticipated 1.25 MAC (1% halothane). On the other hand, an enflurane vaporizer that is 25% full and set to deliver 2% (1.19 MAC) enflurane filled to 100% with halothane has an output of 2.43% (3.03 MAC) halothane and 0.96% (0.57 MAC) enflurane. This represents a total MAC of 3.60—more than three times the intended amount.

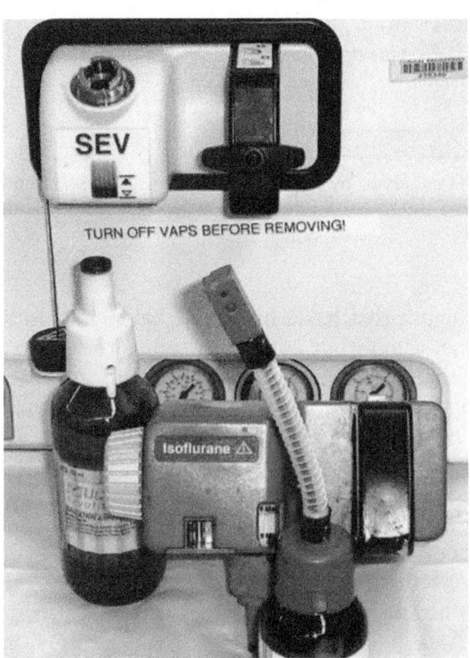

FIGURE 3-12 ■ Agent-specific filling devices for sevoflurane (*yellow;* Quik-Fil, Abbott Laboratories, Abbott Park, IL) and isoflurane (*purple;* Key-Fill, Harvard Apparatus, Holliston, MA).

If a vaporizer filling error is suspected, the vaporizer should be emptied and flushed using 5 L/min of oxygen (in the case of the Tec 4), with the concentration dial set to the maximum output, until no trace of the contaminant is detected in the outflow.[15,16] The vaporizer's temperature should then be allowed to stabilize for 2 hours before it is used clinically, and with great caution. If the contaminant is not volatile, such as with water, the vaporizer should be returned to the manufacturer for servicing.

Contemporary anesthetic vaporizers now incorporate agent-specific filling devices designed to prevent erroneous filling and to reduce contamination of the atmosphere in the operating room while the vaporizing chamber is being filled.

Filling of Vaporizers

Vaporizers should be filled only in accordance with their manufacturer's instructions. Overfilling or tilting a vaporizer—that is, either tilting a freestanding unit or tilting the whole anesthesia machine—may result in liquid agent entering parts of the anesthesia delivery system designed for gases and vapor only, such as a vaporizer bypass. This could lead to the delivery of lethal concentrations of agent to the patient circuit. If a vaporizer has been tilted, liquid agent may have leaked into the gas delivery system. A patient must never be left connected to such a system. Once the machine has been withdrawn from clinical service, the proper procedure is to purge the vaporizer with a high flow rate of oxygen from the flowmeter of the anesthesia machine or workstation—not the oxygen flush, which bypasses the vaporizer—and with the vaporizer concentration dial set to the *maximum* concentration.[12,15] The maximum concentration dial setting ensures the highest possible oxygen flow through the inflow and outflow paths of the vaporizing chamber and through the bypass. A calibrated anesthetic agent analyzer is essential to check the efficacy of the flush procedure before the vaporizer is returned to clinical service. In contemporary practice, it is probably prudent to withdraw the workstation and vaporizer from clinical use until both have been declared safe by authorized service personnel.

TABLE 3-5 **Vaporizer Output After Incorrectly Refilling from 25% Full to 100% Full**

			Vaporizer Output						
			Halothane		*Enflurane*		*Isoflurane*		
Vaporizer	Setting (%)	Refill Liquid	%	MAC	%	MAC	%	MAC	Total MAC
Halothane	1.0	Enflurane	0.33	0.41	0.64	0.38	—	—	0.79
	1.0	Isoflurane	0.41	0.51	—	—	0.90	0.78	1.29
Enflurane	2.0	Halothane	2.43	3.03	0.96	0.57	—	—	3.60
Isoflurane	1.5	Halothane	1.28	1.60	—	—	0.57	0.50	2.10

MAC, minimum alveolar concentration.
From Bruce DL, Linde HW: Vaporization of mixed anesthetic liquids. *Anesthesiology* 60:342-346, 1984.

Table 3-2 shows that 1 mL of liquid volatile agent produces approximately 200 mL of vapor at 20° C. The theoretical derivation of this volume is presented later in this chapter (see Preparation of a Standard Vapor Concentration). Thus it is easy to see how very small volumes of liquid agent entering the gas delivery system might produce lethal concentrations. For example, if 1 mL of liquid isoflurane entered the common gas tubing, some 20 L of fresh gas would be required to dilute the resulting volume of vapor (195 mL) down to a 1% (0.87 MAC) concentration.

Effect of Carrier Gas on Vaporizer Output

The carrier gas used to vaporize the volatile agent in the vaporizing chamber can also affect vaporizer output because the viscosity and density of the gas mixture change as the mixture changes. Figure 3-13 shows the output concentration from an enflurane variable bypass vaporizer set to deliver 1% enflurane. For the first 10 minutes, the carrier gas is 70% nitrous oxide and 30% oxygen and the vaporizer delivers 1% enflurane. After 10 minutes, the carrier gas is changed to nitrogen and oxygen; at approximately 20 minutes, the vaporizer output is seen to increase to a peak of about 2.6%; at 30 minutes, it decreases to 1%, at which point it stabilizes. At 40 minutes, the carrier gas is changed back to nitrous oxide and oxygen, and the vaporizer output concentration transiently decreases to 0.75%. By 55 minutes, it gradually returns to 1%. At 60 minutes, the carrier gas is changed back to nitrogen and oxygen and the vaporizer output again increases.

The effect of carrier gas on vaporizer output can be explained by the solubility of nitrous oxide in a liquid volatile anesthetic agent. Thus, when nitrous oxide and oxygen begin to enter the vaporizing chamber, some nitrous oxide dissolves in the liquid agent, and the vaporizing chamber's output *decreases* until the liquid agent has become saturated with nitrous oxide. Conversely, when nitrous oxide is withdrawn as the carrier gas, the nitrous oxide dissolved in the liquid anesthetic comes out of solution and represents, in effect, additional nitrous oxide gas flow to the vaporizing chamber.

The solubility of nitrous oxide in liquid anesthetics is approximately 4.5 mL per milliliter of liquid anesthetic[17]; therefore 100 mL of enflurane liquid, when fully saturated, can dissolve approximately 450 mL of nitrous oxide. When nitrous oxide is discontinued because it is added (by coming out of solution) to the vaporizing chamber flow over a brief period, the volume of nitrous oxide causes the observed *increase* in vaporizer output concentration.

Dräger vaporizers are calibrated using air as the carrier gas. When 100% oxygen is used, the output concentration, when compared with air, increases by 10% of the set value and by not more than 0.4 vol%. When a mixture of 30% oxygen and 70% nitrous oxide is used, the concentration falls by 10% of the set value at most and by not more than 0.4 vol%.[11] Tec series vaporizers are calibrated at 21° C with oxygen as the carrier gas. In these vaporizers, when air or nitrous oxide is the carrier gas, the output concentration is less than with oxygen. The effect is greatest when nitrous oxide is the carrier gas, but using nitrous oxide decreases the required concentration of volatile agent, thereby somewhat mitigating the decrease in output concentration.[18]

Effects of Changes in Barometric Pressure

Vaporizers are most commonly used at an ambient pressure of 760 mm Hg (1 atm at sea level). They may, however, be used under hypobaric conditions, such as at high altitudes, or under hyperbaric conditions, such as in a hyperbaric chamber.[5]

Vaporizing Chamber Flow Controlled at Inlet

When used at pressures above or below 1 atm, the location of the variable orifice controlling flow into or out from the vaporizing chamber affects vaporizer performance.

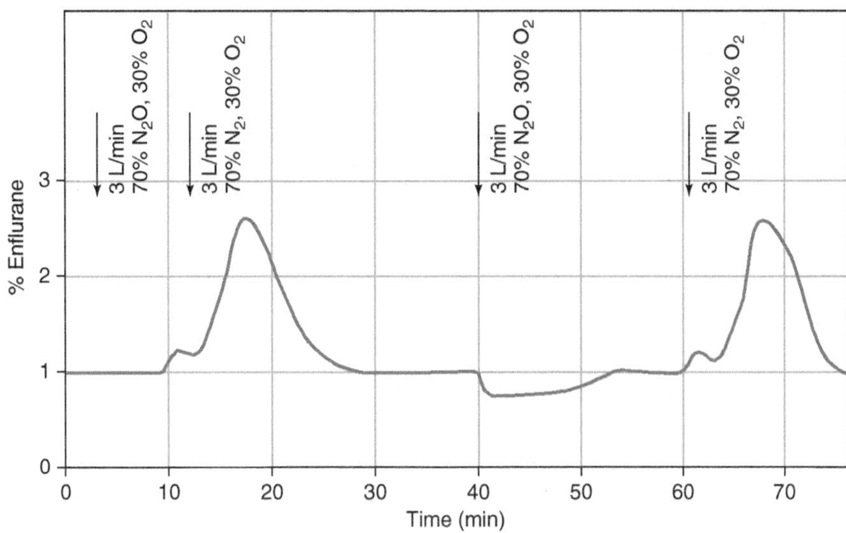

FIGURE 3-13 ■ Effect of changing the carrier gas composition (nitrous oxide vs. nitrogen) on vaporizer output in a variable bypass enflurane vaporizer. (From Scheller MS, Drummond JC: Solubility of N_2O in volatile anesthetics contributes to vaporizer aberrancy when changing carrier gases. *Anesth Analg* 1986;65:88-90. Reproduced by permission of the International Anesthesia Research Society.)

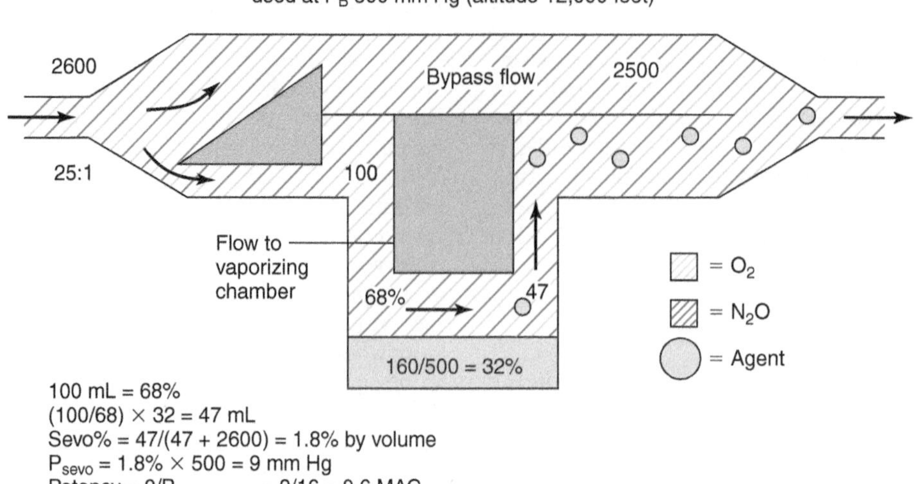

FIGURE 3-14 Use of a concentration-calibrated variable bypass sevoflurane vaporizer under hypobaric conditions. MAC, minimum alveolar concentration; P_B, barometric pressure; P_{MAC1}, partial pressure of a potent inhaled agent at a concentration of 1 MAC.

Hypobaric Conditions

Few reports are available concerning the use of vaporizers under hypobaric conditions.[6] This discussion therefore focuses on theoretical considerations applying to such use.

Consider a variable bypass vaporizer set to deliver 1% sevoflurane (0.5 MAC at 760 mm Hg atmospheric pressure) at an ambient pressure of 500 mm Hg, equivalent to an altitude of approximately 12,000 feet above sea level, and at a temperature of 20° C (Fig. 3-14). In the vaporizing chamber, sevoflurane has an SVP of 160 mm Hg at a temperature of 20° C; however, this now represents 32 vol% (160/500) of the atmosphere there. Set to deliver 1% under normal conditions, for the incoming fresh gas the vaporizer creates a splitting ratio of 25:1 between bypass and vaporizing chamber flows.

If the total gas flow to the vaporizer is 2600 mL/min (Fig. 3-14), 100 mL/min of carrier gas flows through the vaporizing chamber. This now represents 68% of the volume there because sevoflurane represents the other 32 vol% (100% − 68%). Emerging from the vaporizing chamber is 100 mL/min of carrier gas plus 47 mL/min of sevoflurane vapor ([100/68] × 32). When the vaporizing chamber and bypass flows merge, the 47 mL/min of sevoflurane vapor are diluted in a total volume of 2647 mL/min (2500 + 100 + 47 mL), giving a sevoflurane concentration of 1.8% of the atmosphere *by volume*. This appears to be almost twice (1.8 times) the dialed-in concentration in terms of volumes percent.

To determine the potency of this 1.8% sevoflurane concentration, however, partial pressure must be considered because it is the *tension* of the anesthetic agent that determines potency. If sevoflurane represents 1.8% of the gas mixture by volume, its partial pressure in the emerging mixture is 1.8% × 500 mm Hg, or 9 mm Hg. In terms of anesthetic potency, this represents 0.6 MAC (9/16) because the P_{MAC1} of sevoflurane is 16 mm Hg (see Table 3-1). Thus, in theory, a variable bypass sevoflurane vaporizer used at an ambient pressure of 500 mm Hg (at 12,000 feet above sea level) with the dial set to 1% (vol/vol) delivers 1.8 times the dialed-in concentration in terms of volumes percent but only 1.2 times the anesthetic potency in terms of MAC (0.6/0.5).

To summarize, when used at atmospheric pressures below 760 mm Hg (sea level), a variable bypass vaporizer, whose vaporizing chamber gas flow is controlled by a variable orifice at the inlet of the vaporizing chamber, will have an output concentration that is greater than that set on the dial in volumes percent, but potency increases by a lesser amount.

Hyperbaric Conditions

Anesthesia vaporizers are occasionally used under hyperbaric conditions. This can occur in a hyperbaric operating chamber or at altitudes below sea level. Consider the same variable bypass sevoflurane vaporizer set to deliver 1% sevoflurane (0.5 MAC at 760 mm Hg atmospheric pressure) (in which gas flow to the vaporizing chamber is controlled by a variable orifice at the vaporizing chamber inlet). The vaporizer is to be used at 20° C under conditions of 3 atm (3 × 760 = 2280 mm Hg), such as might be created in a hyperbaric chamber (Fig. 3-15).

In the vaporizing chamber, the SVP of sevoflurane is 160 mm Hg and the sevoflurane concentration is 7% by volume (160/2280). A variable bypass sevoflurane vaporizer set to deliver 1% creates a splitting ratio of 25:1 for the fresh gas inflow. If the total gas flow to the vaporizer is 2600 mL/min, 100 mL of carrier gas enters the vaporizing chamber per minute (see Fig. 3-15). This 100 mL represents 93% of the atmosphere there (100% − 7%); the remainder is sevoflurane vapor. The amount of sevoflurane vapor evolved is [100/93] × 7, or 7.5 mL/min. This 7.5 mL is diluted to a total volume of 2607.5 mL (2500 + 100 + 7.5), giving 0.29% (7.5/2607.5) sevoflurane vapor by volume. This is 0.29 (0.29/1) times the vaporizer dial setting in terms of volumes percent.

What about potency? The partial pressure of sevoflurane in the emerging gas mixture is 6.6 mm Hg (0.29% × 2280 mm Hg). Dividing by the P_{MAC1} for sevoflurane of

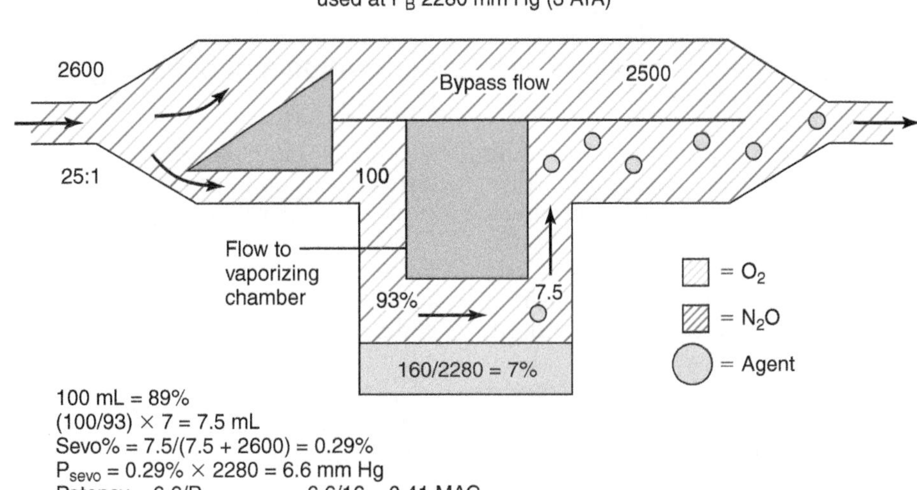

FIGURE 3-15 Use of a concentration-calibrated variable bypass sevoflurane vaporizer under hyperbaric conditions. ATA, absolute atmospheric pressure; MAC, minimum alveolar concentration; P_B, barometric pressure; P_{MAC1}, partial pressure of a potent inhaled agent at a concentration of 1 MAC.

16 mm Hg gives a potency output of 0.41 MAC (6.6/16). Thus a variable bypass sevoflurane vaporizer set to deliver 1% (0.5 MAC under conditions of 1 atm 760 mm Hg) delivers 0.41 MAC at 3 atm, or approximately 0.8 times the anesthetic potency expected (see Fig. 3-15).

To summarize, when used at atmospheric pressures greater than 760 mm Hg (sea level), a variable bypass vaporizer output concentration that is less than that set on the dial in volumes percent, but potency decreases by a lesser amount.

These examples show that although changing ambient pressure affects the output of a variable bypass vaporizer to a significant degree in terms of volumes percent, the effect on anesthetic potency (i.e., MAC multiple) is less dramatic. In the examples discussed, it was assumed that ambient pressure has a negligible effect on SVP. It is also assumed that the set splitting ratios remain constant as ambient pressure changes. In reality, however, changes in gas density occur with changes in ambient pressure and may affect the splitting ratios slightly (see Appendix). From a clinical point of view, however, the anesthetic potency output expected for any given vaporizer dial setting changes little, even though vapor concentration (vol/vol) may be altered considerably. Again, it must be emphasized that vaporizer output concentration expressed in volumes percent is of limited value unless converted to an MAC multiple according to the concept of MAPP, as previously described.

Vaporizing Chamber Flow Controlled at Outlet

The potency output of a variable bypass vaporizer in which the vaporizing chamber gas flow is controlled by a variable orifice located at the vaporizing chamber outlet is unaffected by changes in barometric pressure. With this design, the exit split ratio will apply and is unchanged. Consider the design of a vaporizer used to create 1% sevoflurane. In Figure 3-8, the exit split ratio to create 1% sevoflurane is 20:1. Under the same hypobaric conditions as in the previous section, PB is 500 mm Hg. In the vaporizing chamber, the sevoflurane vapor concentration is 160/500 = 32% by volume. A flow of 100 mL/min of 32% sevoflurane is mixed with a bypass flow of 2000 mL/min; the sevoflurane concentration will be 32/2100 = 1.52% by volume. The partial pressure of sevoflurane will be 1.52% × 500 = 7.6 mm Hg, which is the same partial pressure/potency as 1% sevoflurane at 760 mm Hg.

Under hyperbaric conditions of 2280 mm Hg, in the vaporizing chamber the sevoflurane vapor concentration is 160/2280 = 7% by volume. A flow of 100 mL/min of 7% sevoflurane is mixed with a bypass flow of 2000 mL/min. The sevoflurane concentration will be 7/2100 = 0.33% by volume.

Arrangement of Vaporizers

Very old, now-obsolete models of anesthesia machines had up to three variable bypass vaporizers arranged in series, making it possible for carrier gas to pass through each vaporizer, albeit all through a bypass chamber, to reach the common gas outlet of the anesthesia machine. Without an interlock system, which permits only one vaporizer to be in use at any one time, it was possible to have all three vaporizers turned on simultaneously. Apart from potentially delivering an anesthetic overdose to the patient, the agent from the upstream vaporizer could contaminate agents in any downstream vaporizer.[16] During subsequent use, the output of any downstream vaporizer would be contaminated. The resulting concentrations in the emerging gas and vapor mixture would be indeterminate and possibly lethal.

When such a serial arrangement of vaporizers was present, it was important to ensure that a vaporizer designed for a less volatile agent—such as methoxyflurane, with a low SVP—was not placed downstream relative to more volatile anesthetics, such as halothane. In such a case, halothane upstream would dissolve in the less volatile agent downstream. If during subsequent use the methoxyflurane vaporizer were set to deliver 1% (6 MAC), more than 6% halothane (8 MAC) could have been delivered from the methoxyflurane vaporizer.[19] The most desirable serial sequence of vaporizers from flowmeter manifold to common gas outlet was therefore methoxyflurane, sevoflurane, enflurane, isoflurane, then halothane.

These principles would also apply if a freestanding vaporizer were to be placed in series between the machine common gas outlet and the breathing circuit. Such arrangements, configured by the user and never by the machine manufacturer, are potentially dangerous and should not be used.[20] In addition to the contamination problem by agents upstream, such vaporizers are more easily tipped over, and use of the machine oxygen flush with the freestanding vaporizer turned on could pump a bolus of agent into the patient circuit, while disconnection of the vaporizer tubing could result in hypoxia in the patient circuit (see Chapter 30). Nevertheless, freestanding vaporizers are routinely used in conjunction with pump oxygenators for cardiopulmonary bypass. In such situations, the vaporizer should be securely mounted to the pump (see Fig. 3-16), and correct directional flow of gas through the vaporizer must be confirmed. Such vaporizers are subject to the same routine maintenance and calibration procedures as are all other anesthesia vaporizers.

With contemporary anesthesia workstations, only one vaporizer can be on at any given time. To prevent cross-contamination of the contents of one vaporizer with those of another, the ASTM standards require that a system be in place to isolate the vaporizers from one another and prevent gas from passing through more than one vaporizing chamber.[3] This specification is met by an interlock system. All contemporary anesthesia workstations incorporate manufacturer-specific interlock/vaporizer exclusion systems; these are described in subsequent sections concerning specific vaporizer models.

Calibration and Checking of Vaporizer Outputs

Vaporizers should be serviced according to the manufacturer's instructions, and their output should be checked to ensure that no malfunction exists. The vaporizer dial is set to deliver a certain concentration of the agent; the actual output concentration is measured by a calibrated anesthetic agent analyzer that analyzes gas sampled at the common gas outlet of the anesthesia machine. Currently available methods for practical vapor analysis are described in Chapter 8.

Preparation of a Standard Vapor Concentration

Although the physical methods for measurement described in Chapter 8 may be used to check vaporizer output, the agent analyzers themselves require calibration. For this purpose, standard vapor concentrations must be prepared and made available for use as the calibration gas standards. Standard mixtures are available from commercial suppliers.

Consider the preparation of a standard mixture of isoflurane in oxygen. Avogadro's volume states that 1 g molecular weight of a gas or vapor will occupy 22.4 L at standard temperature and pressure (STP, which is 760 mm Hg pressure, 0° C, or 273 K). Because the molecular weight of isoflurane is 184.5 Da, it would occupy 22.4 L at STP, and 1 g would occupy 22.4/184.5 L.

Charles' law states that the volume of a fixed mass of gas is proportional to absolute temperature if pressure remains constant; therefore 1 g of isoflurane occupies 0.13 L ([22.4 L/184.5 g] × [293 K/273 K]) at 20° C, or 293 K).

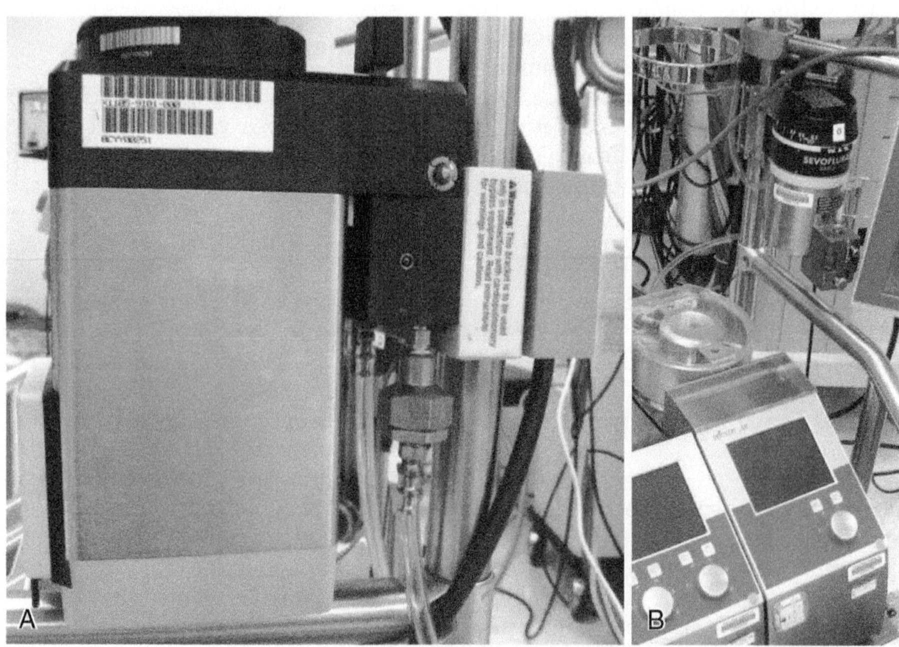

FIGURE 3-16 ▪ Freestanding vaporizer mounted on a pump oxygenator. Note the warning label on the mounting bracket in **A,** which reads, "This bracket is to be used only in conjunction with cardiopulmonary bypass equipment. Read instructions for warnings and caution."

One milliliter of liquid isoflurane weighs 1.5 g (specific gravity of 1.5; see Table 3-2); 1 mL of liquid isoflurane therefore generates 0.195 L of vapor ([22.4/184.5] × [293/273] × 1.5). Thus, 1 mL of liquid isoflurane produces 195 mL of vapor at 20° C.

By this type of calculation, a predetermined volume of liquid agent can be measured accurately and vaporized in a chamber of known volume to produce a calibration-standard gas mixture. As previously discussed, if a vaporizer is tipped on its side and liquid agent enters the bypass chamber or fresh gas piping, small volumes of liquid agent can generate very large volumes of vapor.

The above calculation by which volumes of liquid agent can be related to volumes of vapor at known temperatures and ambient pressures can be used to calculate the cost of an inhaled anesthetic. For example, an anesthetic of 1% isoflurane in 2 L/min N_2O and 1 L/min O_2 requires delivery of 30 mL/min (1% × 3 L), or 1800 mL/h of isoflurane vapor. This can be expressed as 1800/195, or 9.23 mL/h of liquid isoflurane. If, for example, a 100-mL bottle of isoflurane costs $10, the isoflurane anesthetic cost would be $0.92/h ([9.23/100] × $10).

EFFECT OF USE VARIABLES ON VAPORIZER FUNCTION

Fresh Gas Flow Rate

The output of a concentration-calibrated vaporizer is normally a function of fresh gas inflow rate. Because 1 mL of liquid agent produces approximately 200 mL of vapor, the hourly consumption of liquid agent can be estimated by the following formula:

$$3 \times \text{Vaporizer dial setting (vol\%)} \times \text{Fresh gas flow (FGF) rate (mL/min)}$$

The derivation of this approximation is as follows:

$$\text{vol\%} \times \text{FGF}(1000 \text{ mL/min}) = \text{mL/min of vapor used}$$

$$1\% \text{ of } 1000 \text{ mL} = 10 \text{ mL}$$

$$10 \text{ mL} \times 60 \text{ min} = 600 \text{ mL/h}$$

Divided by 200 (*approximate* number of mL vapor/mL liquid agent) = 3

Hence, the factor of 3 is used in the formula. Thus an isoflurane vaporizer set to deliver 1.5% at a flow rate of 4 L/min consumes approximately 18 mL/h (3 × 1.5 × 4) of liquid agent.

The output concentrations of contemporary concentration-calibrated vaporizers are virtually independent of the fresh gas flow rate when used with flows and vaporizer settings in the normal clinical range. At high concentration settings and with high fresh gas flows, output is slightly less than that set on the dial. Under these conditions, evaporation of the agent may be incomplete and temperature in the vaporizing chamber will fall. Thus, saturation of gas flowing through the vaporizing chamber is incomplete and output falls. The effects of flow rate on vaporizer output are shown for the Dräger Vapor 19.1 (Fig. 3-17). Again, note that these effects are of little clinical significance in most situations.

Fresh Gas Composition

As previously noted, changing the composition of the carrier gas, especially by adding or removing nitrous oxide, temporarily alters vaporizer output.[17] In the case of nitrous oxide, this effect is mainly due to solubility of nitrous oxide, although changes in gas density and viscosity also contribute to changes in output by affecting the flow split between vaporizing chamber and bypass gas flows.

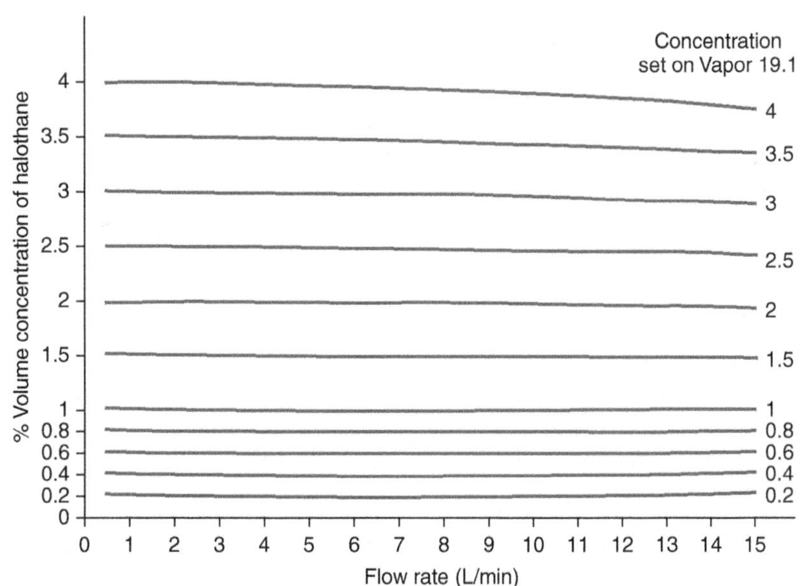

FIGURE 3-17 Effect of airflow rate on output concentration of a Dräger Vapor 19.1 halothane vaporizer (Dräger Medical, Telford, PA) at 22° C.

GE vaporizers are calibrated using 100% oxygen as the carrier gas.[18] If the carrier gas is changed to air or nitrous oxide, the vapor output decreases at low flow rates. At high flow rates and low concentration dial settings, the output may increase slightly.

Dräger Vapor 19.n vaporizers are calibrated with air as the carrier gas.[12] If 100% oxygen is used, the delivered output concentration is approximately 5% to 10% greater than the dial setting (air calibration value). When a mixture of nitrous oxide and oxygen (70:30) is used, the output is 5% to 10% lower than the dial setting. In this model of vaporizer, deviations from the dial setting increase with lower fresh gas flows, small amounts of agent in the vaporizing chamber, higher concentration dial settings, and extreme changes in the composition of the carrier gas.[11]

Effects of Temperature

As previously described, concentration-calibrated vaporizers are temperature compensated. The effects of changes in temperature are negligible under usual conditions of use. However, if the ambient temperature exceeds the vaporizer's specified range of performance, the vaporizer's output may become high. For example, the Dräger Vapor 19.n vaporizer is specified as accurate between 15° C and 35° C.[12] This is because as temperature increases, the vapor pressure of the anesthetic increases in a nonlinear manner, whereas the temperature compensation is linear. Indeed, the output may become unpredictable and uncontrolled if the boiling point of the agent is reached. Conversely, if the temperature falls below the specified range for use, the output may be unpredictably low.

Fluctuating Backpressure

A problem with older model vaporizers was that fluctuating or intermittent backpressure, the so-called *pumping effect*, may be applied to the vaporizer by changes in pressure downstream. Such pressure changes could be caused by intermittent positive-pressure ventilation (IPPV) in the patient circuit or operation of the oxygen flush control. These changes could produce changes in gas flow distribution within the vaporizer, which could lead to increased output if no compensatory mechanism existed. The effects of intermittent pressurization are greatest at low flow rates, low concentration settings, when small amounts of liquid agent are present in the vaporizer, and with large and rapid changes in pressure. Higher flow rates, higher dial settings, larger volumes of liquid agent in the vaporizer, and smaller, less frequent changes in pressure minimize the pumping effect.

Of the several explanations offered for the pumping effect, the most probable is that during pressurization, gas is compressed in the vaporizer in both the vaporizing chamber and the bypass. When the pressure decreases, anesthetic vapor leaves the vaporizing chamber, through both the normal exit pathway and the vaporizing chamber inlet, to enter the bypass flow. The intermittent addition of vapor to the bypass flow results in the observed intermittent increase in vaporizer output.

Contemporary vaporizers incorporate certain design features that minimize the significance of the pumping effect (discussed in the following section). Some older models, such as the Ohio Medical calibrated vaporizers, have a check valve in the vaporizer outlet to prevent transmission of increases in downstream pressure (see Fig. 3-11).[8] Certain models of GE anesthesia machines use a check valve just upstream of the common gas outlet to prevent retrograde transmission of downstream pressures (see Chapter 2). However, while the check valve is closed, the pressure upstream of it—and hence, that in the vaporizers—increases because of continuous fresh gas flow from the machine flowmeters. Thus the use of check valves can limit, but not totally eliminate, the pumping effect. For this reason, the newest anesthesia machine models do not use check valves in their design (see Chapter 2).

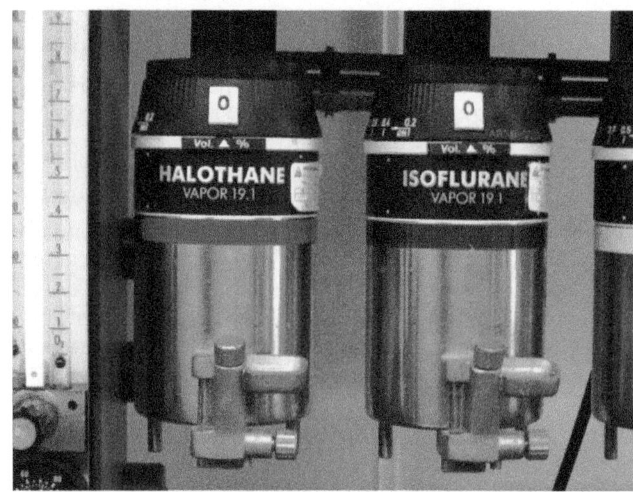

FIGURE 3-18 ■ Dräger Vapor 19.1 vaporizers (Dräger Medical, Telford, PA). Note the funnel-fill design, which has been superseded by an agent-specific key-fill design.

Contemporary Vaporizers

Dräger Vapor 19.n

The Dräger Vapor 19.n vaporizer is used on many contemporary Draeger Medical anesthesia workstations (Fig. 3-18). Up to three such vaporizers may be mounted on the back bar of the workstation and are connected to an interlock system designed to ensure that only one vaporizer or agent is in use at any time. When one vaporizer is turned on, the dials on the others cannot be turned from zero. Because failures have been reported,[21] the interlock system's function must be checked periodically (see Chapter 30).

A schematic of the Dräger Vapor 19.1 vaporizer is shown in Figure 3-19.[11] Its operation is fairly straightforward. With the concentration knob in the zero position, the on/off switch is closed. Fresh gas enters the vaporizer at the fresh gas inlet and leaves via the fresh gas outlet without entering the vaporizing parts of the unit. In this off state, the inlet and outlet ports of the vaporizing chamber are connected and vented to the atmosphere by a hole. The venting prevents pressure buildup in the vaporizing chamber, thereby preventing vapor from being driven under pressure into the fresh gas flow. Dräger specifies that venting results in a loss of only 0.5 mL/day of anesthetic into the operating room

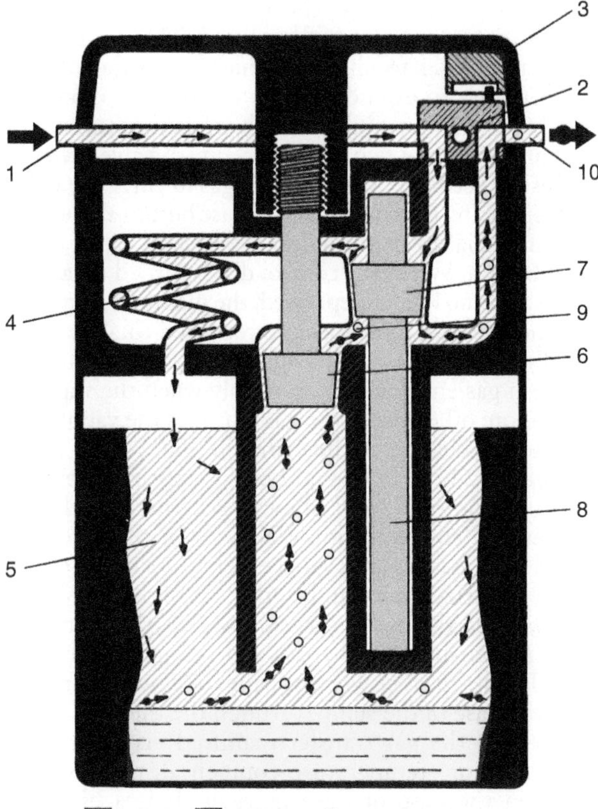

FIGURE 3-19 Schematic of Dräger Vapor 19.1 vaporizer. *1,* Fresh gas inlet; *2,* ON/OFF switch; *3,* concentration dial; *4,* pressure compensator; *5,* vaporizing chamber; *6,* control cone; *7,* bypass cone; *8,* expansion element; *9,* mixing chamber; *10,* fresh gas outlet. See text for details of operation. (Courtesy Dräger Medical, Telford, PA.)

atmosphere at a temperature of 22° C. The vaporizer can be filled only in the off state.[11]

When the concentration knob is turned to any concentration above 0.2 vol%, the on/off switch opens automatically, allowing the fresh gas to enter the interior of the vaporizer. The gas is immediately divided and follows two different routes: part of the fresh gas moves through a thermostatically controlled bypass, which compensates for temperature changes and maintains the correct volumes percent output as selected by the concentration knob. The remaining fresh gas moves through a pressure compensator, which prevents pressure changes that arise either upstream or downstream from being transmitted into the vaporizer and affecting the vapor output. From the pressure compensator, the gas continues into the vaporizing chamber, which contains the liquid anesthetic agent that is absorbed and evaporated by a special wick assembly. As the fresh gas moves through the vaporizing chamber, it becomes fully saturated with anesthetic vapor. The saturated gas leaves the chamber through a control cone, which is adjustable using the concentration knob. The saturated vapor and the fresh gas that did not pass through the vaporizing chamber are combined and leave through the fresh gas outlet. The combination of the bypass opening and the control cone opening determines the volumes percent of the vapor output. The output of this vaporizer is unaffected by changes in barometric pressure.

In this vaporizer, the pumping effect is prevented by the design of the long, spiral inlet tube, the pressure compensator. When the vaporizing chamber becomes decompressed, some anesthetic vapor does enter this spiral, but because of the spiral's length, the vapor does not reach the bypass gas flow.

Temperature compensation is achieved by the bypass cone and the expansion element. When temperature rises, bypass flow increases. Sudden changes in temperature require a compensation time of 6 min/° C for concentration output to be maintained within specifications.[11]

In the past, the Dräger Vapor 19.1 was available with either a funnel-type or an agent-specific filling device even though overfilling was not possible because the liquid level was limited by the position of the filling mechanism. The capacity of the vaporizing chamber is approximately 200 mL with dry wicks and 140 mL with wet wicks. This vaporizer does not include an antispill mechanism and should not be tilted more than 45 degrees. If tilted more than this, it should be flushed with a gas flow of 10 L/min with the concentration dial set to *maximum* before clinical use, similar to when the vaporizer has been tipped. Dräger states that a flushing time of 5 minutes is usually adequate if the vaporizer has been tilted only briefly and then immediately righted. If it has been tilted for a longer time, a minimum flush period of 20 minutes is required, during which it is advisable to drain liquid anesthetic from the vaporizing chamber.[11] The manufacturer stipulates that the vaporizer should be inspected and serviced every 6 months by qualified personnel and that an official maintenance record be kept.[11]

Whether in the off or on position, the Dräger 19.1 vaporizer is designed to limit the pressure of the fresh gas supply to a maximum of approximately 18 psig. Thus, if the anesthesia machine's common gas outlet becomes occluded and the oxygen flush is operated, a pressure of 45 to 55 psig could be transmitted retrograde from the common gas outlet back to the flowmeters if not relieved through the vaporizer. When more than one vaporizer is present (up to three are possible), pressure relief usually occurs through the one closest to the common gas outlet. Thus, even when the vaporizer is turned off, fresh gas continues to flow through the vaporizer unit, albeit not to the vaporizing sections, and is therefore subject to the pressure-limiting mechanism described above.

Dräger Vapor 2000

The Dräger Vapor 2000 uses the same operating principles as the Vapor 19.1, but it incorporates a number of improvements (Fig. 3-20). The sump has an increased capacity (300 mL) for liquid agent. In the United States, the Vapor 19.n vaporizers are bolted to Dräger machines and are not intended to be removed by the anesthesia caregiver. This is to prevent the problems associated with a vaporizer being tipped more than 45 degrees. If the vaporizer is to be transported, it first must be drained of any agent. The Vapor 2000 is designed so that no emptying is required before transportation, and the unit can be removed by the anesthesia caregiver. The spill-proof design ensures that even violent shaking cannot cause any liquid anesthetic to enter the concentration control

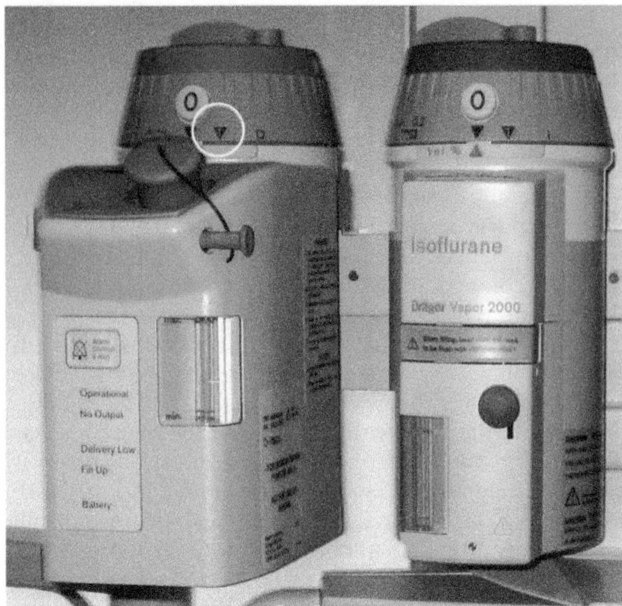

FIGURE 3-20 ■ Dräger Vapor 2000 vaporizers (Dräger Medical, Telford, PA). The *white circle* indicates transport mode (T) on the concentration dial.

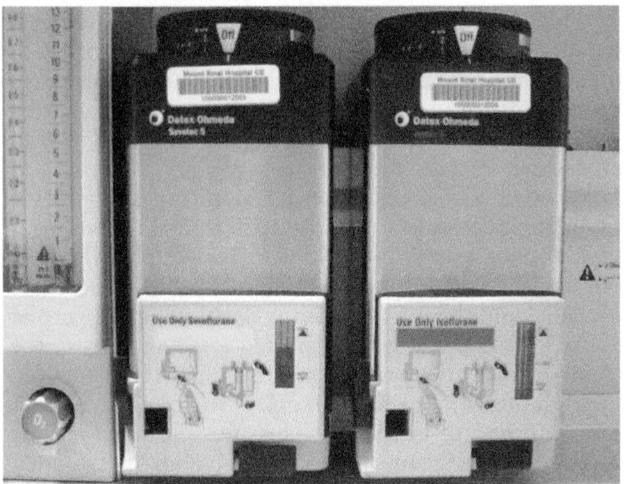

FIGURE 3-21 ■ Datex-Ohmeda Tec 5 vaporizers (GE Healthcare, Waukesha, WI) with a key-fill system.

elements or the atmosphere. To remove a Vapor 2000 from its mount on the machine, the control dial must first be turned to the T position, or transport mode, in which the vaporizer sump is isolated from the rest of the vaporizer (Fig. 3-20). The Vapor 2000 has an extended temperature range (15° C to 40° C) compared with 15° C to 35° C for the Vapor 19.n. The Vapor 2000 can be mounted on the Dräger plug-in system or the GE Select-a-tec system.

Tec 5

The Tec 5 vaporizer is used on recent GE Healthcare Datex-Ohmeda anesthesia machines (see Fig. 3-21).[18] Up to three vaporizers may be mounted and locked on a special, patented Selectatec manifold.

Each Tec 5 vaporizer is locked to the manifold by a Select-a-tec locking lever. Unless this lever is in the locked position, the concentration control dial release cannot be activated (Fig. 3-22). Once the lever is in the locked position, the dial release can be depressed. This operates the vaporizer interlock mechanism, which causes the interlock extension rods to extend laterally to adjacent vaporizers, minimizing the possibility of them being turned on. Simultaneously, the two Select-a-tec port valve actuating spindles are activated to allow fresh gas to enter the vaporizer. Depressing the control dial release button also enables the control dial to be turned to the desired vapor output concentration. When the control dial is turned off and the dial release is no longer depressed, the manifold port valves close and the extension rods are retracted to allow selection of another vaporizer. Thus, in the Select-a-tec system, fresh gas enters a vaporizer only when the vaporizer is turned on; otherwise, fresh gas bypasses the vaporizer(s) via a separate channel in the manifold (Fig. 3-23).

Figure 3-24, *A*, shows a Tec 5 vaporizer flow diagram, and Figure 3-24, *B*, shows a schematic of the Tec 5. When the concentration dial is set in the zero position, all gas passages are closed except for a channel linking the vaporizer inlet and outlet. As shown in Figure 3-24, *B*, when the dial is turned past 0%, the carrier gas stream is split between bypass and vaporizing chamber flows. Bypass gas flows vertically downward from *a*, across the base of the sump, through the thermostat to *c*, and back up the gas transfer manifold via *d* to *e*. The thermostat or temperature-compensating device is located in the base of the vaporizer. It is a bimetallic strip design, which increases bypass flow as temperature rises and decreases bypass flow as temperature falls.

The Tec 5 incorporates an IPPV chamber to minimize the pumping effect. The fresh gas flowing to the vaporizing chamber flows through an IPPV assembly designed to minimize the pumping effect before it reaches the vaporizing chamber and wick assembly system. There the gas becomes saturated with anesthetic vapor and flows onward to combine with the bypass gas flow and exit the vaporizer.

In the Tec 5 vaporizer, temperature compensation is achieved by a bimetallic strip valve rather than a bypass cone and expansion element. The vaporizer incorporates a keyed fill system, but some older models may still have a funnel-fill design. Although the Tec 5 incorporates an antispill mechanism, if the vaporizer is inverted, it is recommended that it be purged with carrier gas at 5 L/min for 30 minutes with the dial set to 5%.[18]

The Tec 5 vaporizer has a liquid agent capacity of 300 mL with dry wicks and 225 mL with wet wicks. The vaporizer is calibrated at 22° C with oxygen at 5 L/min. As previously discussed, changes in carrier gas composition may affect agent output concentration.

The operator's manual recommends that the vaporizer be serviced every 3 years at an authorized service center.[18] Service should include complete disassembly; thorough cleaning; inspection for wear and damage; renewal of wicks, seals, and any worn components; replacement of discontinued parts with more current parts; checking of output; and recalibration if necessary.

Tec 7

The Tec 7 (see Fig. 3-25) is essentially the same as the Tec 5 (see Fig. 3-21) but has an improved ergonomic design, a 300-mL capacity for liquid agent, and an improved

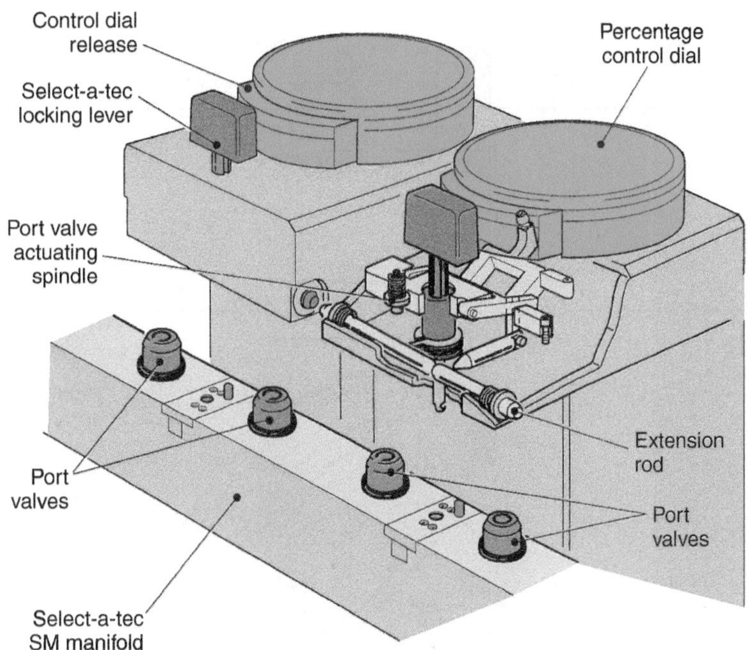

FIGURE 3-22 ■ GE Datex-Ohmeda Select-a-tec vaporizer interlock system. SM, series-mounted manifold. (Courtesy GE Healthcare, Waukesha, WI.)

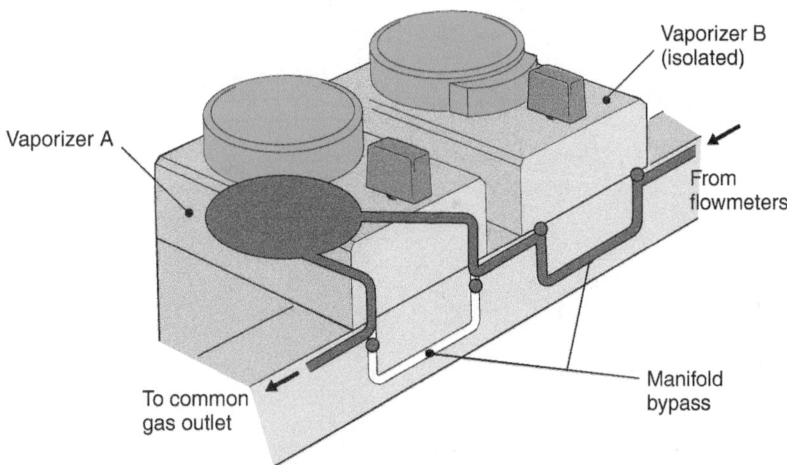

FIGURE 3-23 ■ GE Datex-Ohmeda series-mounted manifold gas circuit. Fresh gas from the machine flowmeters enters the manifolds, which incorporate pairs of series-connected, two-way port valves. When a Tec 5 vaporizer is locked onto the manifold and turned on (vaporizer A), both associated port valves are opened. Fresh gas from the manifold then flows into the vaporizer through the inlet port valves, and the gas-agent mixture exits via the outlet port valve. When the vaporizer is turned off (vaporizer B), or if no vaporizer is fitted to the manifold, each port valve is closed to allow gas to bypass the vaporizer via the manifold bypass circuit. (Courtesy GE Healthcare, Waukesha, WI.)

nonspill system to protect internal components if the vaporizer is moved or tilted and it does not require scheduled factory service.

Limitations of Earlier Selectatec Systems. As previously discussed, the Select-a-tec vaporizer extension system relies on vaporizers being adjacent to one another so that extrusion of the extension rods of one vaporizer prevents the other from being turned on. In earlier designs, the Select-a-tec system could be defeated. Thus, if the middle of the three vaporizers was removed, the remaining two, now nonadjacent, could both be turned on. In such a situation, one of the two outer vaporizers should be moved to the center position so that the vaporizers are adjacent. However, Select-a-tec systems manufactured after 1987 are designed so that when the middle vaporizer is removed, extrusion of the lateral rod of one vaporizer is transmitted to the other via vertical plates joined by a communicating bar. With this Select-a-tec system, the vaporizer interlock is therefore effective even if the center vaporizer is removed.

Desflurane Vaporizers

Tec 6

Desflurane (Suprane, Baxter Health Care Products, Deerfield, IL) is a potent, inhaled, volatile anesthetic approved for use by the U.S. Food and Drug Administration (FDA) in 1992. The physical properties differ considerably from those of other agents in clinical use (see Table 3-2). With an SVP of 669 mm Hg at 20° C and a boiling point of

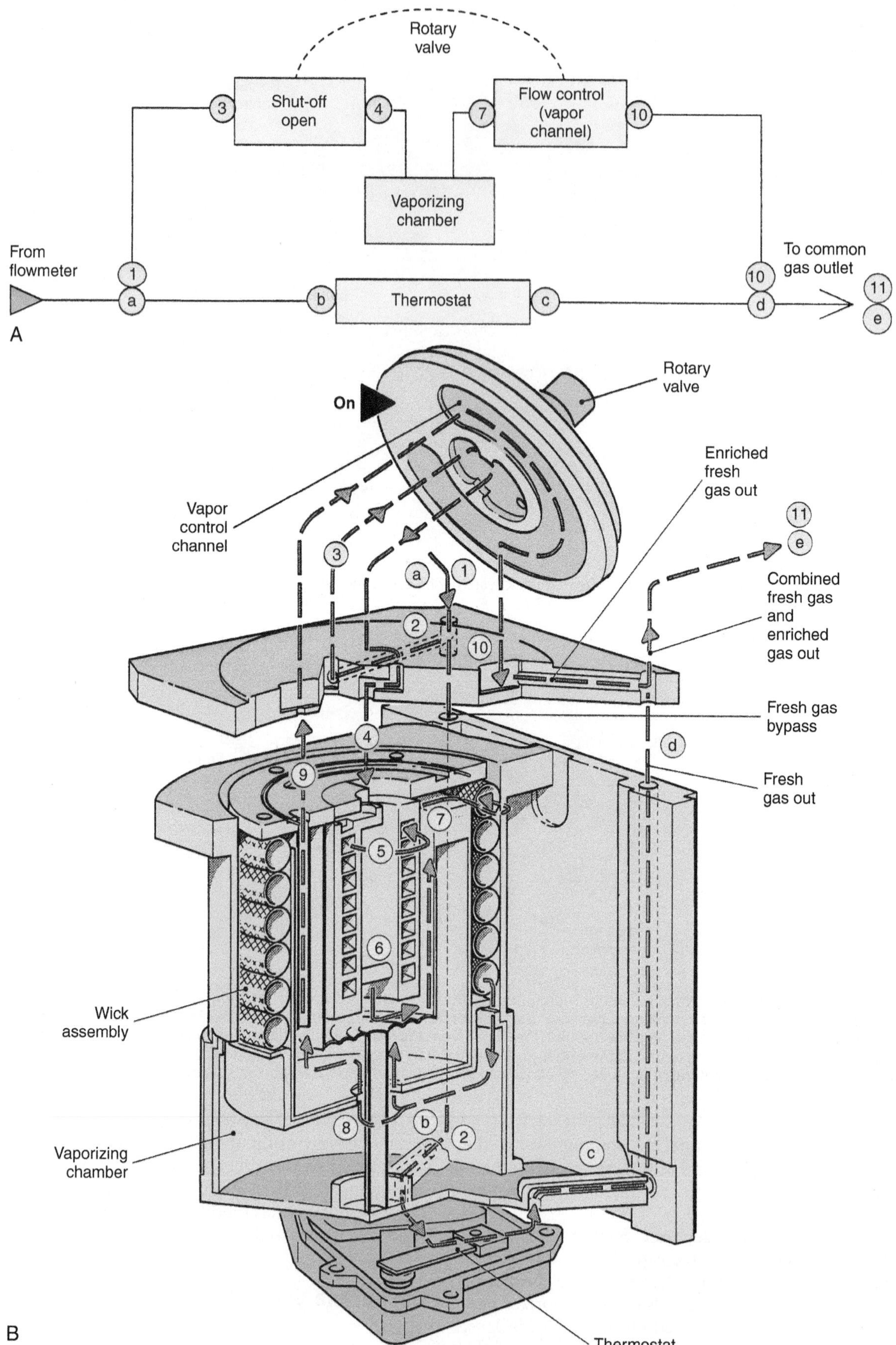

FIGURE 3-24 ■ **A,** GE Datex-Ohmeda Tec 5 vaporizer flow diagram. **B,** Schematic of Tec 5 vaporizer. Gas flow enters the vaporizer (*1*) and is split into two streams: the bypass circuit and the vaporizing chamber. Gas flows downward through the bypass circuit from *a,* across the sump base *b,* through the thermostat to *c,* and back up the gas transfer manifold via *d* to *e.* Gas flowing to the vaporizing chamber flows from *1* across the sump cover (*2*), where it is diverted via *3* through the central cavity of the rotary valve and back through the intermittent positive pressure ventilation (IPPV) assembly via *4, 5,* and *6.* Gas then flows from the IPPV assembly via *7* down the tubular wick assembly, where vapor is added; it then flows across the base of the vaporizing chamber above the liquid agent to *8.* From here the gas-vapor mixture flows via *9* through the sump cover to the proportional radial drug control groove of the rotary valve and back into the sump cover (*10*), where it merges with gas from the bypass circuit. The total flow then exits the vaporizer into the outlet port of the Select-a-tec manifold. (Courtesy GE Healthcare, Waukesha, WI.)

22.8° C at 1 atm, this agent is extremely volatile, which presents certain problems when it comes to vaporization and production of controlled concentrations of vapor. This agent clearly cannot be administered with the conventional mechanical variable bypass vaporizer design used for halothane, enflurane, isoflurane, and sevoflurane. If a variable bypass vaporizer were somehow filled with desflurane, an increase in temperature to above 22.8° C would result in the desflurane boiling in the vaporizing chamber and would lead to uncontrolled output of desflurane vapor from the vaporizer. The consequences of misfilling contemporary agent-specific variable bypass vaporizers with desflurane at 22° C have been predicted.[22] Thus, at 22° C, an enflurane vaporizer set to deliver 3 MAC (~5%) enflurane would deliver 16 MAC (~96%) desflurane.

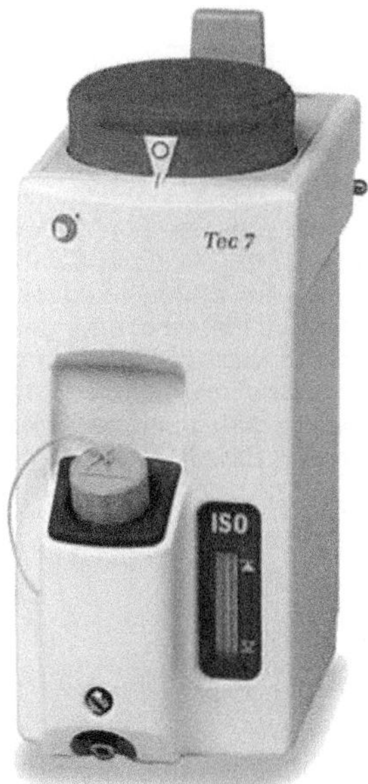

FIGURE 3-25 ■ Tec 7 isoflurane vaporizer (GE Healthcare, Waukesha, WI).

The Tec 6 concentration-calibrated vaporizer was specifically developed for the controlled administration of desflurane (Fig. 3-26). It was designed to make the practical aspect of the clinical administration of desflurane no different from that of other potent inhaled agents with the Tec series of vaporizers. The principle of operation of the Tec 6 is that liquid desflurane is heated in a chamber, or sump, to 39° C to produce vapor under pressure (~1500 mm Hg, or 2 atm absolute pressure). As Figure 3-27 illustrates, this is analogous to having a reservoir of compressed gas in a tank. The vapor leaves the sump via a variable pressure–regulating valve, the opening of which is continuously adjusted based on the output from a pressure transducer to ensure that the pressure of the desflurane vapor entering the rotary valve in the user-controlled concentration dial is the same as the backpressure generated by the fresh gas inflow from the anesthesia machine flowmeters into a fixed restrictor. The concentration dial and rotary valve control the quantity of desflurane vapor added to the fresh gas flow so that what emerges from the vaporizer outlet is the dialed-in concentration of desflurane. In the Tec 6, unlike other concentration-calibrated vaporizers, no fresh gas enters the desflurane sump. In addition, the Tec 6 is calibrated by the manufacturer with 100% oxygen as the fresh gas.

As the oxygen enters the vaporizer, it flows through a fixed restrictor (see Fig. 3-27). This is a device that offers a fixed *resistance*, defined as change in pressure per unit of flow. The resistance is approximately 10 cm H_2O/L/min over a wide range of gas flows. The backpressure created by gas flowing through the fixed restrictor is therefore proportional to the main gas flow as set on the machine flowmeters; this backpressure changes according to Poiseuille's law for laminar flow:

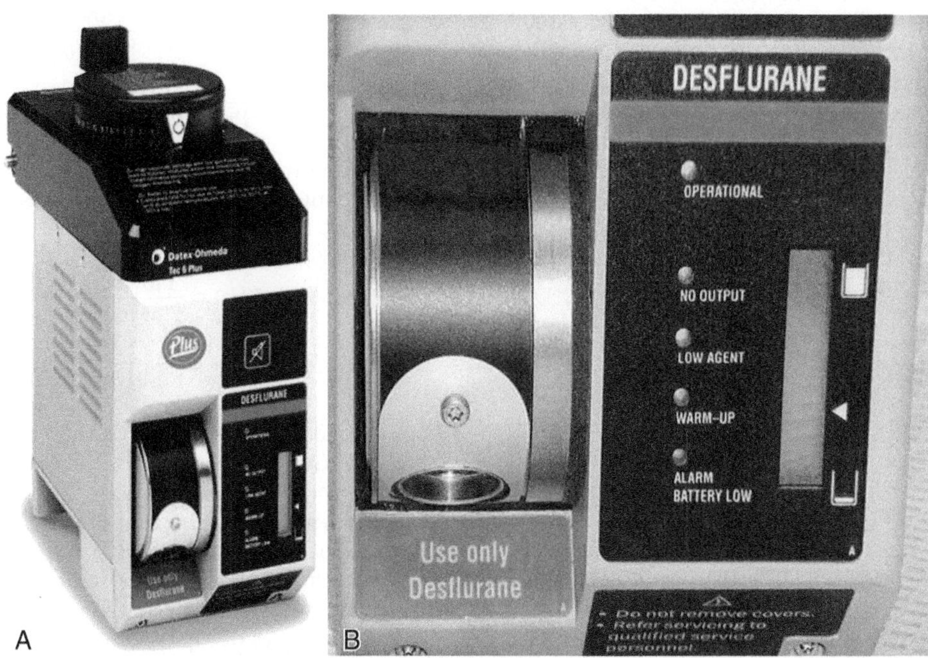

FIGURE 3-26 ■ **A,** GE Healthcare (Waukesha, WI) Tec 6 vaporizer for desflurane. **B,** Close-up of front panel shows status lights and display for agent fill status.

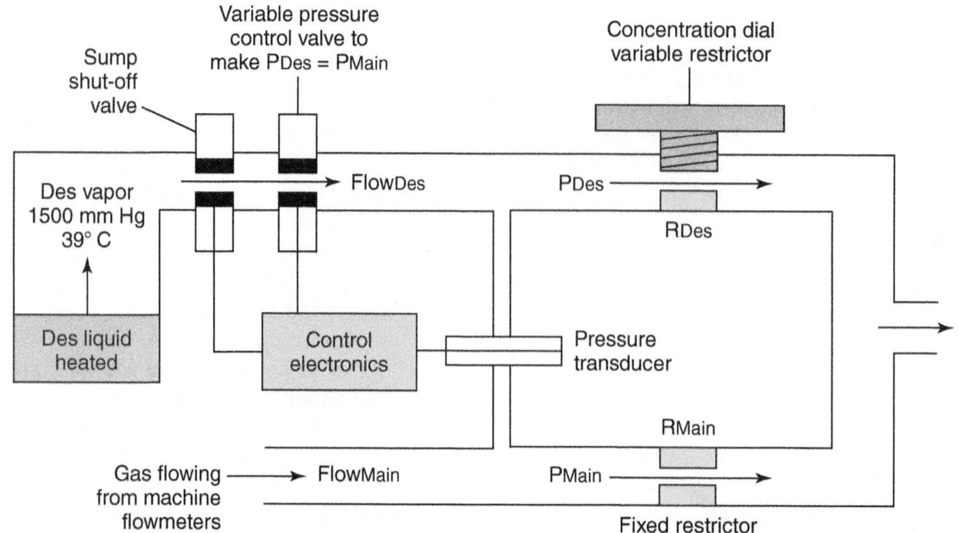

FIGURE 3-27 Simplified schematic of the Datex-Ohmeda Tec 6 vaporizer (GE Healthcare, Waukesha, WI). Liquid desflurane (*Des*) is heated in the sump to 39° C to produce vapor under pressure (~1500 mm Hg). The variable pressure control valve is continuously adjusted by an output from the differential pressure transducer to ensure that the pressure of the desflurane vapor upstream of the rotary valve (concentration dial variable restrictor) is the same as the pressure of the fresh gas inflow to the fixed restrictor. The concentration dial and rotary valve control the quantity of desflurane vapor added to the fresh gas flow so that what emerges from the vaporizer outlet is the dialed-in concentration of desflurane. No fresh gas enters the desflurane vaporizing chamber; this is in contrast to the other Tec series vaporizers, which are of the variable bypass design. *FlowDes,* flow of desflurane vapor; *FlowMain,* gas flow from the machine flowmeters (O_2, N_2O, air); *PDes,* pressure of desflurane vapor flowing into concentration dial variable restrictor; *PMain,* pressure of gas flowing into fixed restrictor; *RDes,* resistance to flow of desflurane created by variable restrictor; *RMain,* resistance of fixed restrictor.

$$\text{Flow} = \frac{(\pi \times P \times r^4)}{(8 \times \eta \times L)}$$

where π is 3.142, P is the pressure difference across the resistor, r is the radius of the resistor, η is the viscosity of the gas flowing, and L is the length of the resistor. That is, flow is directly proportional to pressure. By sensing this backpressure via a pressure transducer and ensuring that the pressure of the desflurane vapor entering the variable restrictor is always made equal to this pressure via the control electronics and variable pressure control valve, the variable restrictor provides a means to control the concentration of desflurane (Figs. 3-27 and 3-28). Thus,

$$\text{Resistance} = \frac{\Delta\ \text{Pressure}}{\Delta\ \text{Flow}} \tag{3-1}$$

For the main gas flow of oxygen entering the fixed restrictor,

$$\text{Resistance (main)} = \frac{\text{Pressure (main)}}{\text{Flow (main)}}$$

or

$$\text{Flow (main)} = \frac{\text{Pressure (main)}}{\text{Resistance (main)}} \tag{3-2}$$

But Resistance (main) is a fixed resistor and is therefore constant (K in equation 3-4, or 10 cm H_2O per L/min), so Flow (main) $\propto$ Pressure (main).

For the desflurane flow entering the concentration dial variable restrictor,

$$\text{Flow (des)} = \frac{\text{Pressure (des)}}{\text{Resistance (des)}}$$

$$\text{Concentration (des)} = \frac{\text{Flow (des)}}{\text{Flow (main)} + \text{Flow (des)}} \tag{3-3}$$

If Flow (des) is low compared with Flow (main), Flow (des) in the denominator of equation 3-1 can be ignored; thus,

$$\text{Concentration (des)} = \frac{\text{Flow (des)}}{\text{Flow (main)}} = \frac{\text{Pressure (des)} \times \text{K}}{\text{Pressure (main)} \times \text{Resistance (des)}} \tag{3-4}$$

The pressure transducer, control electronics, and variable pressure control valve ensure that Pressure (des) = Pressure (main); therefore,

$$\text{Concentration (des)} = \frac{\text{Flow (des)}}{\text{Flow (main)}} \propto \frac{1}{\text{Resistance (des)}}\ \text{(approximately).} \tag{3-5}$$

Thus, it becomes apparent that the variable restrictor in the concentration dial—that is, the resistance to the flow of desflurane—can be calibrated in terms of desflurane concentration. The calibration of the variable restrictor is not linear, however; equation 3-3 above is only an approximation because the Flow (des) value in the denominator of equation 3-3 cannot always be ignored.

Some examples of vaporizer concentration dial and gas flow settings are presented to illustrate the application of these principles.

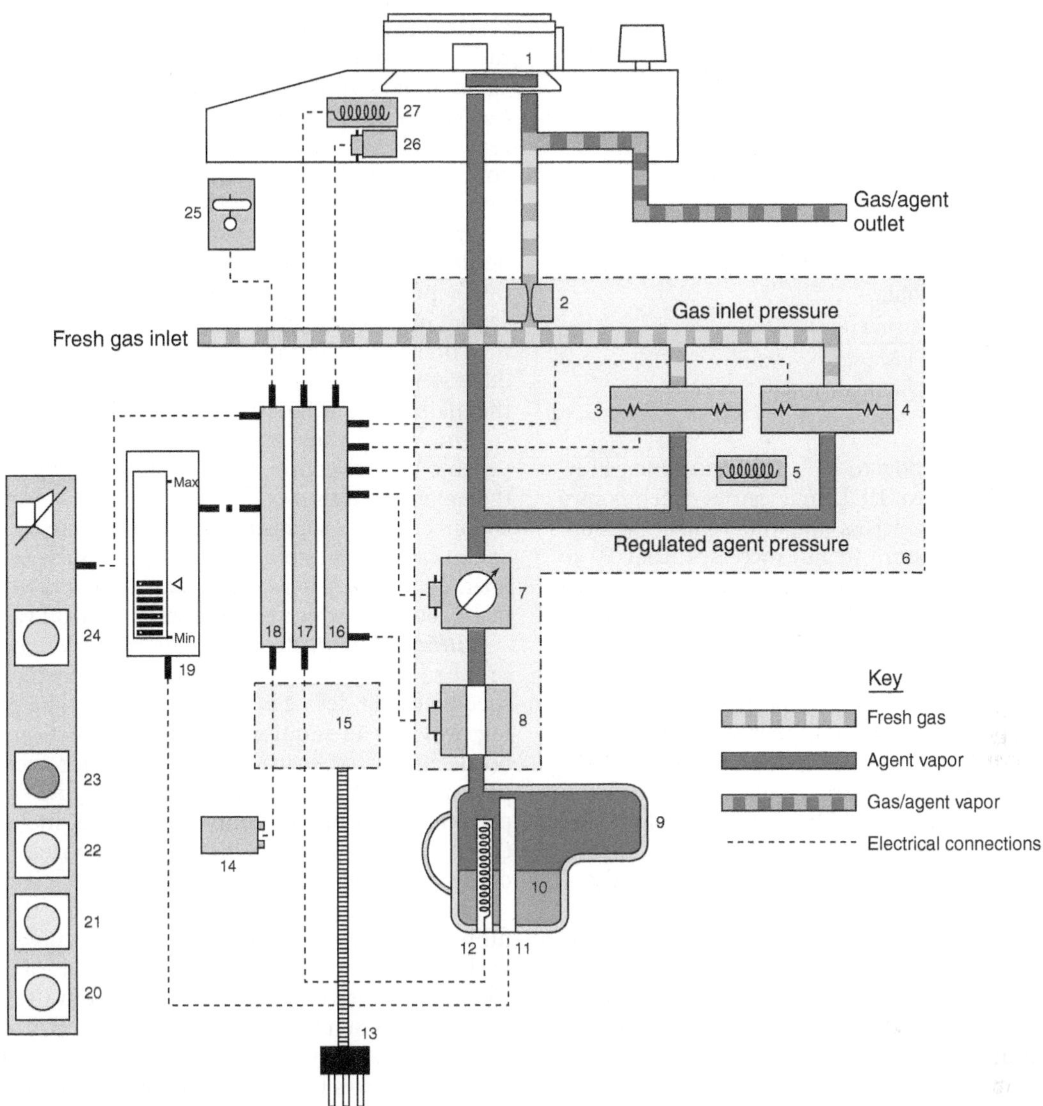

FIGURE 3-28 Detailed schematic of the GE Datex-Ohmeda Tec 6 desflurane vaporizer. *1,* Concentration dial and rotary valve; *2,* fixed restrictor; *3,* pressure transducer; *4,* pressure monitor; *5,* heater to prevent condensation of desflurane; *6,* vapor control manifold assembly; *7,* pressure regulating valve; *8,* shut-off valve; *9,* sump assembly; *10,* liquid desflurane; *11,* level sensor; *12,* sump heater to heat desflurane to 39° C; *13,* power cord; *14,* backup battery for alarms; *15,* power supply; *16,* control electronics printed circuit board; *17,* heater electronics; *18,* alarm electronics circuit board; *19,* liquid crystal sump agent level display; *20,* "alarm battery low" light-emitting diode (LED); *21,* "warm up/operational" LED; *22,* "low agent" warning LED; *23,* "no output" warning LED; *24,* "operational" LED; *25,* tilt switch (shuts down vaporizer if tilted excessively); *26,* solenoid dial lock; *27,* heater to prevent condensation of desflurane in valve plate (From *Ohmeda Tec 6 vaporizer operation and maintenance manual.* Madison, WI, 1992. Courtesy GE Healthcare, Waukesha, WI.)

Examples of Vaporizer Concentration Settings. Consider a Tec 6 vaporizer set to deliver 10% desflurane at a fresh gas flow of 5 L/min O_2.

$$\text{Concentration (des)} = \frac{\text{Flow (des)}}{\text{Flow (main)} + \text{Flow (des)}}$$

$$10\% = 0.10 = \frac{\text{Flow (des)}}{5000 + \text{Flow (des)}}$$

$$\text{Thus,}\quad 0.10 \times (5000 + \text{Flow (des)}) = \text{Flow (des)}$$

$$0.9 \times \text{Flow (des)} = 500 \text{ mL}$$

$$\text{Flow (des)} = \frac{500}{0.9} = 556 \text{ mL/min} \qquad (3\text{-}6)$$

Thus, at a 5 L/min flow of O_2 set to deliver 10% desflurane, the Tec 6 adds 556 mL/min of desflurane vapor to the main gas flow; in effect,

$$\frac{556}{5000 + 556} = \frac{556}{5556} = 0.10 = 10\% \qquad (3\text{-}7)$$

Once the main flow, in this case 5 L/min O_2, and the desflurane flow (calculated as above) are known, the ratio of resistances of the variable resistor, Resistance (des) in the concentration dial, to the fixed resistor, Resistance (main) in the main gas flow, may be calculated. Thus,

$$\text{Resistance (des)} = \frac{\text{Pressure (des)}}{\text{Flow (des)}}$$

$$\text{Resistance (main)} = \frac{\text{Pressure (main)}}{\text{Flow (main)}} \qquad (3\text{-}8)$$

But, Pressure (des) = Pressure (main); therefore,

$$\frac{\text{Flow (main)}}{\text{Flow (des)}} = \frac{\text{Resistance (des)}}{\text{Resistance (main)}} = \frac{5000}{556} = 9{:}1 \quad (3\text{-}9)$$

Resistance (des) may also be calculated as follows:

Pressure (des) = Pressure (main), which is 50 cm H_2O (because main gas flow is 5L/min)

Flow (des) = 556 mL/min

$$\text{Resistance (des)} = \frac{\text{Pressure (des)}}{\text{Flow (des)}} = \frac{50}{0.556} \quad (3\text{-}10)$$

$$= 90\,\text{cm}\ H_2O/\text{L/min}$$

Now increase fresh gas flow to 10 L/min. Increasing Flow (main) from 5 L/min to 10 L/min causes a temporary imbalance of pressures across the differential pressure transducer because Pressure (main) increases from 50 to 100 cm H_2O (see Figs. 3-27 and 3-28); bear in mind that Resistance (main) is 10 cm H_2O/L/min. The pressure imbalance is sensed by the differential pressure transducer, and the control electronics cause the variable pressure control valve to open wider—that is, to decrease its resistance to desflurane vapor flowing from the sump at a pressure of 1500 mm Hg—so that the flow of desflurane vapor into the concentration dial variable restrictor increases until Pressure (des) is also 100 cm H_2O. The increase in Flow (des) and thereby Pressure (des) ensures that the Tec 6 continues to deliver the 10% concentration as set on the dial.

Now increase the concentration dial setting from 10% to 15% while maintaining gas flow of 10 L/min. Increasing the concentration dial setting to 15% causes a decrease in Resistance (des). The resulting decrease in Pressure (des) relative to Pressure (main) is sensed by the differential pressure transducer, and the control electronics cause the variable pressure control valve to open wider—that is, to decrease its resistance to desflurane vapor flowing from the sump—so that Pressure (des) is increased to again be equal to Pressure (main). The resulting increase in Flow (des) ensures that the vapor concentration increases.

Now decrease the concentration dial setting from 15% to 5% at 10 L/min gas flow. Changing the concentration dial setting from 15% to 5% creates an increase in Resistance (des), which causes an increase in Pressure (des). The latter is sensed by the differential pressure transducer because Pressure (des) is now greater than Pressure (main), and the control electronics cause the variable pressure control valve to decrease its opening—that is, to increase its resistance to desflurane vapor flowing from the sump—thereby decreasing Flow (des) until Pressure (des) once again equals Pressure (main).

Special Considerations

Design Features of the Tec 6. The design of the Tec 6 is shown in Figures 3-26 and 3-27.[23,24] The sump, when full, contains 450 mL of desflurane. Because the sump is pressurized to 1500 mm Hg, the agent level is sensed electronically and is shown on a liquid crystal display (LCD) rather than the sight glass used in variable bypass vaporizers. When the vaporizer is energized by connecting the power cord to an electrical outlet, a heater in the sump heats the agent to 39° C and maintains that temperature via thermostatic controls. While the agent is being heated, the sump shut-off valve is held closed, thus keeping the agent in the sump. The vaporizer is not operational during the warm-up period because the sump shut-off valve remains closed, and a solenoid locking device prevents the concentration dial from being turned to ON. Once operational (at 39° C), the dial lock is released and, when the dial is turned on, the sump shut-off valve is opened to permit desflurane vapor to flow to the pressure-regulating valve.

To prevent condensation, or "rain out," of desflurane vapor, in addition to the heater in the sump, heaters in the rotary valve and in the vicinity of the pressure transducers, which sense the backpressures that result from the main gas flow and the flow of desflurane.

The Tec 6 thus differs considerably from mechanical variable bypass vaporizers; none of the fresh gas flow enters the vaporizing chamber. The Tec 6 requires electrical power and incorporates sophisticated electronics to ensure normal operations and a display panel to inform the user about its operational status. It also has alarms to alert personnel to any malfunction, in which case the sump shut-off valve closes.

Filling System. Because of its high SVP, desflurane is supplied in plastic-coated glass bottles to which an agent-specific filling device is firmly attached. The plastic coating provides an additional layer of protection if the glass bottle breaks or shatters. The vaporizer incorporates a patented, agent-specific filling system (SAF-T-FIL) that permits filling of the sump at any time, including when the vaporizer is in use. This may be important because of desflurane's low blood-gas partition coefficient.

During filling, the bottle is locked to the vaporizer filling system and the high pressure of vapor in the sump at 39° C is transmitted to the interior of the bottle, which helps drive liquid desflurane from the bottle into the sump. When filling is complete, the bottle is disconnected from the vaporizer fill system and the valve on the bottle closes to avoid loss or spillage of agent. At this time the bottle contains vapor at 39° C and a pressure of 1500 mm Hg. As the bottle and its contents cool to room temperature, the pressure in the bottle decreases toward atmospheric pressure (760 mm Hg at 22.8° C).

Draining the Vaporizer. The Tec 6 can be drained before returning it for service, but a special draining kit is required and the accompanying instructions must be followed carefully. The manufacturer warns that failure to follow the instructions may result in rapid loss of pressure and/or agent, which could cause injury to personnel.[24]

Effect of Fresh Gas Composition on Performance. The Tec 6 is calibrated by the manufacturer with 100% O_2. Performance accuracy at 5 L/min oxygen is specified as ±0.5% of delivered agent or ±15% of the dial setting, whichever is greater.[24]

From Poiseuille's law, laminar flow through a resistor is determined as follows:

$$\text{Flow} = \frac{\pi \times P \times r^4}{8 \times \eta \times L} \quad (3\text{-}11)$$

where π is 3.142, P is the pressure difference, r is the radius, η is viscosity, and L is length. Thus,

$$\text{Flow} \propto \frac{\text{Pressure}}{\text{Viscosity}},\ \text{or Pressure} \propto \text{Flow} \times \text{Viscosity} \quad (3\text{-}12)$$

The Tec 6 design uses backpressure from gas flow through the fixed resistor to measure flow (see Fig. 3-27). If the viscosity of the gas flowing through the fixed resistor were to decrease, the same flow would result in a lower backpressure. This backpressure is used to determine the pressure of desflurane in the variable resistor in the concentration dial. A lower pressure results in a lower flow of desflurane vapor through the variable resistor.

Of the gases on the anesthesia machine, oxygen is the most viscous and nitrous oxide is the least viscous. Thus changing the main gas flow composition from oxygen to oxygen/nitrous oxide decreases gas viscosity; the output concentration of desflurane from that setting on the dial therefore decreases. Differences between the actual concentration produced and the dial setting are greatest, up to 20% of dial setting, with high concentrations of nitrous oxide at low gas flow rates. The clinical implications of this are minimal, however, because the anesthetic effect lost by the decrease in desflurane is offset by the anesthetic effect of the nitrous oxide.[24,25]

Effects of Changes in Altitude on Output. The Tec 6 accurately delivers the dialed-in concentration of desflurane in terms of volumes percent, even at altitudes other than sea level. At sea level, 7% desflurane (1 MAC) creates a desflurane partial pressure of 53 mm Hg (7% of 760 mm Hg, the P_{MAC1}). At high altitude, if the ambient pressure were 500 mm Hg, the same 7% desflurane creates a desflurane partial pressure of only 35 mm Hg (7% of 500 mm Hg), which is only 0.66 of the P_{MAC1}. To compensate for this decrease in potency output at increased altitude, a higher concentration (10.4%) must be set on the dial because 10.4% of 500 mm Hg renders a desflurane partial pressure of 52 mm Hg. Conversely, at higher ambient pressures, such as those at altitudes below sea level, a lower concentration dial setting would be indicated to create the same potency (MAC equivalent) output. Recommendations as to how the dial setting should be adjusted at various altitudes are provided in the operator's manual.[24]

Interlock System. Although the Tec 6 is manufactured by GE Healthcare and is therefore mountable on a Selectatec manifold on a Datex-Ohmeda anesthesia machine, a version is also available for mounting on Dräger Medical workstations.

Tipping the Vaporizer. The Tec 6 incorporates a tilt switch. If the Tec 6 is tilted while in operational mode, the tilt switch activates an audible alarm, the sump shutoff valve closes (see Fig. 3-27), the vaporizer stops delivering vapor, and the red NO OUTPUT warning indicator flashes (see Fig. 3-26, *B*).

D-Vapor

The Dräger D-Vapor desflurane vaporizer by is an adjunct to the company's Vapor 2000 series of vaporizers (Fig. 3-29).[25] The operating principles are the same as those of the Tec 6, but the D-Vapor weighs significantly less. Similar to other vaporizers in the Vapor 2000 series, the D-Vapor is hermetically sealed when removed from an anesthesia system, allowing transport in any position, even when filled. The 300 mL reservoir capacity of the tank can hold the entire contents of a standard desflurane bottle. Like the Tec 6, the D-Vapor is electrically powered, but it also features 5 minutes of emergency battery operation to ensure that dose

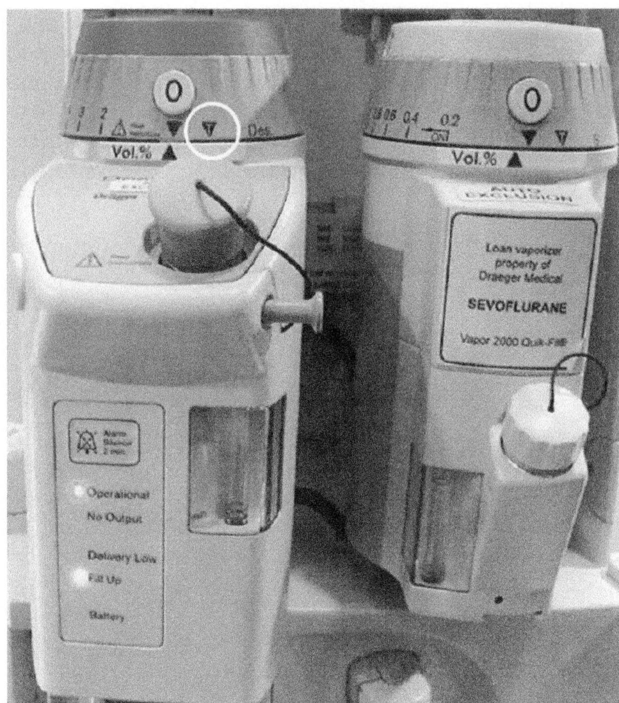

FIGURE 3-29 *Left,* Dräger D-Vapor vaporizer for desflurane (Dräger Medical, Telford, PA). *Right,* Dräger Vapor 2000 sevoflurane vaporizer. The *white circle* indicates transport (T) setting.

settings remain constant even during a brief power failure. Another difference is that the D-Vapor has a conventional sight glass to assess the level of liquid agent in the sump rather than the liquid crystal display of the Tec 6.

Penlon Sigma Alpha

Penlon Limited (Abingdon, United Kingdom) has also added a desflurane vaporizer, the Sigma Alpha, to their Sigma series of vaporizers (Fig. 3-30). The principle of operation differs from that of the Tec 6 and D-Vapor, however.

Special Considerations

Operating Characteristics. The Alpha vaporizer operates by dosing a controlled flow of vaporized desflurane into the fresh gas. It achieves this by maintaining a constant vapor pressure in a small heated chamber and using that vapor pressure to drive the vapor through a microprocessor-controlled proportional valve into the fresh gas system.

Figure 3-31 shows the schematic of this vaporizer, which consists of a number of elements: the reservoir, heater assembly, dosing valves, control mechanism, and redundant backup monitor/control system.

Startup. During switch-on and start-up procedures, the vaporizer control system performs a self-check of all internal systems and then calibraties the two fresh gas flow sensors and the backup vapor flow sensor. At this point the user can zero the "Agent Volume Used" display in preparation for logging if that information is required. The heater in the vaporizing chamber is turned on and brings the desflurane vapor chamber up to its operating temperature.

To provide a force to enable the liquid desflurane to be transferred from the reservoir to the heater assembly, a small mechanical pump is used to generate a pressure in the reservoir by pumping filtered room air into the reservoir. With fresh desflurane a small volume of air is dissolved into the desflurane; the reservoir pressure is therefore constantly monitored to ensure that the pressure is maintained at a minimum level to guarantee adequate pressure, and hence adequate desflurane delivery, at all times. In some operational environments, the temperature of the vaporizer in general ensures that the minimum pressure is achieved in the reservoir without assistance from the pump.

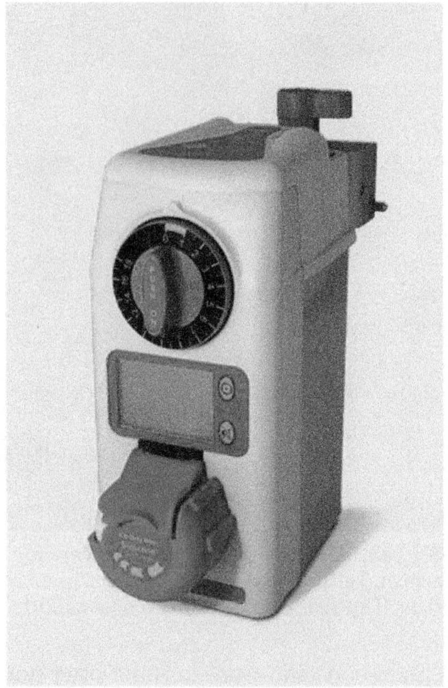

FIGURE 3-30 Penlon Sigma Alpha vaporizer for desflurane. (Courtesy Penlon, Abingdon, United Kingdom.)

Agent Vaporization. When the vaporizer is required to deliver desflurane after the initial start-up period, the liquid on/off valve is opened, and liquid desflurane flows into the heater chamber and vaporizes rapidly, raising the pressure in the heater chamber to at least that of the reservoir pressure to prevent further delivery of liquid desflurane. If the vapor pressure in the heater chamber falls, more liquid desflurane is forced into the heater chamber from the reservoir, allowing more vaporization of the liquid desflurane and raising the pressure again. If pressure exceeds that in the reservoir, the pressure is vented back to the reservoir through the liquid desflurane delivery line, either as vapor or as a condensed liquid.

Once running, this pressure system is self-controlling because the heater chamber temperature, and hence vapor pressure, is kept constant.

Agent Delivery. When in use, the required desflurane concentration is set using the rotary control dial on the front of the vaporizer. The user selects a desired concentration, and the vaporizer inlet and outlet fresh gas flow sensors monitor the fresh gas flow and N_2O concentration. The microprocessor then notes the pressure of the vaporized desflurane and the fresh gas flow rate and sets the calibrated delivery proportional valve to the correct opening to deliver the dialed-in desflurane concentration for that fresh gas flow. The vaporizer delivers desflurane vapor into the fresh gas flow at the required flow rate for

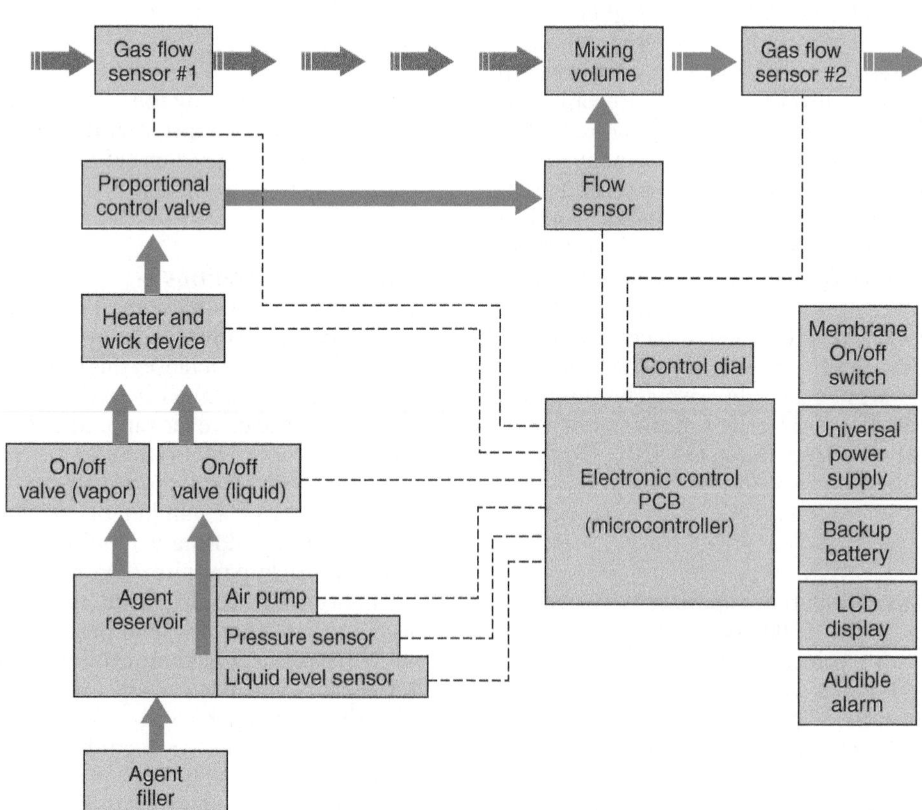

FIGURE 3-31 Schematic of Penlon Sigma Alpha desflurane vaporizer to show principles of operation. *LCD,* liquid crystal display; *PCB,* printed circuit board. (Courtesy Penlon, Abingdon, United Kingdom.)

the selected concentration, and a separate closed-loop control circuit measures the direct flow of desflurane to confirm correct desflurane vapor flows. Only the desflurane needed for vaporization is heated and maintained in a vapor form. The vapor pressure is automatically maintained because the vapor delivered into the fresh gas will be replaced by more vaporized liquid desflurane, and pressure will be maintained in the reservoir either by the excess pressure from the vapor chamber or by the external pump; this control system ensures a self-controlling and energy-efficient system.

Mixing Vaporized Agent into the Fresh Gas Supply. Fresh gas inlet and outlet flows are measured by flow-measuring devices. The gas flow sensors also detect the presence of nitrous oxide in the fresh gas supply and calculate the concentrations of oxygen and nitrous oxide. When desflurane is being delivered, the inlet and outlet flow sensors provide differential flow readings relative to the desflurane concentration irrespective of the fresh gas composition. This independent desflurane concentration measurement is used to provide a second redundant check for safe concentration delivery.

Vaporizer Filling. When the Penlon Sigma Alpha is used for desflurane administration, liquid desflurane is filled into the agent reservoir using a manufacturer-specific vaporizer filler connector design that is fully compatible with the standard desflurane closure and valve assembly attached to the SAF-T-FILL bottle top. The Alpha filler has no traditional sight glass but relies on a capacitive electronic level indicator to display the desflurane liquid level in the reservoir on the front panel display.

The vaporizer filler system contains several valves that open in sequence while the desflurane bottle is inserted and locked into the vaporizer filler by rotation of the vaporizer external filler knob. During the first part of the bottle insertion process, the bottle filler is sealed into the vaporizer filler with an O-ring seal, ensuring an airtight working environment. At this stage, the external filler knob is rotated clockwise and the bottle is drawn and locked into the vaporizer filler, opening the upper filling valve. Further rotation of the external filler knob will open the lower filling valve to the liquid chamber to allow the liquid desflurane to fill via the filling ports; an air return pathway allows a return of air to the emptying bottle. Toward the end of the rotation of the external filler knob, an air bleed valve opens briefly to equalize pressure throughout the filler and reservoir. Finally, on the last revolution of the external filler knob, the bottle valve is opened to allow liquid desflurane to flow into the vaporizer chamber.

When the desflurane liquid level in the reservoir is at its maximum, an air trap occurs in the air return (vapor return) line to the bottle and prevents further liquid desflurane being filled into the vaporizer in a manner similar to that of any traditional vaporizer filler system.

The bottle removal process is a reversal of the filling process. Note that by initially closing the bottle, the bottle and its internal volume, which may be under pressure, are isolated from the filler to minimize the spillage of desflurane vapor when the bottle is removed. The air bleed valve opens briefly again to break the air trap to ensure that pressures throughout the filler and reservoir are equalized. While both the upper and lower filling valves are still open, any liquid desflurane between the bottle and vaporizer filler drains from the bottle filler port and prevents leakage or pooling of desflurane above the vaporizer upper filling valve on final removal of the bottle. The upper and lower filling valves are closed just before the external filler knob reaches the bottle insertion/removal position.

Aladin Vaporizing System

Advances in technology and computerization of the workstation have led to development of the newly designed variable bypass, electrically powered Aladin vaporizing system used in the GE Datex-Ohmeda AS/3 Anesthesia Delivery Unit (ADU), Avance, and Aisys workstations (Fig. 3-32). The principles of operation differ from those of mechanical variable bypass vaporizers and from the Tec 6 design discussed above.

The Aladin vaporizer consists of two separate parts that must be joined to produce a functioning vaporizer. One is a sump, the detachable Aladin cassette that holds up to 250 mL of liquid anesthetic agent. Each anesthetic agent, including desflurane, has its own cassette with a unique agent-specific filling system (e.g., SAF-T-FILL for desflurane and key fill or Quick-Fil [Abbott Laboratories, Abbott Park, IL] for other agents) (Figs. 3-32 to 3-34). Five different cassettes are available, one for each of the currently available potent inhaled agents. The second part of the vaporizer is an integral component of the anesthesia workstation and contains the concentration control hardware and software. The agent-specific cassette identifies itself to the workstation by the arrangement of signature magnets at the top of the cassette (Fig. 3-35, *A*). The Aladin system monitors and controls gas and vapor at several points and also regulates flow through the nitrous oxide, oxygen, and air flowmeters; it will not permit the delivered oxygen concentration to fall below

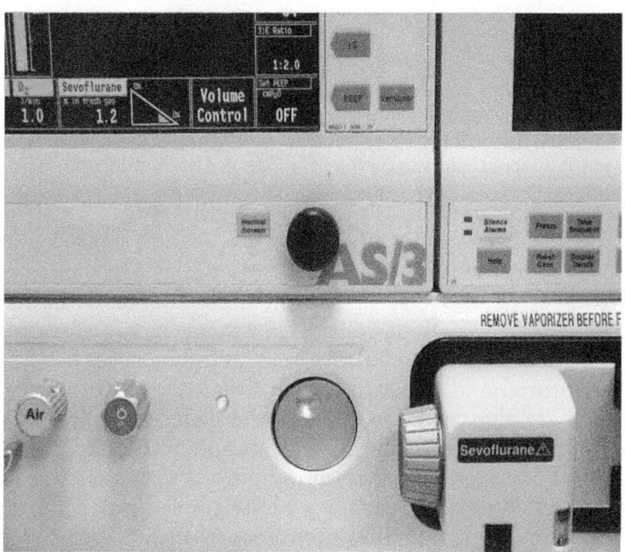

FIGURE 3-32 ▪ Aladin vaporizer system (GE Healthcare, Waukesha, WI) used on the AS/3 Anesthesia Delivery Unit and Aisys workstations.

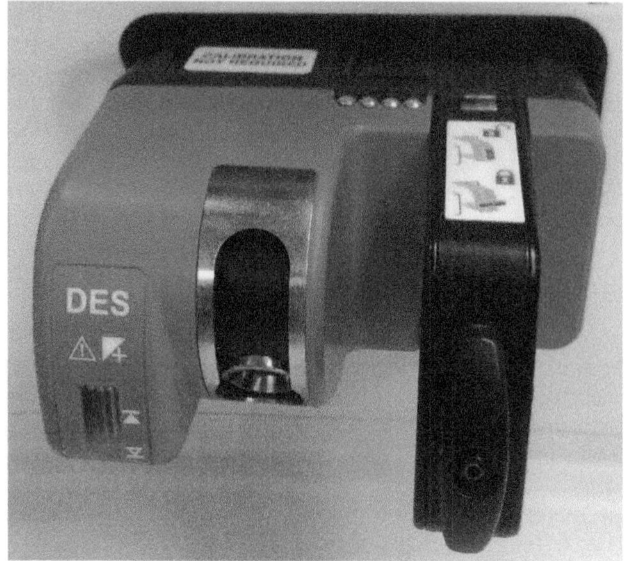

FIGURE 3-33 ■ Aladin vaporizer system (GE Healthcare, Waukesha, WI) cassette for desflurane.

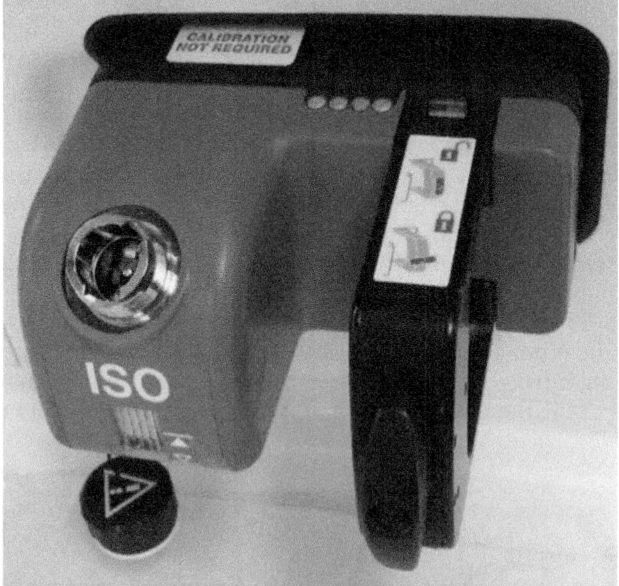

FIGURE 3-34 ■ Aladin vaporizer system (GE Healthcare, Waukesha, WI) isoflurane cassette. The workstation recognizes the agent-specific cassette by the arrangement of identification (signature) magnets (see Fig. 3-35).

25% at the machine's common gas outlet when nitrous oxide is in use. Gas flow from these sources is either delivered to or bypasses the anesthetic in the cassette. The flow issuing from the cassette and the bypass flows is monitored and adjusted by hardware and governed by software algorithms to produce the dialed-in concentration of anesthetic. The algorithms take into account the anesthetic agent, temperatures, and gas pressures in the cassette and bypass; each is separately measured.

Figures 3-35 and 3-36 show a schematic and principles of operation of the Aladin vaporizer.[26] The agent wheel, an electronic control on the front panel of the ADU (see Fig. 3-32; or ComWheel on the front panel of the Aisys Carestation), is used to set the desired concentration of agent to be delivered to the breathing system. A green light-emitting diode (LED) indicates that the vaporizer is on. The vaporizer is controlled by a central processing unit (CPU), and the flow restrictor in the bypass causes fresh gas from the gas flow controls to be split into a bypass flow and a flow that passes through a unidirectional valve, which prevents backflow from the Aladin cassette. The latter is an agent-specific cartridge that contains liquid anesthetic at its SVC at the ambient temperature (e.g., ([160/760] × 100% = 21 volume percents for sevoflurane at 20° C). Continuous monitoring of temperature and pressure in the cassette means that the agent vapor concentration there is always known. The concentration of anesthetic vapor delivered to the common gas outlet of the machine is determined by the concentration of agent vapor in the cassette and the ratio of cassette outflow to the bypass flow, both of which are continuously measured. The delivered concentration is controlled by the position of the agent proportional valve (see Fig. 3-36), which is continuously set according to information from the agent controller (the CPU).

Each Aladin cassette is essentially a flow-over vaporizer because it contains liquid agent that is vaporized as fresh gas flows between the agent-soaked wicks and baffles (see Fig. 3-35). It is equivalent to the sump of a traditional variable bypass vaporizer, but because it does not incorporate bypass flow channels, tilting the cassette during handling, changing, or filling is not hazardous.

The Aladin cassette for desflurane (see Fig. 3-33) incorporates an electronic liquid level measuring device; if less than 10% liquid desflurane (<25 mL) remains, an alarm message is displayed. If the temperature is below 22.8° C, the boiling point of desflurane, fresh gas must enter the cassette for vapor to be delivered via the exit connection. If the temperature is above 22.8° C, no fresh gas inflow is needed and the desflurane vapor is released by controlling the outflow valve. A fan is mounted inside the fresh gas control unit beneath the Aladin cassette housing and is required to heat the cassette when large amounts of agent are being vaporized. The fan operates when the cassette temperature is below 17° C and stops when it rises above 20° C.

The Aladin vaporizing system offers certain advantages, the greatest of which is that the CPU can control the concentration of any of the potent inhaled anesthetic agents. Separate vaporizers, or at least their individual flow-splitting mechanisms, are not required for each agent. Compared with Tec-type variable bypass vaporizers, the Aladin cartridges are relatively lightweight and easily exchanged, and there is no risk of agent spilling if the cartridge is tilted. An obvious disadvantage is that in the event of a prolonged power loss, such as after the workstation's back-up battery has been depleted, delivery of the volatile agent will cease. In contrast, conventional mechanical variable bypass vaporizers will function as long as there is a source of compressed gas to the machine.

APPENDIX: SPLITTING RATIOS

Leigh[27] has published a formal mathematical derivation of the splitting ratio (R) and a formula for calculating the

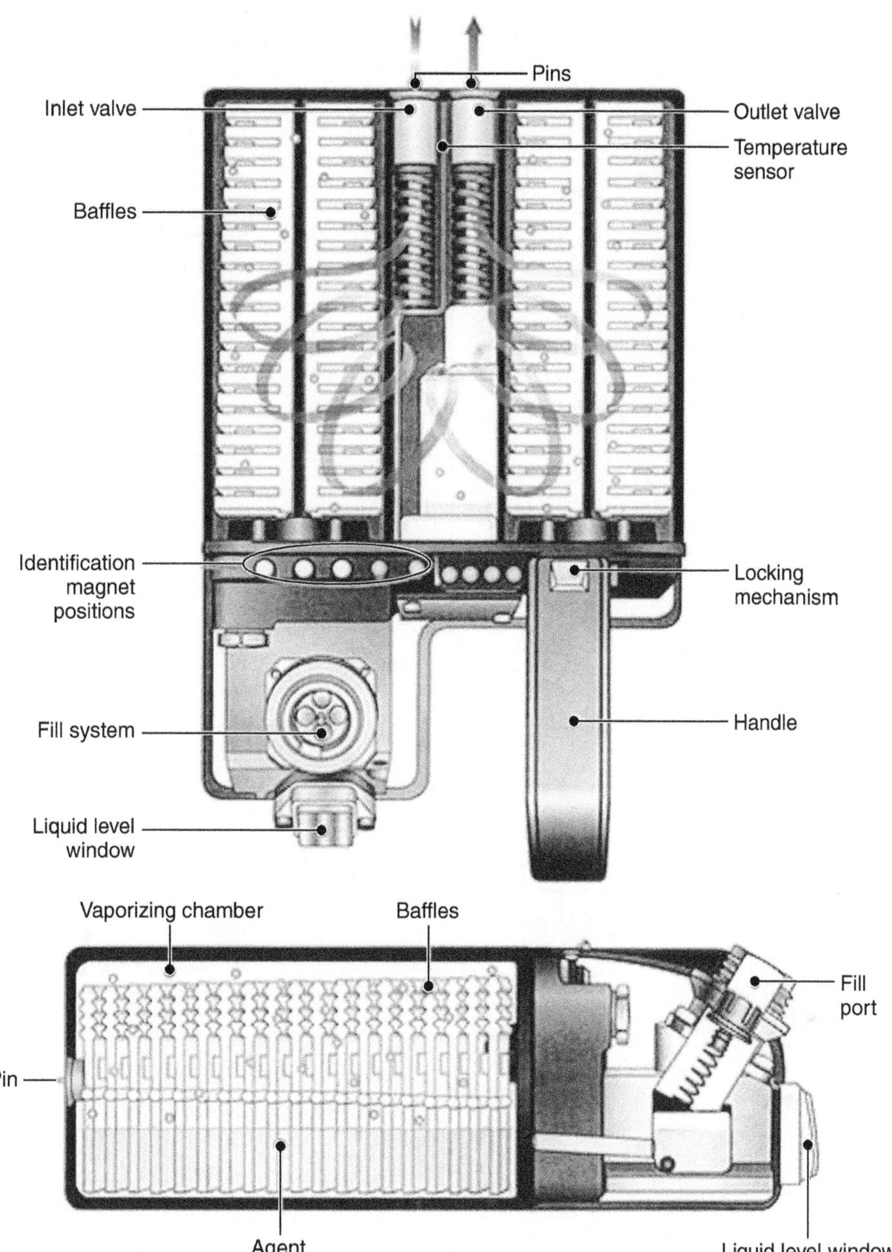

FIGURE 3-35 Schematic of Aladin vaporizer system cassette, which is the equivalent of the vaporizing chamber in a variable bypass vaporizer. Fresh gas flows over wicks and baffles containing liquid anesthetic agent. (Courtesy GE Healthcare, Waukesha, WI.)

splitting ratio for a given fractional concentration (*F*) of agent:

$$R=[(S/F)-1]/1-S$$

where *S* is the saturated vapor concentration of the agent (as a fractional concentration). Thus, for 1% isoflurane, F = 0.01, S = 0.31, and

$$R=[(0.31/0.01)-1]/1-0.31=30/0.69=44:1$$

The fractional concentration of agent (*F*) produced by a given splitting ratio (*R*) is

$$F=S/[R(1-S)+1]$$

Thus, for sevoflurane (S = 0.21) in a vaporizer set to a splitting ratio of 12:1:

$$F=0.21/[12(1-0.21)+1]=0.21/[12\times 0.79)+1]$$
$$=0.21/10.48=0.02,\ \text{or } 2\%$$

Compare these equations with the values in Table 3-3, which were derived from first principles. Furthermore, Dorrington[28] provides reasoning that changes in gas density that accompany changes in barometric pressure have no effect on splitting ratios.

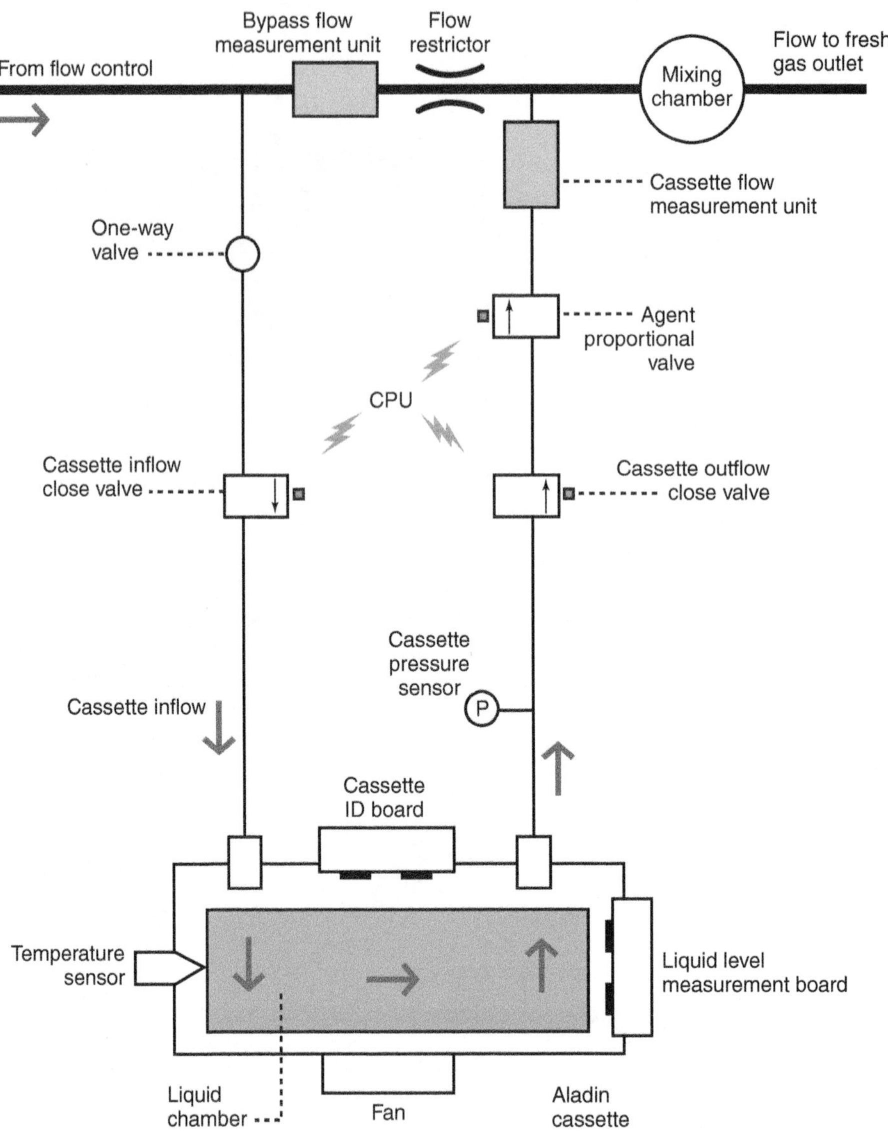

FIGURE 3-36 Schematic of Aladin vaporizer system to show principles of operation. CPU, central processing unit; ID, identification. (Courtesy GE Healthcare, Waukesha, WI.)

REFERENCES

1. Hill DW: *Physics applied to anaesthesia* ed 4, Boston, 1980, Butterworth, p 220.
2. *Minimum performance and safety requirements for components and systems of anesthesia gas machines, ASTM F1161-88,* Philadelphia, 1989, American Society for Testing and Materials.
3. *Standard specification for particular requirements for anesthesia workstations and their components, ASTM F-1850-00,* West Conshohocken, PA, 2000, American Society for Testing and Materials.
4. Parbrook GD, Davis PD, Parbrook EO: *Basic physics and measurement in anesthesia*, ed 4, Oxford, UK, 1995, Butterworth-Heinemann.
5. Fink BR: How much anesthetic? *Anesthesiology* 34:403–404, 1971.
6. James MFM, White JF: Anesthesia considerations at moderate altitude, *Anesth Analg* 63:1097–1105, 1984.
7. Keenan RL: Volatile agent overdose is potential cause of catastrophe, *Anesthesia Patient Safety Foundation (ASPF) Newsletter* 3(2):13, 1988.
8. *Operations and maintenance manual, Ohio calibrated vaporizers for ethrane, halothane and forane.* Madison, WI, 1980, Ohmeda (formerly Ohio Medical Products).
9. *Understanding the Tec 4 vaporizer,* Steeton, UK, 1985, Ohmeda.
10. *Dräger Vapor 19.1 operating instructions.* Lübeck, Germany, 1992, Drägerwerk AG.
11. *Dräger Vapor 2000 Anaesthetic Vaporizer: instructions for use*, ed 2, Lübeck, Germany, 1998, Dräger Medical.
12. *Dräger Vapor 19.n Anaesthetic Vaporizer*, ed 16, Lübeck, Germany, 1991, Dräger Medical.
13. Bruce DL, Linde HW: Vaporization of mixed anesthesia liquids, *Anesthesiology* 60:342–346, 1984.
14. Korman B, Ritchie IM: Chemistry of halothane-enflurane mixtures applied to anesthesia, *Anesthesiology* 63:152–156, 1985.
15. *Ohmeda Tec 5 continuous flow vaporizer: operations and maintenance manual*, Madison, WI, 1989, Ohmeda.
16. *Tec 4 continuous-flow vaporizer: operations and maintenance manual*, Madison, WI, 1989, Ohmeda.
17. Scheller MS, Drummond JC: Solubility of N_2O in volatile anesthetics contributes to vaporizer aberrancy when changing carrier gases, *Anesth Analg* 65:88–90, 1986.
18. *Tec 5 continuous flow vaporizer: operation and maintenance manual*, Madison, WI, 1998, Datex Ohmeda.
19. Murray WJ, Zsigmond EK, Fleming P: Contamination of in-series vaporizers with halothane-methoxyflurane, *Anesthesiology* 38:487–489, 1973.
20. Marks WE, Bullard JR: Another hazard of freestanding vaporizers: increased anesthetic concentration with reversed flow of vaporizing gas, *Anesthesiology* 45:445, 1976.
21. Silvasi DL, Haynes A, Brown ACD: Potentially lethal failure of the vapor exclusion system, *Anesthesiology* 71:289–291, 1990.
22. Andrews JJ, Johnson RV, Kramer GC: Consequences of misfilling contemporary vaporizers with desflurane, *Can J Anaesth* 40:71, 1993.
23. Weiskopf RB, Sampson D, Moore MA: The desflurane (Tec 6) vaporizer, *Br J Anaesth* 72:474, 1994.
24. *Tec 6 vaporizer: operation and maintenance manual*, Madison, WI, 1992, Ohmeda.
25. *D-Vapor: instructions for use*, ed 2, Telford, PA, 2004, Dräger Medical.
26. Hendrickx JFA, De Cooman S, Deloof T, et al: The ADU vaporizing unit: a new vaporizer, *Anesth Analg* 93:391–395, 2001.
27. Leigh JM: Variations on a theme: splitting ratios, *Anaesthesia* 40:70–72, 1985.
28. Dorrington KL: Splitting ratio, *Anaesthesia* 40:704, 1985.

CHAPTER 4

BREATHING CIRCUITS

Scott G. Walker • Theodore Craig Smith • George Sheplock • Michael A. Acquaviva • Nicole Horn

CHAPTER OUTLINE

THE ANESTHESIA MACHINE

The anesthesia machine serves to create a desired mixture of anesthetic gases, vapors, oxygen, and air (as well as other gases such as helium and carbon dioxide, albeit less frequently). The patient is the recipient of these prepared gas mixtures of known composition, and the breathing circuit is the interface between the anesthesia machine and the patient. This circuit delivers the gas mixture from the machine to the patient as it removes carbon dioxide, excludes operating room (OR) air, and conditions the gas mixture by adjusting its temperature and humidity. It converts continuous gas flow from the anesthesia machine to the intermittent flow of breathing, facilitates controlled or assisted respiration, and provides other functions such as gas sampling and pressure and spirometric measurements.

The desirable characteristics of a breathing circuit include 1) low resistance to gas flow, 2) minimal rebreathing of the preceding alveolar expirate, 3) removal of carbon dioxide at the rate at which it is produced, 4) rapid changes in delivered gas composition when required, 5) warmed humidification of the inspirate, and 6) safe disposal of waste gases. The components of a breathing circuit include the breathing tubing; respiratory valves; reservoir bags; carbon dioxide absorption canisters; a fresh gas inflow site; a pop-off valve leading to a scavenger for excess gas; a Y-piece with a mask or tube mount; and a face mask, laryngeal mask, or tracheal tube. Other devices that may be included are filters; humidifiers; valves for positive end-expiratory pressure (PEEP); and detecting mechanisms for airway pressure, spirometry, and gas analysis. Although these circuit components can be assembled in many ways, contemporary systems are usually configured by the manufacturer and permit little intervention by the user in regard to their configuration. Understanding the advantages and limitations of the different configurations allows the user to select the most appropriate type for varying clinical settings.

HISTORY OF DEVICE DEVELOPMENT

Breathing circuits have been an important concern from the start. Because of a delay in the production of his inhaler, Morton was late to his first public exhibition of the "Somniferon" (ether) in 1846. The earliest circuits were mechanically simple; differences among them were related to the characteristics of the primary anesthetic agent. Because nitrous oxide and ether anesthetic mixtures were weak (less potent) or slow to produce anesthesia, it was necessary to exclude air and helpful to include oxygen enrichment. The rapid onset of action and potency of chloroform, on the other hand, demanded precise control. It became apparent that the unique features of each agent were important. The ability to assist respiration was advantageous, as was conservation of costly agents and avoidance of large leaks of flammable ones.

In the twentieth century, a large number of relatively small but more highly engineered improvements were made as other demands on the breathing circuit were recognized. In 1915, Dennis Jackson described the first carbon dioxide absorber to save on the cost of nitrous oxide for animal studies.[1] Ralph Waters brought the idea into the OR, designing a to-and-fro absorption canister that used soda lime.[2,3] Bryan Sword introduced the first circle breathing circuit in 1930.[4] Thus low-flow absorption systems were already in use when cyclopropane made them essential. A return to high flows in the United States was brought about by the poor performance of vaporizers for halothane in the 1950s, with the demonstration that such flows could eliminate carbon dioxide without the use of soda lime.[5,6]

Stimulated by Magill's use of a number of pieces of apparatus put together in differing configurations for differing purposes, Mapleson described a variety of Magill circuits.[7] The original Ayre's T-piece was modified by numerous practitioners; the Jackson-Rees circuit represents one such example.[8] A variety of proprietary nonrebreathing valves were introduced, and the circuits named for them included the Stephen-Slater,[9] the Fink,[6] the Ruben,[10] and the Frumin.[11]

Partial rebreathing and functionally nonrebreathing circuits—such as the Bain,[12] Humphrey ADE,[13] and Lack[14] systems—found various proponents. Ingenious switching valves permitted transfiguration from one circuit to another,[13] which led to difficulty in remembering which circuit was optimal for what purpose.

Today, in addition to factors of convenience and economy, circuits are used to control heat and humidity; to measure patient variables such as tidal volume, respiratory frequency, airway pressure, and inspired and expired gas concentrations; and to control contamination of the OR environment by the agents themselves. The 150-year history of the development of the breathing circuit offers the practitioner a number of choices. All commonly used circuits accomplish their goals more or less equivalently, but the simple act of increasing fresh gas flow, for example, may markedly increase the work of breathing.[15] Therefore it is vital that the anesthesiologist understand the functional characteristics of each circuit.

CLASSIFICATIONS OF BREATHING CIRCUITS

A widely used nomenclature was developed that classified circuits as *open*, *semiopen*, *semiclosed*, or *closed*, according to whether a reservoir is used and whether rebreathing occurs. An *open system* has no reservoir and no rebreathing; a *semiopen system* has a reservoir but no rebreathing; a *semiclosed system* has a reservoir and partial rebreathing; and a *closed system* has a reservoir and complete rebreathing. Variations on this classification included the type of carbon dioxide absorber and unidirectional valves used.

Because of confusion with this traditional nomenclature, Hamilton recommended its abandonment in favor of both a description of the hardware (e.g., circle filter system, coaxial circuit, T-piece) and the gas flow rates being used.[16] Identifying the circuits by eponym—such as Adelaid, Bain, Hafnia, Humphrey, Jackson-Rees, Lack, Magill, and Waters—did not help in understanding the function or application of the circuit. Almost all anesthesia machines are equipped with some form of a circle breathing circuit with the ability for carbon dioxide absorption during low-flow anesthesia and elimination through the pop-off valve during high-flow anesthesia. Because an understanding of how circuits work is essential, breathing circuits in this chapter are organized by method of carbon dioxide elimination. Methods for removal of carbon dioxide are discussed.

Chemical Absorption of Carbon Dioxide

Semiclosed and closed systems (i.e., circle and to-and-fro) rely on chemical absorption of carbon dioxide. Exhaled carbon dioxide is absorbed, and all other exhaled gases are rebreathed. The quantities of fresh oxygen and anesthetics equal those lost as a result of uptake, metabolism, and circuit leaks.[3,17,18]

Dilution with Fresh Gas

Because of the intermittent nature of carbon dioxide excretion (during exhalation only) and the continuous inflow of fresh gas, the choice of inflow rate—as well as the locations of the inflow site, reservoir bag, and pop-off valves—contributes to the efficiency of carbon dioxide removal. When fresh gas flows are 1 to 1.5 times the minute volume (approximately 10 L/min in an adult), dilution alone is sufficient to remove carbon dioxide.[17,19-23] Such systems then behave the same as a nonrebreathing system.

Use of Valves to Separate Exhaled Gases from Inhaled Gases

Systems that use nonrebreathing valves are examples of this method of carbon dioxide removal.[6,9,11,24,25] A circuit that by virtue of high flows behaves as if it were nonrebreathing is not considered a nonrebreathing circuit in this analysis.

Use of Open-Drop Ether or a T-Piece Without a Reservoir to Release Exhaled Carbon Dioxide into the Atmosphere

Although similar to the second method above, systems that used open-drop ether or a T-piece without a reservoir were not truly breathing circuits. The T-pieces with an expiratory reservoir rely on dilution of carbon dioxide by both fresh gas and room air for its removal; these have been included in semiclosed circuits below.[26]

COMPONENTS OF A BREATHING CIRCUIT

The circuits described above have many features in common; they connect to the patient's airway through a face mask, laryngeal mask, or tracheal tube adapted to the breathing circuit through a Y-piece or elbow. The system may include valves to permit directional gas flow, and a reservoir bag is almost always present, which can be used to manually force gas into the lungs. Fresh gas must be supplied to the circuit, and excessive gas must be allowed to escape. In some, carbon dioxide is absorbed in a chemical filter. A variety of ancillary devices may also be present, such as humidifiers, spirometers, pressure gauges, filters, gas analyzers, PEEP devices, waste gas scavengers, and mixing and circulating devices.

Connection of the Patient to the Breathing Circuit

Either an anesthesia mask, supraglottic device, or a tracheal tube connects the circuit to the patient. Masks are made from rubber or clear plastic to make secretions or vomitus visible (Fig. 4-1). Most have an inflatable or inflated cuff, a pneumatic cushion that seals to the face. Masks are available in a variety of sizes and styles to accommodate the wide variety of facial contours. For example, a prominent nasal bridge may prevent a tight fit if the mask's cuff is flat at that point. A prominent chin (mentum) with sunken alveolar ridge causes a leak at the corner of the mouth, and the volume of the mask contributes to apparatus dead space. The mask should fit between the interpupillary line over the nose and in the groove between the mental process and the alveolar ridge (Fig. 4-2). The average length of this area is 85 to 90 mm in adults. The newest disposable plastic masks are available in a wide range of sizes, intended

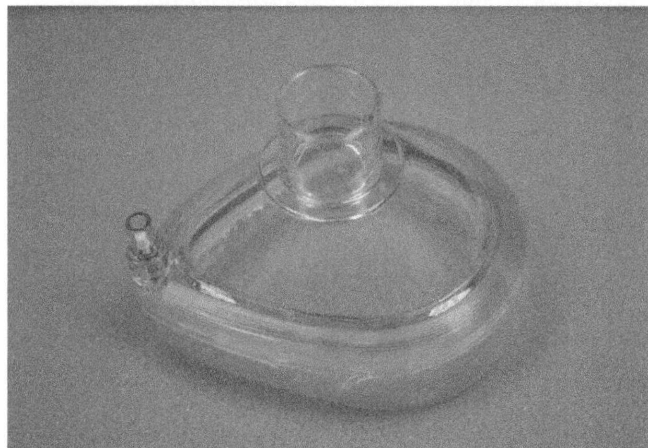

FIGURE 4-1 ■ The modern, clear plastic anesthesia mask. (Courtesy K. Premmer, MD.)

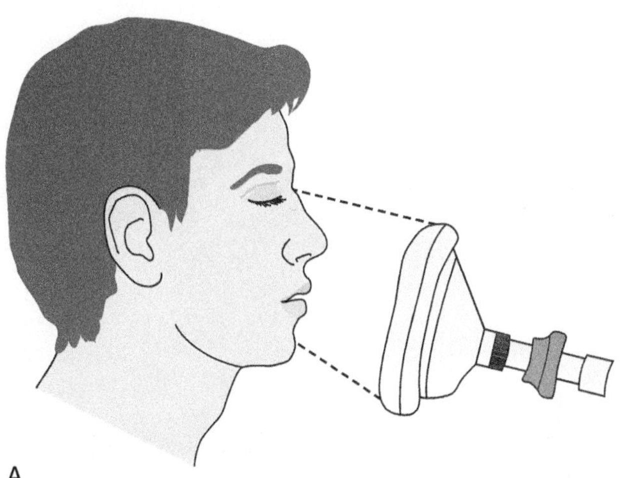

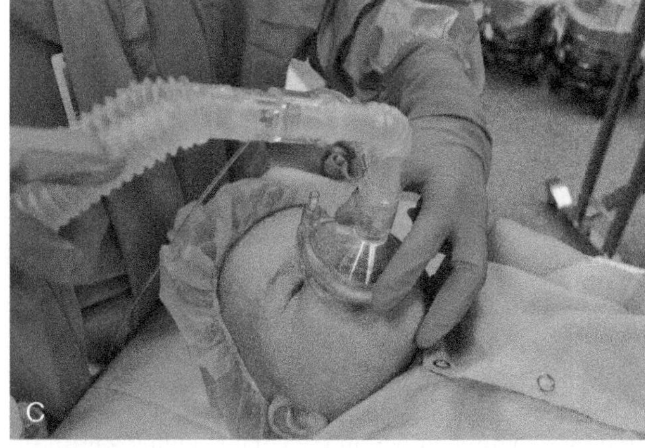

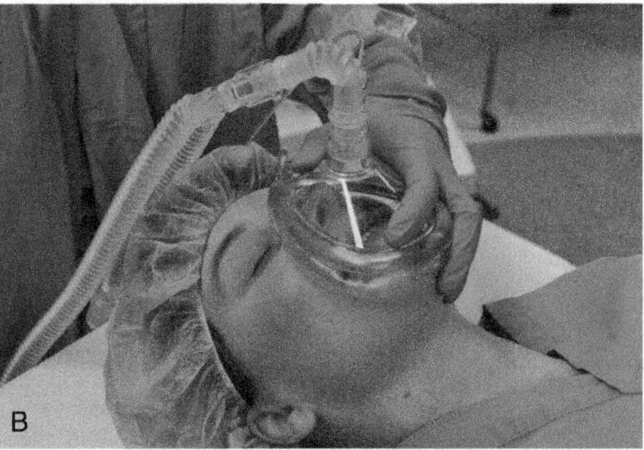

FIGURE 4-2 ■ **A to C,** The mask's cushion fits over the nose at the interpupillary line and above the mental process. (Courtesy K. Premmer, MD.)

to fit the faces of small children and large adults equally well. Choosing from a selection of mask sizes and styles is more rational than a "one size fits all" approach because a poorly fitting mask can result in trauma to the patient. This is especially true when the mask must be positioned above the eyebrows because it can cause pressure on, and possibly damage to, the optic and supraorbital nerves. Masks often have a set of prongs for attachment to a rubber mask holder or head strap; however, if pulled too tight, this mask holder may obstruct the airway. Masks connect to the Y-piece or elbow via a 22-mm (⅞-inch) female connection.

Breathing Tubing

The tubing used in breathing circuits typically is approximately 1 meter in length, has a large bore (22 mm) to minimize resistance to gas flow, and has corrugations or spiral reinforcement to permit flexibility without kinking. The internal volume is 400 to 500 mL/m of length. Although these tubes were formerly made of conductive rubber, disposable plastic tubing has almost completely replaced rubber. Electrical conductivity is no longer necessary when breathing tubing is used with nonflammable agents. The advantage of plastic is that it is lightweight; however, it is not biodegradable and thus is disposable by design although not by use. Plastic tubing for a breathing circuit is supplied sterile despite the lack of convincing epidemiologic data to support the necessity of sterile tubing.[27,28] On occasion, it is necessary to pass a breathing circuit on to the sterile surgical field (e.g., during an ex utero intrapartum treatment procedure). By convention, the ends of the tubing are 22 mm in internal diameter (ID) and are identical in design. Tubing should be inspected before use because manufacturing errors can result in obstruction of the lumen.[29,30] Compliance of the tubing varies from nearly 0 to more than 5 mL/m/mm Hg of applied pressure, and plastic tubing has lower values than rubber (Table 4-1). Apparent distensibility is even greater because compression of gas under pressure, to the order of 3% of the volume, occurs at typical inflation pressures. Inflation of a patient's lungs to 20 cm H_2O peak inspiratory pressure compresses 30 to 150 mL of gas in the tubing.[31] This volume is not delivered to the patient's lungs, but some fraction of it may be measured by a spirometer within the circuit, adding a form of apparatus dead space to the system. The exact fraction depends on where the spirometer is placed in the circuit with respect to the unidirectional valves.

TABLE 4-1 **Compliance of Ohio Anesthesia Breathing Circuits**

Circuit Pressure (cm H_2O)	Volume (mL)	
	Conductive Rubber	Disposable Plastic
10	80	30
15	130	100
20	210	190
25	290	320

From *Fluidically controlled anesthesia ventilator operation and maintenance manual.* 1974, Ohio Medical Products (now GE Healthcare, Waukesha, WI).

Resistance to gas flow in standard, corrugated breathing tubes is exceedingly small—less than 1 cm H_2O/L/min of flow.[32] When it is desirable to have the anesthesia machine at some distance from the patient's head, several tubes may be connected in series with connectors 22 mm (⅞ inch) in outside diameter (OD). Alternatively, extra-long tubing is available, including tubing that can be compressed to 200 mL of volume in approximately 50 cm of length or that can be stretched to nearly 2 m with an 800-mL volume. These "concertina" extensions do not increase the resistance of the system by any appreciable amount and affect the apparatus dead space only by their compliant volume (Fig. 4-3).

The pattern of gas flow through the circuit is almost always turbulent because of the corrugations in the tubing, which promote both radial mixing and longitudinal mixing.

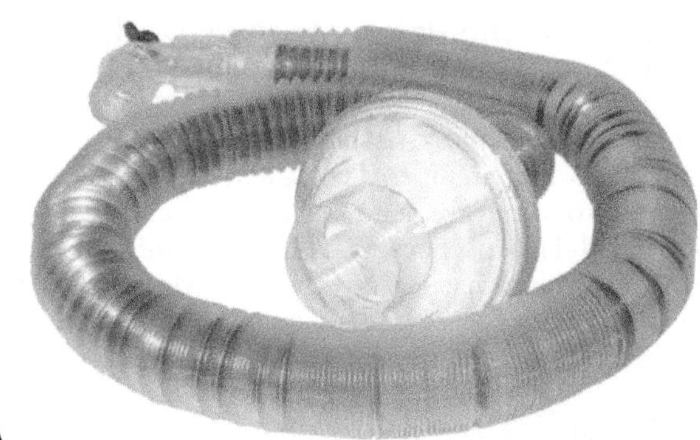
A

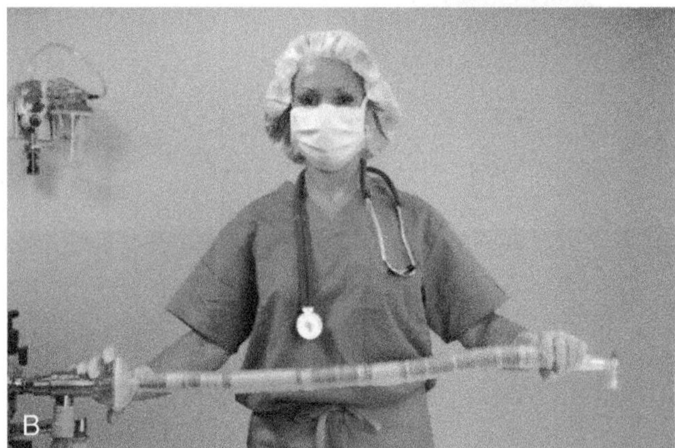

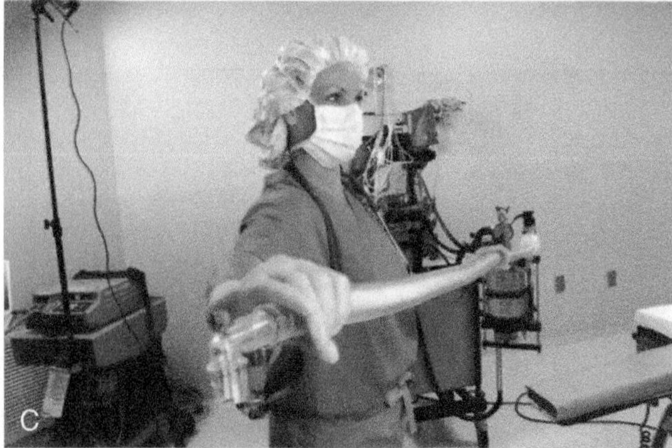

FIGURE 4-3 "Concertina" style breathing circuit tubes can be or compressed (**A** and **B**) or stretched (**C**) to change in length and volume without significantly affecting apparatus dead space. (Courtesy King Systems, Noblesville, IN.)

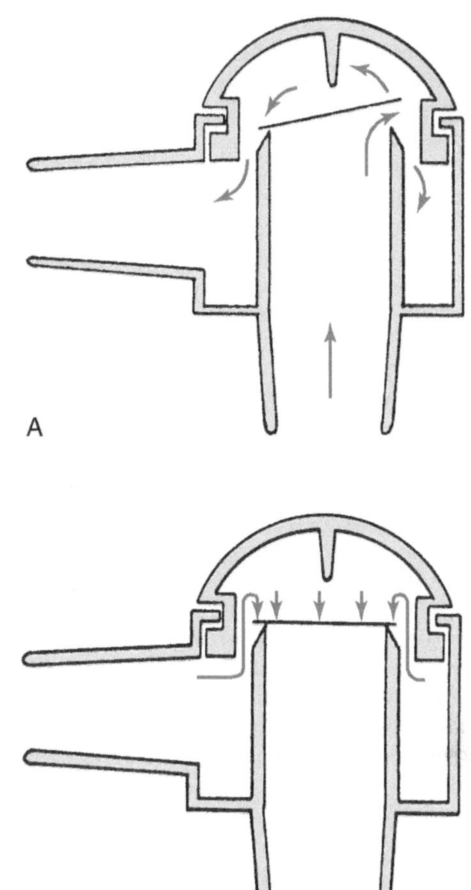

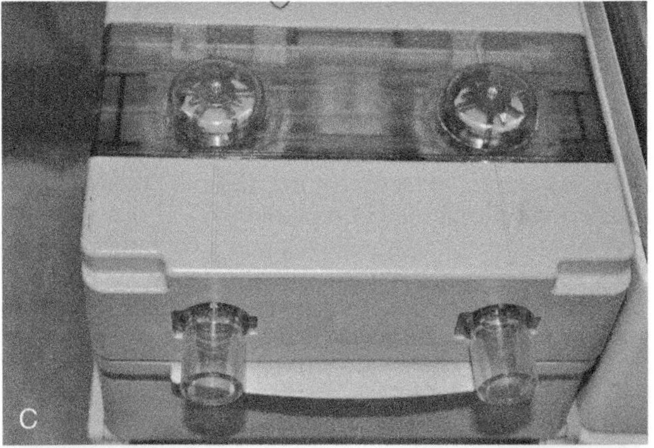

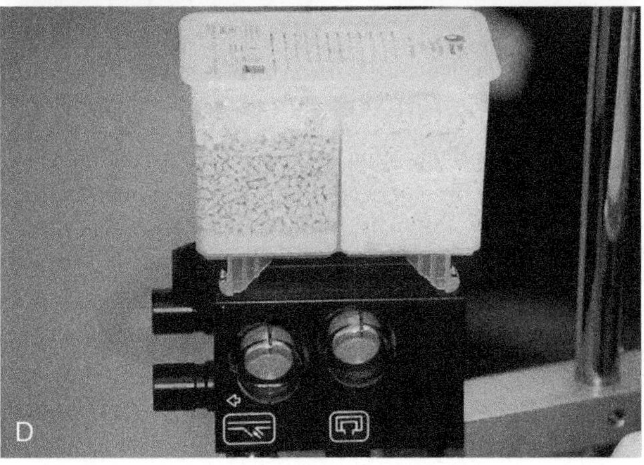

FIGURE 4-4 ■ **A,** Typical dome valve incorporated into a circle absorber housing. The valve is in the open position with gas flowing. **B,** Because of backpressure, the plastic disk seats on the knife edge and the valve is closed. **C,** One-way valves on the Datex-Ohmeda machine (GE Healthcare, Waukesha, WI). **D,** Datex-Ohmeda ADU absorber block showing unidirectional valves mounted vertically. (Courtesy K. Premmer, MD.)

In documenting performance of one circuit, Spoerel[33] demonstrated complete mixing of dead space and alveolar gas after gas had passed through 1 m of such tubing. A change in gas composition at one end, such as when the delivered gas is altered at the anesthesia machine, completes a change in the inspired concentration at the patient connection within two to three breaths. The change in inspired concentration is nearly exactly the change in delivered concentration when high fresh gas flows are used (≥10 L/min). The change decreases to nearly imperceptible as inflow is decreased toward that of closed systems.

Lengths of breathing tubing are sometimes used to connect ventilators to the bag mount and to connect to scavenging devices. Optimally, either a 19- or 30-mm diameter ends on the scavenger mounts prevent inappropriate connections. Tubing of smaller diameter is made for use in circle systems designed specifically for infants and children, and their resistance to gas flow is insignificantly increased. With less compression volume, measured ventilation is more accurate.

Reusable rubber tubing is connected to the mask or tube by a separate Y-piece. Disposable sets often incorporate a Y that may or may not be detachable. Such a Y may be rigid, and it may incorporate an angle elbow or a pair of swivel joints. Although the swivel joints are convenient, they offer a greater chance of leaking; most connectors have negligible leakage, but those with swivels are twice as likely to leak.[34] Any circuit should be tested before use by determining the oxygen inflow required to maintain 30cm H_2O of pressure in the circuit (see also Chapter 32).

Unidirectional Valves

Unidirectional valves are incorporated into a breathing circuit to direct respiratory gas flow. They are commonly disks on knife edges or rubber flaps or sleeves. The essential characteristics of respiratory valves in breathing circuits are low resistance and high competence.[35,36] The valves must open widely with little pressure and must close rapidly and completely with essentially no backflow.

Circle and nonrebreathing systems use two nearly identical valves: the *inspiratory valve* opens on inspiration and closes on expiration, preventing backflow of exhaled gas in the inspiratory limb. The *expiratory valve* works in a reciprocal fashion to prevent rebreathing. These valves can be mounted anywhere within the inspiratory and expiratory limbs of the circuit. The only critical feature of their location is that one must be placed between the patient and the reservoir bag in each limb. Properly positioned and functioning, they prevent any part of the circle system from contributing to apparatus dead space.[37] Thus the only apparatus dead space in such a circuit is the distal limb of the Y-connector and any tube or mask between it and the patient's airway. The respiratory valves on most modern anesthesia machines are located near, or incorporated into, the carbon dioxide absorber canister casing along with a fresh gas inflow site and excess gas (pop-off) valve. In the past, unidirectional valves have been incorporated into the housing of the Y-piece to decrease the apparatus dead space effect of compliance volume, but they have fallen into disfavor because of the weight they add to the mask. More importantly, they cause an obstruction to respiration if they are accidentally incorporated backward to the conventional valves in the circle.[38] When valved Y-pieces were used, it was recommended that circle system valves be removed. Failure to reinsert the circle system valves when a normal nonvalved Y-piece was used has caused needless complications.

The common valves in anesthetic circuits are dome valves consisting of a circular knife edge occluded by a very light disk of slightly larger diameter (Fig. 4-4). The disk lifts off the knife edge when flow is initiated by the patient's inspiratory effort, when positive pressure is applied to the reservoir bag, or when the ventilator bellows empties. The disk is contained either by a small cage or by the dome itself. It must be hydrophobic so that water condensation does not cause it to stick to the knife edge and thereby increase the resistance to opening. Most modern disks are made of hydrophobic plastic and are light and thin. When properly functioning, the disk in a unidirectional valve can be lifted with a circuit pressure of 0.31 cm H_2O or less. Most unidirectional valves are mounted vertically, with the disk oriented horizontally, so that it will fall properly into the closed position and seal the circuit from backflow. The valve disks also can be oriented vertically, as on the absorber block of the Datex-Ohmeda ADU workstation (GE Healthcare, Waukesha, WI; see Fig. 4-4, D). Failure to seal converts a large volume of the circuit into apparatus dead space, resulting in rebreathing. The top of the valve is covered by a removable clear plastic dome so that the disk can be easily seen and periodically cleaned or replaced.

A nonrebreathing system requires two appropriately placed one-way respiratory valves (Fig. 4-5). Nonrebreathing valves permit the patient to inspire fresh gas from a reservoir and exhale alveolar gas into the room or into a scavenger. Such valves usually consist of a pair of leaflets in the same housing: one opens during inspiration, the other opens during expiration. The early nonrebreathing valve designs, such as the Digby-Leigh or Steven-Slater, required the anesthesiologist to occlude the expiratory valve with a finger if assisted or controlled ventilation was needed (Fig. 4-5, *A*).[9,24] Modern designs that use springs, magnets, or flaps automatically close the expiratory valve when respiration is controlled.[39-44] Other designs use the pressure difference across the inspiratory valve to inflate a mushroom-shaped balloon (Frumin) valve (Fig. 4-5, *B*),[11] or to depress a dome-shaped cover on the expiratory (Fink) valve.[6] Resistance is negligible in both designs, but the Frumin valve has the marked advantage of collapsing if the inspiratory supply is inadequate, permitting inspiration of room air. The Frumin valve also is lighter and more compact than the others. Some nonrebreathing valves are position sensitive and must be

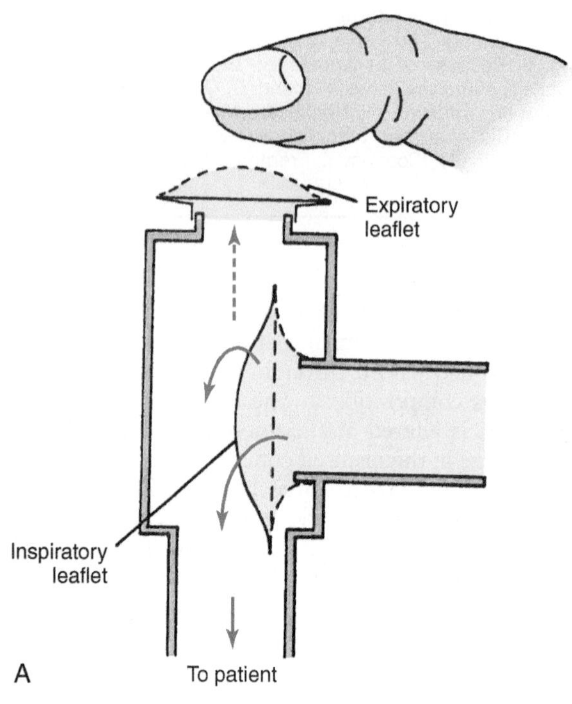

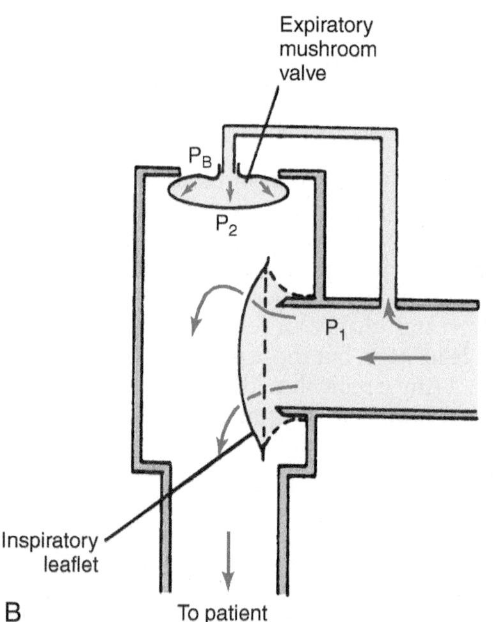

FIGURE 4-5 ■ These nonrebreathing valves incorporate two leaflets that open alternately on inspiration or expiration. **A,** In the simplest form, the valve functions well during spontaneous ventilation (*solid arrows*), but an attempt to inflate the patient's lungs manually blows open both inspiratory and expiratory leaflets (*dotted arrow*) unless the anesthesiologist simultaneously occludes the expiratory valve with a finger. Several nonrebreathing valves have been designed to overcome the necessity for manual assistance of valve function. **B,** Whenever gas flow opens the inspiratory leaflet, the pressure at point P_1 is greater than at point P_2 or P_B. This pressure difference inflates the mushroom-shaped expiratory balloon, sealing the expiratory limb. If no gas is supplied to the inspiratory limb, spontaneous effort on the part of the patient lowers both P_1 and P_2 well below atmospheric pressure (P_B) so that the mushroom valve collapses and the patient inspires room air.

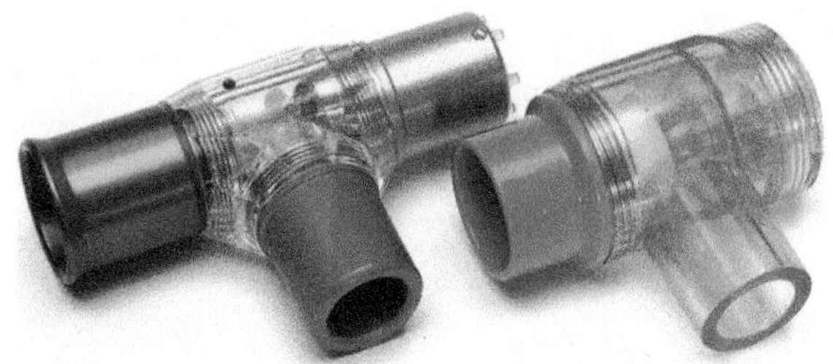

FIGURE 4-6 ■ The Ruben nonrebreathing valve (*left*) and Ambu E-2 valve (*right*). (Courtesy the Sheffield Department of Anaesthesia Museum, Sheffield, United Kingdom.)

vertically oriented to function properly.[45] Those that use flexible rubber leaflets or collapsible rubber tubing to provide the sealing function are not positional. Most nonrebreathing valves connect to masks and/or tracheal tubes, but a valve can be built into a mask.[44]

Self-inflating resuscitators for air or air-oxygen mixtures use similar pairs of valves to control gas flow.[10,46,47] The Ruben valve has an expiratory bobbin-shaped structure that, when open, occludes the inspiratory limb (Fig. 4-6). Anesthetic vapors and secretions tend to expand this bobbin slightly, causing it to jam.[47] Such resuscitator valves should not be used in anesthesia, nor should they be used for transporting patients who are still exhaling anesthetic agents.

Breathing Bags

Breathing bags, also known as *reservoir bags* or *counterlungs*, have three principal functions: 1) they serve as a reservoir for anesthetic gases or oxygen, from which the patient can inspire; 2) they provide the means for a visual assessment of the existence and rough estimate of the volume of ventilation; and 3) they serve as a means for manual ventilation. A reservoir function is necessary because anesthesia machines cannot provide the peak inspiratory gas flow needed during normal spontaneous inspiration. Although the respiratory minute volume of an anesthetized adult is rarely more than 12 L/min, the peak inspiratory flow rate may reach 50 L/min, with 20 L/min not uncommon. For example, assume a patient is breathing at a rate of 20 breaths/min with a tidal volume of 500 mL and a minute volume of 10 L/min. If the inspiratory to expiratory ratio (I:E) is 1:2, each breath takes 1 second for inspiration and 2 seconds for exhalation. The tidal volume of 500 mL inspired in 1 second is an average inspiratory flow (volume per unit time) of 500 mL/sec or 30 L/min. This is many times greater than the commonly used fresh gas flows. The peak flow in mid-inspiration may be 30% to 40% higher.

Assessment of the presence and volume of spontaneous ventilation is affected by the fresh gas flow. In low-flow techniques, virtually all the gas inhaled by the patient comes from the reservoir bag, and its excursion thus reflects tidal volume. If the fresh gas inflow rate from the machine exceeds 10 L/min, most of the gas inhaled by the patient comes from the fresh gas supply, and the reservoir bag shows little excursion. In a spontaneously breathing patient with a circuit gas inflow rate of 6 L/min, nearly half the tidal volume comes from the fresh gas inflow, halving the apparent tidal volume as indicated by movement of the bag.

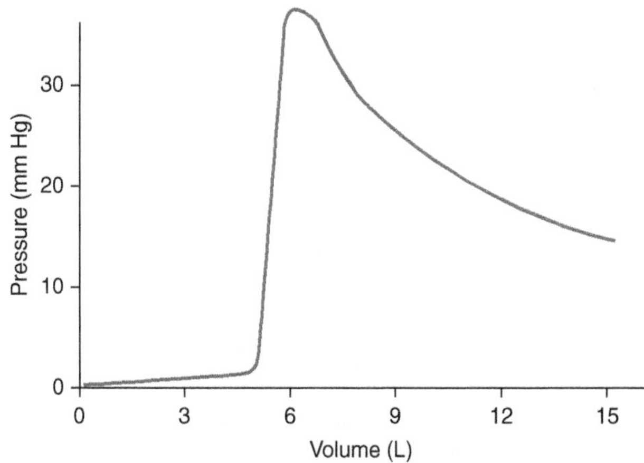

FIGURE 4-7 ■ As an anesthesia reservoir bag is filled from its evacuated volume to its nominal volume, the pressure increases little; as the rubber is slightly stretched, however, a small increase in volume rapidly raises the pressure to some maximum, depending on the shape and wall thickness of the bag. Further increase in the bag's volume causes a decrease in pressure. The falling pressure with rising volume follows Laplace's law: P = 2T/r, where *P* is pressure, the constant *T* is a function of the bag's thickness and material, and *r* is the radius.

Reservoir bags for anesthesia machines usually are ellipsoid so they can be easily grasped with one hand. They are made of nonslippery plastic or latex in sizes from 0.5 to 6 L. To improve grip, some have an hourglass shape or a textured surface; nonlatex bags are available for use with patients who have a latex sensitivity. The optimally sized bag can hold a volume that exceeds the patient's inspiratory capacity; that is, a spontaneous deep breath should not empty the bag. For most adults, a 3-L bag meets these requirements and is easy to grasp. Bags with a nipple at the bottom for use as an alternate pop-off site are available but are rarely used.

In circle systems, the breathing bag usually is mounted at or near the carbon dioxide absorbent canister via a T-shaped fitting, usually near the pop-off valve. The bag also may be placed at the end of a length of corrugated tubing leading from the T-connector to provide some freedom of movement for the anesthesiologist. The pressure-volume characteristics of overinflated bags become important if the pop-off valve is accidentally left in the closed position and gas inflow continues (Fig. 4-7). Rubber bags become pressure limiting with maximum pressures of 40 to 50 cm H_2O, although prestretching may favorably lower the maximum distending pressure.[48-50] Disposable bags may reach twice the pressure of rubber bags and then rupture abruptly.

Gas Inflow and Pop-off Valves

Gases are delivered from the anesthesia machine common gas outlet to the circuit via thick-walled tubing connected to a nipple incorporated into the circuit. In circle systems this gas inflow nipple is incorporated with the inspiratory unidirectional valve or the carbon dioxide–absorbent canister housing. The preferred fresh gas inflow site is between the carbon dioxide absorber and the inspiratory valve. The location for other circuits depends

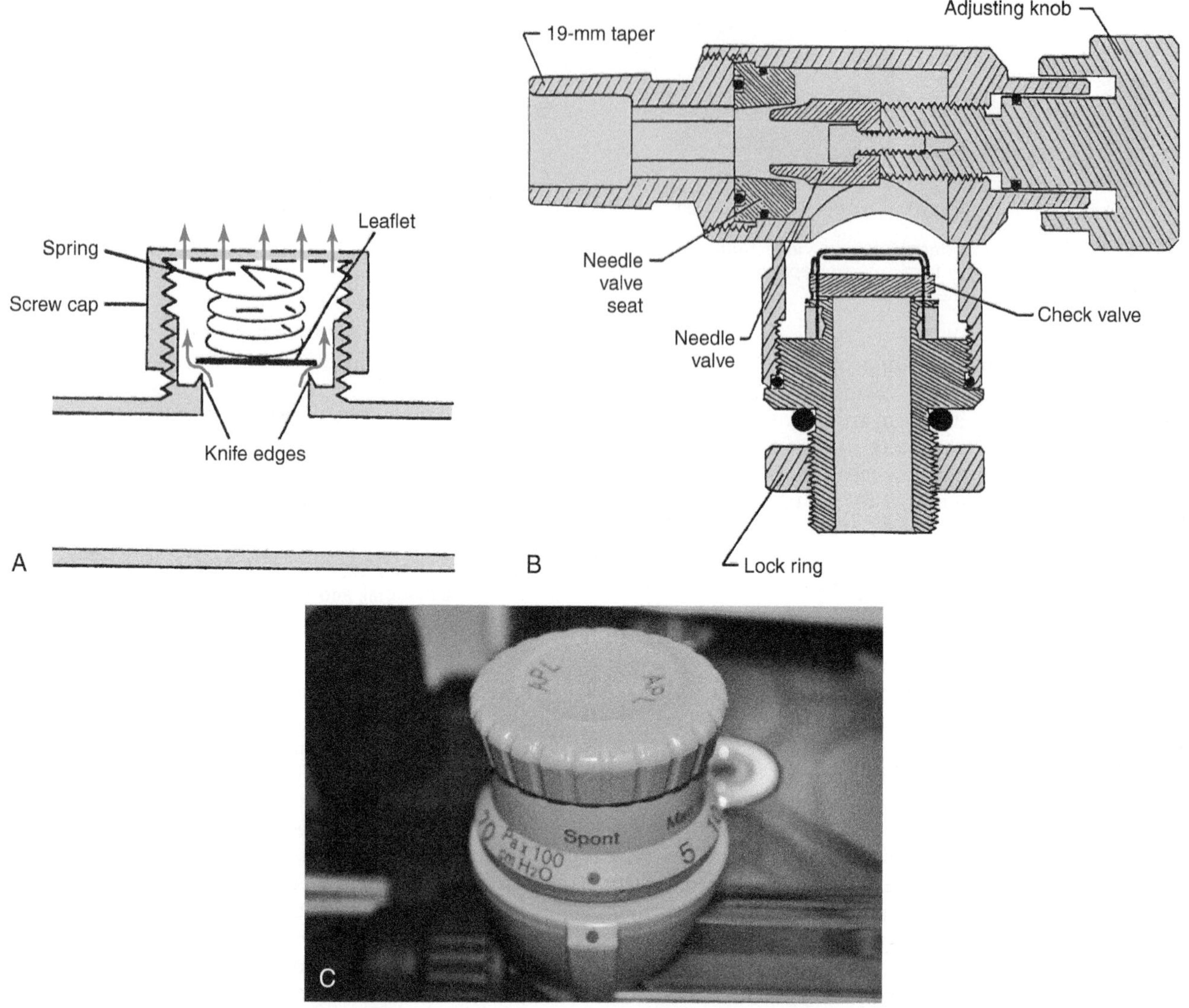

FIGURE 4-8 ■ Adjustable pressure-limiting (APL) or "pop-off" valves. **A,** Spring-loaded design. When the cap is fully tightened down, the spring is compressed enough to prevent the valve leaflet from lifting at *any* airway pressure. When the top is loosened and the spring is not compressed, the valve opens at a pressure equal to the weight of the leaflet divided by its area, usually <1 cm H_2O. **B,** The Dräger Medical (Telford, PA) APL valve design is an adjustable needle valve, the opening of which determines gas flow into the scavenger system. The check valve prevents reverse flow of gas from the scavenger into the patient circuit. **C,** A pop-off valve from a Dräger Apollo anesthesia workstation. This APL valve is similar to that in **A** and has approximate calibrations. (A and B, Courtesy Dräger Medical, Telford, PA. **C,** Courtesy K. Premmer, MD.)

on whether breathing is spontaneous, assisted, or controlled because the type of breathing influences the efficiency of carbon dioxide elimination.

Pop-off valves—also known as *overflow, outflow, relief, spill,* and *adjustable pressure-limiting* (APL) valves—permit gas to leave the circuit, matching the excess to the inflow of fresh gas. The efficiency of an APL valve is related in part to the placement of the fresh gas inflow. There are many different designs, but most are constructed like a dome valve loaded by a spring and screw cap (Fig. 4-8). The valve should open at a pressure of less than 1 cm H_2O. As the screw cap is tightened down, more and more gas pressure in the circuit is required to open it, permitting PEEP during spontaneous ventilation or pressure-limited controlled respiration. The number of clockwise turns from fully open to fully closed should be one or two: fewer turns make it difficult to set a desired circuit pressure accurately, whereas more make it tedious to use. The exhaust from any of the commonly used pop-off valves can be collected by scavenging system transfer tubing connected at this point.[51]

The Datex-Ohmeda GMS absorber uses an APL valve similar in design to that shown in Figure 4-8, which basically is a spring-loaded disk. When the spring is fully extended, it exerts a pressure of approximately 1 cm H_2O on the disk to hold the valve closed. This is necessary because the waste gas scavenging interface is connected downstream of the APL valve and transfer tubing. If an active scavenging system is used—that is, if suction is applied to the interface—the negative pressure could potentially be applied to the patient circuit (see Chapter 5). To prevent this, the Ohmeda scavenger interface uses a negative-pressure relief ("pop-in") valve that opens at a pressure of –0.25 cm H_2O to allow room

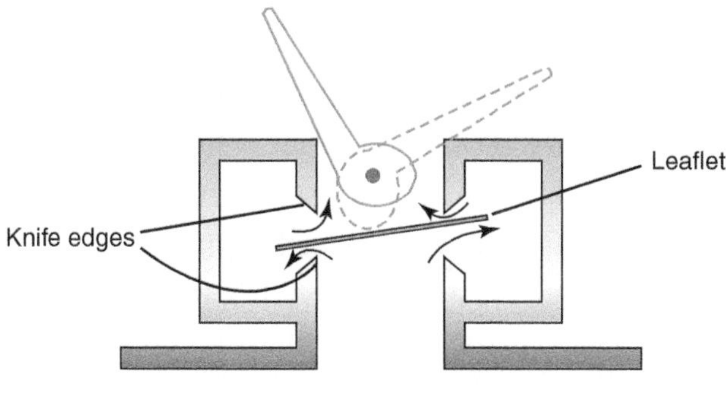

FIGURE 4-9 The Steen valve permits gas to exit from a circuit under the slight pressure that occurs during exhalation. However, a sudden rise in pressure, such as occurs during an assisted or controlled inhalation, seals the leaflet against the upper circular knife edge. A lever-operated eccentric cam defeats this effect if desired and turns the valve into an ordinary pop-off valve that is not spring loaded.

air to enter the interface. Thus the greatest negative pressure needed to open the APL valve (−0.25 cm) is less than the least spring tension needed to keep the valve closed (~1 cm H_2O). This arrangement, with the use of an active scavenging system, protects against application of excess negative pressure to the breathing circuit. In the fully closed position, the maximum spring pressure applied to the Datex-Ohmeda APL valve disk is 75 cm H_2O. Thus, in the manual/bag mode, the circuit pressure in an Datex-Ohmeda breathing system is limited to 75 cm H_2O. Note that in the ventilator mode, the circuit pressure is limited by high pressure-limit settings on the Datex-Ohmeda ventilator (up to 100 cm H_2O with the Datex-Ohmeda 7800 and 7900 ventilators; see Chapter 6).

In Dräger Medical (Telford, PA) anesthesia delivery systems, the design of the APL valve differs from those described above (see Fig. 4-8, *B*). This design uses a needle valve instead of a spring-loaded disk, and adjusting the knob varies the size of the opening between the needle valve and its seat, which in turn adjusts the amount of gas permitted to flow to the scavenger system. A check valve prevents gas from the scavenging system from entering the breathing system. With this design, the needle valve can be totally closed; it therefore does not function as a true pressure limiter.

Special types of pop-off valves permit spontaneous or assisted respiration without tedious adjustment.[40,52-54] The simplest is the Steen valve (Fig. 4-9), which essentially is two knife-edge valves of the dome type, one inverted over the other, that share a common disk.[24] A relatively slow flow of gas during the latter part of exhalation, up to 10 L/min, lifts the valve disk at one side only so that the exhaled gas escapes around the disk. An abrupt increase in pressure lifts the valve vertically, seals it against the upper knife edge, and closes the circuit so that no gas is lost. The Georgia valve adds a light spring loading to the same design, which increases the range of gas flows it can exhaust; this is necessary for use with mechanical ventilators.[55] Most current anesthesia ventilators have such an automatic pop-off valve built in so that gas is exhausted only at end exhalation (see also Chapter 6).

CARBON DIOXIDE ABSORPTION

In partial rebreathing and nonrebreathing systems, carbon dioxide is vented to room air. When a closed system is used, however, the exhaled carbon dioxide must be otherwise removed. Carbon dioxide in the presence of water is hydrated to form carbonic acid. When carbonic acid reacts with a metal hydroxide, the reaction is one of neutralization that results in the formation of water and a metal bicarbonate or carbonate and the generation of heat. This reaction is used in anesthesia for carbon dioxide absorption.[56] In the reactions shown below, only the molecular forms of the reactants are written. The reactions actually proceed by initial ionization in the thin film of water at the surfaces of the absorbent. In soda lime:

$$CO_2 + H_2O \rightarrow H_2CO_3 \quad (4\text{-}1)$$

$$H_2CO_3 + 2NaOH \rightarrow Na_2CO_3 + 2H_2O \quad (4\text{-}2)$$

$$H_2CO_3 + 2KOH \rightarrow K_2CO_3 + 2H_2O \quad (4\text{-}3)$$

$$Na_2CO_3 + Ca(OH)_2 \rightarrow 2NaOH + CaCO_3 \quad (4\text{-}4)$$

$(\text{or } K_2CO_3)$ $(\text{or } 2KOH)$

In barium hydroxide lime—or Baralyme, which is no longer being produced (see Chapter 30)—$Ba(OH)_2$ replaces the NaOH and KOH in equations 4-2, 4-3, and 4-4, with $BaCO_3$ the product.

Wet soda lime is composed of calcium hydroxide (~80%), sodium hydroxide and potassium hydroxide (~5%), water (~15%), and small amounts of inert substances such as silica and clay for hardness. The potassium hydroxide and sodium hydroxide function somewhat like a catalyst to speed the initial reaction, forming sodium and potassium carbonates. The sodium and potassium carbonates react over the course of minutes with the calcium hydroxide to form calcium carbonate and water, regenerating sodium and potassium hydroxides. Soda lime is exhausted when all the hydroxides have become carbonates. Soda lime can absorb 19% of its weight in carbon dioxide[5]; thus 100 g of soda lime can absorb approximately 26 L of carbon dioxide.

A novel carbon dioxide absorbent was created in 1999. Calcium hydroxide lime (Amsorb) is composed of calcium hydroxide (70%); a compatible humectant, calcium chloride (0.7%); and two setting agents, calcium sulfate (0.7%) and polyvinylpyrrolidine (0.7%), to improve hardness and porosity; and water (14.5%).[57] By adding calcium chloride as a humectant, the calcium hydroxide remains damp and eliminates the need for sodium or potassium hydroxide. With removal of the strong alkali, calcium hydroxide lime has potential benefits that include decreased formation of compound A with sevoflurane use, minimal formation of carbon monoxide when exposed to desflurane or isoflurane, and minimal destruction of inhaled agents.[58]

Indicator Dyes

Organic dyes are added to soda lime and barium hydroxide lime to provide a visual indication of its state. As carbonate is formed from the hydroxide, the pH becomes less alkaline and the granules change color: ethyl violet changes from white to blue violet with exhaustion, ethyl orange from orange to yellow, and cresyl yellow from red to yellow. Ethyl violet is the dye most commonly used because the color change is vivid and of high contrast at a pH intermediate between NaOH and $CaCO_3$. It can be bleached by intense light, but in the usual OR setting this is not a problem. A slight fading of color can be seen in the zone of active absorption when use stops. This so-called *regeneration* occurs where the lime is nearly exhausted of calcium hydroxide but has all alkaline hydroxides neutralized.

The color changes only because of the regeneration of a small amount of sodium and potassium hydroxide. At the next use, the expended nature of the soda lime rapidly becomes evident. There is no true regeneration of activity, and the color change of indicator lime is not to be relied on. The anesthesiologist must know what color change is expected of the absorbent being used, allow for the effects of regeneration, be cognizant of the effects of preferential gas flow at the surface between the smooth plastic canister and the irregular granules (channeling), and understand the effects of the fresh gas flows chosen based on how long a given charge of soda lime can be expected to last. No indicator or rules offer absolute predictions, but the use of capnometry to detect increasing inspired carbon dioxide remains the gold standard for assessing adequate carbon dioxide removal.

Mesh Size and Channeling

Soda lime is precisely manufactured to maximize its absorptive qualities and to minimize resistance to gas flow.[5] The granules are sized 4 to 8 mesh (i.e., they will pass through a strainer having 4 to 8 wires per inch) and have a rough, irregular surface that maximizes the surface/volume ratio that facilitates the rapid diffusion of carbon dioxide through the pores to the voids within the granules.[56,59-62] Approximately half the volume of a packed canister is gas. The gas volume of the voids is inversely proportional to the water content of the granules and is 1 to 2 times that of the volume between granules. Soda lime is supplied either in quart cartons that fill a canister, disposable canisters, or bulk containers ranging from 5 pounds to 5 gallons. The volume between granules can be reduced by overzealous packing at the risk of creating fine particles and dust that are irritating. Channeling, or flow moving preferentially along the sides of the canister and within the absorbent itself, was a problem with to-and-fro canisters that were often horizontal and improperly packed. This problem can be minimized by the use of baffles, placement so that gas flow is vertical, permanent mounting to avoid frequent canister movement, use of prepackaged cylinders, and avoidance of overly tight packing. Modern carbon dioxide–absorbent canisters (Fig. 4-10) follow the design of the Roswell Park absorber with double chambers to promote efficient use, circular baffles to minimize channeling, and mixing space at the top and bottom.[19,56] Although most have clear plastic walls, some are tinged blue for the purpose of enhancing the appearance of color change in the indicator dye.

Other Reactions with Absorbents

Sevoflurane did not gain U.S. Food and Drug Administration (FDA) approval for use until 1995 despite its use in Japan and elsewhere since the 1970s. When sevoflurane was first described, early testing revealed the production of fluoromethyl-2,2-difluoro-1-(trifluoromethyl) vinyl ether, better known as *compound A*, when sevoflurane is exposed to various alkalis, including soda lime.[63] This reaction occurs when hydrogen fluoride is eliminated from the isopropyl moiety of sevoflurane. Concern arose over evidence that compound A is nephrotoxic—and, at higher concentrations, lethal—in rats.[64-66] Although studies of the nephrotoxicity of compound A in humans have had conflicting results,[67-69] sevoflurane has been administered with apparent safety for several years.[68] What is clear is that certain factors related to the breathing system can contribute to the production of compound A during anesthesia with sevoflurane. These include increasing inspired sevoflurane concentration, increasing absorbent temperature, decreasing absorbent water content (desiccation), and a decreasing fresh gas flow rate.[70,71] Hypotheses to explain the effect of low flows on compound A production include increased contact of exhaled gas with carbon dioxide absorbent, increased rebreathing of compound A, and increased absorbent temperature. Current sevoflurane labeling indicates that whereas a fresh gas flow from 1 to 2 L/min may be used safely for fewer than 2 minimum alveolar concentration (MAC) hours, flows less than 2 L/min should not be used for more than 2 MAC hours, and flows below 1 L/min are not recommended for any duration with this agent. The choice of absorbent, whether barium hydroxide lime or soda lime, does not seem to significantly influence production of compound A (Fig. 4-11).[70,72]

Desiccation of carbon dioxide absorbents is known to be related to another potential hazard, that of carbon monoxide production. The notion that carbon monoxide could be found in detectable amounts in anesthesia breathing circuits containing soda lime was first reported with the use of trichlorethylene and during closed-circuit anesthesia secondary to endogenous production.[73] More recently, it has been recognized that difluoromethyl ethers in common use today, including desflurane and isoflurane, can liberate carbon monoxide during destruction of these agents by carbon dioxide absorbents.[74] Difluoromethyl ethers are fluorinated volatile anesthetics that contain an –O–CHF_2 moiety. Early case reports of unexplained carboxyhemoglobinemia during enflurane anesthesia pointed to an association with "first case on Monday morning" anesthetics[75] or with older absorbents.[76] This has been explained by invitro studies that revealed a marked association between dryness of the absorbent and production of carbon monoxide.[74] It is theorized that high oxygen flows over the absorbent canister during the weekend, or after prolonged absorbent

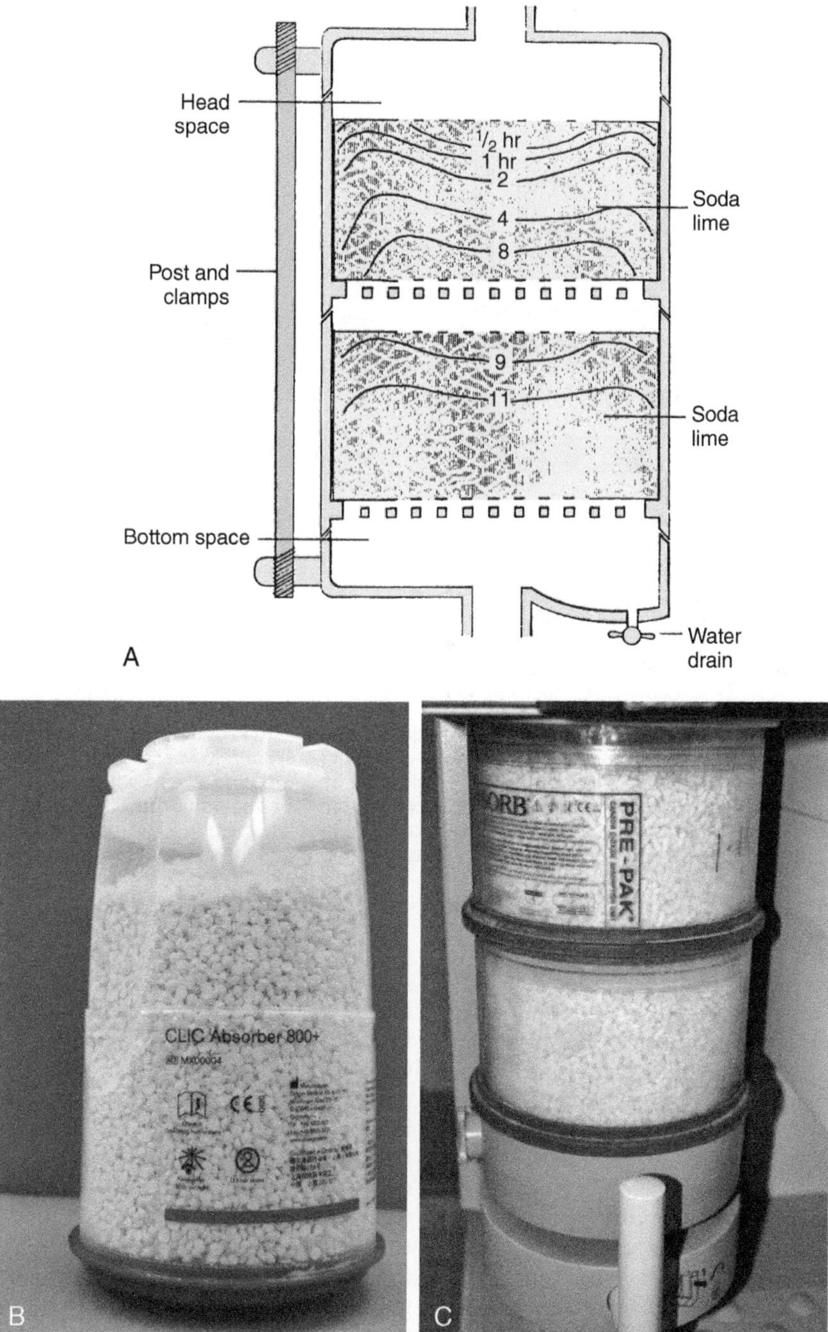

FIGURE 4-10 ■ **A,** Schematic of modern carbon dioxide absorbent canister. Originated by Elam and Brown, these transparent twin-chambered canisters are now supplied by all producers. Permanently mounted with a vertical gas-flow axis, they eliminate dusting, channeling, and packing problems. Used as intended, changing the exhausted canister only when the second half is exhausted, they use the absorptive capacity of soda lime fully, as shown by the lines illustrating patterns of exhaustion. Drop-in, prepacked containers add convenience. The nearly standard shape is 8 cm high and 15 cm in diameter. Because water condensate may collect at the bottom and form a caustic lye solution with the dust, a drain valve is an important component. Convenience of opening, closing, and sealing varies with design, but most now have a single-action clamp mechanism. The casting for the top and bottom should be resistant to alkaline corrosion and may incorporate other components of the breathing circuit (e.g., bag mount, inflow site, and valve housings. **B,** Prefilled single-chamber canister. **C,** Twin canister on Datex-Ohmeda Aestiva machine. (GE Healthcare, Waukesha, WI). (B and C, Courtesy K. Premmer, MD.)

use, desiccate the absorbent. The type of anesthetic is important, with the order of carbon monoxide production being desflurane, which produces the most, followed by enflurane then isoflurane. Sevoflurane and halothane lack an $-O-CHF_2$ moiety and do not appreciably produce carbon monoxide in the presence of carbon dioxide absorbents. Barium hydroxide lime seems to cause greater carbon monoxide liberation than does soda lime, but both absorbents produce more carbon monoxide with increasing temperatures and with increasing concentrations of anesthetic.[74] Recognition of the presence of carbon monoxide in an anesthesia breathing circuit in which

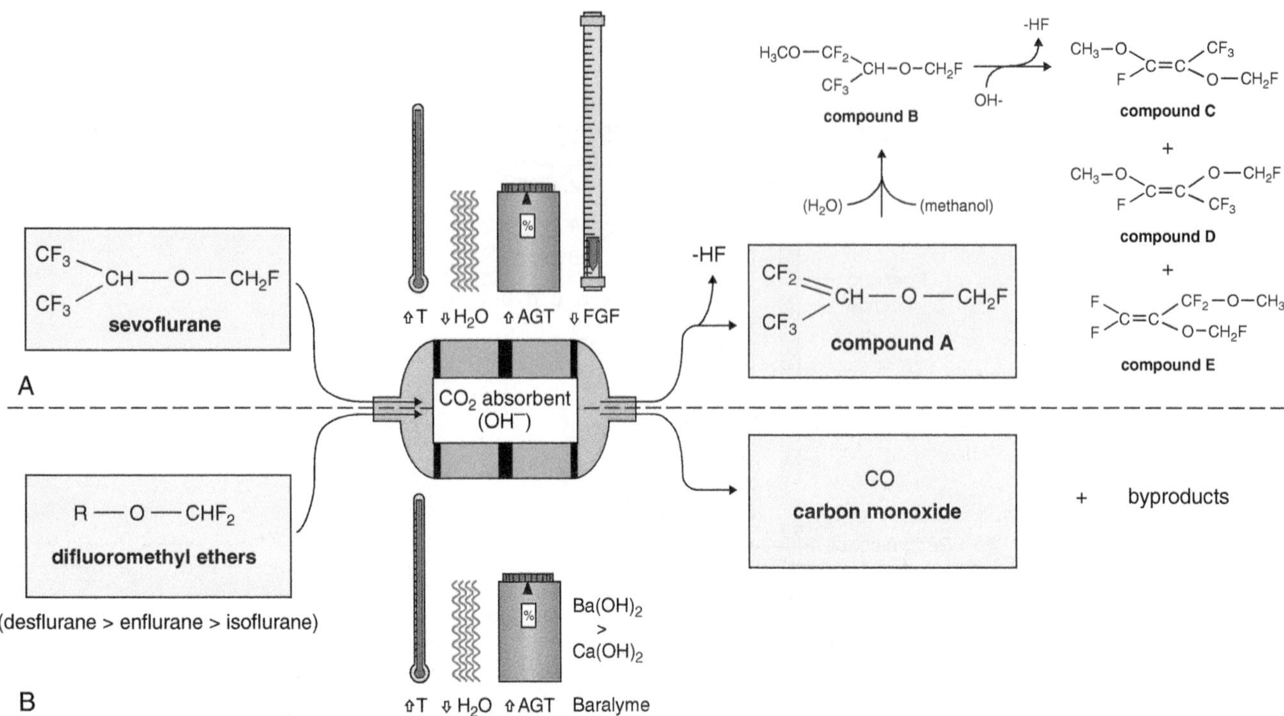

FIGURE 4-11 The degradation of volatile anesthetics by carbon dioxide absorbents. **A,** Production of compound A from sevoflurane is promoted by warmer, drier absorbent and by higher concentrations of agent (*AGT*) and lower fresh gas flows (*FGF*). In the presence of water, sevoflurane produces methanol, which promotes the breakdown of compound A into compound B and other low-toxicity products C, D, and E. **B,** The phenomenon of carbon monoxide (CO) production from the difluoromethyl ethers (desflurane, enflurane, and isoflurane) is often the result of prolonged high gas flows, which dry out the absorbent. Higher temperatures (*T*) and agent concentrations increase CO production in this setting, and the use of barium hydroxide lime (Baralyme) results in more CO production than the use of soda lime.

desflurane or isoflurane is being used may be facilitated by the use of a multiwavelength pulse oximeter (pulse CO-oximeter; see Chapter 11) that can continuously measure carboxyhemoglobin. Such devices are available and used in emergency departments but are not yet widely used in the operating room.[77-78] It is recommended that absorbent that is known or suspected to be desiccated not be used, especially with desflurane, isoflurane, or enflurane. The FDA recommends replacement of any absorbent suspected of contributing to the presence of carbon monoxide in the breathing circuit, although some investigators have suggested rehydration of existing absorbent as a practical and more cost-effective alternative.[79]

Alternatives to soda lime are available. For example, lithium hydroxide offers a little more carbon dioxide absorption capacity per unit of volume but more than three times per unit of weight; it is therefore used in submarines. Barium hydroxide lime contains 20% $Ba(OH)_2$ and little alkali. Its dust is slightly less alkaline when dissolved in water, and it is a suitable alternative to soda lime.[80] The end products are barium carbonate and calcium carbonate. It is initially pink but turns blue-gray with exhaustion because of two indicator dyes, Mimosa Z and ethyl violet. Barium hydroxide is as efficient as soda lime per unit of volume, but because of its density, it is half as efficient per unit of mass.

Methods of carbon dioxide removal other than chemical reaction with metal hydroxides have also been investigated. Much of the research in this area has originated from aviation, space, and submarine technology. One method of particular interest is a molecular sieve that uses synthetic zeolites, crystalline hydrated aluminosilicate materials, arranged in a three-dimensional tetrahedral framework that contains entry pore sites and cavities.[81] Gases that enter the sieve separate on the basis of size and polarity. Carbon dioxide is a polar molecule and is retained in certain zeolites by the action of Van der Waal forces. Because chemical bonding does not take place, the process can be reversed by slight changes in pressure and temperature, thus allowing regeneration of saturated zeolite. This technology has already been used extensively in industry for petroleum refining, water purification, and drying of gases and liquids. It has also been used for aviation and medical purposes in oxygen generators.[82,83] Advantages suggested for the use of molecular sieves in anesthesia breathing systems include lack of compound A in the presence of sevoflurane, avoidance of carbon monoxide production, removal of nitrogen dioxide in circuits that deliver nitric oxide, and cost savings as a regenerative process.[84,85]

Mixing Devices

Resistance to gas flow in a modern circle system is less than 1 cm H_2O/L/min of gas flow, one half of a person's normal airway resistance to gas flow.[35,36] Patients, including infants and children, may safely breathe spontaneously from a circle system for prolonged periods. However, before circuit designs permitted such low resistances, attempts were made to decrease resistance to breathing by providing a continuous flow of gas around the circle, thereby causing the inspiratory and expiratory valves to float open rather than open and close with each breath. Both pumps and Venturi devices driven by fresh gas flow were designed, the most prominent of which was the Revell circulator.[86,87] Although these devices can decrease dead space and resistance in the apparatus, the potential benefit is slight; in some circumstances these devices can backfire, actually increasing the work of breathing. If the low resistance of modern equipment is still a concern, it can be eliminated by controlled ventilation. Ways to reduce the mean airway pressure during controlled ventilation have been suggested but are not commonly used.[88]

Mixing of the expirate is required to measure carbon dioxide production and physiologic dead space. Standard physiologic testing usually collects all the expired gas for several minutes to mix and measure the mixed expired gas concentrations needed in these calculations (see also Chapter 8). Simply averaging a continuous capnogram will not do; this yields a time-weighted average instead of the required volume-weighted average. To understand the difference, consider what happens toward the end of a respiratory cycle. While the carbon dioxide is increasing slightly, the flow is rapidly decreasing and may become zero at the end-expiratory pause. Carbon dioxide excretion should be the integral of concentration with respect to flow; when flow falls to zero, so does carbon dioxide excretion, but the increased end-tidal value continues to increase the time-weighted integral of the capnogram. Special volume mixing devices can be used, but suitable sites for such measurements may include the breathing bag, the ventilator bellows, or the expiratory port of the ventilator pressure relief valve at its connection with the scavenging system.

BACTERIAL FILTERS

There is little doubt that anesthesia breathing systems are susceptible to contamination from the patient and the environment.[89] What is less clear is what risk this poses to subsequent patients and whether bacterial filters are necessary. Despite a recent resurgence of interest, in part related to a hepatitis C outbreak among patients sharing a common breathing system in an OR in New South Wales in 1993,[90] an international consensus on the use of bacterial filters in anesthesia systems remains elusive. However, the American Society of Anesthesiologists concludes in its recommendations for infection control that a "bacterial filter with an efficiency rating of more than 95% for particle sizes of 0.3 μm should be routinely placed in the anesthesia circuit, where it will protect the machine from contamination with airborne infectious diseases."[91]

Multiple invitro studies of various filters have demonstrated bacterial filtration efficiencies (BFEs) in the range of greater than 99.9% and viral filtration efficiencies (VFEs) of 96.43% to 99.84%.[89] These efficiencies are achieved in the myriad commercial filters now available by the use of one of two fiber arrangements. The first consists of a small-pore compact matrix with a high airflow resistance offset by pleating to create a larger surface area. The second is a less dense, larger pore size arrangement that has less resistance to accommodate a smaller surface area. Some filters possess a permanent electrical polarity designed to enhance the Van der Waal forces that hold organisms within the matrix. Some are also considerably hydrophobic, which prevents water penetration and subsequent increased resistance and loss of efficiency. A few have combined roles as filters and heat and moisture exchangers (HMEs). These filters generally are placed at the Y-piece and serve as both an inspiratory and expiratory barrier, whereas standard filters usually are placed on the expiratory limb.

Considering the favorable evidence regarding filtration efficiency, the question of whether to use filters might be simpler if they were free of problems. Complications reported with the use of breathing system filters are in general related to either obstruction or leakage. Obstruction has been described when filters become saturated with circuit humidity as a result of sputum,[92,93] edema fluid,[94] nebulized aerosols,[95] or malpositioning of the filter.[96] In one case, a leak in the housing of a gasline filter resulted in patient hypoxia.[97] Another consideration is cost; at least one author advocates the use of disposable or autoclavable circuits, carbon dioxide absorbers, and ventilator bellows—all components in contact with the patient's breathing circuit—based in part on cost advantage because filters become unnecessary.[98] Also of concern is the lesser efficiency of bacterial filters with regard to viruses. After discussing the efficiency of bacterial filters and the low likelihood of cross-contamination during their use, Hogarth,[89] in his excellent review of the subject, concludes that "the use of filters within the breathing system adds a known risk to the patient, against which must be balanced the unknown risk of viral contamination and cross-infection by agents both known and unknown."

In addition to bacterial filters, the breathing circuit also may incorporate a spirometer to measure ventilation, a humidifier to provide warmth and moisture, sampling sites for gas analysis, and scavenging devices to control atmospheric contamination by waste gases in the OR. These subjects are discussed in Chapters 5, 7, 8, 9, and 20.

ANALYSIS OF SPECIFIC CIRCUITS

Circle Breathing Systems

The basic components of a circle breathing system are an inspiratory and expiratory limb, each with a unidirectional valve, and a reservoir bag or counterlung that moves reciprocally with the patient's lungs. The system may be divided into quadrants (Fig. 4-12). The patient and counterlung, but not the absorber, separate the inspiratory and expiratory limbs of the system; the valves separate the patient from the bag side of the system. The position of the valves within the limbs is not necessarily fixed; they may be anywhere between the patient and the bag with little practical difference in function. They usually are incorporated with the bag mount, pop-off valve, and absorber for manufacturing ease and durability. Even if the valves are moved to other locations, it is convenient to think of four quadrants when analyzing circle systems.

For practical anesthesia, it is necessary to add three other components: a carbon dioxide absorber, a fresh gas inflow site, and a pop-off valve for venting excess gas. Each of the three may be placed in any of the four quadrants. There are hundreds of different ways to place three components in four quadrants, but only a few are used.[99] Different manufacturers have used different arrangements, and older designs allowed the user to change the configuration with slight change in function. The optimal configurations for spontaneous and controlled ventilation are different,[18] and most current designs are optimal for controlled ventilation.

This analysis emphasizes a frequently overlooked or misunderstood point: The bag, not the absorber, is on the opposite side of the circle from the patient. Most schematics and diagrams of breathing circuits perpetuate this misconception by showing symmetrical circuit limbs on either side of the absorber. The position of the bag is at neither the inspiratory limb nor the expiratory limb; rather it *separates* the two.[37]

Placement of the Carbon Dioxide Absorber, Fresh Gas Inflow, and Pop-off Valve

The carbon dioxide absorber may be placed in any of the four quadrants but is almost invariably placed in the inspiratory limb on the bag side so that apparatus resistance to inspiration may be overcome with assisted or controlled ventilation (Fig. 4-13). Placement on the expiratory side (Foregger circles) adds a mild degree of expiratory resistance that, like PEEP, may be beneficial for oxygen exchange but increases the risk of barotrauma. A bypass valve to permit carbon dioxide to build up was considered desirable by a majority of anesthesiologists but not by those who build the apparatus.[100] The carbon dioxide absorber is absolutely necessary in a low fresh gas flow technique because no other method is available to remove carbon dioxide; that is, it is removable neither by dilution nor exclusion from reinspiration. As fresh gas flow is increased above gas uptake rates, the other methods become increasingly effective. This is noted by the anesthesiologist as longer intervals before the indicator in the absorbent suggest that it be replaced. At a 5 L/min fresh gas flow, the absorbent lasts more than twice as long as at 500 mL/min. This is not cost effective because the extra anesthetic gases and vapors cost more than the absorbent saved. In addition to saving on agents, the absorbent has two other beneficial effects: both expired humidity and heat are partially conserved, and both are optimized as flow decreases.[101,102] The risks of absorbent (e.g., soda lime) include airway reaction to inspired alkaline dust, which can be minimized by good design and technique; alkaline "burns" from condensed water and/or dust spilled from the canister housing; and a breathing circuit with more connections and pieces, which provides more opportunity for user error.

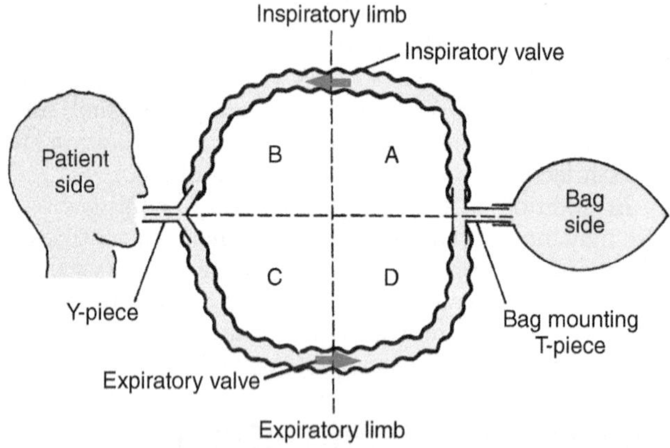

FIGURE 4-12 The four quadrants of a basic circle system. Two corrugated breathing tubes connect the patient and the counterlung (a bag or a ventilator bellows). One-way valves are located in the inspiratory limb and in the expiratory limb. The circle is therefore bisected twice, dividing it into four quadrants: A, B, C, and D. To make a practical circuit for anesthesia, three more essential components must be added: a fresh gas inflow site, a pop-off valve, and a carbon dioxide absorber.

Although the inflow site for fresh gas may be physically placed in any of the four quadrants, efficiency and manufacturing convenience also are factors in placement.[18,103] The inflow site usually is incorporated with the other components; that is, the absorber, bag mount, and valves. If the inflow site is located on the patient side of the inspiratory valve (quadrant B, Fig. 4-13), gas flows continuously around the circle throughout the respiratory cycle. Thus spirometry in the expiratory limb is inaccurate unless total gas flow is shut off.[104] If inflow is located on the patient side of the expiratory valve (quadrant C, Fig. 4-13), any carbon dioxide–containing alveolar gas between the Y-piece and the patient is washed into the patient's lungs during inspiration at the rate of the fresh gas flow. This may be negligible during closed-system anesthesia, but it can produce rebreathing of up to half of the previously exhaled alveolar gas at total flows of 10 L/min. Placement in quadrant D is simply inefficient because some fresh gas will be lost to the pop-off valve in most circles.

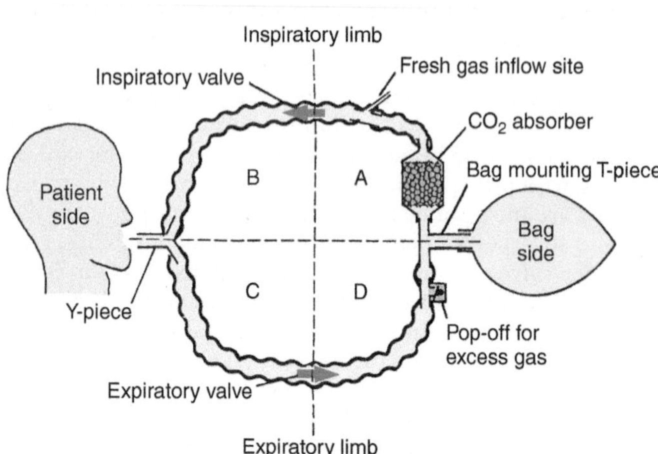

FIGURE 4-13 Placement of the carbon dioxide absorber, fresh gas inflow, and pop-off valve. The typical site for the absorber is in the inspiratory limb on the bag side, that is, in quadrant A. The inspiratory valve typically is mechanically attached to the canister but is shown here as it was in Figure 4-12 for ease of analysis. Fresh gas inflow usually is on the bag side in the inspiratory limb (quadrant A), downstream from the carbon dioxide absorber. The pop-off valve typically is downstream from the expiratory valve, near the bag. It is shown here in quadrant D but could be in A, before the carbon dioxide absorber.

Recommended placement for the fresh gas inflow is on the bag side of the inspiratory limb between the inspiratory valve and absorber (quadrant A, Fig. 4-13). If the absorber housing has appreciable head space, as is common, this inflow site stores the continuously delivered fresh gas during exhalation. Gas flows down the inspiratory limb only during inspiration. During exhalation, fresh gas flows backward toward the absorber, bag, and pop-off valve. Thus fresh gas provides most of or all the respired gas with high-flow techniques, or it enriches the oxygen and anesthetic-depleted expiratory gas with low-flow techniques.

The pop-off valve may be placed anywhere in the circle, but some locations are more rational than others. Locating the valve in the inspiratory limb (quadrants A and B, Fig. 4-13) tends to vent fresh anesthetic and carbon dioxide–free gas. Furthermore, locations in the inspiratory limb on the patient side (quadrant B) permit some carbon dioxide–containing exhaled gas to enter the inspiratory limb during the end of a spontaneous breath. This rebreathing is clearly undesirable. It is mechanically convenient to place the pop-off valve between the expiratory valve and the bag mount, or opposite the bag mount, before the absorber (i.e., in quadrants D or A, but close to the bag mount). Incorporating the pop-off valve into a one-piece absorber/bag mount/expiratory valve/pop-off valve assembly provides convenience and durability.

There is at least theoretic value to locating the pop-off valve on the patient side at the Y or next to it (quadrant C, Fig. 4-13). During spontaneous inspiration, the pressure at this site is below atmospheric pressure and the pop-off valve is closed. During exhalation, the pressure is just slightly above atmospheric pressure, and gas flows to the reservoir bag until it is distended to its nominal volume. Then the pressure in the entire circuit increases as fresh gas inflow and exhalation from the patient continue, opening the pop-off valve. The gas vented is primarily carbon dioxide–rich, oxygen-depleted, and anesthetic-depleted end-tidal gas. However, the situation is reversed during assisted or controlled ventilation. During inspiration, the pressure in the circuit at the Y-piece is positive with respect to atmospheric pressure. A pop-off valve located at the Y-piece would dump fresh gas, and one near the bag would dump a mixture of dead space gas and end-tidal gas. Two pop-off valves on the same circuit double the risk of hypoventilation when ventilation is changed to manual because the anesthesiologist may fail to close both valves. For this reason, pop-off valves at the Y-piece are no longer used.

Flow and Concentration

The gas mixture inspired by a patient breathing from a circle system is determined by the fresh gas inflow, the configuration of the circle, the respiratory pattern, and the uptake by the patient of oxygen and anesthetics. At fresh gas inflow rates that exceed minute ventilation, the circle behaves similar to a nonrebreathing system. The concentration of inspired gas closely approaches that being delivered from the gas flowmeters on the machine. As flow is progressively decreased, a disparity between fresh gas inflow and actual inspired concentration of anesthetics increases.

In a closed system, in which inflow matches loss from the system, the composition of reinspired gas is not predictable from the inflow concentration of gases.[105] Inspired and exhaled gases differ because of uptake of oxygen and anesthetic and excretion of carbon dioxide. Oxygen concentration in mixed exhaled gas usually is 4% or 5% lower than that in inspired gas. Although oxygen uptake remains relatively constant during anesthesia (approximately 250 mL/min standard temperature and pressure dry [STPD]) in the average adult, provided that body temperature does not change appreciably, anesthetic uptake varies; it is greatest at the start of anesthesia and decreases with time. If oxygen concentration is maintained constant during closed-system anesthesia, the flowmeter values reflect oxygen consumption and anesthetic uptake by the patient rather than inspired concentrations. When nitrous oxide is used in closed-system anesthesia, the oxygen tension or concentration in the circle must be continuously monitored because nitrous oxide uptake declines but oxygen uptake does not. The inspired gas mixture may become hypoxic if the nitrous oxide inflow is not gradually decreased. Whether it is necessary to measure the concentration of potent volatile anesthetics during closed-system anesthesia remains controversial. Some believe that it is necessary, and others prefer to monitor anesthetic depth and patient responses clinically (see also Chapter 26).

Semiclosed Systems: Mapleson Classification

Mapleson configurations of Magill circuits are characterized by a reservoir that can be filled by fresh gas, exhaled gas, or both. They may or may not have a pop-off valve, but if one is present it does not prevent rebreathing. Carbon dioxide, eliminated by both dilution with fresh gas and by efficient arrangement of the circuit components, is critically affected by total fresh gas flow and the pattern of respiration. The pattern of respiration includes the respiratory rate, tidal volume, dead space, I:E ratios, and inspiratory and expiratory flow patterns. The earliest semiclosed systems consisted of a bag attached to a mask by an elbow or a length of breathing tubing if it was desirable to move the large bag away from the face. The inlet for fresh gas was through a nipple on the elbow or through the tail of the bag, and a pop-off valve was placed either at the bag's tail or at the elbow. The bag ideally contained a volume approximating the patient's inspiratory capacity, about 3 L in an adult, to permit spontaneous deep breaths without the feeling of suffocation. Gas flows totaling 1 to 2 times the minute volume were used.[8,101] Mapleson organized the various configurations into five typical models and later added a sixth (Fig. 4-14).[7,26] Each of these breathing systems may be thought of as part of the continuum shown in Table 4-2.

In Table 4-2, the far right situation represents complete rebreathing and is of use only in the study of respiratory control. The original Mapleson B and C configurations lie midway on the continuum and are judged to have no particular merit, except perhaps for brief procedures or to transport patients while supplemental oxygen is administered and breathing is augmented.

None of the Mapleson systems meets the requirements on the far left of Table 4-2, but with optimal configuration and high fresh gas flow, they may approach the function of

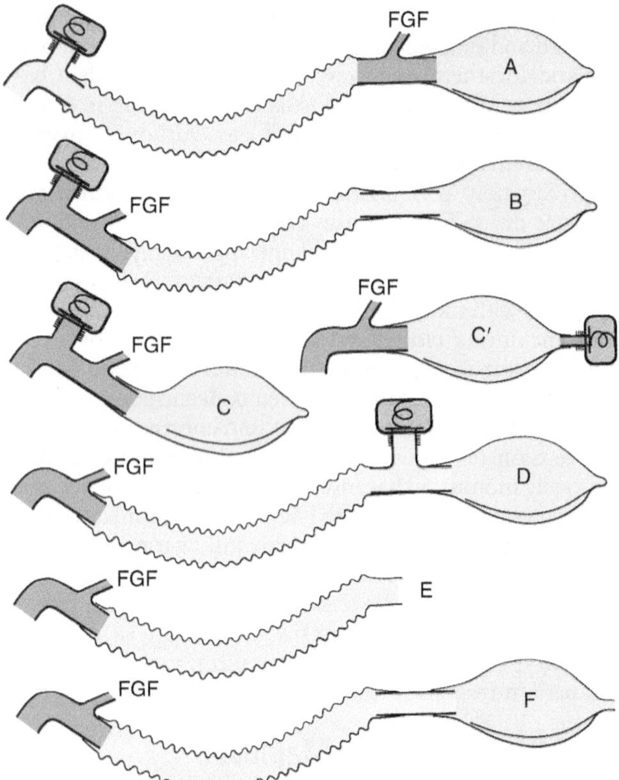

FIGURE 4-14 Mapleson classification of breathing systems. Note that the semiclosed systems (top four) contain most of the components of a circle system: tubing, connectors, bag, fresh gas inflow (*FGF*), and pop-off site. They lack carbon dioxide absorbers because carbon dioxide is lowered by the addition of fresh gas and elimination of carbon dioxide–rich gas preferentially through the pop-off valve. They also lack separate inspiratory and expiratory limbs; one tubing serves both purposes. The Mapleson A system (Magill attachment) is optimal for spontaneous respiration. The Mapleson C system is a simple bag and mask. Moving the pop-off to the bag tail is a major improvement (C'), because this permits more mixing of fresh and exhaled gas than the Mapleson C (this modification, not one of Mapleson's, has been added by the author). The B circuit is wasteful of fresh gas in both spontaneous and controlled respiration. The D circuit is similar to the A except that it exchanges the inflow and pop-off sites. A is optimal for spontaneous breathing, and D is best for controlled breathing. The Mapleson E system is essentially an Ayre's T-piece with an added reservoir. If the reservoir is short, it is an open, not a semiclosed, system. This system is simple but lacks the convenience of a bag for ventilatory assistance or control. A bag can be added to it (*F*, or Jackson-Rees modification), which may or may not possess an adjustable pop-off valve to help assist or control ventilation. All these circuits share a common advantage. Vigorous hyperventilation cannot reduce the patient's carbon dioxide tension much below normal if FGF is kept between one and two times the patient's normal respiratory minute volume.

an open system. Efficiency of the systems in this context can be translated as the lowest fresh gas flow that will ensure normal removal of carbon dioxide, thereby minimizing rebreathing. There is normally a partial pressure difference for carbon dioxide such that alveolar CO_2 (P_ACO_2) is greater than mixed expired CO_2 ($P_{\bar{E}}CO_2$), which is greater than inspired CO_2 (P_ICO_2).

$$\text{Alveolar} > \text{Mixed expired} > \text{Inspired}$$

$$P_ACO_2 > P_{\bar{E}}CO_2 > P_ICO_2$$

TABLE 4-2 Spectrum of Carbon Dioxide Elimination

Maximum Carbon Dioxide Elimination	To	Maximum Carbon Dioxide Retention
No mixing of fresh and alveolar gas occurs.	Complete mixing of fresh and alveolar gas occurs.	No missing of fresh and alveolar gas occurs.
Fresh gas goes to the patient.	The mixture is inhaled.	Alveolar gas is rebreathed.
Alveolar gas goes to the pop-off valve.	Fresh gas and mixed gas are "popped off" simultaneously.	Fresh gas goes to the pop-off valve.
DESIRABLE	ACCEPTABLE	UNDESIRABLE

The most efficient configurations place the pop-off valve where the highest concentration of carbon dioxide is found during the phase of breathing in which the circuit pressure is above atmospheric pressure. This occurs at end expiration during spontaneous breathing and during inspiration with manually assisted or controlled breathing.

A great deal of attention has been devoted to determining the lowest gas flow that can be safely used in clinical anesthesia. A variety of claims have been made for the various circuits and for proprietary modifications of the circuits, such as Bain, Lack, Humphrey ADE, and Mera F circuits. Unfortunately much of the published work has one or more of the following flaws:

1. Theoretical analyses embody unrealistic assumptions about mixing and breathing patterns, especially the I:E ratio and expiratory flow.
2. Model studies embody nonphysiologic states, particularly lack of responsiveness to carbon dioxide and simplified flow patterns.
3. Studies were done in awake volunteers, whose metabolic rates and physiologic responses differ from those of anesthetized patients.
4. Imprecise endpoints were used, such as rebreathing of carbon dioxide identified by capnography rather than by an increase in alveolar or arterial carbon dioxide concentration.

However, consensus has been reached in one regard: systems classified as Mapleson A (Magill attachment, Lack, and Humphrey A) are most efficient for spontaneous, unassisted ventilation, and those classified as Mapleson D, E, or F (Jackson-Rees, Bain, Humphrey DE) are most efficient for assisted or controlled ventilation.

A general criticism of the published analyses of breathing circuits is a failure to distinguish between the quantity of reinspired carbon dioxide and minimum inspired carbon dioxide tension. The most common tool, a capnograph, displays a signal of airway concentration as a function of time. Thus, if airway carbon dioxide falls slowly with inspiration, just reaching zero near end inspiration, it is interpreted as no rebreathing, even though a significant amount of carbon dioxide has been reinspired. Conversely, if airway carbon dioxide falls to a low but nonzero concentration for all of inspiration, carbon dioxide excretion may be adequate despite perceived rebreathing if total ventilation is increased. Inspired carbon dioxide is properly calculated as the integral of instantaneous flow multiplied by instantaneous carbon dioxide concentration, which is difficult or impossible to measure with simple instrumentation. (See also sections on volumetric capnography in Chapters 8 and 10.) A better analysis is based on the equation of defining alveolar ventilation ($\dot{V}_A$):

$$\dot{V} = \frac{\dot{V}_{CO_2}}{F_{A}CO_2} \quad (4\text{-}5)$$

$$\dot{V}_A = \dot{V}_E - (V_{DS} \times f) \quad (4\text{-}6)$$

Equation 4-5 states that alveolar ventilation is the quotient of carbon dioxide production and alveolar fractional concentration of carbon dioxide. Because the fractional volume of alveolar carbon dioxide (F_ACO_2) is proportional to the partial pressure of alveolar carbon dioxide (P_ACO_2), a specific PCO_2 defines one and only one $\dot{V}_A$ in a given patient. Equation 4-6 demonstrates that any increase in dead space ventilation ($V_{DS} \times f$) can be accommodated by an equivalent increase in minute volume ($\dot{V}_E$), keeping alveolar ventilation, and hence carbon dioxide elimination, constant. Any amount of carbon dioxide may be rebreathed, at a concentration equal to or below alveolar carbon dioxide, if an increase in minute volume maintains alveolar ventilation.

Even if instantaneous PCO_2 reaches zero near end inspiration, a significant volume of carbon dioxide may be rebreathed, requiring an appropriate increase in minute volume. A numerical example may help clarify this. Consider a patient in need of 4 L/min of $\dot{V}_A$ with F_ACO_2 of 0.05 (5%) and a current $\dot{V}_E$ of 6 L/min with a respiratory rate (f) of 20 breaths/min. The patient could rebreathe 2.5% carbon dioxide and keep F_ACO_2 at 5% if the apparent alveolar ventilation doubled to 8 L/min. If the dead space ventilation did not change—it probably would, but not much, depending on whether tidal volume or f were increased—a total minute volume of 10 L would suffice. Clearly, an inspired carbon dioxide load can be compensated for. Note that the ventilatory response to carbon dioxide of an awake person (slope of 2 L/min/mm Hg) would require a rise of less than 2 mm Hg P_ACO_2. However, at a sensitivity to carbon dioxide frequently seen in an anesthetized person (e.g., 0.5 L/min/mm Hg), the carbon dioxide tension would have to rise nearly 8 mm Hg. Thus a significant difference is apparent between spontaneous breathing, for which ventilation is set by the patient's P_ACO_2 and responsiveness, and controlled ventilation, for which minute volume is set by the anesthesiologist.

Any gas mixture that contains carbon dioxide can be considered to consist of a fraction of carbon dioxide–free gas and a fraction of alveolar gas. Any rebreathing of alveolar gas is simply added dead space and can be compensated for by increasing overall ventilation. For example, given 4 L/min of alveolar ventilation and 2 L/min of dead space ventilation, what will happen if a patient suddenly inspires 1% carbon dioxide? Each unit of alveolar ventilation now holds only four-fifths of the previous level of newly produced carbon dioxide, so increasing alveolar ventilation by 125% will result in the same degree of carbon dioxide elimination.

Mapleson A Configurations and Carbon Dioxide Removal

Consider first the Mapleson A circuit shown in Figure 4-15. The assumptions for this model include spontaneous breathing with a rate of 20 breaths/min, tidal volume (VT) of 400 mL, I:E ratio of 1:2, a sinusoidal inspiratory flow averaging 24 L/min, a near exponential expiratory flow with a half-time of less than 0.5 second, a functional residual capacity (FRC) of 2400 mL, a fresh gas flow of 6 L/min, a bag of 3 L nominal volume at the pop-off valve opening pressure, and a corrugated tube of 500 mL volume. The top diagram shows the condition at end inspiration, after the lung has inspired 400 mL over 1 second, consisting of 100 mL of fresh gas flow and 300 mL from the circuit. All of the circuit has been flushed with fresh gas, and carbon dioxide

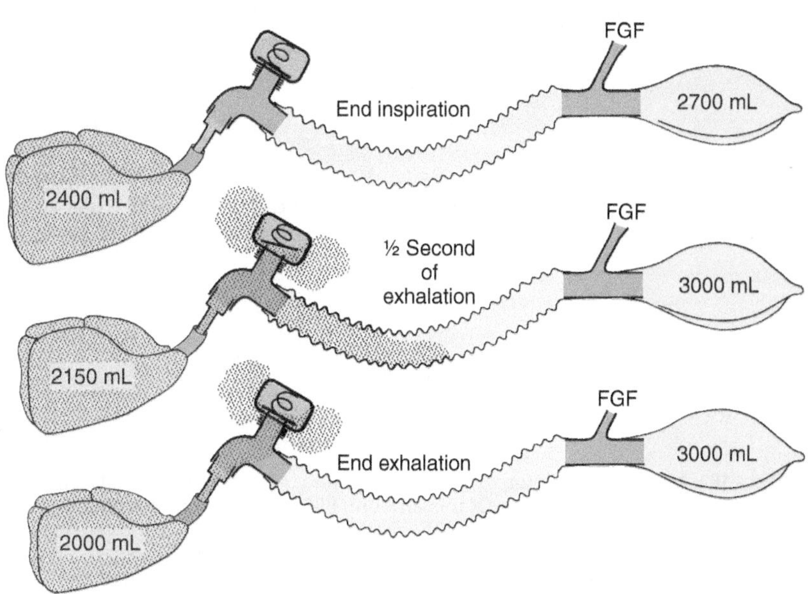

FIGURE 4-15 ■ Mapleson A circuit, spontaneous breathing. Stippled areas indicate carbon dioxide–containing gas. *Top,* The end of a normal spontaneous inspiration for a normal adult patient. As the patient begins to exhale, carbon dioxide–free gas flows from the upper dead space, then carbon dioxide–rich gas flows into the corrugated tube and, together with continuing fresh gas flow (*FGF*), fills the bag a half second later (*middle*). The rest of the expirate goes out through the pop-off valve, along with carbon dioxide–containing gas in the tubing, which is pushed toward the pop-off valve by the fresh gas flow. Optimally, at end exhalation (*bottom*), the circuit has largely been flushed of carbon dioxide.

is found only in alveolar gas (stippled area). In the first 0.5 second of exhalation, 250 mL of gas are exhaled and, together with 50 mL of fresh gas, have distended the reservoir bag to 3 L and have just opened the pop-off valve (see Fig. 4-15). Carbon dioxide–containing alveolar gas has penetrated partway down the breathing tube, but the exact distance depends on the dead space; the shape and volume of zones I and II of the capnogram (see Chapter 10 for capnogram zones); and the longitudinal mixing, or conical flow pattern, in the tube. In the next 1.5 seconds of exhalation, the rest of the expired alveolar gas (150 mL) has exited the pop-off valve, and 150 mL of fresh gas has flushed the carbon dioxide–containing expirate in the breathing tube back and out through the pop-off valve. If the sum of the fresh gas flow (150 mL) and the carbon dioxide–free dead space gas from zone I exceeds the penetration of zone II and alveolar gas, the situation at the end of exhalation, as shown in the bottom diagram of Figure 4-15, is the result. This generally is true when fresh gas flow exceeds 55% of the respiratory minute volume.[106,107] In this particular model, about 100 mL of fresh gas exits the pop-off valve with each breath along with the carbon dioxide–containing alveolar expirate. In studies of anesthetized patients, the fresh gas flow that maintains carbon dioxide homeostasis in Mapleson A circuits used with spontaneous breathing has been found to be 70% to 100% of the minute volume, depending on the many variables.[107-109]

During assisted or controlled ventilation, two different things happen to decrease efficiency. First, the bag must be squeezed during inspiration, both to deliver the entire tidal volume (400 mL) and to vent the fresh gas flow that comes in over an entire respiratory cycle (in this case, 1/20 of 6 L/min, or 300 mL). Now all the exhaled tidal volume flows into the breathing tubing, followed by the continued fresh gas flow during the end-expiratory pause. During the next compression, some alveolar gas may reenter the airway until the circuit pressure rises to the threshold of the pop-off valve. Thereafter, some carbon dioxide and some fresh gas go both to the lung and to the pop-off valve. Understandably, the effect would depend on the rate of compression of the bag, that is, the inspiratory flow, lung and chest wall compliance, airway resistance, volume of dead space, I:E ratio, and fresh gas flow. Thus, during assisted ventilation, the Mapleson A circuit is far less efficient than during spontaneous ventilation in terms of preventing rebreathing.

Mapleson D Configurations and Carbon Dioxide Removal

A typical circuit for controlled ventilation is shown in Figure 4-16. The assumptions for this model are a fresh gas flow of 6 L/min; a minute volume of 10 L, using a VT of 1000 mL and respiratory rate of 10; an FRC of 2000 mL; an expiratory flow nearly exponential with a 0.5-second half-time; an I:E ratio of 1:2; and a peak inspiratory gas flow rate of 30 L/min. At inspiration the bag is squeezed to deliver 1000 mL to the patient in 2 seconds and to blow 600 mL out the pop-off valve. A total of 200 mL of fresh gas entered in these 2 seconds, which results in the state shown in the top panel of Figure 4-16.

Two seconds after exhalation begins, the patient has exhaled 900 mL, which is diluted with 200 mL of fresh gas as it enters the circuit. This has refilled the bag to 2700 mL. In the next 2 seconds of exhalation, the rest of the tidal volume, 100 mL, and 200 mL more of fresh gas have filled the breathing tubing, and the bag has regained its initial volume of 3 L. The lungs now contain 6% carbon dioxide because this gas has been slowly increasing as a result of continued carbon dioxide delivery to a progressively smaller alveolar volume. The bag contains 3% carbon dioxide, but in the breathing tubing the concentration falls toward zero, the fresh gas fraction of inspired carbon dioxide ($FiCO_2$). In fact, if two thirds of the fresh gas flow is washed into the

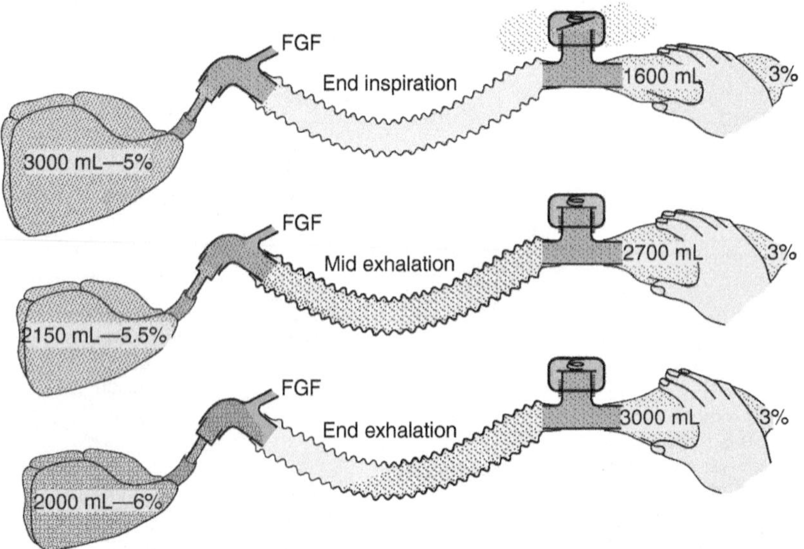

FIGURE 4-16 Mapleson D circuit, controlled breathing. At end inspiration, the anesthesiologist has squeezed the bag from its nominal volume of 3 L down to 1600 mL. Of this amount, 800 mL went into the patient's lungs along with 200 mL of fresh gas; 600 mL of the bag's contents, with about 3% carbon dioxide, left the circuit through the pop-off valve (*top*). During the next 2 seconds, the patient exhales nearly all of the tidal volume (900 mL); this, with the continuing fresh gas flow (*FGF*), fills the bag (*middle*). Because of the fresh gas flow, the bag's carbon dioxide concentration content is diluted below alveolar gas. Furthermore, the patient's expiratory flow diminishes toward the end-expiratory pause, and the fresh gas flows into the patient end of the circuit. This is the gas that will enter the patient's lungs first on the next inspiration (*bottom*).

lungs, it will provide 4 L/min of carbon dioxide–free alveolar ventilation, and the P_ACO_2 will be normal despite obvious rebreathing of some carbon dioxide. In fact, studies of anesthetized patients show normal carbon dioxide homeostasis with a fresh gas flow of 70% of total minute ventilation in Mapleson D circuits during controlled breathing, if minute volume is 150 mL/kg or greater.[12,110]

Proprietary Semiclosed Systems

Although a variety of pieces of anesthesia hardware can be used to assemble Mapleson circuits A through F, several specific circuits with eponymous identities have been introduced that offer specific advantages. These include the Jackson-Rees, Bain, Lack, Mera F, and Humphrey ADE. The last four are conveniently coaxial; they have a tube-within-a-tube arrangement that moves the physical location of the fresh gas inflow and/or the expiratory valve away from the patient connection elbow while preserving the advantages of the A, D, or F circuits. The Bain and Lack circuits are shown in Figure 4-17.

The Bain circuit is basically a coaxial Mapleson D design. Instead of a separate small-bore tube for delivery of fresh gas to the patient elbow, the delivery tube enters the corrugated expiratory tube near the bag mount and pop-off valve and runs coaxially to the patient end, where the end is secured by a plastic "spider" in the center of the tube. Thus fresh gas is delivered at the patient end, and the pop-off valve exhausts gas at the bag end of the corrugated tube, a Mapleson D arrangement. Various recommendations for fresh gas flow have been published. One commercial brand has a package insert that recommends a fresh gas flow of 100 mL/kg/min. Such recommendations often were based on an instantaneous inspired carbon dioxide concentration of zero for some portion of the cycle. However, with suitably augmented minute ventilation—150 mL/kg or more, instead of the 90 mL/kg for a normal person at rest—adequate carbon dioxide elimination results from a fresh gas flow of 70 mL/kg/min during assisted or controlled ventilation.[12,33,110] Although not recommended for prolonged periods, spontaneous ventilation requires a greater fresh gas flow, up to 150 mL/kg/min.[25,111,112]

The Bain circuit may malfunction if the central tube (fresh gas delivery) becomes disconnected, either where it enters the corrugated outer tube or from its retaining spider at the patient end. Either disconnection effectively increases the apparatus dead space, and for any given minute volume, it reduces alveolar ventilation accordingly.[113] Disconnection at the bag end is by far the more serious problem, and visual inspection alone may not identify the problem. Because of this, two tests have been proposed: one uses a very low oxygen flow (50 mL/min) and occlusion of the inner tube with a finger or plunger from a small disposable syringe[114]; the flowmeter bobbin should fall with occlusion of the inner tube. Alternatively, filling the reservoir bag with gas and operating the oxygen flush will normally create a Venturi effect that partially empties the bag.[115]

The Lack circuit (coaxial Mapleson A) appears similar to the Bain circuit externally. Near the bag are both a pop-off valve and a fresh gas inflow nipple. However, the central tube is larger in diameter and serves as an expiratory limb, leading from a spider that centers it coaxially to the pop-off valve.[14] The circuit is long enough that this central tube has a volume of 500 mL. Fresh gas flows between the external corrugated tube and the central tube to the patient connection end. This is essentially a Mapleson A circuit and is optimal for spontaneous breathing. Figure 4-17 shows the Lack system at end expiration. The first part of exhalation has passed retrograde between the corrugated hose and inner tube toward the bag, which is simultaneously filling with fresh gas. Because this first part contains little or no carbon dioxide, little carbon dioxide is found in the outer channel. When the bag reaches its nominal volume, the pressure rises enough to open the pop-off valve; for the rest of exhalation, carbon dioxide–rich gas passes into the inner channel. If expiratory flow falls to nearly zero at the end-expiratory pause, fresh gas flows toward the patient through the outer channel and even into the inner tube, pushing alveolar gas out through the pop-off valve. Any carbon dioxide remaining in the inner tube is not rebreathed during the subsequent inspiration because the expiratory valve closes, and little gas flows backward in the inner (expiratory) tubing. Reports that the Lack system is more efficient, equally efficient, or less efficient than a Magill attachment may be found in the literature, but the differences are always slight.[108,116,117] Fresh gas flow at 70% of minute volume results in negligible carbon dioxide rebreathing. It is important to note that with spontaneous breathing, increasing fresh gas flow is of little value in lowering arterial PCO_2, which is set by the patient's intrinsic respiratory control centers.

The original Humphrey ADE circuit was available as a coaxial volume or as a parallel circuit.[118] A fixed, machine-mounted valve assembly with one control lever permitted selection of either a Mapleson A or D configuration.

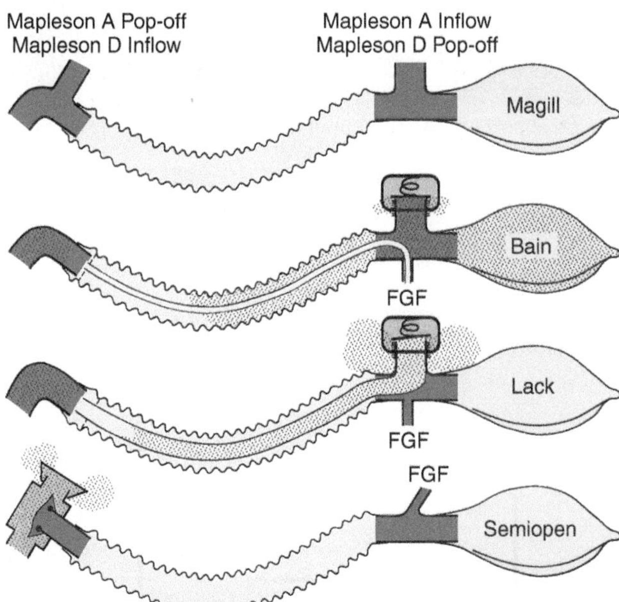

FIGURE 4-17 ▪ Comparison of the Mapleson A and D circuits with the Bain, Lack, and semiopen circuits. *From the top,* A schematic of the Mapleson A and D circuits with an indication for placement of the inflow and pop-off valves that distinguish A from D. The Bain circuit, shown at end expiration, uses a small-bore fresh gas delivery tube to deliver fresh gas to the patient end of the circuit. The Lack circuit looks similar externally, but the inner tube is now an expiratory limb that delivers exhaled gas to the pop-off valve at the bag end. In a semiopen circuit, the breathing tube is inspiratory and all exhaled gas exits at the valve. Only fresh gas is found in the tubing. FGF, fresh gas flow.

With modern anesthesia ventilators that exhaust excess gas at end expiration, the system in D mode becomes equivalent to a Mapleson E circuit, hence the suffix ADE.[118] In the parallel setup, the Humphrey ADE can be used with or without a carbon dioxide absorber (Fig. 4-18). The disadvantage of forgetting to switch the lever and the ubiquitous circle systems in U.S. hospitals have led to greater interest outside than inside the United States. A notable exception is the work of Artru and Katz,[119] who studied patients and used a rise in end-tidal rather than inspired carbon dioxide concentration as the criterion for rebreathing. They found that with an appropriate lever setting, an FGF of 66 mL/kg/min prevented an increase in end-tidal carbon dioxide during both spontaneous and controlled ventilation.

Since the original concept of combining the benefits of the Magill, Lack, Bain, and T-piece into one universal unit in 1984, there have been significant improvements to the design and function of the Humphrey ADE system. A new exhaust valve has significantly improved function for spontaneous respiration and eliminated the necessity for a D mode (Fig. 4-19). This new valve also has allowed the T-piece mode for children to be superseded by use of the system in the much more efficient Mapleson A system. A detachable soda lime canister has been added, turning the system into a multipurpose apparatus.

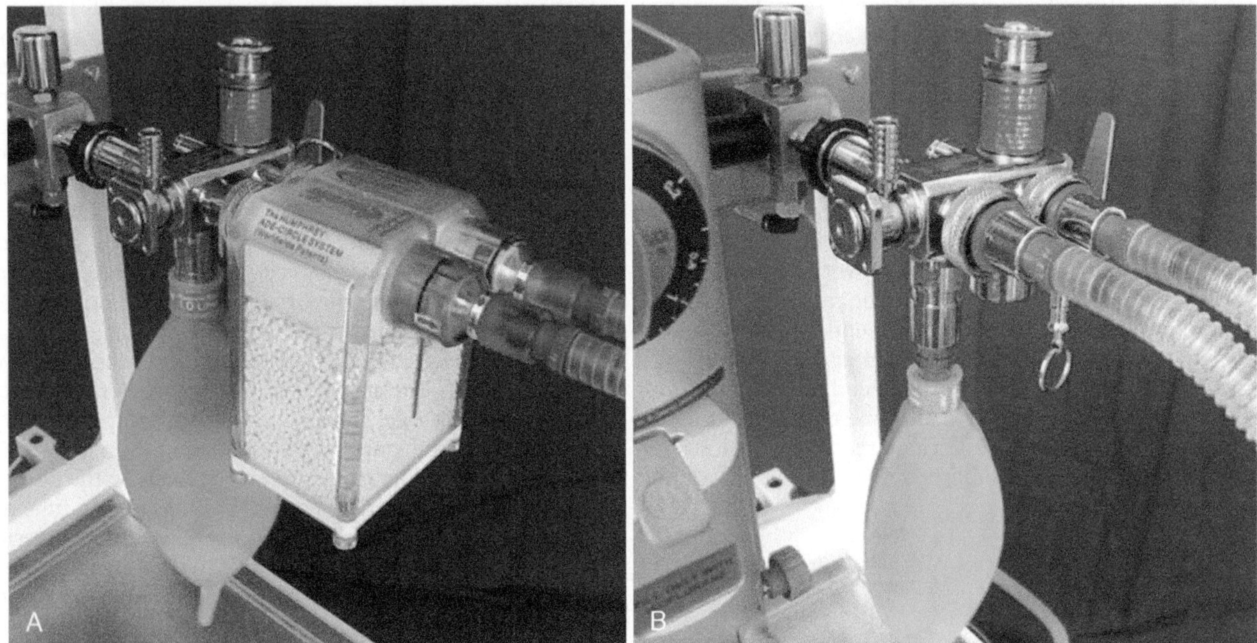

FIGURE 4-18 ■ The Humphrey ADE system can be used with carbon dioxide absorbent (**A**) or without (**B**). (Courtesy Dr. D. Humphrey.)

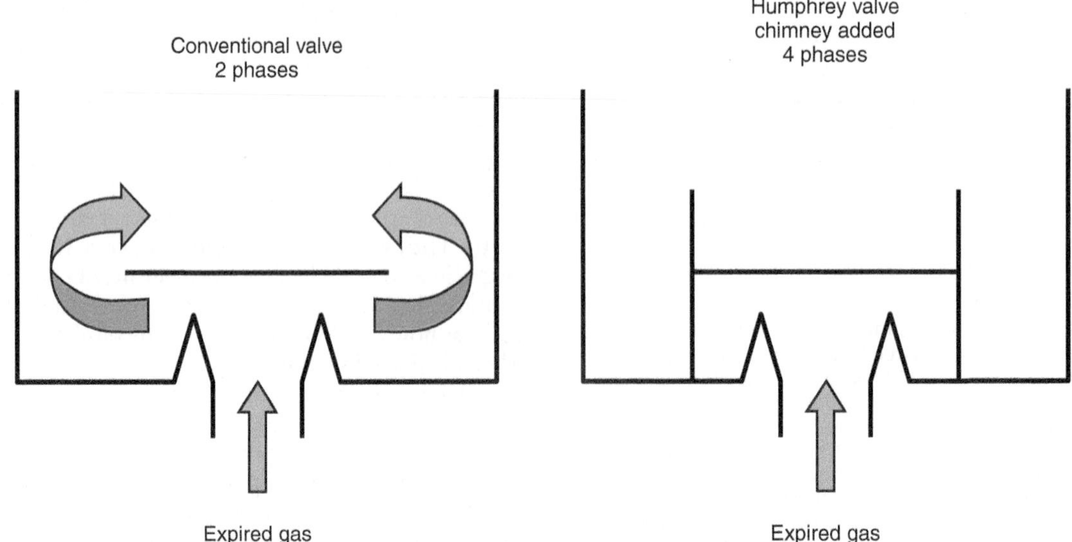

FIGURE 4-19 ■ Cross-sections through a conventional and the Humphrey ADE exhaust valve.

The efficiency of Mapleson A systems for spontaneous respiration depends on the preservation of unused dead space gas within the system during the early phase of exhalation and elimination of alveolar gas in the second half. Standard exhaust valves often open unpredictably, with significant loss of dead space gas, and there can be significant contamination by alveolar gas at the mixing interface within the tube. To prevent the loss of dead space by premature opening of the exhaust valve, a valve was designed that functions in four phases rather than two (i.e., simply open or closed).

The new valve is designed to always ensure that no exhaled gas is vented until the reservoir bag on the inspiratory limb is completely full, whether in the Mapleson A mode or with the soda lime canister. It has a 5-mm chimney encircling the knife edge on which the valve seat rests and a spring that exerts approximately 1 cm H_2O pressure on the seat. When the patient exhales, any pressure within the system lifts the valve seat into the chimney, but the spring keeps it closed (phase 1). In the Mapleson A mode, the expiratory limb remains closed in phase 1, and all dead space gas consequently is preserved along the inspiratory limb, as is fresh gas within the reservoir bag. In mid-exhalation, alveolar gas now flows into the inspiratory limb; at this point, the bag fills completely and the pressure rises within the system. The valve seat now lifts above the chimney to open the valve, allowing it to vent what is now alveolar gas (phase 2). Once open, the valve acts a variable orifice offering almost no resistance to flow. At this stage, mixing at the interface between alveolar gas and dead space is reduced by the use of 15-mm parallel smooth bore tubes (less turbulence and mixing) rather than coaxial or corrugated tubing. A "flip-flop" design Y-patient connector also helps direct the flow of alveolar gas into the expiratory limb. Exhalation continues with venting of alveolar gas through the exhaust valve until the falling pressure allows the valve seat to drop back into the chimney to close the valve (phase 3). At this point, there is a small backpressure (PEEP) within the system, preventing possible alveolar collapse that can occur under anesthesia, especially in children and the elderly. Exhalation is now complete. During the inspiratory phase (phase 4) the valve is completely closed, shutting off the expiratory limb. The patient can now breathe only from the inspiratory limb, the first part being warmed, humidified dead space gas. The fresh gas flow required is approximately equal to that needed to vent alveolar gas. Under anesthesia, this can be as low as 50% of respiratory minute volume.

The significant difference from standard valves is that the efficient function of the new valve is ensured and does not vary from patient to patient or with variable respiratory patterns. The valve cap is always fully open because it functions automatically. With almost no impedance to flow and being easy to breathe through, the design of this valve is such that it is appropriate for pediatric anesthesia. The PEEP effect also is beneficial for children. It was a logical step that such a valve could be used in the Mapleson A mode for spontaneous respiration in children.[120] In this more efficient mode, fresh gas flows can be reduced to approximately one fourth of that required for the T-piece,[120] and a scavenging tube is conveniently connected to the exhaust valve well away from the patient. The dead space gas adds beneficial heat and moisture to the system. The ADE system became a standard system for pediatrics in 1996 in the United Kingdom. Consequently, the Mapleson A mode is used for both adults and children, simplifying the concept of a multipurpose system.

To facilitate manual ventilation, the stem of the valve seat has been extended out of the top of the valve. Manual downward pressure on the stem closed off the valve such that the bag could be squeezed to assist ventilation manually without having to screw the valve cap down. Interestingly, the altered gas dynamics within the system proved to be more efficient than the Mapleson D mode.[121] For automatic ventilation, the exhaust valve and reservoir bag are automatically excluded by the lever, which, at the same time, brings in the ventilator connection. This is a safe design because forgetting to switch it causes the ventilator to sound immediately (high pressure obstruction alarm signal).

In summary, in the semiclosed mode, the Humphrey ADE system is now used in the Mapleson A mode for spontaneous respiration and manual ventilation for adults and children, while configuratively it is simply two tubes for automatic ventilation (Mapleson E). (The term *ADE system* is retained to indicate both adult and pediatric use because there is no longer a D mode.) The simplicity of the system is that the lever automatically switches between these modes. The more popular version uses parallel rather than coaxial tubing.

Finally, the introduction of the detachable soda lime canister to the original ADE system in 1999 added a new dimension to allow recycling by the absorption of carbon dioxide and included a better design of the circle system. The four-phase exhaust valve (although fully open) stays closed during exhalation such that exhaled gas is automatically recycled back to the reservoir bag until the bag is fully distended. Only then does it open to vent any excess exhaled gas. By positioning the reservoir bag on the inspiratory limb, fresh gas is efficiently preserved into this bag during the expiratory phase. (In contrast, when the bag is positioned on the expiratory limb on alternative equipment, fresh gas is forced backward through the canister and is potentially lost from the system.) The lever operates in the same way, switching between spontaneous, manual, and controlled ventilation. The anesthesiologist thus has two basic decisions to make: to use the Humphrey ADE system in a semiclosed mode or with the recycling soda lime canister, and to set the system for spontaneous and manual ventilation (lever up) or for automatic ventilation (lever down).

The Mera F system, introduced in Japan in 1978, uses a modern circle canister-valve assembly as the mounting for a coaxial Bain-type circuit. Byrick and colleagues[112] found that at 100 mL/kg/min fresh gas flow, the Mera F functioned as well as the standard Bain circuit. During controlled respiration, this flow kept P_ACO_2 at 45 ± 9 mm Hg during light anesthesia, despite a lower minute volume, because of a slightly improved capture of dead space gas for reinspiration. The Mera F tubing is quite suitable for the Humphrey ADE single-lever hardware.

The Universal F system (King Systems, Noblesville, IN) is essentially equivalent in design and function to the Japanese Mera F and is based on the same patents, but it is manufactured and available in the United States (Fig. 4-20, *A*). It also uses a coaxial arrangement and mounts on standard circle system hardware. Differences from the Mera F include larger diameter inspiratory and expiratory tubing to decrease resistance, corrugation of the inspiratory tube

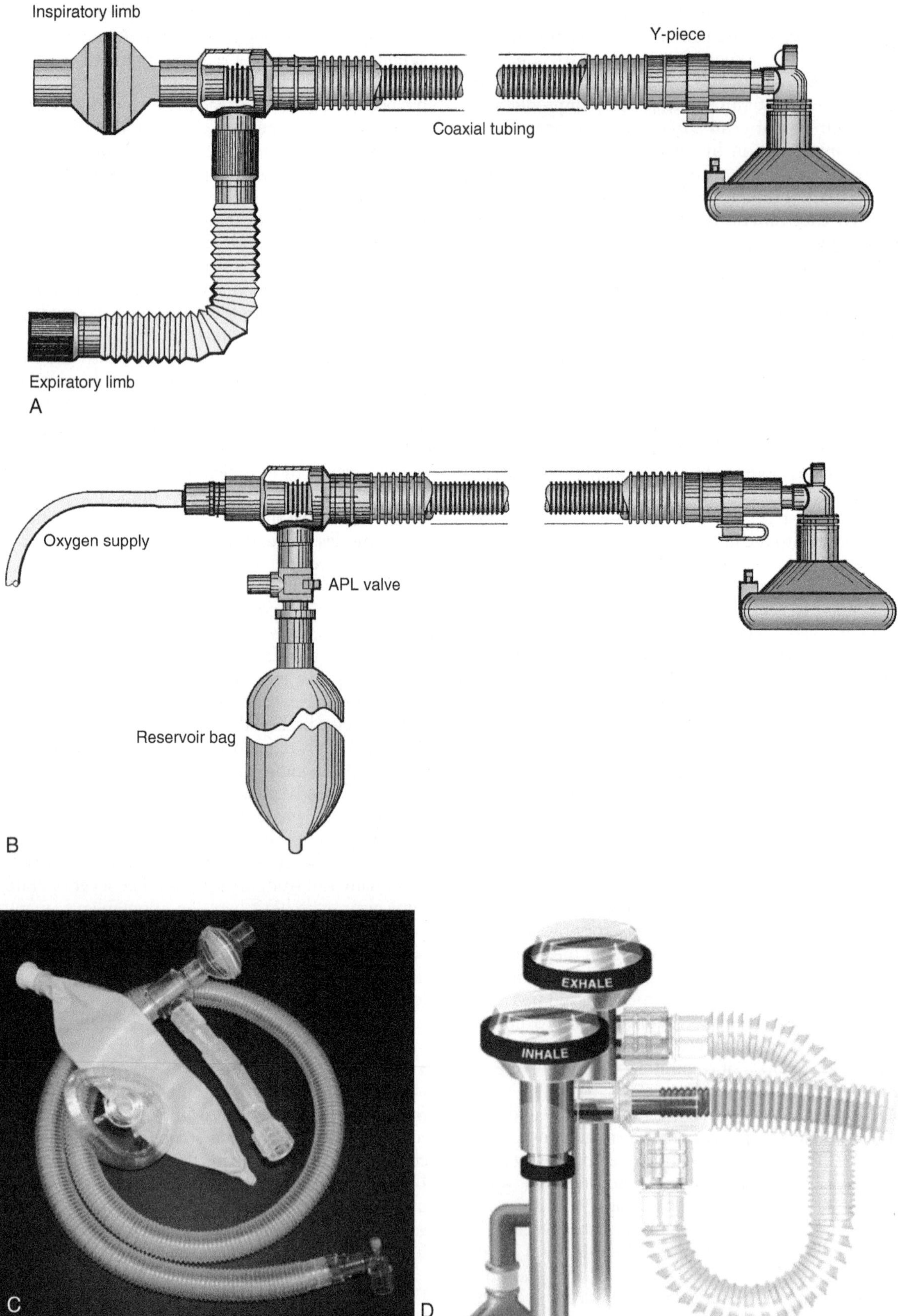

FIGURE 4-20 ■ **A** and **B**, The Universal F circuit, a coaxial system that can be mounted on standard circle system hardware. **C**, Universal F circuit with circle system adaptor tubing. Note the green inner hose carries the inspiratory gases. The circuit can be adapted for patient transport by adding an oxygen supply source to the inspiratory limb and a reservoir bag and pop-off valve to the expiratory limb. **D**, The Universal F circuit attached to the circle system. APL, adjustable pressure-limiting valve. (Courtesy King Systems, Noblesville, IN.)

to prevent kinking, and the ability to be used as a transport system. When used with circle system hardware, the Universal F system is functionally no different than a standard circle system circuit, with the exception that the inspiratory limb is enclosed by the expiratory limb for the purpose of uncluttering the tubing apparatus and providing improved humidification of inspired gas. For patient transport, the Universal F system can be converted to a Bain circuit by the attachment of an oxygen source to the inspiratory limb and a reservoir bag with a pop-off valve to the expiratory limb (Fig. 4-20, *C*). As with a standard Bain circuit, it is important that a fresh gas flow appropriate for the mode of ventilation being used be supplied when using this circuit for transport (70 to 100 mL/kg/min for controlled ventilation and ≤150 mL/kg/min for spontaneous ventilation). Following transport, this system can function as part of a nonrebreathing system on an intensive care unit ventilator.

The Enclosed Afferent Reservoir (EAR) breathing system (Fig. 4-21) reflects an attempt to create a semiclosed system that retains efficiency during both spontaneous and controlled ventilation without the use of switching valves. Use of the term *afferent* denotes a system in which the reservoir is located on the portion of the system closely associated with the fresh gas supply. Mapleson A systems, including the Lack system, are afferent reservoir systems; they preferentially exhaust alveolar gas during the expiratory phase of spontaneous respiration, but with controlled ventilation, the pop-off opens during inspiration as well, which limits efficiency. *Efferent* systems have the reservoir closely associated with the pop-off valve and include Mapleson systems D through F. As previously noted, they are most efficient during controlled ventilation. An *enclosed afferent* system prevents venting of gas from the expiratory valve during controlled inspiration by enclosing the reservoir in a chamber; as pressure in the chamber is increased to deliver a breath, the expiratory valve is forced to close. It has been demonstrated that efficiency during controlled ventilation using the EAR system is similar to that of the Bain.[122] During spontaneous ventilation, the EAR system is essentially identical to the Mapleson A. In adults, it is suggested that a fresh gas flow of 70 mL/kg is sufficient to prevent rebreathing during controlled ventilation with the EAR system.[123] Appropriate fresh gas flow during spontaneous ventilation using the EAR in adults can vary and are best determined by clinical assessment, but in a mathematical model, a value greater than 0.86 times the minute ventilation has been shown to prevent rebreathing.[124] In children, a fresh gas flow equal to 0.6 times the weight of the child has been demonstrated to provide normocapnia to mild hypocapnia regardless of the mode of ventilation.[125]

The Jackson-Rees breathing circuit is a modification of Ayre's T-piece, which is used in pediatric anesthesia worldwide. It adds a corrugated tube, a bag, and sometimes a variable, spring-loaded valve to the expiratory limb of the T-piece. Mapleson added it to his classification system as "F" in 1975.[26] Nightingale and colleagues[23] have pointed out that if the volume of the expiratory limb exceeds the tidal volume, Mapleson D, E, and F systems function identically during spontaneous breathing and should be supplied with a fresh gas flow of 100 mL/kg/min or more. Further, if the Jackson-Rees system is assembled with a spring-loaded valve in the tail of the bag, it becomes a Mapleson D and can be used with controlled ventilation with a fresh gas flow of 70 mL/kg/min.

Semiopen Systems

Semiopen systems, also known as *nonrebreathing systems*, eliminate carbon dioxide by use of two valves that exclude rebreathing. The reservoir bag contains pure fresh gas,

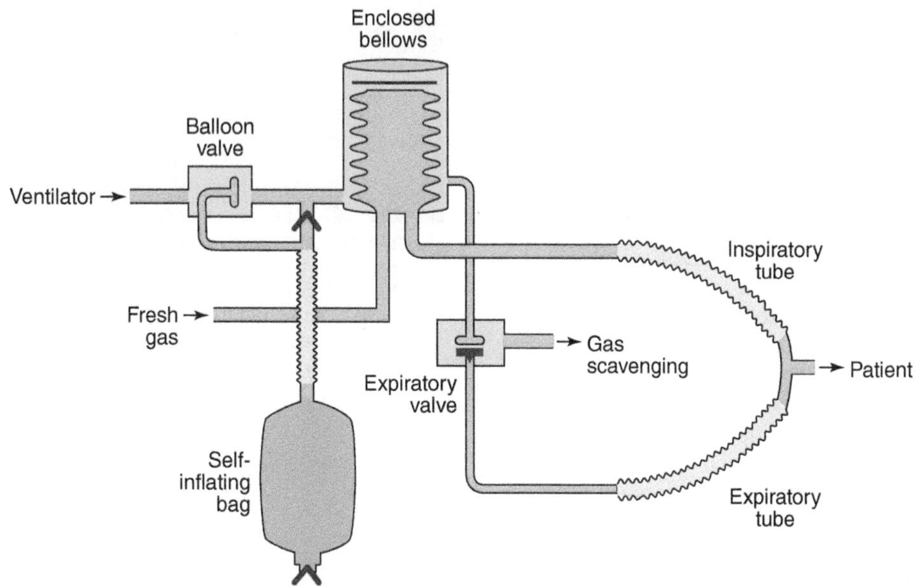

FIGURE 4-21 The enclosed afferent reservoir breathing system. This system functions like a Mapleson A system during spontaneous ventilation, but efficiency during controlled ventilation is improved by closure of the expiratory valve on delivery of a breath from the self-inflating bag, preventing wasting of fresh gas. This occurs because the same pressure increase that forces the bellows downward also inflates a balloon in the expiratory valve, causing the valve to close. (From Droppert PM, Meakin G, Beatty PC, etal: Efficiency of an enclosed afferent reservoir breathing system during controlled ventilation. *Br J Anaesth* 1991;66:638-642.)

which must be supplied at rates at or above the current respiratory minute volume. Apparatus dead space is minimized if the pair of valves, one opening on inspiration and one on exhalation, are incorporated into one small-volume assembly near the mask or tracheal tube (see Fig. 4-5, *B*). The valves must be designed to open with little pressure and to close quickly with the change in gas flow between inspiration and expiration. Clever design permits the pressure gradient across the inspiratory valve to positively close the expiratory valve, making transition from spontaneous to controlled breathing automatic; all the anesthesiologist has to do is squeeze the bag. The Frumin and Fink valves were once commonly used in anesthesia, and Ruben valves and others still find application in self-inflating resuscitator bag valve assemblies. Most mechanical ventilators used postoperatively and in ICUs also use such circuits, actively closing the expiratory valve by the machine pressure generated to start inspiration. Gas masks and scuba gear are other examples of nonrebreathing circuits, as were the intermittent-flow anesthesia machines of earlier times. The major advantages of semiopen circuits were the relative accuracy of flowmeters at high gas flow, ensuring inspired gas concentrations, and the ability to measure respiratory minute volume by setting fresh gas flow to keep the breathing bag just partly distended at each end expiration. With instrumentation currently available, neither advantage is of much value. Semiopen systems could be heated, humidified, and scavenged as readily as could semiclosed systems,[44,126-129] but often they required a higher fresh gas flow, typically 80 to 100 mL/kg/min.

Positive End-Expiratory Pressure

To improve oxygenation, the application of PEEP to a breathing system may be required. PEEP may be achieved either by adding a freestanding mechanical PEEP valve, such as a Boehringer valve (Boehringer Laboratories, Wynnewood, PA) between the expiratory limb of a circle system and the expiratory unidirectional valve (Fig. 4-22) or, in the case of the Datex-Ohmeda 7900 ventilator, by electronically regulating pressure on the expiratory valve by means of precision-controlled gas flow from the bellows. A schematic of a mechanical add-on PEEP valve is shown in Figure 4-23. A weighted ball must be lifted off its seat by the gas flow. The weight of the ball determines the amount of PEEP. Valves are available for application of various levels of PEEP, including 2.5, 5, 10, 15, and 20 cm H_2O. Such valves can be used in series to create any desired level of PEEP. It is essential that they be placed correctly—that is, vertically—in the *expiratory limb* (Fig. 4-23, *B*). Placement in the inspiratory limb would completely obstruct the circuit (see Chapter 30). Also, if not mounted vertically, they can malfunction. The use of add-on mechanical PEEP valves with the 7900 ventilator is not recommended because this could cause errors in the electronic control of PEEP, pressure, and flow by the ventilator.

"Electronic PEEP," as supplied by the 7900 ventilator, is available only during mechanical ventilation because it relies on the function of the bellows to operate. In theory, a mechanical PEEP valve could be added to the circuit during bag-mode ventilation only, but this could result in ventilator errors if the valve is left in place after switching to the ventilator mode. Because the PEEP is controlled precisely by a computer-operated flow control valve, an advantage of electronic PEEP is that any gas leak from the airway can be compensated for by increasing airway pressure from the bellows. The result is a stable, repeatable, calibrated PEEP level.

Dräger Medical offers mechanical PEEP valves as an optional part of their Narkomed anesthesia breathing systems, as does Datex-Ohmeda as part of the 7800 and earlier machines. These valves are purpose-designed and

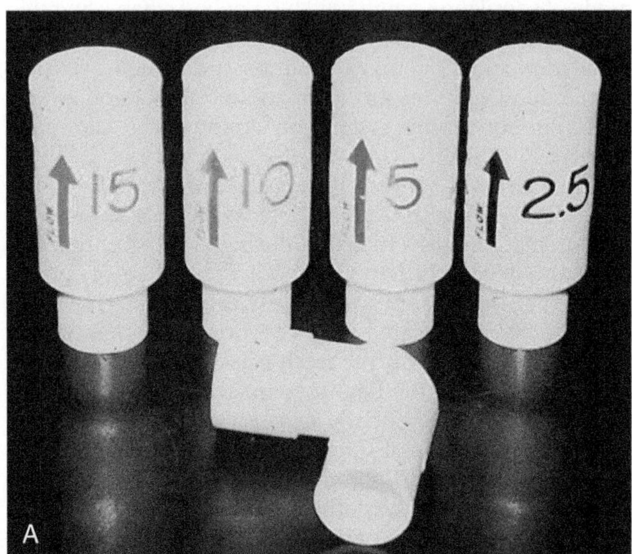

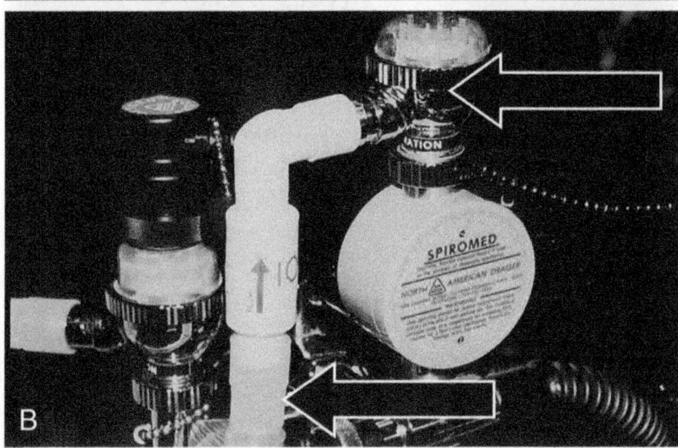

FIGURE 4-22 ■ **A**, Freestanding weighted ball positive end-expiratory pressure (PEEP) valves and elbow adapter. **B**, Freestanding PEEP valve correctly positioned vertically between the expiratory limb of the circuit *(bottom arrow)* and the expiratory unidirectional valve *(top arrow)*.

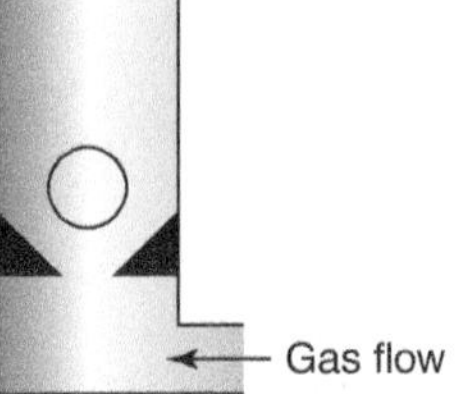

FIGURE 4-23 ■ Weighted-ball design freestanding positive end-expiratory pressure valve. This valve is designed to be mounted vertically in the expiratory limb of a circle just upstream of the exhalation unidirectional valve.

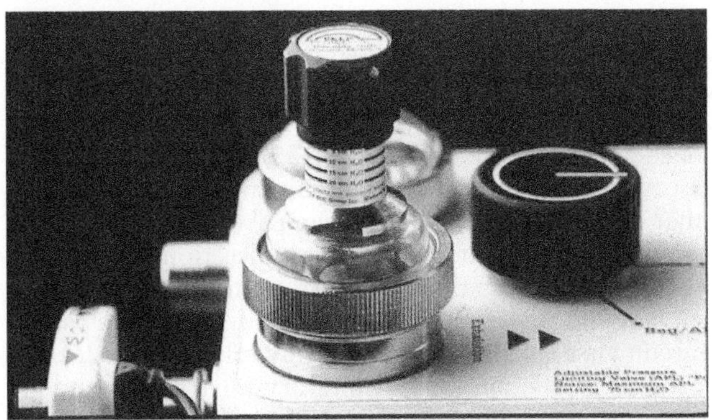

FIGURE 4-24 ■ Ohmeda positive end-expiratory pressure valve (GE Healthcare, Waukesha, WI). It it essentially a spring-loaded expiratory unidirectional valve.

built into the system to prevent erroneous placement. The Ohmeda mechanical PEEP valve is essentially a spring-loaded, expiratory, unidirectional valve that is adjustable between 2 and 20 cm H_2O (Fig. 4-24). It is essential that the PEEP valve be installed only on the exhalation unidirectional valve, never on the inhalation valve. Thus, in Figure 4-4, if an adjustable spring were to be placed between the valve disk and the dome, it would tend to prevent the opening of the disk, thereby requiring a higher pressure upstream for gas to flow across the valve. Adjusting the spring tension with the calibrated knob thereby adjusts the level of PEEP applied to the circuit between the inspiratory valve and the expiratory, unidirectional PEEP valve, as was the case in the old Ohmeda GMS Absorber. In that system, the pressure in the circuit is sensed just downstream of the inspiratory unidirectional valve so that the circuit pressure gauge and any alarms will detect the presence of PEEP in the circuit (see also Chapters 9 and 30).

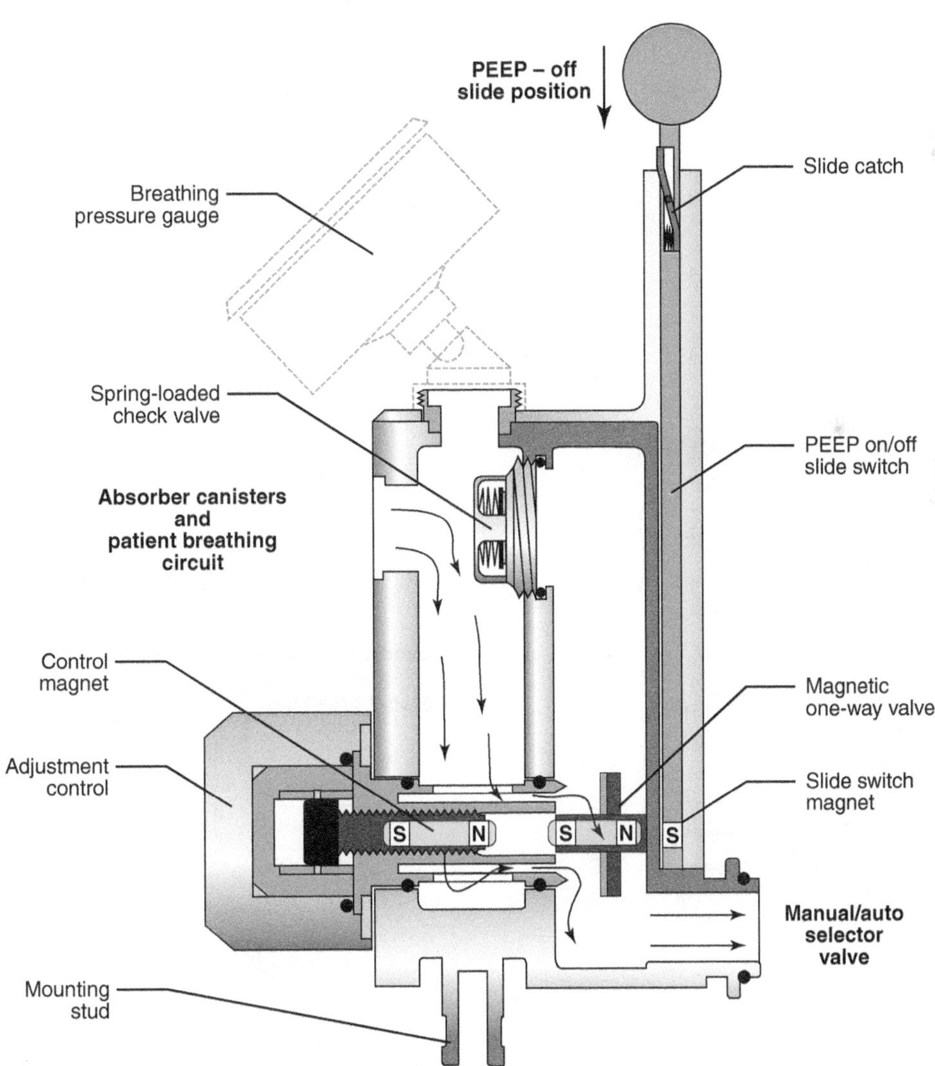

FIGURE 4-25 ■ The Narkomed positive end-expiratory pressure (*PEEP*) valve actually contains two valves, one magnetic and one spring loaded, that affect the flow of gas in the patient breathing circuit during exhalation. In this diagram, the PEEP valve is in the off position because the slide switch is moved down, placing a magnet in opposition to the magnetic one-way valve. Because the slide-switch magnet is stronger than the control magnet, the magnetic one-way valve is held in a fully open position. Thus, during exhalation, gas flows from the patient through the magnetic one-way valve unopposed, creating no PEEP. *N* and *S* refer to the north and south poles of the magnets. (Courtesy Dräger Medical, Telford, PA.)

With an old Ohmeda GMS absorber in the APL or bag mode, and with the patient breathing spontaneously, the setting on the APL valve must be higher than the PEEP setting. If it is not, inadequate tidal volumes may be delivered to the patient during inspiration. Ohmeda also warns that the PEEP valve should be installed into the GMS absorber only when the use of PEEP is anticipated for that case. It should be removed when not in use; otherwise, deposits from the breathing circuit can collect in the valve mechanism and cause it to malfunction (see also Chapter 30).[130] The use of PEEP in the patient circuit may result in a significant decrease in delivered tidal volume. Factors that influence the tidal volume delivered to the patient include patient circuit pressure (affected by PEEP), compliance, and resistance. The ventilation must be appropriately adjusted to compensate for any decrease in tidal volume caused by the addition of PEEP.[131]

The Narkomed delivery systems use a PEEP valve based on magnetic principles. Instead of using the force of a weighted ball or a spring, the force of attraction between two magnets is used to adjust the pressure needed to open the valve (Fig. 4-25). Because this valve is located between the patient circuit and the selector block that houses the switch for manual (bag) or automatic (ventilator) mode, it must permit bidirectional gas flow so that during inspiration gas flows from the reservoir bag or ventilator bellows, through the valve, and to the patient circuit via a spring-loaded, one-way valve (Fig. 4-26). On exhalation, the one-way inspiratory valve closes, and gas pressure must now overcome the force of attraction between the two magnets to open the magnetic valve and flow to the bag or ventilator bellows (Figs. 4-27 and 4-28). This PEEP valve is not calibrated, but the knob is marked to show direction of rotation for increasing or decreasing PEEP. A slide switch is incorporated into the latest version of this valve to control and clearly indicate whether the PEEP valve is on or off (Fig. 4-29).

The location of the PEEP valve in relation to the expiratory unidirectional valve (freestanding valve or Datex-Ohmeda PEEP valve) or in the manual/automatic switch block (Dräger) permits application of PEEP to the patient circuit during all modes of ventilation: spontaneous, assisted, controlled, and automatic. In this location, the

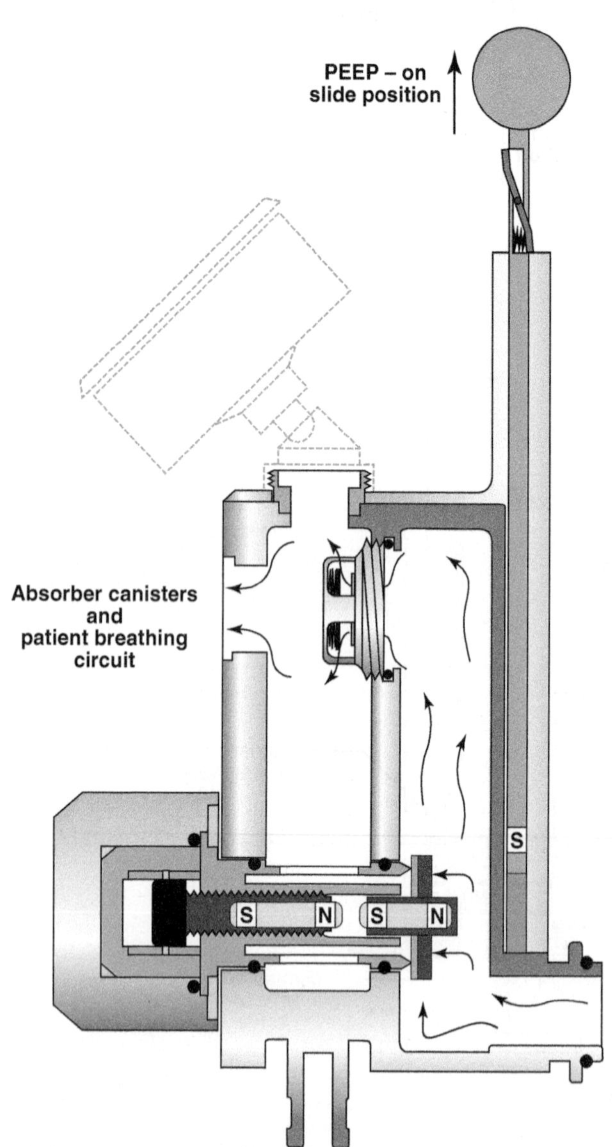

FIGURE 4-26 ■ The Narkomed positive end-expiratory pressure (*PEEP*) valve in the on position during inspiration. Gas cannot flow through the closed magnetic valve and instead flows unopposed to the patient through the one-way check valve. *N* and *S* refer to the north and south poles of the magnets. (Courtesy Dräger Medical, Telford, PA.)

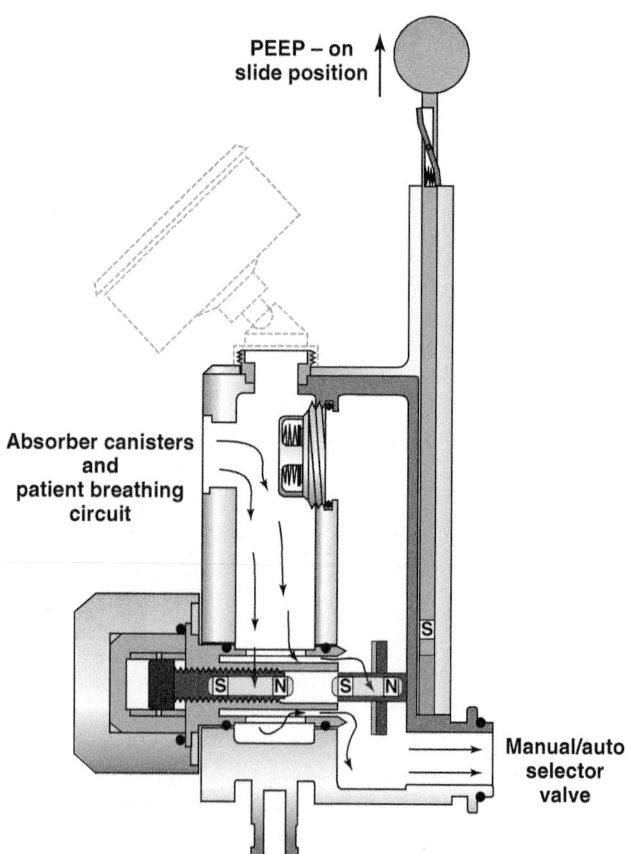

FIGURE 4-27 ■ The Narkomed positive end-expiratory pressure (*PEEP*) valve in the on position at the beginning of exhalation. Gas from the patient cannot flow through the one-way check valve, so it creates pressure in the valve apparatus that eventually forces open the magnetic valve. *N* and *S* refer to the north and south poles of the magnets. (Courtesy Dräger Medical, Telford, PA.)

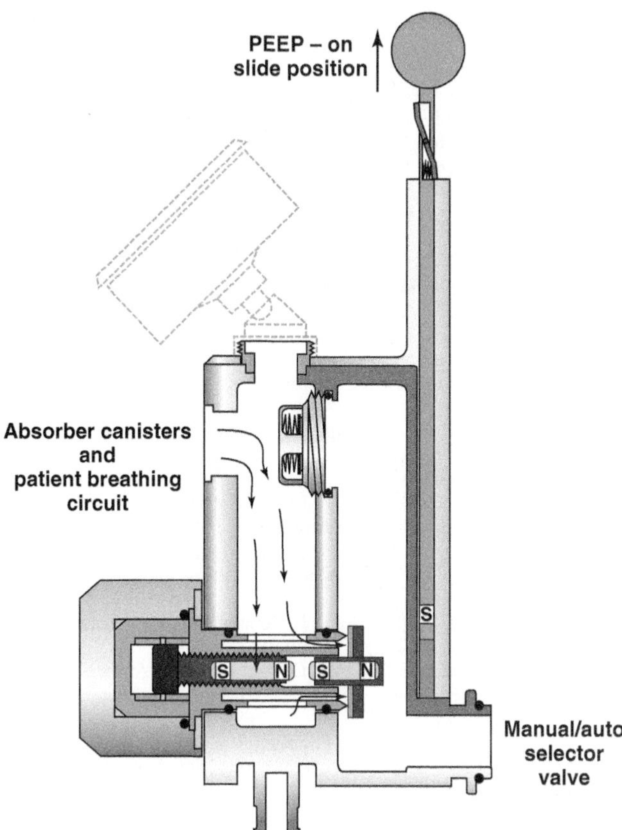

FIGURE 4-28 The Narkomed positive end-expiratory pressure (*PEEP*) valve in the on position at the end of exhalation. When the pressure of the exhaled gases decreases to a level insufficient to oppose the attraction of the control magnet to the magnetic valve, the magnetic valve closes. Gas is no longer allowed to escape from the patient's lungs, creating PEEP. The level of PEEP is increased by turning the adjustment knob such that the control magnet is moved closer to the magnetic valve, increasing the force of attraction and closing the valve earlier in exhalation. *N* and *S* refer to the north and south poles of the magnets. (Courtesy Dräger Medical, Telford, PA.)

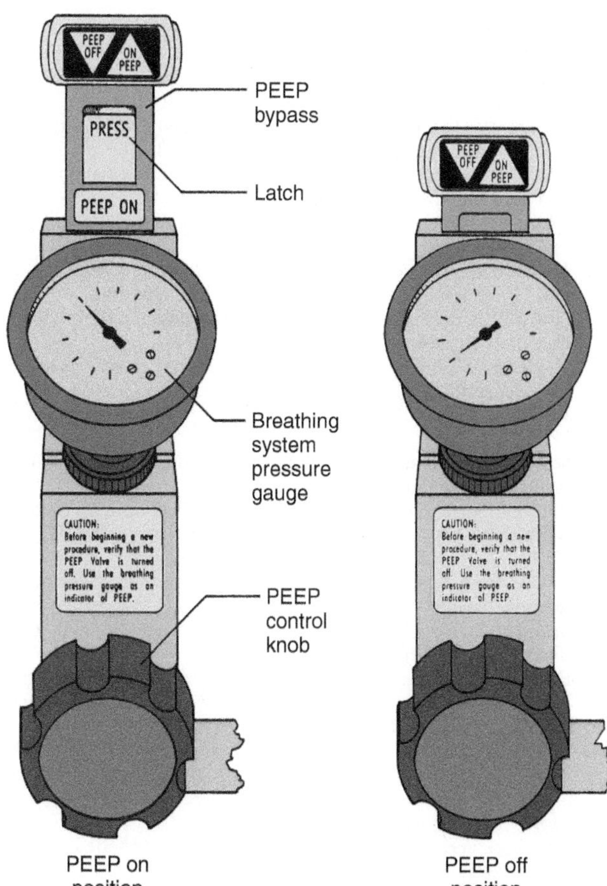

FIGURE 4-29 The Narkomed positive end-expiratory pressure (*PEEP*) valve slide switch to indicate and control the on/off function of the PEEP valve. (Courtesy Dräger Medical, Telford, PA.)

circuit pressure gauge and alarms sensing pressure at the absorber will detect the presence and level of PEEP applied (see also Chapter 30).

CIRCUIT MALFUNCTION AND SAFETY

Despite continued improvement in the design and function of anesthesia machines and related equipment, accidents resulting from their misuse or malfunction continue to occur.[131-134] A 1997 American Society of Anesthesiologists Closed Claims Project analysis of 3791 claims from 1961 to 1994 revealed that the most common source of injury related to gas delivery equipment was the breathing circuit and that the breathing circuit continues to be a source of anesthesia claims.[135] Preventable anesthesia mishaps are largely due to equipment failures or misuse. Despite the relative complexity of anesthesia gas delivery equipment, equipment misuse was found in the ASA analysis to be three times more frequent as a cause of injury than equipment failure. Interestingly, the breathing circuit, a relatively simple component of the gas delivery system, contributed to misuse more than any other component. The majority of claims related to breathing circuit misuse were attributable to either misconnections or disconnections. Rare causes included leak, valve failure, and carbon dioxide absorber defect. As previously mentioned, the bacterial filter has also been implicated as a source of problems within the breathing system.[90-94,96]

From these and similar analyses come important recommendations that anesthesiologists and manufacturers of anesthesia equipment should heed. First, anesthesiologists must be thoroughly familiar with and understand the function of the equipment they use. Second, a routine for checking equipment before using it each time is essential. Third, the design of a piece of equipment should be as simple as possible; needless elaboration may confuse the user and detract from the basic utility of the device. In fact, some have suggested that a fundamental reevaluation of breathing circuit design may be in order.[106] Finally, not all potential equipment malfunctions or errors in their use can be anticipated; anesthesiologists must be constantly vigilant for their possible occurrence and must be prepared to manage their consequences (see also Chapter 30).

Acknowledgment

We thank David Humphrey, MB BS, DA, for his contributions to this chapter.

REFERENCES

1. Jackson DE: A new method for the production of general analgesia and anesthesia with a description of the apparatus used, *J Lab Clin Med* 1:1–12, 1915.
2. Waters RM: Clinical scope and utility of carbon dioxide filtration in inhalation anesthesia, *Anesth Analg* 3:20–26, 1924.
3. Waters RM: Carbon dioxide absorption technique in anesthesia, *Ann Surg* 103:38–45, 1936.
4. Sword BC: The closed circle method of administration of gas anesthesia, *Anesth Analg* 9:198–202, 1930.
5. *The Sodasorb manual of carbon dioxide absorption*. New York, 1974, WR Grace & Co, Dewey and Almy Chemical Division.
6. Fink BR: A non-rebreathing valve of new design, *Anesthesiology* 15:471–474, 1954.
7. Mapleson WW: The elimination of rebreathing in various semi-closed anaesthetic systems, *Br J Anaesth* 26:323–332, 1954.
8. Sykes MK: Rebreathing circuits: a review, *Br J Anaesth* 40:666–674, 1968.
9. Stephen CR, Slater HM: A nonresisting nonrebreathing valve, *Anesthesiology* 9:550–552, 1948.
10. Ruben H: Anaesthesia system with eliminated spill valve adjustment and without lung rupture risk, *Acta Anaesthesiol Scand* 28:310–314, 1984.
11. Frumin MJ, Lee ASJ, Papper EM: New valve for non-rebreathing systems, *Anesthesiology* 20:383–385, 1959.
12. Bain JA, Spoerel WE: A streamlined anaesthetic system, *Can Anaesth Soc J* 19:426–435, 1972.
13. Dixon J, Chakrabarti MK, Morgan M: An assessment of the Humphrey ADE anaesthesia system in the Mapleson A mode during spontaneous ventilation, *Anaesthesia* 39:593–596, 1984.
14. Lack JA: Theatre pollution control, *Anaesthesia* 31:259–262, 1976.
15. Kay B, Beaty PCW, Healy TEJ, etal: Change in the work of breathing imposed by five anaesthetic breathing systems, *Br J Anaesth* 55:1239–1246, 1983.
16. Hamilton WK: Nomenclature of inhalation anesthetic systems, *Anesthesiology* 25:3–5, 1964.
17. Tenpas RH, Brown ES, Elam JO: Carbon dioxide absorption: the circle versus the to-and-fro, *Anesthesiology* 19:231–239, 1958.
18. Eger EI, Ethans CT: The effects of inflow, overflow and valve placement on economy of the circle system, *Anesthesiology* 29:93–100, 1968.
19. Brown ES, Seniff AM, Elam JO: Carbon dioxide elimination in semiclosed systems, *Anesthesiology* 25:31–36, 1964.
20. de Silva AJC: Normocapnic ventilation using the circle system, *Can Anaesth Soc J* 23:657–666, 1976.
21. Keenan RL, Boyan CP: How rebreathing anaesthetic systems control $PaCO_2$: studies with a mechanical and a mathematical model, *Can Anaesth Soc J* 25:117–121, 1978.
22. Ladegaard-Petersen HJ: A circle system without carbon dioxide absorption, *Acta Anaesthesiol Scand* 22:281–286, 1978.
23. Nightingale DA, Richards CC, Gress A: An evaluation of rebreathing in a modified T-piece system during controlled ventilation of anaesthetized children, *Br J Anaesth* 37:762–771, 1965.
24. Steen SN, Chen JL: Automatic non-rebreathing valve circuits: some principles and modifications, *Br J Anaesth* 35:379–382, 1963.
25. Spoerel WE: Rebreathing and end-tidal CO_2 during spontaneous breathing with the Bain circuit, *Can Anaesth Soc J* 30:148–154, 1983.
26. Willis BA, Pender JW, Mapleson WW: Rebreathing in a T-piece: volunteer and theoretical studies of the Jackson-Rees modification of Ayre's T-piece during spontaneous respiration, *Br J Anaesth* 47:1239–1246, 1975.
27. Feeley TW, Hamilton WK, Xavier B, etal: Sterile anesthesia breathing circuits do not prevent postoperative pulmonary infection, *Anesthesiology* 54:369–372, 1981.
28. ParmLey JB, Tahir AH, Dascomb HE, etal: Disposable versus reusable rebreathing circuits: advantages, disadvantages, hazards and bacteriologic studies, *Anesth Analg* 51:888–894, 1972.
29. Berry FA, Eastwood DW: Serious defects in "simple" equipment, *Anesthesiology* 28:471, 1967.
30. Cozantis OA, Tahkuman O: Aneurysm of ventilator tubing, *Anaesthesia* 26:235–236, 1971.
31. Bushman JA, Collins JM: The estimation of gas losses in ventilator tubing, *Anaesthesia* 22:664–667, 1967.
32. Proctor DF: Studies of respiratory air flow: resistance to air flow through anesthetic apparatus, *Bull Johns Hopkins Hosp* 96:49–58, 1955.
33. Spoerel WE: Rebreathing and carbon dioxide elimination with the Bain circuit, *Can Anaesth Soc J* 27:357–361, 1980.
34. Wang JS, Hung WT, Lin CY: Leakage of disposable breathing circuits, *J Clin Anesth* 4:111–115, 1992.
35. Foregger R: The classification and performance of respiratory valves, *Anesthesiology* 20:296–308, 1959.
36. Hunt KH: Resistance in respiratory valves and canisters, *Anesthesiology* 16:190–205, 1955.
37. Eger EI 2nd: Anesthetic systems: construction and function. In Eger EI 2nd, editor: *Anesthetic uptake and action*, Baltimore, 1974, Williams and Wilkins.
38. Dogu TS, Davis HS: Hazards of inadvertently opposed valves, *Anesthesiology* 33:122–123, 1970.
39. Hirano T, Saito T: A new automatic nonrebreathing valve, *Anesthesiology* 31:84–85, 1969.
40. Horn B: Valve for assisted or controlled ventilation, *Anesthesiology* 21:83, 1960.
41. Lewis G: Nonrebreathing valve, *Anesthesiology* 17:618–619, 1956.
42. Newton GW, Howill WK, Stephen CR: A piston-type nonrebreathing valve, *Anesthesiology* 16:1037–1038, 1955.
43. Ruben H: A new nonrebreathing valve, *Anesthesiology* 16:643–645, 1955.
44. Stephen CR, Slater HM: A nonrebreathing mask, *Anesthesiology* 13:226–229, 1952.
45. Loehning RW, Davis G, Safar P: Rebreathing with "nonrebreathing valves." *Anesthesiology* 25:854–856, 1964.
46. Redick LF, Dunbar RW, MacDougal DC, etal: An evaluation of hand operated self-inflating resuscitation equipment, *Anesth Analg* 49:28–32, 1970.
47. Wisborg K, Jacobsen E: Functional disorders of Ruben and Ambu-E valves after dismantling and cleaning, *Anesthesiology* 42:633–634, 1975.
48. Johnston RE, Smith TC: Rebreathing bags as pressure limiting devices, *Anesthesiology* 38:192–194, 1973.
49. Waters DJ: Use and misuse of a pressure-limiting bag, *Anaesthesia* 22:322–325, 1967.
50. Woolmer R, Lind B: Rebreathing with a semiclosed system, *Br J Anaesth* 26:316–322, 1954.
51. Lecky JH: The mechanical aspects of anesthetic pollution control, *Anesth Analg* 56:769–774, 1977.
52. Lee S: A new popoff valve, *Anesthesiology* 25:240–242, 1964.
53. Linker GS, Holaday DA, Waltuck B: A simply constructed automatic pressure relief valve, *Anesthesiology* 32:563–564, 1970.
54. Mitchell JV, Epstein HG: A pressure-operated inflating valve, *Anaesthesia* 21:277–281, 1966.
55. Smith RH, Volpitto PP: Volume ventilator valve, *Anesthesiology* 20:885–886, 1959.
56. Brown ES: Elam JO: Practical aspects of carbon dioxide absorption, *NY State J Med* 55:3436–3442, 1955.
57. Murray JM, Renfrew CW, Bedi A, etal: Amsorb: a new carbon dioxide absorbent for use in anesthetic breathing systems, *Anesthesiology* 91:1342–1348, 1999.
58. Kharasch ED, Powers KM, Artru AA: Comparison of Amsorb, sodalime, and Baralyme degradation of volatile anesthetics and formation of carbon monoxide and compound A in swine invivo, *Anesthesiology* 96:173–182, 2002.
59. Adriani J, Rovenstine EA: Experimental studies in carbon dioxide absorbers for anesthesia, *Anesthesiology* 2:1–19, 1941.
60. Brown ES: The activity and surface area of fresh soda lime, *Anesthesiology* 19:208–212, 1958.
61. Brown ES: Voids, pores and total air space of carbon dioxide absorbents, *Anesthesiology* 19:1–6, 1958.
62. Brown ES, Bakamjian V, Seniff AM: Performance of absorbents: effects of moisture, *Anesthesiology* 20:613–617, 1959.
63. Wallin RF, Regan BM, Napoli MD, etal: Sevoflurane: a new inhalational anesthetic agent, *Anesth Analg* 54:758–765, 1975.
64. Morio M, Fujii K, Satoh N, etal: Reaction of sevoflurane and its degradation products with soda lime: toxicity of the byproducts, *Anesthesiology* 77:1155–1164, 1992.
65. Gonsowski CT, Laster DVM, Eger EI 2nd, etal: Toxicity of compound A in rats: effect of a 3-hour administration, *Anesthesiology* 80:556–565, 1994.
66. Gonsowski CT, Laster DVM, Eger EI 2nd, etal: Toxicity of compound A in rats: effect of increasing duration of administration, *Anesthesiology* 80:566–573, 1994.

67. Eger EI II, Koblin DD, Bowland T, etal: Nephrotoxicity of sevoflurane versus desflurane anesthesia in volunteers, *Anesth Analg* 84:160–168, 1997.
68. Bito H, Ikeuchi Y, Ikeda K: Effects of low-flow sevoflurane anesthesia on renal function: comparison with high-flow sevoflurane anesthesia and low-flow isoflurane anesthesia, *Anesthesiology* 86:1231–1237, 1997.
69. Kharasch ED, Frink EJ, Zagar R, etal: Assessment of low-flow sevoflurane and isoflurane effects on renal function using sensitive markers of tubular toxicity, *Anesthesiology* 86:1238–1253, 1997.
70. Fang ZX, Knadel L, Laster MJ, etal: Factors affecting production of compound A from the interaction of sevoflurane with Baralyme and soda lime, *Anesth Analg* 82:775–781, 1996.
71. Ruzicka JA, Hidalgo JC, Tinker JH, etal: Inhibition of volatile sevoflurane degradation product formation in an anesthesia circuit by a reduction in soda lime temperature, *Anesthesiology* 81:238–244, 1994.
72. Frink EJ, Malan TP, Morgan SE, etal: Quantification of the degradation products of sevoflurane in two CO_2 absorbents during low-flow anesthesia in surgical patients, *Anesthesiology* 77:1064–1069, 1992.
73. Middleton V, Poznak AV, Artusio JF, etal: Carbon monoxide accumulation in closed circle anesthesia systems, *Anesthesiology* 26:715–719, 1965.
74. Fang ZX, Eger EI 2nd, Laster MJ, etal: Carbon monoxide production from the degradation of desflurane, enflurane, isoflurane, halothane, and sevoflurane by soda lime and Baralyme, *Anesth Analg* 80:1187–1193, 1995.
75. Moon RE, Meyer AF, Scott DL, etal: Intraoperative carbon monoxide toxicity [abstract], *Anesthesiology* 73:A1049, 1990.
76. Moon RE, Ingram C, Brunner EA, etal: Spontaneous generation of carbon monoxide within anesthetic circuits [abstract], *Anesthesiology* 75:A873, 1991.
77. Hampson NB: Noninvasive pulse CO-oximetry expedites evaluation and management of patients with carbon monoxide poisoning, *Am J Emerg Med* 30:2021–2024, 2012.
78. Roth D, Herkner H, Schreiber W, et al: Accuracy of noninvasive multiwave pulse oximetry compared with carboxyhemoglobin from blood gas analysis in unselected emergency department patients, *Ann Emerg Med* 58:74–79, 2011.
79. Baxter PJ, Kharasch ED: Rehydration of desiccated Baralyme prevents carbon monoxide formation from desflurane in an anesthesia machine, *Anesthesiology* 86:1061–1065, 1997.
80. Kitborn MG: Preliminary clinical report on a new carbon dioxide absorbent—Baralyme, *Anesthesiology* 2:621–637, 1941.
81. Holloway AM: Possible alternatives to soda lime, *Anaesth Intens Care* 22:359–362, 1994.
82. West JB: Oxygen enrichment of room air to relieve the hypoxia of high altitude, *Respiration Physiology* 99:225–232, 1995.
83. Anonymous: Oxygen concentrators, *Health Devices* 22:3–24, 1993.
84. Fee JPH, Murray JM, Luney SR: Molecular sieves: an alternative method of carbon dioxide removal which does not generate compound A during simulated low-flow anaesthesia. *Anaesthesia* 50:841–845.
85. Poulton BB, Foubert L, Klinowski J, etal: Extraction of nitric oxide and nitrogen dioxide from an oxygen carrier using molecular sieve 5A, *Br J Anaesth* 77:534–536, 1996.
86. Revell DG: An improved circulator for closed circle anaesthesia, *Can Anaesth Soc J* 6:104–107, 1959.
87. Neff WB, Burke SF, Thompson R: A venturi circulator for anesthetic systems, *Anesthesiology* 29:838–841, 1968.
88. Eger EI, Hamilton WK: Positive-negative pressure ventilation with a modified Ayre's T-piece, *Anesthesiology* 19:611–618, 1958.
89. Hogarth I: Anaesthetic machine breathing system contamination and the efficacy of bacterial/viral filters, *Anesth Intens Care* 24:154–163, 1996.
90. Chant K, Kociuba K, Munro R, etal: Investigation of possible patient-to-patient transmission of hepatitis C in hospital, *NSW Pub Health Bull* 5:47–51, 1994.
91. American Society of Anesthesiologists: *Recommendations for infection control for the practice of anesthesiology*, ed 3, 1998, Available at www.asahq.org.
92. Smith C, Otworth D, Kaluszyk P: Bilateral tension pneumothorax due to defective anaesthesia breathing circuit filters, *J Clin Anaesth* 3:9–34, 1991.
93. McEwan A, Dowell L, Karis J: Bilateral tension pneumothorax caused by a blocked filter in the anesthesia breathing circuit, *Anesth Analg* 76:440–442, 1993.
94. Kopman A, Glaser L: Obstruction of bacterial filters by edema fluid, *Anesthesiology* 44:169–170, 1976.
95. Barton R: Detection of expiratory antibacterial filter occlusion, *Anesth Analg* 77:197, 1993.
96. Buckley P: Increase in resistance of in-line breathing filters in humidified air, *Br J Anaesth* 56:637–643, 1984.
97. Schwartz A, Howse J, Ellison N: The gas line filter: a cause for hypoxia, *Anesth Analg* 59:617–618, 1980.
98. Komesaroff D: Disposable and autoclavable circuits: the future is now, *Anaesth Intens Care* 24:173–175, 1996.
99. Harper M, Eger El 2nd: A comparison of the efficiency of three anesthesia circle systems, *Anesth Analg* 55:724–729, 1976.
100. Neufeld PD, Johnson DL: Results of the Canadian Anaesthetists' Society opinion survey on anaesthetic equipment, *Can Anaesth Soc J* 30:469–473, 1983.
101. Chalon J, Kao ZL, Dolorico VN, etal: Humidity output of the circle absorber system, *Anesthesiology* 38:458–465, 1973.
102. Dery R, Pelletier J, Jacques A, etal: Humidity in anesthesiology. II. Evolution of heat and moisture in the large CO_2 absorbers, *Can Anaesth Soc J* 14:205–219, 1967.
103. Molyneux L, Pask EA: The flow of gases in a semiclosed anaesthetic system, *Br J Anaesth* 23:81–91, 1951.
104. Briere C, Patoine JG, Audet R: Inaccurate ventimetry by fresh gas inlet position, *Can Anaesth Soc J* 21:117–119, 1974.
105. Smith TC: Nitrous oxide and low inflow circle system, *Anesthesiology* 27:266–271, 1966.
106. Norman J, Adams AP, Sykes MK: Rebreathing with the Magill attachment, *Anaesthesia* 23:75–81, 1968.
107. Kain ML, Nunn JF: Fresh gas economics of the Magill circuit, *Anesthesiology* 29:964–974, 1968.
108. Humphrey D: The Lack, Magill and Bain anaesthetic breathing systems: a direct comparison in spontaneously breathing anaesthetized adults, *J R Soc Med* 75:513–524, 1982.
109. Ungerer MJ: A comparison between the Bain and Magill anaesthetic systems during spontaneous breathing, *Can Anaesth Soc J* 25:122–124, 1978.
110. Bain JA, Spoerel WE: Prediction of arterial carbon dioxide tension during controlled ventilation with a modified Mapleson D system, *Can Anaesth Soc J* 22:34–38, 1975.
111. Byrick RJ: Respiratory compensation during spontaneous ventilation with the Bain circuit, *Can Anaesth Soc J* 27:96–104, 1980.
112. Byrick JJ, Janssen E: Yamashita, M: Rebreathing and co-axial circuits, *Anaesthesia* 32:294, 1977.
113. Paterson JG, Vanhooydonk V: A hazard associated with improper connection of the Bain breathing circuit, *Can Anaesth Soc J* 22:373–377, 1975.
114. Foex P: Crampton Smith A: A test for co-axial circuits, *Anaesthesia* 32:294, 1977.
115. Pethick SL: *Can Anaesth Soc J* 22:115, 1975, (letter).
116. Barnes PK, Conway CM, Purcell GRG: The Lack anaesthetic system, *Anaesthesia* 35:393–394, 1980.
117. Noh M, Walters F, Norman J: A comparison of the Lack and Bain semi-closed circuits in spontaneous respiration, *Br J Anaesth* 49:512, 1977.
118. Humphrey D, Brock-Utne JG, Downing JW: Single lever Humphrey A.D.E. low flow universal anaesthetic breathing system. Part I, *Can Anaesth Soc J* 33:698–709, 1986. 1986; Part II. *Can Anaesth Soc J* 33:710-718.
119. Artru A, Katz RA: Evaluation of the Humphrey A.D.E. breathing system, *Can J Anaesth* 34:484–488, 1987.
120. Humphrey D: Manual ventilation and the Humphrey ADE breathing system, *Anaesthesia* 47:625, 1992.
121. Orlikowski CEP, Ewart MC, Bingham RM: The Humphrey ADE system: Evaluation in paediatric use, *Br J Anaesth* 66:253–257, 1991.
122. Miller DM, Miller JC: Enclosed afferent reservoir breathing systems: description and clinical evaluation, *Br J Anaesth* 60:469–475, 1988.

123. Droppert PM, Meakin G, Beatty PCW, etal: Efficiency of an enclosed afferent reservoir breathing system during controlled ventilation, *Br J Anaesth* 66:638–642, 1991.
124. Barrie JR, Beatty PCW, Campbell IT, etal: Fresh gas requirements of an enclosed afferent reservoir breathing system in anaesthetized, spontaneously breathing adults, *Br J Anaesth* 70:468–470, 1993.
125. Meakin G, Jennings AD, Beatty PC, Healy TE: Fresh gas requirements of an enclosed afferent reservoir breathing system in anaesthetized, spontaneously ventilating children, *Br J Anaesth* 68:333–337, 1992.
126. Bruce DL: A simple way to vent anesthetic gases, *Anesth Analg* 52:595–598, 1973.
127. Dery R, Pelletier J, Jacques A, etal: Humidity in anesthesiology. III. Heat and moisture patterns in the respiratory tract during anesthesia with the semi-closed system, *Can Anaesth Soc J* 14:287–298, 1967.
128. Gedeon A, Mebius C: The hygroscopic condenser humidifier, *Anaesthesia* 34:1043–1047, 1979.
129. MacKanying N, Chalon J: Humidification of anesthetic gases for children, *Anesth Analg* 53:387–391, 1974.
130. *GMS PEEP valve: operation and maintenance manual*, Madison, WI, 1991, Ohmeda, a Division of BOC Health Care.
131. Wyant GM: *Mechanical misadventures in anaesthesia*, Toronto, 1978, University of Toronto Press.
132. Cooper JB, Newbower RS, Kitz RJ: An analysis of major errors and equipment failures in anesthesia management, *Anesthesiology* 60:34–42, 1984.
133. Eger EI, Epstein RM: Hazards of anesthetic equipment, *Anesthesiology* 25:490–504, 1964.
134. Simon BA, Lovich MA, Sims N, etal: The time has come for evolution of the breathing system, *J Clin Monit* 9:60–63, 1993.
135. Caplan RA, Vistica MF, Posner KL, etal: Adverse anesthetic outcomes arising from gas delivery equipment: a closed claims analysis, *Anesthesiology* 87:741–748, 1997.

CHAPTER 5

WASTE ANESTHETIC GASES AND SCAVENGING SYSTEMS

James B. Eisenkraft • Diana G. McGregor

CHAPTER OUTLINE

TRACE CONCENTRATIONS OF ANESTHETIC GASES

Concern over trace concentrations of anesthetic gases dates back to 1967, when Vaisman[1] reported findings of a survey of 354 anesthesiologists in Russia. All worked in poorly ventilated operating rooms and used nitrous oxide (N_2O), halothane, and ether. Of the total, 303 responded to the survey; and of these, 110 were female. Female responders reported 31 pregnancies, 18 of which ended in spontaneous abortion. One pregnancy resulted in a congenitally abnormal child. Vaisman concluded that these problems in pregnancy—as well as other reported effects, such as nausea, irritability, and fatigue—were due to a combination of long-term inhalation of anesthetic vapors, emotional strain, and excessive workload. Although uncontrolled and largely anecdotal, this study drew attention to the possibility that trace concentrations of anesthetics may be harmful. The matter was taken up by investigators in Europe[2,3] and in the United States.[4-6] Their results, and those from animal studies,[7] gave cause for further inquiry.

In 1970, the U.S. Congress passed the Occupational Safety and Health Act,[8] the purpose of which was to ensure "safe and healthful working conditions for all men and women in the nation." The act established the National Institute for Occupational Safety and Health (NIOSH), which was given the responsibility to conduct and fund research in exposure hazards and to recommend safety standards. The act also established the Occupational Safety and Health Administration (OSHA), which, after due procedure, would enact into law and then enforce NIOSH recommended standards.[9] NIOSH funded a number of studies, one of which was the National Survey of Occupational Disease Among Operating Room Workers, conducted in conjunction with the American Society of Anesthesiologists (ASA) Ad Hoc Committee on Waste Anesthetic Gases. This study surveyed 49,000 people who were potentially exposed—members of the ASA, American Association of Nurse Anesthetists (AANA), Association of Operating Room Nurses (AORN), Association of Operating Room Technicians (AORT)—and 26,000 unexposed personnel, members of the American Academy of Pediatrics and American Nurses Association.[10,11] The results, published in 1974, showed an increased reported incidence among women of spontaneous abortion, liver and kidney disease, and cancer, and a higher incidence of congenital abnormalities in the offspring of exposed women. Among the exposed men, the incidence of cancer did not increase, but that of hepatic disease did. NIOSH sponsored further related studies that included investigation of methods for reducing exposure to waste gases.[12] The organization planned to introduce scavenging of waste anesthetic gases and repeat this survey to determine whether scavenging did indeed reduce these adverse health effects and show an association between trace anesthetic gases and disease.

In March 1977, before a repeat survey was commenced, NIOSH published *Criteria for a Recommended Standard; Exposure to Waste Anesthetic Gases and Vapors*.[13] This report estimated that 214,000 workers were potentially exposed to trace concentrations of anesthetic gases on a day-to-day basis. The document reviewed all the available data and found that, although not definitive, the evidence suggested a relationship between health hazards and trace concentrations of anesthetic gases. No cause-and-effect relationship was established, and no safe exposure levels could be identified. However, the document recommended that risks be minimized as much as possible by maintaining "exposures as low as is technically feasible." The document also recommended measures to reduce exposure and to monitor exposure levels, and it advocated extensive recordkeeping regarding the health of operating room (OR) personnel.

NIOSH recommended environmental limits for the upper boundary of exposure: "Occupational exposure to halogenated anesthetic agents shall be controlled so that no worker is exposed at concentrations greater than 2 ppm [parts per million] of any halogenated anesthetic agent. When such agents are used in combination with N_2O, levels of the halogenated agent well below 2 ppm are achievable. In most situations, control of N_2O to a time-weighted average (TWA) concentration of 25 ppm during the anesthetic administration period will result in levels of approximately 0.5 ppm of the halogenated agent. Occupational exposure to N_2O, when used as the sole anesthetic agent, shall be controlled so that no worker is exposed at TWA concentrations greater than 25 ppm during anesthetic administration. Available data indicate that with current control technology, exposure levels of 50 ppm, and less for N_2O, are attainable in dental offices."

These recommended exposure limits were based on two studies. First, Whitcher and colleagues[11] showed that these levels were readily attainable in the OR when certain precautionary measures were taken. Second, Bruce and Bach[14] found no decrement in the psychomotor capacities of volunteers exposed for 4 hours at the recommended levels. The newer volatile agents, such as sevoflurane and desflurane, were not available at this time, so exposure limits for these agents have not yet been assessed.

To provide a perspective on how small 1 ppm is, consider that the presence of 25 ppm of N_2O in the atmosphere represents a concentration of one four-hundredth of 1% (100% N_2O is 1 million ppm [by volume]):

$$100\%\ N_2O = 10^6\ \text{ppm}$$
$$1\%\ N_2O = 10{,}000\ \text{ppm}$$
$$(1/100) \times 1\%\ N_2O = 0.01\%\ N_2O = 100\ \text{ppm}$$
$$(1/400) \times 1\%\ N_2O = 0.0025\%\ N_2O = 25\ \text{ppm}$$

Similarly, 2 ppm and 0.5 ppm of halothane represent a concentration of one five-thousandth and one twenty-thousandth of 1% halothane:

$$100\%\ \text{halothane} = 10^6\ \text{ppm}$$
$$1\%\ \text{halothane} = 10{,}000\ \text{ppm}$$
$$(1/5000) \times 1\%\ \text{halothane} = 0.0002\% = 2\ \text{ppm}$$
$$(1/20{,}000) \times 1\%\ \text{halothane} = 0.00005\% = 0.5\ \text{ppm}$$

To express this in terms of anesthetic potency, divide the value expressed in parts per million by the minimum alveolar concentration (MAC) of halothane (0.76%) at 1 atmosphere pressure:

$$2\ \text{ppm} = 0.0002\% = \frac{(2 \times 10^{-4})}{(0.76 \times 10^{-2})}\text{MAC},$$
$$\text{or } 0.00026\ \text{MAC halothane}$$

What levels of trace anesthetics may be found in the OR? When no attempt has been made to reduce leakage or to scavenge waste gases, trace gas levels of 400 to 600 ppm of N_2O and from 5 to 10 ppm of halogenated agents may be detected.[12] Effective scavenging alone can reduce these levels more than 10-fold.

The volume of N_2O that must be released into an OR to reach the NIOSH maximum recommended limit of 25 ppm can be calculated by the following equation. Assume the size of an OR is 5 m^2 × 4 m. The volume of the OR is therefore given by:

$$500\ \text{cm} \times 500\ \text{cm} \times 400\ \text{cm} = 100 \times 10^6\ \text{mL} = 100,000\ \text{L}$$

Therefore the NIOSH limit is 25/10^6. If the OR volume is 100 × 10^6 mL, this limit is reached by release of 2500 mL (25 × 100) or 2.5 L of N_2O.

This calculation assumes uniform mixing of all gases and no ventilation or air conditioning of the OR. If it is assumed that the OR ventilation system produces 12 air changes per hour, in the OR described above, a leakage rate of 2.5 L/5 min or 0.5 L/min N_2O would be necessary to maintain the ambient air N_2O level at 25 ppm.

In 2000, OSHA revised its recommendations on waste anesthetic gases in the light of current knowledge.[15] The revised recommendations are published on the Internet for informational purposes only and are regularly updated as information becomes available. The document is not published in the standard OSHA manual on occupational hazards, however. The recommendations are advisory and have not been promulgated as a standard; rather, they are to be seen as guidelines. OSHA recommends scavenging of waste anesthetic gases in all anesthetizing locations and advocates work practices to reduce trace levels of anesthetic gases in the ambient air. A documented maintenance program should be in place for all anesthetic delivery machines, and an ongoing education program for all personnel to inform them of these recommendations must exist. OSHA recommends a program for monitoring trace anesthetic gases and also recommends a preemployment medical examination for all employees. Each institution also should have a mechanism in place for employees to report any work-related health problems.

Contamination with trace concentrations of anesthetic gases also may occur in the corridors of an OR suite, in the anesthesia workroom, and in the N_2O storage area. Poorly ventilated postanesthesia care units (PACUs) also may be contaminated with exhaled anesthetic agents.[16]

SOURCES OF ANESTHETIC GAS CONTAMINATION

Potential sources of anesthetic gas contamination are the adjustable pressure-limiting (APL) or "pop-off" valve, the high- and low-pressure systems of the anesthesia machine, the anesthesia ventilator, cryosurgery units, and other miscellaneous sources.

Adjustable Pressure-Limiting Valve

The APL valve of the anesthesia breathing circuit is the outlet for waste anesthetic gases during spontaneous or assisted ventilation. Depending on the inflow rate of fresh gas, more than 5 L of gas can exit the circuit through this valve every minute. The effect of such spillage on the level of anesthetic contamination in the OR is given by the following equation:

$$C = (L \times 60 \times 10^6)/(NV)$$

where *C* is the OR pollutant level in parts per million, *L* is the pollutant spillage in liters per minute, *V* is the OR total air volume in liters, and *N* is the number of air exchanges per hour. For example, if L = 3 L/min, V = 100,000 L, and N = 10 exchanges per hour, then

$$C = (3 \times 60 \times 10^6)/(12 \times 100,000) = 150\ \text{ppm}$$

Very large volumes of anesthetic gas are discharged through the relief valve of nonrebreathing systems, such as the Bain circuit (Mapleson D) or Jackson-Rees (Mapleson E). Without scavenging and proper room ventilation, N_2O levels as high as 2000 ppm have been found in the breathing zone of anesthesiologists.[17]

High- and Intermediate-Pressure Systems of the Anesthesia Workstation

The high- and intermediate-pressure systems of the anesthesia workstation include the N_2O central supply pipeline and reserve tanks and the internal piping of the machine that leads to the N_2O flowmeter (Fig. 5-1). The pressure in this system can be from 26 to 750 psig; leaks therefore are likely to contribute significantly to the contamination of the OR. Common sources of leaks are defective connectors in the N_2O central supply line "quick connects" (see Fig. 5-1) and defective yokes for the N_2O reserve tanks. In one OR suite, major high-pressure leaks were detected in 50% of the anesthesia machines.[18] When the OR is not being used, background N_2O contamination is primarily caused by high-pressure leaks.

Low-Pressure System of the Anesthesia Machine

The low-pressure system of the anesthesia machine includes the N_2O flowmeter, the vaporizers, the fresh gas delivery tubing from the anesthesia machine to the breathing circuit (Fig. 5-2, *F*), the carbon dioxide absorber (Fig. 5-2, *E*), the breathing hoses (Fig. 5-2, *D*), the unidirectional valves, the ventilator, and the various components of the waste gas scavenging system. Leaks occur

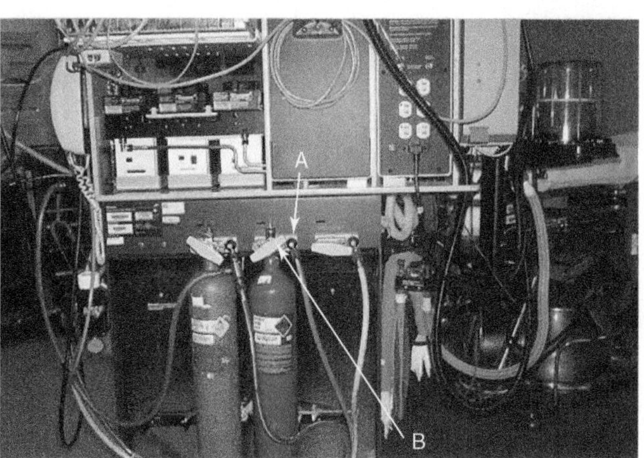

FIGURE 5-1 ■ Sources of leaks in the high-pressure system. *A,* Diameter index safety system. *B,* Yoke of N_2O reserve tank.

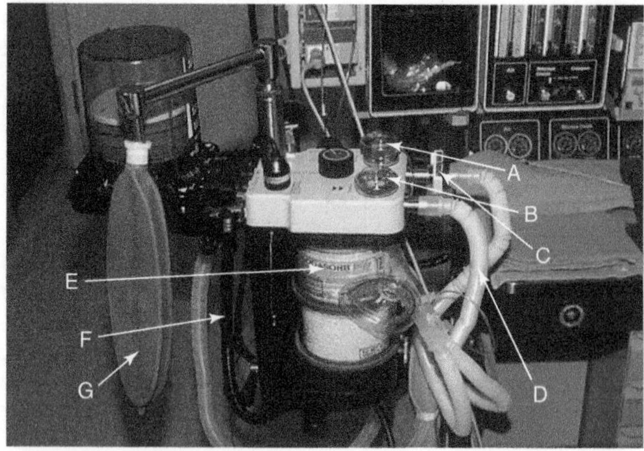

FIGURE 5-2 Sources of leaks in the low-pressure system. *A* and *B*, Domes of unidirectional valves. *C*, Oxygen sensor. *D*, Breathing circuit hoses. *E*, Carbon dioxide absorber canister. *F*, Fresh gas delivery tube. *G*, Breathing system reservoir bag.

most commonly in the carbon dioxide absorber because of loose screws, worn gaskets, granules of absorbent on the gaskets, and an open petcock. Other leaks may occur as a result of breaks in the rubber and plastic components of the breathing circuit, loose domes on the unidirectional valves (Fig. 5-2, *A* and *B*), or a poorly fitting oxygen sensor in the breathing circuit (Fig. 5-2, *C*). Disposable breathing circuits are particularly prone to leakage, especially those of the swivel type, because of imperfections in the manufacturing process.[19] Although vaporizers usually are gas tight, they, too, occasionally leak as a result of loose mounts, defective seals and gaskets, or incompletely closed fill ports.

A direct linear relationship exists between the peak pressure in the breathing circuit and the amount of gas that escapes through a leak in the low-pressure system: the higher the pressure, the greater the leak. Despite effective scavenging, as much as 2 L/min may leak from the breathing circuit, increasing the N_2O concentration in the air by 100 to 200 ppm.

The scavenging system itself may be a source of leakage. The rubber parts and safety valves may leak anesthetic gases, as may improperly sized hoses, such as 22-mm hoses that have been "adapted" to fit the 19-mm or 30-mm scavenger connections. The system also may be overloaded because of inadequate vacuum or ventilation systems; consequently, waste gases are spilled into the OR atmosphere.

Anesthesia Ventilator

The anesthesia ventilator may be a major source of leakage. Some ventilators leak internally and cause anesthetic gases to mix with the nonscavenged driving gas of the ventilator. In one OR, the N_2O level increased from 5 to 80 ppm each time the ventilator was used.

Errors in Anesthesia Technique

With a leak-proofed anesthesia workstation and breathing system and an effective scavenging system, 94% to 99% of all OR anesthetic contamination is caused by errors in anesthesia technique.[11] The following are significant errors in technique:

1. Incorrect insufflation techniques.
2. Turning the N_2O flowmeter and/or a vaporizer on while the breathing circuit is not connected to the patient causes direct loss of anesthetic gases into room air. This often occurs at the beginning and end of anesthesia administration and during intubation. When the breathing circuit is not connected to the patient, the anesthesiologist should turn off the vaporizer and the gas flows; otherwise, anesthetic-laden gas in the circuit will flow into the room.
3. A poorly fitting face mask, laryngeal mask, or other airway device permits leakage of anesthetic gases around the rim.[20]
4. An uncuffed tracheal tube that is too small relative to the tracheal diameter or a poorly seated cuffed tracheal tube may allow anesthetic gases to leak and spill into the room air.
5. At the conclusion of surgery, if a deeply anesthetized patient is disconnected from the breathing circuit, relatively high concentrations of anesthetic gases can be exhaled into the room air.
6. Accidental spillage of liquid volatile anesthetic agent while a vaporizer is refilled adds vapor to room air; each milliliter of spilled liquid adds about 200 mL of vapor.
7. Emptying the breathing circuit of anesthetic gases while the circuit is disconnected from the patient spills anesthetic gases directly into the room air.

Cryosurgery

Cryosurgery is used by gynecologists, ophthalmologists, otolaryngologists, and dermatologists and is a major source of OR contamination.[21] A jet of 20 to 90 L/min of liquid N_2O is used as a surgical tool. The liquid rapidly evaporates and raises the level of N_2O in the air. Air contamination with N_2O is particularly high when cryosurgery is used in a small, poorly ventilated office.[22] These units should be scavenged.

Miscellaneous Sources of Anesthetic Contamination

When a potent volatile anesthetic agent is used during cardiopulmonary bypass, the waste anesthetic vapor is discharged into the room air because scavenging of pump oxygenators affects their performance.[23] Diffusion of anesthetic vapors from rubber and plastic goods in the anesthesia workroom is another cause of anesthetic contamination of the atmosphere. As much as 300 mL of anesthetic vapor may be released from a used rubber breathing circuit.[11] Cardiopulmonary bypass machines are not sold with a scavenging system. Also, any vaporizer must be added in-house. A scavenging system should be set up from the exit port of the membrane oxygenator if inhaled anesthetic agents are used.[24,25]

A minor cause of anesthetic contamination is diffusion of anesthetic gases from the surgical wound and the patient's skin. The concentration of halothane in the air immediately adjacent to the operating field was found to be three to six times higher than in the room air. Higher levels were also found under the surgical drapes, possibly as a result of diffusion of halothane from the patient's skin.[26]

An infrequent cause of OR contamination is accidental crossing of the fresh air intake and exhaust ducts of the OR ventilation system. Also, installing the system exhaust port in a position upwind from the fresh air intake port may result in contamination of all ORs supplied by that ventilation system.

Another cause of OR contamination is failure to scavenge the exhaust from a sidestream-sampling capnograph or multigas analyzer. These monitors generally draw from 100 to 300 mL/min of gas via an adapter at the Y-piece in the breathing system. After it has passed through the analyzer, this gas should be directed either to the waste gas scavenging system of the machine or back into the breathing system.

OPERATING ROOM VENTILATION SYSTEMS

The OR ventilation system is an important factor in reducing anesthetic air pollution. Unventilated ORs may have levels of trace anesthetic gases four times as high as those with proper ventilation. The nine components of a typical OR ventilation system are as follows:

1. Fresh air intake from outside
2. Central pump
3. Series of filters
4. Air conditioning units
5. Manifold that distributes fresh air to the OR
6. Manifold that collects air from the OR
7. Fresh air inflow port in each OR
8. Exhaust port to the hospital air conditioning system in each OR
9. Exhaust port to the outside

The OR fresh air inflow port is located in the ceiling, and the exhaust port is located on an adjacent wall 6 inches above the floor. In general, OR ventilation systems are one of two types: *nonrecirculating* or *recirculating*. The following sections describe the various features of each system.

Nonrecirculating Ventilation System

Most ORs are equipped with a nonrecirculating ventilation system (Fig. 5-3). This type of system pumps in fresh air from the outside and removes and discards all stale air. The number of air exchanges per hour varies significantly, even among ORs in the same suite. A survey of one OR suite revealed that the number of air exchanges varied from less than 5 to more than 30 per hour.

The number of air exchanges per hour is an important determinant of the level of anesthetic contamination in the OR atmosphere. A rate of 10 or more exchanges per hour is recommended. Lower rates might permit creation of *hot spots*, air pockets highly contaminated by anesthetics; higher rates may create air turbulence that may cause discomfort to OR personnel.

The airflow pattern in the OR and the location of the anesthesia workstation in relation to the airflow also influences the level of anesthetic contamination (Fig. 5-4). When airflow generates floor-to-ceiling eddies, causing extensive air mixing, hot spots are reduced in size and number. On the other hand, hot spots are more likely to form with laminar airflow, which reduces air mixing.

Recirculating Ventilation System

A recirculating ventilation system partially recirculates stale air. Each air exchange consists of part fresh outdoor air and part filtered and conditioned stale air. This is more economical than the nonrecirculating systems because it requires less air conditioning. The recirculating system is particularly popular in locations with extremely hot or cold climates. Because filtering does not cleanse air of anesthetic gases, a recirculating system may contaminate clean ORs by recirculating air from contaminated ORs to clean ORs.

The American Institute of Architects published recommendations for ventilation in ORs and PACUs. New ORs are required to have 15 to 21 air exchanges per hour, of which three must be fresh outside air. For PACUs in use, the minimum number of total air changes is six per hour with a minimum of two air changes per hour of outdoor air.[27]

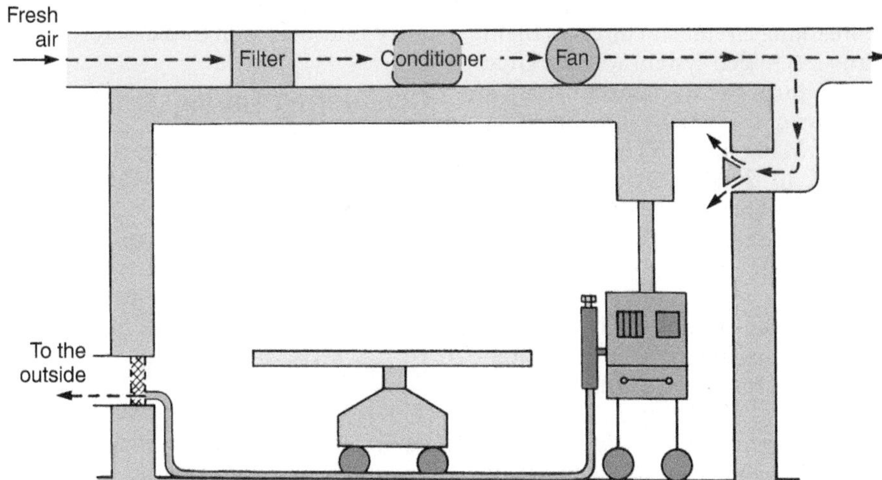

FIGURE 5-3 ■ A nonrecirculating ventilation system serving as a passive disposal route for anesthetic waste gases. (From U.S. Department of Health, Education and Welfare [NIOSH] Publication No. 75-137, Washington, DC, 1975, U.S. Government Printing Office.)

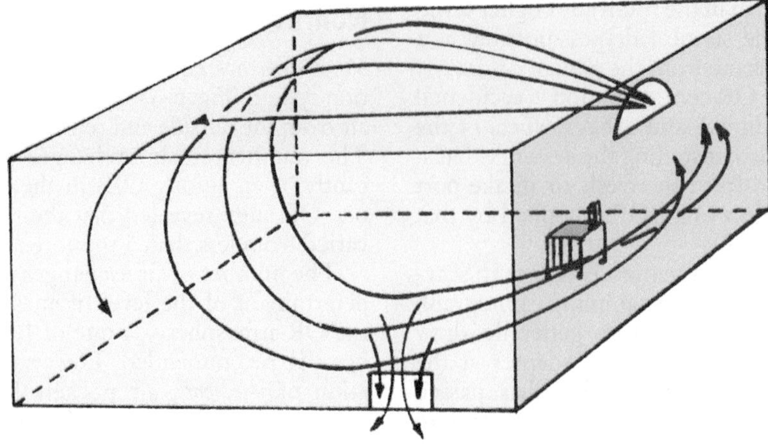

FIGURE 5-4 ■ **Operating room airflow pattern with ceiling-to-floor eddy.** (From Berner O: Concentration and elimination of anaesthetic gases in operating theatres. *Acta Anaesth Scand* 1978; 22:46.)

WASTE GAS SCAVENGING SYSTEMS

Modern anesthesia workstations are factory equipped with scavenging systems. The Joint Commission (TJC; formerly known as The Joint Commission on Accreditation of Healthcare Organizations), requires that all waste anesthetic gases be scavenged using active scavenging methods. Although it is highly unlikely, anesthesia machines not equipped with such systems may still be in use. Some anesthesia personnel discharge the waste anesthesia gases toward the floor, believing that the heavier-than-air anesthetic gases form a layer on the floor and flow out via the OR ventilation system. In reality, waste anesthetic gases are effectively mixed with room air by air eddies created by OR traffic. When the anesthesia machine is equipped with a properly functioning scavenging system, the trace concentrations of waste anesthetic gases and vapors are reduced by 90%.

General Properties of Scavenging Systems

An anesthesia scavenging system collects the waste anesthetic gases from the breathing circuit and discards them. A properly designed and assembled system will not affect the dynamics of the breathing circuit, nor will it affect ventilation and oxygenation of the patient. The American Society for Testing and Materials (ASTM) document F1343-02, last published in 2002, provided standard specifications to serve as guidelines for the manufacturers of equipment that removes excess anesthetic gases from the working environment.[28]

A typical scavenging system consists of four parts: 1) a relief valve by which gas leaves the circuit, 2) tubing to conduct the gas to a scavenging interface, 3) the interface, and 4) a disposal line. Scavenging systems are classified as either active or passive. In an *active scavenging system*, a substantial negative pressure (hospital vacuum) is applied to the disposal line connected to the interface, and waste gas is literally sucked away from the interface. In a *passive scavenging system*, waste gases flow under their own pressure via a wide-bore tube to the OR ventilation exhaust grille.

ADJUSTABLE PRESSURE-LIMITING AND VENTILATOR PRESSURE RELIEF VALVES

When a breathing circuit is in use, the waste anesthetic gases leave the circuit via an APL, or pop-off, valve (Fig. 5-5). The valve is usually spring loaded and requires only minimal positive pressure to open and allow escape of the waste gases from the circuit (see also Chapter 4). The valve has a single exhaust port (Figs. 5-6 and 5-7). To prevent accidental connection to the breathing circuit, this port is usually a 19-mm male fitting with a 1:40 conical shape.

When an anesthesia ventilator is in use, the APL valve is out of circuit and the waste anesthetic gases leave the circuit via the ventilator pressure relief (PR) valve (Fig. 5-5). During inspiration, this valve is held closed by positive pressure transmitted from the ventilator driving gas circuit or some other mechanism, as in the case of piston ventilators. The exhaust port of the PR valve is also 19 mm in diameter, as with the APL valve.

Conducting Tubing

The conducting tubing moves the waste anesthetic gases from the APL and PR valve to the scavenging interface. Tubing usually is specified to be of 19 mm or 30 mm diameter to avoid accidental connection to the breathing circuit, and it is made sufficiently rigid to prevent kinking.[24]

Scavenging Interface

The scavenging interface system is a safety mechanism equipped with relief valves interposed between the breathing circuit and the hospital's vacuum or ventilation system. A scavenging interface system may contain either a closed or an open reservoir.

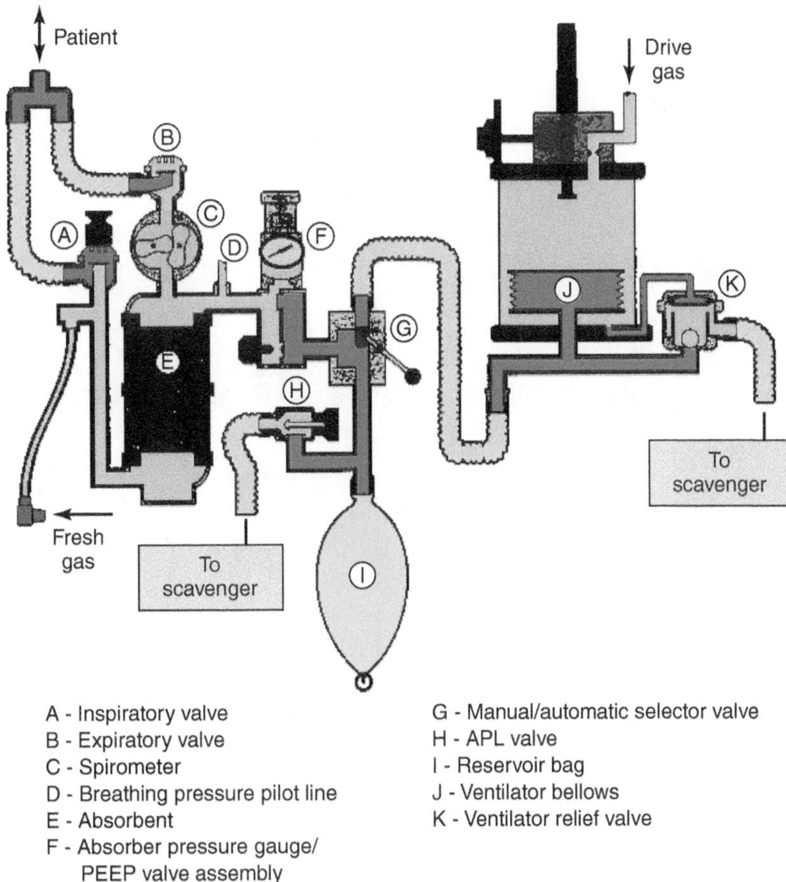

FIGURE 5-5 ■ Points of exit for waste gas from a typical circle system. APL, adjustable pressure-limiting; PEEP, positive end-expiratory pressure. (Courtesy Dräger Medical, Telford, PA.)

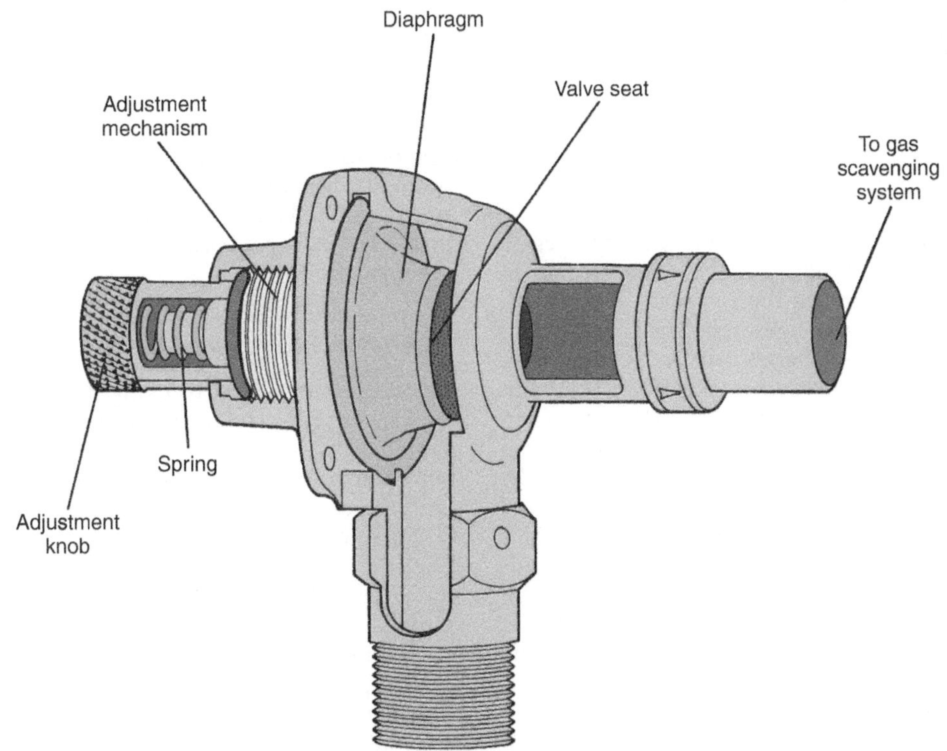

FIGURE 5-6 ■ The Datex-Ohmeda adjustable pressure-limiting valve. (Courtesy GE Healthcare, Waukesha, WI.)

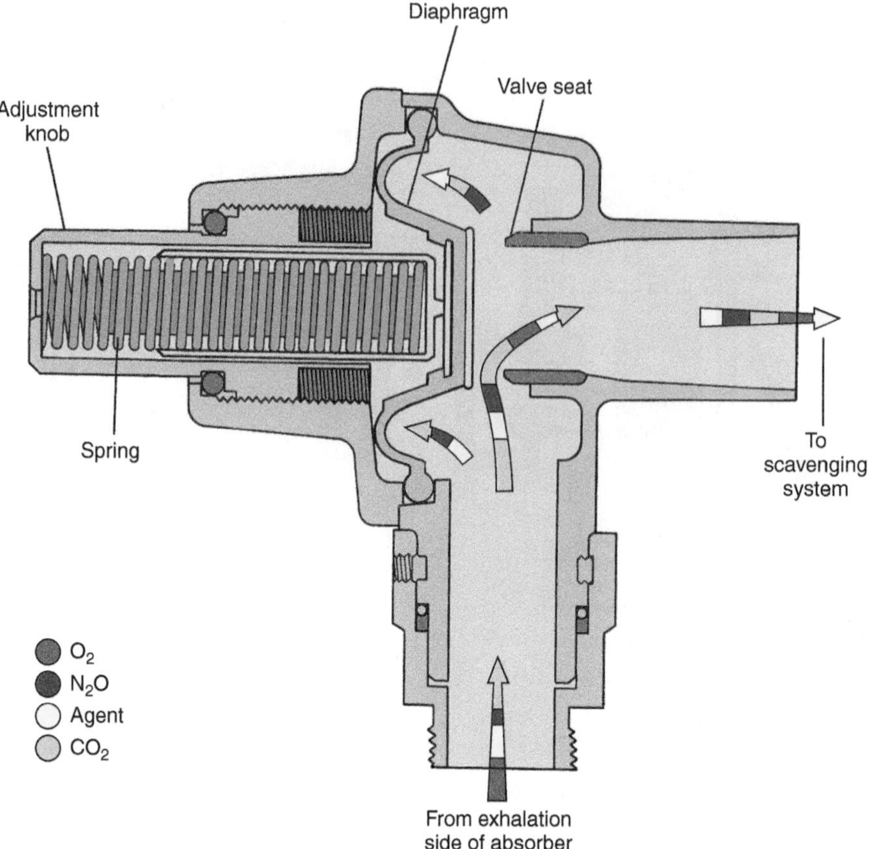

FIGURE 5-7 ■ Schematic of Datex-Ohmeda adjustable pressure-limiting valve. Note that it is a spring-loaded valve in contrast with the needle-valve design used by Dräger Medical. (From Bowie E, Huffman L: *The anesthesia machine: essentials for understanding.* Madison, WI, 1985, Ohmeda. Reproduced by permission of GE Healthcare, Waukesha, WI.)

Closed-Reservoir Scavenging Interface Systems

A closed-reservoir interface system includes a reservoir bag, which contains exhaled waste anesthetic gases, and spring-loaded valves that prevent the hospital evacuation system from exerting excessively high or low pressures on the breathing circuit (Figs. 5-8 and 5-9). The waste gases can be evacuated from the reservoir bag using either the hospital vacuum or ventilation system.

When the hospital vacuum system is used to evacuate waste anesthetic gases, a failure of the system results in excessive pressure buildup in the reservoir, the pop-off valve opens, and the waste anesthetic gases are vented into the room. Such pop-off valves usually open when the positive pressure in the reservoir reaches 5 cm H_2O, but some newer systems, such as the Datex-Ohmeda Aisys systems, open at 10 cm H_2O.[29] In contrast, if the hospital vacuum system generates excessive negative pressure, the negative-pressure relief, or "pop-in," valve will open and allow room air to be sucked into the reservoir. This avoids application of negative pressure to the breathing circuit.

The Datex-Ohmeda closed-reservoir interface system (see Fig. 5-8) has one negative-pressure relief valve, whereas the Draeger system has two (see Fig. 5-9). The negative-pressure relief valves pop inward when the pressure in the reservoir falls below −0.5 to −1.8 cm H_2O.

Figure 5-10 depicts a closed-reservoir interface system evacuated by the hospital ventilation system. No vacuum is connected to the interface, and the needle valve is closed. This is an example of a passive scavenging system.

In addition to containing the waste anesthetic gases during exhalation, the reservoir bag of a closed-reservoir scavenging interface provides a visual indication of whether the scavenging system is functioning properly. An overdistended bag indicates a weak vacuum or occluded disposal route. A collapsed bag indicates excessive vacuum. When the scavenging system is operating properly, the bag fills during exhalation and empties during inhalation.

Open-Reservoir Scavenging Interface Systems

An open-reservoir scavenging interface system (Figs. 5-11) is valveless and uses continually open relief ports to avoid positive or negative pressure buildup. In the Draeger open-reservoir interface, the reservoir canister contains the excess waste gas that arrives from the breathing circuit during exhalation, and the gas is removed from the reservoir by the hospital vacuum. Because this type of interface depends on open ports for pressure relief, care must be taken to ensure that the ports remain unoccluded at all times.[30]

An open-reservoir scavenging interface incorporates a flowmeter to show that gas is being sucked from the interface into the hospital vacuum disposal system. The Dräger interface has a needle-valve adjustment nut;

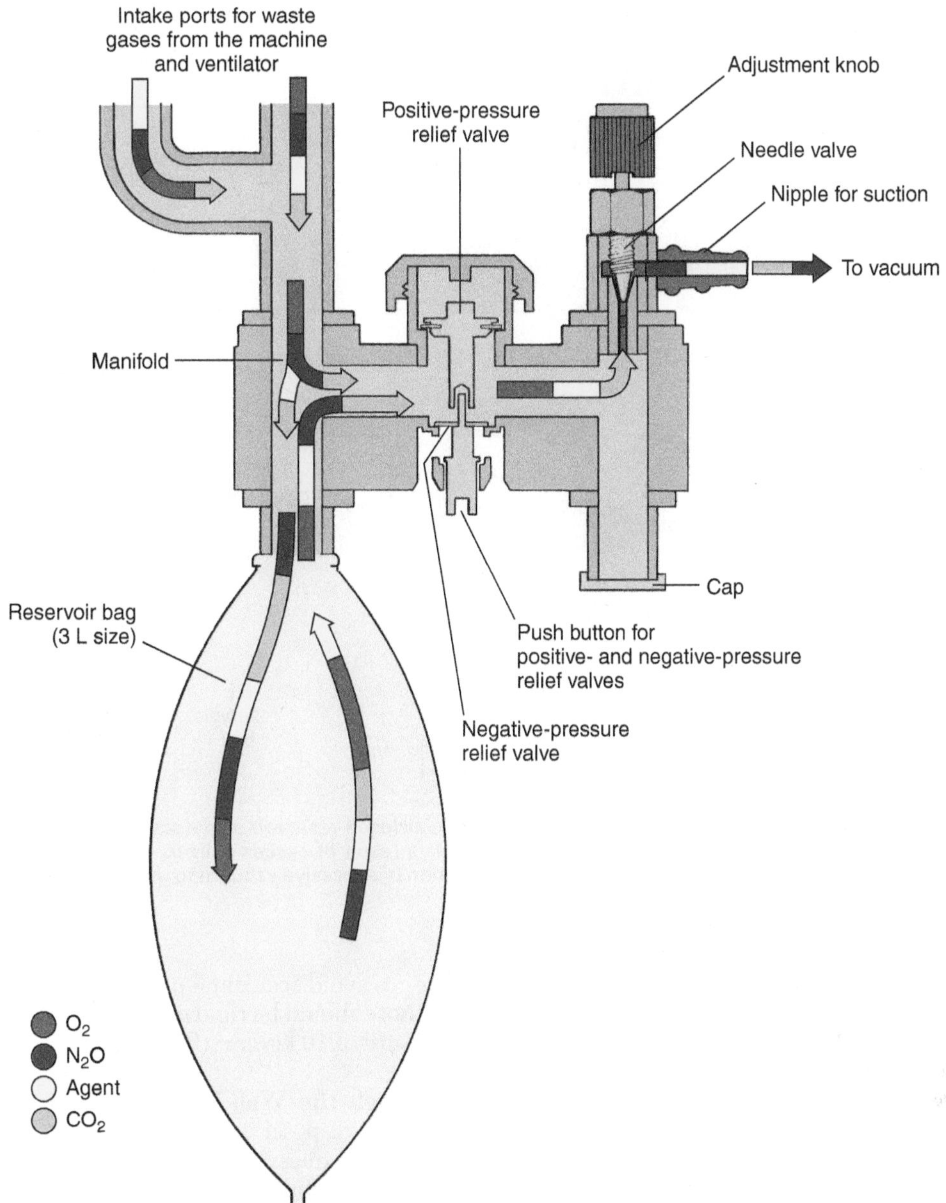

FIGURE 5-8 Datex-Ohmeda closed-reservoir active scavenging safety interface. The negative-pressure relief valve opens at a pressure of −0.25 cm H_2O, and the positive-pressure relief valve opens at 4 to 5 cm H_2O. (From Bowie E, Huffman L: *The anesthesia machine: essentials for understanding.* Madison, WI, 1985, Ohmeda. Reproduced by permission of GE Healthcare, Waukesha, WI.)

when the flowmeter ball "floats" between the two line markings, it indicates that gas is being removed from the interface at a rate of 25 L/min (Fig. 5-12). If waste anesthetic gas leaves the breathing system at 3 L/min (fresh gas flow is approximately 3 L/min), the difference in flow of 22 L/min (25 L/min − 3 L/min) is made up by room air entering via the open ports.

A reservoir bag is sometimes incorporated in the open-reservoir systems for the same reasons it is incorporated in closed-reservoir systems.

Disposal Routes

Waste anesthetic gases may be disposed of by active disposal routes, such as wall suction or a dedicated evacuation system, or by passive disposal routes, either the OR ventilation system or a through-the-wall conduit.

Active Disposal Routes

When waste anesthetic gases are disposed of by way of wall suction, the following requirements should be met:

1. The wall suction should be capable of drawing at least 30 L/min of air.
2. The scavenging interface should be equipped with at least one negative-pressure relief valve (closed reservoir) or ports open to the atmosphere (open reservoir).
3. The exhaust port of the wall suction should be at a safe distance from the breathing zone of personnel.

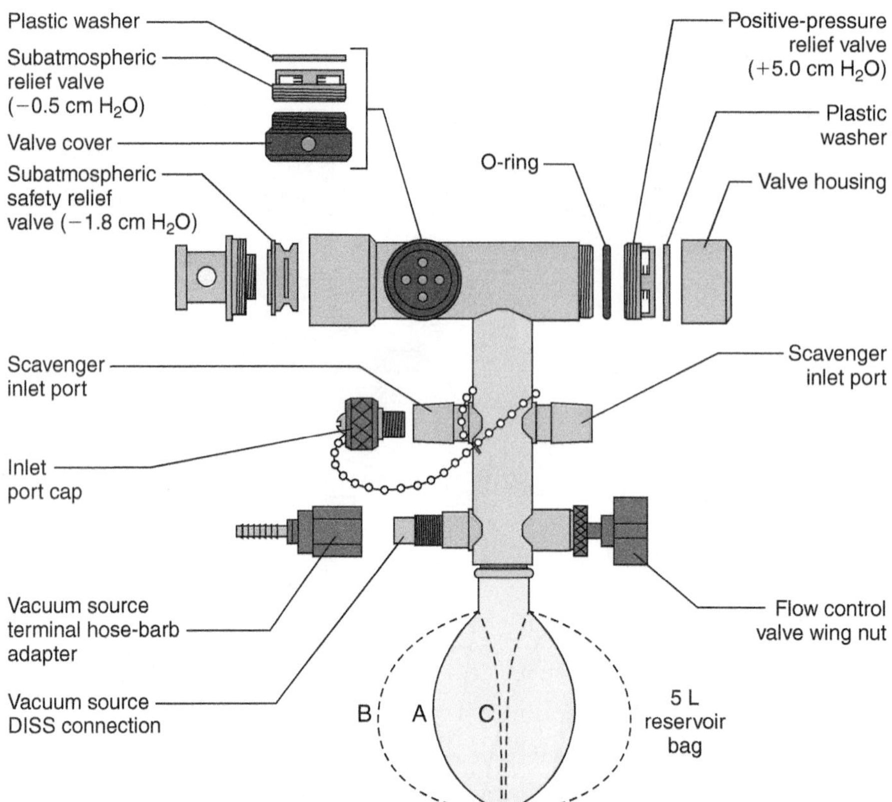

FIGURE 5-9 Schematic of the Dräger scavenging safety interface. This is a closed-reservoir active scavenging system. *A,* Normal state of distension of the scavenger reservoir bag. *B,* Overdistended bag as a result of excess delivery or inadequate removal of waste gases from the interface. *C,* Collapsed position of the bag from application of excessive vacuum to the interface. DISS, diameter index safety system. (Courtesy Dräger Medical, Telford, PA.)

4. Explosive anesthetic gases should not be used (per National Fire Protection Association regulations).

It is preferable to have a separate, dedicated vacuum system for waste anesthetic gases. This is because of two significant disadvantages when the wall suction system is used. First, the strength of the wall suction may not be sufficient to meet the needs of both the anesthesiologist and the surgeon in addition to the needs of the scavenging system. Diverting 20 L/min of air to the scavenging system reduces the intensity of the remaining vacuum by 25%, which may not be adequate to meet the needs of the anesthesiologist. Second, waste anesthetic gases may damage the vacuum system's machinery.

Waste gas scavenging connectors and tubing are purple or yellow, and associated fittings are either 19 mm or 30 mm in diameter (Fig. 5-13, *A* and *B*). The waste gas removal tubing that connects the scavenging interface to the vacuum connection on the wall uses diameter index safety system (DISS) fittings to ensure the connection is appropriate.

Passive Disposal Routes

Operating Room Ventilation System. When used for disposal of waste anesthetic gases, the OR ventilation system should be of the nonrecirculating type and must meet the requirements of the American Institute of Architects. The hose leading from the scavenging interface to the ventilation outflow port should be kept off the floor to avoid accidental occlusion. If placed on the floor, the hose should be rigid enough to remain patent under a pressure of 10 kg/cm^2 (Fig. 5-14).

Through-the-Wall Disposal. With a passive, through-the-wall disposal system, waste anesthetic gases flow through a duct in the wall, window, ceiling, or floor toward the outside. Because OR ventilation results in a slight positive pressure in the OR with respect to the outside, gases flow naturally into disposal ducts connected to the outside. A potential danger of such a disposal route is occlusion of the exhaust port by ice, nesting birds, or insects. In addition, gusting winds may generate positive pressure at the exhaust port that may interfere with disposal of waste anesthetic gases. These problems can be avoided by directing the exhaust port downward and shielding it with a wire screen. Also, an airflow indicator should be installed in the tubing between the anesthesia machine and the wall to confirm the proper direction of gas flow.

Scavenging the Anesthesia Ventilator

Modern anesthesia ventilators are factory equipped with a disposal system that directs waste anesthetic gases to the anesthesia workstation's scavenging system. Older anesthesia ventilator designs, however, often discharge waste anesthetic gases directly into the ambient air or do not have a standard 19-mm scavenging connection. Also,

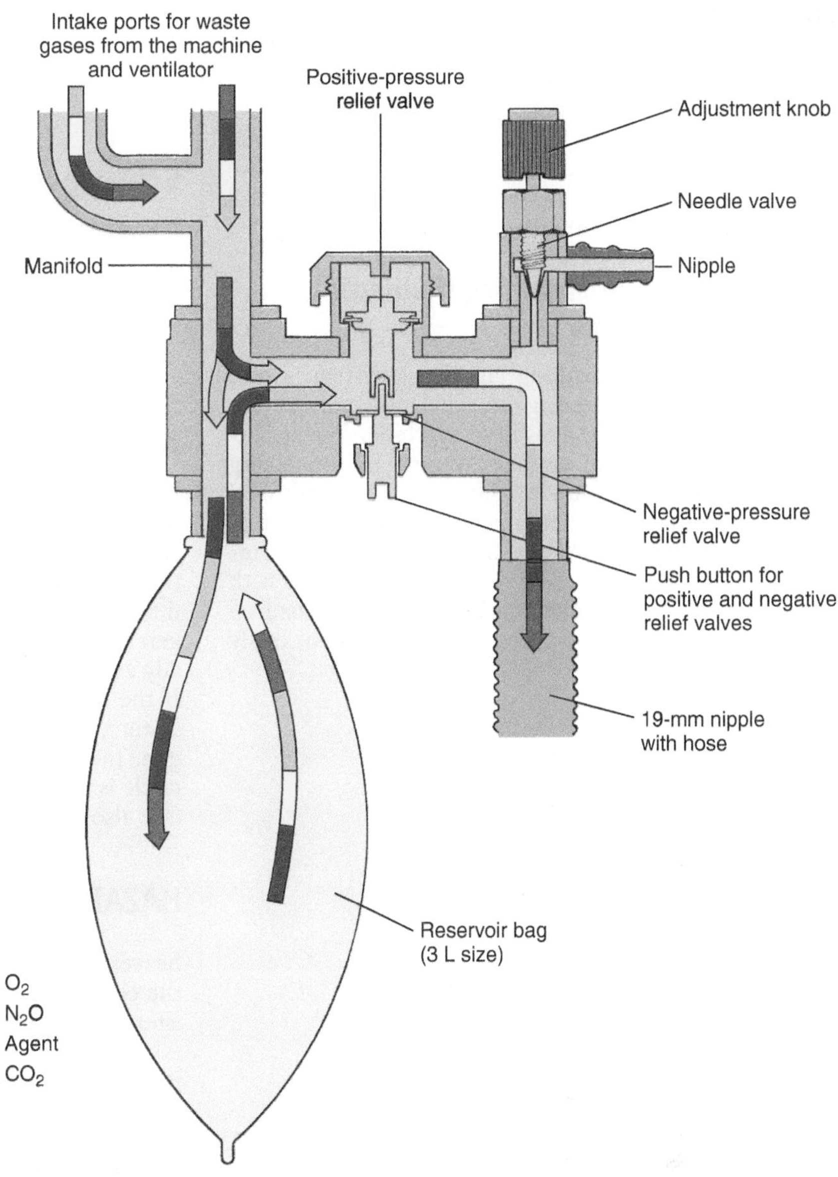

FIGURE 5-10 ■ Datex-Ohmeda closed-reservoir scavenging interface used as a passive system. The vacuum is not connected (compare with Figure 5-9), and gas flows passively to the operating room exhaust ventilation duct. (From Bowie E, Huffman L: *The anesthesia machine: essentials for understanding.* Madison, WI, 1985, Ohmeda. Courtesy GE Healthcare, Waukesha WI.)

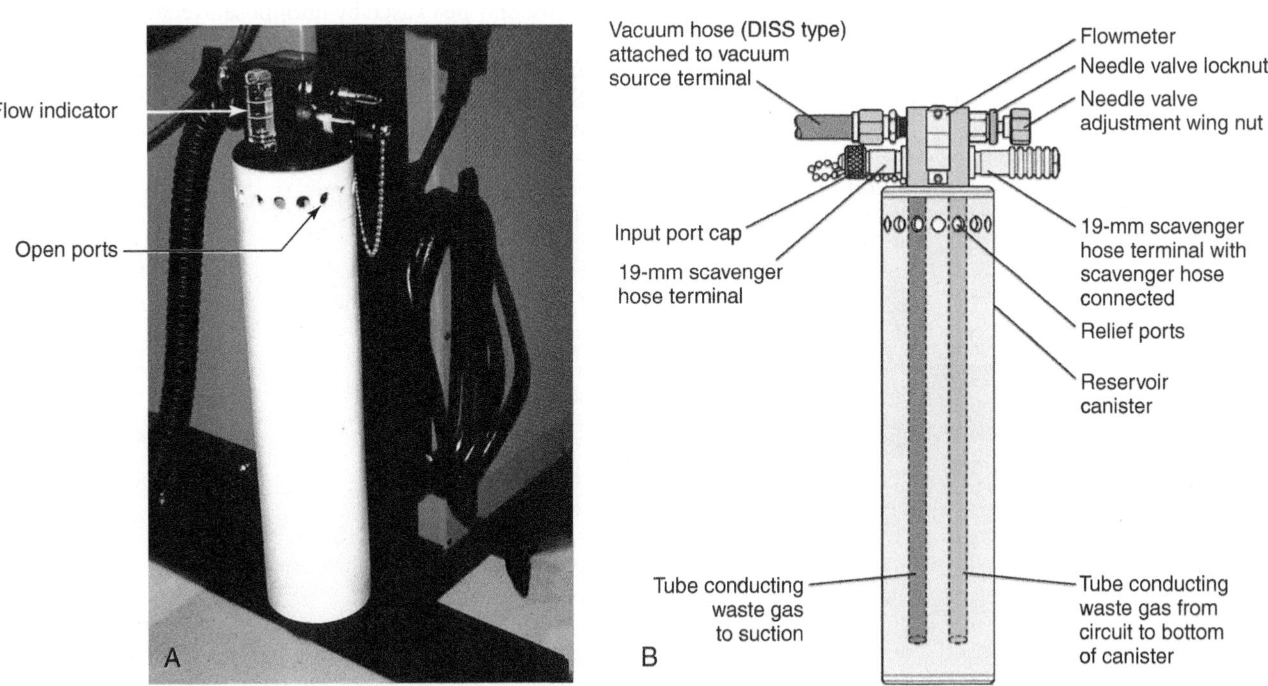

FIGURE 5-11 ■ **A,** An open-reservoir scavenging system. **B,** Schematic. *DISS,* diameter index safety system. (Courtesy Dräger Medical, Telford, PA.)

older ventilators often are fraught with internal leaks, which mix the anesthetic gases with the ventilator's driving gas. This significantly increases the volume of gas that must be disposed of with each breath and might therefore overwhelm the capacity of the scavenging system and result in spillage of anesthetic gases.

Scavenging Nonrebreathing (Pediatric) Anesthesia Systems

Scavenging a nonrebreathing anesthesia system is best accomplished by connecting its exhalation port to the scavenging system of the anesthesia machine. The pediatric Jackson-Rees system can be scavenged by connecting either the open tail of its breathing bag or of the relief valve (if one is used) directly to the scavenging interface of the anesthesia machine. Vital Signs (Totowa, NJ) manufactures a scavenging relief valve that can be used with all Mapleson systems, including the Jackson-Rees pediatric modification (Fig. 5-15). This relief valve can be easily connected to the scavenging interface of the anesthesia machine.

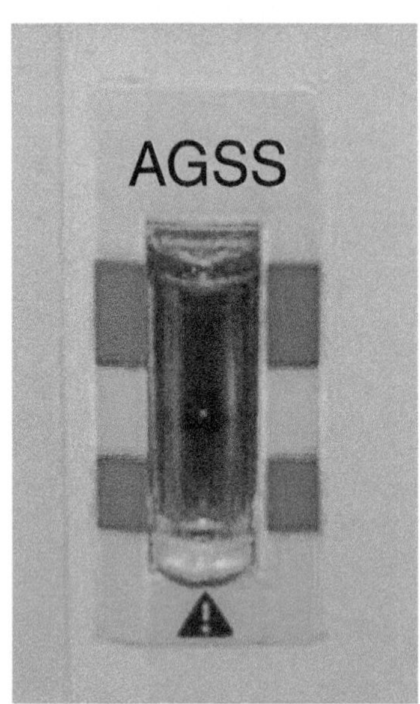

FIGURE 5-12 ■ Flow indicator on open-reservoir scavenging interface.

Scavenging Cryosurgical Units

Newer models of N_2O cryosurgical units are equipped with built-in scavenging systems. Older models, however, do not have scavenging systems and spill large amounts of N_2O gas into the ambient air. Fitting older units with scavenging systems is strongly recommended.

Scavenging Sidestream-Sampling Gas Analyzers

As previously mentioned, the exhaust from the sidestream-sampling gas analyzers should be conducted via tubing to the waste gas scavenging system or returned to the breathing system for scavenging (Fig. 5-16). Of note, if the multigas analyzer incorporates a paramagnetic oxygen analyzer, the analyzer draws a constant stream, usually about 10 mL/min of room air, to use as a reference. If the monitor exhaust gas is returned to the breathing system, this will include an additional 8 mL/min of nitrogen. In most cases this presents no problem, but if the circle is used as a closed system, nitrogen will accumulate (see also Chapter 8).

HAZARDS OF SCAVENGING

Scavenging of the anesthesia breathing circuit increases the complexity, and consequently the hazards, of administering anesthesia. If the scavenging interface were mistakenly bypassed or were to malfunction, excessive positive or negative pressure in the scavenging system could be directly transmitted to the breathing circuit. This might cause cardiovascular embarrassment and pulmonary barotrauma to the patient. Excessive negative pressure may be caused by unopposed vacuum, and excessive positive pressure may be caused by occlusion of the connecting tubing (see also Chapter 30).

Scavenging mishaps typically are the result of user error. In one case, a one-way metallic connector was

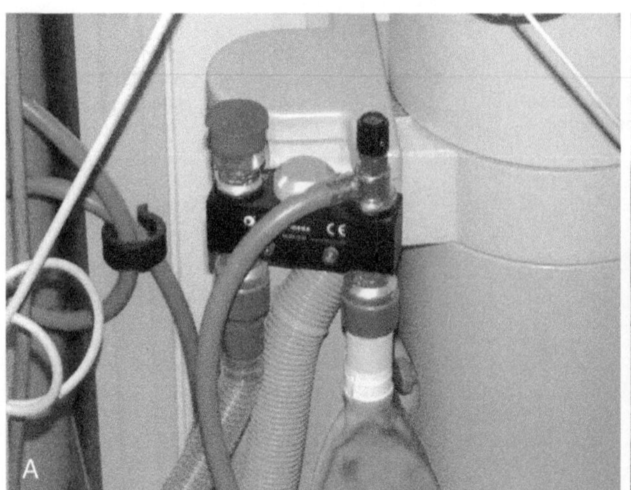

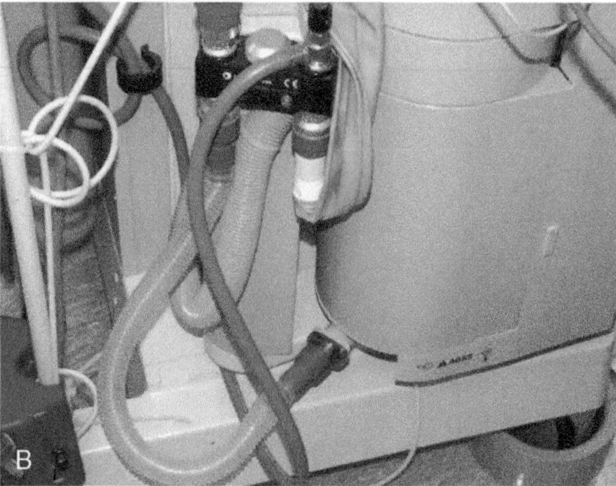

FIGURE 5-13 ■ **A** and **B,** Waste gas tubing and connectors. Yellow and purple colors indicate waste gas scavenging system.

assembled in reverse and obstructed the disposal line, causing excessive positive pressure in the breathing circuit.[31] No PR valve had been incorporated into the system. In another case, the perforated connector of a tube-within-a-tube assembly was accidentally replaced with one that had no perforations.[32] The unopposed negative pressure in the scavenging system shut off the ventilator's exhalation valve and caused excessive positive pressure in the breathing circuit, and the patient sustained bilateral pneumothoraces and subcutaneous emphysema. In yet another case, the expiratory breathing hose was mistakenly connected to the scavenging port of the relief valve and caused an abrupt increase in the pressure in the breathing circuit.[33] Accidental occlusion of the disposal line by the wheels of the anesthesia machine has also been reported (Fig. 5-17).

The inherent vulnerability of scavenging systems has been the cause of some mishaps. In one case, the negative-PR valve failed to open despite excessive negative pressure in the system, causing the patient circuit reservoir bag to collapse.[34] In another case, ice buildup in the exhaust port of a passive through-the-wall disposal route was apparently the cause of pneumothorax and death in a laboratory animal.[35] In yet another case, a plastic bag was sucked in by the perforated connector of an active disposal route,[36] which occluded the perforations and led to unopposed negative pressure in the breathing circuit.

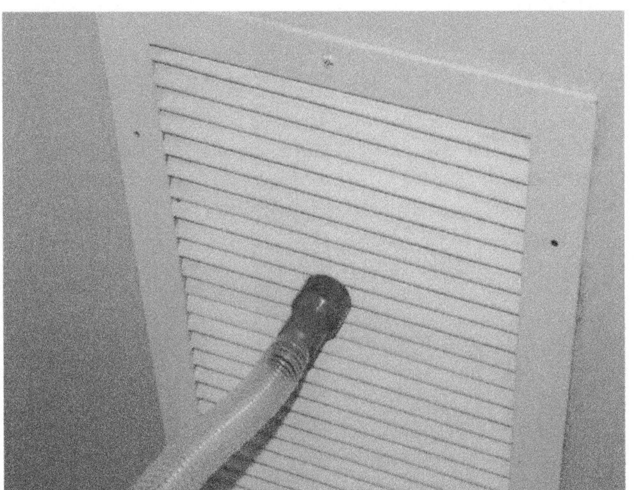

FIGURE 5-14 Exhaust grille adapter for passive disposal of waste anesthetic gases via the operating room ventilation system.

Whenever abnormal pressure exists in the breathing circuit, the scavenging system should be checked for possible malfunction. If a malfunction is suspected, the system should be immediately disconnected from the breathing circuit.

In 2004, fires were reported in engineering equipment rooms that house the vacuum pumps used for waste anesthetic gas evacuation.[37] In some hospitals, waste gases are not directly vented to the outside but may be vented into machine rooms that have vents that open to the outside. In some anesthesia workstations, the ventilator drive gas also is scavenged. This gas is 100% oxygen in most cases and is added to gas leaving the breathing system. As a result, the environments in these machine rooms may become highly enriched with oxygen gas. One sequela of this has been the production of fires in these spaces outside the OR.[37] These sites also may contain equipment or materials, such as petroleum distillates (pumps, oil, or grease) that, in the presence of an oxygen-enriched atmosphere, could be extremely combustible and present a significant fire hazard.

LOW-FLOW SCAVENGING SYSTEMS

Active waste gas scavenging systems draw large volumes of gas—anesthetic waste plus entrained air in the range of 25 to 75 L/min—from each OR. This requires large and costly vacuum pumps; operating continuously, they incur a high energy cost. Some practitioners disconnect the scavenging interface from the vacuum system when the OR is not in use for long periods, such as overnight and on weekends. Most, however, do not; this results in unnecessary operation of the vacuum pumps, as they suck in room air and waste the fuel and energy needed to power them. Recently, in an effort to reduce the carbon footprint associated with running these pumps, a more

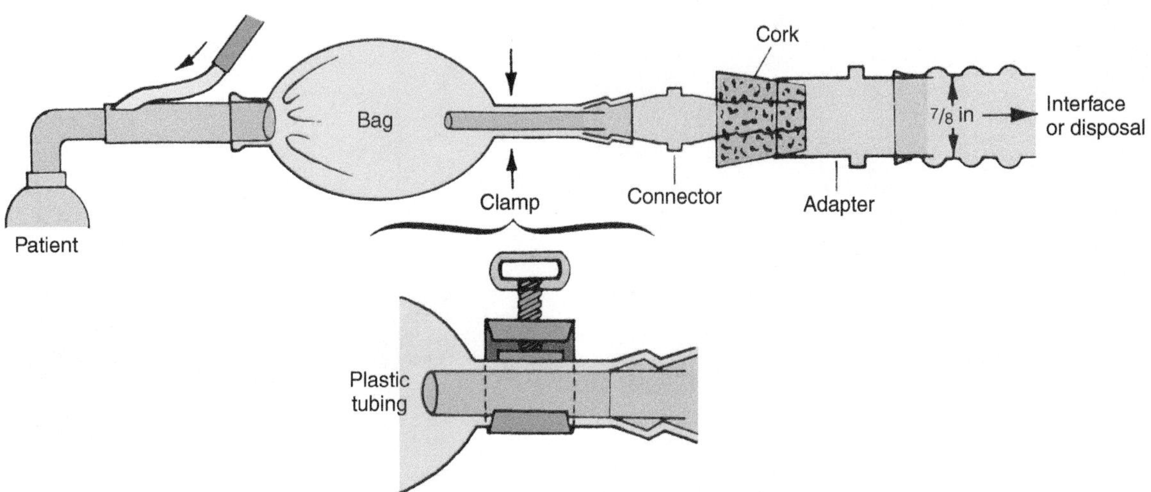

FIGURE 5-15 Connection of scavenging interface to a Jackson-Rees modification of the Mapleson D system. (From U.S. Department of Health, Education and Welfare [NIOSH] Publication No. 75-137. Washington, DC, 1975, U.S. Government Printing Office.)

efficient, low-flow scavenger interface has been designed and evaluated.[38] The Dynamic Gas Scavenging System (DGSS; Anesthetic Gas Reclamation, Nashville, TN; Fig. 5-18) interface is a gas-tight metal container with a 3-L reservoir bag attached to ensure compliance with OSHA recommendations. The design is such that scavenging outflow to the vacuum system remains closed until a pressure of 0.5 cm H_2O from the anesthesia workstation exhaust, via the APL or ventilator PR valve, is sensed in the interface enclosure by a sensitive pressure transducer. A solenoid valve then opens and remains open until the internal pressure reaches –0.5 cm H_2O, thus emptying the interface reservoir bag. In this way the flow to the vacuum system is continuously titrated according to needs.

The DGSS was evaluated in a suite of four ORs and was placed in regular clinical use for 6 months while data were collected on failures, trace gas exposure, and use of the central vacuum pump for the OR suite. No failures of the DGSS were reported. In an anesthetic technique using fresh gas flows of 2 L/min and ventilator drive gas flows of 6 L/min (drive gas was scavenged), the central vacuum pump duty cycle decreased from 92% before installation of the DGSS to 12% when the ORs were in use and from 92% to 1% when the rooms were not in use. The authors suggest that their novel system will produce energy cost savings and may prolong the life of the vacuum pump. Cost savings are greatest when the DGSS is used with workstations that do not vent ventilator drive gas into the scavenging system and in those that use piston ventilators.

The DGSS is commercially available and compatible with many current anesthesia workstations (Fig. 5-19). An added benefit is that by producing a more concentrated flow of waste gases, technologies designed to recover potent inhaled anesthetic agents from the waste-gas flow are facilitated. Such technologies are likely to become more important because the inhaled anesthetics are greenhouse gases with the potential to increase global warming.[39]

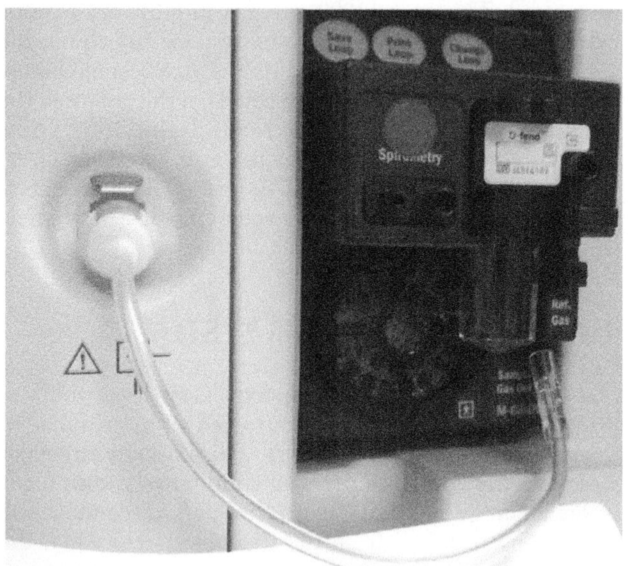

FIGURE 5-16 ■ Exhaust from sidestream gas analyzer directed into scavenging system.

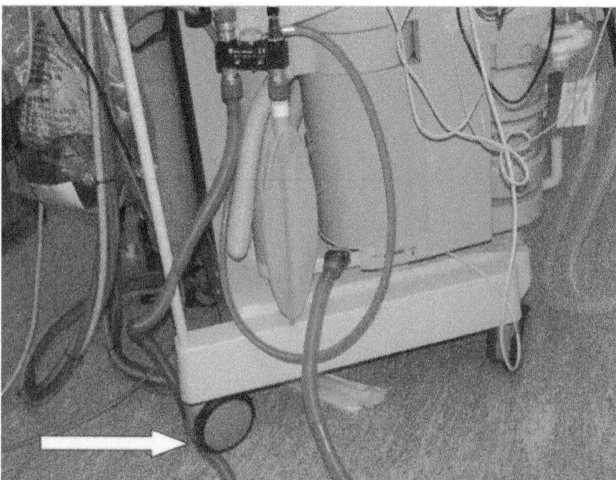

FIGURE 5-17 ■ Occlusion of 19-mm scavenger hose conducting gas from the outlets of the adjustable pressure-limiting and pressure relief valves to the closed-reservoir active scavenging system. Note that the reservoir bag is collapsed. This situation can lead to high pressure in the breathing circuit and barotrauma.

VOLATILE ANESTHETIC RECLAMATION

An estimated 500,000 gallons of anesthetic agents are used annually in the United States, and this volume is subsequently released into the atmosphere. Reclamation of these agents would be of environmental benefit and also potential financial benefit. A system has been described by

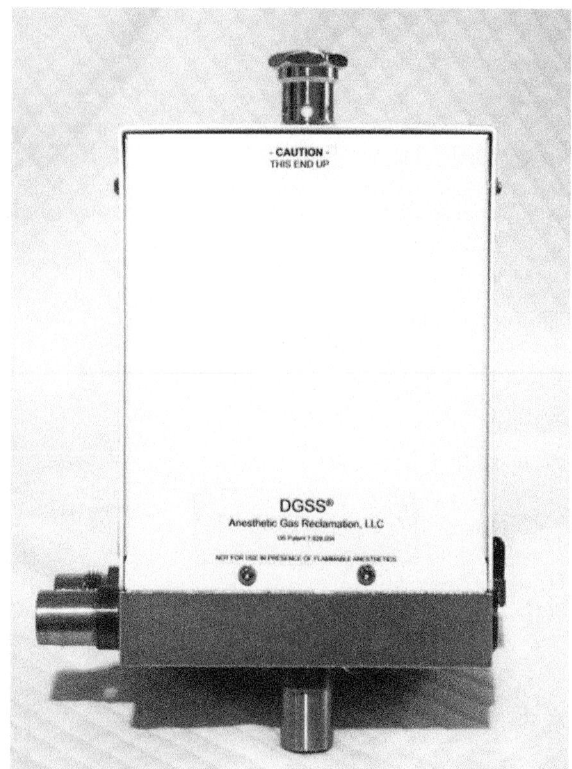

FIGURE 5-18 ■ The Dynamic Gas Scavenging System (DGSS; Anesthetic Gas Reclamation, Nashville, TN.)

which inhaled anesthetic agents could be recovered from a concentrated waste gas stream, such as that produced by the DGSS, by condensation at cryogenic temperatures.[40] The recovery rate of undiluted waste anesthetic gas using a condensation temperature of −100° C reportedly would be approximately 98%.[41]

ANESTHETIC LEAK DETECTION AND WASTE GAS MANAGEMENT

The scavenging system removes waste anesthetic gases captured from only the relief valve. Spillage from other sources is not evacuated by the scavenging system and depends solely on the OR's ventilation system for disposal. As a consequence, trace levels of anesthetic gases in the OR occasionally may be in excess of the levels recommended by NIOSH.

To reduce the level of anesthetic contamination in the OR, the anesthesia workstation should be regularly tested for leaks. Any leaks found should be corrected as soon as possible. Errors in anesthetic technique that lead to spillage of anesthetic gases also should be corrected.

To detect and prevent anesthetic leaks, a waste gas management program should be adopted in every OR suite. Anesthetic equipment should be checked with each use and at specified intervals by a service technician. The results should be documented, and the records should be maintained indefinitely. These records are useful for equipment maintenance follow-up and compliance with recommendations of government agencies and accrediting organizations. The records also can potentially be used for legal defense.

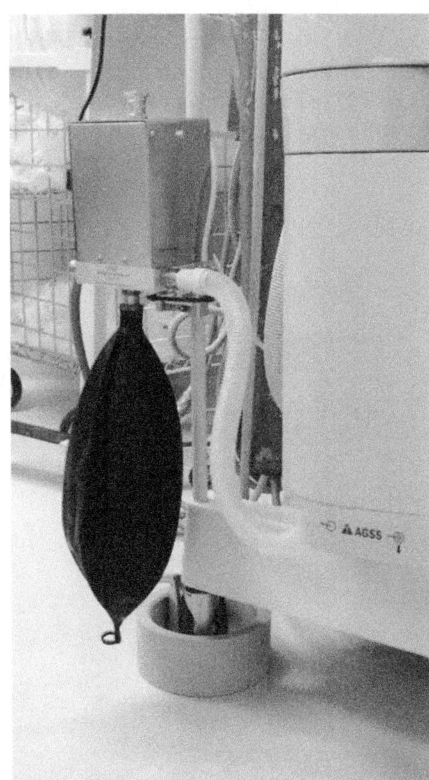

FIGURE 5-19 ■ Dynamic gas scavenging system in use.

WORK PRACTICE RECOMMENDATIONS

Testing the High- and Intermediate-Pressure Systems for Leaks

Testing of the high- and intermediate-pressure systems of the anesthesia machine for leaks begins with the DISS quick connector in the N_2O central supply line. The connector is submerged in water or rinsed with liquid soap; the appearance of gas bubbles indicates a leak. Liquid soap also can be used to detect leaks in the yokes of the reserve N_2O tanks. Faulty quick connectors should be immediately repaired or replaced, the yokes of the reserve tanks should be tightened, and defective washers should be replaced (Fig. 5-20).

Next, the N_2O high-pressure system inside the anesthesia machine is tested. The N_2O central supply hose is disconnected from the machine, a reserve N_2O tank is used to pressurize the N_2O system, and the tank is turned off. The N_2O system pressure indicated by the N_2O pressure gauge is recorded and then rechecked 1 hour later; a significant decrease in pressure suggests a leak inside the machine between the N_2O reserve tank and the N_2O flowmeter.

In one study, significant high-pressure N_2O leaks were detected in 50% of the anesthesia machines.[11] After the leaks were corrected, the background N_2O level in the OR suite decreased from 19 to 0.2 ppm.

Internal N_2O leaks are difficult to correct and should be left to the manufacturer's maintenance service. A high-pressure N_2O system should be serviced by the manufacturer at regular intervals and tested by departmental anesthesia technicians.

Testing the Low-Pressure System for Leaks

The following procedure has been recommended for testing the low-pressure system for leaks:

1. Remove the breathing hoses and bag from the anesthesia breathing circuit.
2. Connect the two unidirectional valves with a short piece of corrugated hose.

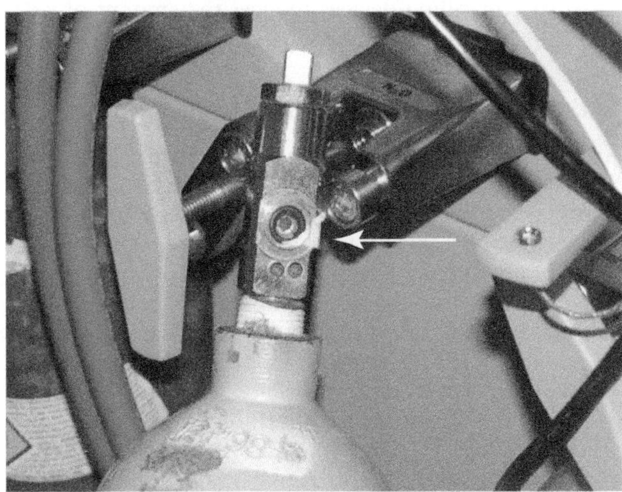

FIGURE 5-20 ■ High-pressure leak caused by a defective washer (*arrow*) on the yoke of a N_2O reserve tank.

3. Close the APL valve tightly, remove the reservoir bag, and occlude the bag mount opening; this minimizes the compliance of the low-pressure system.
4. Slowly turn on the oxygen flowmeter until the breathing circuit pressure gauge indicates 40 cm H_2O.
5. Record the rate of oxygen flow necessary to maintain this pressure for 30 seconds. This rate of flow is equal to the low-pressure system's leak rate. The low-pressure leak rate generally should not exceed 200 mL/min, which would contribute no more than 4 ppm of N_2O air pollution to an average-sized OR.

Correcting Errors in the Anesthesia Technique

The following precautions in anesthetic technique significantly reduce the spillage of anesthetic gases:

1. All gases and vaporizers should be turned off when the patient is not connected to the breathing circuit, such as during intubation.
2. The face mask should be carefully selected and firmly held against the patient's face.
3. The tracheal tube should be carefully selected. Except for pediatric patients, no leak should be allowed around the cuff.
4. Upon conclusion of anesthesia, when the reservoir bag is emptied of anesthetic gases, the breathing circuit should be connected to the patient with the relief valve held wide open. This should direct the contents of the bag into the scavenging system.
5. After completion of surgery, and while still deeply anesthetized, the patient should remain connected to the breathing circuit, breathing 100% oxygen for a few minutes. This will direct the exhaled anesthetic gases to the scavenging system of the anesthesia machine.
6. Vaporizers should be refilled in the evening, when the OR is not being used. This reduces the risk of exposing OR personnel to anesthetic vapors from accidental spillage of volatile anesthetic liquid while the vaporizers are refilled. The careful use of agent-specific filling devices reduces the amount of volatile anesthetic agent spilled (see Chapter 3).

Miscellaneous Preventive Measures

The OR ventilation system should be regularly serviced to ensure optimal function. Hospital engineers should check the filters for cleanliness and the dampers for proper position and balance. If the system is allowed to deteriorate, the number of air exchanges per hour gradually decreases, and the level of anesthetic contamination increases. Also, the function of the hospital vacuum should be checked at regular intervals to ensure adequate negative pressure and flow capacity.

In the PACU, the concentration of N_2O in the air is directly related to room ventilation and the number of patients in the unit. If ventilation is maintained at the rate of 500 m^3 of fresh air per patient per hour, the mean N_2O level in the room is approximately 10 ppm.[26]

MONITORING TRACE LEVELS OF ANESTHETIC GASES

Monitoring the concentration of trace anesthetic gases may be undertaken to 1) determine whether the leak-detecting and waste anesthetic gas program is effective, 2) uncover occult leaks from unexpected sites, and 3) document compliance with OSHA recommendations.

Monitoring Trace Anesthetic Levels in the Operating Room

The levels of both N_2O and halogenated agents in the OR can be determined individually. Infrared (IR) analyzers can measure trace levels of anesthetic agents. These devices are capable of measuring not only N_2O, but all the volatile anesthetics in trace concentrations. The MIRAN SapphIRe series of analyzers (Thermo Environmental Instruments, Franklin, MA) measures N_2O in the range of 0 to 100 ppm and the halogenated agents in a range of 0 to 30 ppm (Fig. 5-21). Because the level of halogenated agents in the OR atmosphere is closely related to that of N_2O, the level of the halogenated agent can be extrapolated from that of N_2O, as follows:

$$\frac{\%\ \text{H in FGI}}{\%\ \text{N}_2\text{O in FGI}} = \frac{\text{ppm H in RA}}{\text{ppm N}_2\text{O in RA}}$$

where *H* is the halogenated agent, *FGI* is fresh gas inflow, and *RA* is room air.

Measurements of trace anesthetic levels are reliable only if the anesthetic gases are evenly distributed in the ambient air. The uniformity of distribution depends on four factors: 1) the number of room air exchanges per hour, 2) the flow pattern of room ventilation, 3) placement of the anesthesia machine in relation to the ventilation flow, and 4) traffic patterns of personnel in the OR. When the number of room air exchanges is greater than

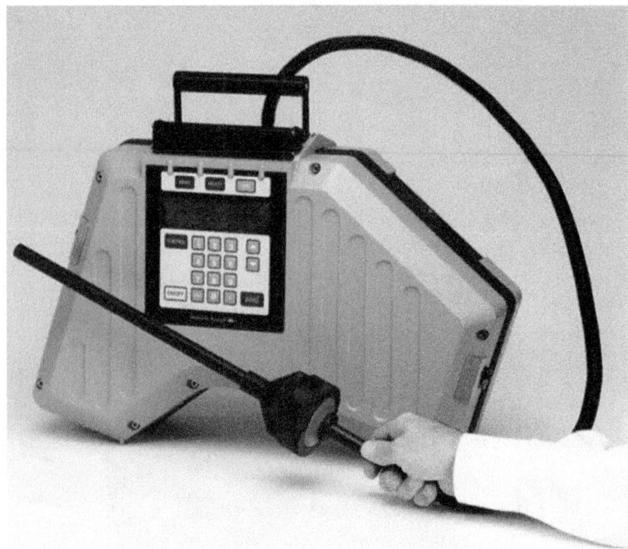

FIGURE 5-21 ■ MIRAN SapphIRe infrared spectrophotometer. (Courtesy Thermo Fisher Scientific, Franklin, MA.)

10 per hour, the anesthetic gases are fairly evenly distributed in room air. The air near the ventilation outflow grille represents the mean level of the trace anesthetic gases in the room.[22]

Optimum reduction of air contamination is achieved by certain control measures that include scavenging and work practices to reduce trace gas levels. Monitoring can determine the efficacy of control measures and leak identification, defects in technique, and documentation of compliance with the recommended standard. OSHA recommends that air sampling for anesthetic gases be conducted every 6 months to measure worker exposures and to check the effectiveness of control measures. Furthermore, OSHA recommends monitoring only the most frequently used agents because proper engineering controls, work practices, and control procedures should reduce all agents proportionately. However, the decision to monitor only selected agents could depend on the frequency of their use as well as the availability of an appropriate analytic method and cost of instrumentation.

The American Society of Anesthesiologists (ASA) emphasizes regular maintenance of equipment and scavenging systems, daily checkout procedures for anesthesia equipment, and education to ensure use of appropriate work practices. The ASA does not consider a routine monitoring program necessary when these actions are being carried out, but rather encourages the use of monitoring when indicated, such as in the event of a known or suspected equipment malfunction. OSHA recommends that monitoring be done either by a knowledgeable person familiar with techniques of sampling or by an industrial hygienist. Monitoring requires both sampling and analysis; the latter may be performed by IR methods or by gas chromatography, either inside or outside the hospital.

Sampling Methods

Two decisions must be made with regard to sampling: where to do it and when to do it. Various methods of sampling are available.

Where to Sample

Monitoring personal exposure by sampling the atmosphere in the face mask area of exposed personnel is not required by NIOSH, although perhaps this method offers the most pertinent information on individual exposure. Sampling in the immediate work area of the most highly exposed person, the anesthesiologist, is recommended. One study has shown that measuring N_2O at the level of the anesthesia machine's shelf correlates well with personal sampling when levels of N_2O are below 35 ppm.[42] Shelf-level measurement is certainly more practical than personal sampling.

General area sampling is valid if complete air mixing has been previously demonstrated in the OR. In a room where all leakage is under effective control, gas concentrations may be uniform, making this kind of sampling appropriate. This type of sampling may be most appropriate in the empty OR to detect background leakage.

When to Sample

The timing of sampling also is critical to obtain representative exposure concentrations. Three types of temporal sampling are 1) grab sampling, 2) TWA sampling, and 3) continuous sampling.

Temporal Sampling

Grab Sampling. Grab sampling is useful for monitoring steady-state conditions—for example, high-pressure leakage from N_2O lines—and to establish baseline N_2O levels. With this technique, an air sample from the empty OR is taken for subsequent analysis. Inert containers are available for this purpose. The container is sealed and mailed to the company for analysis of the contents. Delay in obtaining the results is one disadvantage; another is that the value of such sampling is obviously limited because anesthetic leakage tends to be intermittent.

Time-Weighted Average Sampling. The TWA sample may be obtained by continuously pumping ambient air into an inert bag at a constant low rate of flow, usually around 4 L/h. The bag has a capacity of 20 to 30 L, and five-layer aluminized 5-L gas sampling bags also can be used to collect a sample. The resulting concentration in the bag therefore represents an average exposure over the collection period; commercially available TWA gas sampling systems provide TWA concentrations over periods of 1 to 8 hours.

The sampling pump can be mounted on a pole in the OR, and aliquots of a collected TWA sample can be analyzed in-house or mailed in an inert container to a central testing laboratory. The TWA for personal exposure also can be obtained from a battery-powered sampling pump and collection bag worn by the anesthesiologist. Clearly, wearing a bag and pump is inconvenient; however, knowledge of the TWA concentrations is useful for documentation purposes because the recommended standard refers to a TWA concentration of 25 ppm, although the time period for collection is not specified. The OSHA *Chemical Information Manual,* accessible online, contains current sampling technology for several anesthetic gases.

Nitrous Oxide Time-Weighted Average Sampling. Personal N_2O exposures can be determined by using a passive monitor, such as the Vapor-Trak (Kern Medical Products, Farmingdale, NY). These are sometimes called *passive dosimeters* or *diffusive samplers* (Fig. 5-22). The dosimeter is a lightweight badge that can be worn by personnel to monitor their individual exposure; its sensitivity is 2 ppm. It can also be mounted on a pole for area sampling. The minimum sampling duration for the dosimeter is 15 minutes; however, it can be used for up to 8 hours of passive sampling. At the end of the sampling/exposure period, the dosimeter is mailed to a laboratory for analysis; the results are sent by e-mail to the individual and/or institution.

Sampling of Halogenated Agents. Three chlorofluorocarbon-based anesthetic agents—halothane, enflurane, and

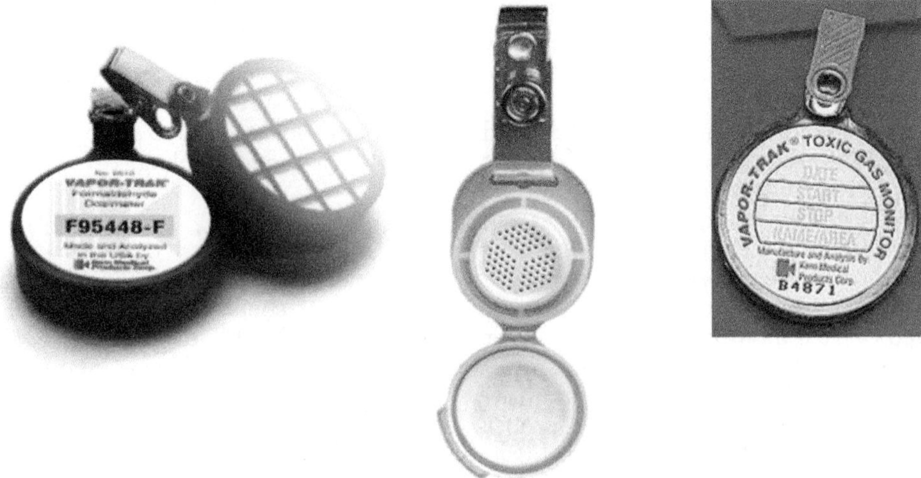

FIGURE 5-22 ■ Personal nitrous oxide samplers.

isoflurane—and one fluorocarbon-based agent, desflurane, are listed in the OSHA *Chemical Information Manual.* The current recommended media sampling for halothane, enflurane, and isoflurane requires an Anasorb tube, and the sample can be taken at a flow rate of 0.5 L/min; total sample volumes not exceeding 12 L are recommended. The current recommended sampling media for desflurane requires an Anasorb 747 tube, and the sample can be taken at a flow rate of 0.05 L/min; total sample volumes not exceeding 3 L are recommended. As with the N_2O dosimeters, the tubes are sent to a laboratory for analysis.

Continuous Sampling. The best method for monitoring the OR atmosphere is with the portable IR spectrophotometer, which is capable of continuous sampling (see Fig. 5-21). Because this device offers a continuous readout, it can be used for detection of leaks, demonstration of errors in anesthetic technique, and determination of trace gas levels. Analyzers operate on the principle that most gases possess unique IR absorbance spectra. For example, the IR absorbance spectrum for N_2O peaks at a wavelength of around 4.5 μm (see Chapter 8).

IR spectrophotometer trace gas analyzers work by action of a pump that perfuses a cell with OR air. To measure N_2O, the IR source generates a light beam that is filtered to pass the IR component at a wavelength of approximately 4.5 μm. The beam is transmitted through the sample cell and is sensed by a detector: the higher the concentration of nitrous oxide, the more IR radiation is absorbed and the less energy is sensed at the detector. The signal is processed and displayed in parts per million N_2O, although IR analysis can detect concentrations in parts per 100 million; the sensitivity of the instrument is a function of the path length of the IR beam through the sample of gas, and path lengths of 20 m or more produce very high sensitivity.

Trace concentrations of anesthetics in question are clearly well below the concentrations used for clinical anesthesia. For this reason, the analyzers used to monitor clinically useful concentrations of anesthetic gases, such as the IR gas analyzers used to measure inspired and end-tidal concentrations in the OR, are not sensitive enough to monitor trace concentrations in the atmosphere.

By using a chart recorder connected to the output of an IR trace concentration gas analyzer, a continuous plot of the N_2O concentration in room air can be obtained during anesthesia. The value of this type of monitoring is quite obvious. Instantaneous peaks on the chart reflect a high level of leakage of the gas, such as that resulting from adjustment of a face mask. Alternatively, the chart may reflect a leak in some other part of the system. Also, because levels of waste gases do fluctuate, this approach is more reliable than a grab sample for measuring concentrations that may be inhaled by personnel in the OR.

TWA concentrations may be obtained from the IR trace concentration gas analyzer by integrating the output; that is, by determining the area under the time-concentration curve and dividing by the time. This can be done by counting the squares (in a chart record) or with a planimeter. The integration for N_2O also can be derived electronically by a relatively inexpensive microcomputer that provides a continuously updated TWA concentration. If a peak concentration suggestive of a leak in the system is sensed, the analyzer, acting as a leak detector, can be used to "sniff out" the source of the leak.

The ideal air monitoring program should measure all anesthetic gases used in the OR. The recommended standard, however, requires monitoring only of the most frequently used agent because following recommended work practices and control procedures will reduce all agents proportionately. Thus N_2O can be monitored and act as a tracer for the potent agents that may be administered along with it in some fixed proportion. However, in rooms where N_2O is rarely used (i.e., cardiac ORs), this technique is not satisfactory. In these rooms the specific halogenated agents must be monitored.

Biological Exposure

Sonander and colleagues[43] attempted to correlate biologic exposure as measured by analysis of urine samples from exposed OR personnel with technical exposure as measured by gas sampling. They studied four anesthesiologists and 25 nurse anesthetists. Urine samples were obtained early in the day, before OR work began, and then 8 hours later during the workday. These personnel also wore personal sampling pumps so that TWA exposure concentrations could be obtained. The N_2O concentrations in the gas above the urine in the collection containers, measured by gas chromatography, showed a good correlation ($r = 0.97$) with technical exposure measurements. The authors suggested that this method of analyzing urine gas provides a useful means of assessing biologic exposure during routine anesthetic work.

Olfaction

Although the anesthesiologist is the ultimate monitor of the patient in the OR, human senses are not very effective at detecting trace concentrations of anesthetics. The olfactory thresholds for N_2O and halothane are 10% to 30% (100,000 to 300,000 ppm) and 0.005% to 0.01% (50 to 100 ppm), respectively.[44]

ARE TRACE CONCENTRATIONS OF WASTE ANESTHETIC GASES HAZARDOUS?

The United States currently has no formal requirements for monitoring the OR atmosphere for waste anesthetic gases, but recommendations do exist.[45,46] Although published in 1977, the limits recommended by NIOSH have not been enacted into law by OSHA, and it is quite likely that they never will be. Such a law has been opposed by both hospitals and anesthesiologists because the recommendations are considered by many to be unreasonable. First, the limits are recommended on the basis of the work of Whitcher and colleagues,[11] who showed that these levels were readily achievable. However, their results have not been duplicated.[47] In 1979, they reported data to the effect that even when all reduction measures were taken, exposure levels strongly depend on the anesthetic technique used. Thus, when a mask was used, mean levels of 180 ppm of N_2O were found. When patients underwent tracheal intubation, mean levels of 16 ppm were achieved. Should all anesthetized patients therefore undergo tracheal intubation so that this arbitrary level can be maintained? Obviously not. Clearly, each technique has its associated degree of atmospheric contamination. An inhalational induction of a pediatric patient would certainly violate the recommended standard, yet it has obvious advantages for the patient. Second, the results of tests of psychomotor activity conducted by Bruce and Bach,[13] which also formed a basis for the recommended standard, have not been substantiated by others, all of whom found no effects at much higher trace concentrations of anesthetics.[48,49] Third, no "safe" trace level has ever been demonstrated for any of the anesthetics in use.

An even more fundamental issue still remains unresolved. Are trace levels of anesthetics really hazardous? Certainly no cause-and-effect relationship has ever been demonstrated.[50,51] The studies to date that have incriminated anesthetics have all been based on questionnaire surveys sent to people who were assumed either to have been exposed to trace anesthetics in the OR, such as members of the ASA or AANA, or those assumed not to have been exposed, such as pediatricians. Such studies are notoriously unreliable; they are open to responder bias, which could explain all the observed differences to date between "exposed" and "unexposed" personnel.

That such bias exists in these studies was very clearly demonstrated by Axelsson and Rylander,[52] who studied 655 pregnancies among workers in one Swedish hospital. Following a postal questionnaire survey, they checked the accuracy of the responses they received against the respondents' medical records. They found that all women who had miscarriages and who worked at sites with exposure to anesthetic gases correctly reported their work sites and miscarriages, whereas one third of all miscarriages by women who were not exposed during pregnancy went unreported in the questionnaire. The authors concluded that their study draws attention to the methodologic difficulties in using questionnaires to study pregnancy outcome and pinpoints the importance of responder bias.

The ASA Ad Hoc Committee on Effects of Trace Anesthetic Agents on Health of Operating Room Personnel retained a group of epidemiologists and statisticians, the Epistat Group, to review all the available data pertaining to health hazards among OR workers. This group reviewed 17 published reports.[53] Four were excluded from further consideration because they did not present data on the specific outcomes under evaluation. Five more were excluded because they did not use comparable control groups. Data from two studies among dentists and dental assistants were also excluded because the exposure of these personnel to anesthetic gases substantially differs from that of OR personnel. Thus data from only six studies were considered worthy of scrutiny. The group's report found that the only health hazard consistently reported among female OR workers was an increased relative risk of spontaneous abortion.

The Epistat Group authors observed that, on the basis of the available data, the relative risk for spontaneous abortion among exposed women is approximately 1.3, or 33% greater than for nonexposed women. The authors further stated that the magnitude of this increase is well within the range that might be due to bias or uncontrolled confounding variables, such as responder bias, and that epidemiologic data currently available are insufficient for developing standards or setting exposure limits. Furthermore, even if this increased relative risk were genuine, it should still be viewed in perspective. For example, maternal smoking of one pack of cigarettes per day increases the spontaneous abortion rate by 80%, and maternal consumption of alcohol may increase the rate by 200%.[40,54]

The report urged that future studies be "prospective cohort studies, with careful documentation of type, amount and duration of exposure, meticulous and uniform follow-up, and thorough ascertainment and confirmation following predefined criteria of outcome events" to avoid previous methodologic errors.

In the same year, Tannenbaum and Goldberg[55] came to a similar conclusion. Their analysis of articles finding adverse health effects from exposure to trace anesthetic gases found that methodologic errors in data collection may have led to inaccuracies in interpretation of the data. They also recommended a prospective study be performed with appropriate epidemiologic methods to avoid bias and confounding variables. Several other reviews have come to the same conclusion.[56]

Spence and Maran[57,58] conducted a prospective study in the United Kingdom. They surveyed 11,500 female medical school graduates younger than 40 years and gathered information on occupational details, work practices, lifestyle, and obstetric and medical history. They found that female anesthesiologists had no greater incidence of infertility compared with other physicians. They also found that the incidence of cancer was unrelated to occupation and that the incidence of spontaneous abortion, and of the development of a congenital abnormality in any infant, was not associated with the occupation of the mother, with working in the OR, or even with the presence of a waste anesthetic gas scavenging system.

Rowland and colleagues[59,60] reported an increased incidence of infertility and spontaneous abortion in female personnel working in unscavenged rooms in the dental operatory where N_2O was administered; levels of N_2O may reach up to 1000 ppm under these circumstances. In any event, no adverse reproductive effects were reported in personnel who worked in areas where scavenging systems for waste anesthetic gases were in place.

In 1999, the ASA published the report of its Task Force on Trace Anesthetic Gases of the ASA Committee on Occupational Health. This informational booklet addresses analysis of the literature, the role of regulatory agencies, scavenging and monitoring equipment, and recommendations.[46] A summary of the report appears below.

Risks

Studies have not shown an association between trace levels of anesthetic gases found in scavenged anesthetizing locations and adverse health effects on personnel.

Recommendations

1. Waste anesthetic gases should be scavenged.
2. Appropriate work practices should be used to minimize exposure to waste anesthetic gases.
3. Personnel working in areas where waste anesthetic gases may be present should be educated regarding current studies on health effects of exposure to waste anesthetic gases, appropriate work practices to minimize exposure, and machine check and maintenance procedures.
4. Evidence is insufficient to recommend routine monitoring of trace levels of waste anesthetic gases in the OR and PACU.
5. Evidence is insufficient to recommend routine medical surveillance of personnel exposed to trace concentrations of waste anesthetic gases, although each institution should have a mechanism for employees to report suspected work-related health problems.

To date, trace concentrations of anesthetics have not been satisfactorily proven to be a cause of health problems in OR workers. However, absence of evidence does not constitute evidence of absence; because the possibility of a hazard may exist, measures should be taken to reduce exposure. This recommendation is made by all concerned agencies, including NIOSH, the American Hospital Association, TJC, and the ASA. Exposure limits for N_2O have been suggested or agreed upon in some countries, namely The Netherlands (25 ppm) and the United Kingdom, Italy, Sweden, Norway, and Denmark (100 ppm).[61-63] The differences illustrate the difficulty in setting standards without adequate data.

The ASA Task Force on Trace Anesthetic Gases of the Committee on Occupational Health of Operating Room Personnel emphasizes that the administration of anesthesia and the safety of the patient are the primary goals, and that atmospheric contamination control must be of secondary concern. This document on waste anesthetic gases emphasizes the use of scavenging and work practices to reduce levels of trace concentrations of waste anesthetic gases and the importance of education. Regular checking and documented maintenance of anesthetic equipment also is recommended. Quality assurance data provide excellent documentation that if the above measures are carried out, levels of trace gases will be below the NIOSH recommendations. In determining adequacy and appropriateness of waste gas scavenging systems, current recommended standards should be reviewed and adopted.

ENVIRONMENTAL CONCERNS

Since the report from the ASA Task Force on Trace Anesthetic Gases of the Committee on Occupational Health of Operating Room Personnel was published in 1999, concern has been growing about the potential global warming effects of chemicals released into the atmosphere. The potent inhaled anesthetic agents isoflurane, sevoflurane, and desflurane are minimally metabolized in the body; once they are released into the atmosphere, they have long lifetimes there.[64] Ryan and Nielsen[39] have calculated the relative impact of inhaled anesthetics as greenhouse gases and on global warming. They concluded that desflurane has a greater potential impact on global warming than either isoflurane or sevoflurane, and that N_2O alone produces a significant greenhouse gas contribution compared with sevoflurane or isoflurane. Their recommendations are to avoid N_2O as a carrier gas if possible and to avoid unnecessarily high fresh gas flow rates, especially when using desflurane. They acknowledge that using low fresh gas flow rates requires increased use of CO_2 absorbents, the disposal of which introduces other environmental concerns. The ideal solution would be to avoid release of waste anesthetic gases into the atmosphere altogether and to reclaim (recycle) them for subsequent use.

Low-Flow (Fresh Gas) Anesthesia

Most of the anesthetic fresh gas flow eventually finds its way into the atmosphere; minimizing such flow therefore offers both economic and environmental advantages.

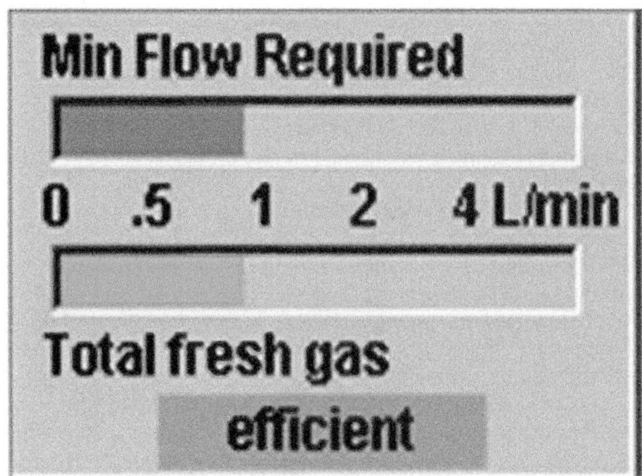

FIGURE 5-23 ■ Dräger Low-Flow Wizard display. The top bar graph shows the loss of volume from the system. The bottom bar graph shows the current fresh gas flow (FGF) setting. If the bottom bar is shorter than the top bar, the display bar is red (too little FGF). If the FGF is less than 1 L/min more than the required flow, then the display bar is green (efficient), as shown. If the FGF is more than 1 L/min more than the required flow, then the display bar is yellow (too much FGF). (Courtesy David Karchner, Dräger Medical, Telford, PA.)

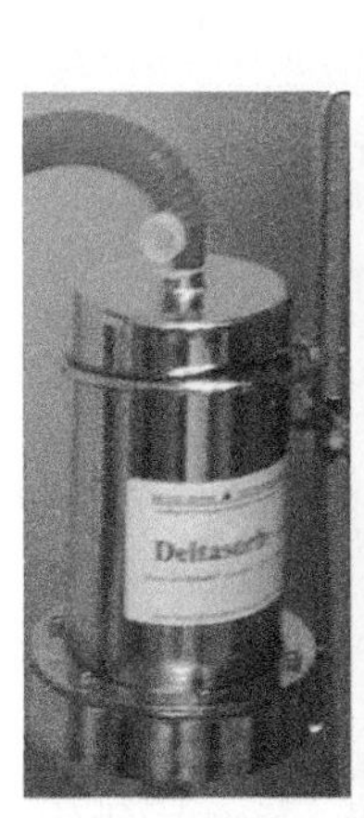

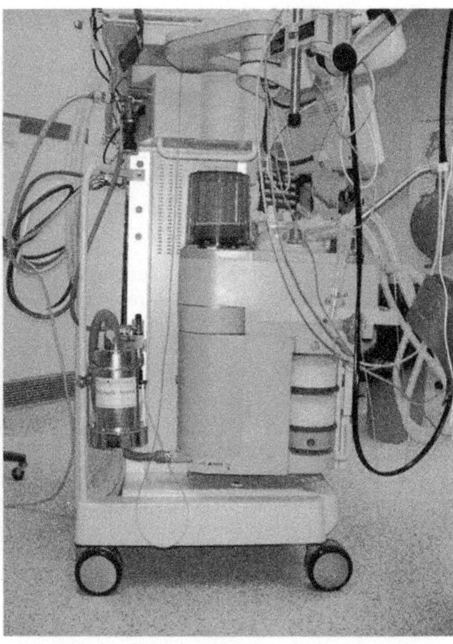

FIGURE 5-24 ■ *Left,* The Deltasorb stainless steel canister contains Deltazite, an anesthetic agent–adsorbing sieve. *Right,* Location of the canister is between the waste gas scavenging interface on the anesthesia machine and the tubing connecting to the hospital's waste gas evacuation system. (Courtesy of Mark Filipovic, Blue-Zone Technologies, Concord, Canada.)

Low-flow anesthesia means different things to different people. Modern anesthesia workstations and their monitoring features facilitate the use of low flows, but a certain amount of education concerning anesthetic uptake and circuit dynamics is required.[65]

To help clinicians optimize fresh gas flow settings in real time, one manufacturer (Dräger Medical) has incorporated a Low-Flow Wizard (LFW) into its Narkomed 6000 series and Apollo workstations. The LFW displays the minimum fresh gas flow required to meet patient uptake and system leakage compared with the currently set total fresh gas flow (Fig. 5-23). The minimum fresh gas flow required is continuously computed as the sum of four variables: 1) any leakage between the inspiratory and expiratory ports of the circle system, 2) oxygen uptake, 3) agent uptake, and 4) N_2O uptake. Items 2, 3, and 4 are determined from the inspired-expired concentration difference and the patient's minute ventilation. The information is displayed as two bar graphs: the top graph shows loss of volume from the system, and the bottom shows the current fresh gas flow setting (see Fig. 5-23).

Anesthetic Capture

An alternative solution to both scavenging waste anesthetic gases and protecting the environment is to insert an anesthetic agent–absorbing filter between the anesthesia machine's waste gas scavenging interface and the hospital waste gas evacuation system in the OR. In 2002, Doyle and colleagues[66] reported that silica zeolite was effective at completely removing 1% isoflurane from exhaled gases for periods of up to 8 hours. They concluded that "the technology shows promise in removing isoflurane emitted from anesthesia machine scavenging systems." This technology is applied in the Deltasorb Anesthetic Collection Service (Blue-Zone Technologies Ltd., Concord, Canada), which uses a portable stainless steel canister that is delivered and exchanged weekly to health care facilities. The canister uses a sieve-like filtering matrix (Deltazite) to selectively adsorb each halogenated anesthetic gas—desflurane, sevoflurane, and isoflurane—as waste gas flows through the canister en route to being vented to the atmosphere. Each canister weighs about 5 lb and can adsorb approximately two full bottles of halogenated anesthetics. When the canister is full, it is shipped to the company's facility, where it is desorbed of contained anesthetic and returned to the hospital for further use (Fig. 5-24). At that time, the reclaimed anesthetic is stored while approval for its reuse is pending (personal communication, Mark Filipovic, Blue-Zone Technologies).

REFERENCES

1. Vaisman AI: Working conditions in the operating room and their effect on the health of anesthetists [in German], *Eksp Khir Anesteziol* 12:44–49, 1967.
2. Askrog V, Harvald B: Teratogenic effects of inhalation anesthetics, *Nord Med* 83(16):498–500, 1970.
3. Knill-Jones RP, Rodrigues LV, Moir DD, Spence AA: Anaesthetic practice and pregnancy: controlled survey of women anaesthetists in the United Kingdom, *Lancet* 1:1326–1328, 1972.
4. Corbett TH, Cornell RG, Lieding K, Endres JL: Incidence of cancer among Michigan nurse anesthetists, *Anesthesiology* 38:260–263, 1973.
5. Corbett TH, Cornell RG, Endres JL, Lieding K: Birth defects among children of nurse anesthetists, *Anesthesiology* 41:341–344, 1974.
6. Cohen EN, Bellville JW, Brown BW Jr: Anesthesia, pregnancy, and miscarriage: a study of operating room nurses and anesthetists, *Anesthesiology* 34:343–347, 1971.
7. Fink BR, Shepard TH, Blandau RJ: Teratogenic activity of nitrous oxide, *Nature* 214:146–148, 1967.
8. Congress of the United States. Occupational Safety and Health Act of 1970.
9. All About OSHA. U.S. Department of Labor and Occupational Safety and Health Administration. 2012, OSHA publication 3302.

10. Anonymous: Occupational disease among operating room personnel: a national study. Report of an Ad Hoc Committee on the Effect of Trace Anesthetics on the Health of Operating Room Personnel, American Society of Anesthesiologists, *Anesthesiology* 41:321–340, 1974.
11. Cohen EN, Brown BW, Bruce DL: Occupational disease among operating room personnel: a national study, *Anesthesiology* 41:321–340, 1974.
12. Whitcher CE, Piziali R, Sher R, Moffat RJ: Development and evaluation of methods for the elimination of waste anesthetic gases and vapors in hospitals. Cincinatti, 1975, U.S. Department of Health, Education and Welfare, Public Health Service, Centers for Disease Control, NIOSH. Publication No. (NIOSH) 75-137.
13. NIOSH: Criteria for a recommended standard: occupational exposure to waste anesthetic gases and vapors. Bethesda, MD, 1977, US Department of Health, Education, and Welfare, Public Health Service, Centers for Disease Control, National Institute for Occupational Safety and Health.
14. Bruce DL, Bach MJ: Effects of trace anesthetic gases on behavioural performance of volunteers, *Br J Anaesth* 48:871–876, 1976.
15. OSHA: *Anesthetic Gases: Guidelines for Workplace Exposure. OSHA Directorate of Technical Support and Emergency Management [formerly Directorate of Technical Support]*; July 20, 1999 revised May 18, 2000. Accessed 2012 Feb 20 at, http://www.osha.gov/dts/osta/anestheticgases.
16. Pfaffli P, Nikki P, Ahlman K: Concentrations of anaesthetic gases in recovery rooms (letter), *Br J Anaesth* 44:230, 1972.
17. Mehta S, Burton P, Simms JS: Monitoring of occupational exposure to nitrous oxide, *Canad Anaesth Soc J* 25:419–423, 1978.
18. Lecky JH: The mechanical aspects of anesthetic pollution control, *Anesth Analg* 56:769–774, 1977.
19. Cottrell JE, Chalon J, Turndorf H: Faulty anesthesia circuits: a source of environmental pollution in the operating room, *Anesth Analg* 56:359–362, 1977.
20. Hoerauf KH, Hartmann T, Acimovic S, et al: Waste gas exposure to sevoflurane and nitrous oxide during anaesthesia using the oesophageal-tracheal Combitube small adult, *Br J Anaesth* 86:124–126, 2001.
21. Wray RP: A source of non-anesthetic nitrous oxide in operating room air, *Anesthesiology* 52(1):88–89, 1980.
22. ECRI: *Nitrous oxide exhausted from cryosurgical units:* Plymouth, PA, 1979, Emergency Care Research Institute.
23. Blokker-Veldhuis MJ, Rutten PM, De Hert SG: Occupational exposure to sevoflurane during cardiopulmonary bypass, *Perfusion* 26:383–389, 2011.
24. Hoerauf K, Harth M, Wild K, Hobbhahan J: Occupational exposure to desflurane and isoflurane during cardiopulmonary bypass: is the gas outlet of the membrane oxygenator an operating theatre pollution hazard? *Br J Anaesth* 78:378–380, 1997.
25. Mierdl S, Byhahn C, Abdel-Rahman U, et al: Occupational exposure to inhalational anesthetics during cardiac surgery on cardiopulmonary bypass, *Ann Thorac Surg* 75:1924–1927, 2003. discussion 1927–1928.
26. Berner O: Concentration and elimination of anaesthetic gases in recovery rooms, *Acta Anaesth Scand* 22:55–57, 1978.
27. American Institute of Architects: *Guidelines for construction and equipment of hospitals and medical facilities*, Washington, DC, 1992, American Institute of Architects.
28. *Standard specification for anesthetic gas scavenging systems: transfer and receiving systems.* West Conshohocken, PA, 2002, ASTM International. F1343-02.
29. Wabiszewski J, editor: *Explore! The Anesthesia System, Aisys.* Madison, WI, 2005, Datex-Ohmeda. p 6.6.
30. *Open reservoir scavenger, operation and maintenance manual*, Telford, PA, 1986, North American Dräger.
31. Hamilton RC, Byrne J: Another cause of gas-scavenging-line obstruction [letter], *Anesthesiology* 51(4):365–366, 1979.
32. Abramowitz M, McGill WA: Hazard of an anesthetic scavenging device [letter], *Anesthesiology* 51:276, 1979.
33. Tavakoli M, Habeeb A: Two hazards of gas scavenging, *Anesth Analg* 57(2):286–287, 1978.
34. Mor ZF, Stein ED, Orkin LR: A possible hazard in the use of a scavenging system, *Anesthesiology* 47(3):302–303, 1977.
35. Hagerdal M, Lecky JH: Anesthetic death of an experimental animal related to a scavenging system malfunction, *Anesthesiology* 47(6):522–523, 1977.
36. Patel KD, Dalal FY: A potential hazard of the Dräger Scavenging Interface System for Wall Suction, *Anesth Analg* 58:327–328, 1979.
37. Allen M, Lees DE: Fires in medical vacuum pumps: Do you need to be concerned? *ASA Newsletter* 68:22, 2004.
38. Barwise JA, Lancaster LJ, Michaels D, et al: An initial evaluation of a novel anesthetic scavenging interface, *Anesth Analg* 113:1064–1067, 2011.
39. Ryan SM, Nielsen CJ: Global warming potential of inhaled anesthetics: application to clinical use, *Anesth Analg* 111:92–98, 2010.
40. Berry JM: System for removal of halocarbon gas from waste anesthetic gases. U.S. Patent number 6729329, issued May 2004.
41. Berry JM: *Volatile Anesthetic Reclamation: It's About Time (and Temperature)! Poster presentation*, 2006, Society for Technology in Anesthesia.
42. Kaarakka P, Malischke PR, Kreul JF: Alternative sites for measuring breathing zone nitrous oxide levels (abstract), *Anesthesiology* 55:A139, 1981.
43. Sonander H, Stenqvist O, Nilsson K: Nitrous oxide exposure during routine anaesthetic work: measurement of biologic exposure from urine samples and technical exposure by bag sampling, *Acta Anaesth Scand* 29(2):203–208, 1985.
44. Halsey MJ, Chand S, Dluzewski AR, et al: Olfactory thresholds: detection of operating room contamination, *Br J Anaesth* 49:510–511, 1977.
45. Mazze RI: Waste anesthetic gases and regulatory agencies, *Anesthesiology* 52:248–256, 1980.
46. American Society of Anesthesiologists Task Force on Trace Anesthetic Gases of the Committee on Occupational Health of Operating Room Personnel: *Waste anesthetic gases: information for management in anesthetizing areas and the post anesthesia care unit (PACU).* Park Ridge, IL, American Society of Anesthesiologists, 1999.
47. Whitcher CE, Siukola LVM: Occupational exposure, education and sampling methods, *Anesthesiology* 51(3):S336, 1979.
48. Gambill AF, McCallum RN, Henrichs TF: Psychomotor performance following exposure to trace concentrations of inhalation anesthetics, *Anesth Analg* 58(6):475–482, 1979.
49. Frankhuizen JL, Vlek CA, Burm AG, Rejger V: Failure to replicate negative effects of trace anaesthetics on mental performance, *Br J Anaesth* 50:229–234, 1978.
50. Ferstandig LL: Trace concentrations of anesthetic gases: a critical review of their disease potential, *Anesth Analg* 57:328–345, 1978.
51. Ferstandig LL: Trace concentrations of anesthetic gases, *Acta Anaesth Scand* 75(Suppl):38–43, 1982.
52. Axelsson G, Rylander R: Exposure to anaesthetic gases and spontaneous abortion: response bias in a postal questionnaire, *Int J Epidemiol* 11:250–256, 1982.
53. Buring JE, Hennekens CH, Mayrent SL, et al: Health experiences of operating room personnel, *Anesthesiology* 62:325–330, 1985.
54. Hennekens CH, Colton T, Rosner B, et al: *Evaluation of the epidemiologic evidence for occupational hazards of anesthetic gases*, Park Ridge, IL, 1982, American Society of Anesthesiologists.
55. Tannenbaum TN, Goldberg RJ: Exposure to anesthetic gases and reproductive outcome: a review of the epidemiologic literature, *J Occup Med* 27:659–668, 1985.
56. Ebi KL, Rice SA: Reproductive and developmental toxicity of anesthetics in humans. In Rice SA, Fish KJ, editors: *Anesthetic toxicity*, New York, 1994, Raven Press, pp 175–198.
57. Spence AA: Environmental pollution by inhalation anaesthetics, *Br J Anaesth* 59:96–103, 1987.
58. Maran NJ, Knill-Jones RP, Spence AA: Infertility among female hospital doctors in the UK, *Br J Anaesth* 76:581P, 1996.
59. Rowland AS, Baird DD, Shore DL, et al: Nitrous oxide and spontaneous abortion in female dental assistants, *Am J Epidemiol* 141:531–538, 1995.
60. Rowland AS, Baird DD, Weinberg CR, et al: Reduced fertility among women employed as dental assistants exposed to high levels of nitrous oxide, *N Engl J Med* 327:993–997, 1992.
61. Health Services Advisory Committee: *Anaesthetic agents: controlling exposure under COSHH*, Suffolk, 1995, Health and Safety Executive.
62. Borm PJA, Kant I, Houben G, et al: Monitoring of nitrous oxide in operating rooms: identification of sources and estimation of occupational exposure, *J Occup Med* 32:1112–1116, 1990.

63. Arbejdstilsynet (The Danish National Institute for Occupational Safety): Grænseværdier for stoffer og materialer, *At-anvisning*, 1988. Nr.3.1.o.2 (April).
64. Langbein T, Sonntag H, Trapp D, et al: Volatile anaesthetics and the atmosphere: atmospheric lifetimes and atmospheric effects of halothane, enflurane, isoflurane, desflurane and sevoflurane, *Br J Anaesth* 82:66–73, 1999.
65. Feldman JM: Managing fresh gas flow to reduce environmental contamination, *Anesth Analg* 114(5):1093–1101, 2012.
66. Doyle DJ, Byrick R, Filipovic D, Cashin F: Silica zeolite scavenging of exhaled isoflurane: a preliminary report, *Can J Anaesth* 49:799–804, 2002.

CHAPTER 6

ANESTHESIA VENTILATORS

Raj K. Modak • Michael A. Olympio

CHAPTER OUTLINE

OVERVIEW

Since the 1960s, the use of intermittent positive-pressure ventilation (IPPV) has become widespread. Today's observer might wrongly conclude that the research, development, and methods for mechanical ventilation in the operating room (OR) had occurred only recently. However, much of the necessary experimentation and design took place much earlier.

Anesthesia ventilators are commonly compared with mechanical ventilators used in the intensive care unit (ICU); however, anesthesia ventilators are unique; they not only deliver oxygen and remove carbon dioxide, they also facilitate the delivery of inhalational agents used to render patients unconscious and maintain surgical anesthesia. Modern delivery systems typically are semiclosed systems, which require removal of carbon dioxide and conservation of potent inhalational agents. Low gas flows are commonly used to aid in agent sparing and reduce patient exposure to unheated gases. In contrast, the ICU ventilator typically has an open system because no gases are recirculated through the system; as such, a carbon dioxide absorber is not used. High gas flows can be used because elaborate gas-warming and humidification techniques are available and have proven cost effective in the ICU.

In the past, it was not uncommon to bring an ICU ventilator into the OR for oxygenation and ventilation of patients with extremes of pulmonary pathophysiology because these machines had more options. Recent advances in ventilator technology have made the differences between ICU ventilators and anesthesia ventilators negligible. Outcome data continue to be lacking in the scientific literature regarding differences in modes used in the OR: synchronized intermittent mechanical ventilation (SIMV) or pressure-support ventilation (PSV). However, this has not stopped manufacturers from providing these modes of ventilation, nor has it stopped clinicians from using them while delivering anesthetic during surgery.

In this chapter, the sections on pulmonary mechanics, physiology, and basic principles of mechanical ventilation delineate the technology and contemporary strategies for lung ventilation. Major features of commonly used anesthesia ventilators in the United States are described.

Of note, no chapter can substitute for the detailed information provided by each ventilator manufacturer, which is found in the educational materials and the operator's and service manuals for each piece of equipment. The reader should refer to these documents for the most detailed pneumatic and electrical schematics.

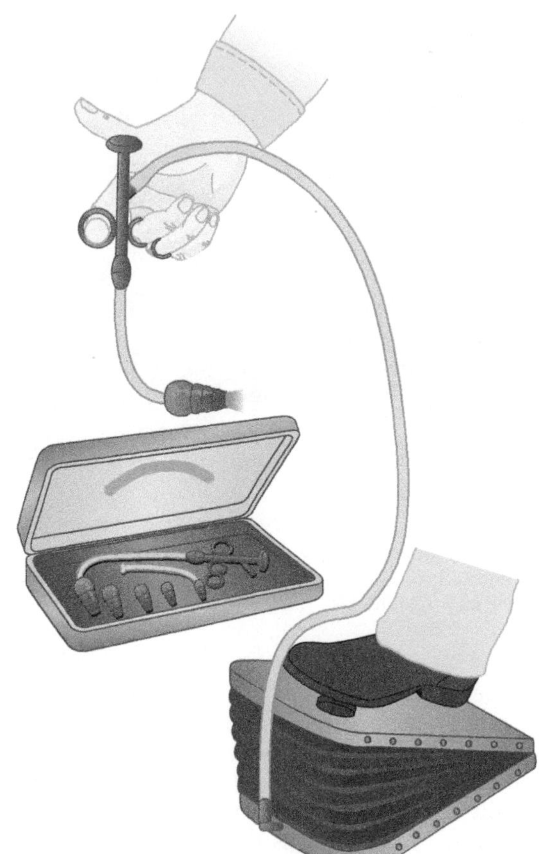

FIGURE 6-1 ■ **Fell-O'Dwyer apparatus.** (From Mushin WW, Rendell-Baker L, Thompson PW, et al: *Automatic ventilation of the lungs*, ed 3, Oxford, UK, 1980, Blackwell Scientific.)

HISTORY

Early recorded attempts to artificially ventilate the lungs of a person date from the 1400s. Baker[1] found records of mouth-to-mouth resuscitation of a newborn in 1472 and of an asphyxiated miner in 1744. Paracelsus is credited with the first use of a bellows in 1530 to artificially inflate the lungs.[2] Open-chest ventilation of a dog via an endotracheal reed was described by Andreas Vesalius in 1555,[3] using mouth-to-tube pressurization, but it was later replaced with bellows ventilation by Robert Hooke in 1667.[4] By the late 1700s, Denmark had initiated a formal campaign and monetary reward for those using a bellows to resuscitate victims of near-drowning. The metal endoral tube, with a conical adapter for the glottic opening, was introduced in 1887 by O'Dwyer for the treatment of patients with diphtheria.[5] This tube was combined with George Fell's manual ventilating bellows and valve device[6] and was used to treat opium overdose in 1891. The resulting Fell-O'Dwyer apparatus[7] (Fig. 6-1) was simplified by removing the valve and placing a hole in the circuit; the hole could be occluded by the thumb during inspiration, thus providing positive-pressure ventilation and passive exhalation. In France in 1896, Tuffier and Hallion[8] were able to partially resect the lung of a patient whose trachea they had intubated blindly with a cuffed tracheal tube and whose lungs they ventilated during the surgical procedure. Finally, in 1898, the first rudimentary anesthesia machine was developed by Rudolph Matas of New Orleans, who added an anesthetic vapor delivery system to the Fell-O'Dwyer apparatus, thus allowing the resection of a chest wall lesion under positive-pressure ventilation with anesthesia.[9]

Attempting to circumvent the difficulties of tracheal intubation, in 1904, Sauerbruch developed a negative-pressure operating chamber that required the patient's head to be sealed outside the chamber. Further development resulted in the electrically powered "iron lung" by Drinker and Shaw in 1928,[10] which was widely used to treat patients with respiratory failure during the polio epidemics. In an alternative approach, in 1905, Brauer provided positive-pressure ventilation via the head, sealed within a chamber and thus eliminating the need for intubation or operating within a chamber (Fig. 6-2).[11]

Modern techniques of endotracheal ventilation during general anesthesia were initiated by Magill in 1928 for head and neck surgery.[12] The beginnings of modern mechanical ventilation are attributed to Engström and his ventilator during the polio epidemics in Denmark circa 1952.[13] This ventilator was later modified for use

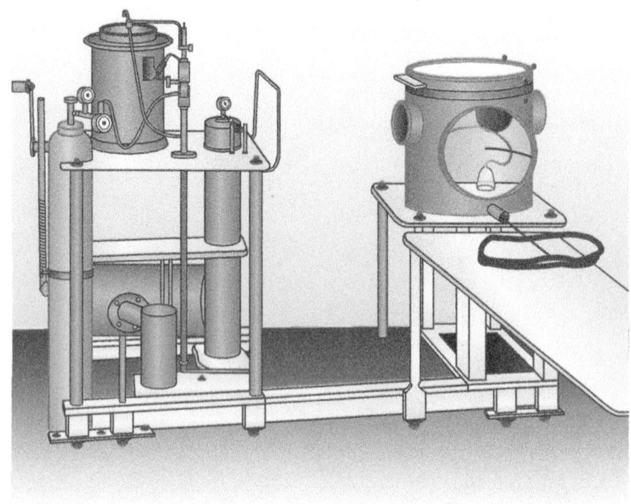

FIGURE 6-2 ■ Brauer's positive-pressure apparatus. (From Mushin WW, Rendell-Baker L, Thompson PW, et al: *Automatic ventilation of the lungs*, ed 3, Oxford, UK, 1980, Blackwell Scientific.)

during general anesthesia,[14] which stimulated the development of a huge number of anesthesia ventilators with a wide diversity of characteristic behaviors, mechanisms, and power sources. Gradually, designs were modified and eventually replaced by pneumatically controlled and fluidically time-cycled systems that were optional accessories for the anesthesia machine. These stand-alone ventilators substituted for the reservoir bag at the connection to the breathing circuit and took on the appearance of modern "bag in a bottle" double-circuit systems.

Contemporary anesthesia machines have replaced these freestanding ventilators by integrating the fresh gas delivery system, scavenging system, and ventilator into one unit. Modern ventilators have electronically controlled circuits and, in some cases, closed feedback loops with microprocessor-regulated flow control valves. Modern ventilators allow digital and graphic displays to aid in ventilator management.

PHYSIOLOGY AND MECHANICAL CONCEPTS

Gas Exchange

The two major functions of the lung are taken into consideration during mechanical ventilation: *ventilation*, the elimination of carbon dioxide (CO_2), and *oxygenation*, the intake of oxygen (O_2). A clear distinction should be made between the elimination of carbon dioxide and the intake of oxygen, even though these two processes are mechanically coupled during natural, spontaneous breathing and are interrelated at the metabolic level. Each is capable of stimulating ventilation.

Carbon dioxide elimination depends on ventilation, which means the lungs are inflated with non–CO_2-containing gases. The carbon dioxide gas of metabolism enters the alveoli of the lungs, and the CO_2-containing gas is expelled from the lungs on exhalation. As such, the achieved ventilation determines the partial pressure of CO_2 in the arterialized blood ($PaCO_2$).

Oxygenation is best represented by the partial pressure of oxygen in the arterialized blood (P_AO_2). Predictable improvements in oxygenation can be facilitated by enriching the inspired gas as dictated by the alveolar gas equation:

$$PaO_2 = FiO_2(P_B - P_{H2O}) - (PaCO_2/R)$$

where P_AO_2 is the partial pressure of alveolar oxygen, FiO_2 is the fraction of inspired oxygen, P_B is barometric pressure, P_{H2O} is partial pressure of water vapor at 37° C, $PaCO_2$ is partial pressure of alveolar carbon dioxide, and R is the respiratory quotient. Increased oxygenation also can be accomplished by increases in airway pressure, which can recruit collapsed alveoli and redistribute alveolar fluid. These changes may be largely independent of ventilation.

Carbon Dioxide Equilibrium

The quantity of carbon dioxide produced normally dictates the minute ventilation. With the exception of using cardiopulmonary bypass or an extracorporeal membrane oxygenator (ECMO), no alternative method has proved satisfactory for eliminating carbon dioxide. Breathing is essential. Normally, in the absence of disease, high altitude, and pharmacologic intervention, spontaneous ventilation results in a $PaCO_2$ of approximately 40 mm Hg. However, the quantitative relationship between CO_2 production and minute ventilation often is poorly understood.

Carbon Dioxide Production

A resting adult weighing 70 kg produces approximately 0.008 gram molecules (moles) of carbon dioxide per minute. At standard temperature (0° C) and pressure (760 mm Hg), one mole of any gas occupies 22.4 L. Therefore, 0.008 moles of carbon dioxide occupy approximately 180 mL. At body temperature (37° C), this is approximately 200 mL.

Carbon Dioxide Elimination

Expressing carbon dioxide production either in moles or in milliliters at atmospheric pressure provides no insight into the volume of ventilation required to maintain homeostasis. More helpful information is provided when the same quantity of carbon dioxide is expressed at different partial pressures, using Boyle's law (Table 6-1).

The volume of carbon dioxide shown at each partial pressure in Table 6-1 is the volume occupied by the metabolic production for 1 minute (0.008 moles). At each pressure, the volume shown is the volume of carbon dioxide produced and therefore is the least alveolar ventilation per minute that is capable of eliminating the carbon dioxide produced. Any lesser alveolar ventilation is insufficient to allow the carbon dioxide to escape at that partial pressure.

The patient's minute volume is made up of both the alveolar and the total dead space ventilation. Normally, the dead space ventilation is one third of the minute

TABLE 6-1 **Metabolic Production of CO_2 Expressed at Different Partial Pressures**

	Partial Pressure (mm Hg)	Volume Occupied (mL)
Normal atmospheric pressure	760	200
One-tenth atmospheric or double alveolar partial pressure	76	2000
Normal alveolar partial pressure	38	4000
Half alveolar partial pressure	19	8000

Each volume represents the minimum alveolar ventilation capable of achieving that partial pressure of carbon dioxide.

volume. For an alveolar minute ventilation of 4000 mL, the required total minute ventilation therefore is approximately 6000 mL. The mixed expired carbon dioxide has a partial pressure of approximately 27 mm Hg.

During IPPV under anesthesia, the total dead space typically increases to approximately 45% of the tidal volume. The same alveolar ventilation of 4000 mL/min thus requires a total minute ventilation of approximately 7275 mL, which will eliminate a mixed expired partial pressure for carbon dioxide of approximately 22 mm Hg.

Oxygen Uptake

At rest, the 70-kg adult human has an oxygen consumption of approximately 250 mL/min. Strictly speaking, ventilation is not essential for oxygenation. When the patient is breathing oxygen, the pulmonary reservoir represents approximately 12 minutes worth of metabolic consumption. Furthermore, if a denitrogenated apneic patient is connected to an oxygen supply (apneic oxygenation), oxygenation theoretically is unlimited.[15] In that case, survival is limited by carbon dioxide accumulation, not by hypoxia.

Net Effect of Respiratory Quotient

Respiratory quotient (RQ) is the ratio between carbon dioxide production and oxygen consumption. The production of carbon dioxide, such as 200 mL/min, normally is slightly less than the oxygen consumption, at 250 mL/min (RQ: 200/250 = 0.8). This discrepancy has interesting implications. With an RQ of 0.8, the sum of the arterial partial pressures for carbon dioxide and oxygen (PaO_2 [100] + $PaCO_2$ [40] = 140 mm Hg) will always be slightly less than the humidified inspired oxygen tension (PiO_2 = 0.21 × [760 − 47] = 149 mm Hg) instead of being exactly equal to it. Because the minute volume inspired is slightly greater than that exhaled, a continuing, small, net inward movement of gas into the lungs is observed. At equilibrium, the partial pressure of nitrogen, or nitrous oxide (N_2O), is slightly greater in the lung than in the inspired gas and, of necessity, this causes an equal reduction in the space that would have been available for the respiratory gases, carbon dioxide, and oxygen.

PHYSICS OF GAS FLOW

Each ventilator discussed in this chapter has a selection of primary variables that the user may set. These may include any of the following:

Inspired pressure:	P_I
Peak inspiratory pressure:	P_{Imax}
Tidal volume:	V_T
Minute volume:	V_M
Inspiratory flow:	Q_I
Frequency:	f
Respiratory cycle time:	T_c
Inspiratory pause time:	T_{plat}
Inspiratory time:	T_I
Expiratory time:	T_E
Inspiratory/expiratory ratio:	I:E

As spontaneous breathing occurs, work is done to move gas into and out of the lung. This work has been designated the *work of breathing* (WOB). Another way to view this is the energy expended to move the gas into and out of the lungs. It is well known that the total work of breathing (WOB_T) is the sum of the work related to overcoming the elastic properties of the lung and chest wall (WOB_E) and the work related to overcoming the resistance aspects of the circuit, endotracheal tube, and large and small airways (WOB_R). Thus,

$$WOB_T = WOB_E + WOB_R$$

Under normal circumstances, the work related to overcome the elastance of the lung and chest wall is nearly 70% of the total WOB; the work related to overcome the resistance of the airways is nearly 25%, and approximately 5% is related to inertial properties of the tissues and gases. *Elastance* (E) of the chest wall is defined as the change of airway pressure (ΔP) divided by the change in volume (ΔV):

$$E = \Delta P/\Delta V$$

Elastance, however, is more commonly described by the inverse, *compliance* (C):

$$C = \Delta V/\Delta P$$

Experimentally derived, formulated, and published in the 1840s by Jean Louis Marie Poiseuille (1797–1869), Poiseuille's law identifies the relationship of gas flow (Q) directly to the pressure gradient (ΔP) and identifies an inverse relationship to the resistance (R) of the system:

$$Q = \Delta P/R$$

This equation can be manipulated to show that:

$$R = \Delta P/Q \text{ and } \Delta P = Q \times R$$

Because the purpose of the ventilator is to perform the work of breathing, it becomes advantageous to examine these physical relationships. In so doing, a method for classifying and understanding ventilator function using the "equation of motion" has emerged.[16]

The force exerted by a ventilator is measured as pressure. This pressure must overcome two distinct impedances to motion during inspiration: *compliance* and *resistance*. Exhalation is passive when mechanical ventilation is used and usually remains unaccounted. The pressure required to overcome the compliance properties of the lung and chest wall can be expressed as:

$$P_C = V_T/C$$

where P_c is pressure compliance. A second element of pressure required to overcome the resistance is found within the breathing circuit, the endotracheal tube, and the conducting airways. The pressure required to overcome this resistance may be expressed mathematically:

$$P_R = Q_I \times R$$

where P_R is pressure resistance and Q_I is inspiratory flow. Because the ventilator exerts pressure to overcome both the compliance and resistance, these two equations may be combined during inspiration:

$$P_T = P_I = P_C + P_R$$

where P_T is total pressure and P_I is inspiratory pressure, or:

$$P_I = ([V_T / C] + [Q_I \times R])$$

Compliance and resistance may be regarded as the "load" facing the inspiratory pressure that results in the two fundamental variables: *tidal volume* and *inspiratory flow*. Changes in inspiratory pressure result in changes in both tidal volume and inspiratory flow. Changes in a desired tidal volume can be achieved by changes in inspiratory pressure and/or flow. Changes in a desired inspiratory flow can be achieved as the result of changes in inspiratory pressure, tidal volume, or both. While using specific ventilator modes, a ventilator attempts to control the inspiratory flow rate to provide a "set" tidal volume *or* inspiratory pressure (Fig. 6-3). When the inspiratory flow is matched to a desired tidal volume, the inspiratory pressure varies to the given load (Fig. 6-4). When the inspiratory flow is matched to a desired inspiratory pressure, the tidal volume varies to the given load (Fig. 6-5).

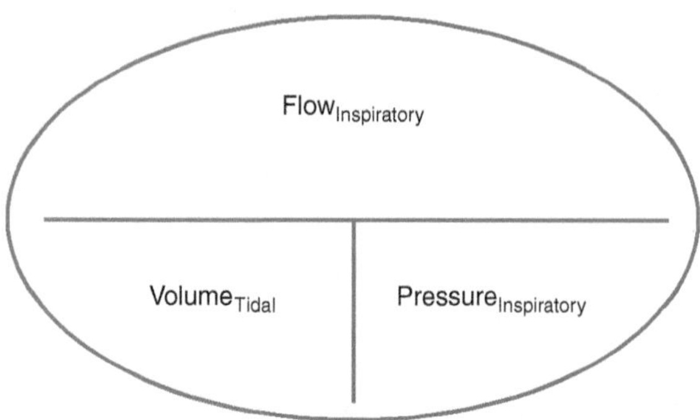

FIGURE 6-3 ■ Triad of ventilator parameters.

Interdependence of Ventilator Settings

Many of these respiratory variables are interdependent, such as minute volume, tidal volume, and respiratory rate ($V_M = V_T \times f$). In some ventilators, the tidal volume is determined by dividing the minute volume by the rate:

$$V_T = V_M / f$$

Tidal volume is also related to the inspiratory flow rate and the inspiratory time:

$$V_T = Q_I \times T_I$$

An inspiratory pause (plateau time [T_{plat}]) is a part of the inspiratory time. Because the inspiratory pause makes no contribution to the tidal volume, the equation for tidal volume may be modified:

$$V_T = Q_I \times (T_I - T_{plat})$$

Clinicians are also concerned about the relationship between inspiratory and expiratory time because the I:E ratio and the absolute times T_I and T_E affect ventilation and oxygenation. This ratio and the absolute time of inspiration are related to frequency and may be expressed mathematically.

Frequency determines time of the respiratory cycle (T_c), usually expressed in seconds, by the following relationship:

$$T_c = 60 / f$$

It follows that 60/f is equal to the inspiratory and expiratory times combined:

$$60/f = T_I + T_E$$

The relationship between T_I and T_E is conventionally expressed as the I:E ratio with 1 as the numerator. This ratio may be derived mathematically as follows, where $R_{I:E}$ equals I:E ratio:

(1) Seconds per minute devoted to inspiration:

$$f \times T_I$$

(2) Seconds per minute devoted to exhalation:

$$60 - (f \times T_I)$$

(3) Dividing (1) by (2), the I:E ratio:

$$R_{I:E} = (f \times T_I) / (60 - [f \times T_I])$$

(4) The frequency and the inspiratory time can be derived by rearranging (3):

$$(60 \times R_{I:E}) - (f \times T_I \times R_{I:E}) = f \times T_I$$

(5) $60 \times R_{I:E} = (f \times T_I) + (f \times T_I \times R_{I:E})$

(6) $60 \times R_{I:E} = (f \times T_I) \times (1 + R_{I:E})$

(7) $f \times T_I = (60 \times R_{I:E}) / (1 + R_{I:E})$

(8) $T_I = (60 \times R_{I:E})/([1 + R_{I:E}] \times f)$

Depending on the manufacturer and the particular model of ventilator, the clinician must choose the $R_{I:E}$ (I:E ratio), mean Q_I (average inspiratory flow rate), or both. The reader is encouraged to study the manufacturer variations shown in Figures 6-6 to 6-13.

The following example demonstrates how frequency, tidal volume, flow, and I:E ratio are interdependent. Assume that in a 60-kg patient V_T is 600 mL and *f* equals 10 breaths/min. As such, the cycle time is fixed at 6 seconds.

By choosing an I:E ratio of 1:2, the inspiratory time becomes fixed at 2 seconds, which *mandates* a mean inspiratory flow rate of 300 mL/sec or 18 L/min (300 mL/sec × 60 sec/min = 18 L/min). Choosing an I:E ratio of 1:1 increases the inspiratory time to 3 seconds, resulting in an inspiratory flow rate of 200 mL/sec or 12 L/min. An I:E ratio of 1:3 reduces the inspiratory time to 1.5 seconds, resulting in an inspiratory flow rate of 400 mL/sec or 24 L/min.

This situation is complicated somewhat by the selection of an inspiratory pause because the respiratory gases are not in transit into or out of the lungs. Exhalation begins when gases start leaving the lungs, so the inspiratory pause is considered part of the inspiratory phase of the respiratory cycle. When incorporated into the original example, with an I:E ratio of 1:2, the inspiratory time of 2 seconds would result in a mean inspiratory flow rate of 300 mL/sec or 18 L/min. In a situation in which T_{plat} equals 25%, T_I is selected, and 25% of the original inspiratory time is added to the inspiratory time. This results in a changed I:E ratio. In this example, the inspiratory time is 2 seconds and 25% of the inspiratory time is 0.5 seconds, which results in a total inspiratory time of 2.5 seconds. Superficial calculations of inspiratory flow rate would suggest 240 mL/sec or 14.4 L/min flows. However, the ventilator would continue to deliver the inspiratory flow at 300 mL/sec or 18 L/min. Inspiratory flow is stopped at 2 seconds, achieving the 600 mL tidal volume, but exhalation occurs 0.5 seconds later. As such, the I:E ratio is changed without affecting the tidal volume, respiratory rate, or inspiratory flow rate. This pause at end inhalation allows for a mild increase in mean airway pressure, increased alveolar recruitment, and improved oxygenation (Fig. 6-14).

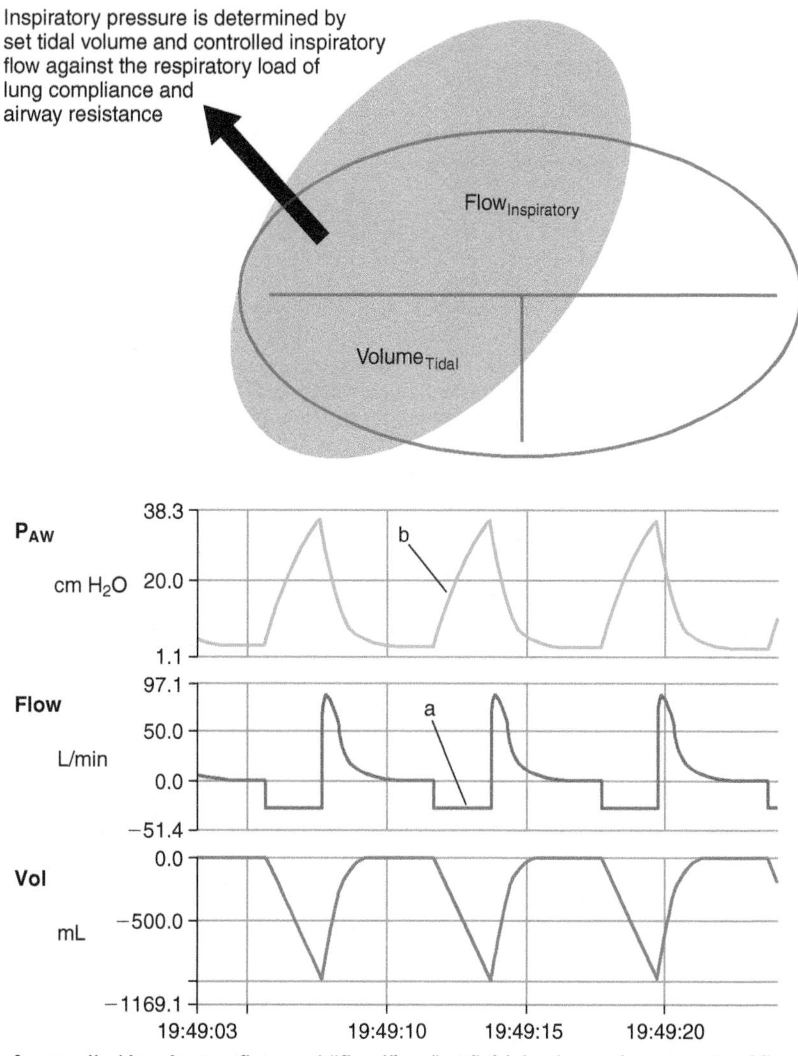

FIGURE 6-4 ■ Relationship of controlled inspiratory flow and "fixed" or "set" tidal volume. An example of fixed flow on a 3-L anesthesia circuit reservoir bag with volume control ventilation settings. Notice inspiratory flow is constant (*a*) and inspiratory pressure rises linearly (*b*). P_{AW}, airway pressure. (From Datex-Ohmeda S/5 Collect, v4.0. 2003. Courtesy GE Healthcare, Waukesha, WI.)

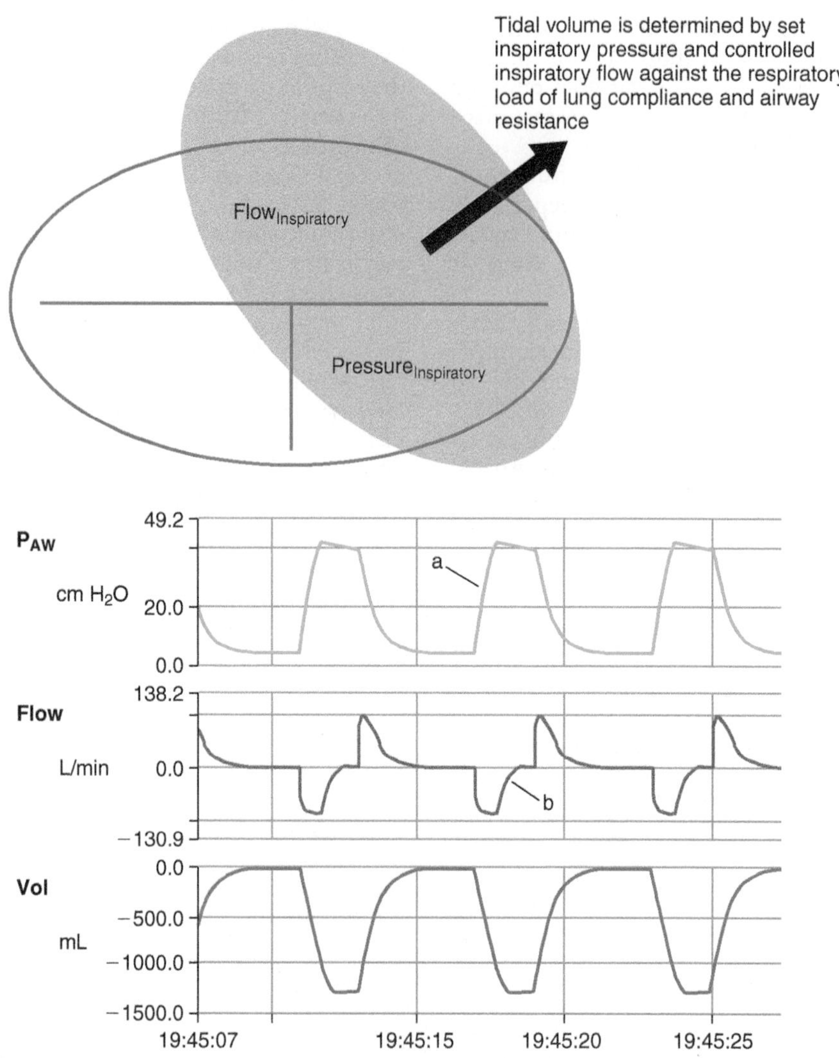

FIGURE 6-5 ■ Relationship of controlled inspiratory flow and "fixed" or "set" inspiratory pressure. An example of a set pressure limit on a 3-L anesthesia circuit reservoir bag with pressure control ventilation settings. Notice inspiratory pressure rises sharply to the set pressure limit (*a*) and inspiratory flow rises sharply, then decays before exhalation (*b*). P_{AW}, airway pressure. (From Datex-Ohmeda S/5 Collect, v4.0. 2003. Courtesy GE Healthcare, Waukesha, WI.)

Primary selection of an inspiratory flow mandates the inspiratory time for the given 600 mL V_T and thus determines the I:E ratio. For example, selecting a flow of 18 L/min (300 mL/sec) mandates an I:E ratio of 1:2 ($V_T/Q_I = T_I$):

$$600 \text{ mL} \div 300 \text{ mL/sec} = 2 \text{ sec}$$

At f = 10, each cycle is 6 seconds. Therefore expiratory time equals 4 seconds. The I:E ratio is 2 seconds relative to 4 seconds, or 1:2.

Some combinations of settings may exceed the capability of the ventilator. For example, a very low flow setting may not be able to deliver the 600 mL within the allotted 6-second cycle time. The alarm "VENT SET ERROR" will appear in the Datex-Ohmeda 7800 ventilator (GE Healthcare, Waukesha, WI) display (Fig. 6-15). In the Datex-Ohmeda 7800, with Q_I equal to 18 L/min, selection of the inspiratory pause of 25% will prolong the T_I to 2.5 seconds, thus changing the I:E ratio to 1:1.4.

Other ventilators allow the selection of the I:E ratio *and* flow simultaneously. Three situations may result: 1) flow will be inadequate to deliver the selected tidal volume, 2) flow can be increased to create a variable end-inspiratory pause, and 3) flow can be just enough to depress the bellows to the bottom, thus delivering the desired tidal volume without a pause.

The final primary variable is the inspiratory pressure (P_I). This variable can be set on some ventilators as a primary variable if the ventilator is in a pressure mode. In so doing, airway pressure increases very rapidly to the set level and is maintained at that level for the duration of the inspiratory period. This behavior must be distinguished from that of an airway pressure limiter, a passive device that does nothing more than prevent airway pressure (P_{AW}) from exceeding a certain value. A Venturi ventilator can be set to function like a pressure generator if the flow is set to a high level and the pressure limiter is carefully adjusted to the desired peak airway pressure.

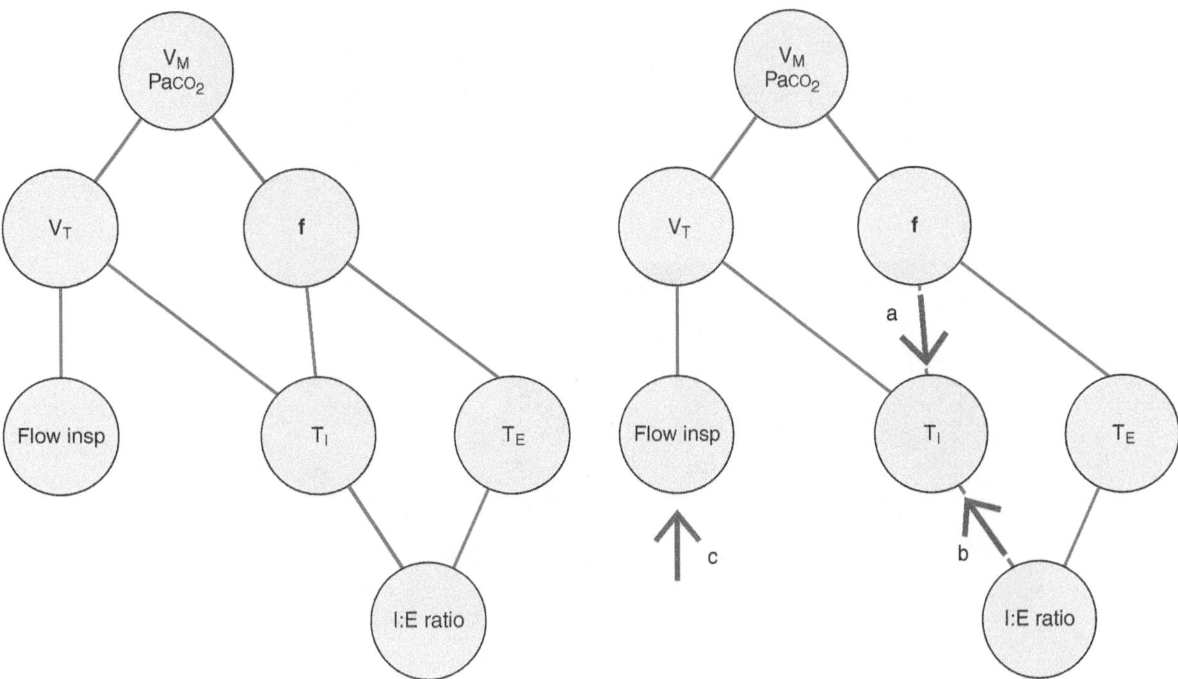

FIGURE 6-6 ■ Interdependence of ventilator settings. V_M, minute ventilation; V_T, tidal volume; *f*, frequency or respiratory rate; *Flow insp*, inspiratory flow; $Paco_2$, partial pressure of arterial carbon dioxide; T_I, inspiratory time; T_E, exhalation time; *I:E ratio*, inspiratory time to exhalation time ratio. Notice that the frequency and the I:E ratio are independent of one another. If tidal volume is fixed, changes in the respiratory rate (*a*) or I:E ratio (*b*) alter the inspiratory time. The inspiratory flow must then be adjusted (*c*) to maintain the fixed tidal volume at the new inspiratory time.

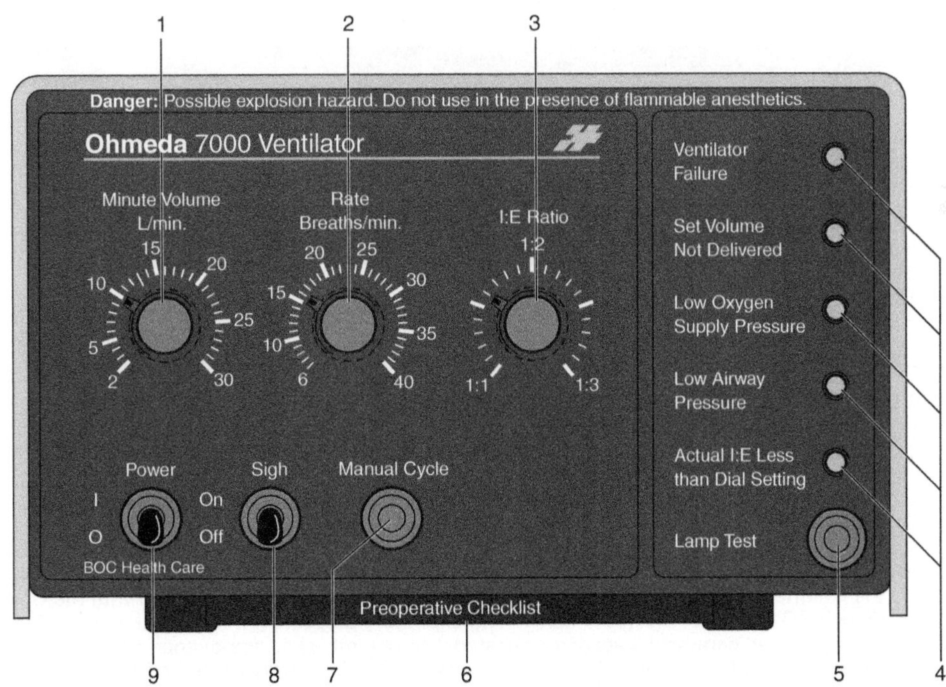

FIGURE 6-7 ■ The Datex-Ohmeda 7000 ventilator (GE Healthcare, Waukesha, WI) requires the user to set minute volume and rate. Tidal volume must be calculated. Numbered components indicate the following: set minute volume (*1*), set frequency (*2*), set I:E ratio (*3*), warning lamps (*4*), switch to test the warning lamps (*5*), ventilator preoperative checklist (*6*), switch to activate one manual cycle (*7*), sigh function on/off (*8*), and power on/off switch (*9*).

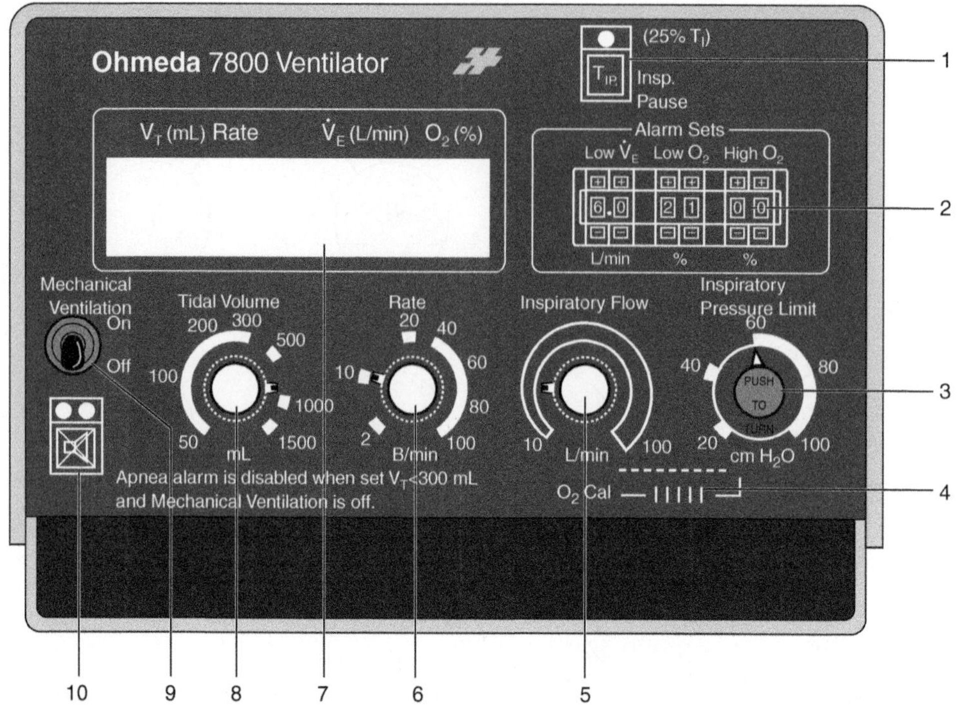

FIGURE 6-8 ■ The Ohmeda 7800 ventilator (GE Healthcare, Waukesha, WI) allows the user to select inspiratory flow (*5*) to determine the rate at which the selected tidal volume is delivered. This selection alters the I:E ratio, which is announced in the liquid crystal display (*7*), which also displays ventilatory parameters and alarms. Compared with the Ohmeda 7000, the Ohmeda 7800 adds a pressure limiter (*3*) and a fixed inspiratory pause option (*1*). Additional numbered components include alarm limit sets (*2*), oxygen calibration dial (*4*), set frequency (*6*), set tidal volume and apnea alarm disable (*8*), power on/off switch (*9*), and alarm silence button (*10*).

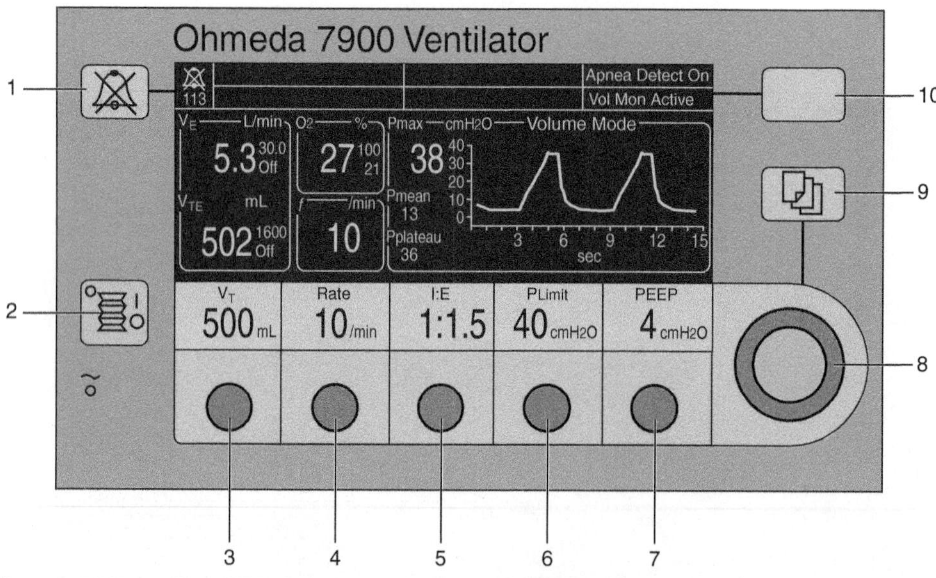

FIGURE 6-9 ■ The Ohmeda 7900 ventilator (GE Healthcare, Waukesha, WI) allows the user to set desired tidal volume (as shown) or inspired pressure (*3*) in the volume-controlled or pressure generator modes, respectively. Compared with the Ohmeda 7800 ventilator, the user selects the I:E ratio (*5*) instead of the flow. Positive end-expiratory pressure (*PEEP; 7*) is an integral feature on the control panel. Dedicated displays of measured parameters are demonstrated. Other numbered components include the audible alarm silence button (*1*), mechanical ventilation on/off switch (*2*), select frequency (*4*), select inspiratory pressure limit (*6*), adjustment knob for the corresponding selection (*8*), select menu (*9*), and select apnea–volume alarm combinations (*10*).

LUNG FUNCTION DURING ANESTHESIA AND MECHANICAL VENTILATION

During anesthesia with a tracheal tube, lung function is adversely affected by many factors. Most of these factors are related to the physical aspect of a tracheal tube: retention of secretions as a result of cough suppression, interference and damage to the mucociliary elevator, increased insensible water loss by lack of humidification, inspissation of secretions by dry gases, and heat loss in exhaled gases. In addition, an increase in ventilation/perfusion (V/Q) mismatching occurs from changes in physiologic and mechanical dead

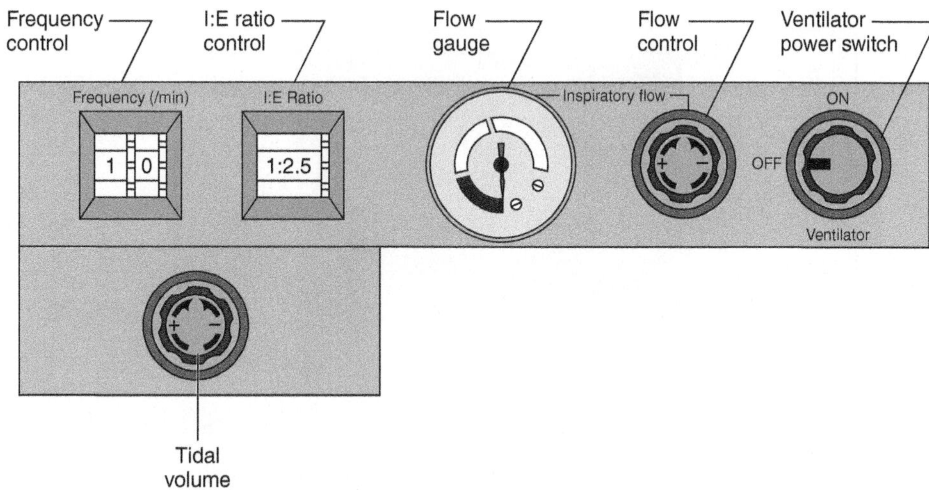

FIGURE 6-10 ■ A unique feature of the Dräger AV ventilators (Dräger Medical, Telford, PA) is that both the inspiratory flow and the I:E ratio may be set by the user, creating a variable inspiratory pause within the preset inspiratory time.

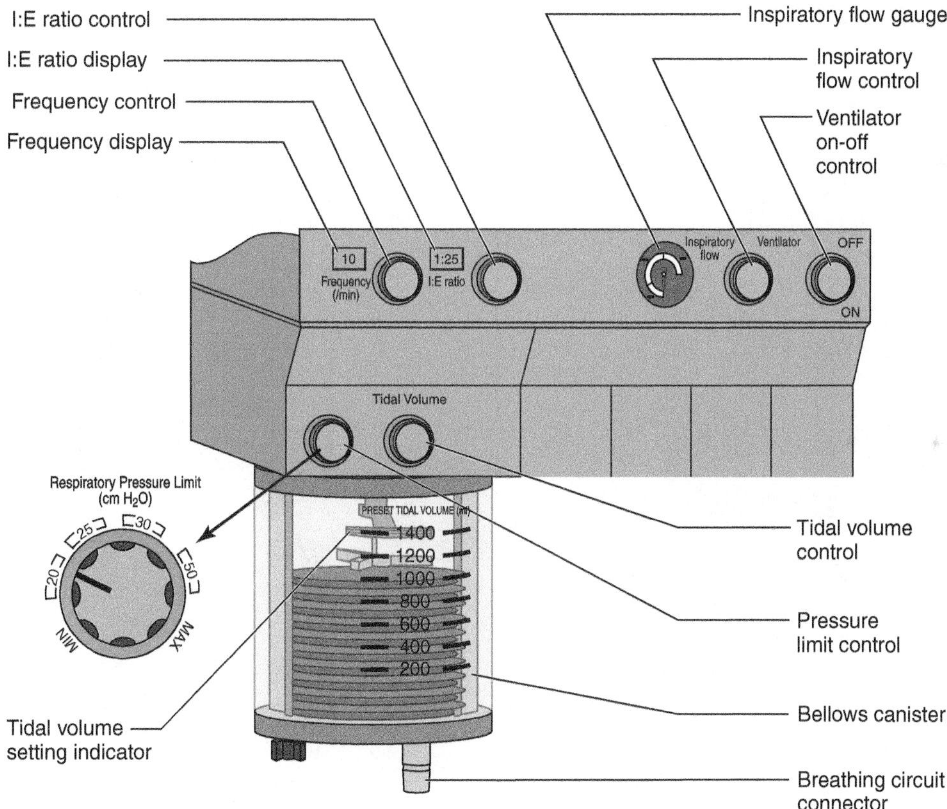

FIGURE 6-11 ■ The Dräger AV-2 ventilator (Dräger Medical, Telford, PA) control panel adds a pressure limiter and digital displays of frequency and I:E ratio. The inspiratory flow and I:E ratio are set by the user, creating a variable inspiratory pause.

space. The work of breathing may be increased from resistance changes to load related to the inner diameter and length of the tracheal tube.

Tracheal suctioning, the solution to the problem of airway secretions, has mixed risks and benefits. The removal of secretions from airways can improve oxygenation and ventilation, but the act of suctioning the secretions can cause negative airway pressure, resulting in atelectasis and entrainment of nitrogen that reduces the fraction of inspired oxygen. In addition, direct airway irritation by instrumentation can cause coughing and straining that can transiently affect the cardiac output and blood pressure.

IPPV causes an increase in intrathoracic pressure during inspiration. Elevated intrathoracic pressures can decrease the blood flow returning to the heart from extrathoracic blood vessels, which in turn decreases cardiac output. Venous return also can be decreased by positive end-expiratory pressure (PEEP), which increases intrathoracic pressure during exhalation.

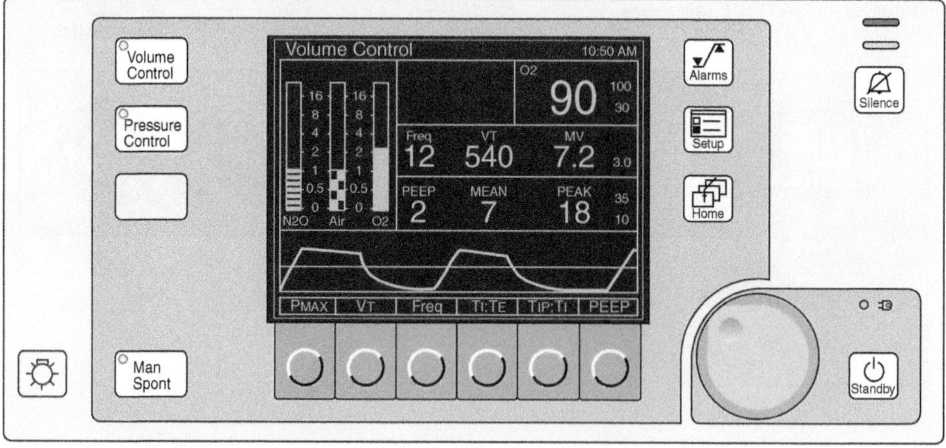

FIGURE 6-12 ■ The Fabius ventilator controls (Dräger Medical, Telford, PA).

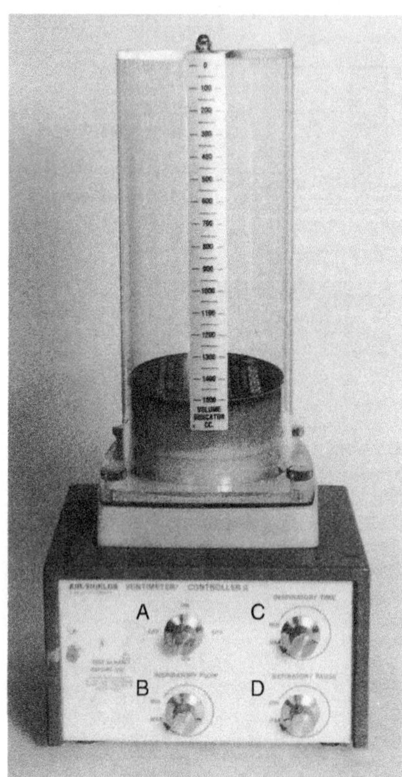

FIGURE 6-13 ■ The Air-Shields Ventimeter Controller II. Shown are the on/off switch (*A*), the inspiratory flow control (*B*), the inspiratory time control (*C*), and expiratory pause control (*D*).

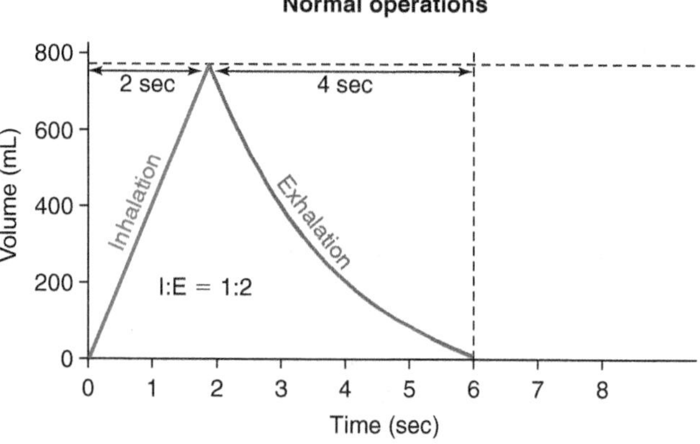

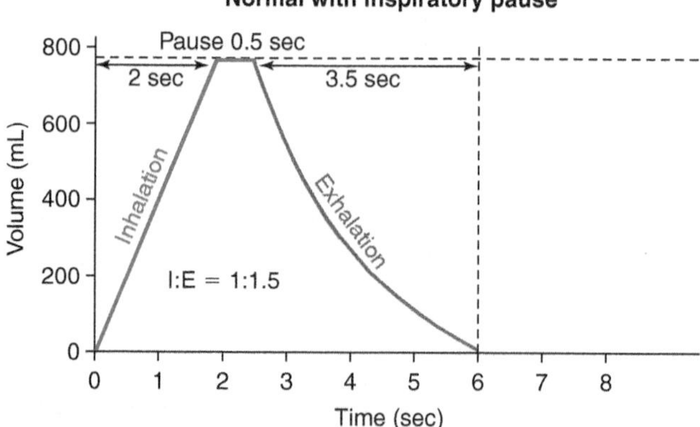

FIGURE 6-14 ■ The effect of the inspiratory pause on the I:E ratio. (From *Explore the anesthesia system.* 1996, Ohmeda [now GE Healthcare, Waukesha, WI], pp 6-18.)

Lung function can be improved by the use of a tracheal tube. Tracheal intubation can protect the airway from oral and gastric secretions, especially if a cuffed endotracheal tube is used, and it can establish a patent conduit for ventilation to occur. The latter occurs when upper airway obstruction is present. Mechanical ventilation can reduce the work of breathing and allow fatigued respiratory muscles a chance to recover. Mechanical ventilation allows consistent and predictable ventilation patterns, which removes the need for an anesthesiologist to ventilate manually for long periods. This also makes it possible to change ventilation strategies in response to changes in the surgical process, patient condition, and indicators of oxygenation and ventilation, such as capnography, oximetry, blood gases, and mechanical parameters that include airway pressure and resistance and lung compliance. In specific circumstances, appropriate modes of ventilation can improve the function of an abnormal lung during anesthesia. Finally, the delivery of medicines such as potent inhalational agents, helium, and other aerosolized substances through the tracheal

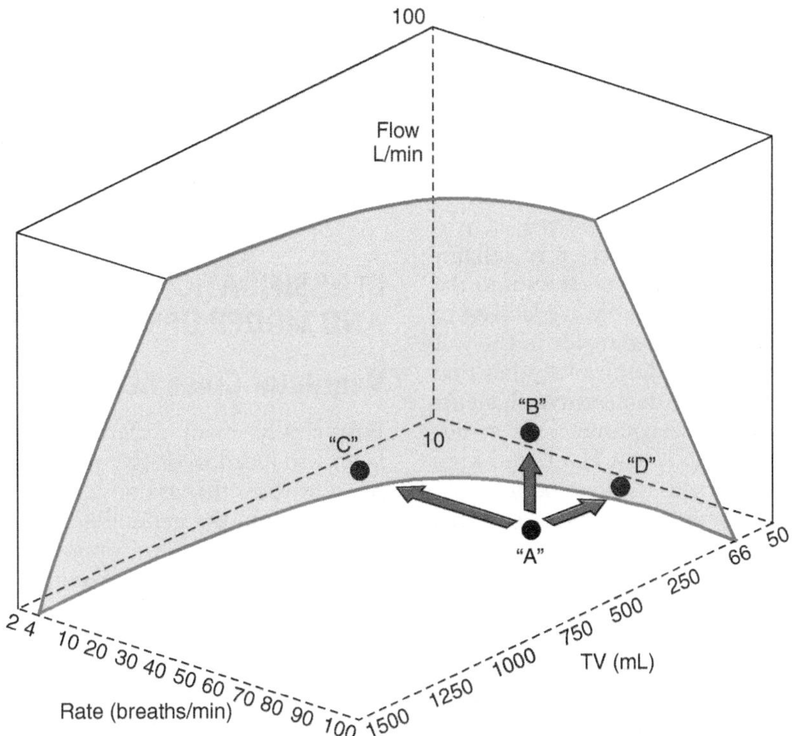

FIGURE 6-15 The limitations of the Datex-Ohmeda 7800 ventilator, illustrating the relationships among flow, frequency, and tidal volume. Only combinations of settings behind the shaded area are possible. In situation *A*, the message "VENT SET ERROR" appears and may be corrected by decreasing the rate *C*, increasing the flow *B*, or decreasing the tidal volume to *D*. (Courtesy GE Healthcare, Waukesha, WI.)

tube with the aid of mechanical ventilation can relieve bronchospasm.

Lung Protection Strategies

Institution of IPPV is associated with the ever-present risk of traumatic lung injury. *Barotrauma*, or injury related to pressure, can be grossly manifested as a pneumothorax or more subtly as physiologic and pathologic changes related to alveolar overstretching. *Volutrauma*, injury related to volume, also can cause alveolar overstretching. Damage related to shear stress from the opening and closing of the alveoli, called *atelectrauma* or *shear trauma*, can be caused by both pressure- and volume-related changes. Airway irritation that causes patient/ventilator dissynchrony—coughing, bucking, and straining—can result in sharp changes in airway pressure, which can cause lung injury. Usage of PEEP can lessen the injury from shear trauma but also can result in increases in physiologic dead space and reduced cardiac output.

Disease states that affect the uniformity of the lung can increase the risk of lung injury. This happens when small segments of the lung have reductions in compliance compared with their normal counterparts. Previous assumptions about the relatively predictable distribution of the volume, pressure, and perfusion to the lung segments may no longer hold true; nondiseased segments receive a greater share of the tidal volume and effects of the inspiratory pressure and PEEP. As a result, these "good" lung segments can be injured, and physiologic changes related to V/Q mismatch maybe exaggerated. This can be seen in patients with congestive heart failure, pneumonia, and acute respiratory distress syndrome (ARDS).

Large tidal volumes (15 to 20 mL/kg) also have been used during anesthesia to maintain alveolar distension. Although this strategy effectively prevents atelectasis and reduces shunt fraction, it is now recognized as a potential cause of barotrauma. Overdistension of healthy alveoli can cause disruptions of the alveolar-capillary membrane and lead to pulmonary interstitial emphysema and pneumothorax. As already stated, the presence of diffuse lung disease may compound injury to remaining healthy alveoli. Tidal volumes of 6 to 8 mL/kg are now recommended, with the addition of PEEP.[17,18]

Complementing the recommendation of normal tidal volumes, safe peak inflation pressures now dominate ventilation strategies. Studies show that maximal alveolar pressures only slightly greater than 30 to 40 cm H_2O may be associated with lung injury.[17] Recent designs of anesthesia ventilators have all incorporated peak airway pressure limiters.

Optimal PEEP recruits collapsed alveoli and maximizes functional residual capacity (FRC). However, increases in PEEP beyond this point may overdistend patent alveoli without further recruitment of others. New strategies analyze static pressure–volume plots to determine optimal PEEP and safe peak inspiratory pressures. Optimal PEEP is usually 5 to 15 cm H_2O.[17]

For the past 10 years, clinicians have been reducing tidal volumes even further for patients with acute lung injury (ALI) or ARDS. A landmark paper from the ARDS Network showed a reduction in mortality rate in a group with lower tidal volumes (6 mL/kg) compared with those in a control group (12 mL/kg).[22] Ventilator settings that result in injury are attributed to diffuse alveolar damage that causes pulmonary edema, activation of inflammatory cells, local production of inflammatory mediators, and leaks of these mediators into the systemic circulation.[23] Prospective studies are lacking to examine the use of lung protective strategies in the OR for non-ALI patients. The few randomized studies that have been done do not confidently demonstrate benefits in the OR, and some authors still recommend the avoidance of high plateau pressures (>20 cm H_2O) and high tidal volumes (>10 mL/kg) in this patient population. The objective of this strategy is to minimize regional end-inspiratory stretch and thereby reduce alveolar injury and inflammation.[23]

Caution with tidal volumes and peak airway pressures is associated with an increased incidence of hypercapnia. Permissive hypercapnia promises to reduce ventilatory complications without adverse effects.[19] Humans seem to tolerate respiratory acidosis well, with an arterial pH of 7.15 and a $PaCO_2$ of 80 mm Hg. This strategy may be contraindicated in patients with increased intracranial pressure, recent myocardial infarction, pulmonary hypertension, or gastrointestinal bleeding.[19] This is because acute increases in $PaCO_2$ increase sympathetic activity, cardiac output, pulmonary vascular resistance, and cerebral blood flow and also may impair central nervous system (CNS) function.[19]

Inverse ratio ventilation (IRV) originated in the early 1970s as a method to improve oxygenation in neonates with hyaline membrane disease[20] and was later extended to adults with ARDS. Although ratios were as high as 4:1, the benefits of this mode depend more on an absolute prolongation of inspiratory time in combination with a decreased peak inspiratory pressure. Typical I:E ratios of 1:2 to 1:4 have been lengthened to 1:1 or greater. The objective is to increase mean airway pressure and minimize peak pressure; the desired outcome is recruitment of collapsed alveoli without overdistension. Mean airway pressure directly corresponds with alveolar recruitment, reduction in shunt fraction, and oxygenation. Clinical evidence supports the contention that shunt fraction is reduced and oxygenation is improved, although modestly.[17] Because pressure control is the desired outcome, this mode of ventilation is more commonly applied with pressure generators. Caution is advised when using IRV because this strategy may not allow adequate alveolar emptying, thus causing "breath stacking" and auto-PEEP. In addition, IRV is contraindicated in obstructive lung disease, such as asthma. It also may cause hypotension from a reduction in venous return since there is a higher inspiratory pressure for a longer portion of the respiratory cycle.

High-frequency ventilation (HFV), defined below, may be an applicable strategy during anesthesia, although some anesthesia ventilators are capable of rates only to 100 breaths/min. The conceptual advantage of HFV is a lower peak airway pressure combined with nonbulk flow of gas to provide a motionless surgical field. This technique has not proven clinically advantageous in patients with respiratory failure, but it is helpful in patients with large pulmonary air leaks. In addition, pulmonary complications in neonates may be reduced with this strategy.[21]

CLASSIFICATION, SPECIAL FEATURES, AND MODES OF VENTILATION

Ventilator Classification

Historically, many different anesthesia ventilators have been produced over the years. Many of them incorporated features that are no longer considered valuable, but these serve in the general description and understanding of ventilator function. Commonly, such things as ventilator mechanisms, cycling parameters, and special clinical features were used to classify anesthesia ventilators.

Power Source

Most ventilators today function in an environment where electricity and compressed gases are readily available. In the past, however, some ventilators were designed to function solely on pneumatic gases. Currently, the only ventilators that function solely on pneumatic gases are not anesthesia delivery systems; these pneumatically powered ventilators are used in patient transport and in magnetic resonance imaging suites. Ventilators that use the bag-in-a-bottle design commonly have a double circuit in which a high-pressure driving gas, electrical circuits, and solenoids are used to achieve ventilator function. Some newer ventilators use electricity exclusively to drive the ventilator, which spares gas use for the patient.

Drive Mechanism

Classification of ventilators has been reduced to those that push or drive the patient gas to the patient, which is done by either a *bellows* or a *piston.*

Bellowed Ventilators. Bellowed ventilators have used two main varieties of bellows designs over the years: the ascending, or standing, bellows and the descending, or hanging, bellows. The designation of ascending or descending was based on bellows movement on exhalation; an *ascending bellows* moves up during exhalation (Fig. 6-16), and a *descending bellows* moves down (Fig. 6-17).

In the event of a circuit disconnect or significant leak, an ascending bellows would not fill or would improperly fill during exhalation. This provides clinicians a visible monitor of ventilator function. Because of the improved patient safety, this type of bellows generally is preferred, but does not represent a standard according to the latest document by the American Society for Testing and Materials (ASTM F1109-90).[24] The ECRI Institute has published a commentary and recommendations for hanging bellows in its Health Devices Alerts (1996-A40).

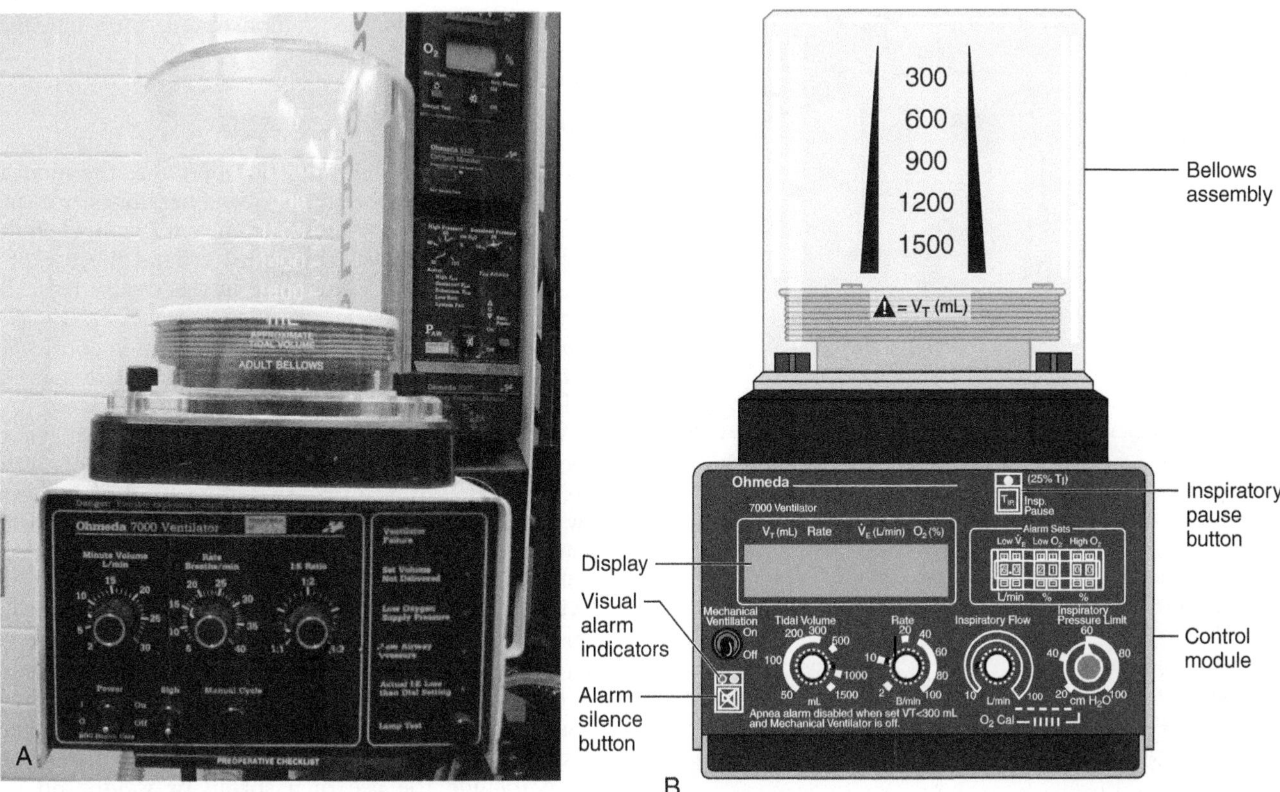

FIGURE 6-16 ■ Bag-in-a-bottle bellows design, ascending bellows variety. Ohmeda 7000 ventilator (*left*); illustration of Ohmeda 7800 ventilator (*right*) (GE Healthcare, Waukesha, WI). The bellows is contained within a clear housing, and a drive gas pushes the gas inside the bellows through the circuit. The bellows displayed in the images are deflated.

The hanging bellows, which typically is weighted, could fill whether a circuit disconnect, leak, or normal exhalation was present. Room air could enter the circuit and allow the bellows the ability to return to its filled position. In association with fresh gas decoupling, hanging bellows ventilators rely on a separate reservoir bag to detect leaks and inadequate fresh gas flow (FGF).

Bellows designs are not without inherent problems. Because a high-pressure gas typically is used to drive the bellows, a hole or perforation in the bellows can subject the patient to driving gas pressures and result in barotrauma. In addition, mixing of the patient circuit gas with the driving circuit gas may cause unpredictable concentrations in oxygen. Typically, 100% oxygen is used as the driving circuit gas. When high oxygen concentrations are undesirable or the potential for an airway fire exists, leaks into the patient circuit gas may cause disastrous consequences. When air is used as the driving circuit gas, unexpectedly low concentrations of oxygen may be observed. In both circumstances, patient awareness may occur because the driving gas may dilute the intended gas concentrations of inhaled anesthetics to be delivered to the patient. In addition, hypoventilation may occur if the bellows is not properly seated inside the bellows assembly.

Piston Ventilators. Piston ventilators rely on a piston-cylinder configuration, in which an electric motor is used to drive or displace the piston within the cylinder to cause gas flow. Tidal volume accuracy is believed to improve because the precise position of the piston during inspiration is monitored from start to finish; the motor returns the piston to the filled position prior to the next delivered breath. The drive motor requires maintenance and usage monitoring for good function because ventilator failure has been reported from worn motor parts. A leak occurring at the piston diaphragm could cause a loss of circuit gases to the room with hypoventilation during inspiration. Entrainment of room air into the patient circuit could occur as the piston returns to the filled position. Some recent designs have placed the piston ventilator within the workstation housing to make visible operation impossible. Piston-driven bellows currently manufactured by Dräger Medical (Telford, PA) have placed the piston in both vertical and horizontal positions in different models. Such systems use fresh gas decoupling with a separate reservoir bag, which is monitored for circuit leaks or inadequate FGF.

Cycling Behavior

Cycling behavior is believed to be one of the most complicated concepts in ventilator classification and description. In a normal ventilator breath, two significant events occur: *inspiration* and *exhalation*. However, cycling behavior describes the event that transitions the ventilator from exhalation to inspiration and from inspiration to exhalation. In sequence, the ventilator cycles from exhalation to inspiration, inspiration occurs, the ventilator cycles from inspiration to exhalation, and exhalation occurs. For most modern anesthesia ventilators, respiratory rate and I:E ratio are set in controlled modes, either

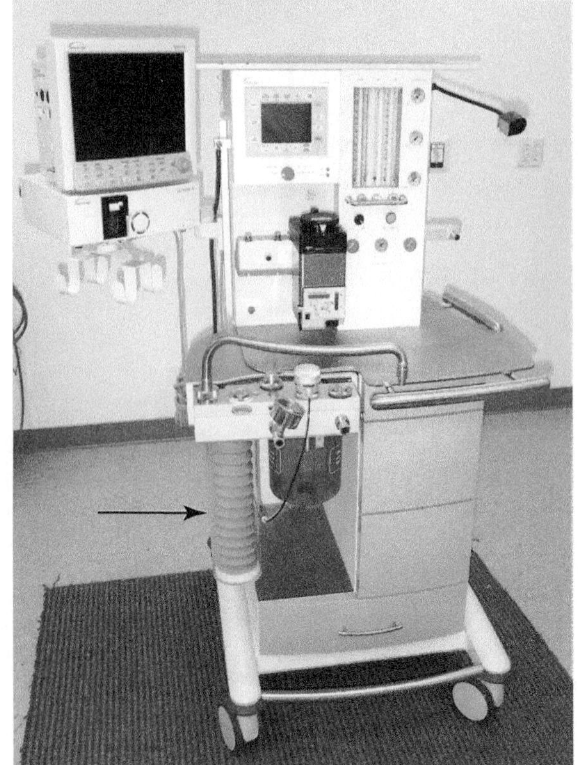

FIGURE 6-17 ■ Bag-in-a-bottle bellows design, descending bellows variety. Shown is the Datascope Patient Monitoring Anestar anesthesia machine (Mindray North America, Mahwah, NJ) with descending bellows. The bellows *(arrow)* are in the inflated position.

by *volume control ventilation* (VCV) or *pressure control ventilation* (PCV); time cycles the breath from exhalation to inspiration and from inspiration to exhalation. A trigger can be used to initiate inspiration on spontaneous patient effort in *pressure support ventilation* (PSV). The trigger, an observed parameter to allow inspiration to occur, can use pressure, volume, or flow values. As will be seen, the method of delivering the inspired breath also can be manipulated. Cycling from inspiration to exhalation can occur as a result of achieving a set volume, pressure, flow, or time.

Exhalation typically is a passive event. Pressures in the airway can be manipulated during exhalation by the addition of PEEP. More recent developments in ventilator cycling allow the cycling from exhalation to inspiration to include uses of airway pressure, volume, and flows in the ICU. However, most anesthesia ventilators still use time as the determinant to cycle from exhalation to inspiration.

Many machines can function in at least two modes; the most common example is the ventilator that normally cycles when a given time or tidal volume is reached. In the Datex-Ohmeda 7800 series, reducing the pressure limit makes the ventilator cycle when a given pressure is reached. By contrast, in the Dräger AV-2+, the inspiratory phase is not ended; the bellows is held in its compressed state by the continuing flow of drive gas, which escapes to the atmosphere through the pressure-limiting valve. These mechanisms afford a poor basis for classification because, as demonstrated, they may not indicate functional behavior.

Inspiratory Flow

The inspiratory flow classification describes the method used to make a breath: either a flow generator or pressure generator. A *flow generator* is used in ventilation when the inspiratory waveform is controlled around the use of a high-pressure source; the source in this case is typically greater than five times the airway pressure. A *pressure generator* is used when the pressure waveform is controlled around the use of a low-pressure source, usually near or moderately higher than the airway pressure.

When a high-pressure source is used, changes in patient compliance and resistance have little effect on the inspiratory flow waveform. As such, a fixed or constant flow can be established to generate a reliable tidal volume breath for a given inspiratory time. This type of ventilator is called a *constant flow generator*.

With a low-pressure source, changes in patient compliance and resistance affect the inspiratory waveform. As a result, the pressure waveform is controlled because it is not affected by patient changes and the use of a low-pressure source. Mechanisms used to achieve this behavior of constant airway pressure during the inspiratory period include the use of a spring or weight on the bellows. This is what is known as a *constant-pressure generator*. On inspiration, a large pressure gradient exists from the ventilator to the alveoli that results in high initial gas flows. Rising gas volumes in the lung slowly equilibrate pressures between the ventilator and lung to cause a diminishing inspiratory flow; the delivered tidal volume is the result of the variable flow related to the equilibrating pressures between the ventilator and lung and the time allotted for inspiration to occur.

Some flow generators can vary the inspiratory flow to provide different flow waveforms; that is, increasing flow (ascending ramp), decreasing flow (descending ramp), or sinusoidal flow may be selected. This type of ventilator is called a *variable-flow generator*. Modern flow generators can provide pressure generator behavior by using negative feedback to vary the orifice of the inspiratory flow control valve during inspiration.

Classification by inspiratory flow should not be confused with the volume- or pressure-control modes of ventilation. Modern ventilators can now switch between flow and pressure generator methods. In addition, both flow and pressure generators can achieve the same modes of ventilation by advances in sensor application and electronic feedback control.

Control of the Pressure and Flow Waveform During Ventilation

The pattern of ventilation occasionally used has a critical influence on lung function. The most common example in the OR is the hypotension that accompanies hyperventilation. In critical care, greater attention is given to optimizing lung function by appropriate selection of the inspiratory waveform. For example, several advantages have been proposed for using a decelerating waveform:

the maximum pressure is minimized, the risk of barotrauma is diminished, alveoli are kept expanded, V/Q ratios are more uniform, and distribution of gas within the lung is facilitated.

Controlled ventilation also tends to affect venous return and cardiac output. To a large extent, the best strategy to optimize cardiac output is the reverse of that which promotes improved lung function. A relatively short inspiratory period, with no time for distribution and no plateau, will have the least effect on the mean intrathoracic pressure and therefore on venous return.

Debate about the potential benefits of variation in the inspiratory waveform has persisted for at least 35 years. The expense and complexity required to achieve such waveforms have been critically discussed since the early 1960s. In the OR, fine control of the inspiratory waveform usually is not provided or needed. To this day, many anesthesia ventilators offer no control of the inspiratory waveform, and the anesthesiologist must occasionally approximate a desired pattern with the equipment available.

Constant Inspiratory Flow

Most anesthesia ventilators are powered by a high-pressure gas source. For practical purposes, flow is not affected by the patient, and it remains constant during the inspiratory period (see Fig. 6-4).

Declining Inspiratory Flow

Declining inspiratory flow allows time for gas redistribution at the end of inspiration. An anesthesia ventilator can be set to approximate this pattern by continuing the normal inspiratory flow rate until the lung is filled and then maintaining a plateau for distribution; this minimizes the time required to fill the lung and maximizes the time for redistribution. Many anesthesia ventilators have this option. It is very rare for a patient to be so dependent on a critical pattern of decelerating inspiratory flow that this approximation does not suffice (see Fig. 6-5).

Accelerating Inspiratory Flow

An accelerating inspiratory flow pattern is intended to achieve ventilation while minimizing the effect on intrathoracic pressure. In a patient in whom this is beneficial, the anesthesia ventilator can approximate this pattern by prolongation of the period for exhalation, followed by a rapid inspiration with no plateau. The prolongation of the expiratory period maximizes the time for venous return. The time devoted to filling the lungs, which adversely affects venous return, is reduced to the minimum. No data supporting the use of accelerating inspiratory flow are available.[18]

Sinusoidal Inspiratory Flow

Once promoted as mimicking normal ventilation, the sinusoidal inspiratory flow pattern was provided by the Engström and Emerson piston ventilators. Some thoracic surgeons preferred this pattern because it provided a smoother transition from inspiration to exhalation and vice versa. Ventilators that offer this pattern of inspiratory flow are no longer in general use.

Improvement in Control

Closed-loop negative feedback can be used to improve performance in a controlled category, such as flow or volume. Some newer machines measure either the machine's delivered flow or the delivered tidal volume; these measures allow more accurate control of the ventilator to improve its performance. Unfortunately, better control of the volume or flow at the ventilator still tends to be offset by the compliance and resistance of the circuit itself because the measurements of flow and volume are not routinely made at the tracheal tube. The most modern technique to date uses automatic self-measurement of the ventilator and breathing circuit compliance; this enables accurate calculation and delivery of flow and tidal volume, as seen in newer GE Healthcare and Dräger workstations. Other preexisting technologies, such as spirometry, use sensors placed at the endotracheal tube that enable accurate measurement of delivered and exhaled volumes, pressure, compliance, and resistance. However, such technologies are not always set up to influence the ventilator automatically.

In units with closed feedback loops, microprocessors attempt to maintain the designated variable constant by processing data hundreds of times per second and by regulating the flow control valve with equal frequency. Feedback may be helpful in the midst of changing clinical conditions such as bronchospasm, secretions, or even a leak in the system. Open-loop systems cannot compensate for these external loads and eventually fail to deliver the prescribed parameter, which requires vigilance and adjustments by the anesthesiologist.

Special Ventilator Features

Many other valuable features may be available on a given ventilator. These features are less suitable as tools to classify ventilators, even though they may be critically important when managing a particular patient.

Inspiratory Manipulation

Inspiratory Plateau or Inspiratory Hold. A tidal volume maintained after the inspiratory flow ceases, a so-called *plateau* or *inspiratory hold*, provides an opportunity for gas to redistribute within the lung. This maintained pressure may also improve gas exchange by keeping alveoli expanded for a longer period, thus reducing shunt fraction. In addition, the pause facilitates the measurement of static lung compliance. The potential penalty of a plateau, particularly in a hypovolemic patient, is that the increased intrathoracic pressure may impede venous return and decrease cardiac output. Inspiratory hold also affects the I:E ratio (see Fig. 6-14).

Inverse Ratio Ventilation. Modern anesthesia ventilators have recently offered IRV as a means of increasing mean airway pressure without increasing peak airway pressure.[25,26] *Inverse ratio ventilation* is defined as an I:E ratio greater than 1:1. It has physiologic effects similar to the inspiratory pause described above. The ratio may be inverted in ventilators that use both flow generator (FG) or pressure generator (PG) modes. When FG-IRV is used, the I:E ratio can be inverted only by decreasing the mean inspiratory flow or by adding an end-inspiratory pause. For the same minute ventilation and I:E ratio, the inspiratory pause provides a greater mean airway pressure than does the lower flow rate of the first option.[25-27] When using IRV, caution is advised to prevent breath stacking and auto-PEEP. This can occur if there is inadequate time for exhalation; using IRV with a PG merely prolongs the inspiratory time.

Expiratory Manipulation

Positive End-Expiratory Pressure. Most anesthesia ventilators now routinely provide PEEP. At the end of each breath, the pressure is commonly maintained at an end-expiratory pressure of 2 to 4 cm H_2O above zero because of the weight of valves and bellows, although some anesthesia ventilators provide a direct control to set additional PEEP. When lung function is less than optimal, PEEP may be added to improve oxygenation by alveolar recruitment. This is a more logical response to desaturation than merely increasing the inspired oxygen concentration because it is better to improve the function of the lung than to conceal the evidence of dysfunction. Because PEEP can affect the venous return to the heart, careful monitoring of the hemodynamics is advised.

Expiratory Retard. The introduction of a constrictive orifice during exhalation can benefit some patients with advanced lung disease. This is due to the fact that expiratory retard will decrease the expiratory flow rate and allow more laminar flow and better emptying of the lung. This modality can be useful in patients with severe bronchoconstriction, such as those with status asthmaticus. It is similar to the pursed-lipped breathing seen in asthmatics; air trapping is minimized, and exhalation may, paradoxically, be improved. This modality is rarely incorporated in anesthesia ventilators today because it carries the risk of incomplete exhalation (breath stacking) if the frequency is suddenly increased, which would cause a potentially dangerous high pressure. The clinician must always be sure that the end-expiratory pressure is zero.

Interactions with the Breathing System

Fresh Gas Flow. In combination with oxygen, anesthetic gas typically flows continuously from the common gas outlet of the anesthesia machine into the breathing circuit. In some ventilators, FGF is directly delivered into the ventilator bellows, which is preloaded under a certain degree of spring tension, called the *working pressure*. These ventilators (e.g., Servo Ventilator 900C [Siemens-Elema AB, Solna, Sweden]) store fresh gas for every cycle, mandating an FGF at least equal to the minute volume. FGF commonly contributes to actual delivered tidal volume if it continues to flow into the breathing circuit during the inspiratory phase. This contribution is measured by:

$$V_{FGF} = (FGF \times T_I) / 60$$

where V_{FGF} is the volume of FGF. For example, at an FGF of 3 L/min and a T_I of 2 seconds, the FGF contribution to tidal volume is calculated as follows:

$$(3000 \times 2)/60 = 100 \text{ mL}$$

New designs of ventilators offer fresh gas uncoupling by electronically interrupting or diverting the FGF during the inspiratory phase. Others compensate for the FGF by first measuring total delivered flow and then adjusting the next breath through servo mechanisms.

Scavenging Systems. Modern dual-circuit ventilators have an integral ventilator pressure relief valve at or inside the bellows that is sealed during inspiration and at the beginning of exhalation, until the ascending bellows has been refilled. This ventilator pressure relief valve provides a minimum mandatory level of PEEP, usually 2 to 3 cm H_2O, and then releases anesthetic gas into the scavenging system once the bellows is full. Typically, this waste gas travels directly to the scavenging system, although newer technologies, such as those designed into the Datex-Ohmeda 7900, incorporate this gas flow into a PEEP-generating mechanism, discussed below. Similarly, ventilator drive gas is commonly vented to the atmosphere, although it may be routed to the scavenger. The Datex-Ohmeda workstations (Avance, Aespire, and Aisys) have an adjustable needle valve in the scavenging system. Improper adjustment of this valve can result in 10 cm H_2O of PEEP being applied to the patient circuit. Unintentional PEEP could result in improved lung function, but also cause hypotension or barotrauma.

CAPABILITIES AND LIMITATIONS OF ANESTHESIA VENTILATORS

Anesthesia Versus Critical Care Ventilators

Historically, the anesthesiologist was limited in the type of ventilation that could be delivered to a patient. A number of reasons allowed for this limitation: 1) most surgical patients did not have pulmonary disease, 2) widespread use of muscle relaxants enabled complete control of ventilation without patient interaction, 3) the anesthesiologist was immediately available to makes changes in the ventilator settings and/or provide manually assisted ventilation, 4) use was intended for short duration, and 5) recirculation of patient gas was desirable. All these factors focused ventilator design to function only in the control mode.

In contrast, critical care ventilators became far more complex because they were used in different conditions. A trend is now apparent: anesthesia ventilators are are being manufactured to mimic the performance of their critical care counterparts while maintaining the simplicity of complete control. However, critical care ventilators offer ever-increasing complexities of flow and pressure waveforms that may not be needed, desirable, or available in anesthesia ventilators.

Ventilator Performance

Perhaps the most distinguishing characteristic of any ventilator is its performance under extremes of load—in effect, under conditions of very poor compliance. Information regarding performance of individual ventilators may not be readily available in the manufacturer's literature and is scarcely available in the scientific literature.[28,29] The American National Standards Institute (ANSI) specifies set values for compliance, resistance, and flow within a test lung as the conditions under which breathing machines for patient use should be tested to determine their performance capabilities.[30] Although the operator's manual may specify certain maximum capabilities, these numbers should be regarded as ideal figures under conditions *without* load. Some manufacturers specify the conditions under which their ventilator is tested, thus giving a basis for reported accuracy data.[31] One study clearly demonstrates the limitations of anesthesia ventilators when subjected to increasing airway pressures.[28] Minute ventilation decreased linearly for some ventilators as airway pressure increased; however, the Siemens 900D maintained its minute volume when the airway pressure was below 60 cm H_2O. This might be attributed to the design of a nonrebreathing system without compression loss in the absorber.

System Compliance and Compression of Gas

As previously stated, gas compression and compliance volume losses caused by expanding hoses explain why delivered tidal volumes are frequently less than desired. Loss of tidal volume is greatest and most variable in machines that have an external ventilator connected to a circuit that includes a soda lime absorber and a humidifier. This is because the compressible volume is large, there is a greater total length of compliant breathing hose, and the change in pressure during each breath affects the gas in the entire circuit, including the bellows. The total volume of the gas that may be compressed in the circuit often exceeds 6 L. The amount lost due solely to gas compression may then be calculated; for every 10 cm H_2O pressure, approximately 1% of the compressible volume is lost from the circuit. Boyle's law ($P_1V_1 = P_2V_2$) explains this phenomenon. Boyle's law can be applied such that the resultant volume (V_2) is calculated by knowing the original volume (V_1) and pressure (P_1) and the secondary pressure (P_2). For example, if compression of V_1 (6000 mL) increases the pressure 10 cm H_2O (1%) above atmospheric pressure (P_1 = 1000 cm H_2O and P_2 = 1010 cm H_2O), the resultant volume (V_2) will be 5941 mL, or approximately 1% less. This would equal a loss of 120 mL at 20 cm H_2O for a 6 L system. Next, the amount lost due to expansion of the system must be calculated by using compliance specifications from the manufacturers of the ventilator and the breathing hose. These losses typically are overcome by default of FGF, which at 3 L/min would add 100 mL to the circuit during a 2-second period of inspiration.

As the complexity of ventilators has increased, their ability to deliver the intended volume has improved. New designs with fresh gas decoupling do not contribute any fresh gas to the delivered inspiratory volume; they have low-volume, noncompliant metallic manifolds, they calculate and sequentially compensate for circuit and patient compliance and gas compression losses, and they may subtract the breathing hose volume compensation from the measured exhaled volume to report an actual exhaled volume.

Atmospheric Pressure Variations

At least one anesthesia ventilator (Siemens Servo 900B) has been tested under hyperbaric conditions (1 to 3 atm), which cause increases in gas density, resistance to flow, and dead space ventilation.[32,33] Minute ventilation was found to decrease linearly as atmospheric pressure increased, but the ventilator functioned well as long as compensation was made to restore the minute ventilation.[34] Different ventilators have variable outputs in flight because of lower barometric pressures, but they may be used under these conditions during military emergencies. Their performance is determined by the type of control circuit, fluidic or electronic, and the method of powering the ventilator because gas density decreases at increased altitude. Differences in the mass versus volume of gas used to control these units are responsible for the alterations in function.[35] In general, effective ventilation at abnormal ambient pressure depends on providing the patient's usual minute volume. Carbon dioxide continues to be eliminated at the usual partial pressure but is accompanied by either a smaller or greater mass of other gases.

Mode Conversion

With the appearance of pressure generator capabilities within the OR, the opportunities for conversion from flow to pressure generator systems will increase. The clinician should first record the tidal volume and frequency; peak, mean and plateau airway pressures; PEEP; and I:E ratios while in flow mode. The emphasis of the conversion is on the maintenance of plateau pressure because inspiratory, peak, and plateau pressures are merged into the square-wave airway pressure profile. Whether desired and set inspiratory pressure is absolute or whether it is a set pressure above PEEP should be noted. Leaving PEEP and frequency the same, the inspiratory time—and therefore the I:E ratio—should now be set to equal the total inspiratory time from the flow generator mode, accounting for inspiratory pause. Next, a change in modes must be initiated and the new parameters are measured; mean airway pressure should be slightly higher, considering the new airway pressure profile. Minor increases in set inspiratory pressure usually are necessary to match tidal volume.[27] For convenience, some modern ventilator designs are able to apply an algorithm automatically on conversion from a volume to pressure mode, or vice versa.

MODES OF VENTILATION

Recently, advances in ventilator technologies have included improved microcircuit designs and applications, pressure and flow sensor enhancements, and better material design and use features that have improved the performance regardless of classification. Precision, accuracy, and reliability lie in the delivery of volume and pressure over great lengths of time and under a variety of clinical conditions. Adjunct technologies in waveform display and monitoring allow the rapid adjustment of ventilator parameters to meet dynamic intraoperative objectives.

In addition, alarms have been designed around these improved sensors and monitors, which in turn allow the delivery of safer mechanical ventilation regardless of the mode of ventilation. As such, the actual *mode* (method) of ventilation may be less important when endpoints of oxygenation (saturation of arterial oxygen [SaO_2], pressure of arterial oxygen [PaO_2]), ventilation (end-tidal carbon dioxide [$ETCO_2$], pressure of arterial carbon dioxide [$PaCO_2$]), tidal/minute volume, or airway pressure are managed. This may be supported by the lack of scientific literature regarding the benefits of specific modes of ventilation in the OR, except in pathophysiologic outliers.

Ventilator modes can be divided into three basic categories: 1) controlled breathing modes, 2) assisted or supported modes, and 3) spontaneous breathing without assistance or support. Division into these categories allows the user to define whether the ventilator is doing *all* of the work of breathing, *some* of the work of breathing, or *none* of the work of breathing, respectively. The vocabulary, however, is difficult and less than perfect—the result of historic developments, imprecise usage, and technologic advances. The use of dual modes of ventilation, especially in ventilator weaning, has added to conceptual difficulties.

Controlled Breathing Modes

In controlled breathing modes of ventilation, the patient cannot contribute any effort toward the work of breathing. Such situations commonly occur with nondepolarizing neuromuscular blocking agents, such as pancuronium. The variable to be *controlled*—fixed, targeted, or limited—defines the mode.

Volume-Control Ventilation

If *volume* is the fixed parameter, then the ventilation mode is volume-control ventilation (VCV). Modern ventilators in VCV mode require the parameters of tidal volume, respiratory rate, and I:E ratio to be set. The ventilator calculates the inspiratory time from the respiratory rate and I:E ratio, and a fixed flow for gas delivery is determined using the set tidal volume and calculated inspiratory time. Airway pressure rises linearly with time as the gas volume is pushed into the lung. The peak airway pressure is directly related to airway resistance and inversely related to lung compliance (Fig. 6-18). As such, worsening airway resistance (bronchospasm, secretions, mucus plugging) and lung compliance (fluid overload, abdominal distension) can place the patient at risk of barotrauma; therefore vigilance should be applied in the monitoring of peak airway pressure when using VCV.

Pressure-Control Ventilation

If *pressure* is the fixed parameter, the ventilation mode is pressure-control ventilation (PCV). In this mode, the peak airway pressure is controlled. The user must set the peak airway pressure, respiratory rate, and I:E ratio. As with VCV, the inspiratory time is calculated using the respiratory rate and I:E ratio; however, in this mode, the flow is varied to match the set peak airway pressure. This is accomplished by variable flow control. High flows are delivered at the start of inspiration, and the flow is rapidly diminished while maintaining the pressure constant. In

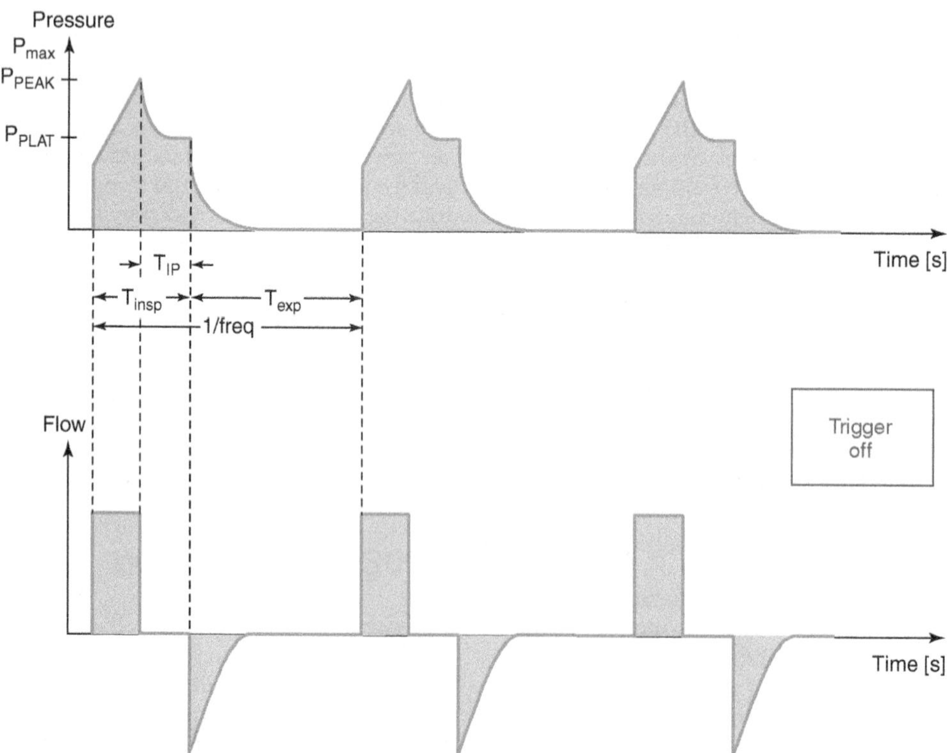

FIGURE 6-18 Graph of pressure and flow traces for volume control ventilation. Shown are time-pressure (*top*) and time-flow (*bottom*) representations. Flow is constant for inspiration. (Courtesy Dräger Medical, Telford, PA.)

addition, the flow tends to drop in an exponential decay over time. The tidal volume is directly proportional to lung compliance and inversely to airway resistance, so worsening airway resistance and lung compliance result in potentially inadequate oxygenation and ventilation (Fig. 6-19). An emphasis is placed on monitoring tidal volume and carbon dioxide when PCV is used because it is difficult to preset appropriate minimum and maximum volume alarms when initiating PCV.

Volume Guarantee Pressure-Control Ventilation

A recent advanced mode of PCV called *volume guarantee PCV*, or *VG-PCV*, seen in Datex-Ohmeda ventilators, allows the ventilator to change the inspiratory pressure dynamically based on the compliance of the respiratory system. In a steady-state system using PCV, a sudden improvement in pulmonary compliance would result in large tidal volumes and hyperventilation. An example of this can be seen during abdominal laparoscopic procedures, when the insufflation pressure is suddenly lost. Large tidal volumes and hyperventilation would occur until the insufflation pressure was reestablished or the anesthesiologist manually adjusted the ventilator. VG-PCV would allow the ventilator to adjust the inspiratory airway pressure dynamically over several breaths to maintain tidal volumes and ventilation parameters at a constant. Alterations in the pulmonary system that result in reduced compliance allow the ventilator to increase the set inspiratory pressure limit, which leads to an increase in the tidal volume and ventilation over several breaths; therefore the clinician must be vigilant in the adjustment of the peak pressure alarm.

Assisted and Supported Modes

In assisted and supported modes of ventilation, both the patient and the ventilator can contribute to the work of breathing. At times, the patient may be doing some or most of the work of breathing; at other times, the ventilator may contribute little to the work of breathing or the ventilator may be doing it all. These modes were developed as a solution for the pulmonary recovery of critically ill patients. As a group, these patients typically required long-standing intubation and mechanical ventilation. In the OR, these modes may allow augmentation of the patient's breathing effort while anesthetized. When native breathing can occur, the patient's effort is assisted, supported, or synchronized with mechanical breathing. Because the mechanical effort occurs while the patient is attempting to breathe, patient-ventilator dissynchrony is minimized, which in turn decreases coughing, bucking, and straining during surgery. The transition from effortless breathing to spontaneous breathing during an anesthetic emergency is commonly associated with risks of hypoxemia, hypercarbia, and dissynchrony. It is believed that these modes facilitate this transition by synchronizing with the patient's effort while maintaining minimum set minute ventilation.

Assist-Control Ventilation

Assist-control ventilation (ACV) is the improvement to assisted ventilation (AV). In AV, the patient's effort to breathe is manifested as a negative deflection in the airway pressure, and a predetermined negative pressure triggers the ventilator to deliver a set tidal volume. The

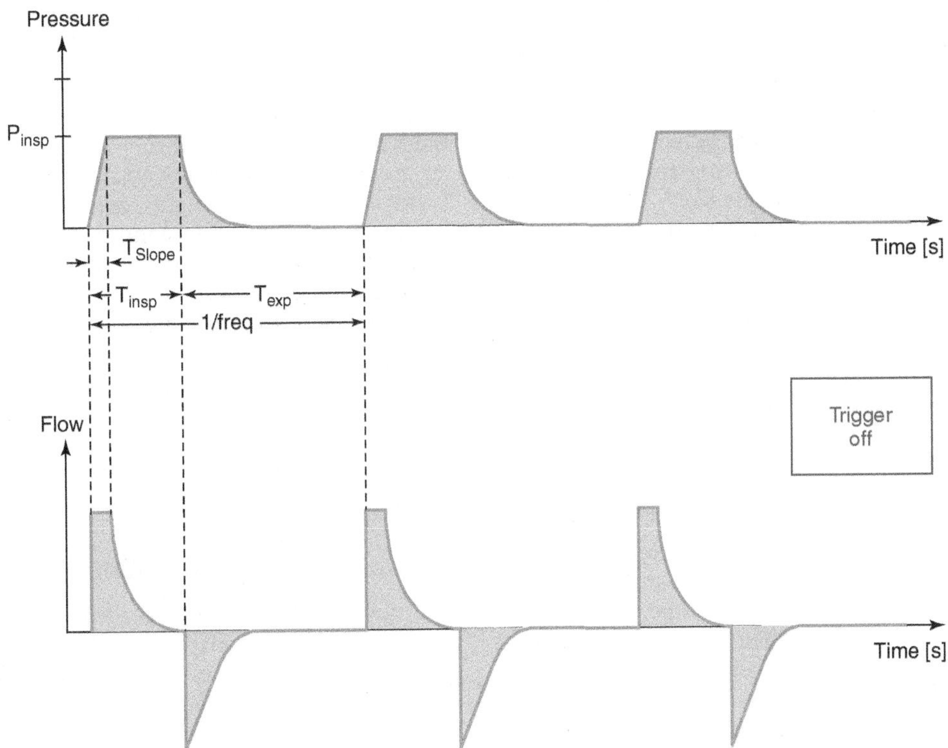

FIGURE 6-19 ▪ Graph of pressure and flow traces for pressure control ventilation. Time-pressure (*upper*) and time-flow (*lower*) representations are shown. The airway pressure rises rapidly to a set pressure limit, and the flow decays over inspiratory time. (Courtesy Dräger Medical, Telford, PA.)

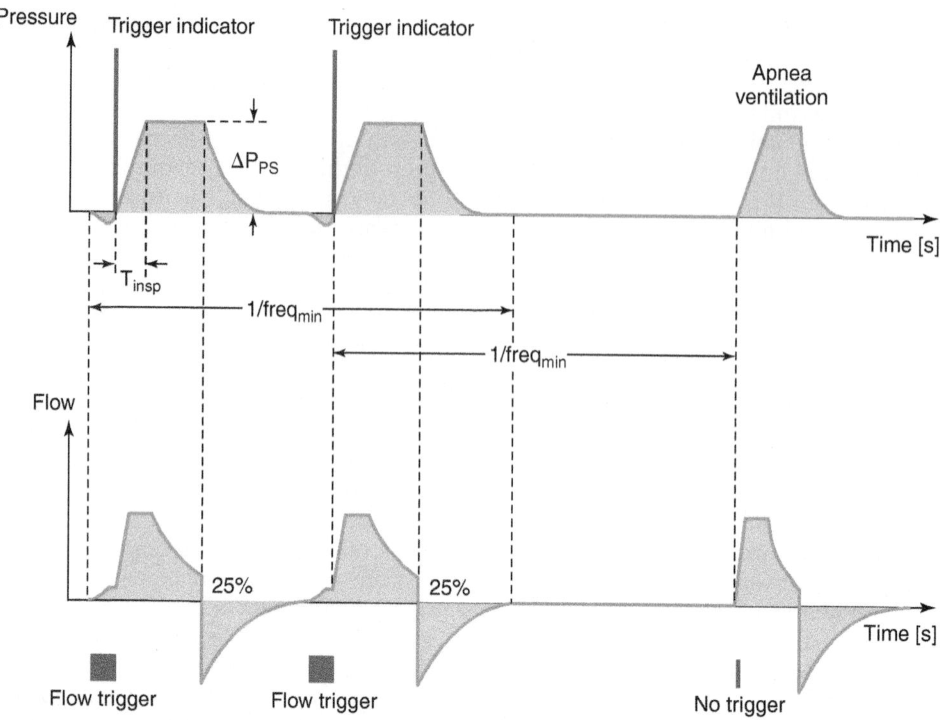

FIGURE 6-20 Graph of pressure and flow traces for pressure support ventilation. Shown are time-pressure (*upper*) and time-flow (*lower*) representations. Pressure or flow can be used to trigger the ventilator to cycle. The pressure trigger is indicated as a negative deflection in the pressure trace prior to inspiration; the flow trigger is indicated as inspiratory flow prior to main inspiratory pressure and flow changes. When no triggering has occurred, the ventilator will cycle without the triggering indices. (Courtesy Dräger Medical, Telford, PA.)

user can set the trigger for small or large efforts based on the magnitude of the negative deflection. Historically, hyperventilation occurred from overtriggering that caused apnea and hypoxemia. The improvement is ACV, in which the technician sets up the ventilator the same as in VCV and the patient is able to trigger the ventilator by respiratory effort. As long as the patient triggers the ventilator more than the interval defined by the set control rate, a control breath will not be delivered. If the patient has a pause or does not breathe, controlled breaths will be delivered to the patient without being triggered, which will make this mode perform exactly like VCV. The minute ventilation is the sum of the delivered control breaths and the patient's triggered breaths. The distinguishing feature between the two breaths (assisted vs. controlled) is the presence or lack of negative deflection in the airway pressure-time waveform, respectively.

Proportional Assisted Ventilation

Few OR ventilators use ACV, although it is not uncommon to place patients on this mode upon arrival to an ICU. For ICU patients going to the OR, VCV will substitute once the patient is anesthetized. Recently, ACV has further evolved into a new mode of ventilation called *proportional assisted ventilation* (PAV). The new feature, proportion, allows the tidal volume to correlate to respiratory effort, and more negative effort is rewarded with greater tidal volumes. In the past, pressure-triggering mechanisms were the only way to trigger the ventilator. Recently, these mechanisms have competed with flow-triggering mechanisms as the trigger of choice.

Pressure Support Ventilation

Pressure support ventilation (PSV) is the pressure equivalent of AV. In PSV mode, the clinician sets the inspiratory time, peak airway pressure to be delivered, and the trigger (Fig. 6-20). Some believe that this mode of ventilation addresses patient load issues related to compliance and resistance better than volume delivery techniques. As such, it could be considered more physiologic. Despite the lack of evidence for this claim, it has become a popular mode of ventilation in ventilator weaning in the ICU. Low-pressure PSV breaths are believed to match the resistance effects of the endotracheal tube. Use in this manner allows clinicians to equate resulting tidal volumes as the patient's own effort and ability to overcome respiratory load. In the OR, this mode has been successfully used in adults and children to support patient breathing efforts during general anesthesia with an endotracheal tube and laryngeal mask airway. An apnea alarm and backup mode are provided for PSV mode in the OR because dynamics of the surgery and anesthetic could unexpectedly alter respiratory effort.

Intermittent Mandatory Ventilation

In *intermittent mandatory ventilation* (IMV), the clinican sets mandatory ventilator breaths by either volume or pressure at a defined rate and inspiratory time. *Mandatory* means that the patient is guaranteed the set mechanical breaths. Between breaths, however, the patient is afforded the luxury of displaying native effort. The effort can be as simple as spontaneous breathing with or

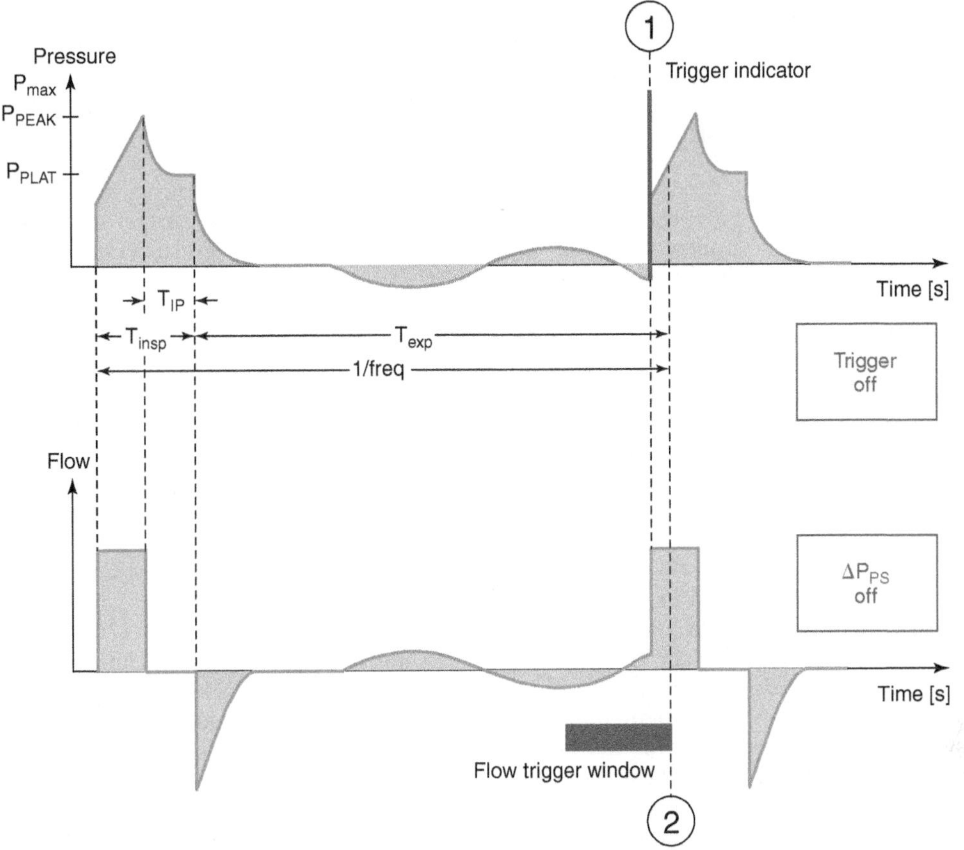

FIGURE 6-21 ■ Graph of pressure and flow traces for synchronized intermittent mandatory ventilation. Shown are time-pressure (*upper*) and time-flow (*lower*) representations. The observational window can use pressure or flow as a monitor of airway status. (Courtesy Dräger Medical, Telford PA.)

without airway pressure. Also, assisted or supported breaths can be delivered between the mandatory breaths. This mode was developed for ventilator weaning and mandates a defined minute ventilation but also affords the patient the ability to exercise respiratory muscles between mandated breaths. The problem with this mode of ventilation is the risk of the patient getting a mandatory breath while not having completed a spontaneous or assisted breath. Resulting breath stacking puts the patient at risk for barotrauma.

Synchronized Intermittent Mandatory Ventilation

To avoid breath stacking, a refined mode of IMV was created called *synchronized intermittent mandatory ventilation* (SIMV). As with IMV, a mandatory volume or pressure, breath rate, and inspiratory time are set by the technician, and respiratory intervals are calculated for the breaths, the rate of which is known. What makes SIMV different than IMV is the ability to give a mandatory breath at the beginning or the end of the interval. This is accomplished by placing a time observation window at the beginning of each respiratory interval. This time window allows the ventilator to monitor the status of the airway for pressure or flow changes from baseline. If the pressure or flow does not exceed the set limit parameters, the mandatory breath is delivered at the beginning of the respiratory interval. If the pressure or flow exceeds the set parameters, the mandatory breath is delivered at the end of the respiratory interval. The clinician sets the pressure or flow limits and the time increment for the observation window (Fig. 6-21).

This observation window is not a trigger as seen in ACV or PSV; it is a sensor or monitor. The rationale revolves around the volume of gas expected in the airway during the window period. Low pressure and flow changes from baseline within the window period are associated with small airway volumes, and high pressure and flow changes from baseline during the window period are associated with large volumes. The delivery of a mandatory breath at the beginning of the cycle is safe if there is no significant gas volume in the airway. Delivery of a mandatory breath when a large gas volume is already in the airway places the patient at significant risk for barotrauma. When airway volumes are predictably high, the ventilator delivers the mandatory breath at the end of the respiratory interval. Although there is still a chance that breath stacking will occur at the end of the interval, breath stacking rarely occurs in this mode.

When a patient is on SIMV mode, it is difficult to determine the ventilator mode simply by observation. Because breaths can occur at the beginning or end of a respiratory interval, consecutive mandatory breaths may appear at intervals of long, intermediate, or short duration. Consecutive breaths may be initiated in four configurations: 1) beginning and end (long interval), 2) beginning and beginning (intermediate interval), 3) end and end (intermediate interval), and 4) end and beginning (short interval). SIMV mode appears the same as VCV or PCV when the patient does not make a respiratory effort.

Spontaneous Breathing Without Assistance or Support

All anesthesia ventilators allow spontaneous ventilation without mechanical assistance or support. The use of a ventilator in this fashion allows continuous monitoring of respiratory parameters while the patient generates all the work of breathing. Pressure, volume, flow, and respiratory rate can be monitored for all phases of anesthetic management in which the patient spontaneously breathes. In steady state, only two possible conditions can occur to change respiratory parameters: the airway pressure can start and end at atmospheric pressure, the so-called *flow-by mode*, or positive pressure can be applied to the airway during breathing, the *continuous positive airway pressure* (CPAP) mode.

CPAP mode is more easily accepted in the ICU as a mode of breathing because it can be set on the ventilator. The CPAP number represents the airway pressure between exhalation and inhalation, when the gas flow within the airway is zero. When the patient inhales, a relative negative pressure is created within the airway compared with the set CPAP number, and gas flows into the patient. On exhalation, the airway pressure exceeds the set CPAP number and causes airway gases to exit the patient. As such, the airway pressure appears to oscillate around the set CPAP number.

On the anesthesia machine, the CPAP setting is manually dialed with the adjustable pressure-limiting (APL) valve. (Modern valves are now pressure *regulators* and not pressure *resistors*.) End exhalation occurs as a fleeting moment on an anesthesia monitor between exhalation and inhalation, which is why most clinicians use peak exhalation pressures as a guide for CPAP when administering an anesthetic. Unless there is vigorous exhalation, the difference between peak exhalation pressure and the end exhalation pressure is only 1 to 2 cm H_2O. In the ICU, the end exhalation pressure correlates to the set CPAP because the ICU ventilators are able to distinguish between peak exhalation pressure and end exhalation pressure.

Confusion regarding this mode commonly occurs if a subatmospheric pressure is generated during a vigorous inhalation. The trough pressure created at maximal inspiratory effort is confused with the terminology *peak inspiratory pressure*, in which the word *peak* is taken to mean "the highest." Most clinicians use the term *peak* to refer to maximal flow or maximal effort. Thus the term *peak inspiratory pressure* means the highest airway pressure when positive pressure ventilation is used to generate a breath and the lowest airway pressure achieved when spontaneous ventilation occurs.

CPAP during anesthesia may serve in alveolar recruitment and facilitate oxygenation. On the pressure-volume curve, CPAP can shift function to the right and allow the best compliance characteristics of the lung to be manifested. In doing so, patients may be able to generate a better tidal volume for a given generated pressure. However, as with all conditions that increase airway pressure, CPAP increases intrathoracic pressure, which in turn decreases venous return and cardiac output. Also, patients with obstructive lung physiology may incur air trapping and worsening oxygenation and ventilation. Flow-by mode is generally used immediately before extubation; and use at this time allows the clinician to judge native respiratory effort and respiratory parameters most consistent with successful extubation.

Other Modes of Ventilation

High-Frequency Ventilation

High-frequency ventilation (HFV) generally is defined as 60 to 3000 breath cycles/min but has been technically defined by the FDA as a rate exceeding 150 breath cycles/min.[36,37] HFV may be classified into three types. The first, *high-frequency positive-pressure ventilation* (HFPPV), uses a nasotracheal tube or catheter without side holes to insufflate a controlled anesthetic gas mixture. Small tidal volumes and rates of 60 to 120 breaths/min are used, inspiration is active, and exhalation is passive. This technique may require specially designed low-compliance ventilators, although most conventional ventilators can be effectively used in this manner. HFPPV has been used successfully in many types of airway and thoracic surgical procedures and during extracorporeal shock wave lithotripsy.[21,38,39] The Datex-Ohmeda 7800 and Dräger ventilators have both been tested under extreme conditions, mimicking ARDS, and were found capable of maintaining minute ventilation fairly well.[40]

High-Frequency Jet Ventilation

The second type of high-frequency ventilation is *high-frequency jet ventilation* (HFJV), but it is not discussed here. The third type is *high-frequency oscillatory ventilation* (HFO). In contrast to the HFJV, HFO uses the highest frequencies, smallest volumes, and an active expiratory phase, through oscillation, using piston pumps or diaphragms that oscillate like loudspeakers. Sinusoidal waveforms are generated with an I:E ratio of 1:1.[21] Rates of 400 to 2400 cyles/min are used. Gas exchange at these frequencies and at volumes less than dead space volume depend on diffusion and coaxial airway gas flow. Special ventilators, such as the Sensormedics 3100A (Sensormedics, Yorba Linda, CA), oscillate a diaphragm by electromagnetic impulses. Precise amounts of potent inhaled volatile anesthetics can be delivered via a vaporizer proximal to the ventilator and require minimal entrainment of room air. Advantages of these techniques include 1) low airway pressures for bullous lung diseases, 2) small excursions for peripheral lung surgery, and 3) prevention of barotrauma in neonates. OR experience with these ventilators is limited.

Airway Pressure-Release Ventilation

Airway pressure-release ventilation (APRV) is a newcomer to the ventilator mode arena, although similar modes are already used as a bridge mode of ventilation for nonintubated patients, as seen in the use of bilevel positive airway pressure (BiPAP). During the inspiratory cycle, high-pressure CPAP (P_{high}) is delivered for a preset period of inspiratory time (T_I). During inspiration, the patient's efforts to breathe can be observed as deflections in the pressure and flow monitors.

At this point, APRV looks like an anesthesia circuit set at high-pressure CPAP using the APL valve; satisfactory alveolar recruitment is achieved, but ventilation depends on the patient's ability to generate a tidal volume. If the ventilator does not release the airway pressure often enough, carbon dioxide concentrations would rise and cause predictable effects.

Once the inspiratory time has been achieved, exhalation occurs, and airway pressure is released to a lower pressure (P_{low}) for the time of exhalation (T_e). The lower airway pressure is PEEP if the exhalation airway pressure is supraatmospheric. However, if the exhalation pressure is equal to atmospheric pressure, it is the P_{low}. To avoid confusion, the term P_{low} is used to refer to the exhalation pressure. Carbon dioxide is removed from the patient during exhalation. Clinically, the inspiratory time is greater than the exhalation time. As such, IRV is a functional characteristic of this mode of ventilation, and I:E ratios as high as 8:1 are commonly observed. More attention is applied to the exhaled tidal volume and its relationship to indicators of satisfactory ventilation.

As with some other modes of ventilation, APRV has not been considered clinically useful in the OR. Scientific literature advocating the superiority of this mode of ventilation for patients undergoing surgery is lacking, and use of this mode of ventilation for patients undergoing surgical procedures in the OR currently is experimental or is reserved for pathophysiologic outliers.

CURRENT DESIGNS OF ANESTHESIA VENTILATORS

The traditional anesthesia machine—composed of the gas mixer, vaporizer, ventilator, and circuit—has evolved to the anesthesia workstation. As such, the workstation as a unit is designed to 1) monitor patients for important parameters, 2) sound an alarm when dangerous events occur, 3) serve as an integrated anesthesia delivery device, and 4) record the significant events of the anesthetic for the permanent record.

Recent events in anesthesia workstation sales have resulted in a merging of manufacturer product lines. In the process of this merging, workhorse technologies have surfaced, and although variation and expression in ventilator design may be reduced, reliable and predictable ventilator products are now in the marketplace. Two major manufacturers are presented to demonstrate current ventilator designs.

GE Healthcare joined forces with Datex-Ohmeda in the production of workstations using the 7100 series of ventilators and their newest ventilator, the 7900 Smartvent. GE Healthcare markets these ventilators in many workstation product lines, including the Aisys, Aespire, Avance, and Aestiva Carestations.

Dräger Medical, the producer of the E-vent piston ventilator, is currently a joint project of the Dräger and Siemens companies. Dräger Medical uses its piston ventilator in the Apollo Anesthesia Workstation and Fabius lines, which include the GS Premium, MRI, Tiro, and Tiro M.

When examining a specific ventilator among these product lines, the actual ventilator design and function do not appear to change. The changes in the product line models occur in the breathing circuit design and sensor systems. The breathing circuit design changes as new ventilators emerge, improvements in materials are applied, and philosophies on safety, oxygenation, ventilation, and lung protection are recognized. The application of sensors for pressure and flow at various locations throughout the circuit ensures proper function of the system, monitoring of critical events, and feedback systems to improve ventilator performance. As circuit design and sensor systems change, appropriate changes in microprocessor control must occur. For proper function, different hardware and/or software may be required to integrate the vast amount of information for the various configurations.

Lastly, workstation manufacturers offer various displays of important parameters. An analog survivor, the circuit pressure strain gauge, allows continuous direct circuit pressure monitoring without the use of electricity. Most displays now offer combinations of numeric and digital waveform information (parameter vs. time). As an example, the airway pressure-versus-time waveform, numeric tidal volume, and numeric peak airway pressure are displayed as a standard for most product lines. Digital parameters allow trending and waveform analysis. The most basic software packages—those set by safety, industry standard, and legislation— usually are included in the base price of the workstation. In addition, advanced spirometry loops have been available for many years. The complexity of the monitoring, trending, alarming, and waveform analysis is a determinant of the cost of the analysis software package.

7900 Smartvent

The Datex-Ohmeda 7900 Smartvent is designed around the bag-in-a-bottle configuration. As such, two different gas circuits are used in ventilation. When the ventilator is in use, the *driving-gas circuit* uses high-pressure air or oxygen (flow-generator classification) to squeeze a visible ascending bellows; this bellows is housed in a clear, hard plastic case and is under microprocessor control. The gas contained inside the bellows is part of the *patient circuit*.

When the bellows is pushed, the gas contained within it is pushed through the carbon dioxide adsorber. This gas mixes with the fresh gas flow just prior to entering the inspiratory limb of the patient circuit on its way to the patient (Fig. 6-22). On exhalation, used gases pass down the expiratory limb of the patient circuit and back to the bellows. Unidirectional valves, just prior to the inspiratory limb and immediately following the exhalational limb of the patient circuit, ensure one-way gas flow through the entire patient circuit (Fig. 6-23).

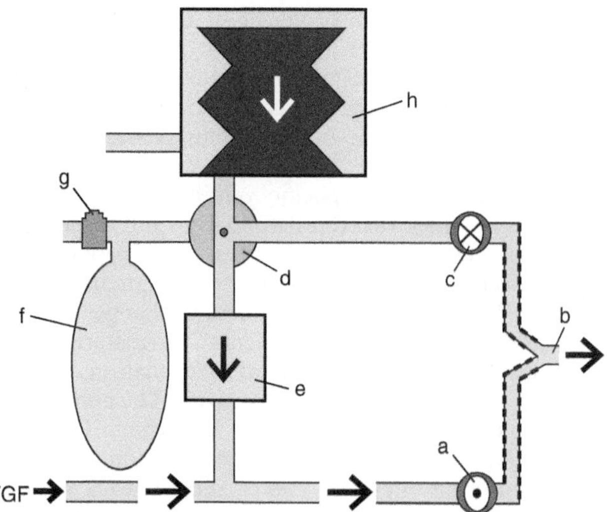

FIGURE 6-22 ■ Ventilator-delivered breath in inspiration with the Datex-Ohmeda 7900 ventilator (GE Healthcare, Waukesha, WI) circuit (simplified schematic). While the bag/ventilator switch (*d*) is in the "ventilator" position, the ventilator (*h*) is activated. Gases within the ventilator bellows are pushed into the ventilator circuit, closing the exhalation valve (*c*). These gases pass antegrade through the CO_2 absorber (*e*) and combine with the fresh gas flow (*FGF*). The mixed gases enter the patient circuit through the inspiratory valve (*a*) to the patient (*b*). A higher pressure within the patient to machine circuit closes the exhalation valve (*c*). *f*, reservoir bag; *g*, adjustable pressure limiting value.

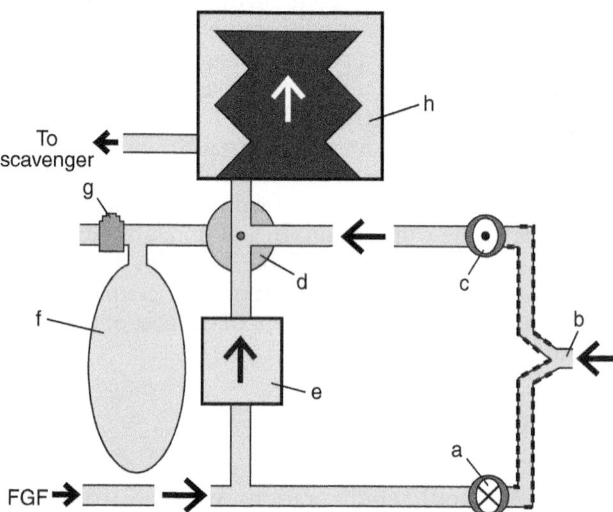

FIGURE 6-23 ■ Ventilator-delivered breath in exhalation with the Datex-Ohmeda 7900 ventilator (GE Healthcare, Waukesha, WI) circuit (simplified schematic). While the bag/ventilator switch (*d*) is in the "ventilator" position, the ventilator (*h*) is activated. Exhaled patient gases (*b*) close the inspiratory valve (*a*) and open the exhalation valve (*c*). Because the inspiration valve is closed, the fresh gas flow (*FGF*) is diverted retrograde through the CO_2 absorber (*e*). Mixed gases from the FGF and exhaled gases reinflate the ventilator bellows. Excess gas volume is eliminated through a low-pressure pop-off valve within the ventilator assembly to the gas scavenger system. *f*, reservoir bag; *g*, adjustable pressure limiting value. (From *Explore the anesthesia system*, 1996, Ohmeda [now GE Healthcare, Waukesha, WI], pp 6-45.)

The drive gas can be either oxygen or air. This is set up by the service technician when the ventilator is first installed; the gas comes from either the anesthesia machine pipeline or cylinder supply. If a cylinder is used to power the ventilator, it will use up the gas supply faster than would be predicted from the flowmeter settings. The gas being used to drive the ventilators can be seen by pushing the *menu* key, selecting *setup/calibration*, then selecting *about ventilator*.

During exhalation, both exhalational gases from the patient and absorber gases being pushed retrograde by the fresh gas flow fill the bellows. Also during exhalation, when the bellows is filled and the pressure exceeds 2.5 cm H_2O, an internal mechanical valve within the bellows assembly opens and redirects the patient circuit gas to the scavenger system (Fig. 6-24). This must occur because gas is constantly being added to the system by the fresh gas flow.

Basic ventilator modes available include spontaneous breathing (Figs. 6-25 and 6-26) with or without CPAP and VCV. Certain GE Healthcare products may include PCV, SIMV, and PSV (Pro series) modalities as a standard build or as an option. The SIMV mode is a volume mode with the ability to deliver PSV between breaths. Interestingly, the PSV Pro mode has an apnea back-up mode using SIMV in pressure mode, with the ability to conduct PSV breaths between controlled breaths. Once the apnea alarm has been triggered, SIMV (pressure) with PSV will be delivered until the PSV Pro mode is selected through the menu system or the ventilator is turned off and on by using the ventilator/bag selector. This ventilator is equipped with electronic PEEP.

The 7900 Smartvent is also capable of providing tidal volume compensation from circuit feedback. This helps provide consistent delivery of set tidal volumes by automatically adjusting for changes in fresh gas flows; changing lung compliance; small system leaks; or compression losses in the ventilator, patient circuit, absorber, or bellows. The manufacturer claims accurate volume delivery to 20 mL of set tidal volume when available. When present, the compensation requires a few breaths to reach a compensated volume.

The set tidal volume range is 20 to 1500 mL for VCV and SIMV (volume) modes. Users may set an inspiratory pause for modes with volume breaths. In PCV modes, inspired pressure can be set from 5 to 60 cm H_2O and from 2 to 40 cm H_2O in PSV modes. For VCV and PCV, the respiratory rate can be set from 4 to 100 breaths/min, and the I:E ratio may be adjusted from 2:1 to 1:8 in increments of 0.5. The inspiratory time may be set to 0.2 to 5 seconds for SIMV and PSV Pro modes. In addition, the flow trigger for PSV Pro can be adjusted. In SIMV modes the observational window period, called a *trigger window* by GE Healthcare, can be adjusted.

GE Healthcare claims less than a 7% and 9% deviation in tidal volume delivery and monitoring, respectively, when set tidal volumes are above 210 mL. Accuracy is improved in delivery and monitoring at lower set tidal volumes. Pressure delivery and monitoring is accurate to ±3 and ±2 cm H_2O, respectively, and delivery of PEEP is accurate to ±1.5 cm H_2O.

Among the common adjustable alarms are *tidal volume* (low and high) and *minute volume* (low and high). In addition, four pressure alarms include *high pressure*, *low pressure*, *negative pressure*, and *sustained pressure;* an apnea alarm and a FiO_2 alarm (low and high) are also adjustable. The priorities of ventilator alarms are *low*, *medium*, and

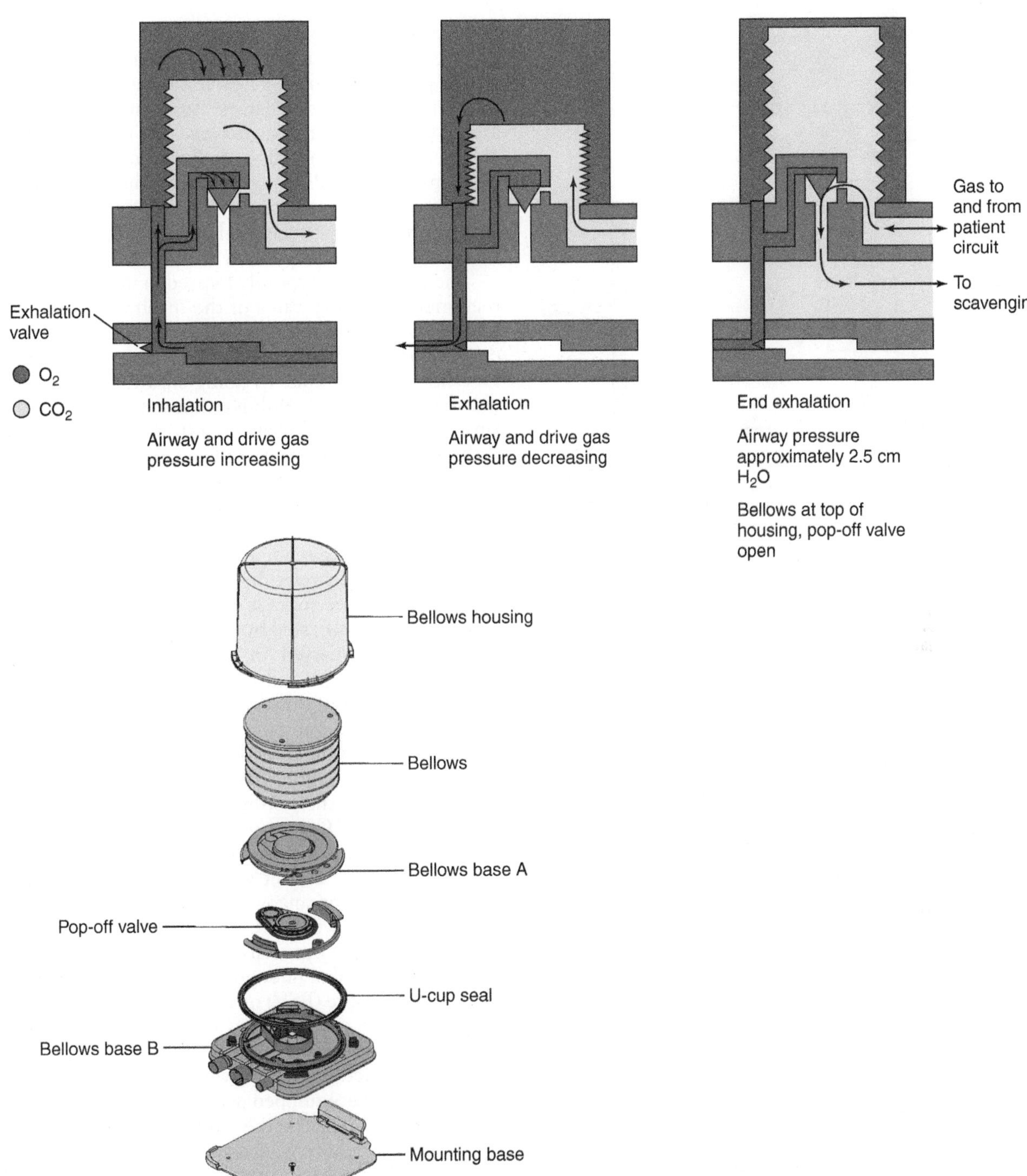

FIGURE 6-24 ■ **Bellows pop-off valve. Figure demonstrates the scavenging of excess airway gases at late exhalation when pressure inside the bellows exceeds 2.5 cm H_2O.** (From *Explore the anesthesia system,* 1996, Ohmeda [now GE Healthcare, Waukesha, WI], pp 6-18.)

high. Low-priority alarms are sounded only once, as a single tone; as priority increases, multiple alarm tones are repeated until disabled by the user or the problem resolves.

Condensation of circuit humidity could foul the normal function of the variable-orifice flow sensors located at the proximal inspiratory and distal exhalation limb of the patient circuit, especially if the clinician does not interpose a disposable heat and moisture exchanger (HME). This problem is magnified in a cold OR; such a malfunction may be heralded by various flow senor alarms, such as *check flow*, *exp reverse flow*, *insp reverse flow*, and *Vte* > *Insp Vt*. A new flow sensor design purportedly minimizes this condensation problem. In addition, holes or perforations in the ventilator bellows may cause the entrainment of driving gas into the bellows. The resulting dilution of the anesthetic agent can cause patient awareness, and the use of air as the drive gas may cause the unintentional delivery of a gas mixture with a lower than expected oxygen concentration, which could lead to hypoxia. Many clinicians appreciate being able to see the ventilator bellows because it affords early detection of ventilator malfunction, disconnect, and circuit leak.

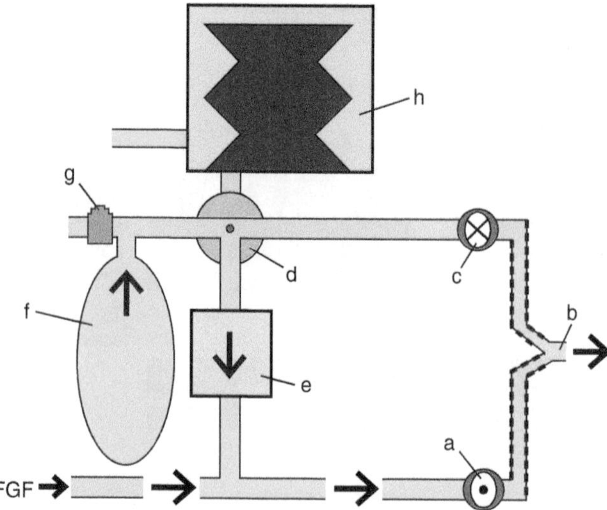

FIGURE 6-25 ■ Spontaneous breath in inspiration with the Datex-Ohmeda 7900 ventilator (GE Healthcare, Waukesha, WI) circuit (simplified schematic). While the bag/ventilator switch (*d*) is in the "bag" position, the machine circuit has access to the reservoir bag (*f*) and the adjustable pressure-limiting (APL) valve (*g*). The ventilator (*h*) is deactivated. A patient-initiated breath (*b*) opens the inspiratory valve (*a*) and closes the exhalation valve (*c*). Gases within the reservoir bag are pulled antegrade through the CO_2 absorber (*e*). These gases mix with the fresh gas flow (*FGF*) while traveling to the patient (*b*).

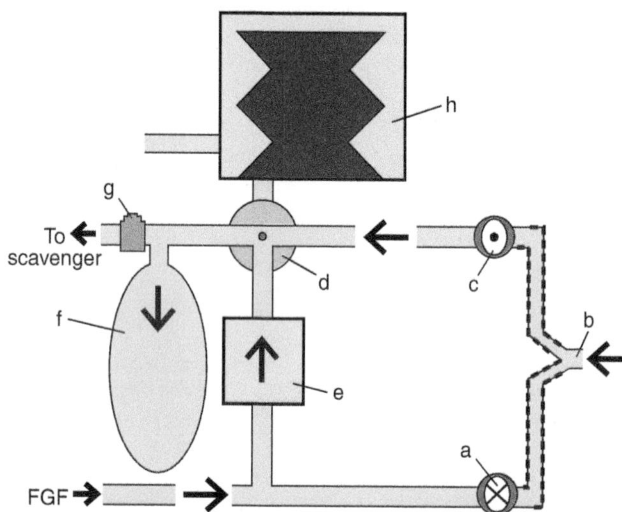

FIGURE 6-26 ■ Spontaneous breath in exhalation with the GE Datex-Ohmeda 7900 ventilator (GE Healthcare, Waukesha, WI) circuit (simplified schematic). While the bag/ventilator switch (*d*) is in the "bag" position, the machine circuit has access to the reservoir bag (*f*) and the adjustable pressure-limiting (APL) valve (*g*). The ventilator (*h*) is deactivated. Exhaled patient gases (*b*) close the inspiratory valve (*a*) and open the exhalation valve (*c*). Because the inspiratory valve is closed, fresh gas flow (*FGF*) is diverted retrograde through the CO_2 absorber (*e*). The mixed gases from the FGF and exhalation fill the reservoir bag. Excess gas volume is removed from the system by the APL valve.

E-vent

The E-vent ventilator deviates from common ventilator designs of the past 40 years by the use of a piston and electrical motor to generate airway pressures, gas flows, and tidal volumes. This system is used in all of the current Dräger Medical workstations. As this piston ventilator produces pressures close to, or only moderately above, airway pressure to move gases, it fits the pressure generator classification of ventilators. Again, its classification as a pressure generator does not exclude its ability to provide reliable, constant flow at fixed volumes (VCV) or constant pressure (PVC) ventilation. Once calibrated, the movements of the piston within the cylinder are well defined and allow precise calculations of the delivered tidal volume, especially in low FGF states.

The ventilator is typically located in front of the unidirectional inspiratory valve of the inspiratory limb of the circuit. The reported advantage of this comes from decreasing the compressible gas volume on the inspiratory side of the circuit. In doing so, the accuracy of the delivered ventilator breath is increased. When the ventilator is cycled, the emptying piston ventilator closes a fresh gas decoupler upstream from the ventilator, which causes two separate events to occur. First, the piston gases are pushed into the inspiratory limb of the circuit to the patient, while the computer closes the PEEP/P_{max} value in the expiratory circuit. At the same time, the closed fresh gas decoupler valve diverts FGF through the carbon dioxide absorber retrograde to the reservoir bag. The reservoir bag is not adjusted by the APL valve because this is automatically bypassed in the mechanical ventilation mode (Fig. 6-27). On exhalation, gases from the patient and exhalation limb exit the circuit and pass through the unidirectional expiratory valve and PEEP/P_{max} valve. These gases combine directly with the residual and fresh reservoir bag gas before passing over the CO_2 absorber with retraction of the piston. Thus, the mixed gases from the reservoir bag, CO_2 absorber, and fresh gas inflow all join together as the piston cylinder fills (Fig. 6-28).

The most basic E-vent ventilator and workstation are provided with a spontaneous mode of breathing (Figs. 6-29 and 6-30) with or without CPAP and VCV. Some models offer as standard or optional modes PCV, PSV, and SIMV (volume) with PSV. The supported breathing mode allows support by pressure (PSV) or volume breaths (AV).

The fresh gas decoupler valve affords the ventilator volume and pressure delivery without interference from the FGF, which improves ventilator accuracy. Some workstations are equipped with an automated start-up procedure that checks the compliance of the circuit before use. In addition, some models can adjust initial ventilator settings based on patient age and weight.

The E-vent ventilator can provide respiratory frequencies from 3 to 80 breaths/min, and the I:E ratio can be adjusted from 1:4 to 5:1. Tidal volumes between 20 and 1400 mL are attainable. In pressure modes, peak pressure can be adjusted to 70 cm H_2O, and the inspiratory time window for SIMV can vary from 0.3 to 6.7 seconds. The inspiratory flow in pressure mode can achieve 150 L/min in some workstations; the flow trigger for PSV can be adjusted from 0.3 to 15 L/min, and maximum deliverable PEEP is 20 cm H_2O. Similar standard alarms are provided compared with the previous manufacturer; however, tones and screen warnings may differ.

An advantage over the gas-driven bellows configuration described above is the motor-driven piston. Because the motor is electrically driven, no oxygen or air is required

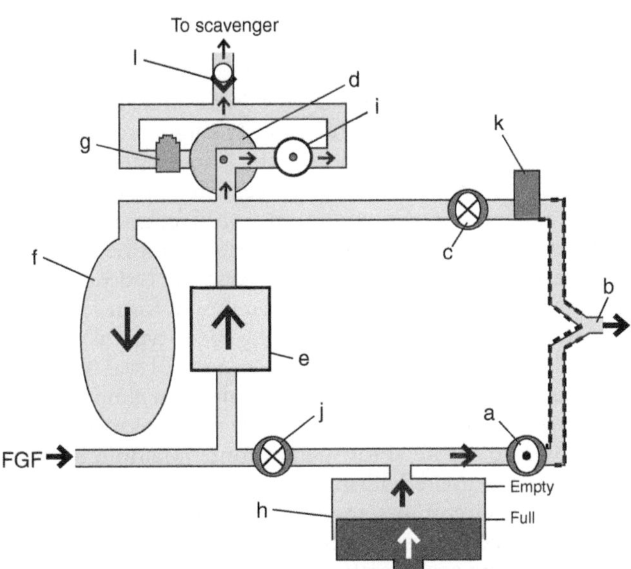

FIGURE 6-27 Ventilator-delivered breath in inspiration with the Apollo and Fabius ventilator (Dräger Medical, Telford, PA) circuits (simplified schematic). While the ventilator switch is on, the ventilator piston (*h*) is activated. In addition, the adjustable pressure-limiting (APL) valve (*g*) is deactivated, and the APL bypass valve (*i*) is actively opened. This functionally diverts (*d*) excess circuit gas across the APL bypass valve toward the scavenger nonreturn valve (*l*). The ventilator piston empties gas contents into the inspiratory limb, closing the fresh gas decoupling valve (*j*) and opening the inspiratory valve (*a*). This allows gas to be pushed into the lungs (*b*). During inspiration, the PEEP/P_{max} valve (*k*) is closed electronically, preventing inspiratory gas from passing across the expiratory valve (*c*). If the patient circuit exceeds the set pressure maximum, the PEEP/P_{max} valve opens to release the excess airway pressure. While the fresh gas decoupler valve is closed, fresh gas flow (*FGF*) is diverted retrograde through the CO_2 absorber (*e*), filling the reservoir bag (*f*). When the reservoir bag is filled, excess pressure causes excess gas volume to pass out of the system through the APL bypass valve and the scavenger nonreturn valve.

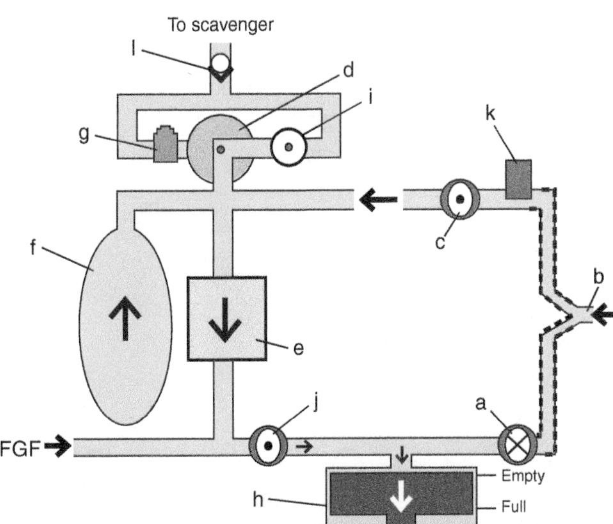

FIGURE 6-28 Ventilator-delivered breath in exhalation with the Apollo and Fabius ventilator (Dräger Medical, Telford, PA) circuits (simplified schematic). While the ventilator switch is on, the ventilator piston (*b*) is activated. In addition, the adjustable pressure-limiting (APL) valve (*g*) is deactivated, and the APL bypass valve (*i*) is actively opened. This functionally diverts (*d*) circuit gas across the APL bypass valve toward the scavenger nonreturn valve (*l*) whenever excess gas fills the reservoir bag (*f*). On exhalation, gas from the lungs (*b*) is first expelled passively into the ventilator circuit across the expiratory valve (*c*) into the reservoir bag by the active opening of the PEEP/P_{max} valve (*k*). (Note that the PEEP/P_{max} valve would only partially open if PEEP were desired.) Exhalation closes the inspiratory valve (*a*). Next, the ventilator piston moves from the empty position to the full position, opening the fresh gas decoupling valve (*j*), and mixed gases from the expiratory limb and reservoir bag are pulled antegrade through the CO_2 absorber (*e*). This gas mixes with the fresh gas flow (*FGF*) while filling the piston.

for its function, which can reduce the costs of compressed and wasted gases. However, the ventilator can fail as a result of worn motor parts. The ventilator piston returning to the filled position could cause negative pressure in the system, with a flat reservoir bag, were it not for negative-pressure entrainment valves. Also, if the reservoir bag were to be torn or removed, or if system leaks occurred, room air could be entrained and thereby dilute the gases to be delivered, causing hypoxia and patient awareness. Some clinicians dislike the workstation design that encloses the ventilator piston within the machine because it occludes the visible function of the ventilator; however, new software displays have been designed that enhance the "visibility" of the piston by revealing its function.

VENTILATOR CONCERNS WITH UTILIZATION

General Concerns with Airway Pressure

Complications of mechanical ventilation have been reviewed by Keith and Pierson.[41] One problem associated with the use of an anesthesia ventilator is overpressurization of the airway, which can occur in several situations: 1) when the patient coughs against the ventilator, 2) when the ventilator's settings are excessive for the first breath, or 3) when the oxygen flush button is depressed during the inspiratory phase. A pressure limit control is available on contemporary anesthesia ventilators; this should be appropriately set because the internal overpressure protection devices may not open until a pressure high enough to cause a pneumothorax is reached. Problem 3 is eliminated by fresh gas–decoupled circuitry.

Some problems arise even during proper operation of the ventilator, such as 1) hypothermia and drying of secretions, usually avoided by using disposable HMEs; 2) hypercarbia or hypocarbia as a result of setting the ventilator incorrectly; 3) hypotension secondary to excessive tidal volume, excessive minute ventilation, or excessive PEEP or auto-PEEP, all of which can reduce preload; 4) barotrauma from excessive transpulmonary pressure; 5) hidden airflow obstruction, particularly from mucous plugging, mainstem intubation, tracheal tube cuff herniation, or bronchospasm; 6) hypoxemia from inadequate ventilator settings; and 7) electromagnetic interference with electronically controlled microprocessors.[41]

As a general rule, when machine malfunction impairs the safe delivery of anesthetic gases, the patient should be immediately disconnected from the anesthesia machine, and a back-up ventilation system should be used instead.

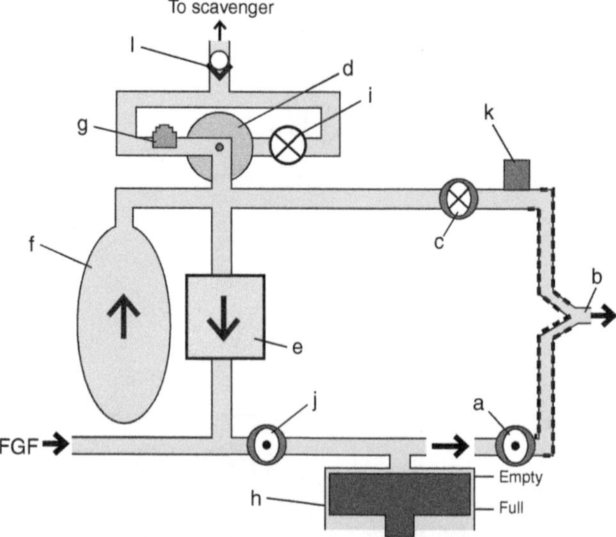

FIGURE 6-29 Spontaneous breath in inspiration with the Apollo and Fabius ventilator (Dräger Medical, Telford, PA) circuits (simplified schematic). While the ventilator switch is off, the ventilator piston (*h*) is deactivated. The ventilator piston stays at the empty, top position (default). In addition, the adjustable pressure-limiting (APL) bypass valve (*i*) is deactivated (default is closed), and the APL valve (*g*) is activated. This functionally diverts (*d*) excess circuit gas across the APL valve toward the scavenger nonreturn valve (*l*). A breath initiated by the patient (*b*) opens the inspiratory valve (*a*) and closes the expiratory valve (*c*). Gases from the reservoir bag (*f*) are pulled antegrade through the CO_2 absorber (*e*) to join the fresh gas flow (*FGF*) while traversing the now open fresh-gas decoupling valve (*j*).

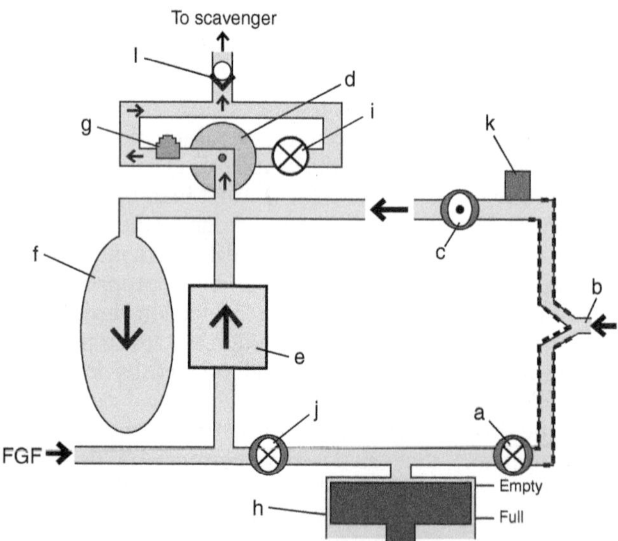

FIGURE 6-30 Spontaneous breath in exhalation with the Apollo and Fabius ventilator (Dräger Medical, Telford, PA) circuits (simplified schematic). While the ventilator switch is off, the ventilator piston (*h*) is deactivated; the ventilator piston stays at the empty, top position (default). In addition, the adjustable pressure-limiting (APL) bypass valve (*i*) is deactivated (default is closed), and the APL valve (*g*) is activated. This functionally diverts (*d*) excess circuit gas across the APL valve toward the scavenger nonreturn valve (*l*). Exhaled gas from the patient (*b*) opens the expiratory valve (*c*) and closes the inspiratory valve (*a*). Exhaled gas joins fresh gas flow (*FGF*) traveling retrograde through the CO_2 absorber (*e*). The mixed gas fills the reservoir bag (*f*). When the reservoir bag is filled, excess pressure closes the expiratory valve and allows excess gas volume to pass out of the system through the APL valve and the scavenger nonreturn valve.

Cross-Infection

Infection risk related to the anesthesia ventilator and circuit was evaluated in the early 1980s. Several authors have studied the risk of cross-infection arising from the use of ventilators and anesthesia circuits. Cross-infection cases have been reported in which the repeated use of the same piece of airway equipment transferred infection among patients.[42] Carbon dioxide absorbers cannot be regarded as a barrier to the transmission of bacteria. Indeed, bacteria such as *Pseudomonas* have been cultured from soda lime absorbers.[43] Nevertheless, with the older type of nondisposable circuits, adequate infection control was achieved by washing with suitable decontamination fluids.[44] The subsequent widespread introduction of disposable circuits has obviated the need for such decontamination; bacteria are not disseminated during quiet breathing, nor does the machine or circuit disseminate organisms.[45,46]

The concern caused by human immunodeficiency virus (HIV) and the even greater risk posed by hepatitis B or C transmission warrant vigilance about controlling cross-contamination in all aspects of anesthesia care. Precautions that prevent cross-contamination appear to offer appropriate safety for airway equipment and anesthesia delivery systems. The use of disposable circuits appears to afford patients adequate safety, although actual sterility is hard to achieve. The GE Healthcare bellows and canister system is easily disassembled and autoclavable; however, the absorber manifold is interposed between the circuit and bellows. Similar to other anesthesia circle breathing systems, it cannot be cleaned effectively without disassembly by trained technicians. The entire Dräger breathing manifold and system are easily removed and autoclavable, which has recently been recommended for the preparation of the machine in patients susceptible to malignant hyperthermia.

CHECK-OUT PROCEDURES

Preoperative Procedures

The 1993 check-out recommendations from the United States Food and Drug Administration (FDA)[47] should be used as a generic checklist for ascertaining the proper function of a ventilator. Specific manufacturer recommendations should always be consulted. The FDA list states that backup manual ventilation must be immediately available and must be tested. These resuscitators typically have a one-way valve that must be properly installed and competent to provide positive-pressure ventilation. The scavenger system and ventilator relief valve (pop-off valve) should be tested together to verify that excess gas will be released once the bellows is full to prevent any distension or sustained pressure. Then, with minimal or no flow, the bellows should remain filled to ascertain a proper seal of the relief valve, proper seating of the bellows, and no holes in the bellows. Next, when the ventilator is activated with a test lung (a second reservoir bag at the patient "Y") and no FGF, the bellows should not lose volume. If it does, the ventilator relief valve may not be sealing under pressure. Furthermore, the volume delivered and motion of the test lung should be appropriate for the set parameters, or a leak in the drive gas circuit should be considered. In the active test mode, external pressure applied to the test lung should appropriately activate the pressure limit safety feature and high-pressure alarm.

Since the 1993 FDA recommendations were made, new check-out procedures have been required to adapt to the changing anesthesia delivery systems. Further, a single check-out procedure is no longer applicable to the various equipment designs. Updated recommendations were developed in 2008 by a multidisciplinary subcommittee of the American Society of Anesthesiologists (ASA) Committee on Equipment and Facilities.[48] The check-out design guideline is also supported as educational information by the FDA's Office of Device Evaluation. Sample check-out procedures have been submitted and approved for inclusion in the ASA library by the ASA Committee on Equipment and Facilities.[49]

Intraoperative Procedures

Vigilance should be maintained whenever a ventilator is in operation. When mechanical ventilation is selected in older workstations, it is essential to change from manual to mechanical ventilation on the ventilator selection switch. The ventilator and pressure limit must be appropriately set for each patient, and the first ventilator-delivered breath must be observed, carefully watching for chest expansion, proper cycling, peak pressure, I:E ratio, airway pressure waveform, plateau pressure, inspiratory pause, and tidal volume before and after adjusting the FGF. Is the bellows compression complete, and does it completely return during exhalation? Is the inspiratory flow adequate to meet ventilatory settings? Once ventilation is established, reset the minute volume and minimum airway pressure alarms, the pressure limiter, PEEP, and the peak airway pressure alarm according to the patient's unique parameters. Listen to breath sounds, despite capnography, to see if they are coincident with, and appropriate for, ventilator sounds. Follow end-tidal carbon dioxide and pulse oximetry as measures of ventilation, breathing circuit valve function, and proper alveolar expansion.

REFERENCES

1. Baker AB: Early attempts at expired air respiration, intubation and manual ventilation. In Atkinson RS, Boulton TB, editors: *The history of anaesthesia*, London, 1987, Royal Society of Medicine, pp 372–374.
2. Gordon AS: History and evolution of modern resuscitation techniques. In Gordon AS, editor: *Cardiopulmonary resuscitation conference proceedings*, Washington, DC, 1966, National Academy of Sciences, pp 7–32.
3. Vesalius A: *De humani corporis fabrica libri septem*, Basileae, 1543, Ex Off. Ioannis Oporini.
4. Mushin WW, Rendell-Baker L: *The principles of thoracic anaesthesia*- Oxford, 1953, Blackwell, pp 28–30.
5. O'Dwyer J: Fifty cases of croup in private practice treated by intubation of the larynx, with a description of the method and of the dangers incident thereto, *Med Rec* 32:557–561, 1887.
6. Fell GE: Forced respiration, *JAMA* 16:325–330, 1891.
7. Hochberg LA: *Thoracic surgery before the 20th century*, New York, 1960, Vantage Press, pp 684–697.
8. Tuffier T, Hallion L: Intrathoracic operations with artificial respiration by insufflation, *C R Soc Biol (Paris)* 48:951, 1896.
9. Matas R: Artificial respiration by direct intralaryngeal intubation with a new graduated air-pump, in its applications to medical and surgical practice, *Am Med* 3:97–103, 1902.
10. Drinker P, Shaw L: An apparatus for the prolonged administration of artificial respiration, *J Clin Invest* 7:229, 1929.
11. Mushin WW, Rendell-Baker L, Thompson PW, et al: *Automatic ventilation of the lungs*, Oxford, UK, 1980, Blackwell Scientific.
12. Magill IW: Development of endotracheal anaesthesia, *Proc R Soc Med* 22:83–88, 1928.
13. Lassen HCA: A preliminary report on the 1952 epidemic of poliomyelitis in Copenhagen with special reference to the treatment of acute respiratory insufficiency, *Lancet* 1:37–41, 1953.
14. Bjork VO, Engstrom CG: The treatment of ventilatory insufficiency after pulmonary resection with tracheostomy and prolonged artificial ventilation, *J Thorac Surg* 30:356–367, 1955.
15. Frumin MJ, Epstein RM, Cohen G: Apneic oxygenation in man, *Anesthesiology* 20:789–798, 1959.
16. Chatburn RL: Classification of mechanical ventilators. In Tobin MJ, editor: *Principles and practice of mechanical ventilation*, New York, 1994, McGraw-Hill.
17. MacIntyre NR: New modes of mechanical ventilation, *Clin Chest Med* 17:411–421, 1996.
18. Slutsky AS: Mechanical ventilation. American College of Chest Physicians' consensus conference, *Chest* 104:1833–1859, 1993.
19. Feihl R, Perret C: Permissive hypercapnia: how permissive should we be? *Am J Respir Crit Care Med* 150:1722–1737, 1994.
20. Marcy TW: Inverse ratio ventilation. In Tobin MJ, editor: *Principles and practice of mechanical ventilation*, New York, 1994, McGraw-Hill, pp 319–331.
21. Schwartz DE, Katy JA: Delivery of mechanical ventilation during general anesthesia. In Tobin MJ, editor: *Principles and practice of mechanical ventilation*, New York, 1994, McGraw-Hill.
22. Acute Respiratory Distress Network: Ventilation with lower tidal volumes as compared with traditional tidal volumes for acute lung injury and the acute respiratory distress syndrome, *N Engl J Med* 342(18):1301–1308, 2000.
23. Schultz MJ, Haitsma JJ, Slutsky AS, Gajic O: What tidal volumes should be used in patients without acute lung injury? *Anesthesiology* 106(6):1226–1231, 2007.
24. ASTM: *Standard specification for ventilators intended for use during anesthesia, F1101-90*, West Conshohocken, PA, 1990, American Society for Testing and Materials.
25. Marini JJ, Ravenscraft SA: Mean airway pressure: physiologic determinants and clinical importance. Part 1. Physiologic determinants and measurements, *Crit Care Med* 20:1461–1472, 1992.
26. Marini JJ, Ravenscraft SA: Mean airway pressure: physiologic determinants and clinical importance. Part 2. Clinical implications, *Crit Care Med* 20:1604–1616, 1992.
27. McKibben AW, Ravenscraft SA: Pressure-controlled and volume-cycled mechanical ventilation, *Clin Chest Med* 17:395–410, 1996.
28. Marks JD, Schapera A, Kraemer RW, Katz JA: Pressure and flow limitations of anesthesia ventilators, *Anesthesiology* 71:403–408, 1989.
29. Marks JD, Katz JA, Schapera A, Kraemer RW: Evaluation of a new operating room ventilator: the Ohmeda 7810, *Anesthesiology* 71(3A):A463 (abstract), 1989.
30. ANSI: *American National Standard for Breathing Machines for Medical Use, ANSI Z79.7*, New York, 1976, American National Standards Institute.
31. *Ohmeda 7900 Ventilator operations and maintenance manual*, Madison, WI, 1996, Ohmeda, The BOC Group.
32. Salzano JV, Camporesi EM, Stolp BW, Moon RE: Physiologic responses to exercise at 47 and 66 ATA, *J Appl Physiol* 57:1055, 1984.
33. Nunn JF, editor: *Nunn's applied respiratory physiology*, ed 4, Oxford/Boston, 1993, Butterworth-Heinemann.
34. Mielke L, Breinbauer B, Kling M, et al: The use of the Servo 900 B for ventilation in hyperbaric chambers [abstract], *Anesth Analg* 82:S315, 1996.
35. Thomas G, Brimacombe J: Function of the Dräger Oxylog ventilator at high altitude, *Anaesth Intens Care* 22: 276–228, 1994.
36. Rouby JJ, Viars P: Clinical use of high frequency ventilation, *Acta Anaesthesiol Scand Suppl* 33:134–139, 1989.
37. Majewski A, Telmanik S, Arrington V: High frequency oscillatory ventilation, *Va Med Q* Fall:230–232, 1994.
38. Malina JR, Nordström SG, Sjöstrand UH: Wattwil, LM: Clinical evaluation of high-frequency positive-pressure ventilation (HFPPV) in patients scheduled for open-chest surgery, *Anesth Analg* 60:324–330, 1981.

39. Heres EK, Shulman MS, Krenis LJ, Moon R: High-frequency ventilation with a conventional anesthetic ventilator during cardiac surgery, *J Cardiothorac Vasc Anes* 9:63–65, 1995.
40. Tessler MJ, Ruiz-Neto PP, Finlayson R, Chartrand D: Can anesthesia ventilators provide high-frequency ventilation? *Anesth Analg* 79:563–566, 1994.
41. Keith RL, Pierson DJ: Complications of mechanical ventilation: a bedside approach, *Clin Chest Med* 17:439–451, 1996.
42. Walter CW: Cross-infection and the anesthesiologist, twelfth annual Baxter-Travenol lecture, *Anesth Analg* 53:631–644, 1974.
43. Dryden GE: Uncleaned anesthesia equipment, *JAMA* 233:1297–1298, 1975.
44. Nielsen H, Jacobsen JB, Stokke DB, et al: Cross-infection from contaminated anaesthetic equipment, *Anaesthesia* 35:703–708, 1980.
45. du Moulin GC, Hedley-Whyte J: Bacterial interactions between anesthesiologists, their patients, and equipment, *Anesthesiology* 57:37–41, 1982.
46. du Moulin GC, Saubermann AJ: The anesthesia machine and circle system are not likely to be sources of bacterial contamination, *Anesthesiology* 47:353–358, 1977.
47. Morrison JL: FDA Anesthesia Apparatus Checkout Recommendations, *American Society of Anesthesiologists Newsletter* 1994(58):25–28, 1993.
48. Recommendations for Pre-Anesthesia Checkout Procedures (2008). Sub-Committee of ASA Committee on Equipment and Facilities. Accessed online at http://www.asahq.org/clinical/FINALCheckoutDesignguidelines02-08-2008.pdf.
49. American Society of Anesthesiologists: Sample checkout procedures. Available at http://www.asahq.org/clinical/checklist.htm.

CHAPTER 7

HUMIDIFICATION AND FILTRATION

Maire Shelly • Craig Spencer

CHAPTER OUTLINE

OVERVIEW

Under normal physiologic conditions, the upper airway adds heat and moisture to inspired air to prevent drying of lower airway secretions, plugging, and mucosal injury. When dry medical gases bypass the upper airway via an endotracheal tube, the normal heat and moisture exchange function of the upper airway is compromised. This function of the upper airway may be replaced in two ways. First, heat and humidity can be actively added with a heated humidifier; second, and more commonly, heat and moisture may be passively retained using a heat and moisture exchanger (HME).

The upper airway also fulfills the function of filtration and expulsion of particles, including bacteria and viruses, from inspired gas. This is achieved by the *mucociliary elevator*. The anesthesiologist is responsible for minimizing the risk of infection from inhaled microorganisms. The use of HME filters (HMEFs) protects patients from inhaled microorganisms and also protects the anesthesia circuit from the patient, thereby allowing its reuse.

PHYSICS OF HUMIDITY

Water vapor is the gas phase of water. The transition from the liquid to the gas phase is called *vaporization*, a process that requires energy. The energy required for this process is the latent heat of vaporization, which is 2.27 MJ/kg water.

Humidity describes the amount of water vapor in air. *Absolute humidity* is the partial pressure of water vapor above its liquid at equilibrium. As such it may be measured in kilopascals (kPa) or other unit of pressure, but in this context it is more commonly referred to as the *mass of water* in a given volume of air (in milligrams per liter). Evaporation occurs at a constant temperature until a critical mass of water in the air is reached and the air is fully saturated. The pressure of the water vapor at this point is the *saturated vapor pressure* (SVP) for water, which increases rapidly with increases in temperature (Fig. 7-1).

At a given temperature, *relative humidity* is the relationship of the absolute humidity to SVP, expressed as a percentage. Air at its SVP has 100% relative humidity. Relative humidity equals the mass of water vapor for a given volume of air for a given temperature, and SVP is the mass of water vapor required to fully saturate that volume. For example, fully saturated air at 20° C contains 17 mg/L water and at 37° C contains 44 mg/L water.

As air is heated, its SVP increases. If no further water mass is added, absolute humidity remains the same while relative humidity decreases. For example, air in a typical operating room (OR) at 20° C contains 10 mg/L of water and has approximately 60% relative humidity. If fully saturated air at 20° C is heated to 37° C without adding further water mass, it is said to have 38.6% relative humidity (17 mg/L ÷ 44 mg/L). If fully saturated air is cooled, it will reach its dew point, at which air can no longer support the mass of water vapor, and water undergoes condensation.

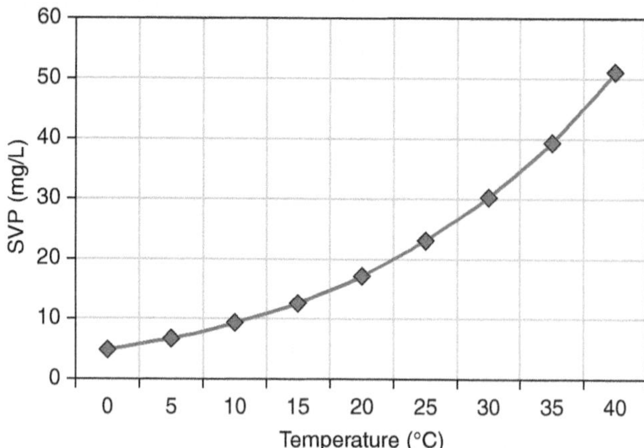

FIGURE 7-1 ■ Saturated vapor pressure (*SVP*) with temperature. (From Mushin W, Jones P: *Physics for the Anaesthetist*, ed 4, Boston, 1987, Blackwell Scientific.)

Measurement of Humidity

Instruments that measure humidity are referred to as *hygrometers.* They typically measure relative humidity. If temperature and SVP are known, absolute humidity can be calculated.

Hair Hygrometer

The hair hygrometer makes use of a hair, or a synthetic membrane with similar properties, that lengthens as relative humidity increases. As the hair lengthens, it moves a pointer to create an analog display of relative humidity. If the temperature is known, absolute humidity may be calculated. Hair hygrometers typically are used in operating theatres and neonatal incubators. Hair hygrometers are most accurate at a relative humidity of 30% to 90%; they have a slow response and are of limited use where humidity changes rapidly.

Wet and Dry Bulb Hygrometer

The wet and dry bulb hygrometer consists of two mercury thermometers: one reads a true ambient temperature, and the other has a water-soaked wick around the bulb that, when exposed to a moving stream of air, produces a cooling effect from the loss of the latent heat of vaporization. With dry ambient air, evaporation is increased, resulting in a greater apparent temperature drop. The difference in the temperature measured between the thermometers (ΔT) is related to the rate of evaporation, which depends on ambient humidity. Relative humidity can be calculated from a table.

Regnault's Hygrometer

Regnault's hygrometer is also known as a *dew point hygrometer*. The original design consisted of a silver tube that contained ether. As air bubbles through, it cools the ether and causes condensation on the silvered exterior of the tube. The formation of condensation indicates the dew point and the SVP at that temperature. The ratio of SVP at dew point to SVP at ambient temperature gives the relative humidity, which may be derived from a chart.

Electric Hygrometer

Electric hygrometers may use an actively cooled, polished metal mirror. Condensation will form on it when ambient gas meets its dew point, indicating SVP. This point can be detected as a result of the change in its reflective properties or a change in another characteristic, such as its electrical conductivity. Other electric hygrometers use substances that change in resistance or capacitance with water vapor pressure. They typically are heated to a set temperature above dew point to avoid temperature dependency. Their small size potentially allows inclusion within the breathing circuit.

PHYSIOLOGY OF HUMIDIFICATION

The upper airway extends from the external nares to the major bronchi. The function of this organ system is to condition inspired gas so that it is warm, humidified, and relatively free of foreign material when it reaches the alveoli. It also has expiratory functions of conservation of heat and humidity, and it facilitates clearance of particulate matter.

Humidification in the Airway

Turbulent flow of inspired gas around the turbinates results in maximal contact of inspired gas with a large mucosal surface area. Particles of all sizes become trapped in the mucous layer; smaller particles may make contact with the mucous layer because they occupy a relatively large apparent space, due to Brownian motion.[1] The large mucous surface area allows efficient transfer of heat and moisture. The majority of heating and humidification has occurred by mid trachea, to approximately 34° C with an absolute humidity of 34 to 38 mg/L (95% to 100% relative humidity).[2] As gas travels distally in the airway and is heated to body temperature, it is further humidified to an absolute humidity of 44 mg/L (100% relative humidity). Transfer of water occurs by evaporation, which is the major energy-requiring process. A lesser amount of energy is required to warm inspired gas by conduction and convection. During the process of heat and moisture exchange, the temperature of the nasal mucosa is reduced to 31° C; consequently, gas cools and loses its capacity to hold water vapor during expiration. Condensation occurs and releases latent heat of vaporization, rehydrating and rewarming the mucosa. Expired air is typically around 32° C to 34° C and 100% relative humidity (38.2 to 42.7 mg/L H_2O). The upper airway effectively forms a countercurrent HME, retaining much of the heat and moisture it imparts to inspired gas to condition it for the alveoli. Under typical physiologic conditions in an adult, the daily net loss from this system is approximately 250 mL of water and 250 kcal.[2,3]

The point in the airway at which inspired gas reaches 37° C and 100% relative humidity is known as the *isothermic saturation boundary* (ISB).[4] This usually lies just below the carina but may vary according to the volume, humidity, and temperature of inspired gas. When the upper airway is bypassed by an endotracheal tube, this boundary is shifted distally. Even under this nonphysiologic condition, the ISB is still achieved before the respiratory bronchioles; this retains a stable humidity in the functional residual capacity.[5]

In cold ambient temperatures, cool inspired air has little capacity to hold water vapor and has a low absolute humidity. The upper airway is required to transfer large amounts of heat and moisture. However, the ISB remains at approximately the same position as the gradients of heat and moisture exchange increase down the airway.[6] In warm ambient temperatures, little heat energy is expired to warm inspired gases. Heat and moisture loss to inspired gas is an important part of body thermoregulation. This potential source of heat loss may be effectively lost in hot, humid conditions and to an extent by mouth breathing. Increased minute volume during exercise may result in high heat and water losses, especially in cold, dry environments. Cool inspired gas may trigger bronchospasm, especially in those with asthma, although the mechanism for this is still poorly understood.

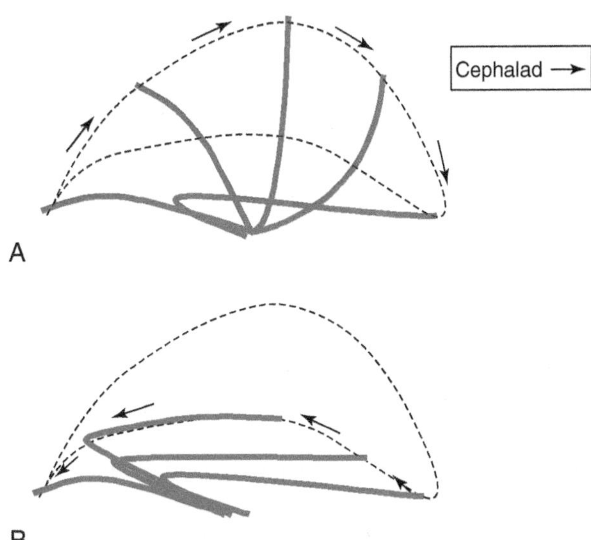

FIGURE 7-2 The cilial beat cycle. **A,** Demonstration of the effective stroke with the cilium erect; the cilial claws grab mucus and propel it cephalad. **B,** The recovery stroke, during which the cilium bends and returns to its rest position through the periciliary fluid layer.

Mucociliary Elevator

The nasopharynx, pharynx, and larynx have squamous epithelia and therefore contribute little to humidification.[7,8] The mucous membranes of the nose, trachea, and bronchi have many mucus glands, and it is here that the majority of humidification takes place. These glands keep the upper airway mucosa moist by direct secretion and transudation of fluid.

Respiratory mucus is formed within goblet cells in response to irritation of the tracheal surface. Mucus is secreted in 1- to 2-µm droplets that absorb water, swell, and coalesce to form a 10-µm film around respiratory cilia. It lies in two layers: the superficial layer is a viscous fluid that contains lipids, glycoproteins, and proteoglycans that trap inspired particles. The deep layer is a more acidic, watery, periciliary layer that contains antibacterial compounds secreted from surface epithelium and glands that, when activated, result in recruitment of inflammatory cells, such as neutrophils and macrophages.[9]

Respiratory cilia are the basic units of the mucociliary escalator. Each ciliated cell has approximately 200 cilia, 5- to 6-µm long projections revealed in cross-section to be formed by a central pair of microtubules surrounded by nine pairs of tubules.[7] Movement is achieved by microtubules sliding against each other by dynein adenosine triphosphatase linking arms. At their tips they have three to seven short, 25- to 35-nm long projections that effectively grip the superficial mucous layer. Cilia beat at approximately 1000 strokes/min in a coordinated fashion, propelling mucus cephalad at a rate of 12 to 15 mm/min.[10,11] Each stroke has two phases, a rapid forward stroke, in which the side "claws" grip the superficial mucous layer and propel it forward, and a recovery stroke, in which the cilia swing slowly back into the starting position through the deep periciliary layer (Fig. 7-2).

Particulate matter transported to the upper airway may be cleared by coughing, which involves rapid inspiration followed by brief closure of the glottis. During this time, elastic recoil and active expiratory contraction increase intrathoracic pressure. When the glottis opens, explosive expiration at over 10 L/sec causes shearing and expectoration of secretions. Effective coughing requires an adequate peak expiratory flow rate and adequately hydrated mucus secretions.

Mucociliary Clearance

Mucociliary clearance may be reduced as a result of abnormal mucus production or cilial activity. In cystic fibrosis, the abnormal transmembrane conductance protein is a chloride ion channel. This results in reduced chloride and water content in the mucus, making it abnormally viscous and thereby reducing clearance and encouraging bacterial colonization.[12] In other inflammatory airway diseases, hypertrophy of mucus glands may result in viscous secretions and a reduced periciliary watery layer that may inhibit the ciliary recovery stroke.

Reduced cilia activity may be congenital in conditions such as primary ciliary diskinesia, in which ciliary ultrastructure is abnormal.[13] The time taken for effective ciliary clearance is approximately doubled in cigarette smokers.[14] Pathogens such as *Pseudomonas aeruginosa* and *Haemophilus influenzae* reduce beat frequency.[15] In addition, ventilated critically ill patients may have reduced mucociliary transport as a result of loss of cilia.[16]

Consequences of Underhumidification

In the presence of inadequate ambient humidity, prolonged excessive mucosal water loss results in viscous mucus that inhibits ciliary movement, especially the recovery stroke in the depleted deep, watery layer. Mucus flow is significantly reduced below a relative humidity of 50% at 37° C (absolute humidity 22 mg/L).[17] Dry membranes have a reduced capacity to humidify inspired gas, and the ISB moves distally, exposing more distal airways to risk of injury. Ciliary loss, mucosal inflammation, epithelial ulceration, and necrosis may eventually occur. Hyperviscous secretion may obstruct bronchi or endotracheal tubes, and encrustation may occur and cause sputum retention, infection, atelectasis, reduced functional capacity, ventilation/perfusion (V/Q) mismatch, and reduced compliance.[18,19] In addition, ventilation with dry gases may exacerbate hypothermia, especially in neonates and children.

Consequences of Overhumidification

When inspired gases are delivered at approaching or exceeding body temperature and fully saturated, the normal humidifying and heating actions of the upper airway cannot occur and may even be reversed. Condensation of water occurs in the airway with consequent reduced mucosal viscosity and risk of water intoxication. Inefficient mucociliary transport results, along with increased airway resistance, risk of pulmonary infection, surfactant dilution, atelectasis, and V/Q mismatch.[2] Hot, humid gases may cause tracheitis by direct thermal injury to the epithelium.[20]

FILTRATION

Inhaled gases commonly carry a suspension of solid or liquid particles known as *aerosols*. Most aerosols are *polydisperse*, meaning they contain a range of particle sizes. Aerosol particles usually firmly attach to surfaces they are in contact with. Particles may make contact with surfaces by five different methods as gas flow is altered around an obstructing surface:

1. *Inertial impaction* occurs when a particle cannot follow a change in gas direction because of its inertia.
2. *Interception* occurs when a particle has low inertia but makes partial contact with a surface because of its large diameter.
3. *Brownian motion* occurs when small particles move in an apparently random pattern under the influence of surrounding gas molecules.
4. *Gravitational settling* typically occurs with large particles as they deviate from a gas stream under the influence of gravity.
5. *Electrostatic deposition* occurs when a particle deviates from the gas stream as a result of electrostatic attraction.

Large particles, those greater than 10 µm in diameter, typically deposit in the larynx or above. In the airways below this level, inertial impaction is the most significant mechanism for large particles in the larger airways, with gravitational settling becoming more important with lower velocities in smaller airways. Brownian motion is important throughout the airways for transportation of small particles.[21]

Artificial filters are generally formed of a mat of fine fibers of paper, glass, or plastic. Because gas flow changes repeatedly as gas flows around the fibers, the chances of contact with the filter increase. An electrostatically charged filter will also benefit from electrostatic deposition. Particles of different sizes make contact with surfaces to different degrees with each mechanism. Intermediate-size particles, those around 0.3 µm, are under the least influence by these five combined forces. In this context, 0.3 µm is regarded as the most penetrating particle size (MPPS) for most filters.[22]

The properties of filters vary enormously. *Filtration efficiency* describes the proportion of test particles prevented from passing beyond a filter. In this context, filtration efficiency is more commonly quoted in terms of *bacterial filtration efficiency* (BFE) or *viral filtration efficiency* (VFE). These terms describe the efficiency of the filter to stop particles of a nonpathogenic test bacterial or viral challenge aerosolized into droplets around 3.0 µm in diameter. Many bacteria have a similar diameter; viruses are smaller, although it must be noted this is a relatively large particle, 10 times the diameter of the MPPS. This large diameter results in a high apparent filtration fraction with this test. An efficiency of 99.97% indicates that 30 particles out of 100,000 aerosolized particles penetrate the filter in testing. Filters with an efficiency of 99.999% of the BFE or VFE are now available. The alternative "salt test" reveals the proportion of aerosolized 0.3-µm diameter sodium chloride particles prevented from penetrating the filter. Because this is the MPPS, this test usually results in a much lower apparent filtration efficiency. The efficiency claims of an individual HME must be understood in the context in which it was tested.[21]

Humidification Devices

As previously discussed, under normal physiologic conditions, much of the work of heating and humidification of inspired gas occurs in the nose. By the time the inspired gas reaches the mid trachea, its temperature is approximately 34° C, and it contains 34 to 38 mg/L water. As gas travels down into the lower airway, it is further heated to 37° C and 100% relative humidity (absolute humidity 44 mg/L). With intubation, the nasopharynx is bypassed. Humidification of dry medical gases now occurs in a more distal region, and the ISB moves distally.

Humidification devices—which may be passive, such as HMEs, or active, such as heated humidifiers—aim to reproduce more normal physiologic conditions in the lower respiratory tract. Achievement of absolute humidity levels of 30 to 35 mg/L in the trachea in clinical practice avoids significant heat and moisture loss and complications of mucosal drying.[2] Overheating of inspired gases must also be avoided. If the gases are overheated, the saturated vapor pressure will increase. If that gas subsequently cools to the patient's temperature as it enters the airway, the saturated vapor pressure will drop, causing water to condense and "rain out."

HEAT AND MOISTURE EXCHANGERS

HMEs consist of an outer casing with an inlet and an outlet with a partial barrier in between. They are placed close to the patient, on the distal end of the endotracheal tube or laryngeal mask airway (LMA). A closed suction unit or flexible extension may be placed between the

HME and the airway, and some HMEs have integral flexible extensions, a piece angled 90 degrees, and a sampling port for sidestream capnography. It must be noted that measured end-tidal carbon dioxide on the machine side of the HME is significantly lower than that measured on the patient side, in both spontaneously and mechanically ventilated patients.[23]

HMEs are a compact, inexpensive, efficient, and non–energy-requiring solution to humidification of relatively cool and dry inspired gases. An HME is, in effect, an "artificial nose"—a passive device or barrier that retains the stored moisture and thermal energy of expired gases—within the lower respiratory tract.

HMEs may be either hygroscopic or hydrophobic. *Hygroscopic HMEs* use a paper or other fiber barrier coated with moisture-retaining chemicals that also may have some electrostatic properties. They may be made of a composite with an intermediate electrostatic membrane between hygroscopic layers. These adsorb water in expiration and release it in inspiration and usually are the most efficient devices for retaining heat and moisture. Being fiber based, they are more prone to becoming saturated, resulting in increased inspiratory/expiratory resistance and reduced heat and moisture retention efficiency.

Hydrophobic HMEs contain a pleated hydrophobic membrane that contains small pores, and they tend to be more efficient filters of pathogens.[24] When using an HME, humidity reaches steady state in the lower respiratory tract within a few breaths. The International Standards Organization (ISO) 9360 standard specifies the lung model, ventilator settings, and absolute humidity standards for HMEs for a standardized 24-hour test.[25]

Potential Hazards and Limitations of Heat and Moisture Exchangers

A range of HMEs is available, with wide variations in properties (Fig. 7-3). A number of factors must be taken into account in selecting an appropriate HME. The internal volume of these devices can vary from approximately 12 to 100 mL, and resistance can be in the range of 0.7 to 3.8 cm H_2O/L/sec.[26] HMEs introduce inspiratory, expiratory, and dead space resistance to the anesthesia circuit. The HME design should aim to reduce this resistance to prevent increased work of breathing and hypercapnea, especially in pediatric patients or when ventilating adults with a low tidal volume strategy. This effect may be overcome in mechanically ventilated patients but may require the addition of up to 5 to 10 cm H_2O inspiratory pressure.[27]

HMEs may become progressively or acutely obstructed, especially by deposition of proteinaceous fluid such as sputum or blood. Acute obstruction is a rare but life-threatening event, so regular visual inspection of the HME is recommended. It is also recommended that the HME be replaced after every 24 hours of use. However, studies of the prolonged use of single filters found they still keep their moisture-retaining efficiency at 7 days without significant increase in resistance.[28]

Tests of HMEs in vivo show that their performance may vary significantly from that quoted for testing in vitro.[29] Efficiency may reduce with large tidal volumes, especially with membrane-based hydrophobic models. The need for a high-efficiency HME may be lessened when using low flows in circle systems. Some of this will be due to rebreathing of expired humidified gas plus the added effect of the heat- and water-generating reaction of CO_2 with soda lime. In pigs ventilated on a circle without an HME, a humidity level of 27 mg/L was noted in the inspiratory limb with an inspiratory flow of 0.6 L/min.[30] The efficiency of this approach seldom matches that of an HME. When using a pediatric circle, a low fresh gas flow (0.5 L/min) is associated with greater relative humidity than a high flow (6 L/min). However, the same low and high flows with an HME are associated with significantly better moisture retention at 20 minutes, and heat retention at 70 minutes, than even low flows without an HME.[31] Without an HME, the lag may be significant, up to an hour, to achieve adequate moisture and humidity even with flows of 1.5 L/min.[32] HMEs have unpredictable performance when used in conjunction with active humidification systems, and their combination generally is not recommended

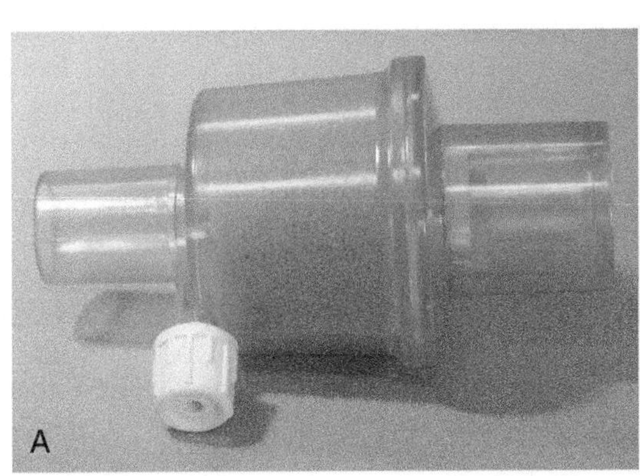

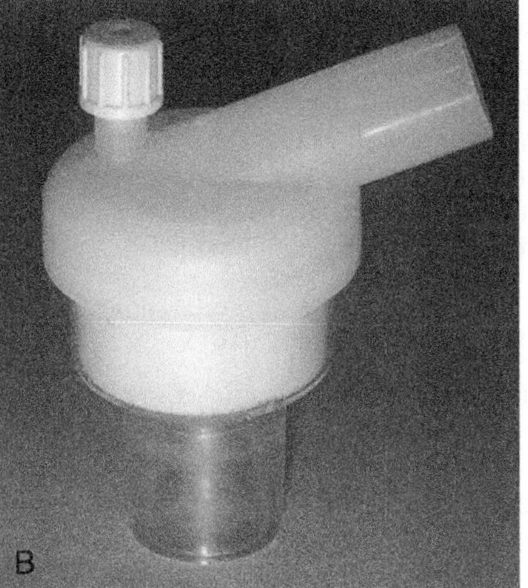

FIGURE 7-3 ■ Portex (**A**) (Smiths Medical, St. Paul, MN) and Hudson RCI (**B**) (Durham, NC) heat and moisture exchangers. Both have a foam element and a port for gas sampling.

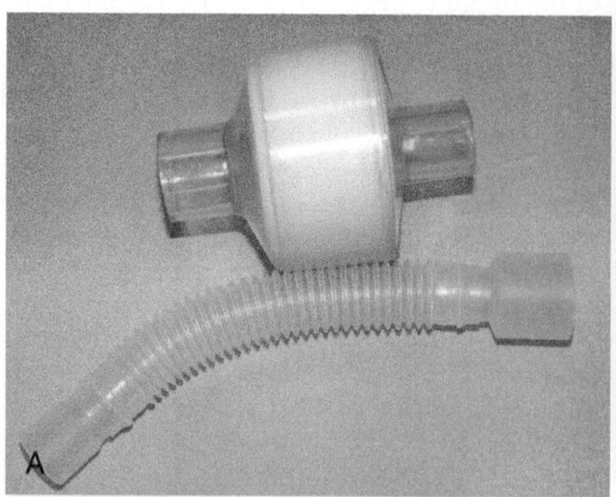

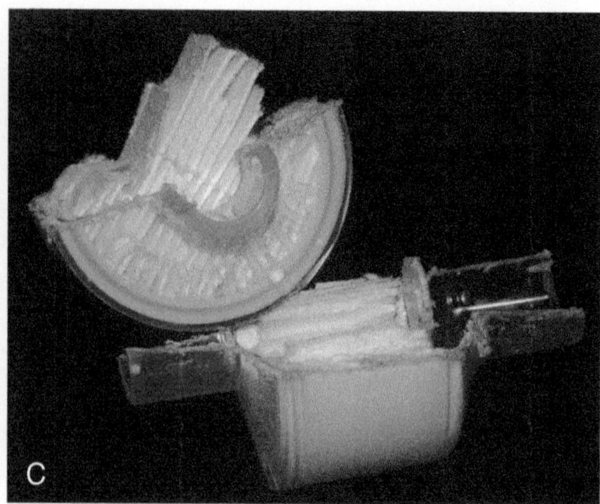

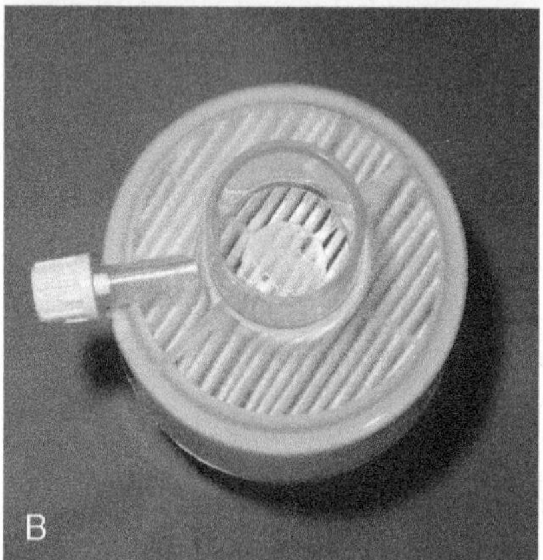

FIGURE 7-4 ■ **A,** A Portex (Smiths Medical, St. Paul, MN) heat and moisture exchanger with a high-efficiency particulate air filter and gas sampling port and optional flex tubing. The medium is a hydrophobic membrane. **B** and **C,** Cutaway of the device to demonstrate the folded design of the membrane, which greatly increases its surface area.

because it may result in saturation of the HME or removal of the hygroscopic coating.

Selecting an appropriate HME in pediatric practice is particularly difficult. Infants and neonates are especially vulnerable to respiratory water and heat loss as a result of a large ratio of minute volume to surface area. This may compound other potential heat losses, such as from a large ratio of skin surface area to volume, and may result in nonshivering thermogenesis in neonates. HMEs with low dead space are preferred, but these often have a lower moisture-retention efficiency. However the applicability to most pediatric practice of quoted in vitro performance at the relatively high test flows of 15 L/min has been brought into question. No HMEs are currently licensed for neonates who weigh less than 3 kg; treatment of such neonates requires the use of active humidifiers.

Heat and Moisture Exchanger Filters

HMEs may be modified to prevent bidirectional passage of both airborne and waterborne pathogens. These modified devices are known as *heat and moisture exchanger filters* (HMEFs), and they are the most commonly used device. HMEFs are designed to remove liquid or solid particles (aerosols) suspended in gas. This is achieved by reducing the pore size of the HME to less than 0.2 μm and/or coating it with a bacteriostatic or electrostatic substance. Larger particles may collide with the filter by direct inertial impaction or interception because the particle cannot follow the path of gas through the obstruction, or they may settle under gravitational influence. Small particles deviate from the gas flow by Brownian motion and make contact with fibers in the filter, and charged particles may be attracted to electrostatic filter fibers. Once in contact with the filter, particles generally adhere firmly (Figs. 7-4 and 7-5).

Potential Hazards and Limitations of Heat and Moisture Exchanger Filters

The HMEF helps the expiratory limb of the breathing circuit stay relatively dry, cool, and free of bacteria. It avoids condensation of water as cooling gas reaches its dew point, at which it may form a reservoir for nosocomial infection. In practice HMEFs are used to protect the patient from the inhaled particles and the anesthesia circuit from the patient to allow reuse. Modern anesthesia circuits are designed as single-use items, but for practical and economic reasons, some anesthesia circuits licensed for single use may be reused for up to 7 days in accordance with manufacturer guidelines, with a change of HMEF with each patient. Certain products have a special indemnity to be used for 7 days, with a new HMEF for each patient, but these should be changed if they become visibly soiled or after use on a known infectious patient.[33]

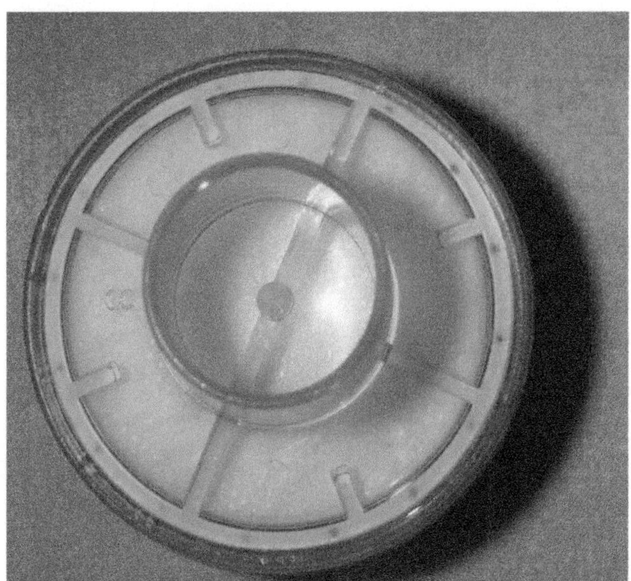

FIGURE 7-5 ■ **A,** Portex (Smiths Medical, St. Paul, MN) bacterial/viral filter without a heat and moisture exchanger, designed for use on the anesthesia circuit. It contains an electrostatically charged polypropylene medium.

No available filter is 100% efficient for all possible particle sizes. Evidence suggests that even bactericidal filters cannot reliably prevent contamination of the machine side of the circuit.[34] The clinical significance of circuit contamination and possible progression to clinical infection in subsequent patients in conjunction with a new HME is hotly debated. Current guidance by Association of Anaesthetists of Great Britain and Ireland is that the breathing circuit can be reused if a new suitable filter is used. Where use of a filter is undesirable, the circuit should be changed after each patient.[31] Guidelines for pediatric practice recommend that the circuit should be changed between each patient,[31] although in practice, circuits are often reused in conjunction with an HMEF. In the United States and Canada, practice is to replace the anesthesia circuit after each patient.[35]

Heated Humidifiers

Active heating and humidification of inspiratory gases may be considered when the mechanical effects of an HME or HMEF are undesirable, such as in neonates; patients with difficult respiratory secretions; or those in whom it is desirable to absolutely minimize heat or respiratory water losses, as with hypothermia.

Heated humidifiers contain a humidification chamber composed of water and a heat source. Gas may be passed over, or bubbled through, the reservoir. A heated wire inside the inspiratory limb may prevent gas cooling below its dew point and causing condensation; if this is not included, a water trap is required. Most heated humidifiers have a sensor at the patient end of the circuit with a servo control that regulates the output of the heating element. If excessive temperature is detected, the heat source power usually is cut as a safety feature. Inspiratory gas typically is heated to between 34° C and 40° C (Fig. 7-6).

Potential Hazards and Limitations of Heated Humidifiers

Heated humidifiers require energy and increased workload for filling, draining, and maintenance; hence, they are more expensive to run than HMEs. Heated humidifiers have a theoretical risk of electrical malfunction or overheating and thermal injury that is not possible with HMEs, and they carry risk of water aspiration from the tubing, water trap, or reservoir. In addition, heated humidifiers are not always more efficient than an HME. An efficient HME may reduce water losses to less than 7 mg/L, which is less than normal lower airway physiologic loss. The ISO minimum standard for the performance of an active humidifier is 33 mg H_2O/L, which would result in a water loss to the patient of 11 mg/L, falling below the efficiency of many HMEs. Heating inspired gas to 34° C does not improve humidification above that of an efficient HME. Only at temperatures of 37° C to 40° C can a heated humidifier reduce respiratory losses below 7 mg/L.

As saturated warm gas cools in the expiratory limb, it may reach its dew point and condense, which may rapidly form a reservoir that may become colonized with bacteria.[36] This is clearly a dangerous source of cross infection that precludes reuse of the circuit with another patient. Whether this reservoir of the patient's own flora can predispose to ventilator-associated pneumonia (VAP) is still under debate. Many individual studies have found no increase in the incidence of VAP with heated humidification, but a meta-analysis of eight randomized controlled trials (RCTs) found a relative risk reduction for VAP of 0.7 with HME use versus a heated humidifier,[37] particularly on patients ventilated for more than 7 days. However, a more recent RCT found an increase in VAP with HMEs and HMEFs over heated humidifiers.[38] With conflicting evidence, it is difficult to establish whether either is more associated with VAP, and this is reflected in a lack of official guidance on the matter.

SUMMARY

Understanding the importance of providing adequate heat and moisture to inspired medical gases to avoid patient harm is increasing. Optimal warmth and humidification can be achieved actively with heated humidifiers or passively with an HME or HMEF. Increasingly, HMEs and HMEFs are becoming the standard for routine humidification in anesthesia, and individual models vary enormously in their efficiency and in their effects on dead space and resistance. Heated humidifiers are expensive, cumbersome, labor intensive, and capable of achieving only a small benefit over HMEs and HMEFs in routine anesthesia. Heated humidifiers do offer some advantages in situations, such as with neonatal anesthesia and low tidal volume ventilation, in which the mechanical effects of HMEs and HMEFs may become significant. Further investigation may be required to determine whether heated humidifiers increase the incidence of VAP.

HMEFs are increasingly used to protect patients from inhaled microorganisms and allow circuit reuse. Although HMEFs have increasingly high filtration efficiencies, and

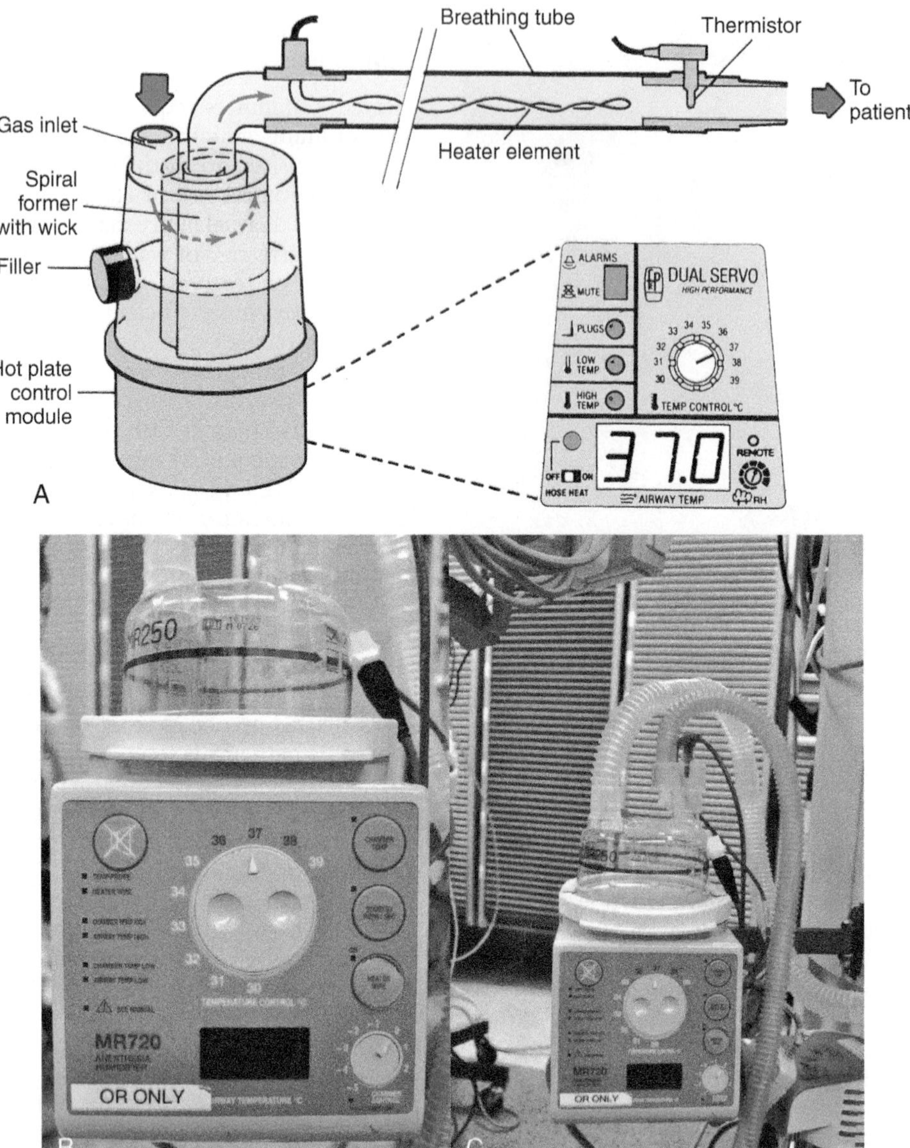

FIGURE 7-6 ■ **A,** Fisher & Paykel Healthcare (Auckland, New Zealand) humidifier system with heater element in the breathing tube. The unit shown has a spiral aluminum scroll and paper wick to increase evaporation during high flows. Also shown are the alarms and relative humidity control. The heated wire keeps the temperature of the gas constant and prevents "rain out." **B,** Fisher & Paykel dual servo heated humidifier, model MR720, for use in the operating room. The temperature and relative humidity can be adjusted. **C,** Humidifier in a breathing circuit. Note the heater wire inside the blue tubing. (A, From Mushin W, Jones P: *Physics for the anaesthetist,* ed 4. Boston, 1987, Blackwell Scientific. B anb C, CourtesyK. Premmer, MD.)

infection with circuit reuse in this way has not been proven, no HMEF provides a complete microbiologic barrier.

REFERENCES

1. Shelly MP: Conditioning of inspired gases. In Marini JJ, Slutsky AS, editors: *The physiological basis of ventilatory support*, New York, 1998, Marcel Dekker, pp 575–593.
2. Sottiaux TM: Consequences of under- and over-humidification. *Respir Care Clin North Am* 12:233–252, 2006.
3. Guyton AC: Partition of the body fluids: osmotic equilibria between extracellular and intracellelular fluids. In Guyton AC, editor: *Textbook of medical physiology*, Philadelphia, 1986, WB Saunders.
4. Dery R, Pelletier J, Jacques A: Humidity in anaesthesiology III. Heat and moisture patterns in the respiratory tract during anaesthesia with the semi-closed system, *Can Anaesth Soc J* 14:287–294, 1967.
5. Dery R: Humidity in anaesthesiology. Part IV: Determination of the alveolar humidity and temperature in the dog, *Can Anaesth Soc J* 18:145–151, 1971.
6 Walker JEC, Wells RE, Merrill EW: Heat and water exchange in the respiratory tract, *Am J Med* 30:259–267, 1961.
7. Sleigh MA, Blake JR, Liron N: The propulsion of mucus by cilia, *Am Rev Resp Dis* 137:726–741, 1988.
8. Negus VE: Humidification of the air passages, *Thorax* 7:148–151, 1952.
9. Widdicombe JH: Regulation of the depth and composition of airway surface liquid, *J Anatomy* 201:313–318, 2002.
10. Conway JH, Holgate ST: Humidification for patients with chronic chest disease, *Probl Respir Care* 4:463–473, 1991.
11 Eckerbom B: The airways during artificial respiration, *Acta Universitatis Upsaliensis, comprehensive summaries of Uppsala dissertations from the faculty of medicine*, vol 5, Stockholm, 1990, Aimqvist & Wiksell International, p 253.

12. Jiang C, Finkbeiner WE, Widdicombe JH, Miller SS: Fluid transport across cultures of human tracheal glands is altered in cystic fibrosis, *J Physiol* 501:637–648, 1997.
13. Rossman CM, Lee RMKW, Forrest JB, Newhouse MT: Nasal ciliary ultrastructure and function in patients with primary ciliary dyskinesia compared with that in normal subjects and in subjects with various respiratory diseases, *Am Rev Respir Dis* 129:161–167, 1984.
14. Stanley PJ, Wilson R, Greenstone MA, et al: Effect of cigarette smoking on nasal mucociliary clearance and ciliary beat frequency, *Thorax* 41:519–523, 1986.
15. Wilson R, Roberts D, Cole P: Effects of bacterial products on human ciliary function in vitro, *Thorax* 40:125–131, 1985.
16. Konrad F, Schreiber T, Brecht-Kraus D, Georgieff M: Mucociliary transport in ICU patients, *Chest* 105:237–241, 1994.
17. Forbes AR: Humidification and mucus flow in the intubated trachea, *Br J Anaesth* 45:874–878, 1973.
18. Noguchi H, Takumi Y, Aochi O: A study of humidification in tracheotomized dogs, *Br J Anaesth* 45:844–847, 1973.
19. Rashad K, Wilson K, Hurt HH, et al: Effect of humidification of anaesthetic gases on static compliance, *Anesth Analg Curr Res* 46:127–133, 1967.
20. Sims NM, Geoffrion CA, Welch PJ, et al: Respiratory tract burns caused by heated humidification of anesthetic gases in intubated, mechanically ventilated dogs: a light microscopic study, *Anaesthesiology* 65:A490, 1986.
21. Thiessen RJ: Filtration of respired gases: theoretical aspects. *Respir Care Clin North Am* 12:183–201, 2006.
22. Demers RR: Bacterial/viral filtration: let the breather beware! *Chest* 120:1377–1389, 2001.
23. Hardman JG, Curran J, Mahajan RP: End-tidal carbon dioxide measurement and breathing system filters, *Anaesthesia* 52:646–648, 1997.
24. Dorsch JA, Dorsch SE: Humidification equipment. In Dorsch JA, Dorsch SE, editors: *Understanding anaesthesia equipment*, ed 5, Philadelphia, 2008, Lippincott, Williams & Wilkins.
25. International Organization for Standardization (ISO): *Anaesthetic and respiratory equipment—heat and moisture exchangers (HMEs) for humidifying respired gases in humans—Part 1: HMEs for use with minimum tidal volumes of 250 mL, ISO 9360-1*, Geneva, 2000, International Organization for Standardization, Geneva Technical Committee.
26. Iotti GA, Olivei MC, Braschi A: Equipment review: mechanical effects of heat-moisture exchangers in ventilated patients, *Crit Care* 3:R77–R82, 1999.
27. Pellosi P, Solca M, Ravagnan M, et al: Effects of heat and moisture exchangers on minute ventilation, ventilatory drive, and work of breathing during pressure-support ventilation in acute respiratory failure, *Crit Care Med* 24:1184–1188, 1996.
28. Ricard JD, Le Miere E, Markowicz P, et al: Efficiency and safety of mechanical ventilation with a heat and moisture exchanger changed only once a week, *Am J Respir Crit Care Med* 161(1): 104–109, 2000.
29. Lemmens MJM, Brock-Utne JG: Heat and moisture exchange devices: are they doing what they are supposed to do? *Anesth Analg* 98:382–385, 2004.
30. Kleemann PP: The climatisation of anaesthetic gases under conditions of high flow to low flow, *Acta Anaesthesiol Belg* 41:189–200, 1990.
31. Nakae Y, Horikawa D, Tamiya K, et al: Humidification during low flow anaesthesia in children, *J Anaesth* 12:175–179, 1998.
32. Kleeman PP: Humidity of anaesthetic gases with respect to low flow anaesthesia, *Anaesth Intensive Care* 22:396–408, 1994.
33. Association of Anaesthetists of Great Britain and Ireland: Infection control in anaesthesia, *Anaesthesia* 63:1027–1036, 2008.
34. Neft MW, Goodman JR, Hlavnika JP, Velt BC: To reuse your circuit: the HME debate, *AANA J* 67:433–439, 1999.
35. Carter JA: The reuse of breathing systems in anaesthesia, *Respir Care Clin* 12:275–286, 2006.
36. Craven DE, Goularte TA, Make BJ: Contaminated condensate in mechanical ventilator circuits: a risk factor for nosocomial pneumonia, *Am Rev Respir Dis* 129:625–628, 1984.
37. Kola A, Eckmanns T, Gastmeier P: Efficacy of heat and moisture exchangers in preventing ventilator-associated pneumonia: meta-analysis of randomised controlled trials, *Intensive Care Med* 31:5–11, 2005.
38. Lorente L, Lecuona M, Jimenez A, et al: Ventilator-associated pneumonia using a heated humidifier or a heat and moisture exchanger: a randomized controlled trial, *Crit Care* 10:R116, 2006.

PART II

SYSTEM MONITORS

CHAPTER 8

RESPIRATORY GAS MONITORING*

James B. Eisenkraft • Michael B. Jaffe

CHAPTER OUTLINE

OVERVIEW

The gases of interest to the anesthesia caregiver include oxygen, carbon dioxide, nitrous oxide, and the potent inhaled anesthetic agents. Other gases that may be relevant in certain situations are nitrogen, helium, nitric oxide, and xenon. Although gas monitors from different manufacturers may appear to offer various options to the user, ultimately, these monitors use one or more of a limited number of technologies to make the analysis and present the data.

The monitoring of respired gases has evolved considerably over the past few years. Contemporary systems are reliable, accurate, have rapid response times, and are becoming less expensive as a result of competition among manufacturers. Early gas monitoring systems were large, stand-alone units that usually were placed on a shelf on the anesthesia machine (Fig. 8-1). As a result of advances in technology and miniaturization, on many contemporary anesthesia workstations, gas analysis is performed in one component module of a modular physiologic

*Parts of this chapter are reproduced by permission from Eisenkraft JB: Respiratory gas monitoring. In Reich DL et al, editors: *Monitoring in Anesthesia and Perioperative Care*, New York, 2011, Cambridge University Press.

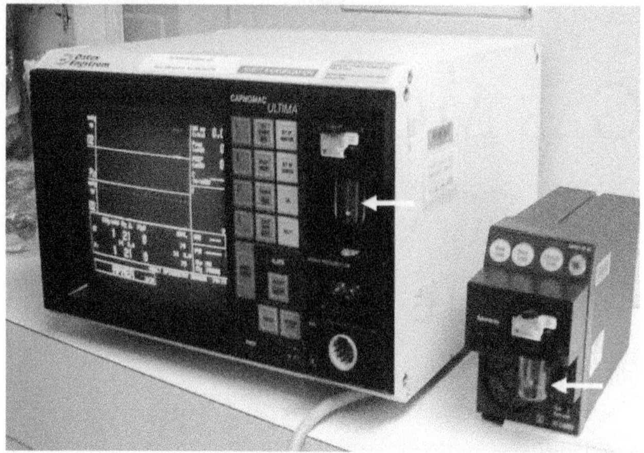

FIGURE 8-1 ■ *Left:* The Datex Capnomac Ultima stand-alone multigas analyzer (GE Healthcare, Waukesha, WI) used infrared analysis for carbon dioxide, nitrous oxide, and anesthetic agents and paramagnetic analysis for oxygen. *Right:* The much smaller GE Compact Airway module uses the same technologies to perform the same functions. *Arrows* indicate water traps.

monitoring system (Fig. 8-2). This chapter is intended to provide a framework for understanding the methods by which respiratory gases are analyzed as well as clinical applications, limitations, and pertinent standards of care.

GAS SAMPLING SYSTEMS

For a respired gas mixture to be analyzed, either the gas must be brought to the analyzer, or the analyzer must be brought to the gas in the airway. A fuel cell oxygen analyzer located in the breathing system by the inspiratory unidirectional valve is one example of bringing the analyzer to the gas in the circuit. Figure 8-3 shows two mainstream analyzer modules. Because gas is not removed from the circuit for analysis elsewhere, this is termed a *nondiverting* or *mainstream* analyzer. Alternatively, and more commonly, the gas to be analyzed is continuously sampled from the vicinity of the patient's airway and is conducted via fine-bore tubing to the analyzer unit (Fig. 8-4). This arrangement is termed a *sidestream* or *diverting* system because the gas is diverted from the airway for analysis elsewhere.

Gas analysis is performed in real time so that changes can be rapidly appreciated by the anesthesia caregiver. It is therefore important to know the *total response time* of the complete system. The total response time is composed of two components: the transit time and the rise time. The *transit time* is the time lag for the gas sample to reach the analyzer; this term applies only to systems that use diverting gas sampling. The *rise time* is the time taken by the analyzer to react to the change in gas concentration. An analyzer's reponse to a sudden (square wave) change in gas concentration is generally sigmoid in shape, so that rise time is specified as the time to change from 10% to 90% of the sudden total change in gas concentration at the analyzer inlet (Fig. 8-5). As an example, the Datex Compact Airway module (GE Healthcare, Waukesha, WI; see Fig. 8-1, *right*) with a 3-meter sampling line and 200 ± 20 mL/min gas sampling rate typically has a sampling delay time of 2.5 seconds and a total response time of 2.9 seconds, which includes the sampling delay and

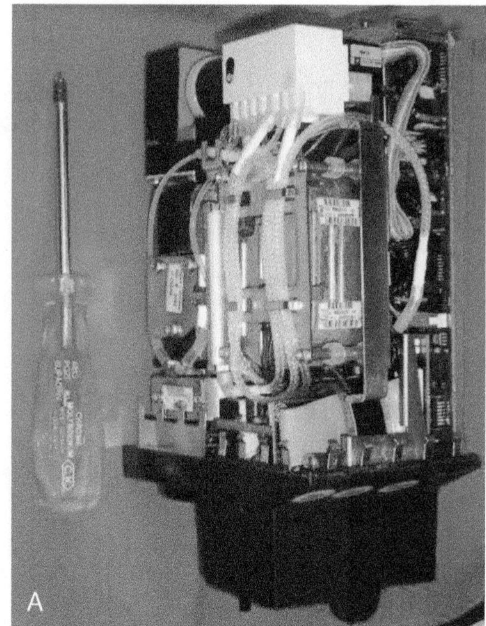

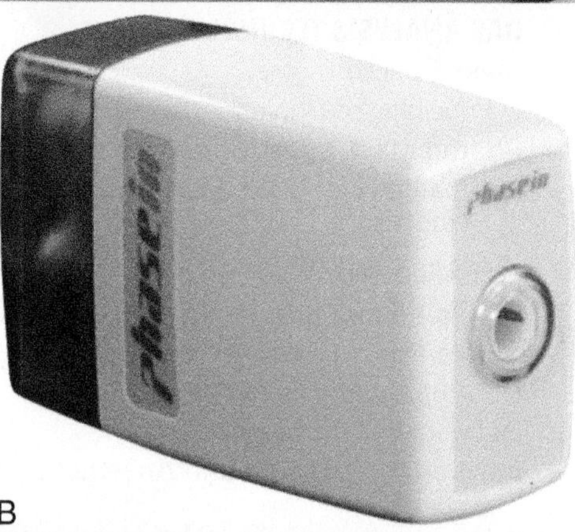

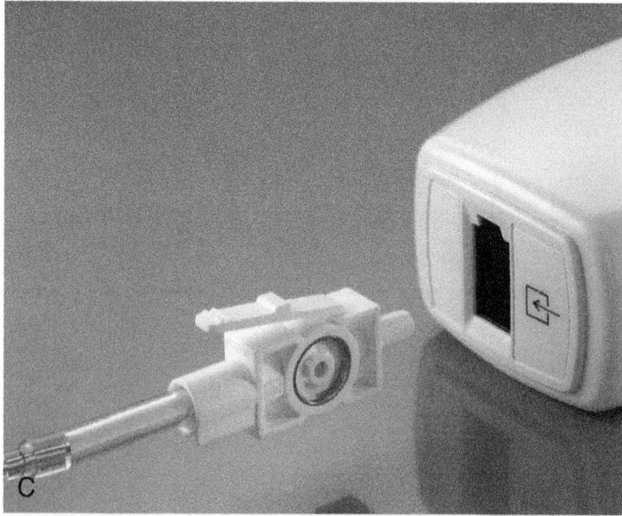

FIGURE 8-2 ■ **A,** GE Compact Airway module (GE Healthcare, Waukesha, WI). **B,** Phasein sidestream-sampling multigas analyzer module. **C,** Philips Respironics LoFlo CO_2 module. (**B,** Courtesy Phasein AB, Danderyd, Sweden; **C,** Courtesy Philips Respironics, Wallingford, CT.)

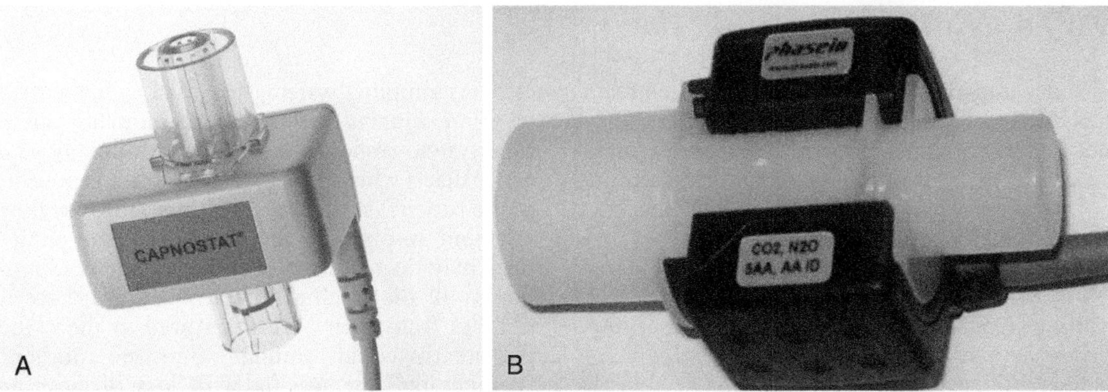

FIGURE 8-3 ■ **A,** Mainstream lightweight Capnostat 5 carbon dioxide sensor. **B,** Mainstream multigas analyzer module that measures carbon dioxide, nitrous oxide, oxygen, and anesthetic agents. The IRMA plug-in and measure are also shown. (A, Courtesy Philips Respironics, Wallingford, CT. **B,** Courtesy Phasein AB, Danderyd, Sweden.)

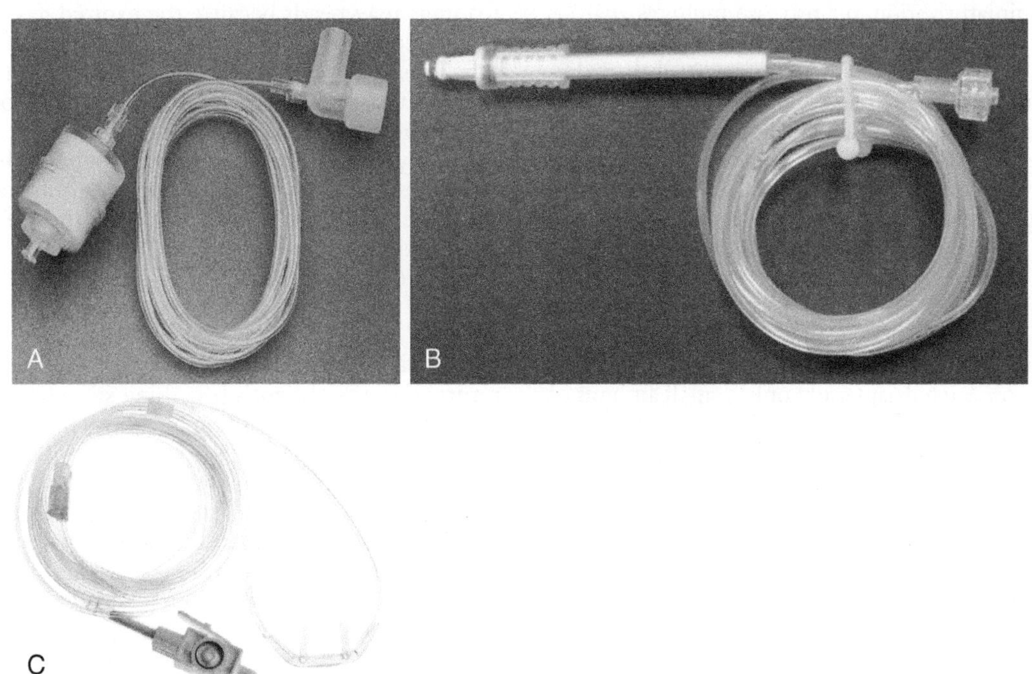

FIGURE 8-4 ■ **A,** Gas-sampling tubing and airway adapter for sidestream-sampling gas analyzers. **B,** Nomoline gas sampling tubing with integral moisture/water removal filter. **C,** Nasal cannula with sampling tubing and integral filter/removable sample cell. (A, Courtesy Phasein AB, Danderyd, Sweden. **B,** Courtesy Philips Respironics, Wallingford, CT.)

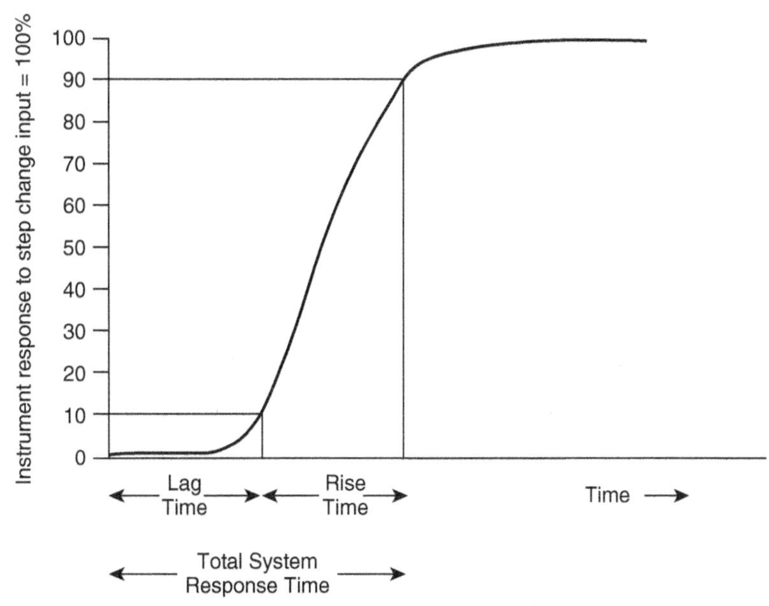

FIGURE 8-5 ■ *Delay time* (lag time) is the time from a step function change in CO_2 concentration at the sampling site to the achievement of 10% of the final CO_2 value in the capnometer. *Rise time* is the time required to achieve a rise from 10% to 90% of the final CO_2 value in the capnometer when a step function change in CO_2 concentration occurs at the sampling site.

rise time.[1] For comparison, the Capnostat 5 mainstream carbon dioxide sensor (Philips Respironics, Wallingford, CT) is specified to have a rise time of less than 60 ms. A rapid total system response time is essential for accurate concentration readings and high-fidelity waveforms.

Nondiverting (Mainstream) Systems

In nondiverting systems, gas flows past the analyzer interface placed in the main gas stream. Until recently, mainstream analysis at the patient's airway was possible only for carbon dioxide using infrared (IR) technology (Mainstream, Philips Respironics) and by the inspiratory unidirectional valve for oxygen using a fuel cell. As a result of advances in miniaturization, mainstream multigas analysis at the patient's airway is now available (Phasein, Danderyd, Sweden); this permits rapid acquisition of breath-by-breath data for carbon dioxide, nitrous oxide, oxygen, and the five potent inhaled anesthetics. Although mainstream analyzers overcome the gas sampling problem, they require a special airway adapter and analysis module to be placed in the breathing system near the patient's airway. From this location, the analyzers produce a sharp concentration-versus-time waveform in real time, but they may be vulnerable to damage with repeated drops onto hard surfaces. New designs are lightweight, such as the Phasein IRMA sensor head, which uses a miniaturized, spinning filter wheel that weighs only 1 oz. Such designs add only a small amount of dead space, and some, such as the Capnostat 5, use solid-state technology. In addition, waste gas scavenging is not necessary with nondiverting systems.

Mainstream analyzer modules are subject to interference by water vapor, secretions, and blood. Because condensed water blocks all IR wavelengths, leaving too low a source intensity to make a measurement, spurious carbon dioxide readings might result. The cuvette's window may be heated (usually to 41° C), or it may be coated with water-repellant material to prevent such condensation and interference. Adding the mainstream analyzer to the breathing system creates two additional interfaces for a potential breathing circuit disconnection. Disposable breathing system adapters are now available, whereas previously, the nondisposable adapters required cleaning between patient uses. In addition, a mainstream carbon dioxide analyzer is now available for patients receiving oxygen via nasal cannula (Cap-ONE, Nihon Kohden America, Foothill Ranch, CA).

Sidestream (Diverting) Systems

Compared with mainstream analyzers, the advantages of diverting analyzers are that, because they are remote from the patient, they can be of any size and therefore offer more versatility in terms of monitoring capabilities. They can be used when the monitor must be remote from the patient, such as in magnetic resonance imaging (MRI) or radiation therapy. The sampled gas is continually drawn from the breathing circuit via an adapter placed between the circuit and the patient's airway (the Y-piece in a circle breathing system); it passes through a filter or water trap (Fig. 8-1, *arrows*) before entering the analyzer. The gas sampling flow rate is usually about 200 mL/min, with a range of 50 to 250 mL/min. Disadvantages include problems with the catheter sampling system, such as clogging with secretions or water, kinking, failure of the sampling pump, slower total system response time (although usually <3 seconds), and artifacts when the gas sampling rate is poorly matched to the patient's inspiratory and expiratory gas flow rates.

Rapid respiratory rates and long sampling catheter lines may decrease the accuracy of the readings and the fidelity of the tracings. This is because there would be samples from many breaths stored in the catheter, and the breaths could "smudge" into one another, thereby "dampening" the tracing with loss of clear peaks and troughs. If a diverting system is used with a very small patient, such as a neonate, and the gas sampling rate exceeds the patient's expiratory gas flow rate, spurious readings may result because the expired gas will be contaminated by fresh gas. Similarly, if an uncuffed tracheal tube is used and a leak develops between the tube and the trachea, the gas sampling pump may draw room air into the tracheal tube and into the analyzer.

Ideally, the gas sampling flow rate should be appropriate for the patient and for the breathing circuit used. Thus the sampling flow rate may limit the use of low-flow or closed-circuit anesthesia techniques. If the gas sampling rate exceeds the fresh gas inflow rate, the potential exists for negative pressures to be created in the breathing system.[2] Once the sampled gas has been analyzed, it should be directed to the waste gas scavenging system or returned to the patient's breathing system.

Leaks in the gas sampling line, both inside the monitor and between the patient's airway and the monitor inlet, will result in erroneous readings that may or may not be obvious. These monitors require calibration using a certified standard gas mixture that is directed into the monitor's gas inlet connection. A leak inside the monitor that allows room air to contaminate the gas sample would result in miscalibration.[3]

In multigas analyzers that incorporate a paramagnetic oxygen sensor, simultaneous room air sampling (10 mL/min) is required to provide a reference. This air is therefore added to the waste gas exiting the monitor at a rate of 10 mL/min; it may then be returned to the patient circuit. This might create a problem during closed-circuit anesthesia because nitrogen, albeit at a rate of about 8 mL/min, would be added to the breathing circuit (see Paramagnetic Oxygen Analyzers later in this chapter).

UNITS OF MEASUREMENT

The respiratory tract and the anesthesia delivery system contain respired gases in the form of molecules that are in constant motion. When the molecules strike the walls of their container, they give rise to *pressure*, defined as force per unit of area; the greater the number of gas molecules present, the greater the pressure exerted for any given temperature. Dalton's law of partial pressures states that the total pressure exerted by a mixture of gases is equal to the arithmetic sum of the partial pressures exerted by each gas in the mixture. The total pressure of all gases in the anesthesia system at sea level is equivalent to approximately 760 mm Hg. Although anesthetic gas monitors may display data expressed in millimeters of mercury (mm Hg), kilopascals (1 kPa = 7.5 mm Hg), or as volumes percent (vol%), it is important to understand in principle how the measurement was made. The reader should understand the difference between *partial pressure*, an absolute term, and *volumes percent*, an expression of a proportion, or ratio.

If the partial pressure of one component of a gas mixture is known, a reading in volumes percent can be computed as follows:

Partial pressure of gas (mm Hg)
÷ Total pressure of all gases (mm Hg) × 100 %

Number of Molecules (Partial Pressure)

An analytic method based on quantifying a specific property of a gas molecule determines in absolute terms—that is, in millimeters of mercury or kilopascals—the number of molecules of that gas that are present. Gas molecules composed of two or more dissimilar atoms—such as carbon dioxide, nitrous oxide, and the potent inhaled anesthetics—have bonds between their component atoms. Certain wavelengths of IR radiation excite these molecules, stretching or distorting the bonds, and the molecules also absorb the radiation. Carbon dioxide molecules absorb IR radiation at a wavelength of approximately 4.3 μm. The greater the number of molecules of carbon dioxide present, the more radiation at 4.3 μm absorbed. This property of the carbon dioxide molecule is applied in the IR carbon dioxide analyzer. Because the total amount of IR radiation absorbed at a specific wavelength is determined by the *number* of molecules present, and the motion of each molecule contributes to the total pressure, the amount of radiation absorbed is a function of partial pressure; thus, an IR analyzer measures partial pressure.

In the analysis of gases by Raman spectroscopy, as was used in the Datex-Ohmeda Rascal II analyzer (GE Healthcare), a helium-neon laser emits monochromatic light at a wavelength of 633 nm. When this light interacts with the intramolecular bonds of specific gas molecules, it is scattered and reemitted at wavelengths different from that of the incident monochromatic light. Each reemission wavelength is characteristic of a specific gas molecule present in the gas mixture and therefore is a function of its partial pressure. Thus Raman spectroscopy also measures partial pressures.

A sufficient number of molecules of any gas to be analyzed—that is, adequate partial pressures—must be present to facilitate gas analysis by the IR and Raman technologies. These systems also must be pressure compensated if analyses are being made at ambient pressures other than those used for the original calibration of the systems.[4]

Measurement of Proportion (Volumes Percent)

Another approach to gas analysis is to separate the molecular component species of a gas mixture and determine what proportion (percentage) each gas contributes to the total (100%). This approach is applied in mass spectrometry. Thus, if 21 molecules of oxygen were in a sample of gas containing 100 molecules, oxygen would represent 21% of the gas sample and therefore might reasonably be assumed to represent 21% of the original gas mixture. The result is expressed as 21 vol% or as a fractional concentration (0.21). This monitor does not measure partial pressures; it measures only proportions. If the system is provided with an absolute pressure reading that is equivalent to 100%, the basic measured proportions can be converted to readings in millimeters of mercury. In the above example, if 100% were made equivalent to 760 mm Hg, oxygen would have a calculated partial pressure of 159 mm Hg (760 × 21%).

These fundamental differences in the approaches to gas analysis and their basic units of measurement are important, particularly when the data presented by these monitors are interpreted in a clinical setting and may affect patient management.

GAS ANALYSIS TECHNOLOGIES

Contemporary respiratory multigas analyzers use some form of IR spectroscopy to measure carbon dioxide, nitrous oxide, and the potent inhaled anesthetic agents. The same multigas analyzers measure oxygen by a paramagnetic, rapid-responding analyzer or by a fuel cell (slow or rapid responding). Although some technologies are no longer in general clinical use, it is worthwhile to review them briefly to appreciate their principles of operation and how monitoring has evolved.

Mass Spectrometry

For many anesthesia caregivers, the term *mass spec* is used as if it were synonymous with respiratory gas analysis. Indeed, many anesthetic record forms still incorrectly include this term, but this technology is no longer in routine clinical use. It was, however, the first multigas monitoring system in widespread clinical use, following a description by Ozanne and colleagues in 1981.[5]

The mass spectrometer is an instrument that allows the identification and quantification, on a breath-by-breath basis, of up to eight of the gases commonly encountered during the administration of an inhalational anesthetic. These gases include oxygen, nitrogen, nitrous oxide, halothane, enflurane, and isoflurane. Other agents—such as helium, sevoflurane, argon, and desflurane—could sometimes be added or substituted if desired. Although the technology of mass spectrometry had been available for many years, analyzer units dedicated to a single patient were too expensive for routine use in each operating room (OR). In 1981, the concept of a shared, or multiplexed, system was introduced.[5] This arrangement allowed one centrally located analyzer to function as part of a computerized, multiplexed system that could serve up to 31 patient sampling locations (ORs and recovery room or intensive care unit [ICU] beds) on a time-share basis.[6] The two multiplexed systems that became widely used were the Perkin Elmer system, which later became the Marquette Advantage system, and the System for Anesthetic and Respiratory Analysis (SARA).

Principles of Operation

The mass spectrometer analyzer unit separates the components of a stream of charged particles (ions) into a

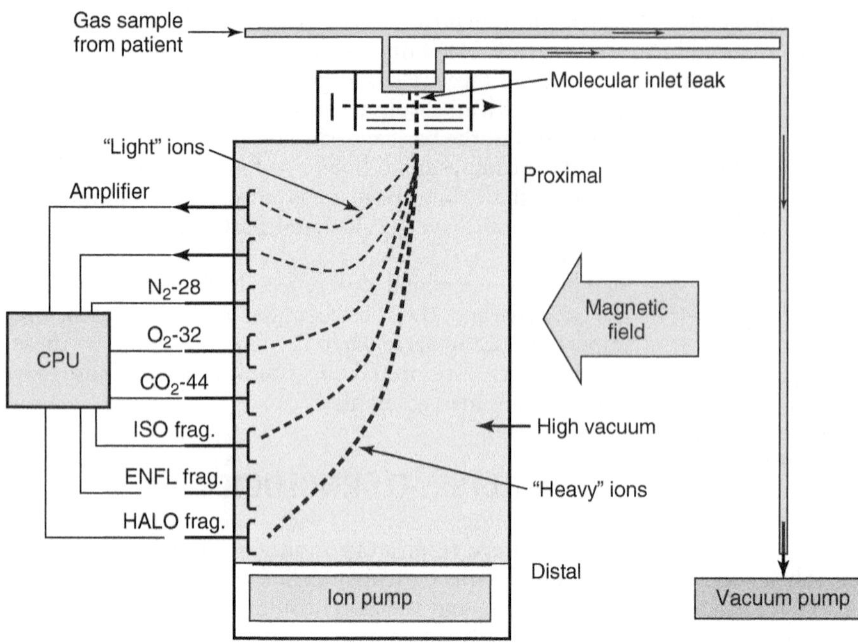

FIGURE 8-6 Schematic of a magnetic sector respiratory mass spectrometer. The respiratory gas is sampled and drawn over a molecular inlet leak. Gas molecules enter a vacuum chamber through the leak, where they are ionized and electrically accelerated. A magnetic field deflects the ions. The mass and charge of the ions determine their trajectory, and metal dish collectors are placed to detect them. The electrical currents produced by the ions impacting the collectors are processed, the composition is computed, and the results are displayed. *CPU,* central processing unit; *ENFL,* enflurane; *frag.,* fragment; *HALO,* halothane; *ISO,* isoflurane.

spectrum according to their mass/charge (m/z) ratios. The relative abundance of ions at certain specific m/z ratios is determined and is related to the *fractional* composition of the original gas mixture. The creation and manipulation of ions is carried out in a high vacuum (10^{-5} mm Hg) to avoid interference by outside air and to minimize random collisions among the ions and residual gases.

The most common design of mass spectrometer was the magnetic sector analyzer, so called because it uses a permanent magnet to separate the ion beam into its component ion spectra (Fig. 8-6). A stream of gas (250 mL/min) to be analyzed is continuously drawn by a sampling pump from an airway connector via a long nylon catheter, an example of a sidestream-sampling system. During transit through the sampling catheter, the pressure decreases from atmospheric pressure, usually 760 mm Hg, in the patient circuit to approximately 40 mm Hg by the inlet of the analyzer unit. A very small amount of the gas actually sampled from the circuit, approximately 10^{-6} mL/sec, enters the analyzer unit's high-vacuum chamber through the molecular inlet leak. The gas molecules are then bombarded by an electron beam, which causes some of the molecules to lose one or more electrons and become positively charged ions. Thus an oxygen molecule (O_2) might lose one electron and become an oxygen ion (O_2^+) with one positive charge. The m/z ratio would therefore be 32/1, or 32. If the oxygen molecule lost two electrons, it would gain two positive charges, and the resulting ion (O_2^{2+}) would have an m/z ratio of 32/2, or 16. The process of electron bombardment also causes large molecules—such as halothane, enflurane, and isoflurane—to become fragmented, or "cracked," into smaller, positively charged ions.

The positive ions created in the analyzer are then focused into a beam by the electrostatic fields in the ion source, directed through a slit to define an exact shape for the beam, and accelerated and directed into the field of the permanent magnet. The magnetic field influences the direction of the ions and causes each ion species to curve in a trajectory whose arc is related to its m/z ratio. The effect is to create several separate ion beams exiting the magnetic field. The separated beams are directed to individual collectors, which detect the ion current and transmit it to amplifiers that create output voltages in relation to the abundance of the ion species detected. The collector plates are positioned so that an ion with a specific m/z ratio strikes a specific collector. The heaviest ions are deflected the least and travel the furthest before striking a collector (see Fig. 8-6). Collectors for these heavy ions are therefore located farthest from the ion source. Summing and other computer software measure the total voltage from all the collector circuits as well as measuring the individual voltages from each collector. Total voltage is considered equivalent to 100% of the analyzed gas mixture.

Individual gas collector circuit voltages are expressed as percentages of the total voltage and are displayed as percentages of the sampled gas mixture. Thus if the voltage from the oxygen collector circuit (m/z ratio = 32) represented 30% of the total voltage from all the collector circuits, oxygen would be read as constituting 30% of the total gas mixture analyzed. The Marquette Advantage and SARA systems used magnetic sector analyzers that had up to eight collectors and therefore were able to detect and analyze up to eight different ion types and their parent gases.

The mass spectrometer functions as a *proportioning* system for the components of a gas mixture. When it displays each of the components of the mixture as a percentage of the total, it makes the assumption that all the gases present have been detected. If ambient (atmospheric) pressure information is entered into the software, the measured percentages or proportions can be converted to readings in millimeters of mercury (i.e., partial pressures). It must be remembered that the mass spectrometer does not *measure* partial pressures; it *calculates* them from the measured proportions and the atmospheric pressure information that must be supplied to it. Thus

Partial pressure (mm Hg) =
Fractional concentration × Total pressure (mm Hg)

Usually, because the mass spectrometer was sampling respired gases from the patient circuit, the total pressure entered into the computer was ambient pressure minus 47 mm Hg, the latter representing the saturated vapor pressure of water at body temperature (37° C). Thus at sea level (760 mm Hg), a pressure of 713 mm Hg would be entered into the mass spectrometer software to be apportioned among the gases present. The mass spectrometer readings, when displayed in millimeters of mercury, represent somewhat of a compromise because inspired gas usually is not fully saturated with water vapor, whereas expired gas usually is. If an incorrect value for total ambient pressure were to be entered into the mass spectrometer software, all readings in millimeters of mercury would be incorrect, but the readings in volumes percent would be correct. For example, assume that end-tidal carbon dioxide is measured as 5% by the mass spectrometer and that ambient pressure is 760 mm Hg. The reading in millimeters of mercury will be 35.65 ([760 − 47] × 5%). If a value of 500 mm Hg is entered instead of 713 mm Hg, the reading will be 25 mm Hg (500 × 5%). In any case of doubt, the astute clinician would revert to the reading in volumes percent; hence the importance of understanding how the displayed value is obtained.

Shared Mass Spectrometry Systems

Multiplexing permitted the sharing of one (rather expensive) mass spectrometer analyzer unit among up to 31 sampling locations, or stations. In a shared system, the gas from each sampling location is directed in sequence by the multiplexing valve system to the mass spectrometer for analysis. In a multiplexed system, the time between analyses at any particular location therefore depended on 1) the number of breaths analyzed from each sampling location (i.e., dwell time), 2) the number of sampling locations in use, 3) the priority settings, and 4) in the case of "stat" samples, the distance between sampling locations and the analyzer, which was up to 300 feet in some installations.

Use of multiplexed mass spectrometry systems led anesthesia caregivers to appreciate the value of continual (i.e., frequently repeated), although not continuous (without interruption), respiratory gas monitoring and the limitations—the main one being that the systems were shared, which meant that data were updated only intermittently.

In October 1986, the American Society of Anesthesiologists (ASA) first approved standards for basic intraoperative monitoring. As the standards evolved, the requirement for *continuous* capnometry was not met by a shared mass spectrometry system. The systems were expensive to install and maintain, and they were not always easily upgradable when the new agents desflurane and sevoflurane were introduced. In addition, the long sampling catheters combined with rapid respiratory rates led to significant artifact; the sampling pump could cause considerable negative pressure in the breathing system, and when the system failed, all the monitored sites were affected.[7,8] Practitioners demanded continuous gas monitoring. The most important functions of a multiplexed mass spectrometry system could be served by other dedicated gas monitors, and the multiplexed, mass spectrometer–based systems became extinct.

Dedicated (Stand-Alone) Mass Spectrometry Systems

A number of smaller stand-alone mass spectrometers were developed for dedicated single-patient use. One model, the Ohmeda 6000 Multigas Analyzer, was a quadrupole-filter mass spectrometer.[9] It worked on the principle that, with regard to the m/z ratio of ions, a controlled electrostatic field can prevent all but a narrow range of charged particles from reaching a target. In the Ohmeda 6000 unit, the gas sampling rate was fixed at 30 mL/min. One advantage of the quadrupole system was that it could be adapted to measure new or additional agents by changes in software only. A number of other stand-alone, quadrupole-filter mass spectrometers were marketed, but their production was discontinued as a result of cost and reliability issues.

INFRARED ANALYSIS

The IR spectrum ranges between wavelengths of 0.40 μm and 40 μm. Measurement of the energy absorbed from a narrow band of wavelengths of IR radiation as it passes through a gas sample can be used to measure the concentrations of certain gases. Asymmetric, polyatomic, polar molecules—such as carbon dioxide, nitrous oxide, water, and the potent volatile anesthetic agents—absorb IR energy when their atoms rotate or vibrate asymmetrically; this results in a change in dipole moment, the charge distribution within the molecule. The nonpolar molecules argon, nitrogen, helium, xenon, and oxygen do not absorb IR energy. Because the number of gas molecules in the path of the IR energy beam determines the total absorption, IR analyzers measure the partial pressure.

IR analyzers are classified as *dispersive* or *nondispersive*. In a *dispersive analyzer*, after passing through the gas sample, the radiation emitted by an IR source is separated, or dispersed, into the component wavelengths and is arranged sequentially. When gas to be analyzed is put in the path of the spectrum of radiation, it absorbs radiation in one or more parts of the spectrum. By examining the entire spectrum, a plot of absorbance versus wavelength is obtained (Fig. 8-7), from which the gas composition can be analyzed and quantified, provided the gases in the mixture have characteristic absorption peaks.

In the *nondispersive analyzer*, radiation from the IR source is filtered to allow passage of only the specific wavelength bands, for which the gases of interest have distinct absorption peaks. The gas sample is placed between the filter and the IR detector (Fig. 8-8) or

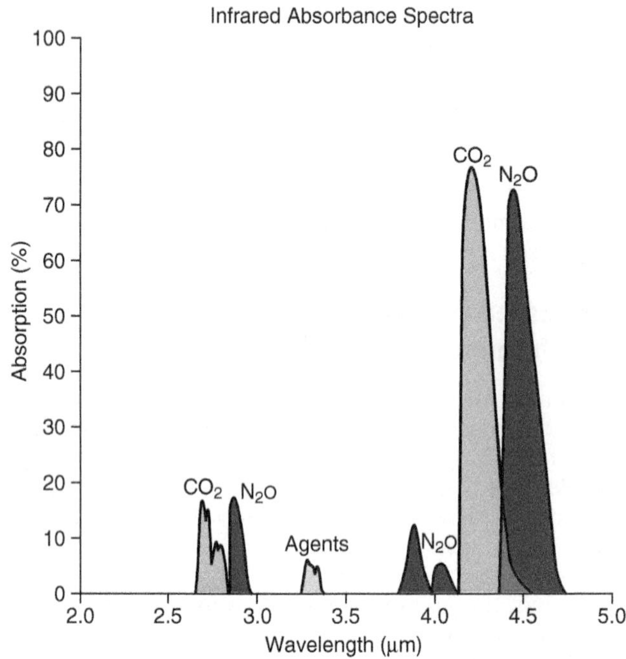

FIGURE 8-7 ■ Absorption bands of respiratory gases in the infrared spectrum. (From Raemer DB: Monitoring respiratory function. In Rogers MC, Tinker JH, Covino BG, Longnecker DE, editors: *Principles and practice of anesthesiology*. St Louis, 1992, Mosby–Year Book.)

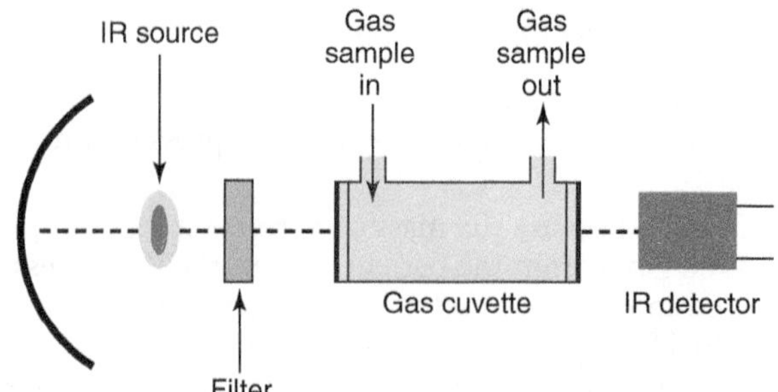

FIGURE 8-8 ■ Block diagram of a simple, single-wavelength, infrared (*IR*) respiratory gas analyzer. An IR source emits a beam that passes through a filter, which passes only the wavelength absorbed by the gas of interest. The respiratory gas from the patient is sampled and passes through the gas cell in the optical path. An IR detector measures intensity of the IR wavelength that has passed through the gas sample; intensity is inversely related to the partial pressure of that gas in the sample cell. The electrical signal from the detector is processed to report the gas composition (in millimeters of mercury); this value can be automatically converted to a reading in volumes percent if the ambient pressure is known.

between the IR source and the filter (Fig. 8-9). With the exception of the Andros, the IR analyzers used clinically are predominantly of the nondispersive type.

Carbon dioxide, nitrous oxide, and anesthetic gases exhibit absorption of radiation at unique bands in the IR spectrum (see Fig. 8-7). Carbon dioxide molecules absorb strongly between 4.2 and 4.4 μm, whereas nitrous oxide molecules absorb strongly between 4.4 and 4.6 μm and less strongly at 3.9 μm. The potent volatile anesthetic agents have strong absorption bands at 3.3 μm and throughout the range 8 to 12 μm.

The close proximity of the nitrous oxide and carbon dioxide absorption bands may cause some analyzers to be affected by high concentrations of nitrous oxide.[10,11] The impact of this cross-interference—that is, the overlapping of absorption bands of other gases—can vary significantly among devices. The use of narrow-band sources or narrow-band filters with sufficiently small bandwidths can effectively reduce the impact of cross interference. The presence of other gases, which may or may not have overlapping absorption bands, can also affect the measurement. This phenomenon is called *collision broadening* or *pressure broadening* because molecular collisions result in a change in the dipole moment of the gas being analyzed; thus the IR absorption band is broadened, and the apparent absorption at the measurement wavelength may be altered.[12] In a typical IR carbon dioxide analyzer, 95% oxygen causes a 0.5% decline in the measured carbon dioxide. Nitrous oxide causes a more substantial increase of approximately 0.1% carbon dioxide per 10% nitrous oxide because of collision broadening. Contemporary multigas analyzers can automatically compensate for the effect of collision broadening if they measure the concentrations of interfering gases.

A simple nondispersive IR analyzer (see Fig. 8-8) consists of the following basic elements:

1. *A source of IR radiation, typically a heated black body.* A black body radiator is a theoretical object that is totally absorbent to all thermal energy that falls on it; it does not reflect any light and therefore appears black. As it absorbs energy, it heats up and reradiates the energy as electromagnetic radiation. Heating the black body causes emission of IR radiation.
2. *A sample cell, or cuvette.* The gas to be analyzed is drawn through the cuvette by a sampling pump.
3. *A detector that generates an output signal.* The signal is related to the intensity of the IR radiation that falls on it.
4. *A narrow-band pass filter.* This filter allows only radiation at the wavelength bands of interest to pass through; it is interposed between the IR source and the cuvette (see Fig. 8-8) or between the cuvette and the detector (see Fig. 8-9). The intensity of radiation reaching the detector is inversely related to the concentration of the specific gas being measured.

A number of sources of IR radiation can be used to produce a broad spectrum of IR radiation. Light sources made of tungsten wires or ceramic resistive materials heated to 1500 to 4000 K emit energy over a broad wavelength range that includes the absorption spectrum of the respiratory gases. The radiation may be pulsed electronically (see Fig. 8-9) or, if constant, may be made intermittent by being interrupted mechanically, or "chopped," such as with a filter wheel (Fig. 8-10). Because energy output of IR light sources tends to drift, optical systems have been designed to stabilize the analyzers. Three common designs are distinguished by their use of single or dual IR beams and by their use of positive or negative filtering.[13]

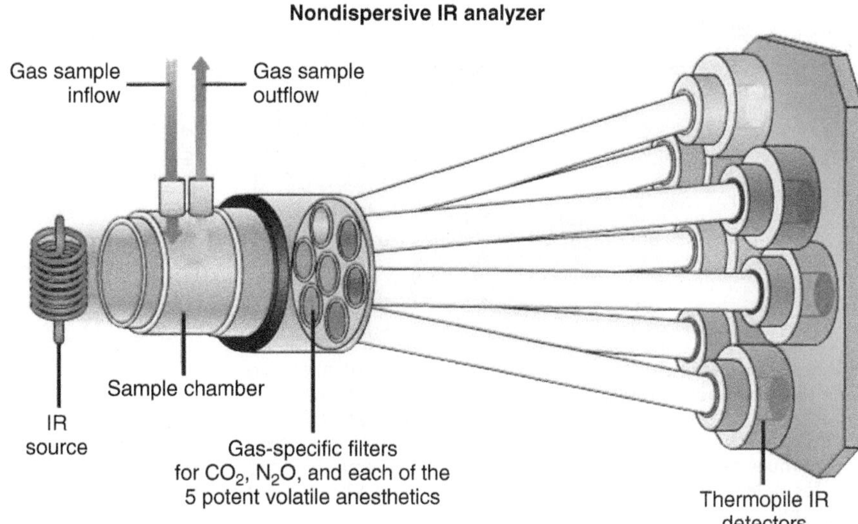

FIGURE 8-9 ■ Principles of the Datex-Ohmeda infrared (*IR*) analyzer in the Compact Airway Module (GE Healthcare, Waukesha, WI). In this design, the IR beam is interrupted electronically, rather than mechanically, by a "chopper" wheel. (From *Explore! The anesthesia system.* Cincinnati, OH, GE Datex-Ohmeda.)

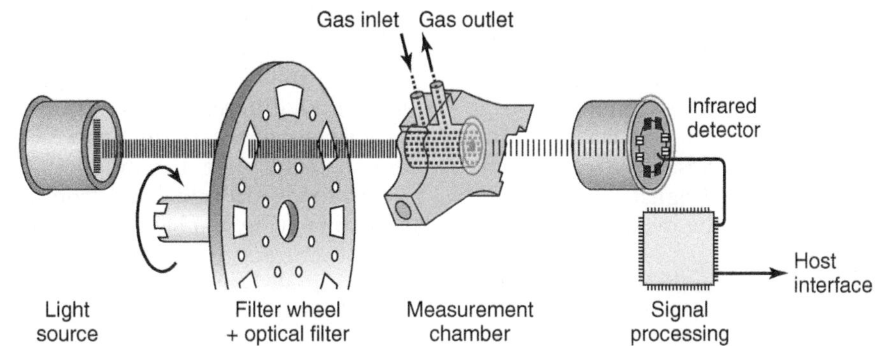

FIGURE 8-10 ■ Diagram of an infrared analyzer with multiple filters on a spinning chopper wheel.

Single-Beam Positive Filter

In single-beam positive-filter designs, the IR beam may be divided in time or in space. If the IR beam is divided in time, precision optical band-pass filters mounted on a chopper wheel spinning at 40 to 250 rpm sequentially interrupt a single IR beam. The beam retains energy at a narrow wavelength band during each interruption. If the IR beam is divided in space, after passing through the cuvette, the beam is divided into separate paths using beam splitters and mirrors before passing through optical filters. For each gas of interest, a pair of band-pass filters is selected at an absorption peak and at a reference wavelength at which relatively little absorption occurs. The chopped IR beam then passes through a cuvette containing the sample gas. The ratio of intensity of the IR beam for each pair of filters is proportional to the partial pressure of the gas and is insensitive to changes in the intensity of the IR source.

Single-Beam Negative Filter

In the single-beam negative-filter design, the filters usually are gas-filled cells mounted in a spinning wheel. During each interruption, the IR beam retains energy at all wavelengths except those absorbed by the gas. The chopped IR beam then passes through a cuvette containing the sample gas. Analogous to the positive-filter design previously described, the ratio of IR beam intensity for each pair of filter cells is proportional to the partial pressure of the gas and is insensitive to changes in intensity of the IR source.

Dual-Beam Positive Filter

In the dual-beam positive-filter design, the IR energy from the source is split into two parallel beams: one passes through the sample gas, the other passes through a reference gas. A spinning blade passes through the beams and sequentially interrupts one, the other, then both. The two beams are optically focused on a single point, where a band pass optical filter selected at the absorption peak of the gas of interest is mounted over a single detector. As before, the ratios of the intensities of the sample and reference beams are proportional to the partial pressure of the gas.

Detectors of Infrared Radiation

To measure carbon dioxide, nitrous oxide, and sometimes anesthetic agents, a radiation-sensitive solid-state material, lead selenide, is commonly used as a detector. Lead selenide is quite sensitive to changes in temperature; it therefore is usually thermostatically regulated (cooled or heated) or temperature compensated.

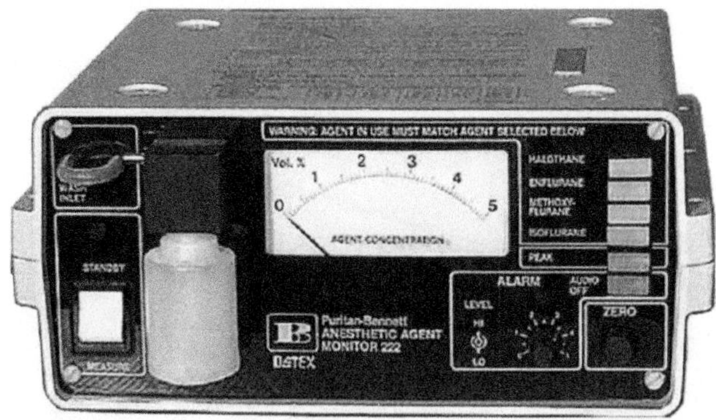

FIGURE 8-11 ■ Datex Puritan-Bennett anesthetic agent analyzer. This analyzer uses a single wavelength, so the agent being measured must be entered into the software by the user; failure to do this results in erroneous readings. Note the warning: "Agent in use must match agent selected below." Keypads on the right are for selection of halothane, enflurane, methoxyflurane, or isoflurane.

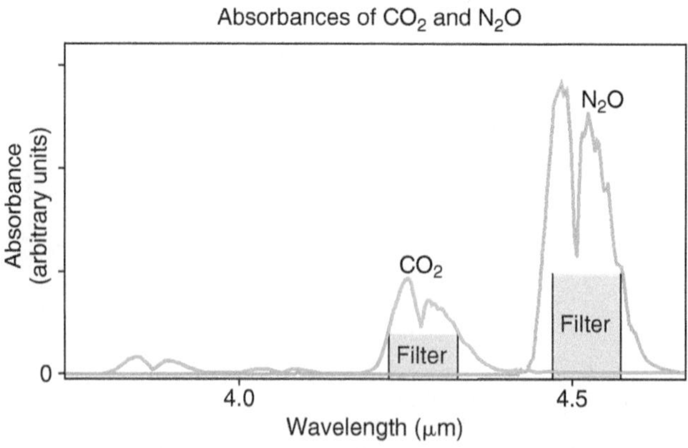

FIGURE 8-12 ■ Absorbance bands for CO_2 and N_2O. (From *Datex-Ohmeda Compact Airway Modules technical reference manual.* Document no. 800 1009-5. Helsinki, 2003, Datex-Ohmeda Division, Instrumentarium.)

Anesthetic agents, carbon dioxide, and nitrous oxide are sometimes measured with another detector called a *Luft cell.* This detector uses a chamber filled with gas that expands as IR radiation enters the chamber and is absorbed. A flexible wall of the chamber acts as a diaphragm that moves as the gas expands, and a microphone converts the motion to an electrical signal.

The signal processor converts the measured electrical currents to display gas partial pressure. First, the ratios of detector currents at various points in the spinning wheel's progress, or from multiple detectors, are computed. Next, electronic scaling and filtering are applied. Finally, linearization according to a reference table for the point-by-point conversion from electrical voltage to gas partial pressure is accomplished by a microprocessor. Compensation for cross-sensitivity or interference between gases can be accomplished by the microprocessor after linearization.

Infrared Wavelength and Anesthetic Agent Specificity

IR analyzers must use a specific wavelength of radiation according to the absorbance peak of each gas to be measured. Early agent analyzers, such as the Datex Puritan-Bennett Anesthetic Agent Monitor (Fig. 8-11),[14] used a wavelength of 3.3 μm to measure the potent inhaled anesthetics. However, use of a single wavelength did not permit differentiation among these agents (see Fig. 8-7). When this system was used, the analyzer had to be programmed by the user for the particular agent being administered. This set the appropriate gain in the software program, and the displayed reading was then accurate for the one agent in use. Obviously, programming such an analyzer for the wrong agent, or the use of mixed agents, would lead to erroneous readings.[15,16]

Modern IR analyzers are agent specific; that is, by measuring each agent with a unique set of wavelengths, they have the capability to both identify and quantify mixed agents in the presence of one another. Contemporary analyzers that can identify and quantify anesthetic agents incorporate individual wavelength filters in the range of 8 to 12 μm. An example is the Datex-Ohmeda Compact Airway Module (GE Healthcare) (see Figs. 8-2 and 8-9), which measures the absorption of the gas sample at seven different wavelengths selected using optical narrow band filters. In this analyzer module, the IR radiation detectors are thermopiles. Carbon dioxide and nitrous oxide are calculated from absorption measured at 3 to 5 μm (Fig. 8-12). Identification and calculation of the concentrations of anesthetic agents are done by measuring absorption at five wavelengths in the 8- to 9-μm band and solving for the concentrations from a set of five equations, one for each agent (Fig. 8-13).[16] A schematic of a multiwavelength analyzer in which the beam of radiation is interrupted mechanically is shown in Figure 8-14.

Sampling Systems and Infrared Analysis

Sidestream-sampling analyzers continuously withdraw between 50 and 250 mL/min from the breathing circuit through narrow-gauge sample tubing to the optical system, where the measurement is made. One of the disadvantages of sidestream monitors is the need to deal with liquid water and water vapor. Water vapor from the breathing circuit condenses on its way to the sample cuvette and can interfere with optical transmission. NAFION tubing, a semipermeable polymer that selectively allows water vapor to pass from its interior to the relatively dry exterior, is commonly used to eliminate water vapor. Also, a water trap often is interposed between the patient sampling catheter and the analyzer to protect the optical system from liquid water and body fluids (see Fig. 8-1). Filters integrated with the sampling tubing have replaced water traps in many of the currently available systems. Three different methods are available; these include 1) *blocking the water*, such as with a hydrophobic filter with large surface area (Oridion Medical, Jersusalem, IL), 2) *absorbing and blocking*, such as with a hydrophilic fibrous element followed by a hydrophobic plug (Philips Respironics, Wallingford, CT), and 3) *active water removal* with a hydrophilic wick, such as an elastomer, described as

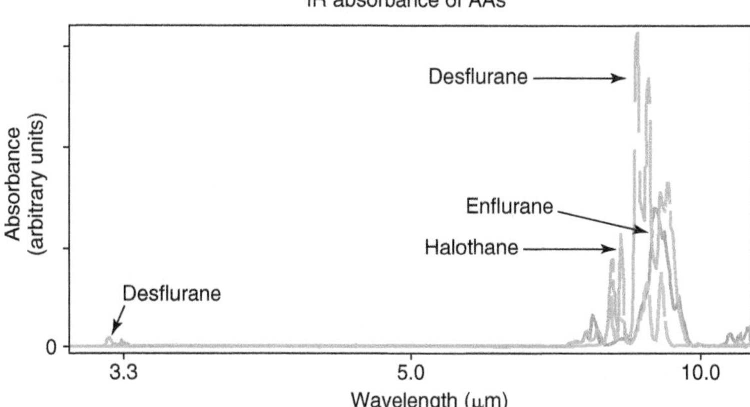

FIGURE 8-13 Absorbance bands for anesthetic agents (*AAs*). (From *Datex-Ohmeda Compact Airway Modules technical reference manual.* Document n. 800 1009-5. 2003, Datex-Ohmeda Division, Instrumentarium.)

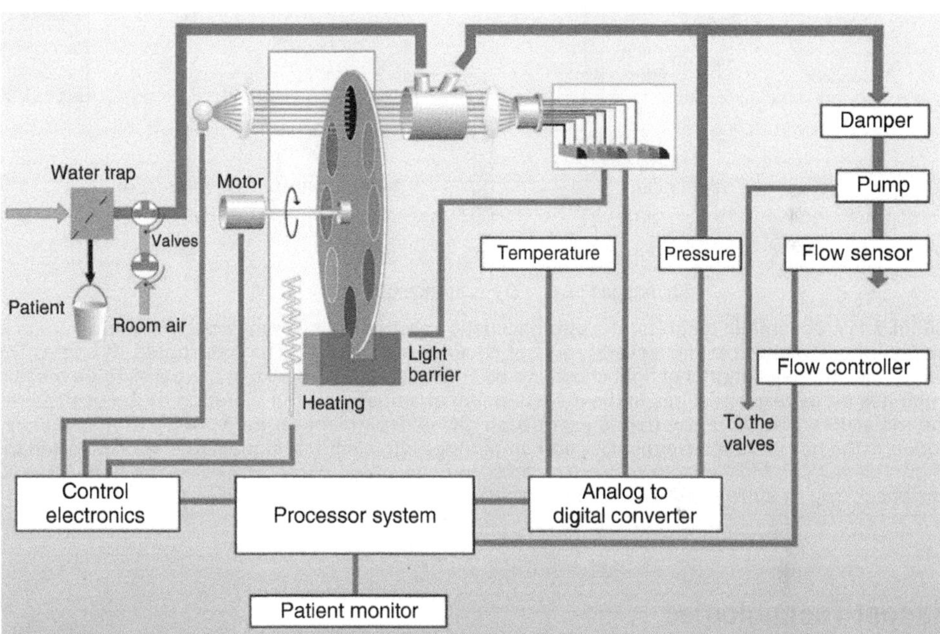

FIGURE 8-14 Schematic of multi-wavelength infrared analyzer with mechanical interruption ("chopping") of infrared beam. (Courtesy Dräger Medical, Telford, PA.)

being able to "sweat" water collected from the gas sample flow to the outer surface of the cover (Nomoline, PhaseIn).

Infrared Photoacoustic Spectrometer

The photoacoustic spectrometer is similar to the basic IR spectrometer (Fig. 8-15). IR energy is passed through optical filters that select narrow-wavelength bands that correspond to the absorption characteristics of the respired gases. Carbon dioxide is measured at a wavelength of 4.3 μm, nitrous oxide at 3.9 μm, and the potent inhaled agents at a wavelength between 10.3 and 13.0 μm.[17] Evenly spaced windows are located along the circumference of a rotating wheel. The optical components are located astride the wheel along one of its radii. A series of IR beams pulse on and off at particular frequencies, according to the rate of rotation of the wheel and the spacing of the windows. The gas flowing through the measurement cuvette is exposed to the pulsed IR beams. As each gas absorbs the pulsating IR energy in its absorption band, it expands and contracts at that frequency, and resulting sound waves are detected with a microphone. The partial pressure of each gas in the sample is then proportional to the amplitude, or "volume," of the measured sound.

The photoacoustic technique has the distinct advantage over other IR methods in that a simple microphone detector can be used to measure all the IR-absorbing gases. However, this device is sensitive to interference from loud noises and vibration. Also, because only one wavelength is used to measure the potent inhaled anesthetics, this monitor is unable to distinguish among the agents, which requires that it be programmed for the agent in use; also, erroneous readings might arise in the presence of mixed anesthetic agents. This technology was used in the Brüel and Kjær Anesthetic Gas Monitor 1304, and it is used currently in atmospheric trace gas monitors, such as the Innova 1412 (LumaSense Technologies, Santa Clara, CA).

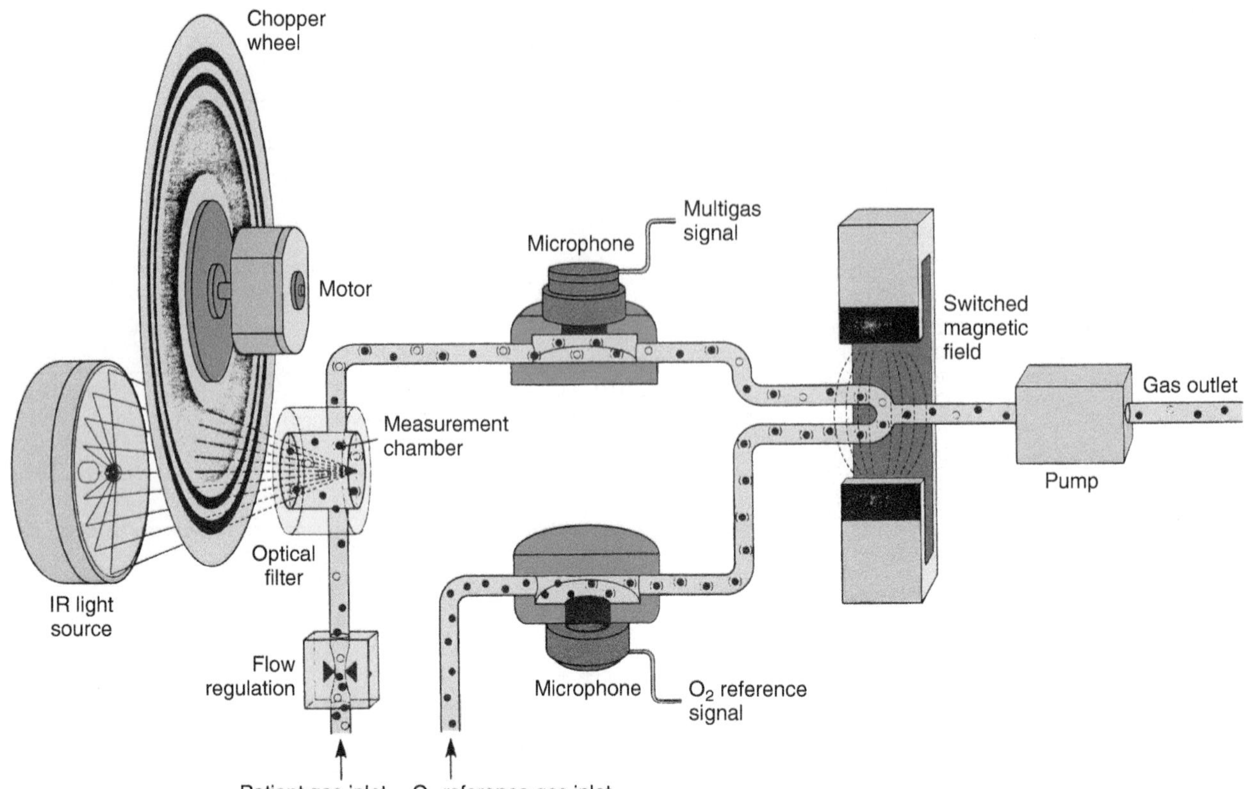

FIGURE 8-15 ■ Schematic diagram of a photoacoustic spectrometer. An infrared (*IR*) source emits a beam that passes through a spinning chopper wheel that has several rows of circumferential slots. The interrupted IR beams then pass through optical filters that select specific wavelengths of light chosen to be at the absorption peaks of the gases to be measured. Each interrupted IR light beam impinges on its respective gas in the measurement chamber, causing vibration of the gas as energy is absorbed and released from the molecules. The vibration frequency of each gas is dependent on the spacing of its slots on the chopper wheel. A microphone converts the gas vibration frequencies and amplitudes into electrical signals that are converted to the gas concentrations for display. (From Raemer DB: Monitoring respiratory function. In Rogers MC, Tinker JH, Covino BG, Longnecker DE, editors: *Principles and practice of anesthesiology.* St Louis, 1992, Mosby–Year Book.)

Recent Technologies

Philips Respironics introduced a flexible monitoring interface, now known as CO_2nnect & Go, which allows the user to choose, based on the patient and environment, which carbon dioxide–monitoring modality should be used, sidestream or mainstream. A complete measurement system is available for both mainstream (Capnostat 5) and sidestream (LoFlo, either external or internal format) modes of gas sampling.

Mainstream multigas IR analysis has recently been introduced by Phasein in their IRMA series of multigas analyzers. The IRMA mainstream probe measures IR light absorption at 10 different wavelengths to determine gas concentrations in the mixture (Fig. 8-16). Adult, pediatric, and infant disposable airway adapters are available. In a bench study, the monitor was found to have a response time for carbon dioxide (96 vs. 348 ms) and oxygen (108 vs. 432 ms) that was significantly less than a contemporary sidestream-sampling gas monitor.[18] The same miniaturized technology is used in Phasein's EMMA Emergency Capnometer, a device that displays respiratory rate and incorporates apnea, high carbon dioxide, and low carbon dioxide audible and visual alarms (Fig. 8-17).

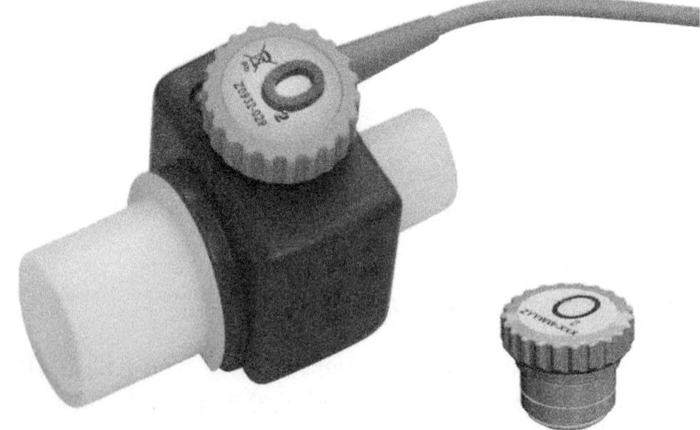

FIGURE 8-16 ■ Mainstream multigas analyzer module that measures carbon dioxide, nitrous oxide, oxygen, and anesthetic agents. Rapid-response fuel-cell oxygen analyzer and IRMA Plug-in and Measure. (Courtesy Phasein AB, Danderyd, Sweden.)

Although Microstream (Oridion Medical) capnography is now used as a generic term to refer to a sampling flow rate of 50 mL/min, a rate now available from several vendors, it also encompasses the unique IR emission

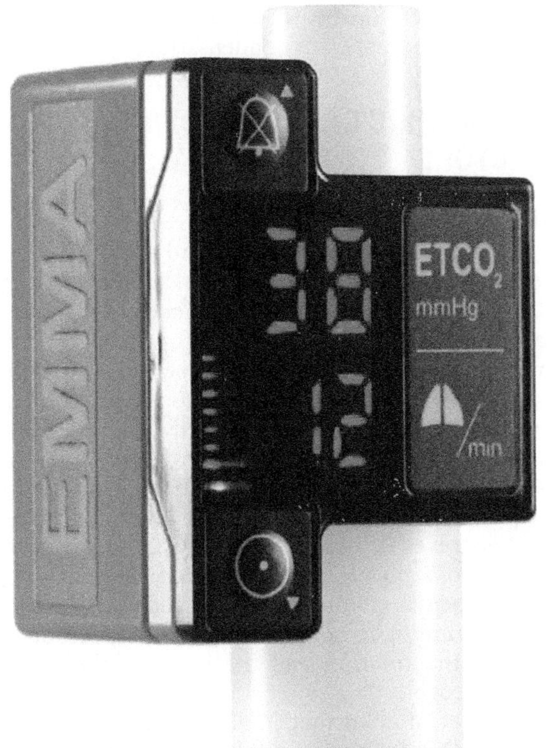

FIGURE 8-17 ▪ EMMA Capnocheck mainstream capnometer Plug-in and Measure. (Courtesy Phasein AB, Danderyd, Sweden.)

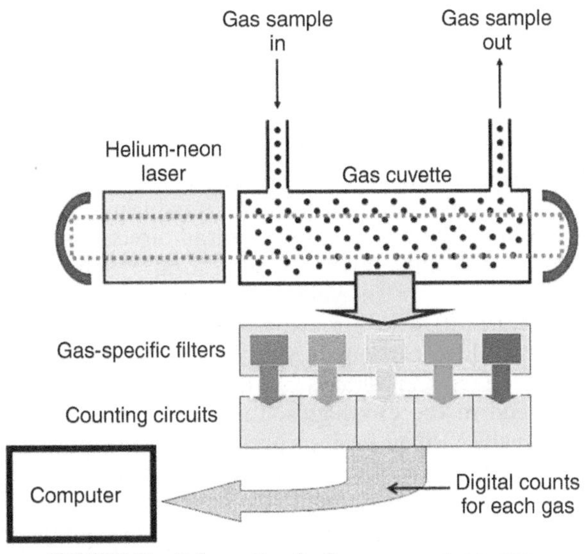

FIGURE 8-18 ▪ Schematic of a Raman spectrometer.

source. This approach is called *molecular correlation spectroscopy* (MCS),[19] and it produces selective emission of a spectrum of discrete wavelengths, approximately 100 discrete lines in the 4.2- to 4.35-μm range, which match those for carbon dioxide absorption. This is compared with the broad IR emission spectrum of black body emitters used with conventional nondispersive IR technology and permits use of a smaller sample cell (15 μL). This technology has been adapted for use in portable carbon dioxide monitors.[20]

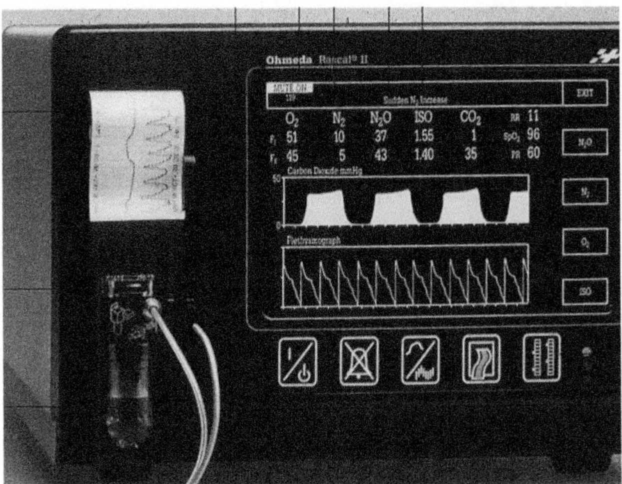

FIGURE 8-19 ▪ Screen of the Ohmeda Rascal II (GE Healthcare, Waukesha, WI). Note the measurements of inspired and end-tidal nitrogen.

RAMAN SPECTROSCOPY

When light strikes gas molecules, most of the energy scattered is absorbed and reemitted in the same direction, and at the same wavelength, as the incoming beam (Rayleigh scattering).[21] At room temperature, about one millionth of the energy is scattered at a longer wavelength, producing a so-called *red-shifted spectrum.* Raman scattering can be used to measure the constituents of a gas mixture. Unlike IR spectroscopy, Raman scattering is not limited to gas species that are polar. Carbon dioxide, oxygen, nitrogen, water vapor, nitrous oxide, and the potent volatile anesthetic agents all exhibit Raman activity. Monatomic gases such as helium, xenon, and argon, which lack intramolecular bonds, do not exhibit Raman activity.

The medical Raman spectrometer used a helium-neon laser (wavelength 633 nm, or 0.633 μm) to produce the incoming monochromatic light beam. The Raman scattered light is of low intensity and is measured perpendicular to the laser beam. The measurement cuvette is located in the cavity of the laser, so that the gas molecules are struck repeatedly by the beam (Fig. 8-18). This results in enough Raman scattering to be collected and processed by the optical detection system. Photomultiplier tubes count the scattered photons at the characteristic Raman-shifted wavelength for each gas. Thus the Raman spectrometer measures the partial pressures of the gases in its measurement cuvette, and measurements are converted electronically to the desired units of measure and are displayed on the screen.

Raman spectroscopy is the principle of operation of the Ohmeda Rascal II monitor (Fig. 8-19). The Rascal II Raman spectrometer has the same capabilities as the mass spectrometer; in particular, it is able to measure nitrogen

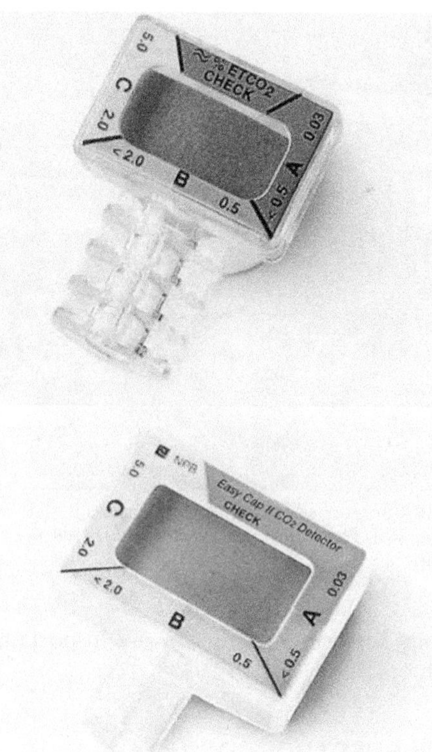

FIGURE 8-20 ■ Nellcor Easy Cap carbon dioxide detector. (Courtesy Covidien, Mansfield, MA.)

for detection of air embolism, and it received a very favorable evaluation.[22] Unfortunately, despite its obvious versatility, this monitor is no longer in production, although a number remain in use.

WATER VAPOR AND ACCURACY OF CAPNOMETERS

Water vapor can be an important factor in the accuracy of a carbon dioxide analyzer. Most sidestream analyzers report ambient temperature and pressure dry (ATPD) values for P_{CO_2} by using a water trap and water vapor–permeable NAFION tubing to remove water vapor from the sample. It has been recommended that carbon dioxide analyzers report their results at body temperature and pressure saturated (BTPS) so that end-tidal values are close to conventionally reported alveolar gas partial pressure.[23] The error in reporting P_{CO_2} at ATPD, when it should be reported at BTPS, is approximately 2.5 mm Hg. Carbon dioxide values reported in ATPD can be converted to BTPS by decreasing the dry gas reading by the fraction $(P_{ATM} - 47)/P_{ATM}$, where P_{ATM} is the atmospheric pressure in mm Hg, and 47 mm Hg is the vapor pressure of water at 37° C.

Mainstream sampling analyzers naturally report readings at the breathing circuit conditions that are typically near BTPS. Depending on these conditions, a small decrease from body temperature may result in the analyzer reading slightly less than BTPS values. Condensation of water can affect the windows of the mainstream airway adapter and cause erroneous readings. These adapters are therefore heated or use coatings on the inside of the windows to prevent condensation.

COLORIMETRIC CARBON DIOXIDE DETECTORS

Carbon dioxide in solution is acidic; pH-sensitive dyes can therefore be used to detect and measure its presence. A colorimetric carbon dioxide detector is designed to be interposed between the tracheal tube and the breathing circuit. Respired gas passes through a hydrophobic filter and a piece of filter paper visible through a plastic window. The originally described detector, the Fenem CO_2 Indicator (Engineered Medical Systems, Indianapolis, IN), consisted of a piece of filter paper permeated with an aqueous solution of metacresol purple, a pH-sensitive dye. Carbon dioxide from the exhaled breath dissolves in the solution, changing the color of the dye from purple to yellow; the degree of color change depends on the carbon dioxide concentration. On inspiration of carbon dioxide–free gas, carbon dioxide leaves the solution and the color of the indicator returns to purple.[24]

A number of colorimetric devices are now commercially available for use in adult and pediatric patients. They may use other carbon dioxide–sensitive dyes and are calibrated to provide an approximate indication of expired carbon dioxide concentration that can be discerned by comparison of the indicator color with a graduated color scale printed on the device's housing. For example, with the Easy Cap II (Covidien, Mansfield, MA), the color changes from purple to yellow to indicate 2% to 5% carbon dioxide (15 to 38 mm Hg) with each exhaled breath. On inspiration the color should change back to purple, indicating absence of carbon dioxide in the inspired gas (Fig. 8-20). A permanent change in color may mislead the uneducated user.[25,26] The following caution appears in the directions for use from the manufacturer: "Interpreting results before confirming six breath cycles can yield false results. Gastric distension with air prior to attempted intubation may introduce carbon dioxide levels as high as 4.5% into the Easy Cap detector if the endotracheal tube is misplaced in the esophagus. Initial Easy Cap detector color (yellow) may be interpreted as a false positive if read before delivery of six breaths." The warnings also further include a statement that "reflux of gastric contents, mucus, edema fluid, or intratracheal epinephrine into the Easy Cap can yield persistent patchy yellow or white discoloration *which does not vary with the respiratory cycle*. Contamination of this type may also increase airway resistance and affect ventilation. Discard device if this occurs."

This type of detector is intended to be used to confirm clinical signs of tracheal intubation when conventional capnography is not available. Both adult and pediatric versions are available. The newest Fenem carbon dioxide indicator is designed to be attached to the exhalation port (19 or 30 mm) of a self-inflating resuscitator bag, where it does not add dead space or resistance to flow (Fig. 8-21).

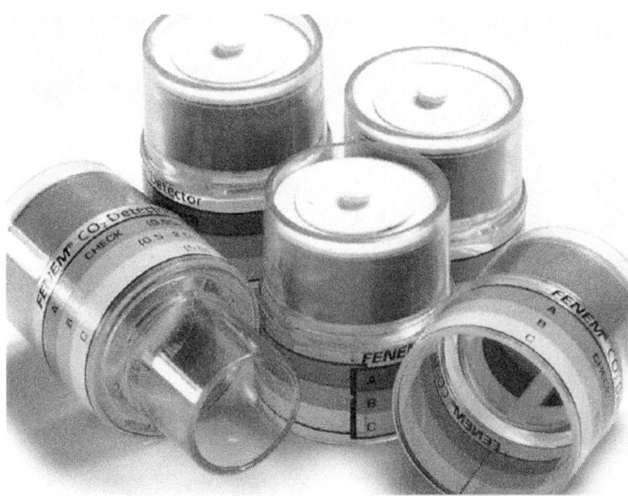

FIGURE 8-21 ■ Fenem CO_2 Detector (Engineered Medical Systems, Indianapolis, IN) designed for exhalation port of self-inflating resuscitation (Ambu) bag.

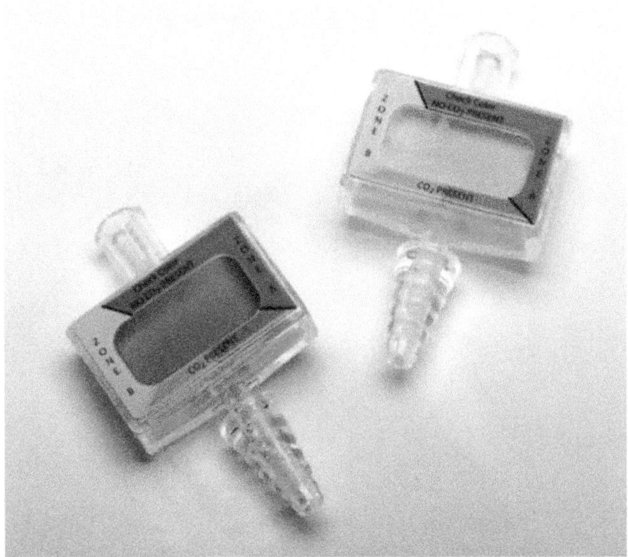

FIGURE 8-22 ■ Colorimetric CO_2 detector designed to ensure the absence of CO_2 for confirming intragastric placement of gastric tube (CO_2nfirm). (Courtesy Covidien, Mansfield, MA.)

Another version of the colorimetric carbon dioxide detector, the CO_2nfirm Now carbon dioxide detector (Covidien), is marketed as a device to confirm intragastric placement of an orogastric or nasogastric tube to avoid intratracheal placement (Fig. 8-22).

OXYGEN ANALYZERS

In all contemporary anesthesia delivery systems, the fraction of inspired oxygen (FiO_2) in an anesthesia breathing circuit is monitored by an oxygen analyzer. Two types of oxygen analyzers are in common use for monitoring: those based on a fuel or galvanic cell principle and the paramagnetic (Pauling) sensor. In the past, in addition to these methods, multigas analyzers that used mass spectroscopy or Raman spectroscopy to measure oxygen were also used.

Fuel Cell Oxygen Analyzer

The *fuel cell* (Fig. 8-23), or *galvanic cell*, is basically an oxygen battery that consists of a diffusion barrier; a noble metal cathode, either gold mesh or platinum; and a lead or zinc anode in a basic, usually potassium hydroxide, electrolyte bath (Fig. 8-24). The sensor is covered by an oxygen-permeable membrane and is exposed to the gas in the breathing circuit. Oxygen diffusing into the sensor is reduced to hydroxyl ions at the cathode in the following reaction:

$$O_2 + 2H_2O + 4e^- \rightarrow 4(OH)^-$$

The hydroxyl ions then oxidize the lead or zinc anode, and the following reaction occurs at the anode:

$$2Pb + 4OH^- \rightarrow 2PbO + 2H_2O + 4e^-$$

The overall reaction is $O_2 + 2Pb \rightarrow 2PbO$

The flow of current depends on the uptake of oxygen at the cathode, according to Faraday's first law of electrolysis, and the voltage developed is proportional to the oxygen partial pressure (PaO_2). No polarizing potential (battery) is needed because the cell produces its own. The fuel-cell sensor voltage is measured and is electronically scaled to units of partial pressure, or equivalent concentration in volumes percent, and is displayed as a readout. Like any battery, the fuel cell has a limited life span, usually several months, depending on its length of exposure to oxygen. For this reason, machine manufacturers have recommended that the cell be removed from the breathing system when not in use. The response time of standard fuel cell oxygen analyzers is slow (~30 seconds); therefore they are best used to monitor the average O_2 concentration in the inspiratory limb of the breathing system.

A faster galvanic oxygen sensor is in development and is designed to be used with the mainstream multigas analyzer (Phasein IRMA; see Fig. 8-16). This sensor claimed to have a lifetime exceeding 100,000 oxygen hours.

Paramagnetic Oxygen Analyzer

The oxygen molecule has two electrons in unpaired orbits, which makes it paramagnetic; that is, it is susceptible to attraction by a magnetic field. Most other gases are weakly diamagnetic and are repelled. The paramagnetic oxygen sensor uses the strong, positive magnetic susceptibility of oxygen in a pneumatic bridge configuration to determine oxygen concentration by measuring a pressure differential between a stream of reference gas (room air at about 10 mL/min) and one of the measured gas, as the two streams are exposed to a changing magnetic field (Fig. 8-25). An electromagnet is rapidly switched off and on (at a frequency of 165 Hz in the GE Healthcare Compact Airway Module[1]), creating a rapidly changing magnetic field between its poles. The electromagnet is designed to have its poles in close proximity, forming a narrow gap. The streams of sample and reference gas have different oxygen partial pressures, and the pressure between the entrance

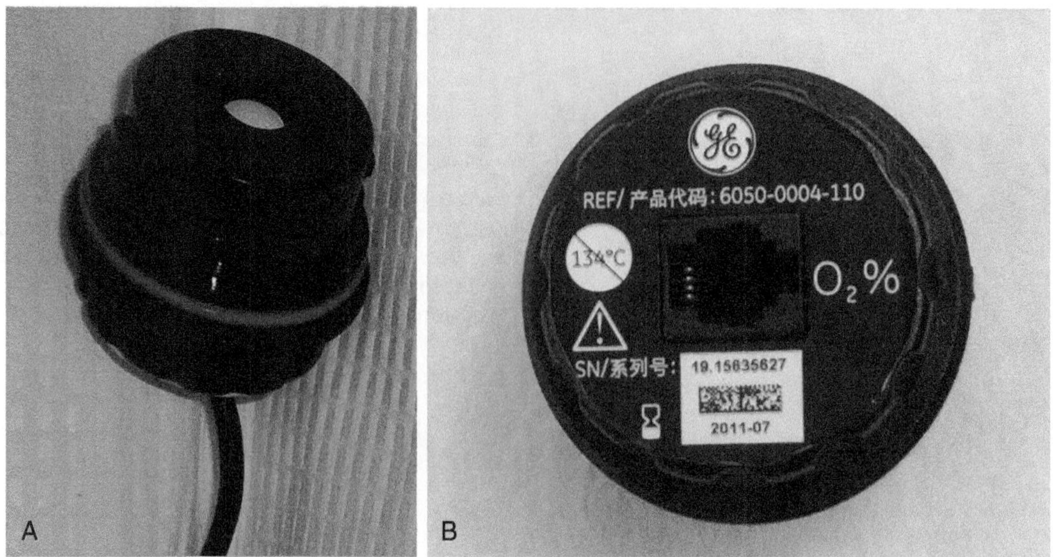

FIGURE 8-23 ■ Fuel cell oxygen analyzer.

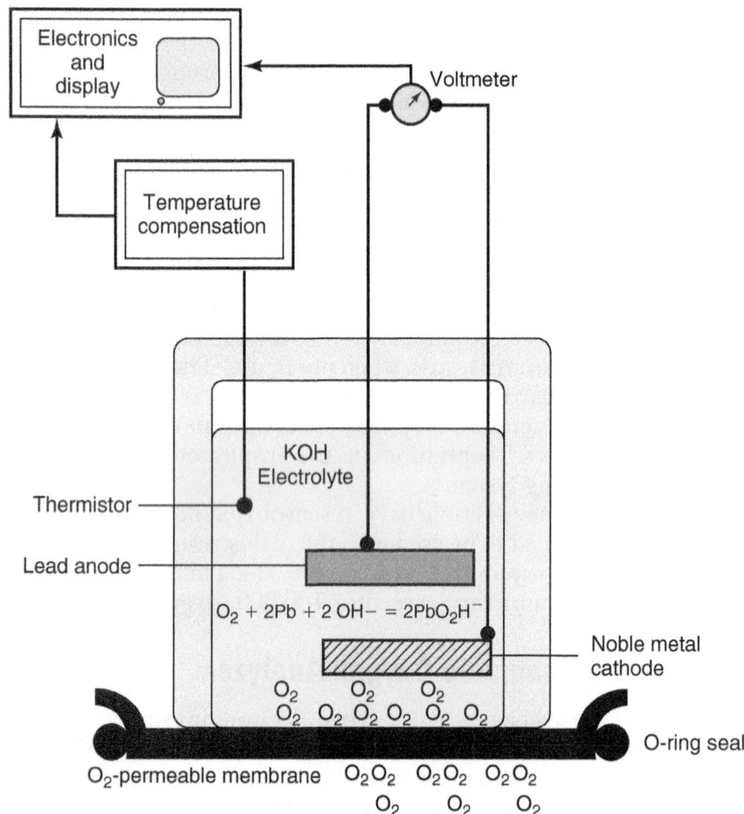

FIGURE 8-24 ■ Principles of fuel cell oxygen analyzer. Oxygen in the gas sample permeates a membrane and enters a potassium hydroxide (*KOH*) electrolyte solution. An electrical potential is established between a lead anode and noble metal cathode as oxygen is supplied to the anode. The measured voltage between the electrodes is proportional to the oxygen tension of the gas sample. Temperature compensation is required for accurate measurement. (From Raemer DB: Monitoring respiratory function. In Rogers MC, Tinker JH, Covino BG, Longnecker DE, editors: *Principles and practice of anesthesiology.* St Louis, 1992, Mosby–Year Book.)

and exit of the respective gas streams differs slightly because of the magnetic force on the oxygen molecules; this generates sound waves from each gas stream. A sensitive pressure transducer (i.e., a microphone) is used to convert the sound waves to an electrical signal. The output signal is proportional to the oxygen partial pressure difference between the two gas streams and should be displayed as the PO_2, but it is more typically displayed as the equivalent concentration in volumes percent. Paramagnetic oxygen analysis is used in most of the contemporary sidestream-sampling multigas analyzers.

The main advantage of paramagnetic analysis over the standard fuel cell is that it has a very rapid response that permits continuous breath-by-breath monitoring of the respired oxygen concentration. The graphic representation of this can be displayed as the *oxygram,* which is essentially a mirror image of the capnogram (Fig. 8-26).

Normally the gas exiting the multigas analyzer is directed to the waste gas scavenging system of the anesthesia delivery system. If a low-flow or closed-circuit anesthesia technique is being used, the gas exiting the

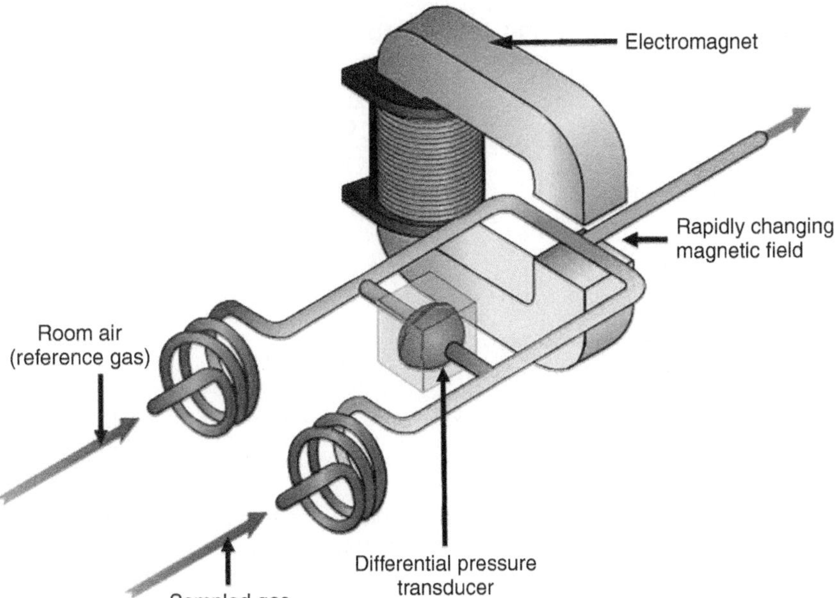

FIGURE 8-25 Schematic of a paramagnetic oxygen analyzer. The sample and reference gas streams converge in a rapidly changing magnetic field. Because the two streams have different oxygen tensions (i.e., different numbers of oxygen molecules), a pressure differential is created across a sensitive pressure transducer. The transducer converts this force to an electrical signal that is either displayed as oxygen partial pressure or converted to a reading in volumes percent. (From Explore Aisys. In *Explore! The anesthesia system.* Cincinnati, OH, GE Datex-Ohmeda.)

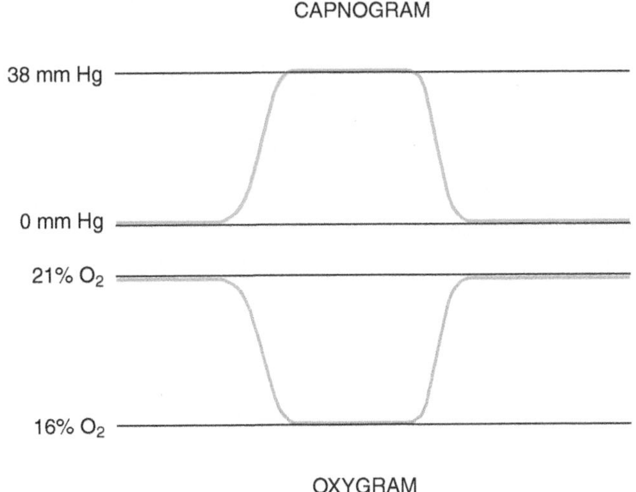

FIGURE 8-26 Capnogram (*top*) and oxygram (*bottom*). The oxygram is almost a mirror image of the capnogram.

analyzer usually is returned to the breathing system. In this case it must be remembered that nitrogen from the room air reference gas stream is being added also, albeit at a low rate (8 mL/min), and will accumulate in the breathing circuit.[27]

Oxigraphy

Another technology used to measure oxygen available from Oxigraf (Palo Alto, CA) uses laser diode absorption spectroscopy in the visible spectrum, similar in principle to the IR absorption methodology used to measure carbon dioxide, nitrous oxide, and the potent inhaled anesthetic agents. The wavelength used to measure oxygen is 760 nm because there is no interference by other gases at this wavelength. The emission line width of the laser and the absorption line width of oxygen are both very narrow (<0.01 nm) compared with the absorption band for carbon dioxide (~100 nm). The laser is thermally tuned precisely to the oxygen line; as the oxygen concentration increases, the intensity of transmitted light is attenuated as energy is absorbed by the oxygen molecules. The response of the photodetector varies linearly with the concentration of oxygen. The analyzer can measure oxygen in the range of 5% to 100% with an accuracy of 0.1% and has an adjustable gas sampling rate of 50 to 250 mL/min. As with the IR analyzers, the Oxigraf analyzer measures the partial pressure of oxygen in the sample chamber. The pressure of the sample at the time of measurement also is needed to convert data from partial pressure to percent oxygen.

Calibration of Oxygen Analyzers

Oxygen analyzers require periodic calibration. Because all analyzers produce an electrical signal proportional to the oxygen partial pressure, the constant of proportionality (gain) must be determined. In general, the electrical signal in the presence of 0% oxygen is known to be near zero; therefore no offset correction is required. In the fuel cell, the gain changes over time because of changes in electrolyte, electrodes (the anode is sacrificial), and membrane; the anesthesia caregiver must therefore calibrate it to display 21% by removing it from the breathing system and allowing equilibration in room air. It must be remembered that the fuel cell is actually measuring the ambient pressure of oxygen (PO_2, normally 159 mm Hg in dry air at sea level), but for convenience, it displays 21 vol%. Therefore, if a fuel cell that has been calibrated to read 21% at sea level is used at a much higher altitude, the readout will show less than 21% because the ambient PO_2 is lower, even though the composition of the atmosphere is still 21% by volume.

The gain of the paramagnetic sensor changes with temperature, humidity, and pneumatic factors. The

TABLE 8-1 **Gas Monitoring Technologies**

	Gas						
Technology	**O_2**	**CO_2**	**N_2O**	**AA Specific**	**N_2**	**He**	**Ar**
Mass spectrometry	X	X	X	X	X	X	X
Raman spectrometry	X	X	X	X	X		
Infrared light		X	X	X			
Infrared acoustic		X	X	X			
Fuel cell	X						
Paramagnetic	X						
Molecular correlation spectroscopy		X					
Laser diode absorption spectroscopy	X						

AA, anesthetic agent; *Ar*, argon; *CO_2*, carbon dioxide; *He*, helium; *N_2*, nitrogen; *N_2O*, nitrous oxide; *O_2*, oxygen.

contemporary paramagnetic oxygen analyzers perform their own periodic computer-controlled automated calibration process.

Gases in the anesthesia delivery system can be analyzed by a number of modern technologies, each of which is based on application of some specific physical property of the gas molecule. The analysis methods and their applications are summarized in Table 8-1. In interpreting gas analysis data, it is important to understand the principles of how the data were obtained so that erroneous data can be identified and, if necessary, rejected.

BALANCE GAS

Contemporary multigas analyzers measure the partial pressure of each gas of interest in a dry gas mixture. They also measure ambient barometric pressure (P_B). The partial pressure of oxygen (PO_2) is measured by paramagnetic analysis, and the partial pressures of nitrous oxide and carbon dioxide (PN_2O and PCO_2) and the anesthetic agent are measured by IR technology. If the sum of these partial pressures is subtracted from the ambient barometric pressure, the result is the partial pressure of unmeasured gases and may be displayed as "Balance Gas" (Fig. 8-27, Box 8-1). In most cases the balance gas is nitrogen, and in the absence of a specific nitrogen gas analyzer (i.e., Raman or mass spectrometer), balance gas has been described as the "poor man's nitrogen." However, if a heliox (75% helium, 25% oxygen) mixture were being analyzed, helium would be read as the balance gas.

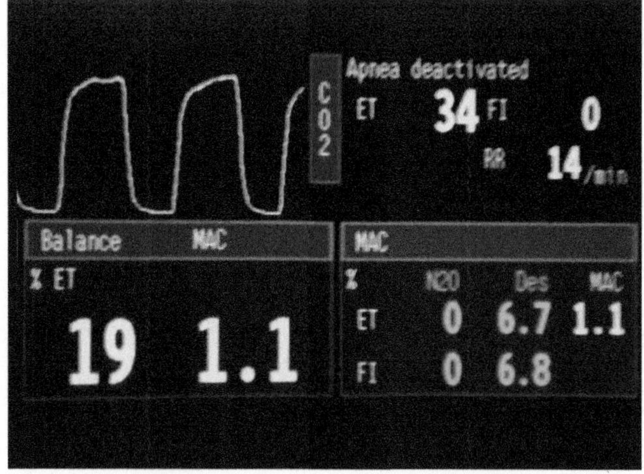

FIGURE 8-27 ■ Screen of the Datex-Ohmeda S5 monitor (GE Healthcare, Waukesha, WI). Balance gas concentration is shown in volumes percent. Measurements are made in millimeters of mercury and then converted to volumes percent using the measured barometric pressure. Capnogram (*top*) and oxygram (*bottom*). The oxygram is almost a mirror image of the capnogram.

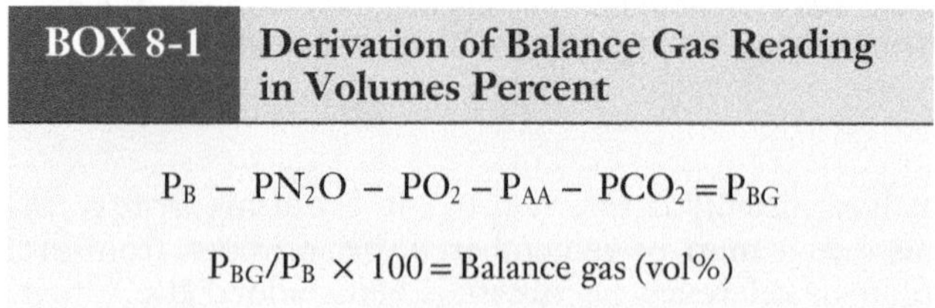

BOX 8-1 Derivation of Balance Gas Reading in Volumes Percent

$$P_B - PN_2O - PO_2 - P_{AA} - PCO_2 = P_{BG}$$

$$P_{BG}/P_B \times 100 = \text{Balance gas (vol\%)}$$

P_B, barometric pressure; P_{BG}, balance gas pressure.

NITRIC OXIDE

Inhaled nitric oxide (NO) is used to treat hypoxemia and pulmonary hypertension associated with acute respirtory failure. A number of nitric oxide delivery systems are commercially available that incorporate or require contemporaneous use of an NO analyzer.

The INOvent delivery system (GE Healthcare) delivers nitric oxide in concentrations of 0 to 40 ppm. Circuit gas is sampled at a rate of 230 mL/min and is analyzed electrochemically (amperometric approach) when nitric oxide reacts with an electrode to induce a current or voltage change. The measurement ranges are 0 to 100 ppm for NO and 0 to 15 ppm for nitrogen dioxide, NO_2.

Chemiluminescence is the emission of light with limited emission of heat (*luminescence*) as the result of a chemical reaction. The concentration of NO can be determined by using a simple chemiluminescent reaction involving ozone[28]; a sample containing nitric oxide is mixed with a large quantity of ozone, and the nitric oxide reacts with the ozone to produce oxygen and nitrogen dioxide. This reaction also produces light (chemiluminescence) that can be measured with a photodetector. The amount of light produced is proportional to the amount of nitric oxide in the gas sample:

$$NO + O_3 \rightarrow NO_2 + O_2 + \text{Light}$$

To determine the amount of nitrogen dioxide in a sample containing no nitric oxide, the NO_2 must first be converted to NO by passing the sample through a converter, before the ozone activation reaction is applied. The ozone reaction produces a photon count proportional to NO, which is proportional to NO_2 before it was converted to NO. In the case of a mixed sample containing both NO and NO_2, the above reaction yields the amount of NO and NO_2 combined in the gas sample, assuming that the sample is passed through the converter. If the mixed sample is not passed through the converter, the ozone reaction produces activated NO_2 only in proportion to the NO in the sample. The NO_2 in the sample is not activated by the ozone reaction. Although unactivated NO_2 is present with the activated NO_2, photons are emitted only by the activated species, which is proportional to the original NO. The final step is to subtract NO from the combined gas sample (NO + NO_2) to yield NO_2.

APPLICATIONS OF GAS MONITORING

Oxygen

The qualitative and quantitative oxygen-specific analyzer in the anesthesia breathing system is probably the most important of all of the monitors on the anesthesia workstation. Before the general use of an oxygen analyzer in the anesthesia breathing system, a number of adverse outcomes from unrecognized delivery of a hypoxic gas had been reported.[29]

To be used correctly, the oxygen analyzer must be calibrated, and appropriate low and high audible and visual concentration alarm limits must be set. Because it samples gas in the inspiratory limb of the breathing system, this analyzer provides the only means of ensuring that oxygen is being delivered to the patient. If a hypoxic gas or gas mixture is delivered, the alarm will go off. Such situations can occur if there is a pipeline crossover (e.g., O_2 for N_2O), an incorrectly filled oxygen storage tank or cylinder, or failure of a proportioning system intended to prevent delivery of a gas mixture that contains less than 25% oxygen. The high oxygen concentration alarm limit is important when caring for patients for whom a high oxygen concentration may be harmful, such as premature infants and patients treated with chemotherapeutic drugs (e.g., bleomycin), who are more susceptible to oxygen toxicity.

Continuous monitoring of inspired and end-expired oxygen is very helpful in ensuring completeness of preoxygenation of the lungs, before a rapid sequence induction of anesthesia, or in patients at increased risk for hypoxemia during induction of anesthesia, such as the morbidly obese.[30-32] During preoxygenation, nitrogen is washed out of the lungs and is replaced by oxygen.[33] Preoxygenation is ideal when the inspired oxygen concentration is 100% and the end-tidal oxygen is 95%, the difference of 5% being the exhaled carbon dioxide. In general, however, an end-tidal oxygen greater than 90% is considered acceptable.

The rapid-response oxygen analyzer makes possible the display of the *oxygram*, a continuous real-time display of oxygen concentration on the y-axis against time on the x-axis. Now that it is possible to accurately measure inspiratory and expiratory gas flows, and therefore volumes (i.e., flow = volume/time), via the airway, the oxygram can be combined with these flow signals to plot inspired and expired oxygen concentrations against volume. This is termed *volumetric oxygraphy*. In theory, the integral of simultaneous flow and oxygen concentration during inspiration and expiration is the inspired and expired volume of oxygen. From the difference between these two amounts, oxygen consumption can be estimated. Barnard and Sleigh[34] used this method (with a Datex Ultima monitor) to measure oxygen consumption in patients under general anesthesia and compared it with that obtained simultaneously using a metabolic monitor. These investigators concluded that the Datex Ultima may be used with moderate accuracy to measure oxygen uptake during anesthesia. The analogous plot for the capnogram, *volumetric capnography*, allows measurement of carbon dioxide production.

The application of this concept is termed *indirect calorimetry*, which is used in the GE Healthcare bedside metabolic module,[35] which has been validated in both the ICU and anesthesia environments.[36] By monitoring flow and measuring the gas concentrations, this module provides measurements of oxygen consumption (VO_2) and carbon dioxide elimination (VCO_2), and it calculates respiratory quotient and energy expenditure (Fig. 8-28).[37] Although the applications may be more pertinent to patients in the ICU, some have found it useful during liver transplantation surgery in predicting the viability of the organ once in the recipient. It might also be useful in the early detection of a hypermetabolic state in a patient under general anesthesia (e.g., malignant hyperthermia) and in distinguishing it from insufflation of carbon dioxide during a laparoscopic procedure.[38] One development worth noting is the trend toward complete in-line measurement of oxygen consumption and carbon dioxide elimination, evidenced by the testing of a prototype in-line system that uses a luminescence quenching sensor for O_2, IR sensing for carbon dioxide, and a fixed orifice for flow sensing.[39]

The oxygen analyzer is one of the most important monitors in the breathing system because it is both qualitative and quantitative. In that location, it helps ensure that the patient does not receive a hypoxic gas mixture. In that regard, it should be noted that if an oxygen delivery device, such as a mask or nasal cannula, is connected to the auxiliary oxygen outlet of the anesthesia workstation—which derives gas from the machine's high-pressure system for oxygen, or to a wall oxygen outlet flowmeter—there is no oxygen monitoring of the delivered gas. Thus if a hypoxic gas were delivered by the oxygen pipeline system

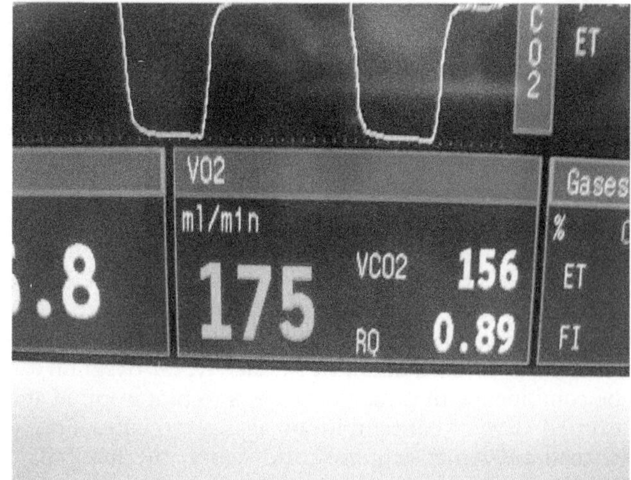

FIGURE 8-28 Screen of Datex-Ohmeda S5 Compact Airway Module monitor (GE Healthcare, Waukesha, WI). Metabolic monitoring data (Vo_2, Vo_2, RQ) are shown from integrating concentration and flow signals.

to the auxiliary oxygen outlet, or an oxygen wall flowmeter were to somehow become connected to a nitrous oxide wall outlet, an adverse outcome could be expected.[40]

Carbon Dioxide

The introduction of carbon dioxide monitoring into clinical practice is one of the major advances in patient safety. Before its introduction, many cases of esophageal intubation were unrecognized and led to adverse outcomes, not to mention increases in malpractice premiums. Detection of carbon dioxide on a breath-by-breath basis is considered to be the best method to confirm endotracheal intubation,[41] and the applications of time and volumetric carbon dioxide monitoring (capnography) are numerous, such that entire textbooks have been devoted to this subject.[42,43]

Time Capnography

The normal capnogram, shown in Figure 8-29, can be divided into four phases. Phase I (A to B) is the inspiratory baseline, which normally is zero. Phase II (B to C) is the expiratory upstroke, which normally is steep. As the patient exhales, fresh gas in the anatomic dead space (with no carbon dioxide) is gradually replaced by carbon dioxide-containing gas from the alveoli. Phase III (C to D) is the expiratory plateau, which normally has a slight upward gradient because of imperfect matching of ventilation and perfusion (V/Q) throughout the lungs. Alveoli with lower V/Q ratios, and therefore higher carbon dioxide concentrations, tend to empty later during exhalation than those with high V/Q ratios. Once exhalation is complete, the plateau continues because exhaled carbon dioxide from the alveoli remains at the gas sampling site until the next inspiration. The end-tidal carbon dioxide concentration ($P_{ET}CO_2$) is considered to be the same as alveolar concentration (P_ACO_2). Phase IV (D to E) is the inspiratory downstroke, as fresh gas replaces alveolar gas at the sampling site. The presence of a

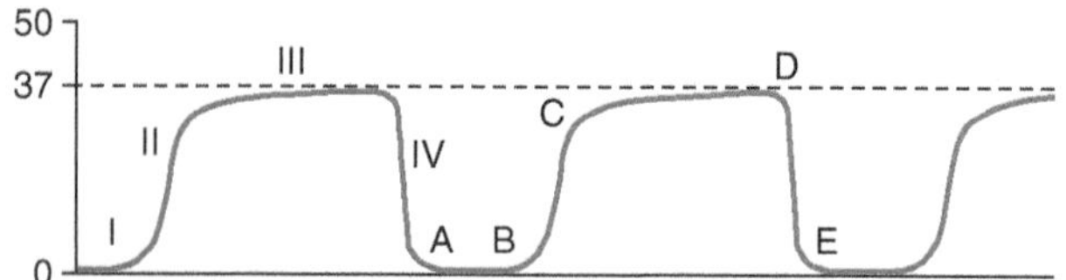

FIGURE 8-29 Normal capnogram. (Courtesy Philips Respironics, Wallingford, CT.)

normal capnogram indicates that the lungs are being ventilated. The ventilation may be spontaneous, assisted, or controlled. The inspired carbon dioxide concentration normally is zero, and the end-tidal volume normally is between 34 and 44 mm Hg. Table 8-2 shows some of the possible causes for values outside of the normal ranges. Table 8-3 lists some other abnormalities in the four phases of the capnogram. Observation of the shape of the capnogram also may be helpful in alerting the caregiver to certain conditions (see Chapter 10 for examples of abnormal capnograms).

The end-tidal carbon dioxide concentration is commonly used as a surrogate for alveolar carbon dioxide tension, which in turn is used to track arterial carbon dioxide, a value that must be obtained invasively. The normal arterial–end-tidal carbon dioxide tension difference is approximately 4 mm Hg. This difference is not constant and is affected by the alveolar dead space (DSA), which is that portion of the alveolar ventilation (V_A) that is wasted.[44] Consider the following example of a patient whose lungs are being ventilated: $PaCO_2$ is 40 mm Hg, end-tidal (alveolar) P_ACO_2 is 36 mm Hg, tidal volume is 500 mL, and anatomic dead space ventilation is 150 mL; therefore alveolar ventilation is 350 mL (500 - 150).

$$\begin{aligned} DSA/VA &= (PaCO_2 - P_ACO_2)/PaCO_2 \\ &= (40 - 36) \div 40 = 10\% \end{aligned}$$

Thus 35 mL (350 × 10%) of the VA is DSA, or wasted alveolar ventilation.

In addition to its use for confirming tracheal, rather than esophageal, intubation and to make adjustments to ventilator settings, end-tidal carbon dioxide monitoring has been found to correlate well with cardiac output during low-flow states. This has been applied in the evaluation of the efficacy of resuscitation efforts in cardiac arrest victims, and several studies have found that low end-tidal carbon dioxide is associated with a poorer prognosis.[45,46]

Volumetric Capnography

Some professional societies, including the ASA, have recognized the important link between carbon dioxide and volume, and although they have not yet mandated the monitoring of expired volume, they have strongly encouraged it. Because the transport of volume is central to the function of the lung, volumetric capnography provides a clearer and more comprehensive picture of the patient than a single-point measure such as an end-tidal value.

TABLE 8-2 **Possible Causes for Abnormal Capnogram Values**

Abnormal Value	Possible Cause
Absent	Capnograph line disconnect No ventilation, circuit obstructed Esophageal intubation, tube misplaced
End-tidal CO_2 increased	Increased production (fever, MH, tourniquet or X-clamp release, bicarbonate, CO_2 administration)
Inspired CO_2 zero	Decreased removal (hypoventilation)
Inspired CO_2 increased	Rebreathing (exhausted absorbent, channeling, incompetent unidirectional valves, CO_2 delivered to circuit in fresh gas flow)
End-tidal CO_2 decreased	Hyperventilation, decreased CO_2 production/delivery to lungs, low CO, V/Q mismatch, increased alveolar dead space, pulmonary embolism, artifact (rapid shallow breaths, gas sampling rate greater than expiratory flow rate, miscalibration of analyzer, air leak into sampling system)

CO, cardiac output; *CO_2*, carbon dioxide; *MH*, malignant hyperthermia; *V/Q*, ventilation/perfusion.

TABLE 8-3 **Possible Capnogram Abnormalities**

Abnormality	Possible Cause
Phase I	
Increased F_iCO_2	Rebreathing of CO_2 (exhausted absorbent, channeling, incompetent inspiratory/expiratory unidirectional valve[s], CO_2 delivered to circuit in fresh gas flow [some machines have CO_2 flowmeters], CO_2 gas being delivered via N_2O pipeline, inadequate fresh gas flow in Mapleson [rebreathing] circuit, Bain circuit inner-tube disconnect, capnograph analyzer not calibrated)
Phase II	
Slow/slanted	Exhalation gas flow obstruction (mechanical or in the patient), kinked tracheal tube, bronchospasm; gas sampling rate poorly matched to exhalation flow rate; exhaled CO_2 more quickly diluted by fresh gas
Phase III	
Irregular	Mechanical impingement on chest or abdomen by surgeon; patient attempting to breathe spontaneously while lungs are being mechanically ventilated ("curare cleft")
Regular	Cardiac oscillations; after complete exhalation, blood pulsating in chest moves gas forward and backward past sampling site. Slow decay of end-tidal value (gas sampling during expiratory pause causes CO_2 to be gradually diluted by fresh gas)
Phase IV	
Widened, slurred downstroke not reaching baseline	Incompetent inspiratory valve; accumulated CO_2 in inspiratory limb mixed with fresh gas, gradually replaced by fresh gas

CO_2, carbon dioxide; *NO_2*, nitrous oxide; *$FiCO_2$*, fractional concentration of inspired carbon dioxide.

The integration of flow or volume signals with the carbon dioxide concentration signal and the measurement of indexes characterizing this curve is widely known as *volumetric capnography*. It has also been referred to as the *single-breath test* for carbon dioxide[47,48] and *carbon dioxide spirography*.[49] It provides information based on physiology using an established and uniform terminology. This terminology was originally used by Fowler to describe the single-breath test for nitrogen (SBT-N_2) curve, with which instantaneous nitrogen concentration is plotted against expired volume.[50] Where instantaneous carbon dioxide fractional concentration is plotted against the expired volume, the resulting curve has been referred to as an *SBT-CO_2 curve*[47] or, preferably, the *volumetric capnogram*.[51] The presentation shown in Figure 8-30 provides a unified framework for such physiologic measures as carbon dioxide elimination, alveolar dead space, and rates of emptying.

This plot of carbon dioxide versus volume has been divided into three phases (Table 8-4).[47] Phase I is the carbon dioxide–free volume, and phase II is the transitional region characterized by a rapidly increasing carbon dioxide concentration resulting from progressive emptying of the alveoli. Phase III, the alveolar plateau, typically has a positive slope that indicates a rising PCO_2. With these three recognizable components of the volumetric capnogram, physiologically relevant measures can be determined, such as the volumes of each phase, the slopes of phase II and III, carbon dioxide elimination (VCO_2), dead space tidal volume, and ratios of anatomic and physiologic dead space.

Under normal conditions, the lungs will excrete carbon dioxide at the same rate as the total body production rate, and no net change in body carbon dioxide stores will occur. Carbon dioxide elimination (VCO_2), which often is incorrectly referred to as *carbon dioxide production*,

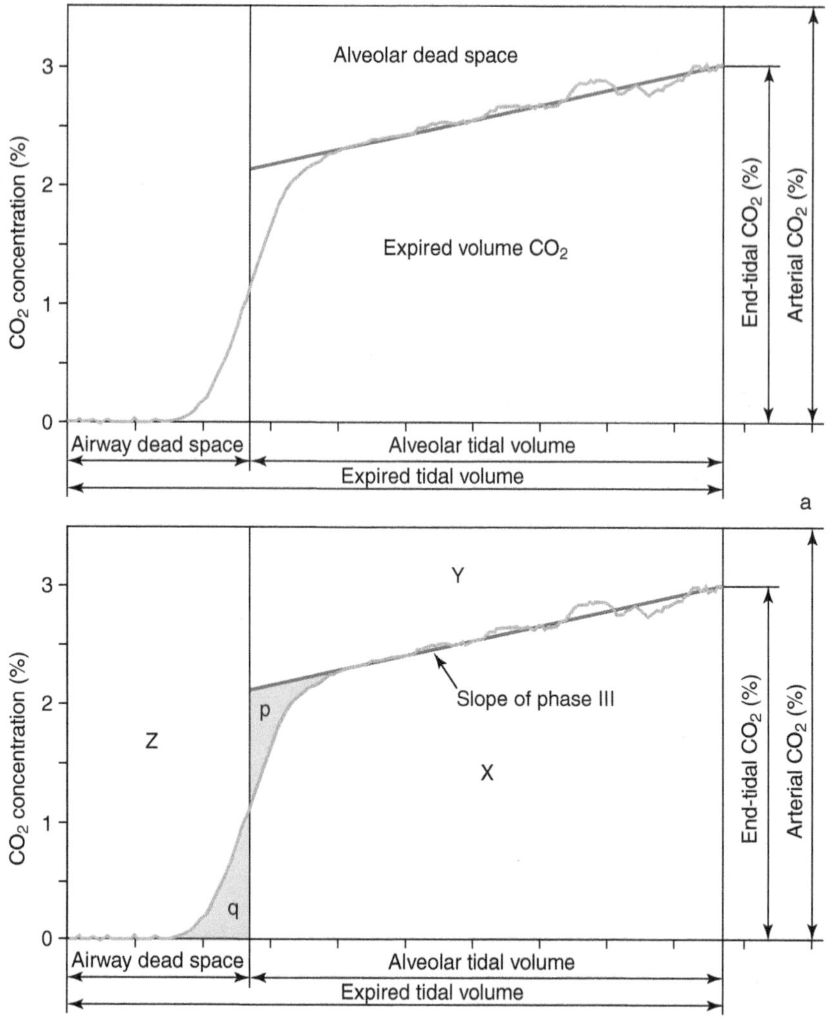

FIGURE 8-30 *Top,* Components of volumetric capnogram (carbon dioxide/volume plot). *Bottom,* Dead spaces shown graphically. Airway dead space, as illustrated by triangles *p* and *q,* are of equal area. Area *X* is the volume of carbon dioxide (CO_2) in the expired breath, and areas *Z* and *Y* are from airway and alveolar dead space (V_{daw} and V_{dalv}). Because it does not contribute to CO_2 elimination, this is wasted ventilation. (Modified from Fletcher R: The single breath test for carbon dioxide [thesis]. Lund, Sweden, 1980; and Arnold JH, Thompson JE, Arnold LW: Single breath CO_2 analysis: description and validation of a method. *Crit Care Med* 1996; 24[1]:96-102.)

is the net volume of carbon dioxide measured at the mouth or airway, calculated as the difference between expired and inspired carbon dioxide volumes normalized to 1 minute. $\dot{V}CO_2$ is computed by taking the integral of the product of the flow and carbon dioxide waveforms over the entire breath cycle and usually is reported at standard temperature and pressure dry (STPD) conditions. For breath-by-breath measurements, it is calculated as follows:

$$\dot{V}CO_2 = \sum FCO_2(t) \times \dot{V}(t) \times \Delta t \times RR$$

where $FCO_2(t)$ and $\dot{V}(t)$ are the sampled individual values of the carbon dioxide and flow waveforms summed over the entire breath, RR is the respiratory rate, and Δt is the sampling interval. When present, inspired carbon dioxide, if not accounted for, could result in an error in the calculation of $\dot{V}CO_2$ of several percent.[52] Figure 8-31 illustrates the multiplication process with the plot of actual flow and carbon dioxide waveforms versus time of a mechanical breath delivered in a volume control mode. If PCO_2 and volume are plotted instead, $\dot{V}CO_2$, the net volume of carbon dioxide eliminated, can be viewed as the area between the expiratory and inspiratory curves (Fig. 8-32). In anesthesia and intensive care, components such as filters, heat-moisture exchangers (HMEs), connecting tubes, elbows, airway adapters, and suction adapters are placed between the tracheal tube connector and Y-piece, causing partial rebreathing and thereby raising the level of the inspired carbon dioxide. Placement of the sampling site more proximally, such as at or near the endotracheal tube, will potentially allow the end-tidal carbon dioxide value to better reflect the alveolar concentration. If the inspiratory carbon dioxide volume is ignored, the overestimation of $\dot{V}CO_2$ will increase with decreases in tidal volume and/or increases in apparatus dead space.

With today's compact systems, measurements of flow and gas partial pressure, or concentration, are undertaken by flow and gas sensors that may or may not be located proximally and in the mainstream flow. Proximal flow measured at the patient's airway can be substantially different from flow measured inside or at the ventilator because the delivered flow in the inspiratory limb of the breathing circuit and the exhaled flow from the expiratory limb typically are measured internally by two separate flow sensors. Gas concentration may be measured at or near the patient airway or distally, away from the patient's airway, or a portion may be sampled and measured by a system located a distance from the sample

TABLE 8-4 **Comparison of Common Measures Available in Volumetric and Time-Based Capnography**

	Volumetric Capnography	Time-Based Capnography
End-tidal CO_2	Time-based average	Time-based average
Inspired CO_2	Various measures computable, including inspired CO_2 volume	Minimum value during inspiratory segment is often calculated and serves as rebreathing indicator
Breathing frequency	May be computed using flow waveform and/or capnogram	Inverse of time between the transition from expiratory to inspiratory segments of successive breaths is measured
Inspiratory/ expiratory time	Timing from start of inspiration and expiration determined from flow waveform	Approximate values may be calculated if dead space and rebreathing are not significant
Mixed expired CO_2 ($PeCO_2$ or $FeCO_2$)	Volume-weighted average of CO_2	Not available
Expired tidal volume	Total volume expired by subject	Not available
CO_2 elimination (VCO_2)	Net volume of CO_2 measured at the mouth or airway and calculated as the difference between expired and inspired CO_2	Not available
Efficiency	Ratio of volume of CO_2 contained in the breath and the volume of CO_2 that would have been eliminated by an ideal lung at the same effective volume and end-tidal fractional CO_2	Not available
Phase I: Carbon Dioxide–Free Gas from the Airways		
Duration	Time from start of expiration to increase in PCO_2	Not available
Volume	Volume from start of expiration to increase in PCO_2	Not available
Phase II: Rapid S-Shaped Upswing on the Tracing Caused by the Mixing of Dead Space Gas with Alveolar Gas		
Duration	Time from end of phase I to intersection of predictive slopes of phase II and III	Approximate measure available
Volume	Volume during phase II	Not available
Slope	Curve fit of central portion of phase II volume	Curve fit of central portion of time-based phase II
Phase III: Alveolar Plateau Representing CO_2-Rich Gas from the Alveoli		
Duration	Time from end of phase II to end of expiration	Approximate measure available
Volume	Volume during phase III	Not available
Slope	Curve fit of central portion of phase III volume	Curve fit of central portion of time-based phase III
α-Angle	Angle between phase II and III	Angle between phase II and III (range, 100-110 degrees)
Dead Space(s)		
Airway ("anatomic")	Volume of the conducting airways at the midpoint of the transition from dead space to alveolar gas	Not available
Alveolar	Dead space that is not airway dead space volume, calculated by subtracting the airway dead space volume from the physiologic dead space	Not available
Physiologic	Total dead spaceis the sum of alveolar, airway, and apparatus dead spaces	Not available
Dead Space Ratios		
Airway	Functional anatomic dead space calculated via Fowler's method divided by expired tidal volume	Not available
Physiologic	Total dead space calculated graphically, with Enghoff-modified Bohr equation or alternate methods	Not available
Alveolar	Alveolar volume divided by expired tidal volume	Not available

Courtesy Philips Respironics, Wallingford, CT.

site. The challenge is to combine the concentration and flow signals in such a way that the temporal relationship between these two variables is accurate. Also, given that frequency response differs among sensors, it is important that the time alignment and frequency response of the flow and carbon dioxide signal be suitably matched (Fig. 8-33).

As noted, the location of gas sampling and flow measurement varies, which can affect the reliability and accuracy of volumetric gas measurements; this applies to both mainstream and sidestream devices. Placement of the gas sampling site more proximally will potentially allow $P_{ET}CO_2$ to better reflect the alveolar concentration.

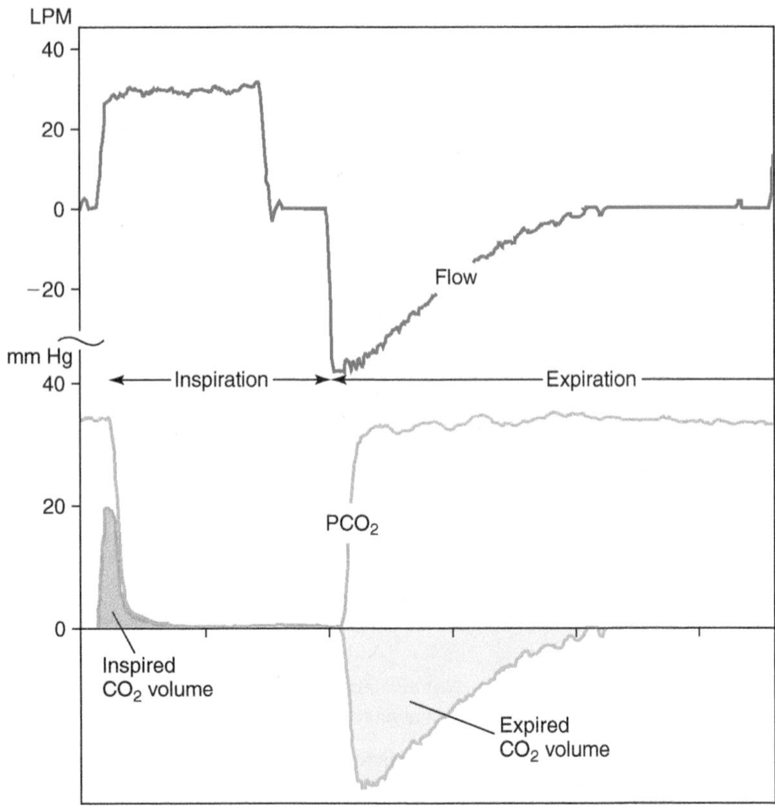

FIGURE 8-31 Plot of flow and CO_2 waveforms for an individual ventilator-delivered breath with cross-product showing inspired and expired CO_2 volumes. Because of apparatus dead space from the mainstream sensor, Y-piece, and other circuit components, a small volume of end-expiratory CO_2 from the previous breath is rebreathed upon the initiation of inspiration. Note that in this patient, the expiratory CO_2 waveform rises rapidly to a plateau, and the CO_2 volume curve follows that of the expiratory portion of the flow waveform. $\dot{V}CO_2$ would then be the difference between the expiratory and inspiratory areas of the dot products. LPM, liters per minute. (Courtesy Philips Respironics, Wallingford, CT.)

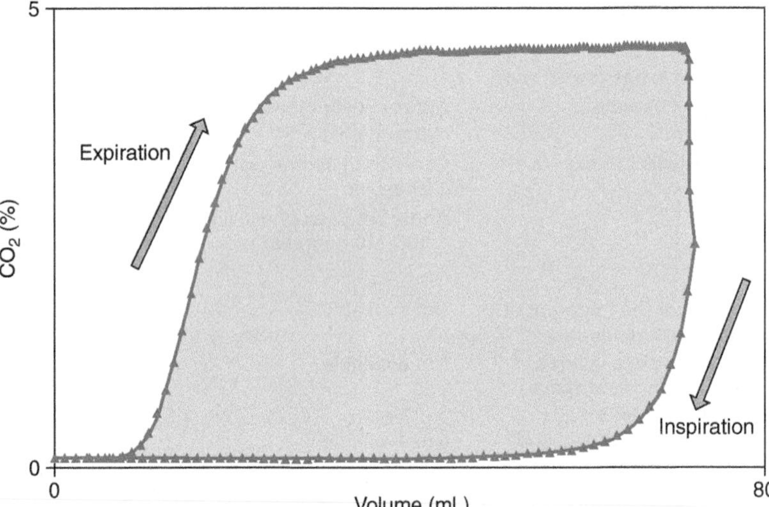

FIGURE 8-32 Plot of CO_2 vs. volume illustrating both the expiratory and inspiratory portions (100 samples/sec) of the breath. Note that the inspiratory portion is usually negligible, and the net CO_2 volume per breath is the difference between the area under the expired and inspired portions of this curve or, similarly, the area within the loop (*shaded portion*). (Courtesy Philips Respironics, Wallingford, CT.)

When leaks are present in the collecting system, or when conditions exist such that all the gas that is considered part of the alveolar ventilation volume cannot be measured, such as a pneumothorax with a leak or a tracheal tube cuff that leaks on exhalation, $\dot{V}CO_2$ may not accurately reflect the underlying physiology. Because of the complex interaction between tidal volume, physiologic dead space, and alveolar ventilation, the volume of carbon dioxide excreted by each breath is variable. The results of several breaths are often averaged in an attempt to decrease the effect of normal breath-to-breath changes in volume. Depending on how $\dot{V}CO_2$ is used (metabolic measurements vs. ventilator adjustments),[53] different averaging intervals may be required that include a range such as 1 breath, 8 breaths, 1 minute, 3 minutes, and longer. Because the body retains a large amount of carbon dioxide relative to the rate at which carbon dioxide is produced, eliminated carbon dioxide can be different from metabolically produced carbon dioxide for a long time—up to 1 hour following a significant change in ventilation. However, changes in $\dot{V}CO_2$ can provide an instantaneous indication of the change in effective alveolar ventilation.[52]

The respiratory dead space, also known as "wasted" ventilation, is considered to be that volume of each breath that is inhaled but does not participate in gas exchange. Airway dead space, a functional surrogate of anatomic dead space,

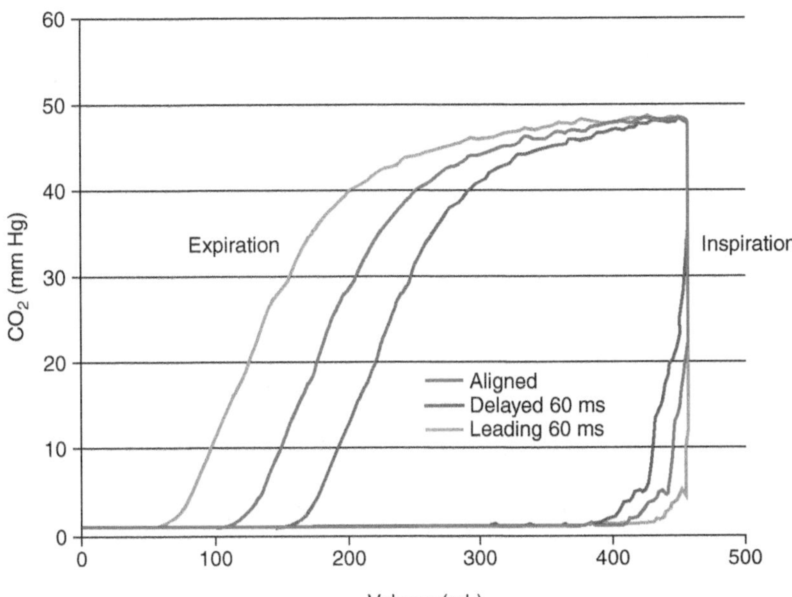

FIGURE 8-33 ■ Volumetric capnogram showing both expiratory and inspiratory limbs and illustrating the effect of time misalignment. Note that if the CO_2 waveform is delayed relative to the volume, the loop gets smaller on both ends; conversely, when the CO_2 waveform is advanced relative to volume, the loop gets larger on both ends. (Courtesy Philips Respironics, Wallingford, CT.)

is calculated from the carbon dioxide volume curve by Fowler's method,[50] which requires that the slope of phase III be estimated. *Physiologic dead space*, the sum of the airway dead space and alveolar dead space, also can be calculated but requires an estimate of the alveolar PCO_2. Arterial PCO_2 usually serves as an estimate of alveolar PCO_2 given the normally close relationship.[54] The portion of the physiologic dead space that does not take part in gas exchange but is within the alveolar space is considered the alveolar dead space. It is considered to be that volume of each breath that is inhaled but does not reach functional terminal respiratory units. The term *functional* has important implications because alveolar ventilation depends on the output of carbon dioxide. A respiratory unit that is ventilated but not eliminating carbon dioxide—that is, it is deprived of its blood flow—is included in the alveolar dead space volume. An increase in the alveolar dead space also occurs when regions of the lung are ventilated but underperfused. Alveolar dead space is affected by any condition that results in a V/Q mismatch, including 1) hypovolemia, 2) pulmonary hypotension, 3) pulmonary embolus, 4) ventilation of nonvascular airspace, 5) obstruction of precapillary pulmonary vessels, 6) obstruction of the pulmonary circulation by external forces, and 7) overdistension of the alveoli.[55]

The ventilation-perfusion relationships of the lung are more accurately reflected in the slope of phase III by a volumetric capnogram, rather than a time-based capnogram, in which the gradient of the phase III slope usually is less obvious and can be misleading. This may be attributed to the small volume of expired gases, approximately the final 15% of expired volume, that often occupies half the time available for expiration. In addition, unlike the volumetric capnogram, the physiologic dead space and carbon dioxide elimination cannot be measured from a time-based capnogram.

In addition, other potentially useful parameters have been calculated from the combination of carbon dioxide and volume, including new surrogates for, and better estimates of, alveolar carbon dioxide, estimates of ventilatory efficiency,[47] and measures of the nonsynchronous emptying of the alveoli with unequal V/Q ratios.[56] Ventilatory efficiency, by definition, requires an arterial blood gas and provides a single value that summarizes the emptying of the lung relative to an ideal lung (see Table 8-4). Alveolar ejection volume has been suggested by Romero et al[56] to serve as a measure of the nonsynchronous emptying of the alveoli with unequal V/Q ratios but is characterized as a misnomer by Fletcher and Drummond.[57] This measure of emptying can be contrasted with physiologic dead space, which can be viewed as reflecting the emptying characteristics of different alveoli.[55] The better understanding of respiratory physiology and related disease processes that volumetric capnography can help provide is only now beginning to be realized.

To properly calculate the various measurements associated with volumetric capnography, the basic measurements of carbon dioxide flow and airway pressure, to allow carbon dioxide to be referenced to in-circuit pressure, are required. It is preferable to measure all these parameters proximally, and a number of different approaches have been pursued over the past 30 years. Clinically acceptable results for carbon dioxide elimination may be obtained with many of the configurations under favorable conditions, if close attention is paid to the measurement, equipment setup, and interpretation of the displayed results. However, as more extremes of ventilator conditions are encountered, only the proximal mainstream flow and gas measurement offer a solution that can provide reliable results under the widely ranging humidity values, pressures, and temperatures seen in the clinical environment.

Commercial Equipment for Volumetric Capnography

Two companies, Philips Respironics and GE Healthcare, offer a family of integrated, disposable airway adapters optimized for different patient populations (Figs. 8-34 and 8-35) that offer volumetric capnography. The combined

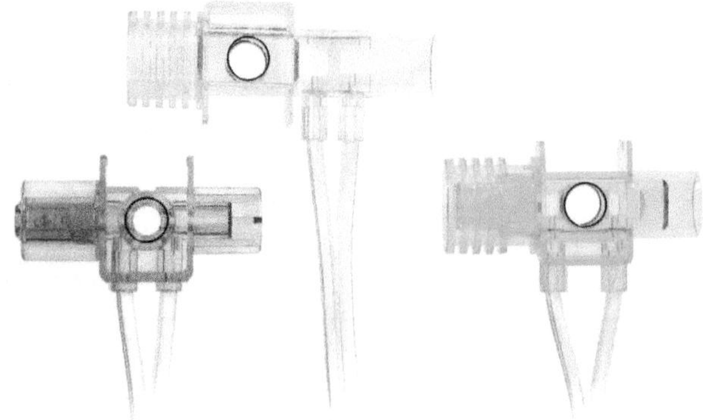

FIGURE 8-34 ■ Adult, pediatric, and neonatal combined CO_2 and fixed-orifice flow sensors. With the adult CO_2 flow sensor (*top*), dead space is less critical; as such, the CO_2 measurement cell and flow measurement portions are separate. With the combined neonatal (*bottom left*) and pediatric (*bottom right*) CO_2 flow sensors, the measurement cell, with small restrictions located on each side of the cell chamber, serves a dual function by adding a differential pressure flow signal to CO_2 measurement. (Courtesy Philips-Respironics, Wallingford, CT.)

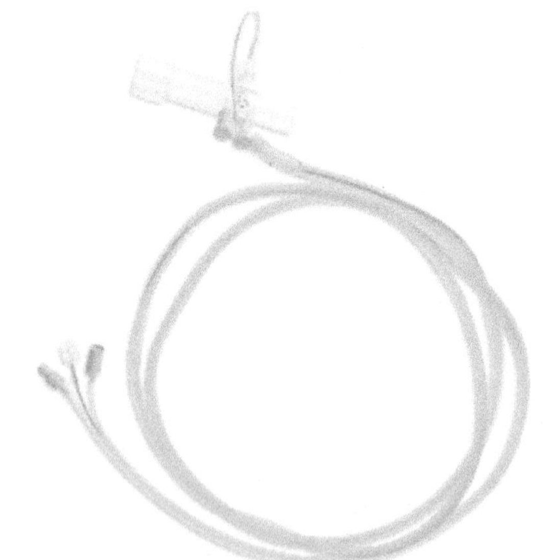

FIGURE 8-35 ■ Combined proximal flow sensor with sidestream gas sampling (D-Lite, GE Healthcare, Waukesha, WI). D-Lite and Pedi-Lite, a pediatric sensor, are available in both reusable (polyphenylsulfone) and disposable (polystyrene) versions. (Courtesy GE Healthcare, Waukesha, WI.)

carbon dioxide flow airway adapters from Philips Respironics are available in neonatal, pediatric, and adult tracheal tube sizes. These interface to an on-airway capnometer and differential pressure–based spirometry measurement module, whereas the GE Datex-Ohmeda adapters use their D-Lite flow sensor, available in adult and pediatric sizes, which has three ports: one for sidestream carbon dioxide gas sampling and two for differential pressure flow measurement.

Applications of Volumetric Capnography

The measured concentration of carbon dioxide is the result of ventilation, perfusion, metabolism, and their interactions and is affected by changes in any of these components. Knowledge of the absolute values and changes in the time-based and volumetric capnograms can assist in the diagnosis of a variety of physiologic and pathologic phenomena, and these serve as a valuable tool during a wide variety of clinical situations.

In some of these clinical situations, accurate knowledge of the end-tidal value may be clinically sufficient, but in other situations, the time-based capnogram is required for proper clinical interpretation. In many clinical scenarios, the time-based capnogram is inadequate as a reliable diagnostic tool or indicator. However, volumetric capnography can serve as a more reliable clinical tool and can be an indicator for a number of clinical situations, including intubation and pulmonary embolism screening. However, the added clinical value of these monitoring modalites often remains unrecognized. The recognized and potential clinical value of both time-based and volumetric capnography are briefly reviewed in Table 8-5 for many of the recognized and developing indications and clinical uses.

Nitrogen

Where available, measurement of nitrogen is useful in following preoxygenation (nitrogen washout), detecting venous air embolism, and detecting air leaks into the anesthesia breathing system. Fortunately, alternative means are now available to perform these functions.

Potent Inhaled Anesthetic Agents and Nitrous Oxide

Contemporary multigas analyzers measure the inspired and end-tidal concentrations of N_2O as well as the potent inhaled anesthetic agents desflurane, enflurane, halothane, isoflurane, and sevoflurane in the presence of one another. Although no study has established the value of this monitoring modality, the possible applications make the potential benefits of its use obvious; it makes possible the monitoring of anesthetic uptake and washout and allows setting high and low alarm limits for agent concentrations.

By adding the minimum alveolar concentration (MAC) values for N_2O and the potent agents to the analyzer software, and because MAC values are additive, once the composition of the gas mixture is known, the total MAC value of the inhaled anesthetic agents can be displayed. This is useful as an indication of anesthetic depth and a form of awareness monitor and has many potential applications.

Monitoring agent levels during uptake permits a safer and more intelligent use of the anesthesia vaporizer to reach target end-tidal concentrations in the patient. A high fresh gas flow and vaporizer concentration dial setting will ensure that the gas composition in the circuit changes rapidly, and the technique of "overpressure" can be used to speed anesthetic uptake. Once the desired end-tidal concentration has been attained, the vaporizer concentration dial setting can be decreased. When equilibrium has been reached—that is, when inspired and end-tidal agent concentrations are almost equal—the fresh gas flow can be decreased to maintain the equilibrium and conserve anesthetic agent. Monitoring of the anesthetic concentration during elimination provides

TABLE 8-5 **Comparison of Clinical Utility of Time-Based and Volumetric Capnography**

Clinical Use	Time-Based Capnography	Selected Refs/ Status	Volumetric Capnography	Selected Refs/Status
Acute Clinical Situations				
Prognosis and adequacy of cardiopulmonary resuscitation	$P_{ET}CO_2$ can guide efforts and indicate patient response; predictive of survival	80-82; accepted	Provides direct assessment of ventilation	83; speculative
Assessment of airway obstruction	Variable	84-86; accepted	Slope of phase III	87, 88; speculative
Screening for suspected pulmonary embolism	Poor; useful only in extreme cases	89, 90; developing	Alveolar dead space and dead space fraction are combined with D-dimer	91-94; developing
Intubation				
Avoiding esophageal intubation during ETT placement	Fast detection of exhaled CO_2 verifies placement; can give false-positive results	75; accepted	Presence of CO_2 and flow strongly indicative of tracheal intubation	76; speculative
Avoiding tracheal intubation during NG tube placement	Fast detection of exhaled CO_2 can be used to verify incorrect placement	77; developing	Lack of CO_2 and flow strongly indicate tube is not in the trachea	Speculative
Avoiding endobronchial intubation during ETT placement	Variable, not sensitive; significant changes in end-tidal levels may be observed	78; developing	Combination of CO_2, flow, airway pressure, and derived measures can assist detection	79; speculative
Routine Monitoring				
Preoperative assessment of respiratory disease	Potential quick screening tool as part of OSA screening	95; developing	See airway obstruction (above)	Speculative
$P_{ET}CO_2$ as a surrogate of $Paco_2$	Normal and constant ET-a gradients result in improved $PaCO_2$ estimates and fewer blood gas samples	109-112; developing	$P_{ET}CO_2$ is predictive of $PaCO_2$ if physiologic dead space is not too large	113, 114; developing
PCBF/cardiac output estimation	$P_{ET}CO_2$ variable	115, 116; developing	VCO_2 surrogate with stable ventilation; partial rebreathing Fick method for PCBF	117-120; developing
Monitoring during transport	Identifies tube displacement, verifies continuous ventilation, and helps optimize ventilation	121-124; accepted	Proximal CO_2, flow and airway pressure (and derived variables) allows continuous assessment of cardiorespiratory status	130; speculative
Intraoperative assessment	Good as front-line monitor	70, 130; accepted	Proximal CO_2, flow and airway pressure (and derived variables) allow continuous assessment of cardiorespiratory status	70, 130; developing
Assessment/safety of sedation/ paralytic therapy	Improved patient safety	125-129; accepted	CO_2 with flow allows better identification of hypoventilation	130; speculative
Mechanical Ventilation				
Detection of circuit leaks and/or rebreathing	Good, but may miss some leaks; rebreathing assessment only qualitative	97; accepted	Monitoring allows quantitative assessment of leaks and rebreathing	96, 98; developing
Detection of disconnection	Monitoring of $P_{ET}CO_2$ *and* waveform in intubated patients helps identify tube displacement	99-100; accepted	Monitoring of capnographic and flow can alert clinician to even partial disconnects	89, 130; developing
Weaning, outcome predictor	Use is self-limited	101-102; developing	Monitoring allows wide range of relevant measures used in protocols to be computed (i.e., VCO_2, RSBI)	53, 103-105; developing
PEEP titration	Arterial end-tidal difference	106; developing	Vco_2, slope of phase III	107, 108; developing

Accepted, widely accepted as standard practice; *CO_2,* carbon dioxide; *developing,* developing application; *ET-a,* end-tidal to arterial; *ETT,* endotracheal tube; *NG,* nasogastric; *OSA,* obstructive sleep apnea; *$PaCO_2$,* partial pressure of carbon dioxide in arterial blood; *PCBF,* pulmonary capillary blood flow; *PEEP,* positive end-expiratory pressure; *$P_{ET}CO_2$,* end-tidal pressure of carbon dioxide; *RSBI,* rapid shallow breathing index; *speculative,* possible, but not confirmed by evidence; *Vco_2,* rate of carbon dioxide.

Courtesy Philips Respironics, Wallingford, CT.

information regarding the state of its washout. The washout rate can then be increased by increasing the fresh gas flow, hence increasing its removal into the waste gas scavenging system.

The anesthetic agent high-concentration alarm can be used to alert the anesthetist to potential anesthetic overdosing. Indeed, the applicable U.S. consensus standard for anesthetic agent monitors requires a high-concentration alarm; a low-concentration alarm is an option.[58] The ASA Closed Claims Project includes several adverse outcomes as a result of anesthetic overdose and other reports of vaporizer malfunction that have led to higher than intended output concentrations.[59,60] The low-concentration alarm can be used to help prevent awareness by maintaining an anesthetic agent concentration that exceeds MACawake, which is the average of the concentrations immediately above and below those that permit voluntary response to command.[61] In general MACawake is approximately one third of MAC.[62] The anesthetic agent low-concentration alarm also serves as a late sign that the vaporizer is becoming empty. An agent analyzer may also alert the anesthetist to an air leak into the breathing system, causing an unintended low-agent concentration.[63]

Assuming that the analyzer has been calibrated according to the manufacturer's instructions, it can be used to check the calibration of a vaporizer as well as detect mixed agents in a vaporizer. Monitoring of N_2O concentrations may be helpful when discontinuing or avoiding its administration; this may apply in patients who have closed air spaces that might expand with the use of N_2O.

The continuous analysis of all of the respired gases by a multigas monitor also facilitates recording of the data by an automated anesthesia information management system. Many anesthesia caregivers record end-tidal concentrations of the gases administered. Monitoring of agent concentration, fresh gas flow, and time facilitates calculation of the consumption of the potent agents, both in liters of vapor and in milliliters of liquid agent. Attention to these data can be used to promote a more economical use of the more expensive anesthetics.

Gas Flow Sensor

Flow measurements in anesthesia are most commonly made with fixed-orifice or variable-orifice flowmeters. The Datex-Ohmeda D-Lite and Pedi-Lite flow sensors allow the qualitative and quantitative monitoring of respired gases using the density of the gas mixture for the computation of flow (see Chapter 9). Thus:

$$\text{Flow} \propto 2\times\sqrt{(\text{Pressure Difference/Density})}$$

Measuring Anesthetic Concentrations in the Blood

In some clinical studies, it may be necessary to measure the partial pressure of anesthetics in the blood. Although end-tidal concentrations are commonly used as a surrogate, they may differ considerably from those in arterial blood; yet it is the arterial levels that reflect the partial pressure of anesthetic perfusing the brain.[64,65] Measurement of blood concentrations of anesthetics usually is performed with a head space equilibration method with gas chromatography. Peyton and colleagues[66] have reported successfully using a conventional IR gas analyzer (Datex-Ohmeda Capnomac Ultima) and double head space equilibration technique to measure the partial pressures of anesthetics in blood; accuracy and precision were comparable to that achieved by studies using gas chromatography.

COMPLICATIONS OF GAS MONITORING

The complications associated with respiratory gas monitoring can be divided into two categories: pure equipment failure and use error.[67] As with any mechanical or electronic piece of equipment, failure can occur, but overall such devices are reliable if properly maintained, which includes any recommended maintenance and calibration procedures. Use error is a much more common problem. The user must understand respiratory physiology as well as monitoring technology to recognize a spurious reading. In addition, the user may misinterpret data,[67] which can lead to an inappropriate change in patient management. A simple example is that a low end-tidal carbon dioxide reading may cause the user to assume that the cause is hyperventilation and to decrease ventilation, when the problem is really a low cardiac output state.

In the event of total failure of the capnograph (electrical, mechanical, optical, etc.), a colorimetric carbon dioxide detector should always be kept as an immediate backup. Because these devices have an expiration date shown on the packaging, they should be checked routinely and replaced as necessary. A battery-powered portable capnometer is an alternative backup; if greater accuracy is needed, an arterial blood sample can be drawn for analysis in a blood gas analyzer.

CREDENTIALING FOR THE USE OF GAS MONITORING

There are no specific credentialing requirements associated with the use of gas monitoring. However, all users should receive in-service training when a new monitor is introduced; in particular, clinicians should understand and use the alarm features. Unfortunately, this is often not the case.[68] An educated user will no doubt derive more benefit than someone who has less understanding of the equipment. To this end, the Anesthesia Patient Safety Foundation (APSF) has sponsored a technology training initiative to promote critical training on new, sophisticated, or unfamiliar devices that can directly affect patient safety.[69]

PRACTICE PARAMETERS

In 1986, the ASA first approved standards for basic anesthesia monitoring. These have undergone periodic review and modification, the most recent being in October 2010.[70] The following sections contain excerpts from Standard II of the ASA Standards for Basic Anesthetic Monitoring,[70] and they pertain directly to the contents of this chapter.

Standard II

During all anesthetics, the patient's oxygenation, ventilation, circulation, and temperature shall be continually evaluated.

Oxygenation

Objective

To ensure adequate oxygen concentration in the inspired gas and the blood during all anesthetics.

Methods

1. *Inspired gas: During every administration of general anesthesia using an anesthesia machine, the concentration of oxygen in the patient breathing system shall be measured by an oxygen analyzer with a low oxygen concentration limit alarm in use.**

The requirement to monitor the F_iO_2 in the breathing system is not only one of the ASA standards, it is also included in the health code regulations of some states, including those of New York[71] and New Jersey. Note that the standard does *not* demand use of any specific technology to make the measurement, nor does it specify where in the inspiratory path oxygen must be monitored. Thus it is common to have a fuel cell located in the inspiratory unidirectional valve housing but downstream, on the patient side of the valve. It is also acceptable to sample gas from a connector by the patient's airway at the Y-piece for analysis in a multigas analyzer.

Ventilation

Objective

To ensure adequate ventilation of the patient during all anesthetics.

Methods

1. *Every patient receiving general anesthesia shall have the adequacy of ventilation continually evaluated. Qualitative clinical signs such as chest excursion, observation of the reservoir breathing bag, and auscultation of breath sounds are useful. Continual monitoring for the presence of expired carbon dioxide shall be performed unless invalidated by the nature of the patient, procedure, or equipment. Quantitative monitoring of the volume of expired gas is strongly encouraged.**
2. *When an endotracheal tube or laryngeal mask is inserted, its correct positioning must be verified by clinical assessment and by identification of carbon dioxide in the expired gas. Continual end-tidal carbon dioxide analysis, in use from the time of endotracheal tube/laryngeal mask placement until extubation/removal or initiating transfer to a postoperative care location, shall be performed using a quantitative method such as capnography, capnometry, or mass spectroscopy.* When capnography or capnometry is utilized, the end-tidal CO_2 alarm shall be audible to the anesthesiologist or the anesthesia care team personnel.**
3. *When ventilation is controlled by a mechanical ventilator, there shall be in continuous use a device that is capable of detecting disconnection of components of the breathing system. The device must give an audible signal when its alarm threshold is exceeded.*
4. *During regional anesthesia (with no sedation) or local anesthesia (with no sedation), the adequacy of ventilation shall be evaluated by continual observation of qualitative clinical signs. During moderate or deep sedation, the adequacy of ventilation shall be evaluated by continual observation of qualitative clinical signs and monitoring for the presence of exhaled carbon dioxide unless precluded or invalidated by the nature of the patient, procedure, or equipment.*

The ASA standards applicable to carbon dioxide monitoring have evolved considerably since they were first written. In particular, they have been revised to include use of the laryngeal mask airway, a supraglottic airway device, and use in regional anesthesia and monitored anesthesia care. Note also in item 3, the capnograph could be considered a disconnect detection device and as such must be used with an audible alarm activated. Catastrophes have been reported when state-of-the-art monitoring has been used with the alarms silenced.[68]

At time of this writing, no ASA standard requires monitoring of nitrous oxide and the potent inhaled anesthetics. However, as use of this monitoring becomes more widespread, it may become a de facto standard.[72] The manufacturers of anesthesia workstations anticipate this trend; the most recent American Society for Testing and Materials (ASTM) voluntary consensus standard requires that the anesthesia workstation be provided with a device to monitor the concentration of anesthetic vapor in the inspired gas.[73] The ASA standards for postanesthesia care, last updated in 2004,[74] do *not* require monitoring of gas concentrations.

AMERICAN SOCIETY OF ANESTHESIOLOGISTS STANDARDS FOR POSTANESTHESIA CARE

Standard IV

The patient's condition shall be evaluated continually in the PACU.

1. *The patient shall be observed and monitored by methods appropriate to the patient's medical condition. Particular attention should be given to monitoring oxygenation, ventilation, circulation, level of consciousness, and temperature. During recovery from all anesthetics, a quantitative method of assessing oxygenation, such as pulse oximetry, shall be employed in the initial phase of recovery.* This is not intended for application during the recovery of the obstetrical patient, in whom regional anesthesia was used for labor and vaginal delivery.*

In many postanesthesia care units, capnometry is used in patients who are tracheally intubated. If a patient requires reintubation, a means to confirm tracheal placement of the tube should be available, and its use must be documented.

*Under extenuating circumstances, the responsible anesthesiologist may waive the requirements marked with an asterisk; it is recommended that when this is done, it should be so stated, including the reasons, in a note in the patient's medical record.

REFERENCES

1. *Datex-Ohmeda compact airway modules technical reference manual:* Document no. 800 1009-5. Helsinki, 2003, Datex-Ohmeda Division, Instrumentarium.
2. Mushlin PS, Mark JB, Elliott WR, et al: Inadvertent development of subatmospheric airway pressure during cardiopulmonary bypass, *Anesthesiology* 71:459–462, 1989.
3. Healzer JM, Spiegelman WG, Jaffe RA: Internal gas analyzer leak resulting in an abnormal capnogram and incorrect calibration, *Anesth Analg* 81:202–203, 1995.
4. Pattinson K, Myers S, Gardner-Thorpe C: Problems with capnography at high altitude, *Anaesthesia* 59:69–72, 2004.
5. Ozanne GM, Young WG, Mazzei WJ, et al: Multipatient anesthetic mass spectrometry, *Anesthesiology* 55:62–67, 1981.
6. Gillbe CE, Heneghan CP, Branthwaite MA: Respiratory mass spectrometry during general anesthesia, *Br J Anaesth* 53:103–109, 1981.
7. Scamman FL, Fishbaugh JK: Frequency response of long mass spectrometer sampling catheters. *Anesthesiology* 65:422–425, 1986.
8. Steinbrook RA, Elliott WR, Goldman DB, Philip JH: Linking mass spectrometers to provide continuing monitoring during system failure, *J Clin Monit* 7:271–273, 1991.
9. Schulte GT, Block FE: Evaluation of a single room dedicated mass spectrometer, *J Clin Monit* 8:179–181, 1991.
10. Severinghaus JW, Larson CP, Eger EI: Correction factors for infrared carbon dioxide pressure broadening by nitrogen, nitrous oxide, and cyclopropane, *Anesthesiology* 22:429–432, 1961.
11. Nielsen JR, Thornton V, Dale EB: The absorption laws for gases in the infrared, *Rev Mod Phys* 16:307–324, 1944.
12. Kennell EM, Andrews RW, Wollman H: Correction factors for nitrous oxide in the infrared analysis of carbon dioxide. *Anesthesiology* 39:441–443, 1973.
13. Raemer DB, Philip JH: Monitoring anesthetic and respiratory gases. In Blitt CD, editor: *Monitoring in anesthesia and critical care medicine*, New York, 1990, Churchill-Livingstone, pp 373–386.
14. *PB 254 owners manual*, Wilmington, Mass, 1985, Puritan-Bennett.
15. Guyton D, Gravenstein N: Infrared analysis of volatile anesthetics: impact of monitor agent setting, volatile mixtures and alcohol, *J Clin Monit* 6:203–206, 1990.
16. Nielsen J, Kann T, Moller JT: Evaluation of three transportable multigas anesthetic monitors, *J Clin Monit* 9:91–98, 1994.
17. Møllgaard K: Acoustic gas measurement, *Biomed Instrum Technol* 23:495–497, 1989.
18. Berggren M, Hosseini N, Nilsson K, Stenqvist O: Improved response time with a new miniaturised main-stream multigas monitor, *J Clin Monit Comput* 23:355–361, 2009.
19. Colman Y, Krauss B: Microstream capnography technology: a new approach to an old problem, *J Clin Monit Comput* 15:403–409, 1999.
20. Casati A, Gallioli A, Passarretta P, Borgi B, Torri G: Accuracy of end-tidal carbon dioxide monitoring using the NPB 75 Microstream capnometer: a study in intubated, ventilated and spontaneously breathing nonintubated patients, *Eur J Anaesthesiol* 17:622–626, 2000.
21. Westenskow DR, Smith KW, Coleman DL, et al: Clinical evaluation of a Raman scattering multiple gas analyzer for the operating room, *Anesthesiology* 70:350–355, 1989.
22. Lockwood GG, Landon MJ, Chakrabarti MK, Whitwam JG: The Ohmeda Rascal II: a new gas analyzer for anaesthetic use, *Anaesthesia* 49:44–53, 1994.
23. Severinghaus JW: Water vapor calibration errors in some capnometers: respiratory conventions misunderstood by manufacturers? *Anesthesiology* 70:996–998, 1989.
24. Sum Ping ST, Mehta MP: Symreng T: Accuracy of the FEF CO_2 detector in the assessment of endotracheal tube placement, *Anesth Analg* 74:415–419, 1992.
25. Srinivasa V, Kodali BS: Caution when using colorimetry to confirm endotracheal intubation, *Anesth Analg* 104:738, 2007.
26. Brackney SM: Caution when using colorimetry to confirm endotracheal intubation, *Anesth Analg* 104:739, 2007.
27. Hendrickx JFA, Van Zundert AAJ, De Wolf AM: Influence of the reference gas of paramagnetic oxygen analyzers on nitrogen concentrations during closed-circuit anesthesia, *J Clin Monit* 14:381–384, 1998.
28. Fontijn A, Sabadell AJ, Ronco RJ: Homogeneous chemiluminescent measurement of nitric oxide with ozone, *Anal Chem* 42:575–579, 1970.
29. Holland R: Wrong gas disaster in Hong Kong, *Anesthesia Patient Safety Foundation Newsletter* 4:25–36, 1989.
30. Machlin HA, Myles PS, Berry CB, et al: End-tidal oxygen measurement compared with patient factor assessment for determining preoxygenation time, *Anaesth Intensive Care* 21:409–413, 1993.
31. Tanoubi I, Drolet P, Donati F: Optimizing preoxygenation in adults, *Can J Anaesth* 56:449–466, 2009.
32. Gadhinglaikar SV, Sreedhar R, Unnikrishnan KP: Oxygraphy: an unexplored perioperative monitoring modality., *J Clin Monit Comput* 23:131–135, 2009.
33. Berry CB, Myles PS: Preoxygenation in healthy volunteers: a graph of oxygen "washin" using end-tidal oxygraphy, *Br J Anaesth* 74:116–118, 1994.
34. Barnard JP, Sleigh JW: Breath-by-breath analysis of oxygen uptake using the Datex Ultima, *Br J Anaesth* 74:155–158, 1995.
35. Takala J, Meriläinen P: *Handbook of indirect calorimetry and gas exchange*, Helsinki, 1991, Datex-Ohmeda, p 30.
36. Stuart-Andrews CR, Peyton P, Robinson GJ, et al: In vivo validation of the M-COVX metabolic monitor in patients under anaesthesia, *Anaesth Intensive Care* 35(3):398–405, 2007.
37. Takala J: *Appliguide: clinical application guide of gas exchange and indirect calorimetry*, Helsinki, 2000, Datex-Ohmeda.
38. Gadhinglajkar SV, Sreedhar R, Unnikrishnan KP: Oxygraphy: an unexplored perioperative monitoring modality, *J Clin Monit Comput* 23(3):131–135, 2009.
39. Orr JA, Brewer LM: Clinical evaluation of an on-airway system to measure oxygen uptake, *Anesthesiology* 109:A281, 2008.
40. Surgery mix-up causes 2 deaths. *New Haven Register*, January 20, 2002.
41. Birmingham PK, Cheney FW, Ward RJ: Esophageal intubation: a review of detection techniques, *Anesth Analg* 65:886–891, 1986.
42. Gravenstein JS, Jaffe MB, Paulus DA: *Capnography: clinical aspects*, New York, 2004, Cambridge University Press.
43. Smalhout B, Kalenda Z: *An atlas of capnography*, ed 2, Utrecht, The Netherlands, 1981, Kerkebosche Zeist.
44. Nunn JF: *Applied respiratory physiology*. Boston, 1977, Butterworths, p 226.
45. Sanders AB, Kern KB, Otto CW, Milander MM, Ewy GA: End-tidal CO_2 monitoring during CPR: a prognostic indicator for survival, *JAMA* 262:1347–1351, 1989.
46. Wayne ME, Levine RL, Miller CC: Use of end-tidal CO_2 to predict outcome in pre-hospital cardiac arrest, *Ann Emerg Med* 25:762–767, 1995.
47. Fletcher R: The single breath test for carbon dioxide [thesis]. Lund, Sweden, 1980.
48. Arnold JH, Thompson JE, Arnold LW: Single breath CO_2 analysis: description and validation of a method, *Crit Care Med* 24(1):96–102, 1996.
49. Breen PH, Bradley PJ: Carbon dioxide spirogram (but not capnogram) detects leaking inspiratory valve in a circle circuit, *Anesth Analg* 85(6):1372–1376, 1997.
50. Fowler WS: Lung function studies. II. The respiratory dead space, *Am J Physiol* 154:405–416, 1948.
51. Ream RS, Schreiner MS, Neff JD, et al: Volumetric capnography in children: influence of growth on the alveolar plateau slope, *Anesthesiology* 82(1):64–73, 1995.
52. Breen PH, Serina ER, Barker SJ: Measurement of pulmonary CO_2 elimination must exclude inspired CO_2 measured at the capnometer sampling site, *J Clin Monit* 12(3):231–236, 1996.
53. Taskar V, John J, Larsson A, Wetterberg T, Jonson B: Dynamics of carbon dioxide elimination following ventilator resetting, *Chest* 108(1):196–202, 1995.
54. Enghoff H: Volumen inefficax: Bemerkungen zur Frage des schädlichen Raumes, *Uppsala LäkFör Förh* 44:191–218, 1938.
55. Lumb AB: *Nunn's applied respiratory physiology*, ed 7, London, 2010, Churchill Livingstone.
56. Romero PV, Lucangelo U, Lopez Aguilar J, Fernandez R, Blanch L: Physiologically based indices of volumetric capnography in patients receiving mechanical ventilation, *Eur Respir J* 10(6):1309–1315, 1997.
57. Fletcher R, Drummond GB: Alveolar ejection volume: a misnomer? *Eur Respir J* 15(1):232–233, 2000.

58. American Society for Testing and Materials: *Medical electrical equipment: particular requirements for the basic safety and essential performances of respiratory gas monitors*. West Conshohocken, PA, 2005, ASTM/ISO 21647.
59. Caplan RA, Vistica MF, Posner KL, Cheney FW: Adverse anesthetic outcomes arising from gas delivery equipment: a closed claims analysis, *Anesthesiology* 87:741–748, 1997.
60. Geffroy JC, Gentili ME, Le Pollès R, Triclot P: Massive inhalation of desflurane due to vaporizer dysfunction, *Anesthesiology* 103:1096–1098, 2005.
61. Stoelting RK, Longnecker DE, Eger EI 2nd: Minimal alveolar concentrations on awakening from methoxyflurane, halothane, ether and fluroxene in man: MAC awake, *Anesthesiology* 33:5–9, 1970.
62. Eger EI II, Weisskopf RB, Eisenkraft JB: *The pharmacology of inhaled anesthetics*, San Antonio, 2002, Dannemiller Memorial Educational Foundation, p 27.
63. Sandberg WS, Kaiser S: Novel breathing system architecture: new consequences of old problems, *Anesthesiology* 100:755–756, 2004.
64. Landon MJ, Matson AM, Royston BD, et al: Components of the inspiratory-arterial isoflurane partial pressure difference, *Br J Anaesth* 70:605–611, 1993.
65. Frei FJ, Zbinden AM, Thomson DA, Rieder HU: Is the end-tidal partial pressure of isoflurane a good predictor of its arterial partial pressure? *Br J Anaesth* 66:331–339, 1991.
66. Peyton PJ, Chong M, Stuart-Andrews C, et al: Measurement of anesthetics in blood using a conventional infrared clinical gas analyzer, *Anesth Analg* 105:680–687, 2007.
67. Barker SJ: Too much technology? *Anesth Analg* 97:938–939, 2003.
68. $16 million settlement Monitoring devices turned off/down; patient suffers irreversible brain damage, *Anesthesia Malpractice Prevention (Newsletter)* 2:3, 1997.
69. Olympio MA: Formal training and assessment before using advanced medical devices in the OR, *Anesthesia Patient Safety Foundation Newsletter* 22:63–65, 2007.
70. American Society of Anesthesiologists: Standards for basic anesthetic monitoring. Approved by the ASA House of Delegates on October 21, 1986; last amended October 20, 2010 with an effective date of July 1, 2011. Available at www.asahq.org.
71. NY State Laws and regulations, Section 405.13. Anesthesia services (b)(2)(iii)(d).
72. Eichhorn JH: Pulse oximetry as a standard of practice in anesthesia, *Anesthesiology* 78:423–425, 1993.
73. American Society for Testing and Materials: *Standard Specification for Particular Requirements for Anesthesia Workstations and their Components ASTM F1850-2005*, West Conshohocken, PA, 2005, ASTM.
74. ASA Standards for Postanesthesia Care, approved by the ASA House of Delegates on October 27, 2004, and last amended on October 21, 2009. Available at www.asahq.org.
75. Knapp S, Kofler J, Stoiser B, Thalhammer F, Burgmann H, Posch M, Hofbauer R, Stanzel M, Frass M: The assessment of four different methods to verify tracheal tube placement in the critical care setting, *Anesth Analg* 88(4):766–770, 1999.
76. Cheifetz IM, Myers TR: Respiratory therapies in the critical care setting. Should every mechanically ventilated patient be monitored with capnography from intubation to extubation? *Respir Care* 52(4):423–438, 2007 Apr.
77. Chau JP, Lo SH, Thompson DR, Fernandez R, Griffiths R: Use of end-tidal carbon dioxide detection to determine correct placement of nasogastric tube: a meta-analysis, *Int J Nurs Stud* 48(4):513–521, 2011.
78. Gandhi SK, Munshi CA, Coon R, Bardeen-Henschel A: Capnography for detection of endobronchial migration of an endotracheal tube, *J Clin Monit* 7(1):35–38, 1991.
79. Mahajan A, Wald SH, Schroeder R, Turner J: Detection of Endobronchial Intubation in Infants and Children Using Spirometry, *Anesthesiology* 97(3):A1268, 2002.
80. Falk JL, Rackow EC, Weil MH: End-tidal carbon dioxide concentration during cardiopulmonary resuscitation, *N Engl J Med* 318(10):607–611, 1988.
81. Levine RL, Wayne MA, Miller CC: End-tidal carbon dioxide and outcome of out-of-hospital cardiac Aarrest, *New Eng J Med* 337(5):301–306, 1997.
82. White RD, Goodman BW, Svoboda MA: Neurologic recovery following prolonged out-of-hospital cardiac arrest with resuscitation guided by continuous capnography, *Mayo Clin Proc* 86(6):544–548, 2011.
83. Terndrup TE, Rhee J: Available ventilation monitoring methods during pre-hospital cardiopulmonary resuscitation, *Resuscitation* 71(1):10–18, 2006.
84. You B, Peslin R, Duvivier C, Vu VD, Grilliat JP: Expiratory capnography in asthma: evaluation of various shape indices, *Eur Respir J* 7(2):318–323, 1994.
85. Yaron M, Padyk P, Hutsinpiller M, Cairns CB: Utility of the expiratory capnogram in the assessment of bronchospasm, *Ann Emerg Med* 28(4):403–407, 1996.
86. Nik Hisamuddin NA, Rashidi A, Chew KS, Kamaruddin J, Idzwan Z, Teo AH: Correlations between capnographic waveforms and peak flow meter measurement in emergency department management of asthma, *Int J Emerg Med* 2(2):83–89, 2009 Feb 24.
87. Almeida CC, Almeida-Júnior AA, Ribeiro MA, Nolasco-Silva MT, Ribeiro JD: Volumetric capnography to detect ventilation inhomogeneity in children and adolescents with controlled persistent asthma, *J Pediatr (Rio J)* 87(2):163–168, 2011 Mar-Apr.
88. Romero PV, Rodriguez B, de Oliveira D, Blanch L, Manresa F: Volumetric capnography and chronic obstructive pulmonary disease staging, *Int J Chron Obstruct Pulmon Dis* 2(3):381–391, 2007.
89. Thys F, Elamly A, Marion E, Roeseler J, Janssens P, El Gariani A, Meert P, Verschuren F, Reynaert M: $P_aCO_2/ETCO_2$ gradient: early indicator of thrombolysis efficacy in a massive pulmonary embolism, *Resuscitation* 49(1):105–108, 2001.
90. Courtney DM, Watts JA, Kline JA: Use of Capnometry to Distinguish Cardiac Arrest Secondary to Massive Pulmonary Embolism from Primary Cardiac Arrest, *Acad Emerg Med* 8(5):433, 2001.
91. Anderson JT, Owings JT, Goodnight JE: Bedside noninvasive detection of acute pulmonary embolism in critically ill surgical patients, *Arch Surg* 134(8):869–875, 1999.
92. Kline JA, Israel EG, Michelson EA, O'Neil BJ, Plewa MC, Portelli DC: Diagnostic accuracy of a bedside D-dimer assay and alveolar dead-space measurement for rapid exclusion of pulmonary embolism: a multicenter study, *JAMA* 285(6):761–768, 2001.
93. Moreira MM, Terzi RG, Cortellazzi L, Falcão AL, Moreno H Jr, Martins LC, Coelho OR: Volumetric capnography: in the diagnostic work-up of chronic thromboembolic disease, *Vasc Health Risk Manag* 25(6):317–319, 2010.
94. Verschuren F, Heinonen E, Clause D, Roeseler J, Thys F, Meert P, Marion E, El Gariani A, Col J, Reynaert M, Liistro G: Volumetric capnography as a bedside monitoring of thrombolysis in major pulmonary embolism, *Intensive Care Med* 30(11):2129–2132, 2004.
95. Block FE Jr, Reynolds KM, Kajaste T, Nourijelyani K: Preoperative oximetry and capnometry: potential respiratory screening tools, *Int J Clin Monit Comput* 13(3):153–156, 1996.
96. Blanch L, Romero PV, Lucangelo U: Volumetric capnography in the mechanically ventilated patient, *Minerva Anestesiol* 72(6):577–585, 2006 Jun.
97. Healzer JM, Spiegelman WG, Jaffe RA: Internal gas analyzer leak resulting in an abnormal capnogram and incorrect calibration, *Anesth Analg* 81(1):202–203, 1995.
98. Breen PH, Bradley PJ: Carbon dioxide spirogram (but not capnogram) detects leaking inspiratory valve in a circle circuit, *Anesth Analg* 85(6):1372–1376, 1997.
99. Kennedy RR, French RA: A breathing circuit disconnection detected by anesthetic agent monitoring, *Can J Anesth* 48(9):847–849, 2001.
100. Tripathi M, Tripathi M: A partial disconnection at the main stream CO_2 transducer mimics "curare-cleft" capnograph, *Anesthesiology* 88(4):1117–1119, 1998.
101. Morley TF, Giaimo J, Maroszan E, Bermingham J, Gordon R, Griesback R, Zappasodi SJ, Giudice JC: Use of capnography for assessment of the adequacy of alveolar ventilation during weaning from mechanical ventilation, *Am Rev Respir Dis* 148(2):339–344, 1993.
102. Saura P, Blanch L, Lucangelo U, Fernandez R, Mestre J, Artigas A: Use of capnography to detect hypercapnic episodes

during weaning from mechanical ventilation, *Intensive Care Med* 22(5):374–381, 1996.

103. Boynton JH, O'Keefe G: The use of VCO_2 in predicting liberation from mechanical ventilation, *Resp Care* 44(10):1243, 1999.
104. Hubble CL, Gentile MA, Tripp DS, Craig D, Meliones JN, Cheifetz IM: Deadspace to tidal volume ratio predicts successful extubation in infants and children, *Crit Care Med* 28(6):2034–2040, 2000.
105. Nuckton TJ, Alonso JA, Kallet RH, Daniel BM, Pittet JF, Eisner MD, Matthay MA: Pulmonary dead-space fraction as a risk factor for death in the acute respiratory distress syndrome, *N Engl J Med* 25:346(17):1281–1286, 2002.
106. Murray IP, Modell JH, Gallagher TJ, Banner MJ: Titration of PEEP by the arterial minus end-tidal carbon dioxide gradient, *Chest* 85(1):100–104, 1984.
107. Böhm SH, Maisch S, von Sandersleben A, Thamm O, Passoni I, Martinez Arca J, Tusman G: The effects of lung recruitment on the Phase III slope of volumetric capnography in morbidly obese patients, *Anesth Analg* 109(1):151–159, 2009.
108. Tusman G, Bohm SH, Suarez-Sipmann F, Scandurra A, Hedenstierna G: Lung recruitment and positive end-expiratory pressure have different effects on CO2 elimination in healthy and sick lungs, *Anesth Analg* 111(4):968–977, 2010.
109. Chan KL, Chan MT, Gin T: Mainstream vs. sidestream capnometry for prediction of arterial carbon dioxide tension during supine craniotomy, *Anaesthesia* 58(2):149–155, 2003.
110. King JC, Boitano LC, Benditt JO: End-Tidal Carbon Dioxide (ETCO2) Accurately Predicts Arterial Carbon Dioxide ($PaCO_2$) in Patients with Neuromuscular Disease, *Am J Respir Crit Care Med* 167(7):A424, 2003.
111. Barton CW, Wang ES: Correlation of end-tidal CO_2 measurements to arterial PaCO2 in nonintubated patients, *Ann Emerg Med* 23(3):560–563, 1994.
112. McDonald MJ, Montgomery VL, Cerrito PB, Parrish CJ, Boland KA, Sullivan JE: Comparison of end-tidal CO_2 and $PaCO_2$ in children receiving mechanical ventilation, *Pediatr Crit Care Med* 3(3):244–249, 2002.
113. Banner MJ: Partial pressure of end-tidal CO_2 in the ICU: Reevaluating old beliefs, *Anesthesiology* SCCA:B8, 2000.
114. McSwain SD, Hamel DS, Smith PB, Gentile MA, Srinivasan S, Meliones JN, Cheifetz IM: End-tidal and arterial carbon dioxide measurements correlate across all levels of physiologic dead space, *Respir Care* 55(3):288–293, 2010.
115. Ornato JP, Garnett AR, Glauser FL: Relationship between cardiac output and the end-tidal carbon dioxide tension, *Ann Emerg Med* 19(10):1104–1106, 1990.
116. Saleh HZ, Pullan DM: Monitoring cardiac output trends with end-tidal carbon dioxide pressures in off-pump coronary bypass, *Ann Thorac Surg* 91(5):e81–e82, 2011.
117. Gedeon A, Forslund L, Hedenstierna G, Romano E: A new method for noninvasive bedside determination of pulmonary blood flow, *Med Biol Eng Comput* 18(4):411–418, 1980.
118. Capek JM, Roy RJ: Noninvasive measurement of cardiac output using partial CO_2 rebreathing, *IEEE Trans Biomed Eng* 35(9):653–661, 1988.
119. Jaffe MB: Partial CO_2 Rebreathing Cardiac Output – Operating Principles of the NICO® System, *J Clin Monit* 15(6):387–401, 1999.
120. Young BP, Low LL: Noninvasive monitoring cardiac output using partial CO_2 rebreathing, *Crit Care Clin* 26(2):383–392, 2010.
121. Ruckoldt H, Marx G, Leuwer M, Panning B, Piepenbrock S: Pulse oximetry and capnography in intensive care transportation: combined use reduces transportation risks, *Anasthesiol Intensivmed Notfallmed Schmerzther* 33(1):32–36, 1998.
122. Bacon CL, Corriere C, Lavery RF, Livingston DH: The use of capnography in the air medical environment, *Air Med J* 20(5):27–29, 2001.
123. Tobias JD, Lynch A, Garrett J: Alterations of end-tidal carbon dioxide during the intrahospital transport of children, *Pediatr Emerg Care* 12:249–251, 1996.
124. Langhan ML, Ching K, Northrup V, Santucci K, Chen L: A Randomized Controlled Trial of Capnography in the Correction of Simulated Endotracheal Tube Dislodgement, *Acad Emerg Med* 18(6):590–596, 2011.
125. McQuillen KK, Steele DW: Capnography during sedation/analgesia in the pediatric emergency department, *Pediatr Emerg Care* 16(6):401–404, 2000.
126. Burton JH, Harrah JD, Germann CA, Dillon DC: Does end-tidal carbon dioxide monitoring detect respiratory events prior to current sedation monitoring practices? *Acad Emerg Med* 13:500–504, 2006.
127. McCarter T, Shaik Z, Scarfo K, Thompson LJ: Capnography monitoring enhances safety of postoperative patient-controlled analgesia, *American Health & Drug Benefits*, June 2008, 28–35.
128. Deitch K, Miner J, Chudnofsky CR, Dominici P, Latta D: Does end tidal CO_2 monitoring during emergency department procedural sedation and analgesia with propofol decrease the incidence of hypoxic events? A randomized, controlled trial, *Ann Emerg Med* 55(3):258–264, 2010.
129. Langhan ML, Chen L, Marshall C, Santucci KA: Detection of hypoventilation by capnography and its association with hypoxia in children undergoing sedation with ketamine, *Pediatr Emerg Care* 27(5):394–397, 2011.
130. Gravenstein JS, Jaffe MB, Gravenstein N, Paulus DA, editors: *Capnography*, ed 2, Cambridge, UK, 2011, Cambridge University. Press, p 488.

CHAPTER 9

MONITORING VENTILATION

James M. Berry • Brian S. Rothman • James B. Eisenkraft

CHAPTER OUTLINE

OVERVIEW

Until the early twentieth century, animal life was defined by the presence of *spontaneous ventilation*. Absence of breathing implied death or impending death, although experiments with resuscitation and artificial ventilation had occurred since the eighteenth century.[1] The defining characteristics of spontaneous ventilation, *depth* and *frequency*, were early indicators of anesthetic action, with profound depression of respiration indicating the deepest plane of ether narcosis.[2]

The most fundamental measure of ventilation is frequency, measured in units of inverse time, usually min^{-1}. Although physiology pundits will remind us that respiration is a cellular phenomenon, the term *respiratory rate* is commonly accepted to denote the frequency of ventilation, either spontaneous or controlled.

RESPIRATORY RATE

Respiratory rate is still commonly assessed by direct observation, either by counting the spontaneous breaths observed in a full minute or by doubling the count in 30 seconds. In the nearly well patient, the frequency at rest is relatively predictable (~14 to 18 min^{-1}),[3] whereas in the critically ill or perioperative patient, it is more variable. In reference to hospital patients in the 1950s, one commentator noted that almost all patients had recorded "respiratory rates" of between 18 and 22 min^{-1}, irrespective of their actual value; this led him to conclude that the routine recording of respiration was not only useless but wasted millions of hours of health care time annually.[4] On the other hand, a more astute observer commented that respiratory rate "is a sensitive clinical parameter in a multitude of pulmonary diseases, especially in the critical care setting."[5]

Although tachypnea has many underlying causes, one common perioperative cause is pain. It is unusual for severe, acute pain not to be accompanied by hyperventilation as a part of a clinical picture of systemic stimulus and sympathetic nervous system activation. Conversely, patients who have recently received opioid analgesics may exhibit bradypnea as one sign of a relative overdose. Thus the frequency of spontaneous ventilation may be a crude but valuable tool in preserving the comfort and safety of perioperative patients in that it may express the balance between acute pain and analgesic effects.[6] In a spontaneously breathing patient, the titration of opioid analgesics to effect is much more difficult without access to this simple, real-time variable.

Automated Determination of Respiratory Rate

Determination of respiratory rate by direct observation is difficult because of interobserver variability, length of time needed for accurate readings (up to 1 minute), and the confounding effects of upper airway obstruction that produce chest wall motion and *apparent* breaths in the absence of gas exchange. The reliable automation of this data gathering is valuable, not only to perioperative caregivers—especially those who perform regional or sedation techniques—but also to nonanesthesiology personnel responsible for patient sedation in more remote or ambulatory locations.

Instrumentation to measure respiration may be *direct*, as in airflow sensors—pinwheels, gas sampling, or thermocouples—or *indirect*, imputing air flow from changes in thoracic dimension or breath sounds. Indirect measurements of chest volume may be via strain gauges, impedance measurements, or electrocardiograph (ECG) analysis. In a fully equipped operating suite, the most convenient method of measurement is with a capnograph. In the tracheally intubated, anesthetized patient and in the awake or sedated patient, exhaled gas flow may be sampled using a number of devices. In the case of the spontaneously breathing patient, a nasal cannula may be configured to both sample exhaled gas and simultaneously deliver supplemental oxygen.[7,8]

Thoracic Impedance and Inductance

An early attempt to automate respiratory rate measurement in the 1960s was based on the theory that the electrical properties of the thorax changed during the respiratory cycle. The resistance to the flow of alternating current, known as *impedance*, was found to change with the inflation and deflation of the lungs; it is increased with inhalation. Because of this, this impedance value could be continuously measured; when it exceeded a set threshold, the occurrence of a breath was recorded by a monitor. Efforts were made to correlate changes in impedance with tidal volume, but this was less successful in awake patients and in those with respiratory disease.[9,10] Significantly, this technique does not measure actual air entry but only measures the changes in the shape of the thoracic cage. Accordingly, it could be fooled by respiratory effort in the presence of upper airway obstruction.[11] In anesthetized and ventilated surgical patients, however, the technique was much more valuable, producing accurate respiratory rate measurements and high correlation of tidal volumes ($r = 0.89$) with Wright's respirometer.[12] In addition, the technique was somewhat sensitive to both airway occlusion and circuit disconnects.

Work has been done to determine the optimal placement of electrode pairs for maximum sensitivity. As expected, maximal separation of electrode pairs provides the most sensitive signal.[13] Interference between respiratory monitors that use thoracic impedance and implanted respiratory rate–sensitive pacemakers has been reported, producing unwanted heart rate changes. The only solution was to disable the respiratory rate monitoring function in the physiologic monitor.[14]

Inductive plethysmography is superficially similar to impedance plethysmography in that electrically active sensors detect chest wall movement. However, the inductive technique uses direct-current sensors in the form of coils of wire around the chest and/or abdomen. The changes in self-inductance (stretch) of these sensors are electrically transmitted and analyzed. These signals can reflect respiratory rate and, after calibration, tidal volume.[15] In a study of infants at risk for apnea, Brouillette and colleagues[16] found that inductive plethysmography was superior to impedance-based measurement in that it recorded fewer cardiac artifacts and was better able to discern upper airway obstruction.

Electrocardiograph-Based Respiratory Monitoring

After the use of continuous ECG monitoring became widespread, attempts were made to use ECG-derived data to record respiratory rate. The ECG may be used through the analysis of changes in both the amplitude of the ECG signal and the changes in the axis of the QRS complex. Amplitude changes in the ECG are caused by the change in overall electrical resistance because of the increased proportion of air, rather than tissue, within the chest cavity during inspiration. This is reflected in a decrease in ECG signal voltage, and thus QRS wave size, that is amenable to analysis.

Inflation of the lungs also produces a change in the axis of the heart, as reflected in the multilead ECG. Using two limb leads, measurements are made of the area under a normal QRS complex. By using these areas as amplitudes of known direction, a vector can be derived as the sum of the two values. These measurements are routinely made by most arrhythmia detection software in current use.[17]

Other Techniques

Acoustic techniques actually "listen" for the sound of airflow at the face, pretracheal neck, or chest. One method uses the sound of air impinging on open-ended tubes positioned near the nostrils and mouth.[18] Although lightweight and immune to upper airway obstruction artifact, this method may suffer from interference from ambient noise. Also, it is a pure respiratory frequency monitor, without any other measure of ventilatory adequacy. A variation of this approach uses a pyroelectric polymer mounted inside a face mask that senses the temperature increase from exhaled air. This signal is electrically amplified and displayed. Inexpensive and relatively simple, it can be incorporated into the construction of a face mask or nasal cannula.[19]

A sophisticated, noninvasive sensor was described by Zhu and colleagues in 2006.[20] A head pillow containing fluid-filled tubes is connected to two sensitive pressure transducers. The pressure signal is processed with a derivation of an algorithm known as *wavelet transformation* and is filtered to produce both pulse and respiratory signals. The technique is, as expected, less effective in the presence of motion artifact and poor head positioning. However, in 13 healthy subjects, both the sensitivity and the positive predictive value of the sensor were above 95% for respiration, compared with simultaneous nasal thermistor recordings.[20] The data were even more favorable with respect to detection of pulse rate. In combination with oximetry, this technique will likely prove valuable both in ambulatory monitoring and in the diagnosis of sleep disorders.

The Rainbow Acoustic Monitoring system (Masimo, Irvine, CA) noninvasively and continuously measures respiration rate using an innovative adhesive sensor with an integrated acoustic transducer that is easily and comfortably applied to the patient's neck. Using acoustic analysis, the respiratory signal is separated and processed to continuously display respiration rate.[21] Box 9-1 summarizes the various methods for automated detection and recording of respiratory rate.

BOX 9-1 Methods for Automated Capture of Respiratory Rate

DIRECT

Airflow Sensors

Pneumotachograph
Thermistor
Differential pressure (Bernoulli)
CO_2 waveform

Acoustics

Mouth/nose
Precordial
  Pretracheal
  Neck (Masimo)

INDIRECT

Chest Wall Motion

Strain gauge
Impedance change

Cardiac Derived

Electrocardiograph voltage variation
Cardiac axis change
  RR interval change
  Blood pressure variability

Other Body Motion

Pillow sensor

AIRWAY PRESSURES

Principles Overview

Pressure is defined as the force per unit area exerted on a surface by an external substance, usually a gas or liquid in medical applications. A molecule of a gas can be envisioned as confined within a cube. This molecule of gas transfers its momentum to a vessel wall during a collision equal to 2 × mv, where *m* is mass and *v* is mean velocity. After bouncing off the opposite wall, the molecule then hits the first wall again after a time equal to 2 × d/v, where *d* is the distance between walls, exerting a force of mv^2/d.

With *N* molecules, one third will hit each pair of sides of the box, yielding a force (*F*) on each wall:

$$F = (Nmv^2/d) \div 3$$

Because pressure is force exerted over an area (d^2), total pressure (*P*) is:

$$P = (Nmv^2/d^3) \div 3$$

or, because d^3 is volume (*V*), then:

$$F = (Nmv^2/V) \div 3$$

This gives the useful fact that, at constant temperature, pressure is inversely proportional to volume (Boyle's law) and directly proportional to the square of molecular velocity.[22]

Determination of atmospheric pressure was the first practical application of pressure gauges. Initially, the force exerted by the weight of the atmosphere was balanced against a column of fluid, either water or mercury. This is an example of an absolute pressure gauge, indicating approximately 30 inches (or 760 mm) of mercury, 101 kPa, or 1.01 bars of pressure at sea level. In contrast, relative or "gauge" pressure indicators read zero at atmospheric pressure and indicate only additional pressure sensed.

Sensors

The history of airway pressure measurement parallels the development of sensitive gauges and meters for atmospheric

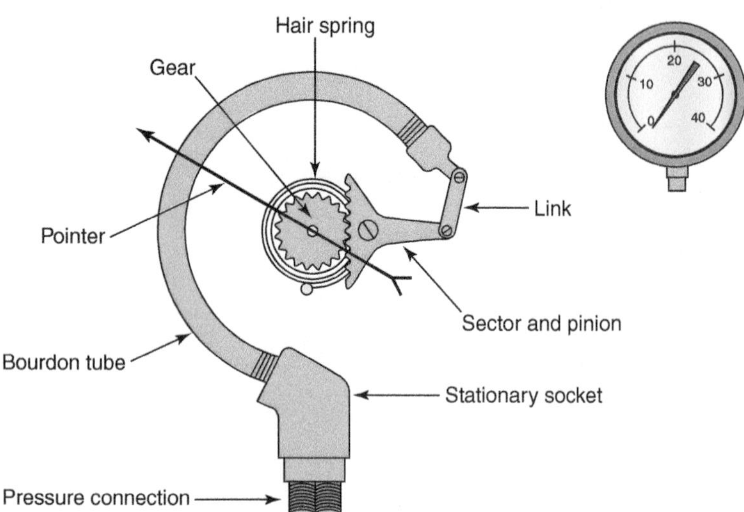

FIGURE 9-1 The Bourdon gauge, representing a mechanical gauge that requires no power. The Bourdon tube is an evacuated compartment.

pressure. Beginning with fluid columns, devices for the estimation of gas pressure rapidly evolved into mechanical linkages translating physical motions—of an evacuated capsule, for example—into displacements of an indicating needle. The Bourdon gauge (Fig. 9-1) uses this principle of change in pressure, translated into motion of an evacuated compartment or tube, and is still a robust and inexpensive mechanism. This mechanical gauge, and others similar to it, require no power, are always on, and have high reliability. Although they do not communicate with data systems or alarms, they are useful backups for modern electronic systems.

Newer electronic sensors use the principle of piezoelectricity, the property of certain crystals, usually quartz, to produce a small electric current when compressed. This output may be calibrated and amplified into a usable signal. A metal or semiconductor whose resistive properties change with strain, a so-called *piezoresistive effect,* also may be used to sense pressure. This additional technologic development has facilitated the evolution and miniaturization of pressure sensors that may be adapted to almost any application. In general, these sensors do require periodic calibration against atmospheric pressure (zero) and occasionally require one other known data point (span) to ensure linearity across their operational range. They are small, lightweight, and generally much more sensitive to small changes.

Applications

Airway pressure is a key component in measuring ventilation. Detecting ventilator-related events (VREs) helps anesthesia providers identify and avoid a majority of serious anesthesia-related events.[23,24] Disconnection of the circuit without occlusion is a significant anesthesia-related event that may lead to adverse patient outcomes.

Pressure sensors have been used to detect other mechanical problems, including tracheal tube disconnection with occlusion, kinking of the inspiratory limb, fresh gas hose kink or disconnection, circuit leaks, high and low scavenging system pressure, continued high circuit pressure, and kinking in the circuit pressure-sensing hose.[25] However, the ability to detect these conditions, especially with older monitors, is not as reliable.

Before the introduction of these sensors, previous techniques included lung auscultation, measures of chest wall movement, use of a precordial or esophageal stethoscope, and measurement of physiologic variables such as pulse, blood pressure, respiration, and skin color. These other monitoring methods, absent end-tidal carbon dioxide and pulse oximetry, often resulted in delayed or failed detection of events.

Ventilation failure events can occur because positive pressure does not always equal tidal volume delivered. Sensors in different locations along the breathing circuit, especially with pressure-based ventilator modes, can give disparate pressure measurements and are thus susceptible to both false-negative and false-positive readings.

Breathing Circuit Low-Pressure Alarms

At a minimum, a low-pressure alarm with an audible alert must be placed in the patient breathing circuit in accordance with the current American Society of Anesthesiologists (ASA) Standards for Basic Anesthetic Monitoring. Pressure-sensitive alarms monitor airway or breathing circuit pressure through a side port and compare it with a preset low-pressure alarm limit. The primary purpose of this alarm is the prompt identification of breathing circuit disconnection. This class of malfunction has been disproportionately associated with adverse outcomes in the intraoperative period and may be almost completely avoided when this relatively simple monitor is used. Although low-pressure alarms are primarily intended to warn of a breathing circuit disconnection when a positive-pressure ventilator is used, it is important to realize that they do not detect some partial disconnections and will likely not detect misconnections or obstructions. However, because 70% of all disconnections occur at the Y-piece,[26] it is an excellent addition to the other sensors used to monitor ventilation.

Sensor Position Within the Breathing Circuit

The location of airway pressure sensors is important to both detect circuit disconnects and accurately reflect distal airway pressures. Sampling location, kinetic energy transfer, and Bernoulli effects all influence final measured pressure. Circuit pressure should be measured at an appropriate site for the particular need and at a right angle to axial flow.[27] The ideal location is at or near the patient Y-piece, but secretions and condensation may cause sensor malfunction. If it is not close enough to the Y-piece, an undetected disconnection (false-negative) may occur as a result of circuit resistance between the measurement site and the distal, now open, end. This will be compounded if a descending bellows ventilator is used, or if the disconnection site is embedded in sheets, blankets, or some other obstructing material.[26]

A sensor inside the circuit, upstream of the inspiratory valve, eliminates any risk of contamination but becomes insensitive under certain conditions. The combination of an inspiratory limb low-pressure monitor with an in-line humidifier, capnometer cuvette, angled tracheal tube connector, or corrugated catheter mount[28] can create backpressure with medium to high flows and may prevent the alarm from being activated. Increased backpressure has also been seen in the Bain (or C-Pram) breathing circuit as a result of circuit tapering and extension of the fresh gas outlet to near the connector at the patient. Lower flows can also prevent the alarm from being activated if moisture builds in the in-line humidifier.[29]

One proposed solution is to place the low-pressure alarm on the expiratory limb to avoid backpressure-induced false-negative events.[30] However, expiratory limb pressure sensors are not without problems. Apnea volume alarms have also been sounded, without the pressure alarm sounding, as a result of loose retaining rings in the expiratory limb not detected during machine leak testing. Interestingly, reverse-flow and minute volume low alarms may trigger without a low-pressure alert.[31] In older anesthesia delivery systems without fresh gas compensation, expiratory valve anemometers routinely overestimated tidal volumes because of high flows of fresh gas passing through the circuit during the expiratory phase.

Pressure sensors within the ventilator obviously are insensitive in machines with a manual/automatic selector switch in the manual position.[26] The placement of pressure sensors in both the circuit and ventilator may provide a solution, but this has been implemented only in the Medical Anesthesia Delivery Unit (ADU) anesthesia machine (GE Healthcare, Waukesha, WI).[32] Recently, ventilation pressure sensors have been placed in both the inspiratory and expiratory circuit limbs.[33,34] The inspiratory limb sensor provides feedback during volume-controlled ventilation. Stress fractures in these sensors may trigger alarms without directing the provider to the site of the fault. The small fracture size prevents detection through low- and high-pressure leak tests. Options include detection through visual inspection, using alcohol-wet hands to detect a small gas leak,[35] or using a second reservoir bag as a test lung to verify sensor integrity.

To improve the rate of detection of true-positive events, the low-pressure limit should be set just below the normal peak airway pressure, and subsequent machine testing should establish that a disconnection would cause the alarm to sound. The disconnection should be performed at the distal (patient) end to ensure that backpressure, flows, and monitor limits are not such that the alarm would fail to sound in the event of a disconnection.[28]

The clinical response to a low-pressure alarm should be rapid and organized. The anesthesiologist must systematically evaluate the gas flow to ensure it is adequate, the breathing circuit to ensure it is not disconnected or leaking, and the ventilator, which may not be driving the bellows or may have a setting error. Working outward from the adjustable pressure-limiting (APL) valve toward the patient helps the anesthesiologist rapidly identify and correct the issue.[26]

Airway Versus Alveolar Pressures

With controlled ventilation, a transpulmonary inflation gradient is provided by positive airway pressure. Generated by a ventilator, this positive pressure gradient may be constant or may vary during the inspiratory phase. The instantaneous pressure during the ventilation cycle is best measured at the distal end of the ventilator circuit, near the connection to the patient.[27] Division of the airway pressure-time product (area under the curve) by total cycle time yields mean airway pressure. In most cases,this average pressure approximates mean alveolar pressure.[36] Mean airway pressure also correlates with alveolar ventilation, arterial oxygenation, hemodynamic performance (venous return), and risk of barotrauma.[27]

Alveolar pressure is clinically of interest, but direct measurement generally is not practical. The measurement requires measurement of airway pressure at the distal portion of the endotracheal tube, as close as possible to the alveoli, whereas clinical airway pressure measurements commonly are at the proximal portion of the endotracheal tube.[37] Measured airway and actual alveolar pressures differ because of proximal dissipation of the frictional inspiratory airway pressure component and the expiratory alveolar pressure resistive contributions. Positive end-expiratory pressure (PEEP) adds to the external circuit pressure throughout the cycle, proportionally increasing the mean airway pressure.[27]

Chest wall and lung compliance, secretions, partial occlusions, and tracheal tube resistance may also affect peak airway pressures. Plateau pressures are measured during an inspiratory pause (no flow) and are affected only by secretions, partial occlusions, and tracheal tube resistance.

Ventilation Mode Effects on Airway Pressures

Volume control will deliver a set tidal volume, and pressure will increase until that volume is reached. In low lung compliance conditions, such as acute respiratory distress syndrome (ARDS), high pressures can be administered in attempts to deliver a set volume.

Pressure control will deliver a set pressure, and the tidal volume will depend on airway resistance and lung and chest wall compliance. Pressure control may be better tolerated in some patients, improving both ventilation and oxygenation. However, if lung compliance decreases, and the same pressure is applied, the tidal volume will decrease. Appropriate volume alarm settings will signal low volumes and avoid undetected hypoventilation.

Pressure support mode delivers a positive pressure that is rapidly achieved and maintained throughout inspiration whenever the patient makes an inspiratory effort. The volume delivered depends on the pressure setting, inspiratory time and effort, and airway resistance and compliance.[38]

Pressure Alarms

Subatmospheric Pressure Alarms

Subatmospheric alarms measure and alert the clinician to a subatmospheric (negative) circuit pressure and the potential for reverse flow of gas. Negative pressures can rapidly cause pulmonary edema, atelectasis, and hypoxia. Commonly, the low pressures result from active (suction) scavenging system malfunctions or patient inspiratory efforts against a circuit that is either blocked or that has inadequate fresh gas flow. Other events detected include suction applied to a gastric tube that has been passed into the trachea alongside the tracheal tube[39] and moisture accumulation in the carbon dioxide absorber that decreases gas flow to the patient.[40]

High-Pressure Alarms

High-pressure alarms are now user adjustable or even automated, but in older monitors, this was not always the case. High respiratory rate, low inspiratory/expiratory ratios, low tidal volume, low flow of inspiration and fresh gas, and high tubing compliance may result in a failure to trigger the alarm. Older machines may generate excessive pressure and put the patient at risk without exceeding their preset level, usually near 40 cm H_2O.[41] Positive inspiratory pressure (PIP) measurement and adjustable alarms are especially valuable in the pediatric population. Endobronchial intubation can be identified rapidly using pressure monitoring before the onset of hypoxia or hypercapnea.[42]

Continuing Pressure Alarms

A continuing pressure alarm is triggered when circuit pressure exceeds 10 cm H_2O for more than 15 seconds, and it alerts the anesthesiologist to more gradual increases in pressure, such as those that result from a ventilator pressure relief valve malfunction (a valve stuck closed) or a scavenging system occlusion. In these situations fresh gas continues to enter the breathing system from the machine flowmeters but is unable to leave. Rate of rise of pressure therefore depends on the fresh gas flow rate.

Modern anesthesia machines now have multiple pressure sensors, as described. In addition to the electronic sensors in the ventilator and the circuit, an analog gauge usually is positioned on the carbon dioxide absorber to serve as a quick reference and as a backup in case of electrical failure.

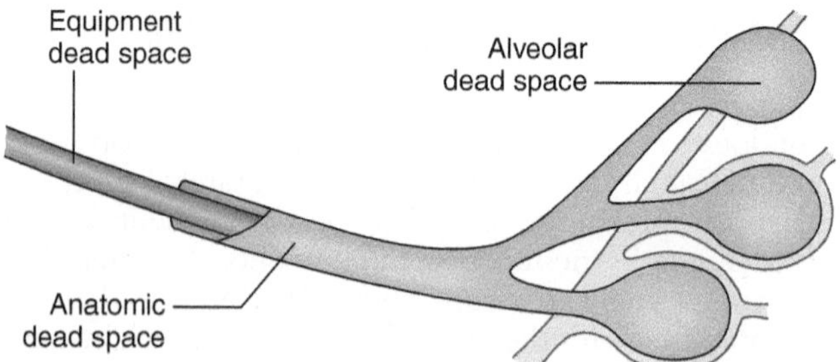

FIGURE 9-2 ■ The relationships among equipment, anatomic, and physiologic dead space.

VOLUME MEASUREMENT

Principles and Requirements

In the management of controlled ventilation, it is important to monitor minute ventilation—the volume of gas delivered to the airway in 1 minute—as a measure of ventilatory "adequacy." This measure is best obtained by measuring tidal (breath) volume and then multiplying by respiratory frequency. Because arterial partial pressure of carbon dioxide is inversely proportional to alveolar minute ventilation,[43] this measurement is important both for initial ventilator setup and subsequent adjustments. Measurements may be made intermittently with manual methods; more commonly, they are made with a device integrated into a ventilator circuit and electronically monitored. This integration may include the derivation and display of minute ventilation, flow-volume loops, and determinations of pulmonary compliance.

Dead Space

Because not all tidal ventilation delivered reaches the alveoli, effective gas exchange occurs only in a fractional part of the tidal volume. The remaining gas occupies the trachea, bronchi, and bronchioles and is referred to as *anatomic dead space*. This volume is relatively fixed in each patient; thus, as tidal volume decreases, it occupies a larger fraction of each breath. At a tidal volume roughly equal to the anatomic dead space, effective alveolar ventilation ceases, with the same gas being transported distally from bronchi to alveoli that was most recently expelled. Also, the distal breathing circuit and patient airway contribute additional mechanical or apparatus dead space to the system (Fig. 9-2).

Measurement of dead space is important to minimize its contribution to total minute ventilation and clearly calculate the relationship between alveolar minute ventilation and arterial carbon dioxide tension. A combination of precise volume measurement and capnography may be used to calculate anatomic dead space using Fowler's method. Initially described using nitrogen as the reference gas, the expired volume was measured from the beginning of exhalation until the onset of the "plateau" of alveolar gas.[43]

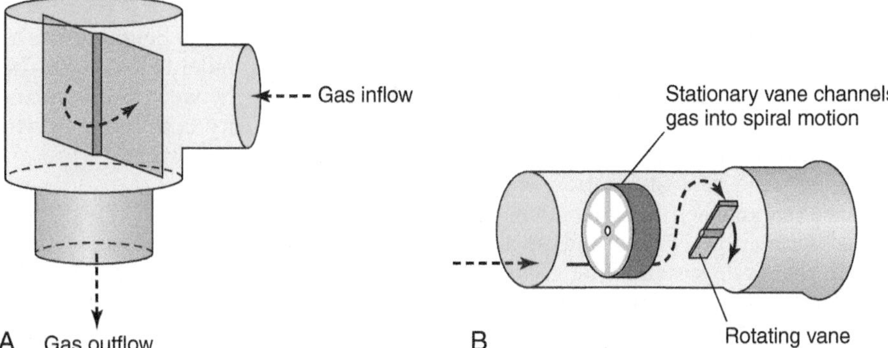

FIGURE 9-3 ■ Rotating vane flow sensors. A conventional Wright respirometer from a MagTrak IV (**A**; Baker Hughes Incorporated, Houston, TX) and an Ohmeda 5400 (**B**; GE Healthcare, Waukesha, WI).

Mechanical Devices

The simplest device for the measurement of gas volume is based on a rotating vane or propeller calibrated against a specific density of gas. The total rotation of the attached shaft correlates with the volume of gas (air) that has passed by. The basic principle is that a force is transmitted to the vanes by the impact of gas molecules, and this force is converted to a rotational (angular) momentum and spins the pinwheel. Optical or mechanical transducers count the rotations and convert the value to an equivalent volume. Critical variables are the gas density—which depends on gas composition, humidity, and altitude—and temperature. At very low flows or volumes, the device may be less accurate as a result of the finite mass and inertia of the vanes.

Wright's Respirometer

Introduced in 1955,[44] this vane anemometer uses a low-mass rotating vane that responds to the force of flowing gas by rotating in proportion to flow. It records tidal volume, which is proportional to total rotations, and it can sum multiple breaths to indicate minute volumes. Manufactured by several companies in both mechanical and optically encoded forms, the overall shortcoming of this device is volume inaccuracy at low flows. Low flow causes the turbine to accelerate more slowly because of inertial effects, so the accuracy is lower. It is considered a very safe monitor, however, because it understates inspired tidal volumes at low volumes[45] and continuous low flows as a result of gas slippage past the vanes,[45] although expired volumes continue to be reliable. Pulsatile flows will cause an overread of tidal volume because of higher peak flow rates and "coasting" of the vane between breaths.[46] The Ohmeda 5400 Volume Monitor (GE Healthcare), an optically encoded turbine, is the exception in this class. It overreads with low flows and underreads with high flows.[46]

The Wright respirometer (Cardinal Health, Dublin, OH) design is not ideal for low-flow anesthesia because it requires a minimum flow of approximately 2 L/min. The monitor is also not appropriate for spontaneously breathing pediatric patients, whose tidal volumes are insufficient to rotate the vane. If pediatric patients are artificially ventilated, the device may be more useful; this is because with expiratory valve opening, the initial flow rates should be sufficient to overcome inertia and rotate the vane.[45] Hatch[47] studied a modified turbine design that is accurate at volumes of 15 to 200 mL; it also is electronically encoded and incorporates an integral apnea alarm.

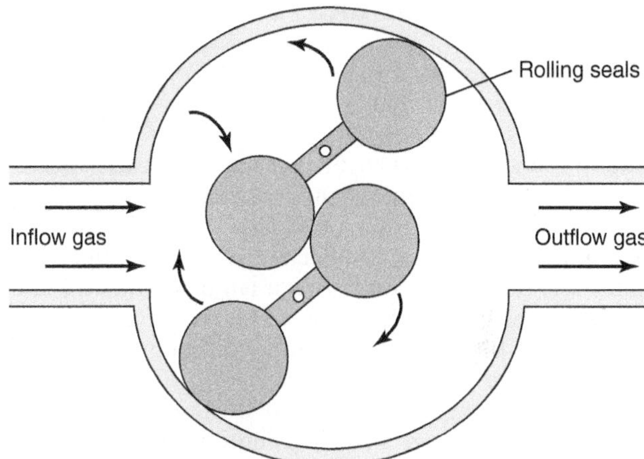

FIGURE 9-4 ■ Schematic of a sealed volumeter. The rotating polystyrene elements seal against the volumeter interior. Fixed volumes of gas flow from the inlet to the outlet and rotate the elements. A mechanical gauge connected to the rotating element shaft (mechanical spirometer) displays the measured volume. Electronic measurements may be read on a remote display. This is the principal of operation of the Drägerwerk AG volumeter (Spiromed; Dräger Medical, Telford, PA).

Several manufacturers have used this technology to measure expiratory volumes at the proximal end of the expiratory limb of a breathing circuit. Head-to-head comparisons of the various devices showed reasonable reliability of this class of tidal volume monitor above minute ventilations of 5 L/min using air, nitrous oxide/oxygen, or humidified air.[46] As minute ventilation decreases, the measured tidal volume will be less than the actual volume delivered; however, the accuracy of the device depends on the transducer used by the manufacturer (Fig. 9-3).[48]

A sealed mechanical volumeter (Fig. 9-4) was used by Dräger Medical (Telford, PA) in some older delivery systems to measure tidal volume and minute ventilation. This device consists of a pair of rotating elements in the gas flow path, configured much like a revolving door at the entrance to a building. A fixed volume of gas is passed across the volumeter with each quarter rotation of the dumbbell-shaped elements. A seal is formed between the polystyrene rotating elements and the interior wall of the tube, and a sealed volumeter provides substantially more resistance to flow than does the vane anemometer. The accuracy of this volumeter is affected by gas density and by the inertia of the rotating elements; however, it is not influenced substantially by the flow pattern of the gas. The number of fixed volumes of gas transferred from inlet to outlet is mechanically measured.

The Dräger Spiromed is an electronic version of the mechanical spirometer. Gas flow through the device determines the rate of rotation of the rotors, which is measured by an electromagnetic sensing system. The Spiromed is direction sensitive and can alert to reversal of gas flow in the circle system. The accuracy of the Spiromed for tidal volumes is ±40 mL and ±100 mL for minute ventilation, or 10% of the reading.

MEASUREMENT OF GAS FLOWS

The flow of any fluid material, liquid or gas, may be described by a set of equations that embody the concepts of *smoothness*, *continuity*, and *conservation of mass*. This description allows for properties such as density, viscosity, compressibility, mass, and volume. As fluids flow, they interact with their surroundings—that is, other fluid or container walls—in predictable ways. An important concept is the distinction between laminar (smooth) and turbulent (chaotic) fluid flow. This is an interesting exception to the normally smooth, continuous nature of fluid transport.

Turbulent flow is characterized by the formation of eddies or vortices on an increasingly small scale. The transition from laminar to turbulent flow is catalyzed by increasing drag on the fluid by friction from interaction with boundary layers, walls, or orifices in the fluid path. It is a chaotic process that depends on a complex combination of fluid density, viscosity, and the size and shape of the obstruction to flow.

Principles

The behavior of fluids and gases depends on whether their flow is laminar (smooth) or turbulent. Flow through a tube with a length greater than the diameter usually is laminar; however, at a critical velocity (V_C), a transition to turbulent flow occurs. This is shown in the following equation, in which r is the radius of the tube, ρ is the density, η is the viscosity of the gas, and k is the critical Reynolds number, which is different for each gas:

$$V_c = k\eta/\rho r$$

This transition to turbulent flow greatly increases the resistance to flow and may be seen in many common scenarios, such as a kink occurring in an otherwise smooth tracheal tube. For flow through an orifice, in which length is less than the radius, turbulent flow is a given. Measured in units of length cubed per unit of time, volume flow may be calculated by detecting a velocity change across a fixed cross-sectional area. Bernoulli's equation makes this possible by measuring a pressure change across this transition:

$$P + \tfrac{1}{2}\rho V^2 + \rho g h = \text{Constant}$$

where P is pressure, g is gravitational acceleration, and h is the height above a reference plane. Note that with turbulent flow, only the gas density affects the relationship between pressure and velocity. Application of a continuity condition, in which gas in equals gas out, gives the following:

$$P_1 - P_2 = \tfrac{1}{2}\rho(V_2^2 - V_1^2)$$

In this case, P_1 and V_1 represent initial pressure and velocity, and P_2 and V_2 represent final values. Rearrangement of this equation allows determination of gas velocity by measurement of pressure change (drop); this is converted into flow by knowing the cross-sectional area (A) of the passage:

$$\text{Flow} = V \times A \text{ (in units of length}^3\text{ time}^{-1}\text{)}$$

Given that flow is proportional to velocity, from the continuity equation we know that flow is also proportional to the square root of the pressure difference (P) across an orifice.[22]

$$\text{Flow} \ \alpha \ P^{1/2}$$

However, for laminar flow, where r and L are the radius and length of the tube, the Hagen-Poiseuille law offers this relationship between flow (F) and pressure drop ($P_1 - P_2$):

$$F = \pi r^4 (P_1 - P_2)/8L\eta$$

This equation allows the laminar flow of a gas to be calculated by determining the pressure drop across a resistance element, not an orifice. Here, in contrast to Bernoulli's equation, gas viscosity is the factor that may contribute to miscalibration or erroneous readings. Also, flow is directly proportional to the pressure difference, rather than to the square root, as with turbulent flow.

Flowmeters

The concept of the flowmeter encompasses two major areas: the metering of gas supplies, usually to a delivery system, and the measurement of tidal (periodic) ventilation in breathing circuits. The use of relatively constant flowmeters requires precise and reproducible settings to control, rather than measure, gas flows. The primary requirement for flowmeters in human breathing is accurate measurement of nonsteady flows.[49]

Rotameters

Variable-orifice rotameters have existed for more than a century; the patent for the initial device was granted to Karl Kuppers in 1909,[50] and commercial production occurred in the same year. The concept of a tapered tube that enclosed a weighted bobbin that rose in the vertical column in response to increases in gas flow was perfectly mated with a controlling needle valve to produce a device to both measure and control gas flow. In 1910, Dr. Maximilian Neu delivered a known volume percentage of nitrous oxide and oxygen during an anesthetic.[51] The introduction of acetylene and of a rotameter calibrated for this gas occurred in 1922.[52] The ability to provide an accurate mixture of gases allows anesthesiologists to more precisely control anesthetic depth. Adoption of this innovation initially was not rapid because it was unable to deliver ether, and nitrous-oxygen-morphine-scopolamine anesthetics did not reliably provide sufficient muscle relaxation for abdominal surgery. Also, nitrous oxide was expensive to produce at the time, whereas ether and its delivery equipment were inexpensive.

Rotameters can measure gas, vapor, or liquid flow. The floating bobbin rotates to avoid friction as gas impinges on its finned head. The tapered outer tube provides what is effectively a variable orifice, as distance between the bobbin and sidewall increases with increasing flow. The float position is read from a calibrated scale on the tube that is specific for that tube, bobbin, gas used, and temperature range. The rotameter must be vertical to avoid friction or collision between the bobbin and the tube walls.[52]

Rotameters typically are used individually for each gas in the fresh gas manifold of an anesthesia machine. Although the glass tubes are normally shielded, cracks or leaks in rotameters do occur, producing the risk of hypoxic mixtures. However, placing oxygen last in the manifold of gases to the patient decreases the risk of hypoxic mixtures. A properly calibrated oxygen analyzer also aids in the detection of hypoxic mixtures.[53] This preferred configuration decreases hypoxic risk but could increase the risk of patient awareness and hypoventilation.

Later changes to the arrangement of rotameters brought nitrous oxide and oxygen together to allow the two to be mechanically "interlocked." This limits the flow of nitrous oxide based on the oxygen flow, which further decreases the risk of a hypoxic mixture delivery. Weakened springs and worn or degraded O-rings have caused intermittent failures not detected on a machine check.[53,54] Empty cylinder yokes also can leak as a result of reverse flow around the rotameter bobbins because the bobbin at zero does not create a seal at the base of the tube. This condition is worsened by ventilator backpressure and is not prevented by pressure regulators or unidirectional valves.[55] The bobbins and tubes are specific to the gas density and viscosity, with the viscosity difference being more significant at low flow rates. At high flow rates, the gas density difference predominates, as it does with the use of helium in an oxygen rotameter.[22] Inadvertent transposition of bobbins and tubes between gas supplies has resulted in both intraoperative patient awareness and hypoxic mixtures.[56,57]

Real-Time Flow Monitoring

Rather than meter gas flows, as with a rotameter, a more interesting application of gas laws is in instantly detecting the velocity and direction of tidal flows, such as might be found in a ventilator circuit. One application of Bernoulli's law is in the pitot tube flowmeter. In this design, the dynamic pressure of gas impacting into a pressure port is compared with the static pressure within the conduit. The pressure difference is proportional to the square of the

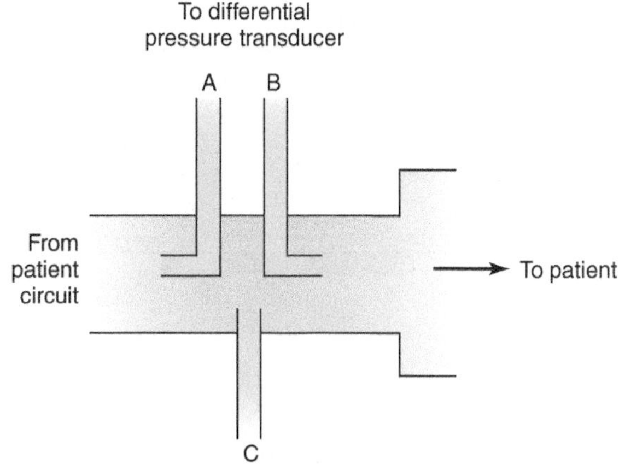

FIGURE 9-5 ▪ A sidestream gas analyzer and spirometry adapter, longitudinal cross section. Using two pitot tubes (*A* and *B*) facing opposite directions, the pressure differential is used to measure inspiration and expiration through flow and flow rate. Absolute pressure is also measured. Port *C* is used to continuously sample respiratory gas for composition, and analysis results are used to correct flow readings for density and viscosity. This technology is used in the Datex Capnomac Ultima Monitor. (Courtesy Datex Medical Instrumentation, Tewksbury, MA.)

flow rate. By using opposing pitot tubes facing in opposite directions, the direction of the flow also may be determined. This technology was developed for use at the distal end of a patient breathing circuit by Datex as the Capnomac Ultima (Fig. 9-5).

Fleisch Pneumotachometer

The principle of operation of the pneumotachometer is to measure the loss of energy of the flowing gas as it passes through a resistive element. The resistive element is designed to ensure that the flow of gas is laminar, so that the energy loss is completely due to viscosity, and the flow is directly proportional to the pressure difference. The energy loss is measured as a pressure difference from the inlet to the outlet of the resistive element. The most common type of resistive element designed by Fleisch[58] consists of narrow, parallel metal tubes aligned in the direction of the flow (Fig. 9-6). Nominally, for laminar flow, the pneumotachometer obeys the Hagen-Poiseuille law:

$$F = (\pi \times r^4 \times [P_1 - P_2])/(8 \times \eta \times L)$$

Here, *F* equals gas flow, *r* and *L* are radius and length of the element, P_1 and P_2 are inlet and outlet pressures, and η represents the viscosity of gas flowing through the device. Measurement of flow is therefore independent of gas density and total pressure.

Fleisch pneumotachometers have been widely used in respiratory physiology and pulmonary function studies and are available in various sizes (resistances) to accommodate the appropriate flow range. The resistance of the element must be chosen so that the pressure difference produced in the flow range of interest is large enough to be measured accurately by the available pressure transducers; too resistive an element will impede ventilation.

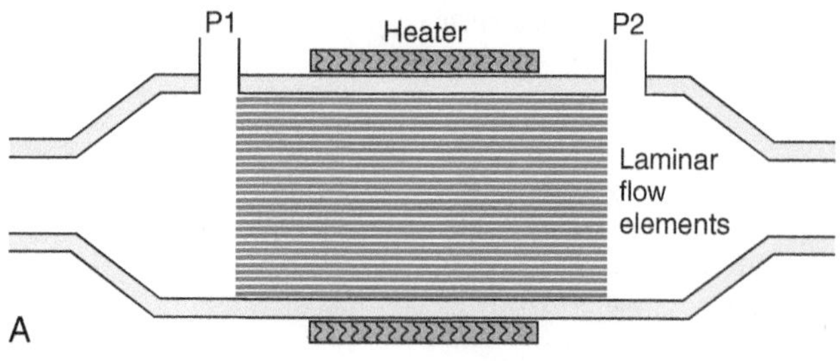

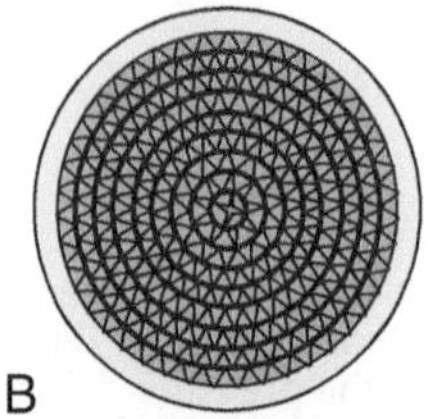

FIGURE 9-6 Fleisch pneumotachometer cross-sectional views. **A,** Longitudinal view: the parallel paths constitute the laminar flow resistance element. *P1* and *P2* (pressure ports) measure the differential pressure across the resistance element. The heating element prevents condensation formation within the elements. **B,** A laminar flow element cross-section. This pneumotachometer is generally bidirectional and constructed from aluminum, and resistance elements are roughly triangular in appearance.

The Fleisch pneumotachometer typically uses a heating element to raise the temperature of the device to approximately 40° C, thus preventing condensation of moisture in expired gas.

The pressure difference across the resistive element, or "head," is measured by a differential pressure transducer with sufficient sensitivity and frequency response. The transducer must be zeroed, or "nulled," electronically by reserving a measurement made with zero flow. The pressure difference is typically in the range of 2 cm H_2O. Pressure transducer output readings tend to drift and the measured signal is small; therefore they must be periodically renulled. For vigorous ventilatory flows, the rate of change in gas flow is great, and the frequency response of the transducer must be adequate to follow these changes.

The respiratory volume is computed by integrating the flow with respect to time because flow equals volume divided by time. The pneumotachometer is calibrated by setting a gain coefficient according to a volume produced by manually emptying a calibrated syringe, usually 1 L in volume, through the device. Often the calibration syringe is emptied several times at different rates to simulate the range of gas flows expected during clinical use. In practice, the characteristics of the Fleisch pneumotachometer depend on the geometry of the tubing on the upstream side of the resistive element. This results in a distinctly nonlinear deviation from Poiseuille's law.[59]

The viscosity of gases in the respiratory mixture must be considered if measurement of flow is to be accurate. Consider that the viscosity of a gas mixture of 88.81% oxygen, 1.61% nitrogen, and 9.58% carbon dioxide is 9.1% greater than that of air. Thus substantial errors can result if gas viscosity is not considered. Temperature is considered to have a linear effect on the viscosity of respiratory gases in the range of 20° to 40° C, although the linear coefficient is different for each gas.

The other disadvantage of the pneumotachometer in an anesthesia circuit is its propensity to accumulate mucus and water in its narrow tubes. It must be repeatedly calibrated because its effective resistance changes with fouling. In addition, the pneumotachometer must be cleaned and sterilized between clinical uses.

Turbulent Flow Fixed-Orifice Flowmeters

The other common alternative to laminar flowmeters for the accurate measurement of ventilatory gas flows is the use of pressure differential between two ports separated by an orifice. This mechanism assumes that gases at low flows have constant density, and it calculates flow from the pressure difference upstream and downstream of a calibrated resistance. Laminar flow is found upstream in a fixed-orifice flowmeter, and it is turbulent downstream; the problem with a fixed-orifice flowmeter is its resistance to high flows and insensitivity to very low flows.

D-Lite Gas Airway Adapter and Flow Sensor

Datex (now part of GE Healthcare) introduced the D-Lite gas sampler and flow-sensor device in 1993. This sensor is evolved from the sensor in the Datex Capnomatic Ultima Monitor (see Fig. 9-5). It measures flow and airway pressure and provides sidestream gas sampling for analysis[60] and sidestream spirometry.[61] This lightweight device attaches between the Y-piece of the circle breathing system and the airway device, such as the tracheal tube, laryngeal mask airway (LMA), and so on. Reliable operation in a humid and secretion-filled environment involves a two-sided pitot-type tube with a robust flow restrictor element.[60] One pressure-sensing port faces "upstream" (Pu), and the other faces "downstream" (Pd). The difference—Pu - Pd, or the dynamic pressure—is proportional to the square of the gas velocity. Across a known cross-sectional area, and assuming laminar flow, velocity converts to flow. Because the ports face in opposite orientation, flow may be measured in both directions with a single, fixed arrangement. Thus

$$(\text{Pu} - \text{Pd})\ \alpha\ (\text{Flow}^2 \times \text{Density}) \div 4$$

$$\text{Flow}^2 \times \text{Density}\ \alpha\ 4 \times (\text{Pu} - \text{Pd})$$

$$\text{Flow}\ \alpha\ 2 \times [(\text{Pu} - \text{Pd}) \div \text{Density}]^{1/2}$$

This is illustrated in Figure 9-7.[61]

The continuous analysis of gas composition supplies the density data required for the flow calculation shown. Flow and pressure measurements—flow rate, peak flow, end-expiratory plateau, and minimum and maximum pressures—are then used to calculate inspiratory and expiratory tidal volume and minute loops as well as compliance and resistance. Low-flow conditions and compensation for pressure and gas fraction variability are handled by monitor calibration and continuous analysis of respired gases (Fig. 9-8).[60]

The sensor head is constructed in a symmetric fashion to measure gas flow in both directions. Connectors are on the outer wall: two sense pressure, and one (Luer Lock) samples gases. Flow resistance is quite low at 1 cm H_2O/L/sec at 30 L/min. Back-and-forth air movement of a precise volume accomplishes calibration while the device is connected to an 8.5-mm tracheal tube, which provides a known resistance. This sensor serves multiple roles in the assessment of patient ventilation: it assesses endobronchial intubation and malposition of double-lumen tubes, and kinks, leaks, and obstructions may also be identified. A pediatric version with a smaller apparatus dead space (Pedi-Lite is 2.5 mL; adult D-Lite is 9.5 mL) partially compensates for the decreased sensitivity to lower flows and volumes.

Because the two sizes have different cross-sectional areas, the user must ensure that the Datex Compact Airway Gas Monitoring Module is set appropriately. Erroneous spirometry data result if the sensor size does not correspond with the appropriate software setting. Helium-oxygen mixtures do not affect the accuracy of this flowmeter.[62]

Variable-Orifice Flowmeters

A novel implementation of flow sensing is found in the Datex-Ohmeda Aestiva, where a variable-orifice flow sensor monitors both inspiratory and expiratory flows and volumes. The problem of nonlinearity and decreased sensitivity at low flows is partially compensated for by the modification of introducing a "flapper" valve between the two pressure sensors. This serves as a variable orifice that increases in size with larger flows. Because flow calibration is different with a variable orifice, each sensor has a unique calibration table stored within the ventilator's electronic memory. This technology is in use in GE Healthcare's latest generation of anesthesia machines, the Medical 7900 Smartvent.[63]

Resistance: Heated Wire

Flow rate can be measured with a heated wire by measuring the cooling of the wire from heat transfer to the gas flowing by. Heat transfer depends on several variables, including gas flow rate, density, heat conductivity, dynamic viscosity, and the temperature difference between the sensor and the gas. With most other variables controlled, heat transfer is a function of the gas velocity from which flow may be derived. This type of flow sensor will always show the flow rate relative to its reference regardless of the pressure, as long as the sensor is in an inelastic tube.[64] In general, because the dynamics of the human respiratory system require that any device measure flow rates from 0 to 2.5 L/sec, the flowmeter should be accurate to within 5% with commonly used

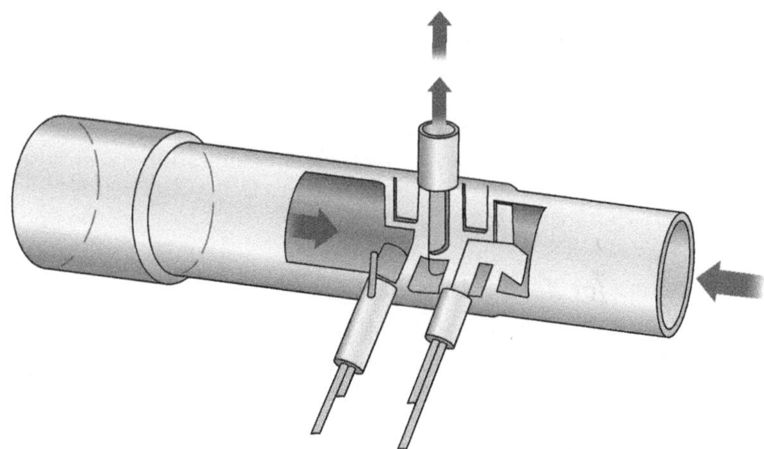

FIGURE 9-7 Section of the D-Lite flow sensor (GE Healthcare, Waukesha, WI) showing the two fixed sidestream resistances and a gas sampling port above.

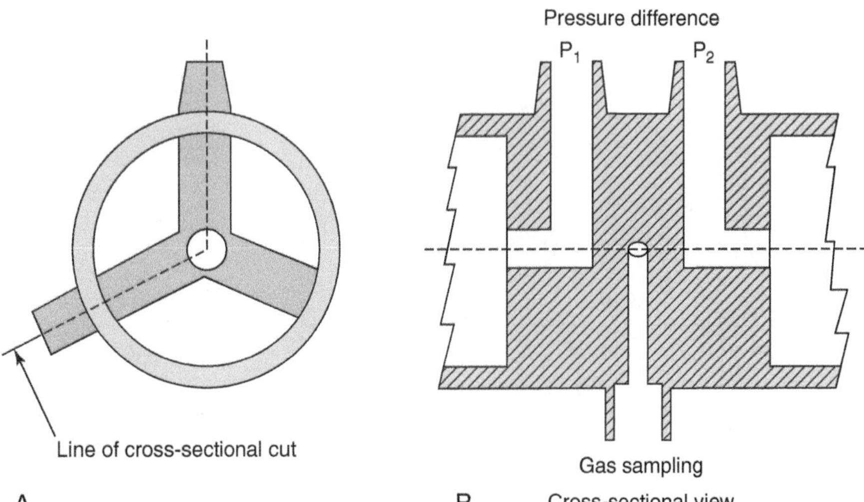

FIGURE 9-8 D-Lite sensor head design (GE Healthcare, Waukesha, WI). **A,** End view through the tube. **B,** Cross-sectional view of holes to measure pressure and sample gas.

gases at typical temperatures and pressures. Minimum flow resistance, dead space, and the ability to detect the direction of the flow also are required.

The heated wire transducer is a tube with a basal temperature sensor and flow rate wires. The design of the device is intentionally small to minimize thermal mass and response time. The two flow-rate sensors are heated, perpendicular to the flow, and connected by a Wheatstone bridge. The temperature of the thin, heated wire is regulated at a constant level; when the airflow rate changes, the induced shift in electrical resistance alters the voltage on one side of the electrically balanced circuit. The limitation of the device is that turbulent flow must be avoided; therefore directional sensors are kept very small so that direction is measured at a point and not at the cross-section of the tube. Baffles at both ends of the sensor prevent laminar flow from becoming turbulent. Dead space is about 5 mL, and an outlet for a pressure transducer is built into the device. The advantage of this type of device over turbines and pressure drop–based devices appears when respiratory flow rates are widely variable. Measuring flows with other devices, such as pressure-based devices, may require several transducers or a variable orifice, which are not as accurate in extreme situations, such as with a high respiration rate, in which errors occur as a result of inertia; with high flow resistance, especially in the setting of spontaneous respiration; and with large dead-space volumes (Fig. 9-9). A new development in this sensor is the addition of vibration to the heated wire sensor. The voltage at constant current varies with gas velocity and allows the sensor to be used with gases of varying composition and temperature. This is useful in the velocity range of 0 to 30 cm/sec and reduces the need for frequent calibration of the hot wire voltage curve. It is likely that this technology will be incorporated in future flow sensors.[65]

Flowmeters for Xenon Anesthetics

The rotating-vane flowmeter is accurate enough for xenon anesthetics because of its insensitivity to gas composition.[48] However, because of the increased density of xenon relative to air, the pitot tube and variable-orifice type flowmeters overestimate tidal volume by a factor of 2. Hot wire anemometers used with xenon would tend to underestimate flows and volumes because of the low thermal conductivity of the gas.

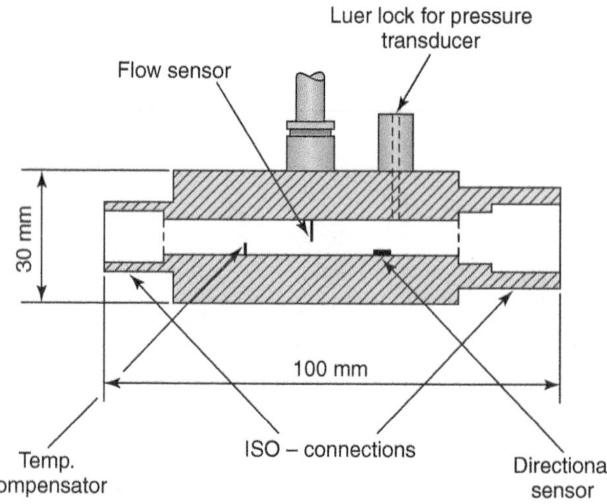

FIGURE 9-9 Transducer mechanical layout for a constant-temperature anemometer. *ISO,* International Organization for Standardization.

Acoustic/Ultrasonic Flow Sensors

A more sensitive flowmeter used for monitoring of variable flows uses ultrasound reflection from moving columns of gas or liquid. Similar to the familiar ultrasound applications to tissue and blood flow imaging, the intrinsic accuracy and compact size of these sensors makes them ideal in the operating room (OR) environment. Initial work on measuring human breathing with ultrasonic flowmeters appeared in the 1980s and was rapidly adopted for measuring many types of ventilation and human populations in and out of the OR.[66,67]

Acoustic/ultrasonic flow sensors use clamp-on or wet transducers and can be applicable to liquids, gases, and multiphase mixtures. Their use has limits, but application to monitoring ventilation can be accomplished with the right combination of technology (Box 9-2).[68]

Within the acoustic domain, various techniques of measurement may be used. Single versus multiple acoustic paths, vortex shedding, and passive and active principles, to name a few, are available, although no single "best" method exists.

Several ultrasonic flowmeters are in current use, including the BRDL flowmeter (Birmingham Research and Development Ltd., Birmingham, UK) and the Spiroson flowmeter (ECO Medics AE, Dürnten, Switzerland). The former has two PVC flowmeters with diagonally opposed flow transducers, and the latter has a single flowhead with two rectangular flow channels, again with diagonally opposed flow transducers. The advantage of these flowmeters is minimal airflow obstruction over a large flow range compared with the traditional Fleisch pneumotachometers (Fig. 9-10).[48,69]

The ultrasonic flow sensor is used on certain models of Draeger anesthesia workstations, such as the Narkomed 6400. Ultrasonic flow measurement uses the transit time principle, by which opposite sending and receiving transducers are used to transmit signals through the gas flow. The signal travels faster when moving with the flow stream rather than against it, and the difference between

BOX 9-2 Unique Qualities of Ultrasonic Flow Sensors

- Ultrasonic flow sensors are easy to use.
- Laminar, turbulent, or transitional flow is possible.
- External transducers are required that either clamp on or are minimally invasive.
- There is no excess pressure drop.
- Accuracy can exceed 0.5%.
- Rapid (millisecond) measurement response is possible.
- Ultrasonic flow sensors are reliable in extreme temperatures.
- Equipment price, installation, and maintenance are reasonable.
- Ultrasonic flow sensors can identify whether the fluid is single-phase or multiphase.

the two transit times is used to calculate the gas flow rate. The device is sensitive to gas flow direction and has no moving parts, and accuracy is independent of gas flow composition.

SPIROMETRY, CURVES, AND LOOPS

Spirometry

Overview

Spirometry is most familiar as an outpatient test for obstructive lung disease, asthma, and other respiratory conditions. Indications include wheezing, cough, stridor, chest tightness, and dyspnea on exertion or at rest. Spirometry can be invaluable in identifying respiratory versus cardiac etiologies, distinguishing between obstructive and restrictive disease, following the progression of neurologic diseases, and evaluating preoperative respiratory risks. As the most widely used test to assess the ventilation portion of the respiratory system, its utility in the OR and the intensive care unit can also be significant.[70] Several approaches to continuous spirometry have been developed, each with advantages and limitations; but the information gathered from spirometry, combined with blood gas measurements, may be used to both optimize care and detect evolving airway issues.[71]

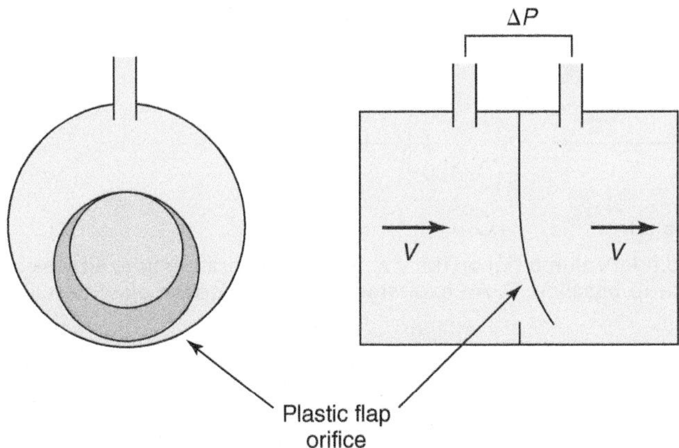

FIGURE 9-10 ■ An Ohmeda 7900 variable-orifice sensor (GE Healthcare, Waukesha, WI). The plastic flap opens with gas flow, causing a pressure decrease across the orifice measured as an index of flow velocity.

Several visual displays are available on modern anesthesia machines. The variables available for two-dimensional displays include *time, volume, flow,* and *pressure.* Time is always on the horizontal (x) axis, and the others are either on the horizontal or vertical (y) axis. If time is on the horizontal axis, the graphic relationship is a curve. If time is not used in the comparison, the visual relationship is a closed curve or loop.

Insufficient studies have been published to compare the utility of the various graphic depictions; currently the choice of display is user dependent.[38]

Spirograms

Spirograms are a visual representation of volume over time. The primary measurements are forced vital capacity (FVC), forced expiratory volume over 1 second (FEV_1), forced inspiratory volume in 1 second (FIV_1), and the calculated value of FEV_1/FVC (Fig. 9-11).[70] Low airway function is measured by the middle 50% of expiratory flow, forced expiratory flow (FEF) 25% to 75%. In an ambulatory setting, testing is performed by the subject taking a maximal inspiratory breath and making a forced maximal exhalation through a mouthpiece. In the OR, the tracheal tube replaces the mouthpiece.

Curves

Curves are a useful depiction of two parameters in a visual format. Traditionally, ventilatory curves use time along the x-axis, and the y-axis can be volume, flow, or pressure.

Volume-Time Curves

Inspirations on volume-versus-time curves are depicted as upslopes; downslopes are exhalations. These curves can identify auto-PEEP, expiratory limb leaks, active (forced) exhalation, and flow transducer miscalbrations (Fig. 9-12).[38]

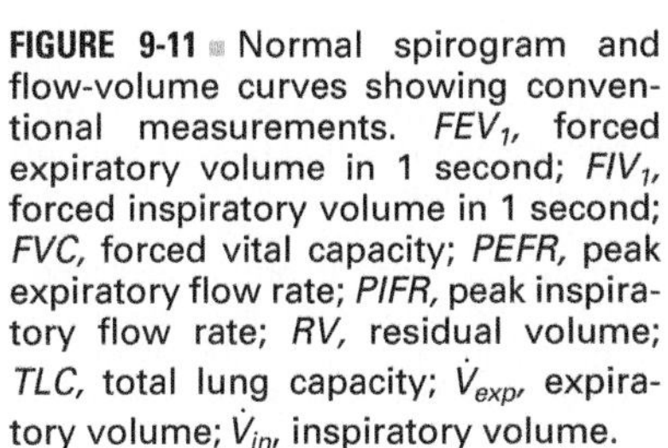

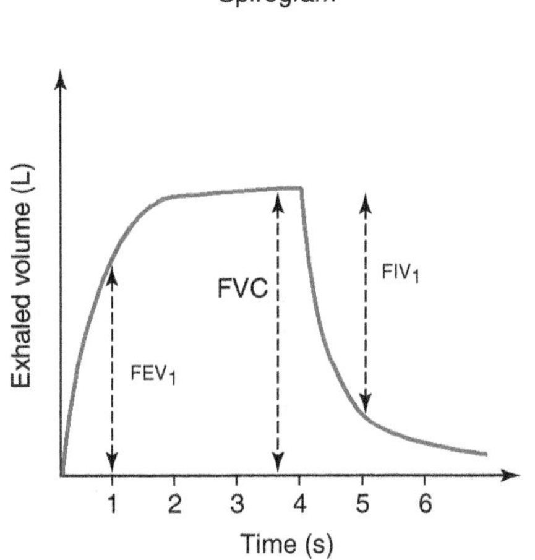

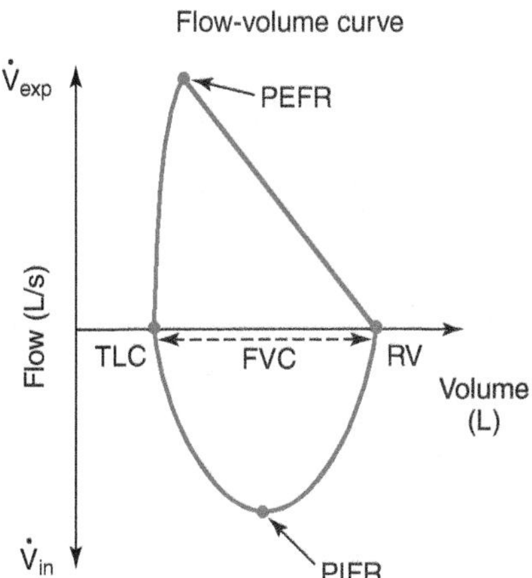

FIGURE 9-11 ■ Normal spirogram and flow-volume curves showing conventional measurements. *FEV_1*, forced expiratory volume in 1 second; *FIV_1*, forced inspiratory volume in 1 second; *FVC,* forced vital capacity; *PEFR,* peak expiratory flow rate; *PIFR,* peak inspiratory flow rate; *RV,* residual volume; *TLC,* total lung capacity; $\dot{V}_{exp}$, expiratory volume; $\dot{V}_{in}$, inspiratory volume.

Flow-Time Curves

When observed with controlled ventilation, these curves may display square, decelerating, descending ramp, or sine flow patterns depending on the type of ventilatory pattern selected. Pressure control and pressure support ventilation curves may be decelerating or descending. Square flows represent constant inspiratory flows that create shorter inspiration time and longer expiration time; higher peak inspiratory pressures (PIP) result from this pattern and increase the risk of ventilator-induced lung injury.[38]

Peak flow is delivered early in both decelerating and descending ramp flows, and it decreases until the target volume or pressure is delivered. Lower PIP is generated, but mean airway pressures can be increased and inspiratory time may be longer. Decelerating flows are recommended in ARDS.[38]

Spontaneous breathing patterns are closest to sine-pattern flows with accelerating then decelerating flows. PIP may be increased and uncomfortable for patients not under general anesthesia (Fig. 9-13).

Loops

Flow-Volume and Pressure-Volume Loops

Flow-volume loops represent flow rates versus inspiratory and expiratory volumes. In forced (spontaneous) breathing, total lung capacity (TLC) and residual volume (RV) are values along the x-axis (zero flow), and the FVC is calculated from the difference of these two values. Peak flow rates at the highest (expiratory) and lowest (inspiratory) points of the loop are at extremes along the y-axis. Flow-volume loops may be used to evaluate compliance changes, effects of bronchodilator therapy (resistance changes), auto-PEEP, air trapping, and air leaks.

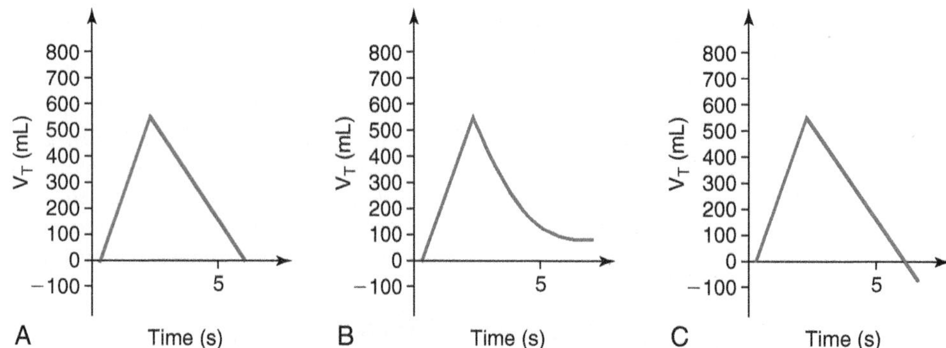

FIGURE 9-12 ■ **A,** Normal volume-time curve, with time on the x-axis and tidal volume (V_I) on the y-axis. **B,** An expiratory limb air leak or positive end-expiratory pressure; the expiratory curve does not return to baseline. **C,** An expiratory curve that goes below baseline because of active exhalation or inaccurate flow transducer calibration.

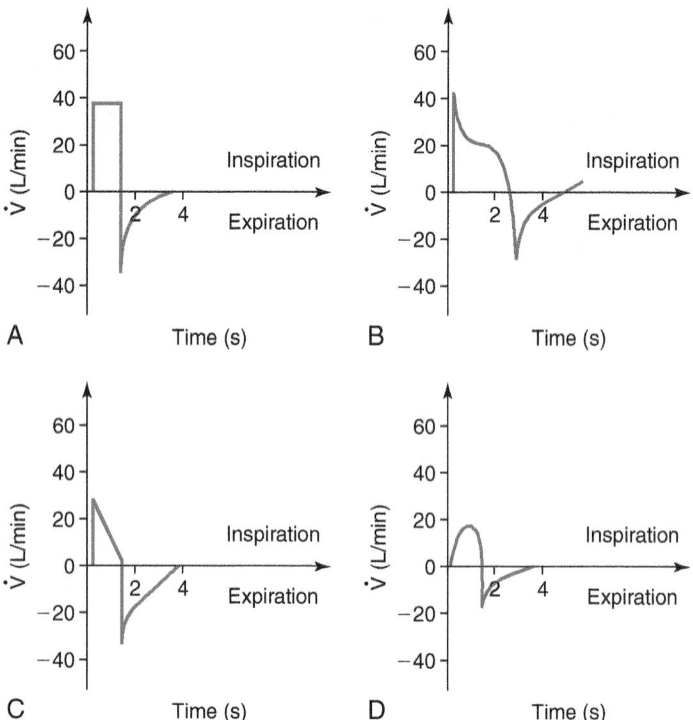

FIGURE 9-13 ■ **A,** Volume control ventilation displays a square flow pattern. Higher positive inspiratory pressure (PIP) and shorter inspiratory times can be seen. **B,** Decelerating ramp seen in pressure control and pressure support ventilation. Lower PIP and longer inspiratory times are seen. **C,** Descending ramp seen in pressure control and pressure support ventilation. Lower PIP and longer inspiratory times are seen. **D,** Sine waveform used in volume control ventilation. Higher PIP can be seen. (Modified from Lian JX: Understanding ventilator waveforms and how to use them in patient care. *Nurs Crit Care* 2009; 4[1]:43-55.)

Normal Loops

Pressure-volume loops have unique characteristics depending on the mode of ventilation. A spontaneous breath loop will show both negative and positive pressures. Negative pressures may be absent if PEEP is applied during the respiratory cycle. The respiratory cycle moves in a clockwise rotation, starting with inhalation and ending with exhalation (Fig. 9-14). Although flow resistance across the tracheal tubes may be seen with vital capacity maneuvers with sizes as large as 7 and 8 mm, normal tidal volume flows are sufficiently low to make such flow limitations minimal.[72] This minimal limitation assumes the absence of secretions, kinking, and other obstructions that would decrease the inner diameter of the tracheal tube and increase flow resistance.[72]

Mechanical ventilation of a paralyzed patient's lungs is different because negative pressure is not generated except in the event of an equipment malfunction. Also, inspiration requires an increase in airway pressure, and exhalation requires a decrement in pressure. The loop cycle thus moves counterclockwise with positive-pressure ventilation (Fig. 9-15).

Although the loops in these figures are idealized, a variety of other loop variations depend on the ventilation mode and the flow pattern selected by the clinician.

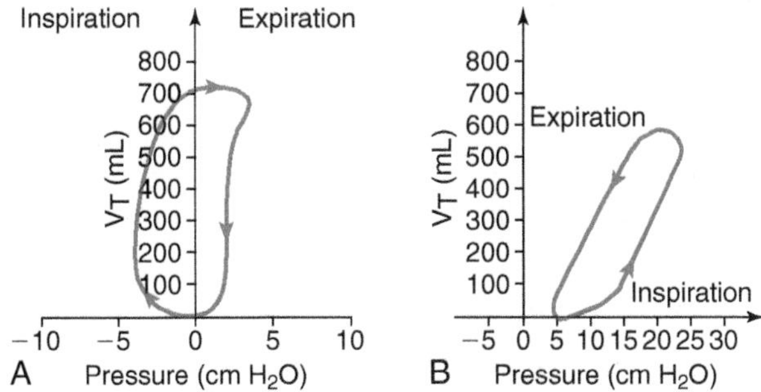

FIGURE 9-14 ■ **A,** The spontaneous breath progresses clockwise, starting at zero, with tidal volume (V_T) on the y-axis. **B,** Ventilator-initiated volume control pressure-volume loop. In this instance, positive end-expiratory pressure is 5 cm H_2O and cycles counterclockwise. (Modified from Lian JX: Understanding ventilator waveforms and how to use them in patient care. *Nurs Crit Care* 2009; 4[1]:43-55.)

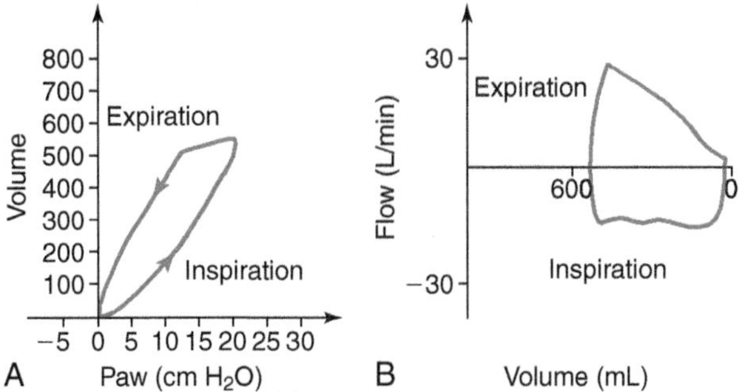

FIGURE 9-15 ■ Normal loops in a mechanically ventilated paralyzed patient, with airway pressure (*Paw*) on the x-axis. **A,** Normal pressure-volume curve. B, Normal flow-volume curve. (Modified from Bardoczky GI, Engelman E, D'Hollander A: Continuous spirometry: an aid to monitoring ventilation during operation. *Br J Anaesth* 1993; 71[5]:747-751.)

Compliance and Resistance Optimization

Pressure-volume loops show bowing and widening as airway resistance increases. The slope of the loop decrease and flatten as compliance decreases (Figs. 9-16 and 9-17).

Compliance is defined as change in volume per unit change in pressure ($\Delta V/\Delta P$) and is not fixed, but rather varies with functional residual capacity (FRC).[73] The application of PEEP to the circuit may increase FRC and improve compliance; this is titrated by examining the pressure-volume loop as PEEP is increased, noting the change in slope of the curve.

Loops Related to Equipment Issues

Equipment issues are independent of patient disease. These can include malposition of the tracheal tube to equipment malfunctions. Using pressure-volume and flow-volume loops continuously can help identify resultant changes in resistance and/or compliance to minimize the potentially negative impact of these events on a patient.

Intubation

Endobronchial Intubation

Endobronchial intubation will demonstrate decreased expiratory flow with single-lung ventilation. The

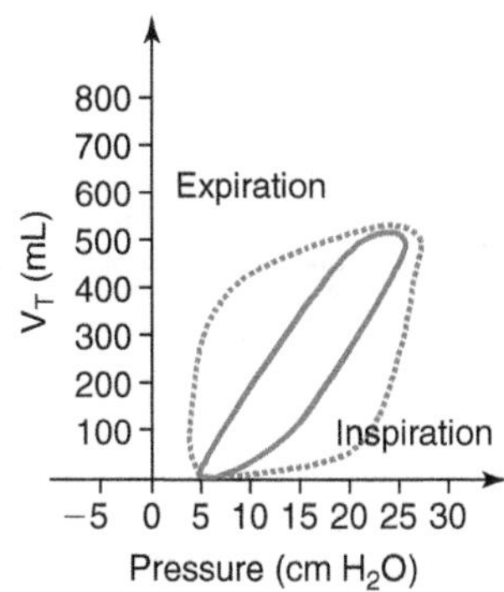

FIGURE 9-16 ■ Pressure-volume loop, with tidal volume (V_T) on the y-axis. The *solid line* is a normal loop and the *dotted line* is a bowed, or widened, loop that signifies an increase in airway resistance.

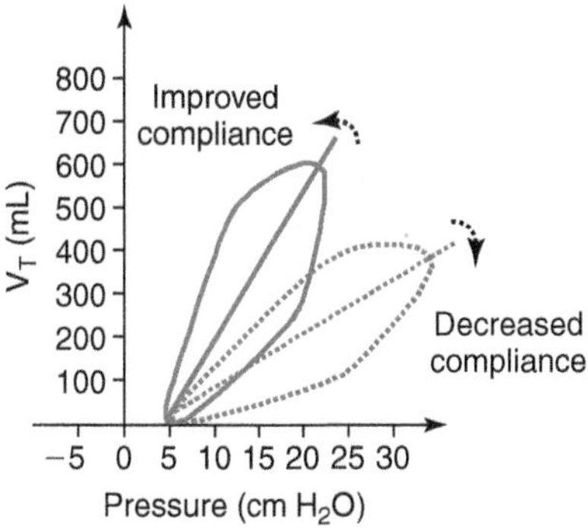

FIGURE 9-17 ■ A comparison of a normal pressure-volume loop (*solid line*) and the *dotted line* loop with a decreased slope, indicating decreased compliance, with tidal volume (V_T) on the y-axis.

pressure-volume curve also behaves as expected with lower volumes and higher pressures (decreased compliance; Fig. 9-18).

Esophageal Intubation

High pressure is accompanied by low volume when attempts are made to ventilate the noncompliant esophagus. The flow-volume loop is irregular with low volume and variable flow (Fig. 9-19).

Kinked Tracheal Tube

Kinking of the tracheal tube decreases the volume delivered and increases the pressure, as shown in the pressure-volume curve. This decrease in volume and flow is shown in the flow-volume loop (Fig. 9-20).

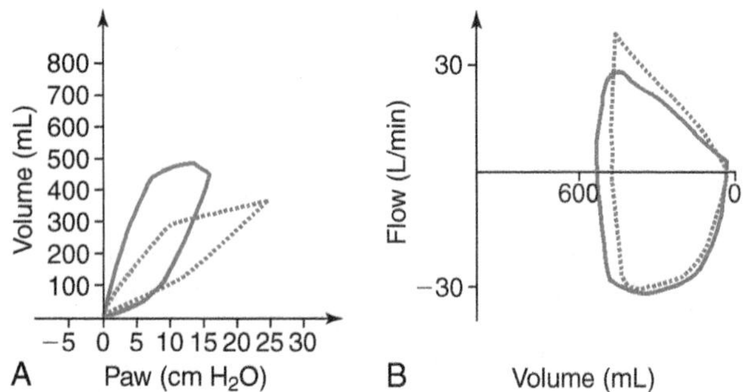

FIGURE 9-18 Volume-pressure and flow-volume loops that demonstrate changes from a right mainstem endobronchial intubation. The *dotted line* loop in **A** shows a right and downward shift in the curve, with airway pressure (*Paw*) on the x-axis. **B** shows decreased expiratory flow. The *solid line* loops show loop correction when the endotracheal tube was withdrawn 3 cm.

CAPNOGRAPHY AND VOLUMETRIC CAPNOGRAPHY

Capnography is the visual, time-based monitoring of carbon dioxide; *capnometry* is the digital display of data. *Volumetric capnography* combines the use of carbon dioxide monitoring and a pneumotachograph. All are used to assess adequacy of ventilation by analyzing exhaled carbon dioxide throughout the respiratory cycle.[74] Although arterial blood gas analysis of carbon dioxide is the gold standard,[75] carbon dioxide levels may change rapidly, and continuous monitoring of this parameter is desirable or, at the very least, comforting. Methods include electrochemical or optical sensors or direct sampling for a gas chromatograph or mass spectrometer.[75] (Time-based capnography is discussed in detail in Chapter 10, and volumetric capnography is covered in Chapter 8.)

Capnographic monitoring of end-tidal carbon dioxide does not detect breathing system disconnects as rapidly as do the pressure alarms, but it identifies problems that are either detected too slowly or not at all. Its ability encompasses esophageal intubation, disconnection, cardiac output changes, inadequate pulmonary circulation, and air embolism. Clinically, its rapid rise is an early indicator of malignant hyperthermia, seen before tachycardia, cyanosis, tachypnea, and other signs and symptoms. Other benefits include detection of valve malfunctions and exhausted carbon dioxide absorbent.[24]

This essential monitor should not be used in isolation. Integrated with other clinical indicators, it can frequently identify patient issues before hemoglobin oxygen desaturation and changes in heart rate and blood pressure are evident.

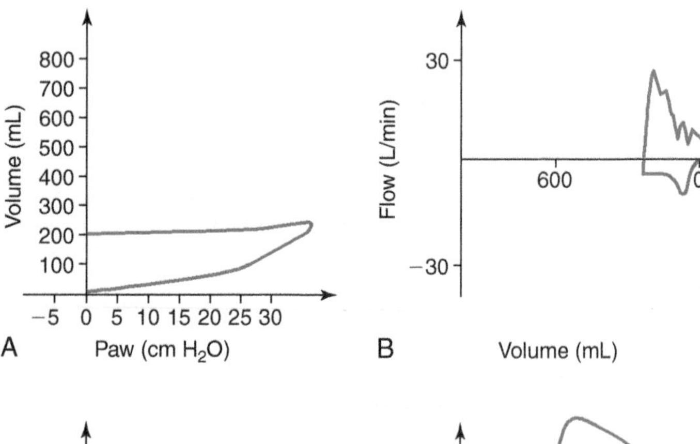

FIGURE 9-19 Endobronchial intubation will cause the pressure-volume loop (**A**) to be enlarged in areas with low volume and high pressure, with volume being delivered to a noncompliant esophagus. The flow-volume loop is irregular in both inspiratory and expiratory phases (**B**). *Paw,* airway pressure.

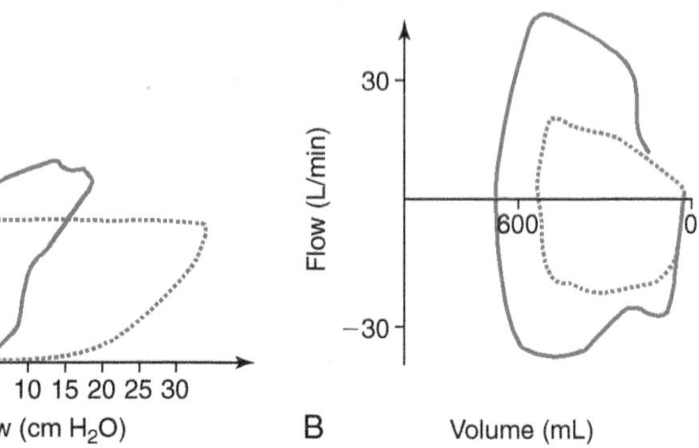

FIGURE 9-20 Endotracheal tube kinking in the *dotted line* pressure-volume loop in **A** shows a right and downward shift with increased loop area and increased inspiratory pressure. **B,** The expiratory and inspiratory portions of the dotted flow-volume loop are diminished. The *solid lines,* or normal loops, were measured during a laparoscopic abdominal procedure. *Paw,* airway pressure.

Apnea and Disconnect Monitoring

As a circuit disconnect alarm, continuous end-tidal carbon dioxide monitoring is considered the most sensitive method to detect a disconnection or cessation of ventilation. It is slower to alarm than the pressure alarms but is an excellent redundant monitor for such a purpose. During general anesthetics and moderate sedation, it alerts faster than other vital sign monitors—such as pulse oximetry and other, later indicators of extubation and obstruction—compared with capnography.

Capnography frequently is used by personnel other than anesthesiologists for monitoring during moderate sedation. Studies conducted in locations such as the endoscopy suite and the emergency department have shown that capnography identifies hypoventilation and apnea that go undetected by care providers before the onset of hypoxia.[76,77]

Continuous Carbon Dioxide Monitoring

End-Tidal Carbon Dioxide

Continuous monitoring of end-tidal carbon dioxide is a noninvasive method of estimating the arterial partial pressure of carbon dioxide ($PaCO_2$) and is derived from a capnographic representation of carbon dioxide relative to time. An algorithm determines the carbon dioxide value at the end of the expiratory plateau. Accuracy depends on accurate sampling of pure expired gas, preferably from a tracheally intubated patient. This measurement method is significantly affected by respiratory disorders that produce diffusion barriers and is also dependent on normal pulmonary perfusion. (For more on continuous carbon dioxide monitoring, see Chapters 8 and 10.)

Transcutaneous Carbon Dioxide Monitoring

Transcutaneous carbon dioxide monitoring has been available since the 1970s. Generally speaking, it uses either electrochemical or optical sensors. A noninvasive, continuous, real-time system for measuring transcutaneous partial pressure of CO_2 ($TcPCO_2$) is commercially available (SenTec AG, Therwil, Switzerland). The SenTec V-Sign sensor is attached to the earlobe and provides $TcPCO_2$ as well as pulse oximeter oxygen saturation (SpO_2) and pulse rate data. An algorithm is used to calculate $TcPCO_2$ from the measured cutaneous PCO_2 ($PcCO_2$), an algorithm that accounts for temperature and metabolic correction factors. The $TcPCO_2$ values displayed by the SenTec digital monitor are corrected and normalized to 37° C and provide an estimate of $PaCO_2$ at 37° C.

Volumetric Capnography and Oxigraphy

With the ability to measure CO_2 concentration and minute ventilation in near real time comes the ability to calculate CO_2 production (VCO_2). The measurement of inspired and expired oxygen concentrations also allows for volumetric oxigraphy and oxygen consumption (VO_2) determination. Dividing the two (VCO_2/VO_2) yields the respiratory exchange ratio (see Chapter 8).

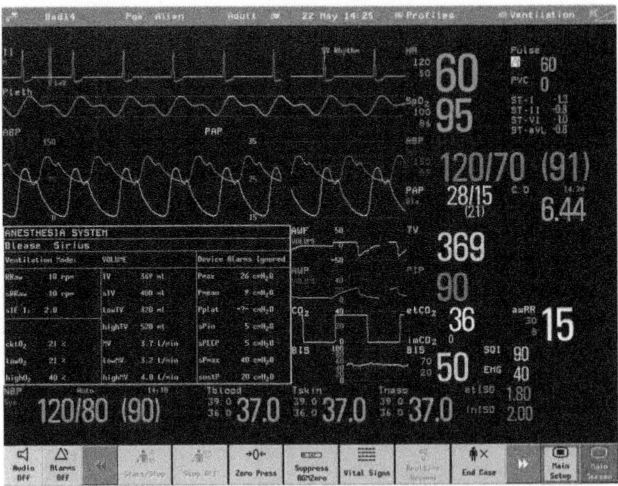

FIGURE 9-21 ■ A combined display demonstrating ventilator and physiologic data on an integrated display. (Courtesy Philips Respironics, Andover, MA.)

DISPLAY OF VENTILATION DATA

Ventilator-Integrated Displays

Most modern anesthesia and critical care ventilators provide, at the very least, a numeric display of commonly used variables such as rate, tidal volume, and inspiratory/expiratory (I:E) ratio. Many also provide a display of airway pressure over time, perhaps also depicting the location of high- and low-pressure alarm limits. These are stand-alone displays, in that they do not depend on other monitors or external devices for their function.

Monitor-Integrated Displays

The next step up in display sophistication integrates the digital output from a ventilator into a combined display, usually in combination with hemodynamic data. Physiologic monitors with modular construction, such as those from Philips Respironics (Wallingford, CT) and Hewlett-Packard (Dayton, OH), allow the insertion of a ventilator monitoring module and the display of volumes and pressures. In addition, they offer the option of visual display of pressure versus time, flow versus time, or other curves. These modular links are specific to the physiologic monitor and normally accept data from the most common anesthesia ventilators (Fig. 9-21).

Data Link from Ventilators

Even today, the output from ventilators, ventilator monitors, and respiratory mechanics sensors proceeds at a relatively low data rate. The most common interfaces are simple serial outputs that typically run at 19,200 Baud or less.[78] This common interface makes data transmission and interface design relatively straightforward and simple. Experiments with Ethernet connectivity have been done, but the future seems to lie with wireless data transmission.[79] The challenges involve data security, verification, and accurate patient identification and tracking as both patients and hardware become more mobile.

BOX 9-3 American Society of Anesthesiologists Standard II: During All Anesthetics, the Patient's Oxygenation, Ventilation, Circulation, and Temperature Shall Be Continually Evaluated

VENTILATION

Objective: To ensure adequate ventilation of the patient during all anesthetics.

METHODS

1. Every patient receiving general anesthesia shall have the adequacy of ventilation continually evaluated. Qualitative clinical signs such as chest excursion, observation of the reservoir breathing bag, and auscultation of breath sounds are useful. Continual monitoring for the presence of expired carbon dioxide shall be performed unless invalidated by the nature of the patient, procedure, or equipment. Quantitative monitoring of the volume of expired gas is strongly encouraged.*
2. When an endotracheal tube or laryngeal mask is inserted, its correct positioning must be verified by clinical assessment and by identification of carbon dioxide in the expired gas. Continual end-tidal carbon dioxide analysis, in use from the time of endotracheal tube/laryngeal mask placement, until extubation/removal or initiating transfer to a postoperative care location, shall be performed using a quantitative method such as capnography, capnometry, or mass spectroscopy.* When capnography or capnometry is utilized, the end-tidal CO_2 alarm shall be audible to the anesthesiologist or the anesthesia care team personnel.*
3. When ventilation is controlled by a mechanical ventilator, there shall be in continuous use a device that is capable of detecting disconnection of components of the breathing system. The device must give an audible signal when its alarm threshold is exceeded.
4. During regional anesthesia (with no sedation) or local anesthesia (with no sedation), the adequacy of ventilation shall be evaluated by continual observation of qualitative clinical signs. During moderate or deep sedation, the adequacy of ventilation shall be evaluated by continual observation of qualitative clinical signs and monitoring for the presence of exhaled carbon dioxide unless precluded or invalidated by the nature of the patient, procedure, or equipment.

*Under extenuating circumstances, the responsible anesthesiologist may waive the requirements marked with an asterisk; it is recommended that when this is done, it should be so stated, including the reasons, in a note in the patient's medical record.

From American Society of Anesthesiologists: *Standards for basic anesthetic monitoring*. Approved by the ASA House of Delegates October 2010 and effective July 1, 2011. Available at www.asahq.org.

PRACTICE PARAMETERS

ASA standards for basic anesthetic monitoring were approved by the ASA House of Delegates on October 21, 1986, and were last amended on October 20, 2010, with an effective date of July 1, 2011. The statements that pertain to pressure and volume monitoring are included Box 9-3. The monitoring equipment needed to meet these standards is now part of every anesthesia delivery system. All contemporary workstations include spirometry for exhaled volume; inhaled volume also is included in many, and all include pressure monitoring and alarms.

As with other monitoring devices and technology, complications may be due to pure device failure or vulnerable monitoring devices, but more commonly they are attributable to user error. Some flow sensors require zeroing or calibration because water accumulation in monitoring tubing may cause spurious readings of flow and volume. Flow sensors commonly are concealed within the workstation; breakage therefore may not be obvious as the source of a breathing circuit leak.

Contemporary ventilation monitoring systems are highly reliable and are integrated with sophisticated, prioritized alarm systems. It is essential that the anesthesia caregiver understand how to use them correctly and how to set appropriate alarm limits and audible alarm volumes, so that critical incidents do not go undetected and adverse outcomes are prevented.

REFERENCES

1. Hunter J: Proposals for the recovery of people apparently drowned, *Philosophical Transactions of the Royal Society of London* 66:412–425, 1776.
2. Guedel AR: *Inhalation anesthesia: a fundamental guide*, New York, 1937, Macmillan.
3. Baker SP, Hitchcock FA: Immediate effects of inhalation of 100% oxygen at one atmosphere on ventilation volume, carbon dioxide output, oxygen consumption and respiratory rate in man, *J Appl Physiol* 10(3):363–366, 1957.
4. Kory RC: Routine measurement of respiratory rate: an expensive tribute to tradition, *JAMA* 165(5):448–450, 1957.
5. Krieger B, Feinerman D, Zaron A, Bizousky F: Continuous noninvasive monitoring of respiratory rate in critically ill patients, *Chest* 90(5):632–634, 1986.
6. Bowdle TA: Adverse effects of opioid agonists and agonist-antagonists in anaesthesia, *Drug Safety* 19(3):173–189, 1998.
7. Ibarra E, Lees D: Mass spectrometer monitoring of patients with regional anesthesia, *Anesthesiology* 63:572–573, 1985.
8. Fukuda K, Ichinohe T, Kaneko Y: Is measurement of end-tidal CO_2 through a nasal cannula reliable? *Anesthesia Progress* 44(1):23–26, 1997.
9. Ashutosh K, Gilbert R, Auchincloss JH, Erlebacher J, Peppi D: Impedance pneumograph and magnetometer methods for monitoring tidal volume, *J Appl Physiol* 37(6):964–966, 1974.
10. Houtveen JH, Groot PF, de Geus EJ: Validation of the thoracic impedance-derived respiratory signal using multilevel analysis, *Int J Psychophysiol* 59(2):97–106, 2006.
11. Wilkinson JN, Thanawala VU: Thoracic impedance monitoring of respiratory rate during sedation: is it safe? *Anaesthesia* 64(4):455–456, 2009.
12. Freundlich JJ, Erickson JC: Electrical impedance pneumography for simple nonrestrictive continuous monitoring of respiratory rate, rhythm and tidal volume for surgical patients, *Chest* 65(2):181–184, 1974.
13. Khambete N, Metherall P, Brown B, Smallwood R, Hose R: Can we optimize electrode placement for impedance pneumography? *Ann N Y Acad Sci* 873:534–542, 1999.
14. Network EUE: Thoracic impedance measurements can interfere with impedance-based rate-responsive pacemakers, *Health Devices* 26:393–394, 1997.
15. Tobin MJ, Jenouri G, Lind B, et al: Validation of respiratory inductive plethysmography in patients with pulmonary disease, *Chest* 83(4):615–620, 1983.
16. Brouillette RT, Morrow AS, Weese-Mayer DE, Hunt CE: Comparison of respiratory inductive plethysmography and thoracic impedance for apnea monitoring, *J Pediatr* 111(3):377–383, 1987.

17. Moody GB, Mark RG, Zoccola A, Mantero S: Derivation of respiratory signals from multi-lead ECGs, *Comput Cardiol* 12:113–116, 1985.
18. Hok B, Wiklund L, Henneberg S: A new respiratory rate monitor: development and initial clinical experience, *Int J Clin Monit Comput* 10(2):101–107, 1993.
19. Dodds D, Purdy J, Moulton C: The PEP transducer: a new way of measuring respiratory rate in the non-intubated patient, *J Accid Emerg Med* 16:26–28, 1999.
20. Zhu X, Chen W, Nemoto T, et al: Real-time monitoring of respiration rhythm and pulse rate during sleep, *IEEE Trans Biomed Eng* 53(12 Pt 1):2553–2563, 2006.
21. Macknet MR, et al: Accuracy and tolerance of a novel bioacoustic respiratory sensor in pediatric patients. Available at www.rcjournal.com/abstracts/2007/?id=aarc07_199.
22. Macintosh R: *Physics for the anaesthetist*, ed 4, Boston, 1987, Blackwell Scientific.
23. Abstracts of the 1998 Joint Meeting of the Society for Technology in Anesthesia and the Rochester Simulator Symposium: Simulation in Anesthesia, *J Clin Monit Comput* 14(7):511–539, 1998.
24. Winter A, Spence AA: An international consensus on monitoring? *Br J Anaesth* 64(3):263–266, 1990.
25. McEwen J, Small C, Jenkins L: Detection of interruptions in the breathing gas of ventilated anaesthetized patients, *Can J Anaesth* 35(6):549–561, 1988.
26. Raphael DT, Weller RS, Doran DJ: A response algorithm for the low-pressure alarm condition, *Anesth Analg* 67(9):876–883, 1988.
27. Marini JJ, Ravenscraft SA: Mean airway pressure: physiologic determinants and clinical importance. Part 2: Clinical implications, *Crit Care Med* 20(11):1604–1616, 1992.
28. Campbell RM, Sheikh A, Crosse MM: A study of the incorrect use of ventilator disconnection alarms, *Anaesthesia* 51(4):369–370, 1996.
29. Milligan KA: Disablement of a ventilator disconnect alarm by a heat and moisture exchanger, *Anaesthesia* 47(3):279, 1992.
30. Slee TA, Pavlin EG: Failure of low pressure alarm associated with the use of a humidifier, *Anesthesiology* 69(5):791–792, 1988.
31. Chung DC, Ho AMH, Tay BA: "Apnea-volume" warning during normal ventilation of the lungs: an unusual leak in the Narkomed 4 anesthesia system, *J Clin Anesth* 13(1):40–43, 2001.
32. Snyders S, Mitton M: Failure of a flow sensor of a Datex Ohmeda S/5 Aespire, *Anaesthesia* 60(9):941–942, 2005.
33. Hari M, Jennings M, Mitton M: Flow sensor fault causing ventilator malfunction, *Anaesthesia* 60(10):1049–1051, 2005.
34. Aldridge J: Leak on Datex Aestiva/5 anaesthetic machine, *Anaesthesia* 60(4):420–421, 2005.
35. Dhar P, George I, Mankad A, Sloan P: Flow transducer gas leak detected after induction, *Anesth Analg* 89(6):1587, 1999.
36. Bowes WA 3rd, Corke BC, Hulka J: Pulse oximetry: a review of the theory, accuracy, and clinical applications, *Obstet Gynecol* 74(3 Pt 2): 541–546, 1989.
37. Bardoczky GI, Engelman EE: Comparison of airway pressures from different measuring sites, *Anesth Analg* 83(4):887, 1996.
38. Lian JX: Understanding ventilator waveforms and how to use them in patient care, *Nurs Crit Care* 4(1):43–55, 2009.
39. Spielman FJ, Sprague DH: Another benefit of the subatmospheric alarm, *Anesthesiology* 54(6):526, 1981.
40. Walker T: Another problem with a circle system, *Anaesthesia* 51(1):89, 1996.
41. Bashein GMD, MacEvoy B: Anesthesia ventilators should have adjustable high-pressure alarms, *Anesthesiology* 63(2):231–233, 1985.
42. Campos C, Naguib SS, Chuang AZ, Lemak NA, Khalil SN: Endobronchial intubation causes an immediate increase in peak inflation pressure in pediatric patients, *Anesth Analg* 88(2):268–270, 1999.
43. West J: *Respiratory physiology: the essentials* ed 8, Baltimore, 2008, Lippincott, Williams & Wilkins, pp 17–19.
44. Wright BM: A respiratory anemometer, *J Physiol (London)* 127:25, 1955.
45. Bushman J: Effect of different flow patterns on the Wright respirometer, *Br J Anaesth* 51(9):895–898, 1979.
46. Ilsley A, Hart J, Withers R, Roberts J: Evaluation of five small turbine-type respirometers used in adult anesthesia, *J Clin Monit Comput* 9(3):196–201, 1993.
47. Hatch DJ, Jackson EA: A new critical incident monitor for use with the paediatric T-piece, *Anaesthesia* 51(9):839–842, 1996.
48. Goto T, Saito H, Nakata Y, et al: Effects of xenon on the performance of various respiratory flowmeters, *Anesthesiology* 90(2):555–563, 1999.
49. Lynnworth LC, Korba JM, Wallace DR: Fast response ultrasonic flowmeter measures breathing dynamics, *IEEE Trans Biomed Eng* 32(7):530–535, 1985.
50. Kuppers K: *An improved apparatus for measuring gases*, Germany, 1909, Deutsches patent and Markenamt.
51. Ball C, Westhorpe R: Maximilian Neu and the first anaesthetic rotameter, *Anaesth Intensive Care* 27:333, 1999.
52. Foregger R: Early use of rotameter in anaesthesia, *Br J Anaesth* 24(3):187–195, 1952.
53. Moore JK, Railton R: Hypoxia caused by a leaking rotameter: the value of an oxygen analyser, *Anaesthesia* 39(4):380–381, 1984.
54. Gupta BL, Varshneya AK: Anaesthetic accident caused by unusual leakage of rotameter [letter], *Br J Anaesth* 47(7):805, 1975.
55. McQuillan PJ, Jackson IJ: Potential leaks from anaesthetic machines: potential leaks through open rotameter valves and empty cylinder yokes, *Anaesthesia* 42(12):1308–1312, 1987.
56. Slater EM: Transposition of rotameter bobbins, *Anesthesiology* 41(1):101, 1974.
57. Cooke R: Transposition of rotameter tubes, *Br J Anaesth* 80(5):699, 1998.
58. Fleisch A: The pneumotachometer [in German], *Arch Ges Physiol* 209:713–722, 1925.
59. Yeh MP, Adams TD, Gardner RM, Yanowitz FG: Effect of O_2, N_2, and CO_2 composition on nonlinearity of Fleisch pneumotachograph characteristics, *J Appl Physiol* 56(5):1423–1425, 1984.
60. Meriläinen P, Hänninen H, Tuomaala L: A novel sensor for routine continuous spirometry of intubated patients, *J Clin Monit Comput* 9(5):374–380, 1993.
61. Bardoczky GI, deFrancquen P, Engelman E, Capello M: Continuous monitoring of pulmonary mechanics with the sidestream spirometer during lung transplantation, *J Cardiothorac Vasc Anesth* 6(6):731–734, 1992.
62. Søndergaard S, Kárason S, Lundin S, Stenqvist O: Evaluation of a pitot type spirometer in helium/oxygen mixtures, *J Clin Monit Comput* 14(6):425–431, 1998.
63. Tham R, Oberle M: How do flow sensors work? *APSF Newsletter* 10–12, 2008.
64. Kann T, Hald A, Jørgensen FE: A new transducer for respiratory monitoring: a description of a hot-wire anemometer and a test procedure for general use, *Acta Anaesth Scand* 23(4):349–358, 1979.
65. Kiełbasa J: Measurement of gas flow velocity: anemometer with a vibrating hot wire, *Rev Sci Instrum* 81(1)015101, 2010.
66. Brusasco V, Beck KC, Crawford M, Rehder K: Resonant amplification of delivered volume during high-frequency ventilation, *J Appl Physiol* 60(3):885–892, 1986.
67. Eberhart RC, Weigelt JA: Respiratory monitoring: current techniques and some new developments, *Bull Eur Physiopathol Respir* 21(3):295–300, 1985.
68. Lynnworth LC, Liu Y: Ultrasonic flowmeters: half-century progress report, 1955-2005, *Ultrasonics* 44(Suppl 1):e1371–e1378, 2006.
69. Kästner SB, Marlin DJ, Roberts CA, Auer JA, Lekeux P: Comparison of the performance of linear resistance and ultrasonic pneumotachometers at rest and during lobeline-induced hyperpnoea, *Res Vet Sci* 68(2):153–159, 2000.
70. Pierce R: Spirometry: an essential clinical measurement, *Aust Fam Physician* 34(7):535–539, 2005.
71. Bardoczky GI, Engelman E, D'Hollander A: Continuous spirometry: an aid to monitoring ventilation during operation, *Br J Anaesth* 71(5):747–751, 1993.
72. Weissman C: Flow-volume relationships during spontaneous breathing through endotracheal tubes, *Crit Care Med* 20:615–620, 1992.
73. Lumb AB: *Elastic forces and lung volumes. Nunn's applied respiratory physiology*, Woburn, MA, 2000, Butterworth Heinemann, p 47.
74. Cheifetz IM, Myers TR: Should every mechanically ventilated patient be monitored with capnography from intubation to extubation? *Respir Care* 52(4):423–438, 2007.

75. Eberhard P: The design, use, and results of transcutaneous carbon dioxide analysis: current and future directions, *Anesth Analg* 105:S48–S52, 2007.
76. Lightdale JR, Goldmann DA, Feldman HA, et al: Microstream capnography improves patient monitoring during moderate sedation: a randomized, controlled trial, *Pediatrics* 117(6):e1170–e1178, 2006.
77. Deitch K, Chudnofsky CR, Dominici P: The utility of supplemental oxygen during emergency department procedural sedation with propofol: a randomized, controlled trial, *Ann Emerg Med* 52(1):1–8, 2008.
78. Respironics Flo-Trak module. Accessed 2012 Oct 5 at http://oem.respironics.com/Downloads/4100306-FloTrak.pdf.
79. Cisco Systems: 802.11ac: The Fifth Generation of Wi-Fi. Available at www.cisco.com/en/US/prod/collateral/wireless/ps5678/ps11983/white_paper_c11-713103_ns767_Networking_Solutions_White_Paper.html. Accessed 4 Nov 2012.

PART III

PATIENT MONITORS

CHAPTER 10

CAPNOGRAPHY

Chris R. Giordano • Nikolaus Gravenstein

CHAPTER OUTLINE

OVERVIEW

The capnograph functions as an "electronic stethoscope" that shows the cyclic appearance and disappearance of carbon dioxide (CO_2): it appears when the lungs are being ventilated, and it disappears when they are not. The American Society of Anesthesiologists (ASA) updated their standards for basic anesthetic monitoring in July 1989, recommending that not only should carbon dioxide be identified in the expired gas to confirm correct placement of an endotracheal tube or laryngeal mask airway, it should also be a standard monitor for assessing ventilation for "every patient receiving general anesthesia."[1] The standards related to carbon dioxide monitoring were again updated effective July 2011 to include carbon dioxide monitoring for any patient undergoing moderate or deep sedation.[2] Carbon dioxide homeostasis involves many organ systems. Most importantly, the clinician skilled in capnography can interpret the capnogram to gain information about a patient's adequacy of ventilation as well as metabolism and the cardiovascular system.

TERMS AND DEFINITIONS

The Greek root *kapnos*, meaning "smoke," is used to form the word *capnometry*, the practice of measuring the carbon dioxide in respiratory gas, and *capnometer*, the instrument used for this purpose. Carbon dioxide can be thought of as the "smoke" of cellular metabolism. The term *capnometer* is used to identify an instrument that provides only digital data—specifically, the minimum and maximum values of carbon dioxide during each respiratory cycle. This is in contrast to a *capnograph*, an instrument that displays, in addition to digital data, a capnogram, the graphic representation of the CO_2 concentration, or partial pressure, over time (Fig. 10-1).

Carbon dioxide levels are most commonly represented as a pressure-versus-time plot, or *time capnography*. An alternative and newer representation is as a pressure-versus-volume plot, or *volumetric capnography* (Fig. 10-2).[3] The physiologic mechanisms responsible for the different phases in time capnography can be translated to the phases represented in volumetric capnography.[4] The tracing of carbon dioxide concentration versus expired volume allows for a real-time continuous calculation and display of anatomic and physiologic dead space ventilation. The alterations of physiologic dead space measured in real time can be used to indicate changes in the alveolar dead space component because the anatomic component usually remains static. In fact, the volumetric capnogram and its derivative calculations may give a more accurate picture of the ventilation/perfusion (V/Q) ratio than the corresponding CO_2-versus-time trace (Table 10-1).[5,6]

Both capnometers and capnographs digitally report carbon dioxide concentrations as "inspired" and "end tidal." Actually, these instruments do not and cannot determine the different phases of respiration; they simply report the minimum and maximum CO_2 values detected during each CO_2 (respiratory) cycle. In certain instances—such as with an incompetent inspiratory valve, a Mapleson-type breathing system, or an erratic breathing pattern—the minimum CO_2 concentration may not always equal the inspired CO_2 concentration. Similarly, the maximum concentration measured may not always be the end-tidal concentration. Thus the terms *minimum inspired* ($P_ICO_2$min) and *maximum expired* ($P_{ET}CO_2$max) partial pressure of CO_2 ($PaCO_2$) are actually more correct. Most time-based capnograph

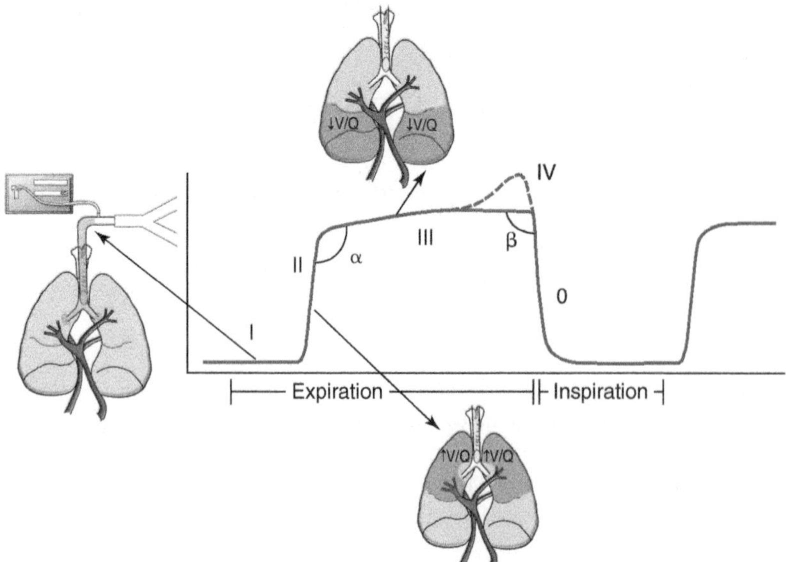

FIGURE 10-1 ▪ A typical capnogram of the upright lung during controlled mechanical ventilation. A capnogram has two segments, *inspiratory* and *expiratory,* that flow seamlessly into one another. The expiratory segment has an α-angle and three, or sometimes four, phases: anatomic dead space reveals an inspiratory baseline (*I*); a mixture of anatomic and alveolar dead space reveals the expiratory upstroke (α-angle) that divides phases II and III and reveals the ventilation/perfusion status of the lung (*II*); the alveolar plateau (*III*); and, occasionally, the terminal upswing (IV). The inspiratory segment includes the β-angle that follows phase III, and phase 0, showing the inspiratory downstroke.

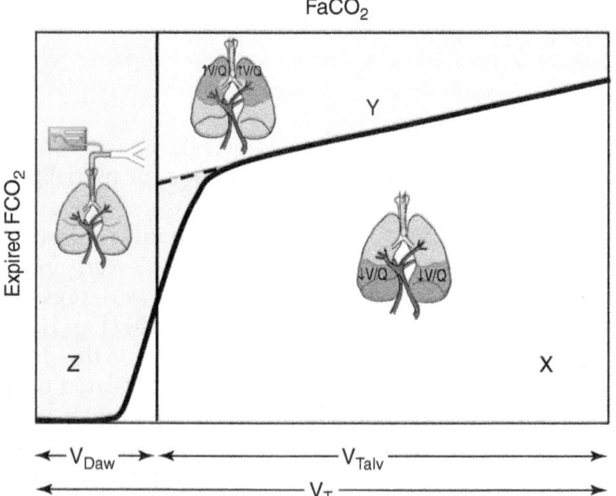

FIGURE 10-2 ▪ Volumetric capnograph of a single breath. $FaCO_2$ represents the fraction of carbon dioxide of gas in equilibrium with arterial blood. Area Z (*blue area*) is the anatomic dead space. Area Y (*yellow area*) is the alveolar dead space, and area X (*white area*) is the volume of carbon dioxide (CO_2) exhaled. The alveolar dead space fraction is Y/(X + Y), and the physiologic dead space fraction is (Y + Z)/(X + Y + Z). V_{Daw}, anatomic dead space; V_T, tidal volume; V_{Talv}, alveolar tidal volume.

TABLE 10-1 Advantages of Time vs. Volume Capnography

Time Capnography	Volume Capnography
Familiar, commonplace	Informs about lung V/Q status
Intubation not required	Provides Vd/Vt composition
Expiratory phase obvious	Provides airway gas flow data

Vd/Vt, dead-space volume to tidal volume; *V/Q,* ventilation/perfusion.

devices can be configured to display the carbon dioxide recorded at two speeds: a *high speed* allows the user to interpret information about each breath, and a *slow speed* enables appreciation of the CO_2 trend.

Two types of capnographs are in use; each has its advantages and disadvantages (Table 10-2). *Sidestream,* or sampling, capnographs aspirate respiratory gas from an airway sampling site at a rate of 50 to 400 mL/min. The sampled gas is transported through a tube to a nearby CO_2 analyzer. *Mainstream,* or in-line, capnographs position the actual CO_2 analyzer on the airway, and respiratory gas is analyzed in situ as it passes through a special adapter. No gas is removed from the airway with a mainstream analyzer.

TABLE 10-2 Comparison of Sidestream and Mainstream Capnographs

	Sidestream (Picture)	Mainstream (Picture)
Small size	Yes	No, but improving
Airway weight	No	Yes
Sampling tubing	Yes	No
Scavenging system	Yes	No
Electrical cord	No	Yes
Response delay	Yes	No
Humidity vulnerability	Minimal	Yes
Neonatal ease	No	Yes
Sterilization need	No	Yes

MEASUREMENT TECHNIQUES

Several analytical techniques can be used to measure respiratory CO_2. Carbon dioxide strongly absorbs infrared (IR) light, particularly at a wavelength of 4.3 μm. Thus most stand-alone capnometers and capnographs use IR light absorption, a relatively inexpensive technique, to measure respiratory carbon dioxide. The IR light absorbed is proportional to the concentration of the absorbing molecules, such as CO_2, and the concentration of the gas can be determined by comparing the measured absorbance against a known standard. IR light absorbs all polyatomic gases; therefore CO_2 concentration may be slightly influenced by the presence of water vapor or nitrous oxide (N_2O). Mass spectrography, molecular

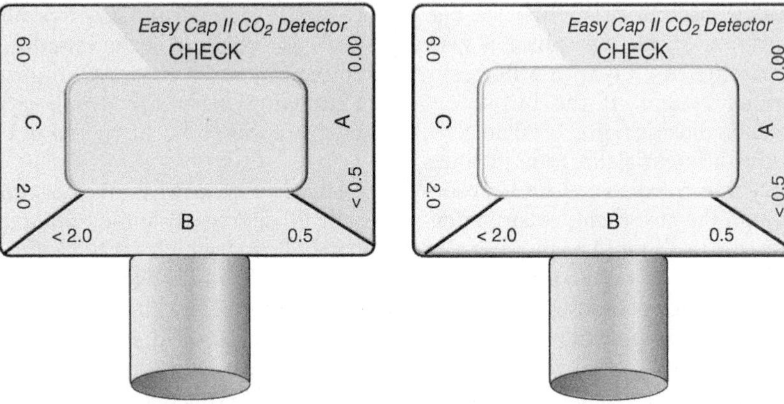

FIGURE 10-3 ■ The color change in the chemical indicator of the Easy Cap II carbon dioxide detector reveals the semiquantitative presence of carbon dioxide (CO_2). The image on the right demonstrates CO_2 in the 2% to 6% range. (Image used by permission from Nellcor Puritan Bennett LLC, Boulder, CO, doing business as Covidien.)

correlation spectrography, Raman spectrography, and photoacoustic spectrography also can be used to measure CO_2 concentration but are expensive and rarely used, or they are no longer available for clinical use. A chemical carbon dioxide indicator, the FEF end-tidal detector (Fenem, New York, NY) is a pH-sensitive chemical paper that changes color on exposure to CO_2.[7] The indicator paper changes color from purple (non–CO_2-containing gas) to yellow (CO_2-containing gas) in a semiquantitative manner (Fig. 10-3). This response is evident with the respiratory cycle as the carbon dioxide appears and disappears. This indicator is very sensitive to even low levels of CO_2, such as may be present in the esophagus[8]; therefore proper intubation must still be recertified by the usual clinical techniques.

SYSTEMATIC INTERPRETATION OF TIME CAPNOGRAPHY

Carbon dioxide analysis can be broken down into three individual components: *numbers* (capnometry), *curves* (capnography), and *gradients* (arterial end-tidal CO_2).[9] When interpreting carbon dioxide values, presumptions of blood CO_2 levels, pulmonary blood flow, and alveolar ventilation can be made; however, assessment of the numbers in conjunction with CO_2 curves assists in correctly identifying clinical situations while taking into proper consideration the adequacy of gas sampling, presence of leaks in the system, and possible malfunction of the CO_2 measuring equipment.

Is there exhaled CO_2? This is the fundamental question for managing every airway. When the capnograph does not register exhaled CO_2 following the patient's exhalation, failure to ventilate the patient's lungs is the most likely explanation, although other etiologies also should be entertained. This differential diagnosis includes esophageal intubation, accidental extubation, disconnection or failure of the sampling line or device, apnea, or cardiac arrest. The importance of capnography in helping to detect esophageal intubation cannot be overemphasized. To avoid misinterpretation of esophageal intubation as endotracheal, clinicians should confirm tracheal intubation not only by the presence, but also the persistent reappearance, of the CO_2 waveform with each respiratory cycle. This repetitive efflux of carbon dioxide from the trachea easily distinguishes itself from CO_2 trapped in the stomach or esophagus because esophageal intubation shows a progressive stepwise decrease in CO_2 with successive ventilation (Fig. 10-4).[10]

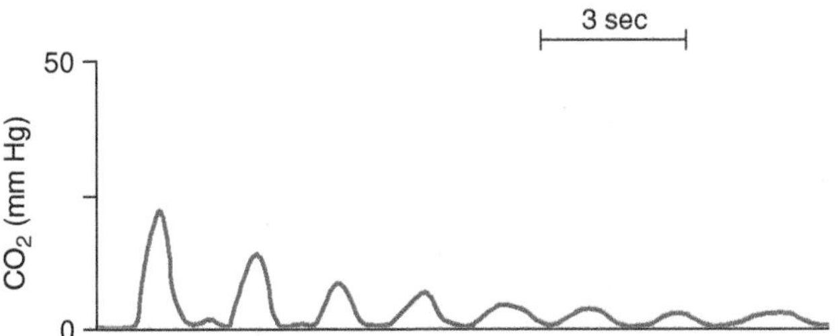

FIGURE 10-4 ■ A typical capnogram from an esophageal intubation. Note the rapid decline of the exhaled CO_2 to nearly zero. Compare this capnogram with the normal capnogram in Figure 10-1.

Interpreting CO_2 in the midst of a cardiac arrest requires additional evaluation to affirm correct airway management. Lack of end-tidal CO_2 or absence of color change on the CO_2 indicator device following intubation alerts the practitioner to a likely incorrect placement of the airway device. However, in the event of a cardiac arrest, little or no end-tidal carbon dioxide ($ETCO_2$) will be detected because no pulmonary blood flow is present to permit gas exchange. Direct visualization of the endotracheal tube passing through the vocal cords or the detection of bilateral breath sounds will aid further decision making.

Disconnection within the breathing system is easily detected with capnography by a flat capnogram and a CO_2 reading of zero. A flat capnogram also is correctly produced by apnea, which may ensue when patients who were previously spontaneously breathing receive agents that hinder respiratory drive. Not until all the above mechanisms have been absolutely ruled out by clinical examination should failure of the capnograph be considered. If the capnograph itself is suspect, the anesthesiologist can quickly disconnect the sampling or sensing adapter and exhale into it to determine whether the capnograph is working and the sampling catheter is patent.

Inspiratory Segment

During mechanical inspiration (*phase 0*), fresh gas with no carbon dioxide flows by the CO_2 sampling or sensing site, and the capnograph traces the inspiratory baseline (see Fig. 10-1). The CO_2 concentration during this phase is zero because there is no rebreathing of CO_2 with a normally functioning circle breathing system. If the inspiratory baseline is elevated and carbon dioxide is greater than zero, CO_2 is being rebreathed; the differential diagnosis includes an incompetent expiratory valve, exhausted CO_2 absorbent, gas channeling through the absorbent, or an imperfectly calibrated capnometer. Also, a rapid respiratory rate combined with a low tidal volume, as is often seen in small children, may exceed the frequency response characteristics of the monitor. The inspiratory baseline may or may not be elevated when the inspiratory valve is incompetent, depending on the size of the breath—that is, if the tidal volume is greater than the volume of the inspiratory hose, it will reach zero; if the tidal volume is less, it will not. Typically, a malfunctioning inspiratory valve and a sidestream capnograph with a high response time show an extension or decrease in the slope of the downstroke.[11-14]

Expiratory Segment

This segment of the capnograph tracing is divided into phases I, II, III, and occasionally IV (see Fig. 10-1).

Phases and Angles

Phase I. Shortly after mechanical inspiration ends, the lungs recoil, gas quickly exits through the trachea, and CO_2-free gas from the apparatus and anatomic dead space, roughly one third of the tidal volume, passes by the IR sensor. Phase I appears as an extension of the horizontal baseline, extending that initiated during phase 0.

Phase II. As the CO_2-free gas from the apparatus and the anatomic dead space is washed out and replaced by CO_2-rich alveolar gas, the expiratory upstroke appears on the capnogram. The upstroke, which should be steep, becomes slanted or S-shaped if gas flow is partially obstructed, the sidestream analyzer is sampling gas too slowly,[15] or the response time of the capnograph is too slow for the patient's respiratory rate.[16] Gas flow may be obstructed in the breathing system, such as by a kinked tracheal tube, or in the patient's airway, as with chronic obstructive pulmonary disease or acute bronchospasm.

α-Angle. Phase II and phase III are separated by the α-angle.[9] Changes in the α-angle correlate with the sequential emptying of the alveoli and thus the overall V/Q matching of the lung. As V/Q matching becomes more heterogenous, the variations in lung time constants increase, and the α-angle increases ($\alpha > 90$ degrees).[17] This is further demonstrated by an increasing slope in phase III.

Phase III. As exhalation continues, the capnogram plateaus, with a slightly increasing slope. If ventilation and perfusion were perfectly matched in all lung regions, alveolar gas would have a constant CO_2 concentration, and the expiratory plateau would be perfectly horizontal. However, ventilation and perfusion are not perfectly matched in all lung units, especially in patients who are supine and whose lungs are being mechanically ventilated with positive pressure.[17] Therefore CO_2 typically continues to increase slowly as a result of cyclic variation in alveolar CO_2 during ventilation, which is greatest during expiration, or because of late emptying of the alveoli with the lowest V/Q ratio, which are therefore the richest in CO_2.

β-Angle. The downstroke that follows phase III is normally 90 degrees (β-angle)[9] and represents the inspiratory phase, during which CO_2-free gas passes over the sampling sensor and is inhaled. Malfunctioning inspiratory valves and rebreathing and a low–tidal volume rapid respiratory rate will increase the β-angle and delay or prevent the inspiratory baseline from returning to zero. Examples of typical abnormal CO_2 capnograms are illustrated in Figures 10-5 to 10-9.

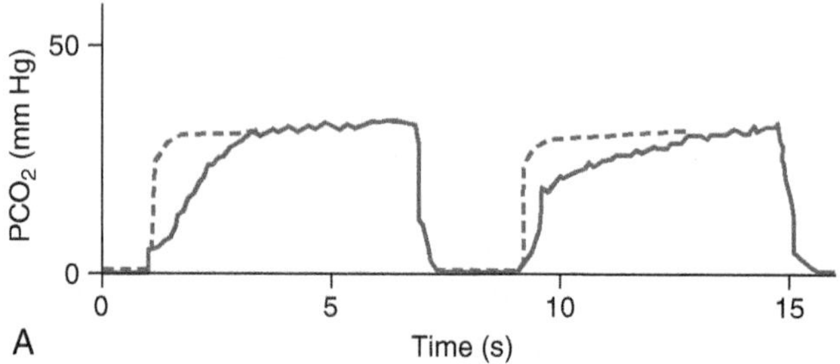

FIGURE 10-5 A capnogram showing increased airway resistance caused by bronchospasm or a kinked tracheal tube. The characteristic abnormal waveform (*solid line*) is superimposed on a normal waveform (*dashed line*). *PCO_2*, partial pressure of carbon dioxide. (From van Genderingen HR, Gravenstein N, van der Aa JJ, et al: Computer-assisted capnogram analysis. *J Clin Monit* 1987; 3:198.)

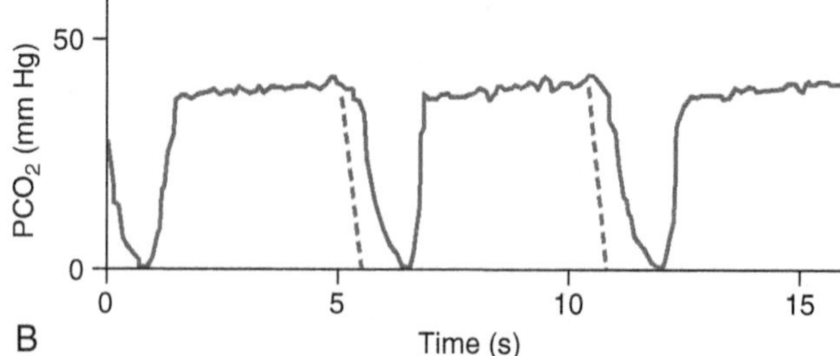

FIGURE 10-6 A capnogram showing an incompetent inspiratory valve, in which part of the expired gas flows back into the inspiratory limb and is inspired with the next breath. The characteristic abnormal waveform (*solid line*) is superimposed on a normal waveform (*dashed line*). *PCO_2*, partial pressure of carbon dioxide. (From van Genderingen HR, Gravenstein N, van der Aa JJ, et al: Computer-assisted capnogram analysis. *J Clin Monit* 1987; 3:198.)

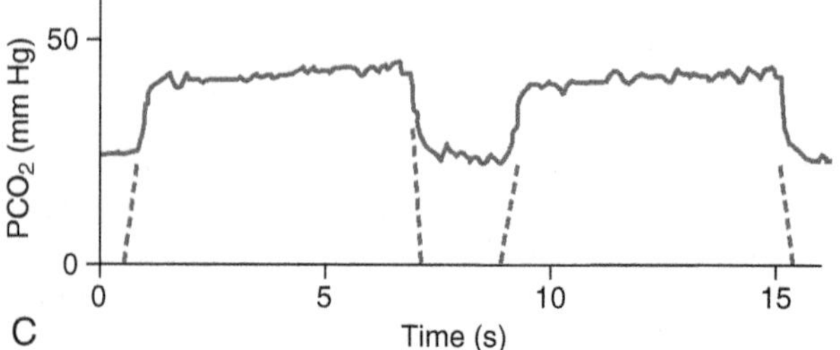

FIGURE 10-7 A capnogram showing an incompetent expiratory valve or soda lime depletion, in which expired gas is reinspired through the expiratory limb. The characteristic abnormal waveform (*solid line*) is superimposed on a normal waveform (*dashed line*). *PCO_2*, partial pressure of carbon dioxide. (From van Genderingen HR, Gravenstein N, van der Aa JJ, et al: Computer-assisted capnogram analysis. *J Clin Monit* 1987; 3:198.)

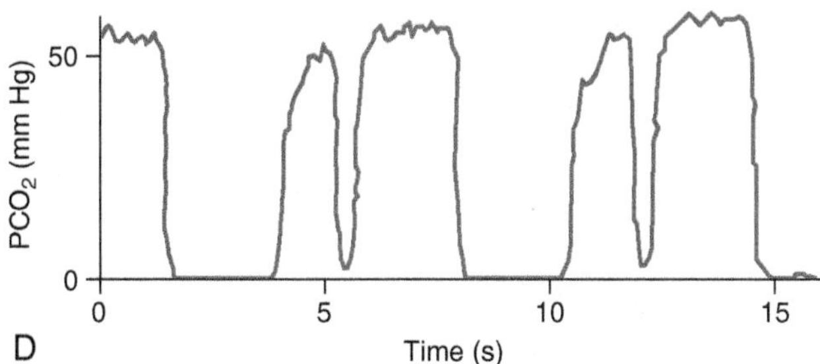

FIGURE 10-8 A capnogram of a patient taking breaths and overriding mechanical ventilation (*solid line*). *PCO_2*, partial pressure of carbon dioxide. (From van Genderingen HR, Gravenstein N, van der Aa JJ, et al: Computer-assisted capnogram analyses. *J Clin Monit* 1987; 3:198.)

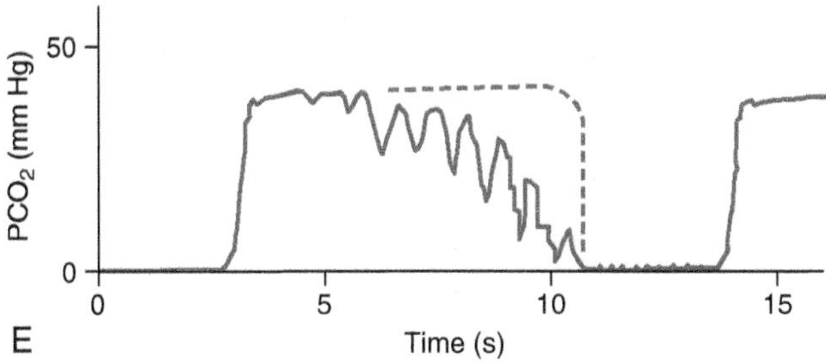

FIGURE 10-9 A capnogram showing cardiogenic oscillations caused by the rhythmic increase and decrease in intrathoracic volume with each cardiac cycle. The characteristic abnormal waveform (*solid line*) is superimposed on a normal waveform (*dashed line*). PCO_2, partial pressure of carbon dioxide. (From van Genderingen HR, Gravenstein N, van der Aa JJ, et al: Computer-assisted capnogram analysis. *J Clin Monit* 1987; 3:198.)

Phase IV. Following the alveolar plateau, a terminal upswing may be seen (phase IV). Barring any intrinsic lung disease, this finding is linked to differing time constants within the lung, indirectly indicating V/Q matching. Phase IV tracings are most frequently seen in pregnant and obese patients because of a decrease in lung compliance and functional residual capacity.[18]

Arterial and End-Tidal Carbon Dioxide Gradient

The best measure of the adequacy of ventilation of the lungs is partial pressure of carbon dioxide ($PaCO_2$). Typically, $PaCO_2$ and $P_{ET}CO_2$ differ in patients without lung disease by approximately 5 mm Hg. This difference is due to V/Q mismatching in the lungs that results from temporal, spatial, and alveolar mixing defects. Several factors cause the normally small difference between $PaCO_2$ and $P_{ET}CO_2$ to increase, and these can be divided into three components (Fig. 10-10):

1. $Paco_2 - P_Aco_2$. The difference between arterial partial pressure of CO_2 and the mixed alveolar partial pressure of CO_2 (P_ACO_2). Mismatching of ventilation (V) and perfusion (Q) increases the difference between $PaCO_2$ and P_ACO_2. Examples are pulmonary embolism and endobronchial intubation. Both increases and decreases in V/Q enlarge the difference between arterial and alveolar CO_2. Consider a simplified, two-unit lung model (Fig. 10-11) with perfect matching of V and Q. Blood with a $PaCO_2$ of 46 mm Hg returns to the lungs, and after equilibration, both the pulmonary capillary blood and the alveolar gas have a $PaCO_2$ of 40 mm Hg. The alveolar gas is exhaled, and the capnograph reports a $P_{ET}CO_2$ of 40 mm Hg. The $PaCO_2$ is also 40 mm Hg, so in this simplified model the difference between $PaCO_2$ and $P_{ET}CO_2$ is zero.

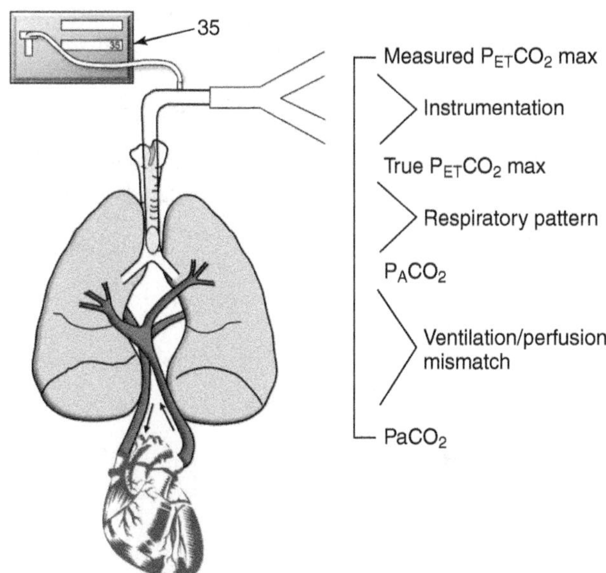

FIGURE 10-10 Components of the difference between partial pressure of carbon dioxide (*$PaCO_2$*) and maximum concentration of end-tidal carbon dioxide (*$P_{ET}CO_2$ max*).

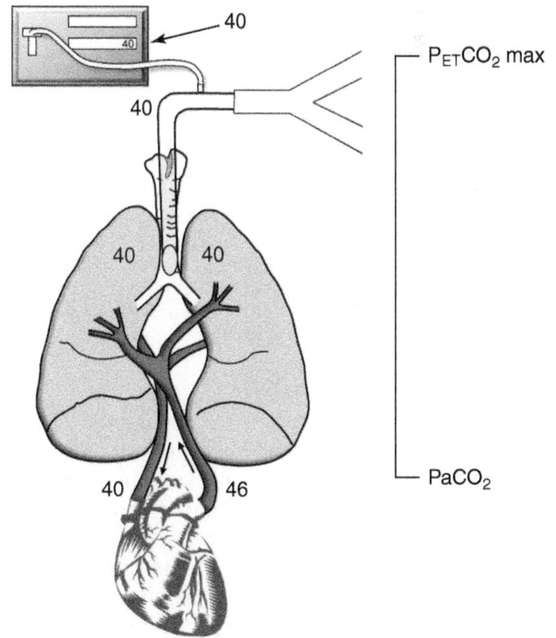

FIGURE 10-11 An idealized two-unit lung model demonstrates how ventilation/perfusion (V/Q) mismatching increases the difference between partial pressure of arterial carbon dioxide (*$PaCO_2$*) and maximum concentration of end-tidal carbon dioxide (*$P_{ET}CO_2$ max*). This figure shows perfect V/Q matching, in which the V/Q ratio equals 1; $PaCO_2$ and $P_{ET}CO_2$ max are both 40 mm Hg.

Endobronchial intubation is an extreme example of V/Q less than 1 (Fig. 10-12). All the blood flowing through the nonventilated lung represents shunt. As before, mixed venous blood with PCO_2 of 46 mm Hg returns to the lungs; gas is exchanged in the ventilated lung, and pulmonary blood and alveolar gas in this lung unit end up with a $PaCO_2$ of 40 mm Hg. The nonventilated lung unit allows no exchange of alveolar gas, so both pulmonary blood and alveolar gas eventually equilibrate at a $PaCO_2$ of 46 mm Hg. Assuming equal distribution of blood flow, after pulmonary blood from the two lung units mixes, the resultant $PaCO_2$ is 43 mm Hg ([46 + 40]/2). Alveolar gas from the ventilated lung unit only is exhaled and reaches the capnograph, which reports a $P_{ET}CO_2$ of 40 mm Hg. In this simplified lung model, a decreased V/Q increases the difference between $PaCO_2$ and $P_{ET}CO_2$ from 0 to 3 mm Hg.

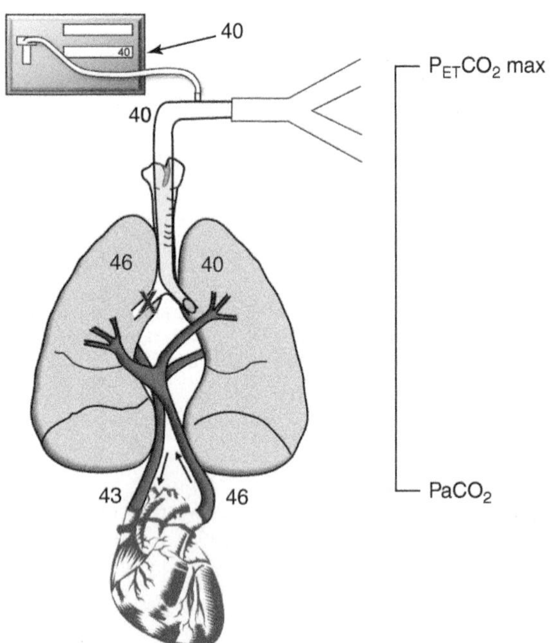

FIGURE 10-12 ▪ The effect of a large increase in shunt from a mainstem intubation. The ventilation/perfusion ratio is less than 1 because part of the lung is perfused but not ventilated. In this case, there is a 3 mm Hg difference between partial pressure of arterial carbon dioxide (*$PaCO_2$*; 43 mm Hg) and the end-tidal carbon dioxide (*$P_{ET}CO_2$ max*; 40 mm Hg).

In contrast, the much greater effect of a V/Q greater than 1 is illustrated by pulmonary embolism (Fig. 10-13). This is an example of increased dead space ventilation. Blood returning to the lungs has a $PaCO_2$ of 46 mm Hg and can flow to only one lung unit because of the embolus. Thus alveolar gas in the nonperfused lung unit has a $PaCO_2$ of zero. Pulmonary capillary blood and alveolar gas equilibrate in the perfused lung unit at a $PaCO_2$ of 40 mm Hg, and the resulting $PaCO_2$ is 40 mm Hg. Assuming equal ventilation of both lung units, the resultant $P_{ET}CO_2$ is 20 mm Hg (from [40 + 0]/2). In this simplified lung model, an increased V/Q, such as that caused by pulmonary embolism, markedly increases the difference between $PaCO_2$ and $P_{ET}CO_2$ to 20 mm Hg. This increase is consistent with the difference between $PaCO_2$ and $P_{ET}CO_2$ measured in patients with acute pulmonary embolism.[19,20]

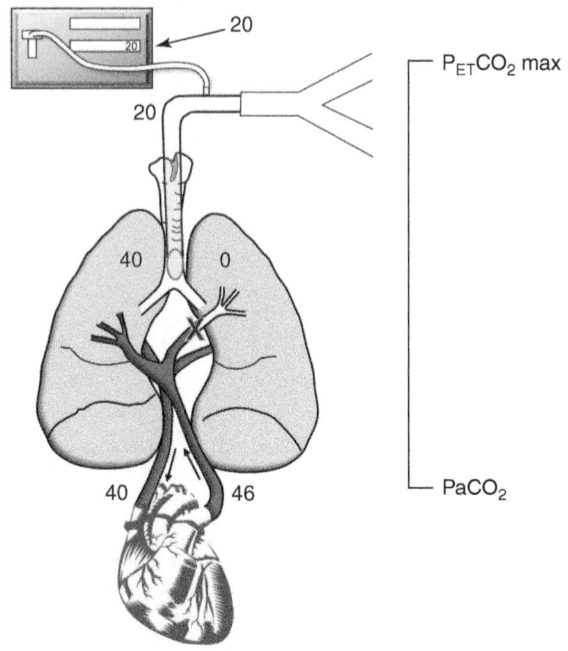

FIGURE 10-13 ▪ The effect of a large dead space from a pulmonary embolus. The ventilation/perfusion ratio is greater than 1 because part of the lung is ventilated but not perfused. In this case, a 20 mm Hg difference is seen between partial pressure of arterial carbon dioxide (*$PaCO_2$*; 40 mm Hg) and the end-tidal carbon dioxide (*$P_{ET}CO_2$ max*; 20 mm Hg).

2. P_ACO_2 - true $P_{ET}CO_2$. The difference between P_ACO_2 and the true partial pressure of CO_2 delivered to the upper airway, or actual CO_2 at the sensing or sampling site (true $P_{ET}CO_2$). Breathing patterns that fail to deliver undiluted alveolar gas to the upper airway increase the difference between P_ACO_2 and true $P_{ET}CO_2$. An example is the higher frequency ventilation that occurs in neonates and infants. If the patient has a rapid respiratory rate and is breathing erratically or is not exhaling completely—such as in Figure 10-8, with chronic obstructive pulmonary disease or acute bronchospasm—a fully mixed alveolar gas sample may not be delivered to the upper airway. The alveolar sample not only must be delivered to the upper airway and then the CO_2 sensor, it also must remain there long enough for the capnometer to measure it. Capnometry in neonates and small children typically results in a larger $PaCO_2$ - $P_{ET}CO_2$ gradient than in adults. Factors that contribute to this increase include a low tidal volume/equipment dead space ratio, a rapid respiratory rate, a high rate of fresh gas flow, and a rate of sampling by CO_2 analyzer higher than the expiratory flow rate of these small subjects at

the time of end exhalation.[21] Uncuffed tracheal tubes, which are used in neonates and infants, compound the problem because exhaled gas escaping around the tube is not seen by the CO_2 sensor in the capnometer.

3. True $P_{ET}CO_2$ – measured $P_{ET}CO_2$. The difference between true $P_{ET}CO_2$ and measured $P_{ET}CO_2$ reported by the capnograph. Problems with the capnograph itself can increase this component of the $PaCO_2$ minus $P_{ET}CO_2$ gradient. Examples are sampling catheter leaks, calibration error, and slow instrument response time relative to the breathing pattern. Even if a mixed alveolar gas sample reaches the CO_2 sensing or sampling site, problems with the capnograph itself, such as a miscalibrated unit, may result in inaccurate CO_2 measurement. Small inaccuracies can arise if the processing algorithms in the capnograph do not accurately account for water vapor.[22] IR analyzers must also compensate for high concentrations of nitrous oxide and oxygen. A capnograph with a slow response time increases the apparent inspired CO_2 and decreases the $P_{ET}CO_2$, thereby increasing the true $P_{ET}CO_2$ – measured $P_{ET}CO_2$ difference. *Response time* refers to how fast the instrument can measure a step change in CO_2 concentration. For example, if the CO_2 or sampling site is exposed to room air (CO_2 free) and suddenly is flooded with 5% CO_2, how long does it take for the capnograph to report a CO_2 value of 5%? A typical IR 10% to 90% carbon dioxide analyzer response time is in the range 100 to 150 ms, which means it takes one tenth of a second for the device to go from measuring 10% of the CO_2 concentration to 90% of the sampled concentration. The response time effect is operational both during inspiration and expiration. Because the inspiratory time is often shorter than the expiratory time, such as if the inspiratory/expiratory (I:E) ratio is 1:3, the artifactual appearance of inspired CO_2 with rapid respiratory rates is easy to understand.

   Why is response time clinically important? If the capnograph has a slow response time and the patient has a rapid respiratory rate, the respiratory gas may not remain at the CO_2 sensing site long enough to be completely measured. The more rapid the response time, the more likely it is that the capnograph will accurately measure CO_2 when the respiratory rate is high.[23]

A subtle problem with sidestream capnographs that leads to an increase in the true $P_{ET}CO_2$ – measured $P_{ET}CO_2$ difference is partial obstruction of the sampling system. For example, if the water filter becomes saturated or extra filters are inserted, resistance to gas flow increases, and the pressure within the CO_2 analyzing chamber may become subambient.

Attempting to protect a sidestream analyzer from moisture by routinely inserting an extra filter may create a systematic error that increases the $PaCO_2$ to $P_{ET}CO_2$ difference in all patients. A solution to this moisture problem is to interpose a heat and moisture exchanger (HME) between the tracheal tube and the CO_2 sampling site or to use a section of Nafion tubing (which is semipermeable to water vapor and reduces the moisture burden presented to the analyzer) for sampling linear to the airway

CLINICAL APPLICATIONS

Maintenance of Normocarbia

It is difficult to find scientific data that support the notion that anesthesia is inherently safer when $PaCO_2$ is kept in the normal range (between 35 and 45 mm Hg). An objective during virtually every routine administration of anesthesia, however, is to maintain the patient's vital signs and physiologic parameters as near as possible to preanesthetic values. This is certainly the goal for heart rate and blood pressure, and it makes intuitive sense to do this for carbon dioxide as well.

The physiologic consequences of hypercarbia and hypocarbia are well recognized. Increased $PaCO_2$ causes respiratory acidosis, increases cerebral blood flow and intracranial pressure in susceptible patients,[24] increases pulmonary vascular resistance, and causes potassium to shift from the intracellular fluid into the serum. Conversely, hypocarbia caused by excessive mechanical ventilation of the lungs causes respiratory alkalosis, decreases cerebral blood flow, decreases pulmonary vascular resistance, and causes potassium to shift from the serum to the intracellular fluid. For certain patients, each of these situations can have hazardous effects. The human body has the capacity to buffer 120 L of CO_2,[25] but during a prolonged anesthetic state in which the lungs are hyperventilated, this buffer becomes progressively depleted. Following emergence from anesthesia, metabolically produced CO_2 is sequestered in this buffer. Consequently, $PaCO_2$ increases at a slower rate than normal. In the same patients, the hypoxia-driven urge to breathe is blunted by residual anesthetics and also shifts the CO_2 ventilatory drive curve to the right. Thus the patient can hypoventilate, or even become apneic, with neither a strong oxygen or carbon dioxide stimulus to breathe. With capnometry and an estimation of the difference between $PaCO_2$ and $P_{ET}CO_2$, the parameters for mechanical ventilation can be adjusted to better maintain normocapnia and avoid the adverse sequelae of either hyperventilation or hypoventilation.

Cardiopulmonary Resuscitation

Capnography is emerging as an important monitor during cardiopulmonary resuscitation (CPR), during which $P_{ET}CO_2$ is low; this reflects the decreased pulmonary blood flow generated by chest compression when compared with that during normal cardiac contraction. Return of spontaneous circulation and increased pulmonary blood flow immediately and significantly increases $P_{ET}CO_2$,[26] which often makes this the earliest sign of successful resuscitation. In one study of 10 patients who had out-of-hospital cardiac arrests, the mean $P_{ET}CO_2$, which was 1.7% ± 0.6% (12.1 mm Hg ± 4.3 mm Hg) during chest compression, rose rapidly to 4.6% ± 1.4% (32.8 mm Hg ± 10 mm Hg) following the return of spontaneous circulation.[27] Noting the difficulty in palpating peripheral arterial pulses during CPR, some investigators use $P_{ET}CO_2$ to assess the hemodynamic responses to CPR noninvasively.[28] Unlike the electrocardiogram (ECG), invasive pressure manometer, and pulse palpation, the capnograph does not require interruption of chest compressions, nor is it vulnerable to the mechanical artifacts of chest compressions. Therefore $P_{ET}CO_2$ can be assessed without interrupting CPR.

Other studies have examined whether $P_{ET}CO_2$ can be used to differentiate cardiac arrest patients likely to be resuscitated from those unlikely to be resuscitated. In one study, Callahan and Barton[29] found that following tracheal intubation, an initial $P_{ET}CO_2$ greater than 15 mm Hg during CPR predicted the eventual return of pulsatile circulation with a sensitivity of 71% and a specificity of 98%. Similarly, Sanders and colleagues[30] demonstrated that a $P_{ET}CO_2$ greater than 10 mm Hg during CPR helped predict those patients who would eventually be resuscitated. The investigators in each study cautioned, however, that a few patients with low $P_{ET}CO_2$ were eventually resuscitated, so the clinician must incorporate all other available clinical data when deciding whether or not to continue CPR. If the patient's $P_{ET}CO_2$ is greater than 10 or 15 mm Hg during stable minute ventilation, this indicates that CPR is achieving some pulmonary blood flow. Because of a higher probability of the return of pulsatile circulation, CPR should be continued in these patients.

A persistently low or progressive decrease in $P_{ET}CO_2$ during CPR requires consideration of several, possibly concurrent diagnoses that include 1) esophageal intubation, 2) cardiac tamponade, 3) tension pneumothorax, 4) massive pulmonary embolus, 5) hypovolemia, 6) hyperventilation, and 7) ineffective CPR.

A low or absent $P_{ET}CO_2$ is not necessarily diagnostic of esophageal intubation; however, during CPR, this possibility must still be ruled out by clinical assessment. Hypovolemia, cardiac tamponade, pneumothorax, and pulmonary embolus can each create a V/Q ratio greater than 1 by interfering with cardiac filling and pulmonary blood flow, causing a low $P_{ET}CO_2$; ineffective CPR may have a similar effect and may be the result of poor technique (compression location, compression depth, or compression/relaxation) or resuscitator fatigue.[31] Alveolar hyperventilation is common during CPR when an enthusiastic resuscitator manually hyperventilates the lungs of a patient who already has a markedly decreased pulmonary blood flow. Keeping constant and normal minute ventilation is essential to derive maximum benefit from airway CO_2 monitoring during CPR.

Ventilatory Management

Intensivists have long sought a noninvasive method to guide the weaning of patients from mechanical ventilation. Can capnography be used in lieu of blood gas analysis? Two studies showed that, although changes in $P_{ET}CO_2$ parallel changes in $PaCO_2$, the large and often variable difference between $PaCO_2$ and $P_{ET}CO_2$ in patients in the intensive care unit (ICU) renders capnograph relatively insensitive to hypercarbia in this setting.[32,33] For example, in one case, a patient had a 10 mm Hg increase in $PaCO_2$ with no change in $P_{ET}CO_2$.[32] Thus, although capnography is useful for detecting many critical incidents in the ICU, at present, unless $PaCO_2 - P_{ET}CO_2$ is known and stable, periodic blood gas analysis remains the method preferred by most intensivists for weaning patients from mechanical ventilation.

The insensitivity to hypercarbia in many ICU patients is also a shortcoming of capnography in the operating room (OR). Therefore, regardless of the setting, if it is important to know a patient's precise $PaCO_2$, blood gas analysis is still needed. Once the relationship between $PaCO_2$ and $P_{ET}CO_2$ for a patient has been quantified, the value serves as a useful guide for future clinical management. Any time a significant change is seen in blood pressure, tidal volume, continuous positive airway pressure, or any other parameter that can alter a patient's V/Q, its effect on $PaCO_2$ and $P_{ET}CO_2$ must be considered. Some investigators have used changes in $PaCO_2/P_{ET}CO_2$ to define recovery from pulmonary disease and to guide therapy.[34] Even in patients with a large $PaCO_2 - P_{ET}CO_2$ gradient, if maximal exhalation is actively or passively performed, or if the peak $P_{ET}CO_2$ encountered over several minutes is used, the $PaCO_2/P_{ET}CO_2$ gradient becomes very small.[35] A patient's metabolic rate may be evaluated with $P_{ET}CO_2$ once it is correlated with the arterial value, and appropriate ventilator settings can be applied for CO_2 elimination.[36] This can further help guide decisions on the likelihood of successful extubation in light of high metabolic rates, such as occurs with sepsis.

Capnography is also increasingly used in the ICU, or during transport to and from the ICU, for the same purpose as in the OR: to alert the clinician to life-threatening problems such as disconnection,[37] failure of the mechanical ventilator, and severe hypercapnia or hypocapnia. In patients dependent on stable ventilation, such as those with elevated intracranial pressure, the capnograph is an indispensable real-time monitor that is especially relevant during transport.[24]

An additional application of capnography is to maximize the benefits of positive end-expiratory pressure (PEEP) in acute respiratory distress syndrome (ARDS). By minimizing the arterial to end-tidal CO_2 gradient, excessive development of "West zone 1" in the lung will be limited.[38] This titration of PEEP can assist in 1) restoring lung volume, 2) decreasing pulmonary vascular resistance, 3) decreasing dead space (Vd/Vt), and 4) improving V/Q matching. Recognizing the ventilation of alveolar dead space led Hubble and colleagues[39] to devise predictions of successful extubation. One predictor of successful extubation is a difference between dead space and tidal volume (Vd/Vt) of 0.5 or less, and a Vd/Vt of 0.65 or greater was associated with a need for additional respiratory support. Nuckton and colleagues[40] found that patients with a Vd/Vt of 63% or greater were at a significant risk of death; therefore this (arterial–end-tidal) CO_2 parameter is of particular clinical interest for patient management.

Pulmonary Embolism

Capnography has been used to aid in the diagnosis of embolisms of all types. A pulmonary embolism represents an increase in pulmonary dead space that results from a sudden decrease in pulmonary perfusion without ventilatory change. These nonperfused alveoli (Vd/Vt) mix with the exhaled gas from perfused alveoli and result in a decreased $P_{ET}CO_2$ relative to the $PaCO_2$. The magnitude of the decrease in $P_{ET}CO_2$ resulting from an embolism has been shown to correlate with the severity of the size of the perfusion deficit and pulmonary artery pressure.[41]

A definitive diagnosis of pulmonary embolism by capnometry often is limited by the lack of a known baseline alveolar dead space for each patient and other pathologic mechanisms that decrease pulmonary perfusion and increase dead space. A common clinical situation that mimics alveolar dead space development is pulmonary arterial hypotension stemming from hemorrhagic, septic, or cardiogenic shock. Pulmonary artery hypotension is also exacerbated by positive-pressure ventilation, which further confounds the issue.

Untoward Events

Clinicians use capnography intraoperatively to detect untoward events that might injure the anesthetized patient if undetected and uncorrected. A number of studies support the premise that capnography can detect many of the problems most likely to injure an anesthetized patient and help guide clinical management. For example, when the technique of critical incident analysis was adapted to study human error and equipment failure in anesthesia, disconnection of the breathing circuit during mechanical ventilation was the most frequently identified critical incident.[42] Capnography readily detects disconnection within the breathing system. Of the 25 most frequent critical incidents identified in this study, more than 40% could have been identified with data from the capnometer.

Another study that strongly supports the intraoperative use of capnography is the ASA's closed claim study.[43] In this study, experts reviewed closed malpractice claims against anesthesiologists. After reviewing 1541 cases, they identified "respiratory events" as the single largest class of problems that resulted in litigation. More than one third (34%) of the adverse outcomes were associated with respiratory events. Of these, 35% were attributed to inadequate ventilation of the patient's lungs, 18% to esophageal intubation, and 17% to difficult tracheal intubation. Both inadequate ventilation of the patient's lungs and esophageal intubation are readily detected with capnography.

Noninvasive Capnography for Sedation

Providing sedation for patients undergoing minor procedures is an increasingly common clinical practice. Of particular concern for the provider is maintaining appropriate oxygenation for these spontaneously breathing patients. Vargo and colleagues[44] studied outpatient endoscopy patients and found that unrecognized apnea is a constant risk that is detectable via pulse oximetry, auscultation, or clinical observation less than half the time. Closed claim analysis of dental procedures performed in 1991 showed that an "avoidable" ventilatory depression or airway obstruction that led to hypoxia was primarily responsible for the majority of catastrophic complications.[45] In fact, ventilatory depression is such a frequent occurrence during monitored sedation that in many procedures, it represents a greater danger than the procedure itself.[46]

Detecting respiratory obstruction and insufficiency is a key element in the utility of capnography for spontaneously breathing patients undergoing sedation. If patients are breathing supplemental oxygen, pulse oximetry may lag behind ventilatory deficiency long enough to allow drastically elevated $PaCO_2$ levels to occur.[47,48] Noninvasive capnography can provide an early warning signal to detect respiratory obstruction or insufficiency, which affords the provider the time to implement interventions to avert ensuing hypoxia. The American Society of Gastrointestinal Endoscopy published guidelines for the use of deep sedation and anesthesia for gastrointestinal endoscopy, acknowledging that "capnography more readily identifies patients with apneic episodes and, when used to guide sedation, results in less CO_2 retention."[44]

The provider should consider the cardiovascular status and pulmonary disease of the patient when interpreting the $P_{ET}CO_2$ during noninvasive monitoring. The alveolar/end-tidal CO_2 gradient is easily altered by conditions of hypoventilation, mouth breathing, poor respiratory effort, and coadministration of high-flow oxygen; thus attention to the details of acquiring a good expiratory gas specimen are particularly important in this setting. Regardless, the trend of end-tidal carbon dioxide and the respiratory rate as reported by the capnometer both alert the provider to respiratory obstruction or insufficiency. Subsequently, the utility of capnography has been extended to monitor patients with acute bronchoconstriction,[49] obstructive sleep apnea,[50] neuromuscular disease,[51] and diabetic ketoacidosis[52] as well as those receiving emergency medical technician and ambulance services and emergency department procedures.[53,54]

The success of capnography to detect inadequate ventilation and thwart hypoxia has led the ASA to mandate the monitoring of ventilation with capnometry during procedural sedation: "During moderate or deep sedation the adequacy of ventilation shall be evaluated by continual observation of qualitative clinical signs and monitoring for the presence of exhaled carbon dioxide unless precluded or invalidated by the nature of the patient, procedure, or equipment."[55]

COMMON PITFALLS

The clinician using the capnograph must avoid three common pitfalls. First, capnography is not a substitute for maintaining sharp clinical skills (inspection, palpation, and auscultation). The capnometer is a very reliable electrical, optical, and mechanical instrument, but it will still occasionally fail; therefore data from the capnography and clinical assessment should be combined to serve as a check-and-balance system so that even in the event of instrument failure, competent monitoring will continue. Second, clinicians using a capnograph must do more than assess the end-tidal CO_2 value reported; they must also interpret the capnogram. Third, and most important, the effective use of capnography depends on understanding the relationship between $PaCO_2$ and $P_{ET}CO_2$. Table 10-3 summarizes common problems that can be diagnosed completely or in part with the capnograph.

TABLE 10-3 **Untoward Situations Detected with Capnography**

Little or no exhaled CO_2	Esophageal intubation Tracheal extubation Disconnection of capnograph or gas source Complete obstruction (by equipment or pulmonary disease) Apnea
Elevated inspiratory baseline (phase I)	Open CO_2 bypass Partially exhausted CO_2 absorbent Channeling through CO_2 absorbent Incompetent expiratory valve
Prolonged expiratory upstroke (phase II)	Obstruction (by equipment or pulmonary disease) Slow gas sampling or slow instrument response
Upsloping alveolar plateau (phase III)	Obstruction (by equipment or pulmonary disease)
Prolonged inspiratory downstroke (phase 0)	Incompetent inspiratory valve Slow gas sampling or slow instrument response
Hypercapnia	Hypoventilation (leak, obstruction of airflow, inadequate ventilation) CO_2 rebreathing Increased CO_2 production or delivery (malignant hyperthermia, fever, CO_2 insufflation, bicarbonate administration, release of tourniquet or cross-clamp)
Hypocapnia	Hyperventilation Decreased CO_2 production or delivery (hypothermia, decreased cardiac output) Increased gradient of arterial to maximum expired CO_2 (V/Q mismatching, endobronchial intubation, pulmonary embolism [air, fat, thrombus, amniotic fluid], shallow or rapid breathing, instrument or sampling problems, miscalibration)

V/Q, ventilation/perfusion.

From Good ML: Capnography: uses, interpretation, and pitfalls. In Barash PG, Deutsch S, Tinker J, editors: *ASA refresher courses in anesthesiology*, vol 18, Philadelphia, 1991, JB Lippincott.

REFERENCES

1. American Society of Anesthesiologists. Standards for Basic Anesthetic Monitoring. Approved by the House of Delegates 21 October 1986 and last amended on 15 October 2003.
2. American Society of Anesthesiologists. Standards for Basic Anesthetic Monitoring. Approved by the House of Delegates 21 October 1986 and last amended on October 20, 2010.
3. Romero PV, Lucangelo U, Lopez Aguilar J, Fernandez R, Blanch L: Physiologically based indices of volumetric capnography in patients receiving mechanical ventilation, *Eur Respir J* 10:232–233, 2000.
4. Schmmitz BD, Shapiro B: Capnography, *Resp Care Clin North Am* 1:107–117, 1995.
5. Hoffbrand BI: The expiratory capnogram: a measure of ventilation-perfusion inequalities, *Thorax* 21:518–523, 1966.
6. Bhavani-Shanker K, Kumar AY, Moseley H, Hallsworth RA: Terminology and the current limitations of time capnography: a brief review, *J Clin Monit* 11:175–182, 1995.
7. Goldberg JS, Rawle RP, Zehnder JL, et al: Colorimetric end-tidal carbon dioxide monitoring for tracheal intubation, *Anesth Analg* 70:191–194, 1990.
8. Puntervoll SA, Soreide E, Jacewicz W, Bjelland E: Rapid detection of esophageal intubation: take care when using colorimetric capnometry, *Acta Anaesthesiol Scand* 46:455–457, 2003.
9. Bhavani-Shanker K, Philip JH: Defining segments and phases of a time capnogram, *Anesth Analg* 91:973–977, 2000.
10. Good ML, Modell JH, Rush W: Differentiating esophageal from tracheal capnograms, *Anesthesiology* 69:A266, 1988, (abstract).
11. van Ganderingen HR, Gravenstein N, van der Aa JJ, Gravenstein JS: Computer-assisted capnogram analysis, *J Clin Monit* 3:194–200, 1988.
12. Berman LS, Pyles ST: Capnographic detection of anesthesia circle valve malfunctions, *Can J Anaesth* 35:473–475, 1988.
13. Pascucci RC, Schena JA, Thompson JE: Comparison of sidestream and mainstream capnometers in infants, *Crit Care Med* 17:560–562, 1989.
14. Kumar AY, Bhavani-Shanker K, Moseley HSL, Delph Y: Inspiratory valve malfunction in a circle system: pitfalls in capnography, *Can J Anaesth* 39:997–999, 1992.
15. Gravenstein JS: *Gas monitoring and pulse oximetry*, Boston, 1990, Butterworths.
16. Gravenstein N: Capnometry in infants should not be done in lower sampling rates [letter], *J Clin Monit* 5:63, 1989.
17. Hess D: Capnometry and capnography: technical aspects, physiologic aspects, and clinical applications, *Resp Care* 35:557–576, 1990.
18. Fletcher R, Jonson B, Cumming G, Brew J: The concept of deadspace with special reference to the single breath test for carbon dioxide, *Br J Anaesth* 53:77–88, 1981.
19. Hatle L, Rokesth R: The arterial to end-expiratory carbon dioxide tension gradient in acute pulmonary embolism and other cardiopulmonary disease, *Chest* 66:352–357, 1974.
20. Warwick WJ: The end-expiratory to arterial carbon dioxide tension ratio in acute pulmonary embolism, *Chest* 68:609–611, 1975.
21. Badgewell JM, Heavner JE, May WS: End-tidal PCO2 monitoring in infants and children ventilated with either a partial rebreathing or a non-rebreathing circuit, *Anesthesiology* 66:959–964, 1987.
22. Severinghaus JW: Water vapor calibration errors in some capnometers: respiratory conventions misunderstood by manufacturers, *Anesthesiology* 70:996–998, 1989.
23. Brunner JX, Westenskow DR: How carbon dioxide analyzer rise time affects the accuracy of carbon dioxide measurements, *J Clin Monit* 4:134, 1988.
24. Kerr ME, Zempsky J, Serika S, Orndoff P, Rudy E: Relationship between arterial carbon dioxide and end-tidal carbon dioxide in mechanically ventilated adults with severe head trauma, *Crit Care Med* 24:785–796, 1996.
25. Nunn JF: *Applied respiratory physiology*, ed 3, London, 1987, Butterworths, p 226.
26. Falk JL, Rackow EC, Weil MH: End-tidal carbon dioxide concentration during cardiopulmonary resuscitation, *N Engl J Med* 318:607–711, 1988.
27. Garnett AR, Ornato JP, Gonzalez ER, et al: End-tidal carbon dioxide monitoring during cardiopulmonary resuscitation, *JAMA* 257:512–515.
28. Weil MH, Gazmuri RJ, Kette F, et al: End-tidal PCO_2 during cardiopulmonary resuscitation, *JAMA* 263:814–815, 1990.
29. Callaham M, Barton C: Prediction of outcome from cardiopulmonary resuscitation from end-tidal carbon dioxide concentration, *Crit Care Med* 18:358–362, 1990.
30. Sanders AB, Kern KB, Otto CW: Prediction from outcome of cardiopulmonary resuscitation: a prognostic indicator for survival, *JAMA* 262:1347–1351, 1989.
31. Kalenda Z: The capnogram as a guide to the efficacy of cardiac massage, *Resuscitation* 6:259–263.
32. Healey CH, Fedullo AJ, Swinburne AJ, et al: Comparison of noninvasive measurement of carbon dioxide during withdrawal from mechanical ventilation, *Crit Care Med* 15:764–768, 1987.

33. Niehoff J, del Guercio C, LaMorte W, et al: Efficacy of pulse oximetry and capnography and capnometry in positive ventilatory weaning, *Crit Care Med* 16:701–705, 1988.
34. Chopin C, Fesard P, Mangaloaboyi J, et al: Use of capnography in diagnosis of pulmonary embolism during acute respiratory failure of chronic obstructive respiratory disease, *Crit Care Med* 18:353–357, 1990.
35. Weigner MB, Brimm JE: End-tidal carbon dioxide as a measure of arterial carbon dioxide during intermittent mandatory ventilation, *J Clin Monit* 3:73–79, 1987.
36. Tasker V, John J, Larsson A, Wetterberg T, Johnson B: Dynamics of carbon dioxide elimination following ventilator resetting, *Chest* 8:196–202, 1995.
37. Palmon S, Maywin L, Moore L, Kirsch J: Capnography facilitates tight control of ventilation during transport, *Crit Care Med* 24:608–611, 1996.
38. Rose JT, Banner MJ: Effects of positive end-expiratory pressure (PEEP) on physiologic deadspace volume to tidal volume ratio (Vd/Vt) [abstract], *Crit Care Med* 28:A86, 2000.
39. Hubble CL, Gentile MA, Tripp DS, et al: Dead space to tidal volume ratio predicts successful extubation in infants and children, *Crit Care Med* 38:2034–2040, 2000.
40. Nuckton TJ, Alonso JA, Kallet RH, et al: Pulmonary dead-space fraction as a risk factor for death in the acute respiratory distress syndrome, *N Engl J Med* 346:1281–1286, 2002.
41. Kline JA, Kubin AK, Patel MM, Easton EJ, Seupal RA: Alveolar dead space as a predictor of severity of pulmonary embolism, *Acad Emerg Med* 7:611–617, 2000.
42. Cooper JB, Newbower RS, Kitz RJ: An analysis of major errors and equipment failures in anesthesia management: considerations for prevention and detection, *Anesthesiology* 60:34–42, 1984.
43. Caplan RA, Posner K, Ward RJ, et al: Adverse respiratory advents in anesthesia: a closed claims analysis, *Anesthesiology* 72:828–833, 1990.
44. Vargo J, Waring P, Faigel D, et al: Guidelines for the use of deep sedation and anesthesia for GI endoscopy, *Gastrointest Endosc* 56:613–617, 2002.
45. Jastek JT, Peskin RM: Major morbidity or mortality from office anesthetic procedures: a closed-claim analysis of 13 cases, *Anesth Prog* 38:39–44, 1991.
46. Galandiuk S, Ahmad P: Impact of sedation and resident teaching on complications of colonoscopy, *Dig Surg* 15:60–63, 1998.
47. Croswell RJR, Dilley DC, Lucas WJ, Vann WF: A comparison of conventional versus electronic monitoring of sedated pediatric dental patients, *Pediatric Dent* 17:332–339, 1995.
48. Hart LS, Berns SD, Houck CS, Boenning DA: The value of end-tidal CO2 monitoring when comparing three methods of conscious sedation for children undergoing painful procedures in the emergency department, *Pediatr Emerg Care* 13:189–193, 1997.
49. Toubas PL, Duke JC, Seakr KC, McCaffree MA: Microphonic versus end-tidal carbon dioxide nasal airflow detection in neonates with apnea, *Paediatrics* 6:950–954, 1990.
50. Magnan A, Philip-Joet F, Rey M, et al: End-tidal CO2 analysis in sleep apnea syndrome: conditions for use, *Chest* 102:129–131, 1993.
51. Kotterba S, Patzold T, Malin JB, Orth M, Rasche K: Respiratory monitoring in neuromuscular disease, *Clin Neurol Neurosurg* 103:87–91, 2001.
52. Garcia E, Abramo TJ, Okada P, et al: Capnometry for noninvasive continuous monitoring of metabolic status in pediatric diabetic ketoacidosis, *Crit Care Med* 31:2539–2543, 2003.
53. Miner JR, Heegaard W, Plummer D: End-tidal carbon dioxide monitoring during procedural sedation, *Acad Emerg Med* 9:275–280, 2002.
54. McQuillen KK, Steele DW: Capnography during sedation/analgesia in the pediatric emergency department, *Pediatr Emerg Care* 16:401–404, 2000.
55. Practice Guidelines for Sedation and Analgesia by Non-Anesthesiologists. Approved by the House of Delegates on October 25, 1995 and last amended October 17, 2001.

CHAPTER 11

PULSE OXIMETRY

Steven J. Barker*

CHAPTER OUTLINE

OVERVIEW

No monitor of oxygenation has had as much impact on the practice of anesthesiology as the pulse oximeter. Unknown in the operating room (OR) before the 1980s, the pulse oximeter is now a minimum standard of care for all patients who receive anesthetics, whether general, regional, or local. Its operation requires no special skill or training, and its use is noninvasive and therefore almost risk free. The pulse oximeter gives continuous, real-time estimates of arterial hemoglobin saturation, which can warn of hypoxemia from many causes, including loss of airway patency, loss of oxygen supply, and increases in venous admixture. As illustrated in Figure 11-1, pulse oximetry provides a monitor of the second of four stages of the oxygen transport process. This important advance goes beyond the first stage of inspired gas monitoring, but it does not ensure the third stage of adequate oxygen delivery to vital organs.

This chapter reviews the historic development of pulse oximetry, its underlying physical and engineering principles, and recent improvements such as artifact reduction and multiwavelength processing. An understanding of these principles will enable the reader to predict sources of measurement error. Pulse oximeter accuracy, response, clinical applications, limitations, and future potential are also discussed.

*Dr. Barker is a member of the Scientific Advisory Board of Masimo Corporation (Irvine, CA) and a community member of their Board of Directors. He is not an employee or a paid consultant of Masimo or any other company involved in pulse oximetry.

HEMOGLOBIN SATURATION AND OXYGEN TRANSPORT

The pulse oximeter provides a noninvasive estimate of arterial hemoglobin saturation, a variable directly proportional to the oxygen content of arterial blood. Two definitions of hemoglobin saturation are in current use. The older definition, called *functional saturation*, or SaO_2, is related to the concentrations of oxyhemoglobin (O_2Hb) and deoxygenated, or "reduced," hemoglobin (RHb) as follows:

$$SaO_2 = [(O_2Hb)/(O_2Hb + RHb)] \times 100\% \qquad (11\text{-}1)$$

Additional species of hemoglobin are often present in adult blood, including carboxyhemoglobin (COHb) and methemoglobin (MetHb). This leads to the definition of *fractional hemoglobin saturation*, or $O_2Hb\%$, which is the ratio of oxyhemoglobin to the total concentration of *all* hemoglobin species:

$$O_2Hb\,\% = [O_2Hb/(O_2Hb + RHb + COHb + MetHb)] \times 100\,\% = (O_2Hb/Hb) \times 100\,\% \qquad (11\text{-}2)$$

In this formula, *Hb* is the total hemoglobin, the sum of all species present. Fractional saturation is sometimes called *oxyhemoglobin fraction* or *oxyhemoglobin percent*.[1] Fractional arterial hemoglobin saturation is related to

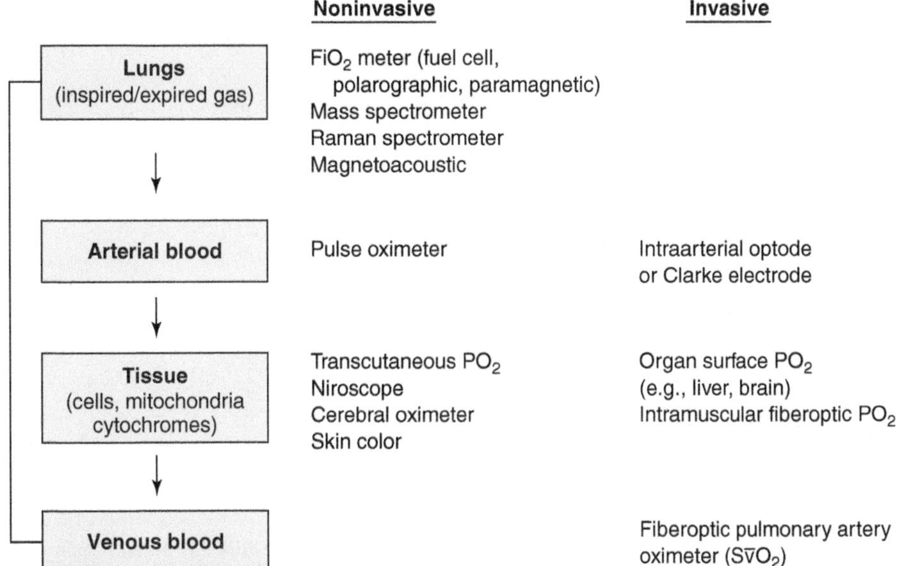

FIGURE 11-1 The four stages of the oxygen transport system, showing that the pulse oximeter monitors oxygen at the level of the arterial blood. Respired gas monitors can confirm only that oxygen is being delivered to the lungs, but the pulse oximeter also monitors the function of the lungs in transporting this oxygen to the arterial blood. Pulse oximetry does not guarantee that oxygen is being delivered to or used by the tissues; this can be determined only by monitors that function further down the oxygen transport chain. *FiO_2*, fractional concentration of inspired oxygen; *PO_2*, oxygen tension; *$S\bar{v}O_2$*, mixed venous oxygen saturation.

the arterial oxygen content, CaO_2, by the following formula:

$$CaO_2 = (1.37 \times Hb\ [O_2Hb\%/100]) + (0.003 \times PaO_2) \quad (11\text{-}3)$$

Here PaO_2 is the arterial oxygen tension in millimeters of mercury. The first expression in brackets in Equation 11-3 represents the oxygen bound to hemoglobin, which under normal conditions (Hb = 15 g/dL and $O_2Hb\%$ = 98) equals approximately 20 mL oxygen per 100 mL blood. The second expression represents oxygen dissolved in plasma, which equals 0.3 mL per 100 mL for a PaO_2 of 100 mm Hg. Plasma-dissolved oxygen usually does not play a significant role in oxygen transport. Equation 11-3 shows that arterial oxygen content is directly proportional to both total hemoglobin (Hb) and fractional saturation. $O_2Hb\%$ and PaO_2 are related by the oxyhemoglobin dissociation curve, shown in Figure 11-2. Under normal conditions, this relationship predicts a hemoglobin saturation for adults of 50% at a PaO_2 of 27 mm Hg, 75% at a PaO_2 of 40 mm Hg (the typical venous blood value), and 90% at a PaO_2 of 60 mm Hg. This normal dissociation curve is shifted to the right by acidosis, hypercarbia, hyperthermia, and increases in 2,3-diphosphoglycerate (2,3-DPG) concentration. Note that for PaO_2 values greater than 90 mm Hg, $O_2Hb\%$ is nearly independent of PaO_2. This saturation property of hemoglobin has important implications in the clinical interpretation of pulse oximeter data, discussed below.

The amount of oxygen delivered to the tissues by the arterial blood (O_{2del}) is simply the product of the arterial oxygen content (CaO_2) and the cardiac output, or

$$O_{2del} = CaO_2 \times \text{Cardiac output} \times 10 \quad (11\text{-}4)$$

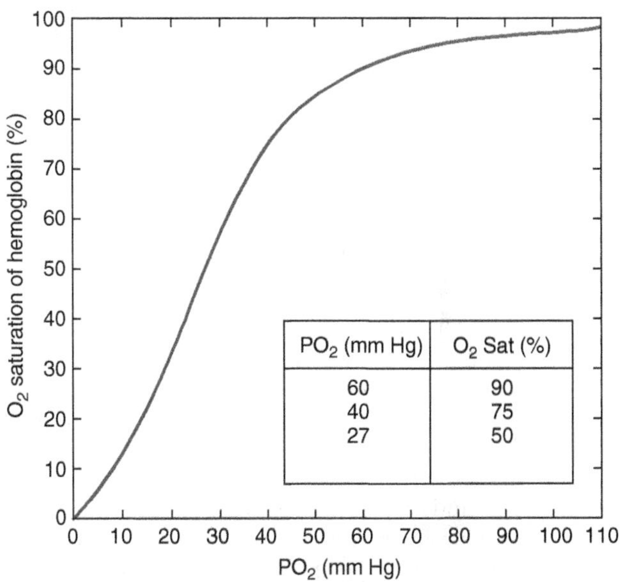

FIGURE 11-2 The oxyhemoglobin dissociation curve. Hemoglobin saturation is plotted as a function of arterial oxygen tension (*PaO_2*) in millimeters of mercury. Under normal conditions for adults, a PaO_2 of 27 mm Hg yields a saturation of 50% (P_{50}). The curve is shifted to the right by acidosis, hypercarbia, increases in 2,3-diphosphoglycerate (2,3-DPG), and hyperthermia.

The factor of 10 appears because CaO_2 is measured in milliliters per deciliter, whereas cardiac output is measured in liters per minute. The quantity of oxygen consumed per minute is then the difference between the arterial oxygen delivery (O_{2del}) and the venous oxygen return (O_{2ret}):

$$VO_2 = O_{2del} - O_{2ret} = (CaO_2 - CvO_2) \times \text{Cardiac output} \times 10 \quad (11\text{-}5)$$

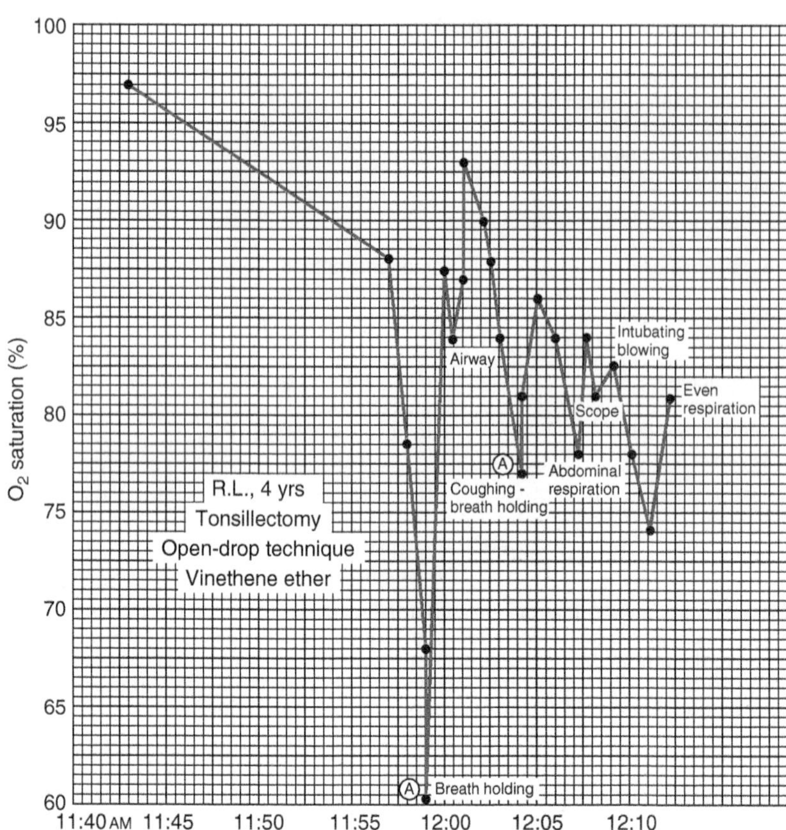

FIGURE 11-3 ▪ Ear oximeter hemoglobin saturation plotted as a function of time. Graph for a 4-year-old child undergoing general anesthesia for tonsillectomy under open-drop ether with no supplemental oxygen. Note the significant desaturation associated with breath holding during induction of anesthesia. Saturation does not return to its preinduction baseline value at any time during the record. (From Steven RC, Slater HM, Johnson AL, et al: The oximeter: a technical aid for the anesthesiologist. *Anesthesiology* 1951;12:548.)

Arterial oxygen content and mixed venous oxygen content (CvO_2) in this form of the *Fick equation* can be replaced by corresponding expressions in terms of hemoglobin saturation from Equation 11-3:

$$VO_2 = 13.7 \times \text{Cardiac output} \times (O_2Hb\,\%_a - O_2Hb\,\%_v)/100 \qquad (11\text{-}6)$$

Subscripts *a* and *v* denote arterial and mixed venous fractional hemoglobin saturations, respectively. The small contributions of plasma-dissolved oxygen have been neglected in this form of the Fick equation. Equation 11-6 describes the relationship between oxygen consumption, arterial and mixed venous hemoglobin saturations, total hemoglobin, and cardiac output. An understanding of this equation is vital to the interpretation of data from pulse oximeters and other oxygen monitors and to understanding their relationship to other hemodynamic variables.

HISTORY OF PULSE OXIMETRY

Although the pulse oximeter became a monitoring standard in the OR in the 1980s, in vivo oximeters date to the 1930s. In 1935, Carl Matthes developed the first instrument that measured hemoglobin oxygen saturation by transilluminating tissue. Matthes's device used two wavelengths of light, one visible and one infrared (IR), much like the modern pulse oximeter. This instrument could follow saturation trends but was difficult to calibrate. J.R. Squires developed a similar instrument that calibrated itself by compressing the ear to eliminate blood, a technique used later in the first commercially marketed in vivo oximeters.

Glenn Millikan created the first lightweight ear oximeter in the early 1940s for aviation research. Millikan coined the term *oximeter* to describe his device, which measured hemoglobin saturation in pilots flying at high altitudes. Similar devices developed in the 1940s were used by Wood and others in the OR. The first perioperative application of an in vivo oximeter to appear in the anesthesiology literature was published in 1951.[2] Figure 11-3 shows a record of the hemoglobin saturation obtained from an ear oximeter plotted against time during a tonsillectomy. Even though this record shows a dramatic fall in saturation during the induction of anesthesia, curiously described as "breath holding" in the original figure, the device drew little attention from anesthesiologists until much later.

The lack of acceptance of early in vivo oximeters was mostly due to their serious limitations. They were delicate instruments that required technician support for calibration and operation. In addition, the earpiece sensor was large and cumbersome, and it produced enough heat to cause occasional burns. Hewlett-Packard (HP) made a major advance in ear oximetry in the 1970s, when it marketed a self-calibrating, eight-wavelength ear oximeter. The HP oximeter was reasonably accurate for intraoperative monitoring, but it was still burdened by the size and bulky nature of the sensor as well as the expense of the instrument.[3] Although the HP oximeter became a standard tool in pulmonary function laboratories, it had virtually no impact in the OR.

The first true pulse oximeter was invented by Takuo Aoyagi in 1975.[4] While investigating a method to measure intravenous dye washout curves using light transmission through the ear, Aoyagi discovered that his data on light

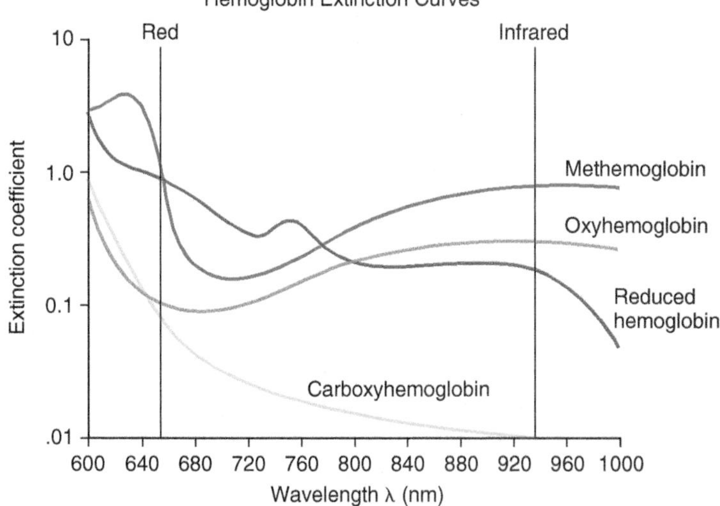

FIGURE 11-4 Extinction coefficient (ε) plotted versus light wavelength in nanometers for the four most common hemoglobin species: oxyhemoglobin (O_2Hb), reduced hemoglobin (RHb), carboxyhemoglobin (COHb), and methemoglobin (MetHb). The absorbance of COHb is very similar to that of O_2Hb in the visible red wavelengths. MetHb has a high absorbance over a broad spectrum, giving it a characteristic brown color. (Modified from Tremper KK, Barker SJ: Pulse oximetry: applications and limitations. In *Advances in oxygen monitoring: International Anesthesiology Clinics*. Boston, 1987, Little, Brown, pp 155-175.)

absorbance versus time contained fluctuations caused by the arterial pulse. In dealing with this "artifact," he discovered that the relative amplitudes of the fluctuations at the two light wavelengths varied with arterial hemoglobin saturation. This fortuitous discovery led him to the creation of the first two-wavelength pulse oximeter, which was developed and marketed by Nihon Kohden Corporation. However, Aoyagi's oximeter used filtered light sources and fiberoptic transmission cables between the instrument and the earlobe sensor, rendering it somewhat awkward for use in the OR.

The next breakthrough in technology came in the late 1970s, when Scott Wilbur of the Biox Corporation (later Ohmeda) developed the first ear sensor that used light-emitting diodes (LEDs) and solid-state photodetectors built into the sensor itself. The fiberoptic cables of Aoyagi's pulse oximeters were thereby replaced by a thin electrical cable.[5] The accuracy of the pulse oximeter was also improved by the incorporation of digital microprocessors into the instrument. Further electronic improvements were made by Biox and Nellcor in the early 1980s, and the pulse oximeter was ready to take its place as a standard perioperative monitor.

The success of Nellcor in marketing its N-100 pulse oximeter to anesthesiologists in the mid-1980s brought these devices into the OR in large numbers. The instrument had now become fairly reliable and easy to use as well as relatively inexpensive. It gained rapid acceptance and became a standard of care in the OR by 1986. Today, no anesthesiologist would feel comfortable inducing general anesthesia without a functioning pulse oximeter. An excellent review of the history of pulse oximetry and the development of blood gas analysis has been written by Severinghaus and Astrup.[4]

PHYSICS AND ENGINEERING OF PULSE OXIMETRY

Spectrophotometry

Spectrophotometry uses the measurement of light absorbance to determine the concentrations of various solutes in clear solutions. Carl Matthes used this technique to determine hemoglobin oxygen saturation as early as the 1930s.[4] The measurement is based on the Lambert-Beer law, which relates solute concentrations to the intensity of light transmitted through a solution:

$$I_{trans} = I_{in} e^{(-dC\varepsilon)} \quad (11\text{-}7)$$

I_{trans} represents the intensity of light transmitted through solution, I_{in} is the intensity of incident light, d is the distance light is transmitted through the solution (optical path length), C is the concentration of the solute, and ε is the extinction coefficient of the solute.

The extinction coefficient ε determines the tendency of a given solute to absorb light at a specific wavelength or color. Equation 11-7 shows it as the natural logarithm of the ratio I_{in}/I_{trans} for a solution whose concentration C and thickness d are both unity. The extinction coefficient is a known constant for a given solute at a specified wavelength. If a solute of known extinction coefficient (ε) is in solution in a cuvette, a transparent measurement chamber of known dimensions, the solute concentration can then be calculated using Equation 11-7 and the measured intensities of incident and transmitted light. If multiple solutes are present, the exponent in Equation 11-7 is simply the sum of similar expressions for each solute; for example, if there are two solutes, it is $dC_1\varepsilon_1 + dC_2\varepsilon_2$. The extinction coefficients of the four most common hemoglobin species in the red to IR wavelength range are shown in Figure 11-4.

Laboratory in vitro blood oximeters, usually called *CO-oximeters*, use spectrophotometry to determine the concentrations of several common hemoglobin species by measuring light transmitted through a cuvette filled with a hemoglobin suspension produced from lysed red blood cells.[1] The analysis above assumes 1) that both the solvent and the cuvette are transparent at the wavelengths used, 2) the light path length is exactly known, and 3) no unknown light-absorbing substances are present in the solution. It is difficult to meet these requirements precisely in clinical devices; hence CO-oximeters theoretically based on the Lambert-Beer law require empirical corrections to improve accuracy.

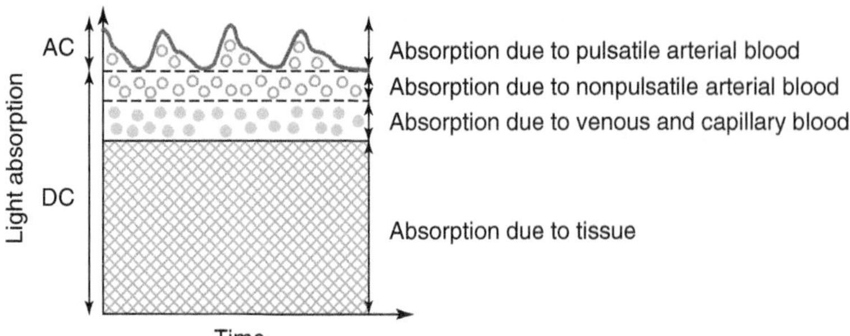

FIGURE 11-5 Schematic of the light absorbances of living tissue plotted versus time. The fixed direct current (*DC*) absorbance results from solid tissues, venous and capillary blood, and nonpulsatile arterial blood. The alternating current (*AC*) component is caused by pulsations in the arterial blood volume. (Modified from *Ohmeda Pulse Oximeter Model 3700 service manual.* Boulder, CO, 1986, Ohmeda, p 22.)

Engineering Principles

Conventional pulse oximeters estimate arterial hemoglobin saturation by measuring the transmission of light at two wavelengths through a pulsatile vascular tissue bed. The pulse oximeter effectively uses the finger, ear, or other tissue as a "cuvette" containing hemoglobin. However, living tissue contains a number of light absorbers other than arterial hemoglobin; these include skin, soft tissue, bone, and venous and capillary blood. Early in vivo oximeters, such as Millikan's, compensated for these additional tissue absorbances by compressing the soft tissues to eliminate all blood during a calibration cycle. The absorbance of the bloodless tissue was then used as a baseline. Some of these oximeters heated the tissue during measurement to render it hyperemic and thus obtain an absorbance more dependent on arterial blood.

The pulse oximeter distinguishes arterial blood from other light absorbers in the tissue in a novel way. As shown in Figure 11-5, light absorbance in tissue can be divided into a constant or *direct current* (DC) component and a pulsating or *alternating current* (AC) component. The AC component of absorbance is almost exclusively the result of arterial blood pulsations; this was Aoyagi's original hypothesis. These pulsations are caused by the systolic volume expansion of the arteriolar bed, which produces an increase in optical path length and thereby increases the absorbance (Equation 11-7). Conventional pulse oximetry thus assumes that arterial blood is the only pulsatile absorber; any other fluctuating light absorbers will constitute sources of error. The consequences of and recent modifications to this assumption are discussed below (see Motion Artifact and Adaptive Digital Signal Filtering).

Most pulse oximeters use the same two wavelengths of light: 660 nm (red) and 940 nm (near IR). The pulse oximeter measures the AC component of the light absorbance at each wavelength and then divides it by the corresponding DC component (see Fig. 11-5), yielding the pulse-added absorbances $S_{660} = AC_{660}/DC_{660}$ and $S_{940} = AC_{940}/DC_{940}$. The pulse-added absorbances at the two wavelengths are independent of the intensity of the incident light. The oximeter then calculates the ratio (R) of the two pulse-added absorbances:

$$R = [AC_{660}/DC_{660}]/[AC_{940}/DC_{940}] \qquad (11\text{-}8)$$

The Lambert-Beer law implies that in the absence of dyshemoglobins (e.g., COHb, MetHb), the ratio R is uniquely related to the arterial hemoglobin saturation.

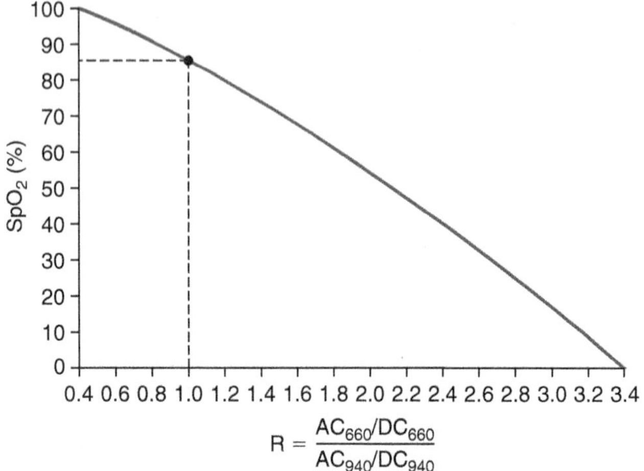

FIGURE 11-6 A typical pulse oximeter calibration algorithm, in which estimated oxygenation (*SpO_2*) is plotted against the ratio *R* from Equation 11-8. The value of R varies from roughly 0.4 at 100% saturation to 3.4 at 0% saturation. Note that an R value of 1.0 corresponds to an SpO_2 reading of 85%. This calibration curve is a best fit of experimental data obtained on healthy volunteers. *AC,* alternating current; *DC,* direct current. (Modified from Pologe JA: Pulse oximetry: technical aspects of machine design. In Tremper KK, Barker SJ, editors: *Advances in oxygen monitoring: International Anesthesiology Clinics.* Boston, 1987, Little, Brown, p 142.)

Although the pulse oximeter saturation estimate SpO_2 can be mathematically derived from the value of R via the Lambert-Beer law, the pulse oximeter uses an empirical calibration curve to relate SpO_2 to this ratio. A typical calibration is shown in Figure 11-6. This curve, as for all other pulse oximeter calibrations, is based on experimental data from human volunteers. The calibration data are stored in the oximeter's microprocessor memory; pulse oximeters do not require user calibration because they assume one calibration algorithm for the entire human race. This does not imply that the instrument "calibrates itself for each patient," as is sometimes erroneously stated.

To summarize these engineering principles, conventional two-wavelength pulse oximetry requires three implicit assumptions regarding human physiology: 1) that the two and only two light absorbers in human blood are oxyhemoglobin and reduced hemoglobin; 2) that all pulsations in light absorbance are caused by fluctuations in the local volume of arterial blood; and 3) that one empirical, experimental calibration curve—the relationship between the ratio R and SpO_2—is valid for the entire human race.

SOURCES OF ERROR

Given the physics and engineering principles of pulse oximetry, as well as the three assumptions noted above, the major sources of error in SpO_2 readings are predictable. This section examines the common sources of error as well as some design approaches and new developments aimed at reducing errors. The wise user of pulse oximetry must be aware of these problems and be able to anticipate erroneous data.

Dyshemoglobins and Intravenous Dyes: Conventional Pulse Oximetry

Because the conventional pulse oximeter measures light absorbance at two wavelengths, it can deal with unknown concentrations of only two solutes, that is, the two hemoglobin species O_2Hb and RHb. If any light-absorbing substance other than O_2Hb and RHb is present, violating the first assumption above, the pulse oximeter cannot accurately estimate saturation. As shown by the light absorbance spectra in Figure 11-4, both carboxyhemoglobin (COHb) and methemoglobin (MetHb) absorb light at one or both of the wavelengths commonly used by the pulse oximeter. Significant concentrations of either dyshemoglobin will therefore produce erroneous SpO_2 values. The fact that *functional saturation* (SaO_2) does not depend explicitly on dyshemoglobin concentrations (Equation 11-1) does not imply that SaO_2 can be determined by a two-wavelength oximeter. In the presence of additional hemoglobins, an oximeter cannot measure the concentrations of *any* hemoglobin species using only two wavelengths of light (Equation 11-7).

The effects of COHb on SpO_2 values were first determined experimentally in dogs in 1987.[6] Figure 11-7 shows SpO_2 from conventional pulse oximetry, as well as fractional saturation O_2Hb% determined by in vitro CO-oximetry, plotted as functions of COHb%. Even when COHb% increases to levels greater than 70%, the displayed SpO_2 values remain greater than 90% at all times. COHb% levels above 50% are considered potentially lethal in humans. The pulse oximeter thus interprets COHb as though it were composed mostly of O_2Hb, a fact that can be predicted from the absorbance spectra in Figure 11-4. At the red wavelength of 660 nm, COHb has roughly the same absorbance as O_2Hb; at 940 nm, COHb is relatively transparent. This is consistent with the clinical observation that patients with carboxyhemoglobinemia exhibit a bright pink skin color.

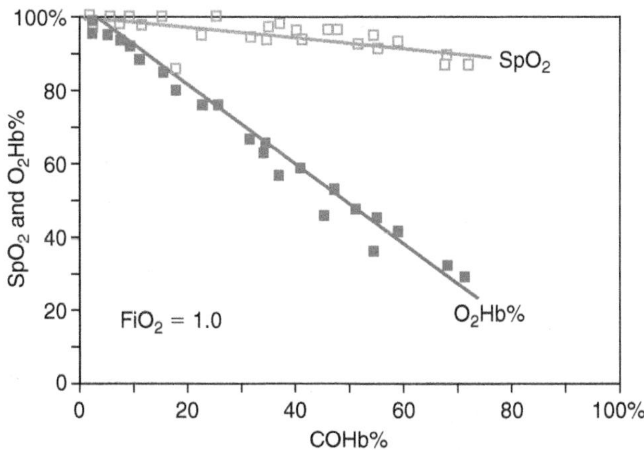

FIGURE 11-7 Estimated oxygen saturation (*SpO_2*) and fractional saturation (*O_2Hb%*) plotted against carboxyhemoglobin level (*COHb%*) for dogs inhaling carbon monoxide at 200 ppm. SpO_2 seriously overestimates arterial fractional hemoglobin oxygen saturation in the presence of COHb and remains greater than 90% even for a COHb% of 70. The pulse oximeter "sees" COHb as though it were mostly O_2Hb. (From Barker S, Tremper K: The effect of carbon monoxide inhalation on pulse oximetry and transcutaneous PO_2. *Anesthesiology* 1987;66:677-679.)

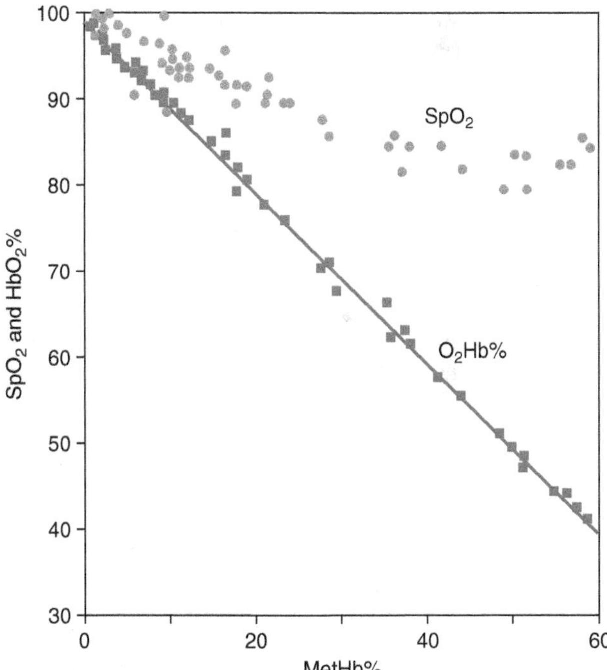

FIGURE 11-8 Estimated oxygen saturation (*SpO_2*) and fractional saturation (*O_2Hb%*) vs. methemoglobin level (*MetHb%*) for dogs with benzocaine-induced methemoglobinemia. Although SpO_2 shows a downward trend with increasing MetHb%, O_2Hb% is consistently overestimated, and it appears that a plateau is reached at an SpO_2 of 85%. When fractional concentration of inspired oxygen (FiO_2) is varied during this experiment, SpO_2 measures neither functional nor fractional saturation. (From Barker SJ, Tremper KK, Hyatt J: Effects of methemoglobinemia on pulse oximetry and mixed venous oximetry. *Anesthesiology* 1989;70:112-117.)

The effects of MetHb on conventional SpO_2 values were similarly evaluated in animal experiments in 1989.[7] Figure 11-8 shows SpO_2 and O_2Hb% determined by CO-oximetry and plotted as functions of MetHb%. As in the case of COHb, the presence of MetHb causes the pulse oximeter to overestimate fractional hemoglobin saturation. However, unlike the behavior of SpO_2 with COHb, here the SpO_2 values tend to decrease with increasing MetHb until they reach a plateau at approximately 85%. For MetHb% values greater than roughly 30%, there is little further decrease in SpO_2 (see Figure 11-8). This fact is again consistent with the light absorbance spectra in Figure 11-4, which shows that MetHb has high absorbance values at both wavelengths used by the pulse oximeter. This high absorbance, which tends to give MetHb its characteristic brown color, adds to both the numerator and denominator of the ratio R in Equation 11-8. Increasing both the numerator and denominator of this ratio by a fixed amount tends to drive the value of R toward 1.0. The pulse oximeter calibration curve of Figure 11-6 shows that an R value of 1.0 corresponds to an SpO_2 value of 85%. This may explain why the pulse oximeter tends to read near 85% saturation in the presence of high MetHb levels.[7] A case report of methemoglobinemia caused by herbal medicines illustrates this phenomenon.[8]

Fetal hemoglobin (HbF) appears to have little effect on the accuracy of conventional pulse oximetry. This is because the extinction coefficients of HbF at the two usual pulse oximeter wavelengths, 660 and 940 nm, are similar to the corresponding values for adult hemoglobin (HbA). This is fortunate because the percentage of HbF present in neonatal blood varies with gestational age and is not very predictable. HbF also produces small errors in multiwavelength in vitro CO-oximeters. The oxygenated state of HbF is interpreted by some older laboratory oximeters as consisting partially of COHb.[9]

Theoretical considerations suggest that sickle hemoglobin (HbS) should also have little effect on pulse oximeter accuracy, but this is difficult to confirm experimentally. It would be unethical to subject sickle cell patients to intentional hypoxemia to study pulse oximeter accuracy. A few clinical case reports have involved sickle cell patients, either under healthy conditions or during a sickle cell crisis; however, these have produced conflicting results. One issue is that there is no clear gold standard for comparison of SpO_2 values in sickle cell patients. One study, which concluded that SpO_2 overestimated SaO_2 with a bias of 6.9%, used a CO-oximeter as the gold standard.[10] However, laboratory CO-oximeters are generally designed to function in the presence of only four types of hemoglobin: 1) reduced Hb, 2) O_2Hb, 3) COHb, and 4) MetHb. Accuracy in the presence of HbS is not specified. Some studies have used as a standard the SaO_2 calculated from the PaO_2, which is measured by a blood gas electrode (Clarke electrode). This method is dubious because it must assume a "normal" oxygen-hemoglobin dissociation curve (see Fig. 11-2), when it is well known that sickle cell patients have right-shifted dissociation curves. At least two studies have measured the O_2 dissociation curves of individual sickle cell patients and then used these to calculate SaO_2 from PaO_2.[11,12] These studies concluded that pulse oximeter accuracy is maintained in sickle cell disease as long as differences in O_2 dissociation curves are accounted for. Other abnormal hemoglobins, such as hemoglobin Bassett, also have produced erroneous SpO_2 readings.[13]

The ratio R, and hence the SpO_2 value, can be affected by any substance present in the blood that absorbs light at 660 or 940 nm. Dyes injected intravenously for diagnostic purposes can have significant effects on SpO_2. For example, intravenous methylene blue produces sudden large decreases in SpO_2 values in normal subjects.[14] Indigo carmine yields small decreases in SpO_2, and indocyanine green has an intermediate effect. The extinction coefficients of these three dyes are plotted against light wavelength in Figure 11-9.[14] A comparison of these absorbance spectra with those of hemoglobin (see Fig. 11-4) predicts the relative effects of the three dyes on SpO_2 values. Bilirubin, another common pigment found

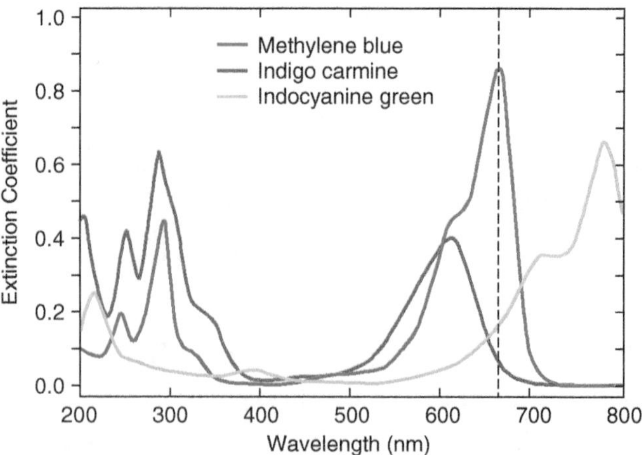

FIGURE 11-9 ■ Extinction coefficient (ε) versus wavelength (λ) in the range 200 to 800 nm for three dyes: methylene blue, indigo carmine, and indocyanine green. (Modified from Scheller MS, Unger RJ, Kelner MJ: Effects of intravenously administered dyes on pulse oximetry readings. *Anesthesiology* 1986;65[5]:550-552.)

in blood, appears to have no significant effect on SpO_2 at concentrations seen clinically.[15]

Nail polish has variable effects upon SpO_2 values and usually produces falsely low readings.[16] Highly opaque, acrylic nail coverings can prevent the pulse oximeter from detecting any pulsatile absorbance at all. This problem can usually be averted by rotating the fingertip sensor 90 degrees so that the coated fingernail does not fall within the optical path.

Multiwavelength Pulse Oximetry

Until 2005, only a few investigations had been made into the possibilities of multiwavelength pulse oximetry. Aoyagi, the inventor of pulse oximetry, performed experiments with three-wavelength sensors in 2002.[17] Although his purpose in using an additional wavelength was to improve the accuracy of the SpO_2 value, he noted that "Dyshemoglobins (e.g., COHb and MetHb) can be measured with a multiwavelength system." A four-wavelength pulse oximeter that estimated total hemoglobin was reported by Noiri and colleagues in 2005.[18] However, this device was never commercially produced and did not see widespread clinical use. Several investigators have used multiwavelength IR in vivo oximetry to estimate hemoglobin saturation in the internal jugular vein or in brain tissue, but again, only the ratio of oxyhemoglobin to total hemoglobin was measured.[19,20]

In 2005, the Masimo Corporation (Irvine, CA) announced the development of their Rainbow technology Rad-57 pulse oximeter. This device uses eight wavelengths of light to measure SpO_2, SpCO (pulse oximeter estimate of COHb%), and SpMet (pulse oximeter estimate of MetHb%). The handheld, battery-powered Rad-57 was later followed by a bench-top version, Radical-7. The first human study of the performance of the Rad-57 was published in 2006.[21] Twenty healthy volunteers were instrumented with radial artery catheters, electrocardiograms (ECGs), sphygmomanometers, and Rad-57 sensors on the fingers. In the COHb arm of the study, volunteers were exposed to inspired CO at 150 ppm until their COHb%

levels reached 15%. Arterial blood samples were analyzed by CO-oximetry, and the resulting COHb% values were compared with the SpCO readings. The bias—that is, the mean difference between SpCO and COHb% by CO-oximeter—was -1.22%, and the precision (standard deviation [SD] of the difference) was 2.19%. These values are nearly the same as the manufacturer-specified uncertainties for conventional pulse oximeters in the measurement of SpO_2. This volunteer study obviously could not investigate the more pathologic COHb% levels found in smoke-inhalation injuries.

Subjects in the MetHb arm of the study were given 300 mg of intravenous sodium nitrite, a drug approved by the Food and Drug Administration (FDA) for treatment of cyanide toxicity; this resulted in methemoglobin levels of up to 13%. The comparison of SpMet with simultaneous CO-oximeter values of MetHb% yielded a bias of 0.00% and a precision of 0.45%. These uncertainties for SpMet are approximately one fourth of those measured for SpCO. This greater accuracy is a result of the fact that MetHb has a high light absorbance at all wavelengths in the range of interest; hence it provides a larger absorbance signal for the pulse oximeter's processing algorithm.

Laboratory volunteer studies cannot predict a monitor's performance in clinical conditions, nor can they establish its effects on patient outcome. For this we rely on clinical studies and case reports, a number of which have been published in the past few years. Coulange and colleagues[22] measured SpCO from Rad-57 and simultaneous values of COHb% from blood CO-oximetry in smoke-inhalation victims. In data from 12 patients, they found a bias of -1.5% and a precision of 2.5%. Layne and colleagues measured SpCO and COHb% (Avox 400 CO-oximeter) in 130 outpatients, both smokers and nonsmokers.[23] They found a bias of -0.65% and a precision of 1.8% in a COHb range from 0% to 31%. Both of these clinical studies found SpCO uncertainties to be essentially the same as in the Barker volunteer study.[21]

Numerous case reports have been published on the use of Rad-57 to detect and measure COHb levels. Some authors have used SpCO as a screening tool to identify smokers and track smoking cessation.[24,25] Another promising application for the handheld device is in fire departments and for emergency medical services (EMS) responders. Hostler and colleagues[26] showed that SpCO could be used as a diagnostic tool for firefighters who respond to CO alarm activations. They found that patients who require transport to the emergency department had mean SpCO levels of 27.8%, whereas patients not in need of treatment had mean levels of 3.2%. A similar study of 149 patients by the New York Fire Department concluded that the Rad-57 "can be used as a screening tool to uncover cases of CO poisoning in which the diagnosis is not suspected."[27] Firefighters themselves have been screened with SpCO in other investigations.[28] Case reports from emergency departments have shown the value of SpCO monitoring for tracking the progress of carbon monoxide poisoning victims and in the detection of CO poisoning in unsuspected cases.[29-31] Figure 11-10 shows an example of SpCO trend monitoring and response to treatment in an 81-year-old woman who was trapped in a house fire.[29]

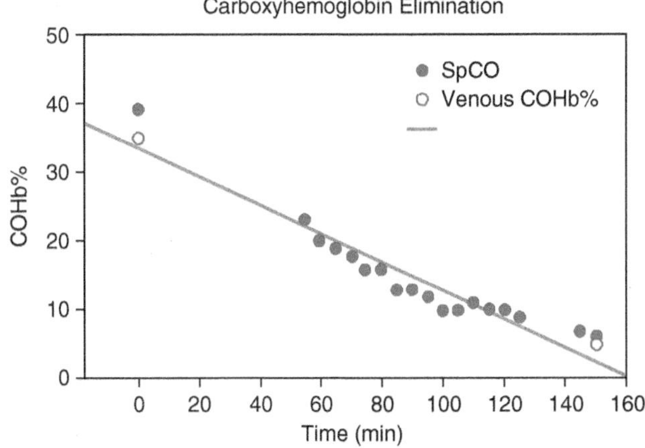

FIGURE 11-10 Carboxyhemoglobin (*COHb%*) and its pulse oximetry estimate (*SpCO*) plotted vs. time in an 81-year-old victim of smoke inhalation. (From Plante T, Harris D, Savitt J, et al: Carboxyhemoglobin monitored by bedside continuous CO-oximetry. *J Trauma* 2007;63[5]:1187-1190.)

Several case reports were published of Rad-57 being used to detect and monitor methemoglobinemia. Many life-threatening methemoglobinemia cases reported involve the use of topical benzocaine.[32] This is one of a large number of commonly used drugs that induce methemoglobinemia as a side effect, a problem that undoubtedly has been underdiagnosed in the past.[33] Macknet and colleagues presented a case of severe benzocaine-induced methemoglobinemia during transesophageal echocardiography, in which the Rad-57 was used to make the diagnosis and to monitor treatment with methylene blue.[34] Barker and colleagues reported a similar case in the OR following topical benzocaine for awake intubation.[35] In both of these cases, the multiwavelength pulse oximeter played a major role in diagnosis and treatment; in vitro laboratory CO-oximeter values were delayed too much to guide treatment.

The current versions of the Masimo Rad-57 and Radical-7 have two limitations. First, they still use a conventional two-wavelength red-over-IR algorithm to calculate the SpO_2 value. Thus, when levels of either COHb or MetHb are significant, the displayed SpO_2 is subject to the same errors described above.[6,7] Of course, the presence of a displayed SpCO or SpMet value would alert the user to the likelihood of this SpO_2 error. The second limitation is the existence of "crosstalk" between the MetHb and COHb measurement channels. That is, in the presence of significant MetHb levels, the instrument will display a falsely elevated SpCO value while also displaying a correct SpMet value. This situation is detected by the device, which will display an error message indicating that the SpCO value may not be accurate.

In March 2008, Masimo announced another innovation in multiwavelength pulse oximetry: the noninvasive measurement of total hemoglobin. Macknet and colleagues[36] published the first clinical validation study, in which 30 surgical patients and 18 healthy volunteers were monitored with the new prototype. The subjects followed a hemodilution protocol in which one unit of blood was withdrawn and replaced with normal saline. Arterial blood was sampled periodically and analyzed for total hemoglobin (Hbt) by a Radiometer ABL-735 CO-oximeter, and

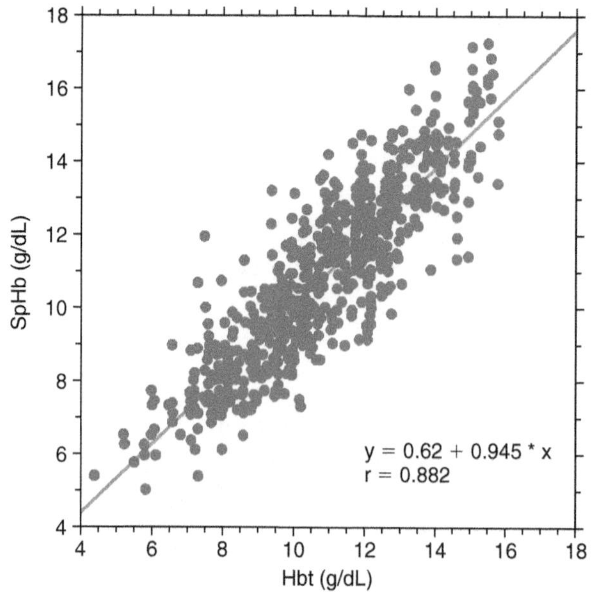

FIGURE 11-11 ■ Radical-7 (Masimo Corporation, Irvine, CA) measurement of total hemoglobin (*SpHb*) plotted against simultaneous laboratory CO-oximeter value. Included were 48 subjects and 802 data points. Bias was 0.03 and precision was 1.12. *Hbt,* total hemoglobin. (From Macknet M, Norton S, Kimball-Jones P, et al: Continuous non-invasive measurement of hemoglobin via pulse CO-oximetry. *Anesth Analg* 2007;105[6]:S-108.)

the values obtained were compared with the simultaneous Radical-7 measurements of hemoglobin (SpHb), as shown in Figure 11-11. In a range of Hbt values from 4.4 to 15.8 g/dL, this comparison revealed a bias and precision of 0.03 and 1.12 g/dL, respectively. Macknet and colleagues[36a] published a similar study in 20 healthy volunteers and concluded that pulse CO-oximetry–based SpHb measurement was accurate to within 1.0 g/dL compared with laboratory CO-oximeter measurements.

A presentation at the 2008 World Congress of Anesthesiology described a case in which casual screening with the Radical-7 revealed an abnormally low SpHb (11 g/dL) in a 72-year-old man.[37] This led to further testing, which yielded the early diagnosis of an asymptomatic esophageal carcinoma. The early complete surgical excision resulted in the probable cure of a highly lethal disease. The noninvasive measurement of Hbt by pulse oximetry is very new, and more case reports and clinical outcome studies can be expected in the future.

Multiwavelength pulse oximetry is now capable of the continuous, noninvasive measurement of MetHb, carboxyhemoglobin, and total hemoglobin. Technology has made real progress in correcting one of the chief weaknesses of pulse oximetry: performance in the presence of abnormal hemoglobin species. Clinical studies and case reports have already documented the importance of these new developments, and it is hoped that further developments will lead to the continuous measurement of other substances in the blood.

Wavelength Variability

The LED used as a light source by the pulse oximeter is not an ideal monochromatic (single-wavelength) radiator. The LED emits light over a narrow but finite range of wavelengths. The center wavelength, or wavelength of peak energy radiation, varies by as much as 15 nm among diodes of the same specification. Figure 11-4 shows that such a variation in wavelength can yield a significantly different extinction coefficient, particularly at the 660-nm wavelength. Manufacturers use at least two approaches to this problem. The simplest method is to measure the center wavelength of all LEDs and reject those that fall outside a specified range, for example, 660 (±5) nm. This method is effective but expensive because of the large number of LEDs that must be discarded. The second method is to store multiple calibration algorithms in the pulse oximeter software, corresponding to different LED center wavelengths. The electrical connector on the sensor cable is then pin coded so that only the appropriate algorithm can be selected for a given sensor. Neither method entirely eliminates the effect of center frequency variation. This variability does not affect the pulse oximeter's ability to follow changes in saturation, but it does produce differences between sensors in the absolute value of SpO_2.[38]

Signal/Noise Ratio

The amplitude of the fluctuating (AC) component of the light absorbance can be much less than 1% of the amplitude of the DC component (see Fig. 11-5). Any influence that decreases the AC component, increases the DC component, or adds an artifactual AC component not related to arterial pulsations will worsen the signal/noise ratio. For example, the AC signal is decreased in low perfusion states, such as shock; the DC signal is increased when ambient room light reaches the detector; and artifactual AC signals are caused by patient motion, such as shivering.

The photodiode light detector in the pulse oximeter sensor cannot discriminate one wavelength of light from another—it is effectively color blind. The detector therefore responds to ambient room light and to light from either of the LED sources. In most two-wavelength pulse oximeters, this problem is solved by activating the red and infrared LEDs in an alternating sequence. During one part of this sequence, both LEDs are turned off, and the photodetector measures the ambient background light. This sequence is repeated many times per second (e.g., 480 Hz) in an attempt to eliminate light interference from rapidly changing ambient sources. Despite this ingenious design, ambient light artifact can create problems with the signal/noise ratio; however, this difficulty can be minimized by covering the sensor with an opaque shield of some sort, such as a surgical drape or towel.

If the peripheral pulse is weak, the AC absorbance signal becomes smaller compared with the DC signal. The pulse oximeter uses an automatic gain control that adjusts either the LED intensity or the photodetector amplifier gain to compensate for changes in AC signal amplitude. Unfortunately, this process also amplifies background noise from all sources, including ambient light. At the highest amplifier gain setting, the pulse oximeter may interpret background noise as a pulsatile absorbance and may generate an SpO_2 value from this artifact.[4] This phenomenon could be demonstrated in early pulse oximeters by inserting a piece of paper between the photodetector and the LEDs. Some of these pulse oximeters would amplify background noise and display a pulse and saturation value from the paper.

This signal/noise ratio problem is also illustrated by the *penumbra effect*.[39] If a finger sensor is partially dislodged or malpositioned in such a manner that light passes through the fingertip at a grazing incidence, the pulse oximeter may display a correct heart rate but an erroneous SpO_2 value. The SpO_2 value from a malpositioned sensor is usually falsely low during normoxemia, but it may be falsely high during moderate hypoxemia.[40] This behavior may be another example of the R = 1.0 phenomenon (Equation 11-8).

Most pulse oximeters display some sort of visual indicator of pulsatile absorbance signal, usually in the form of an absorbance-versus-time plethysmogram. This displayed waveform usually represents the AC signal after amplification and therefore does not directly correspond to the actual amplitude of the absorbance pulsations. However, a few manufacturers display a waveform whose height actually *does* represent pulsatile absorbance amplitude before amplification. The user must therefore determine what the waveform of the pulse oximeter in use measures; in general, it is not safe to assume that waveform amplitude represents pulse amplitude. The plethysmograph is not a quantitative monitor of peripheral perfusion, and it cannot be relied upon to warn of impending ischemia, despite claims to the contrary.

The behavior of first-generation pulse oximeters during shock or low-perfusion states has been studied in both humans and animals.[41-45] During hemorrhagic shock, pulse oximeters may display no SpO_2 value at all, or they may give falsely low saturation estimates. Loss of signal is likely with hypothermia, severe anemia, low cardiac output states, and extremes in systemic vascular resistance. An early study of failure rates in the OR found that pulse oximeters (Nellcor N-100, Ohmeda 3700) failed in 1.12% of all patients.[46] Higher failure rates were associated with poor preoperative physical status, long operations, and elderly patients. A later study used computerized anesthesia records and found that 9% of all cases (n = 9203) had gaps in SpO_2 data of 10 minutes or more.[47] Higher failure rates were associated with higher ASA physical status number and with hypotension and hypothermia. The largest failure rate study was done by Moller and colleagues,[48] in which more than 20,000 surgical patients were followed. Interestingly, this controlled study found little difference in postoperative outcome between patients monitored with pulse oximetry and unmonitored patients, but it did find a very significant variation in failure rate with ASA physical status, shown in Figure 11-12. The failure rate for ASA-4 patients was more than five times that for ASA-1 patients; these higher failure rates in sicker patients have led some to describe the pulse oximeter as a "fair-weather friend."

Several studies have determined thresholds for loss of signal during low-perfusion states. Lawson and colleagues[41] produced gradual occlusion of blood flow with a blood pressure cuff while monitoring flow at the fingertip using a Doppler flow probe. They found loss of signal when blood flow had decreased to an average of 8.6% of its baseline value, which occurred at a cuff pressure of 96% of systolic pressure. On cuff deflation, the signal returned at a blood flow of only 4% of baseline. Severinghaus and colleagues[49] studied pulse oximeter behavior during various types of reduction in extremity blood flow, including via blood pressure cuff, brachial artery pressure clamp, and extremity elevation. Failure occurred at higher mean arterial pressures with the arterial clamp than with gravitational hypotension, showing the importance of blood volume pulsatility. These studies demonstrate that the pulse oximeter functions over a wide range of blood flows and blood pressures in the extremity. Because the pulse oximeter is designed to function independently of changes in flow or pressure, loss of signal cannot be used to determine the adequacy of peripheral perfusion, even though this has been attempted.[50] (See also the related discussion of the plethysmograph above.)

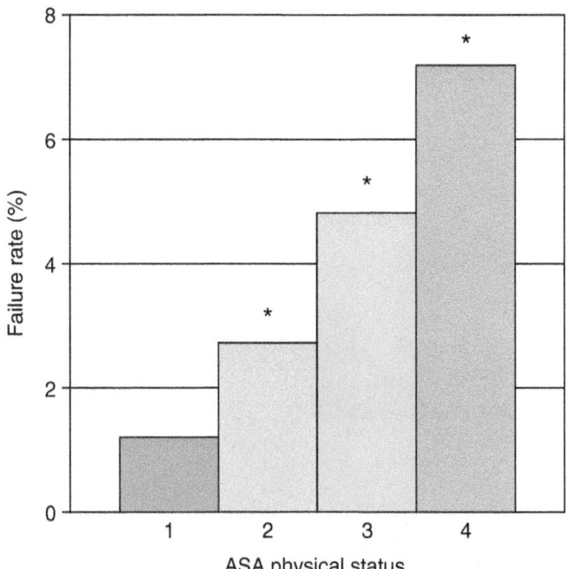

FIGURE 11-12 Pulse oximeter failure rates as a function of American Society of Anesthesiologists (*ASA*) physical status. Data shown are from both the operating room and postanesthesia care unit in 10,312 patients. Failure rate increased from 1% to more than 7% as physical status worsened. Asterisks denote significance. (From Moller JT, et al: Randomized evaluation of pulse oximetry in 20,802 patients. *Anesthesiology* 1993;78:436-453.)

The electrosurgical unit (ESU) is another source of artifact. The intense, high-frequency, electromagnetic radiation from the ESU electrode fills the OR whenever the device is activated. The electrical cable from the pulse oximeter sensor acts as an antenna that receives the ESU radiation. Earlier generations of pulse oximeters were essentially shut down by ESU activation and required up to 30 seconds to recover. More recent pulse oximeters—that is, those made after the year 2000—are much improved in this respect and usually continue to display and update SpO_2 and heart rate values during ESU use. However, some pulse oximeters display their last "valid" SpO_2 value for up to 30 seconds during loss-of-signal periods. In these instruments, the user can be certain that the pulse oximeter is measuring SpO_2 during ESU activation only if a reasonable plethysmograph waveform is observed.

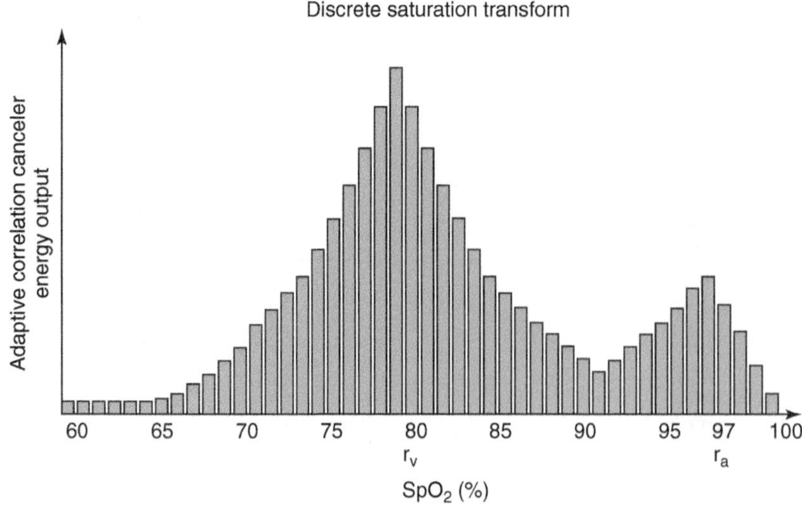

FIGURE 11-13 An example of a discrete saturation transform during patient motion. The signal strength calculated by the algorithm is plotted against saturation for all possible estimated pulse oximetry (*SpO_2*) values. The peak at 97% corresponds to the saturation of arterial blood (*r_a*); the peak at 79% represents venous blood (*r_v*).

Motion Artifact and Adaptive Digital Signal Filtering

Artifacts caused by patient motion have plagued pulse oximetry, particularly in the recovery room, intensive care unit (ICU), and emergency settings. Although loss of signal or erroneous readings as a result of motion are infrequent in the OR (1% to 2%), they can cause a false alarm incidence that exceeds 50% in recovery room and ICU settings.[51] Patient motion, especially shivering, causes a large, fluctuating absorbance artifact that is incorrectly interpreted by the pulse oximeter algorithm. Much of this artifact results from venous blood volume pulsations created by the motion, thus violating the second assumption of conventional pulse oximetry, that the light path length is exactly known.

Until fairly recently, manufacturers used two approaches to this problem: increased signal averaging time and ECG synchronization. In the first approach, the value of the ratio R is stored on a beat-to-beat basis and averaged for several seconds. This running average is less sensitive to patient motion but is also slower to respond to sudden saturation changes. The reduction in the false-alarm rate resulting from motion is thus accompanied by a slower response to true alarms, which is particularly risky in pediatric or neonatal applications. The second approach, ECG pulse rate synchronization, was developed by Nellcor and applied in their N-200 pulse oximeter.[52] Although this "C-lock" feature seemed to be a useful innovation, it was not particularly successful and was abandoned in later models.

A recent, more elegant solution to motion artifact is to determine the "noise signal" and subtract it from the total signal, leaving a noise-free signal from which to calculate the SpO_2. Masimo has used this "adaptive digital filtering" approach to develop an algorithm called signal extraction technology (SET), which improves pulse oximeter performance in the presence of motion artifact.[53-55] The method makes two assumptions, the first being that most of the noise associated with motion artifact is produced by pulsations in venous blood volume, which produce the SpO_2 errors described above. In fact, errors from venous pulsations were documented in an early volunteer study that showed that SpO_2 may decrease by 8% when the arm is moved from a raised to a dependent position.[56] The second assumption is that the saturation values from the venous pulsations will be less than arterial values, which seems rather obvious. The Masimo SET electronically scans all possible values of the ratio R that correspond to saturations of 0% through 100%, and it calculates the signal intensity at each possible R value, as shown in Figure 11-13. In this example of a *discrete saturation transform* curve, two intensity peaks occur at 79% and 97% saturation: the higher peak corresponds to the arterial pulsations and is used to calculate SpO_2, and the lower peak at 50% presumably represents the venous pulsations. The entire sequence is repeated once per second on the most recent 6 seconds of raw data. The displayed SpO_2 value thus represents a 6-second running average of arterial hemoglobin saturation, updated every second.

This new technology has been evaluated in two volunteer experiments in which motion was induced in one hand while the other hand served as a stationary control.[53,54] In both of these experiments, done 5 years apart, the latest version of Masimo SET was compared with the current versions of other manufacturers' instruments, most of which claimed to be "motion resistant." The results of the more recent study are summarized in Table 11-1. These findings are supported by several clinical studies conducted on patients in postoperative care units.[55,57,58] Additional studies will determine whether this approach yields improved performance in clinical settings of low perfusion, such as with shock or after cardiopulmonary bypass.

CLINICAL APPLICATIONS: ACCURACY, RESPONSE, AND LIMITATIONS

This section reviews clinical applications of pulse oximetry and its physiologic limitations, that is, the clinical changes that can and cannot be detected by saturation monitoring. In reviewing studies of pulse oximeter accuracy, simple statistical tools are needed. Studies of pulse oximeter accuracy are generally methods-comparison studies, in which two independent methods are used to measure the same variable simultaneously. One of the two

TABLE 11-1 **Performance of Several Pulse Oximeters During Mechanically Controlled Hand Motion**

Pulse Oximeter	Performance Index (%)	Sensitivity (%)	Specificity (%)
Masimo SET	93	99	97
Viridia/24C	84	78	90
Hewlett-Packard CMS-B	80	70	83
Nellcor N-395	73	70	73
Datex-Ohmeda 3900	68	60	52
Nova Mars	58	40	42
Nellcor N-295	55	39	53

Performance index is the percent of time during which estimated oxygenation by pulse oximetry on the hand in motion is within 7% of the simultaneous value on the stationary (control) hand. Sensitivity and specificity for detection of hypoxemia (saturation values <90%) are also shown. All instruments except the N-295 claim to be "motion resistant."

From Barker SJ: "Motion-Resistant" pulse oximetry: a comparison of new and old models. *Anesth Analg* 2002;95:967-972.

methods usually is a new or unproven technique—in this case, pulse oximetry—and the other method is considered a gold standard. The most common gold standard for pulse oximeter studies is a multiwavelength in vitro CO-oximeter used to analyze arterial blood samples. These laboratory devices claim an uncertainty on the order of ±1% (1 SD) for measurements of fractional saturation (Equation 11-2). Because the accuracy of current pulse oximeters is comparable to this figure (generally ±2%), it must be noted that both methods in all comparison studies are subject to uncertainty; a true gold standard of absolute accuracy for any monitor is rare.

The most commonly used statistics for evaluating methods-comparison studies are *bias* and *precision* as defined by Bland and Altman.[59] *Bias* is defined as the mean of the differences between simultaneous measurements by the two methods, and *precision* is the standard deviation of this difference. (We have suggested calling the latter quantity the *imprecision* because a larger value implies a less precise measurement.) This text defines the difference between measurements as the pulse oximeter SpO_2 value minus the CO-oximeter $O_2Hb\%$ value; however, in some of the literature, the opposite sign is used. The bias indicates systematic error; that is, it shows the tendency of one of the two methods to consistently overestimate or underestimate one value relative to the other. The precision represents the variability or random error between the two methods. If both the systematic and random errors are within acceptable clinical limits, the methods-comparison study suggests that one method can replace the other. Unfortunately, many published methods-comparison studies do not include bias and precision values. Reported statistics often include a correlation coefficient r and a linear regression slope and intercept of the scatterplot, or a graph of method A versus method B values. Correlation coefficient is not a measure of agreement between two variables; rather, it is a measure of their association and is affected by the range of values covered by the data as well as agreement between the two methods. Similarly, linear regression slope and intercept may be meaningless if the data points fall within a narrow range of values.

Accuracy Studies

Most pulse oximeter manufacturers claim an uncertainty of ±2% (1 SD) for SpO_2 values between 70% and 100%. This uncertainty increases to ±3% for SpO_2 values between 50% and 70%; no accuracy is specified for SpO_2 values below 50%. This implies that for saturations above 70%, the SpO_2 value should be within 2% of the actual saturation 68% of the time and within 4% (2 SDs) 95% of the time. These accuracy specifications have not changed since the mid-1980s. The seemingly generous 2% uncertainty is the direct result of the third assumption for pulse oximetry as stated above: one empirical calibration curve—that is, the relationship between the ratio R and SpO_2—fits the entire human race.

In the 1980s and 1990s, a number of studies of pulse oximeter accuracy were done that included both laboratory volunteer tests and clinical trials.[60,61] Three of the studies from this era are of special interest because they evaluated not only accuracy but also response times to sudden changes in hemoglobin saturation.[62-64] These studies found some significant errors in pulse oximeter calibrations, which were subsequently revised by the manufacturers. As a result of such "aftermarket" software revisions, seemingly identical pulse oximeters may actually perform differently. Experimental study reports must therefore specify the software version and the pulse oximeter manufacturer and model used.

The volunteer studies of Severinghaus and Naifeh compared the performance of various pulse oximeters during severe, transient desaturations.[62,64] Subjects underwent brief (45 seconds) desaturations to an $O_2Hb\%$ value of 40% to 70%. Pulse oximeter response times to these sudden saturation changes were much shorter for earlobe sensors than for finger sensors (Figure 11-14). The time for a 50% response to rapid desaturation, or "resaturation," ranged from 10 to 20 seconds for the earlobe sensor; for the finger sensors, it varied between 24 and 50 seconds. A similar result was obtained in another study that compared response times of finger sensors to those of both earlobe sensors and reflectance sensors on the forehead.[65] Both of these studies showed wide variations among subjects in response times for finger sensors, reflecting a wide range of lung-to-finger circulation times. These physiologic time delays and their interpatient variability should be considered in the selection of sensor sites in clinical settings, in which SpO_2 can change rapidly (e.g., the OR). However, clinical studies have also found that finger sensors are the most reliable in obtaining SpO_2 values during periods of hemodynamic instability.[66]

The pulse oximeter's response to sudden saturation changes is also affected by the signal-averaging time of the instrument, which is often user selectable. The displayed SpO_2 value represents a running average of data obtained over the most recent averaging time period, which may range between 1 and 15 seconds. The SpO_2 value will respond more quickly to a sudden change in

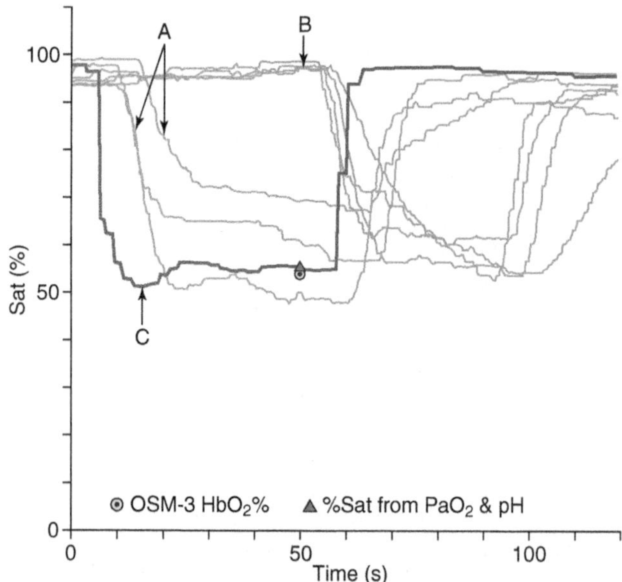

FIGURE 11-14 Tracings of pulse oximetry values plotted against time for seven pulse oximeters during a rapid, brief desaturation in a healthy volunteer. Tracings labeled *A* represent three earlobe sensors, tracings labeled *B* are four finger sensors, and tracing *C* is the pulmonary venous saturation calculated from exhaled oxygen tension measured by mass spectrometry. The earlobe sensors register the desaturation with a 10- to 15-second time lag, whereas the finger sensors show a 50-second time lag in this volunteer. *Hb,* hemoglobin; *OSM-3,* CO-oximeter; *PaO_2,* arterial oxygen tension; *Sat,* saturation. (Modified from Severinghaus JW, Naifeh KH: Accuracy of response of six pulse oximeters to profound hypoxia. *Anesthesiology* 1987;67:553.)

SaO_2 if a short averaging time is selected. On the other hand, if the signal/noise ratio is marginal or artifacts are present, such as with patient motion, a longer averaging time will yield better accuracy. The user must determine the most appropriate averaging time for the clinical setting. The default averaging time, which is the value applied when the power is turned on, varies among manufacturers; hence, the user must know the default value of the particular instrument in use.

Clinical studies of accuracy usually combine data from multiple patients to determine the SpO_2 uncertainty. This procedure yields a more pessimistic view of accuracy than would be obtained by studying results for individual patients. If a sensor is placed on a patient, and the SpO_2 value is 95%, the probability is 68% that the patient's true saturation lies between 93% and 97% (±1 SD). On the other hand, if the displayed SpO_2 on that same patient decreases from 95% to 93%, the amount by which the saturation has decreased is more certain than the original absolute SpO_2 value. In other words, trend accuracy is greater than absolute value accuracy. Variability among patients is a price we pay for the convenience of having the pulse oximeter precalibrated with a universal algorithm (see the third pulse oximetry assumption). The calibration algorithm is a best fit of data from a large number of healthy adult volunteers. Alternatively, manufacturers could have chosen to require user calibration on each individual patient. This would have improved absolute accuracy, but it would have lost an important advantage of pulse oximetry, namely, the absence of a need for user calibration.

Plethysmograph Variability Applications

In 1873, Kussmaul proposed that respiratory variation of the pulse intensity is an important sign of various physiologic derangements, including pericardial tamponade.[67] Nearly 100 years later, Kussmaul's observation led to the measured association between pulsus paradoxus and intravascular volume status.[68] This concept evolved into a relationship between "arterial pulse pressure" from the arterial cannula and fluid responsiveness, addressing the basic clinical question of whether the patient would benefit from additional intravascular fluids.[69,70] Numerous studies over the years have shown that the traditional "static" parameters, including central venous pressure and pulmonary artery occlusion pressure, are of limited value in answering this question. Perhaps "dynamic parameters" such as pulse-pressure variation can be more predictive.[71]

Meanwhile, other investigators had already extrapolated this pulse-variation principle to the dependence of pulse oximeter plethysmograph variations on intravascular volume.[72] These early efforts to use pulse oximetry for the estimation of volume status were interesting but found little clinical use because they were neither sensitive nor specific. However, more recent advances in pulse oximeter signal processing have made this noninvasive possibility more promising. Masimo has developed a new parameter called the plethysmograph variability index (PVI), which is defined as

$$PVI = 100 \times (PI_{max} - PI_{min})/PI_{max} \quad (11\text{-}9)$$

where PI_{max} is the maximum value of the perfusion index, the ratio of AC to DC absorbance signal during the respiratory cycle, and PI_{min} is the minimum value during the cycle. This parameter can be continuously displayed by the pulse oximeter, thus quantifying the respiratory variation of the plethysmograph amplitude. Higher values of PVI are suggestive of lower intravascular volume status and a stronger probability of a positive hemodynamic response to fluid infusion.

Clinical studies of PVI have shown that it correlates strongly with arterial pulse pressure variations during positive-pressure ventilation.[73] More importantly, recent studies have found that PVI is predictive of response to intravascular volume infusion, with a sensitivity and specificity superior to those of either central venous pressure or wedge pressure.[74,75] Figure 11-15 shows typical plethysmograph waveforms and PVI trend plots for patients who are fluid responders and nonresponders.[75] As intravascular fluids are infused, the PVI falls dramatically in fluid responders, but it changes little in the nonresponders.

Plethysmograph variability, like pulsus paradoxus, is sensitive to a number of physiologic factors other than volume status (Box 11-1). The astute clinician must consider all possible causes for changes in PVI. Additional clinical data must be used to distinguish hypovolemia from tamponade, bronchospasm, or pneumothorax for example. Nevertheless, early studies suggest that pulse oximeter plethysmograph variability has excellent potential for monitoring hemodynamics in OR and critical care settings.

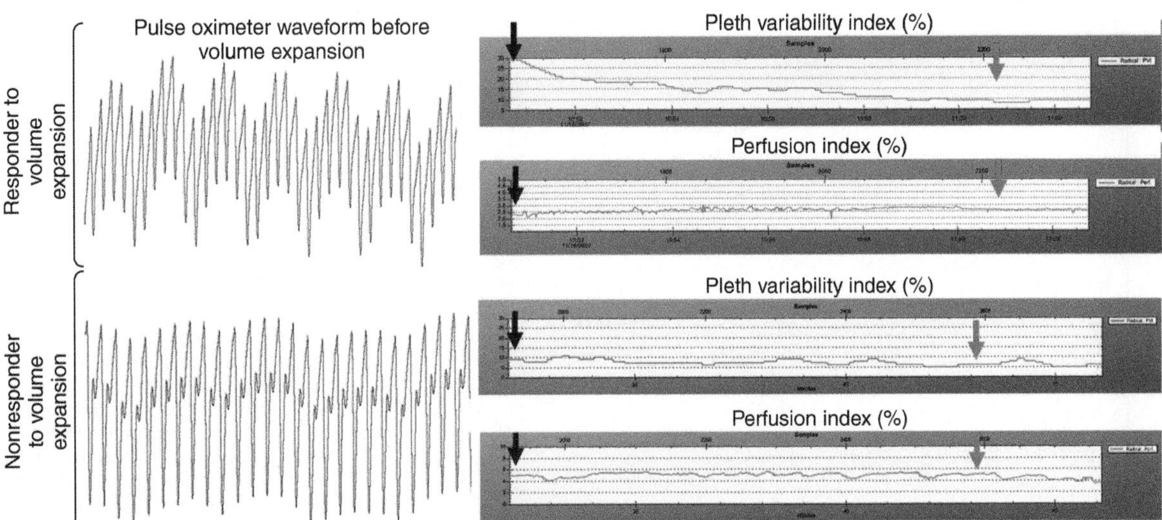

FIGURE 11-15 ■ Plethysmograph (*Pleth*) waveforms and plethysmograph variability index trend plots for patients who are fluid responders and nonresponders. (From Canneson M, Desebbe O, Rosamel P, et al: Pleth variability index to monitor the respiratory variations in the pulse oximeter plethysmographic waveform amplitude and predict fluid responsiveness in the operating theatre, *Br J Anaesth* 101[2]:200-206, 2008.)

BOX 11-1 Physiologic Changes that Can Affect Plethysmograph Variability

CARDIAC

- Cardiogenic shock
- Pericardial tamponade
- Pericardial effusion
- Constrictive pericarditis
- Restrictive cardiomyopathy
- Acute myocardial infarction

PULMONARY

- Asthma
- Tension pneumothorax
- Pulmonary embolism
- Bronchospasm
- Airway obstruction

NONCARDIAC, NONPULMONARY

- Hypovolemia
- Septic shock
- Anaphylactic shock
- Diaphragmatic hernia
- Superior vena cava obstruction
- Extreme obesity

Limitations of Pulse Oximetry

Since the pulse oximeter became a minimum standard of care in the OR in 1986,[76] it has been unethical to perform randomized controlled studies of its clinical effectiveness in that setting.[77] Before that time, several such studies were performed. Coté and colleagues[78] studied 152 pediatric patients during anesthesia and surgery. In half of these patients, the SpO_2 data were unavailable to the anesthesiologist. The study found that "major events," defined as SpO_2 below 85% for more than 30 seconds, occurred significantly more often in the patients for whom the SpO_2 values were hidden, and most of these events occurred in patients younger than 2 years. On the other hand, none of these controlled studies demonstrated a statistically significant difference in patient outcomes—that is, morbidity and mortality—and this includes the Moller study[48] of more than 20,000 patients cited above. This merely shows the difficulty of performing outcomes studies in anesthesiology. When a study cannot disprove the null hypothesis of no difference between treatments, it does not mean that the null hypothesis is true. This basic fact of statistics is too often overlooked in interpretations of clinical studies.

Since becoming an intraoperative standard of care in the 1980s, the pulse oximeter also has had major impact in other clinical settings. Two studies monitored SpO_2 during transport from the OR to the recovery room; both found a high incidence of desaturations with SpO_2 values below 90% in patients who did not receive supplemental oxygen.[79,80] These studies strongly support a uniform policy of transport to the postanesthesia care unit (PACU) with supplemental oxygen for all patients. Similar studies suggest that SpO_2 should be continuously monitored in most patients in the recovery room. One study of postoperative pediatric patients showed no correlation between SpO_2 and a traditional postanesthesia score based on motor activity, respirations, blood pressure, mental status, and color.[81] The authors concluded that postoperative pediatric patients should be monitored by pulse oximetry or be given supplemental oxygen regardless of their apparent state of wakefulness. Another study found that 14% of adult PACU patients had SpO_2 values below 90% and that significant desaturations were associated with obesity, extensive surgery, advanced age, and poor physical status.[82] In fact, most patients are more likely to have hypoxemia in the PACU than in the OR. Recovery room patients no longer have a protected airway and are not receiving mechanical ventilation, yet they have not fully recovered from the depressant effects of anesthesia and surgery.

The pulse oximeter warns of developing hypoxemia, but at the increased inspired oxygen fractions typically used in the OR, SpO_2 may not provide an early warning

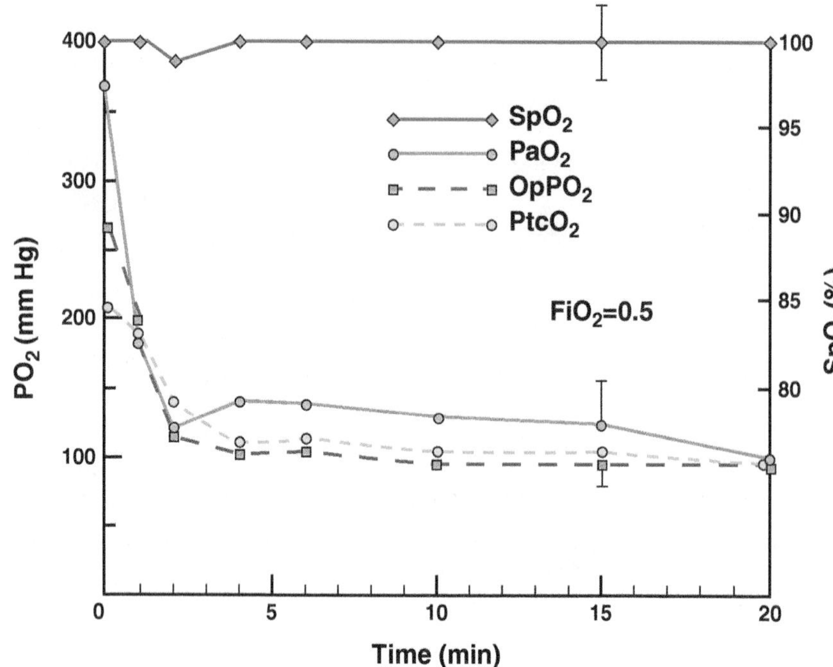

FIGURE 11-16 ■ Four oxygenation variables plotted against time from the onset of endobronchial intubation in a dog at a fraction of inspired oxygen (*FiO_2*) of 0.5. Arterial oxygen tension (*PaO_2*), optode intraarterial oxygen tension (*$OpPO_2$*), and transcutaneous oxygen tension (*$P_{TC}O_2$*) all decreased rapidly during the first 2 minutes following endobronchial intubation, whereas the pulse oximetry value (*SpO_2*) did not change significantly at any time. (From Barker SJ, Tremper KK, Hyatt J, et al: Comparison of three oxygen monitors in detecting endobronchial intubation. *J Clin Monit* 1988;4:241.)

of decreasing arterial oxygen tension. The oxyhemoglobin dissociation curve (see Fig. 11-2) shows that PaO_2 must decrease to less than 80 mm Hg before SaO_2 falls significantly. A good example of this limitation is in the detection of inadvertent endobronchial intubation.

Figure 11-16 shows data from four different oxygenation monitors plotted as functions of time for an animal undergoing general anesthesia at an fractional concentration of inspired oxygen (FiO_2) of 0.5.[83] In addition to SpO_2, the plot shows PaO_2 values from sequential arterial blood samples, transcutaneous oxygen tension ($P_{TC}O_2$), and oxygen tension from an intraarterial fiberoptic "optode" blood gas sensor ($OpPO_2$). At 0 minutes on the time axis, the endotracheal tube was advanced from the trachea into the left mainstem bronchus. Within 3 minutes, the PaO_2 decreased from 360 mm Hg to 120 mm Hg, and the $P_{TC}O_2$ and $OpPO_2$ values also fell significantly. However, SpO_2 never fell below 98% during the entire experiment. In this situation, the pulse oximeter provided no indication that an endobronchial intubation had taken place, whereas the other monitoring techniques all showed significant changes. Only when the experiment was repeated for FiO_2 values of 0.3 or less did the pulse oximeter display consistent SpO_2 decreases of 6% or more. This illustrates an important physiologic limitation of saturation monitoring: when increased FiO_2 is used, the PaO_2 value must decrease far below its baseline before the pulse oximeter will alert the clinician. Metaphorically speaking, the pulse oximeter is a sentry standing on the edge of the cliff of desaturation (see Fig. 11-2), and it gives no warning as we approach the edge; it only sounds an alarm when we have fallen off.

Finally, no discussion of a clinical device is complete without a description of the risks and complications of the monitoring process. Because the pulse oximeter is noninvasive and typically does not produce heat or radiation, these risks might be expected to be nonexistent. Because of human error, however, this is unfortunately not true. In a case report, a Physio-Control (Redmond, WA) pulse oximeter sensor was mistakenly connected to an Ohmeda (now GE Healthcare) instrument.[84] The two oximeters used the same electrical connector for the sensor, but the internal pin connections were different; this resulted in severe thermal burns to both the finger and the earlobe of a newborn infant. The lesson from this case is that compatibility between sensor and instrument must be ensured before a sensor is placed on a patient. This risk has been reduced in more recent designs, but the clinician should never assume that just because the plug fits, it is acceptable to interconnect sensors and instruments of different manufacturers.

The pulse oximeter is unquestionably the most important advance in oxygen monitoring since the development of the blood gas analyzer. It is the only oxygen monitor that provides continuous, real-time, noninvasive data on arterial oxygenation without the need for user calibration. Because it is noninvasive and *almost* risk free, the pulse oximeter should be used in all clinical settings in which risk of arterial hypoxemia is present. It is a minimum standard of care in the OR and is rapidly becoming a standard in most other critical care settings. Hypoxia remains the most common cause of anesthesia-related preventable death.[85,86] Therefore the prudent use of pulse oximetry is a fundamental responsibility of the anesthesiologist.

The pulse oximeter is not an ideal instrument because it is subject to both measurement error and physiologic limitations.[87-95] With an understanding of the physics and engineering principles of pulse oximetry as outlined in this chapter, the astute clinician will be aware of measurement errors and when they are likely to occur. The impact of these errors also can be minimized by obtaining appropriate supportive data. For example, a smoke inhalation victim should have carboxyhemoglobin levels determined by in vitro CO oximetry or be monitored with a multiwavelength pulse oximeter capable of measuring COHb.[21] The pulse oximeter signal/noise ratio should be optimized by careful sensor application, prevention of ambient light from reaching the sensor, and consideration of alternative sensor sites in patients who are shivering or who have diminished peripheral pulses. The avoidance of hypoxia is a fundamental goal of every anesthesiologist, and an understanding of the physics and physiology of arterial saturation monitoring by pulse oximetry will help accomplish this task.

REFERENCES

1. Brown LJ: A new instrument for the simultaneous measurement of total hemoglobin, % oxyhemoglobin, % carboxyhemoglobin, % methemoglobin, and oxygen content in whole blood, *IEEE Trans Biomed Eng* 27:132–138, 1980.
2. Stephen CR, Slater HM, Johnson AL, et al: The oximeter: a technical aid for the anesthesiologist, *Anesthesiology* 12:541–555, 1951.
3. Knill RL, Clement JL, Kieraszewicz HT, et al: Assessment of two noninvasive monitors of arterial oxygenation in anesthetized man, *Anesth Analg* 61:582–586, 1982.
4. Severinghaus JW, Astrup PB: History of blood gas analysis. VI, Oximetry, *J Clin Monit* 2:270–288, 1986.
5. Wukitsch MW, Tobler D, Pologe J, et al: Pulse oximetry: an analysis of theory, technology and practice, *J Clin Monit* 4:290–301, 1988.
6. Barker SJ, Tremper KK: The effect of carbon monoxide inhalation on pulse oximetry and transcutaneous PO_2, *Anesthesiology* 66:677–679, 1987.
7. Barker SJ, Tremper KK, Hyatt J: Effects of methemoglobinemia on pulse oximetry and mixed venous oximetry, *Anesthesiology* 70:112–117, 1989.
8. Chui J, Poon W, Chan K, Chan A, Buckley T: Nitrite-induced methemoglobinaemia: aetiology, diagnosis, and treatment, *Anaesthesia* 60:496–500, 2005.
9. Cornelissen PJH, van Del WC, de Jong PA: Correction factors for hemoglobin derivatives in fetal blood as measured with the IL282 CO oximeter, *Clin Chem* 29:1555–1556, 1983.
10. Craft JA, Alessandrini E, Kenney LB, et al: Comparison of oxygenation measurements in pediatric patients during sickle cell crises, *J Pediatr* 124:93–95, 1994.
11. Rackoff WR, Kunkel N, Silber JH, et al: Pulse oximetry and factors associated with hemoglobin oxygen desaturation in children with sickle cell disease, *Blood* 81:3422–3427, 1993.
12. Weston Smith SG, Glass UH, Acharya J: Pearson TC: Pulse oximetry in sickle cell disease, *Clin Lab Haematol* 11:185–188, 1989.
13. Das A, Sinha S, Hoyer J: Hemoglobin Bassett produces low pulse oximeter and co-oximeter readings, *Chest* 131:1242–1244, 2007.
14. Scheller MS, Unger RJ, Kelner MJ: Effects of intravenously administered dyes on pulse oximetry readings, *Anesthesiology* 65:550–552, 1986.
15. Veyckemans F, Baele P, Guillaume JE, et al: Hyperbilirubinemia does not interfere with hemoglobin saturation measured by pulse oximetry, *Anesthesiology* 70:118–122, 1989.
16. Coté CJ, Goldstein EA, Fuchsman WH, et al: The effect of nail polish on pulse oximetry, *Anesth Analg* 67:683–686, 1988.
17. Aoyagi T, Miyasaka K: The theory and applications of pulse spectrophotometry, *Anesth Analg* 94:S93–S95, 2002.
18. Noiri E, Kobayashi N, Takamura Y, et al: Pulse total hemoglobinometer provides accurate noninvasive monitoring, *Crit Care Med* 33: E2831, 2005.
19. Petrov Y, Petrova I, Patrikeev I, Esenaliev R, Prough D: Multiwavelength optoacoustic system for noninvasive monitoring of cerebral venous oxygenation: a pilot clinical test in the internal jugular vein, *Optics Letters* 31:1827–1829, 2006.
20. Nelson L, McCann J, Loepke A, Wu J: Development and validation of a multiwavelength spatial domain near-infrared oximeter to detect cerebral hypoxia-ischemia, *J Biomed Opt* 11(6), 2006. 064022.
21. Barker S, Curry J, Redford D, Morgan S: Measurement of carboxyhemoglobin and methemoglobin by pulse oximetry, *Anesthesiology* 105:892–897, 2006.
22. Coulange M, Barthelemy A, Hug F, Thierry A, DeHaro L: Reliability of new pulse CO-oximeter in victims of carbon monoxide poisoning, *Undersea Hyperb Med* 32(2):1–5, 2005.
23. Layne T, Snyder C, Brooks D, Enjeti S: *Evaluation of a new pulse CO-oximeter: non-invasive measurement of carboxyhemoglobin in the outpatient pulmonary lab and emergency departments.* Presented at the 52nd Annual Meeting of the American Association for Respiratory Care (AARC), Las Vegas, December 2006.
24. Hampson N, Ecker E, Scott K: Use of noninvasive pulse CO-oximeter to measure blood carboxyhemoglobin levels in bingo players, *Resp Care* 51(7):758–760, 2006.
25. Light A, Grass C, Pursley D, Krause J: *Carboxyhemoglobin levels in smokers vs. non-smokers in a smoking environment.* Presented at the 52nd Annual Meeting of the American Association for Respiratory Care (AARC), Las Vegas, December 2006.
26. Hostler D, Roth R, Kaufman R, et al: The incidence of carbon monoxide poisoning during CO alarm investigations, *Pre-Hospital Emergency Care* 12(1):115, 2008.
27. Ben-Eli D, Peruggia J, McFarland J, et al: Detecting CO: FDNY studies prehospital assessment of COHb, *JEMS* 32(10):S36–S37, 2007.
28. Dickinson E, Mecham C, Thom S, Shofer F, Band R: The noninvasive carboxyhemoglobin monitoring of firefighters engaged in fire suppression and overhaul operations, *Pre-Hospital Emergency Care* 12(1):96, 2008.
29. Plante T, Harris D, Savitt J, et al: Carboxyhemoglobin monitored by bedside continuous CO-oximetry, *J Trauma* 63(5):1187–1190, 2007.
30. Li Z, Gao C, Huang X, Wang G, Ge H: Clinical analyses of 429 cases of acute CO poisoning, *Anesthesiology* 107: A1490, 2007.
31. Suner S, Partridge R, Sucov A, et al: Non-invasive pulse CO-oximetry screening in the emergency department identifies occult carbon monoxide toxicity, *J Emerg Med* 34(4):441–450, 2008.
32. Throm M, Stevens M, Hansen C: Benzocaine-induced methemoglobinemia in two patients: interdisciplinary collaboration, management, and near misses, *Pharmacotherapy* 27(8):1206–1214, 2007.
33. Ash-Bernal R, Wise R, Wright S: Acquired methemoglobinemia: a retrospective series of 138 cases at two teaching hospitals, *Medicine* 83(5):265–273, 2004.
34. Macknet M, Kimball-Jones P, Applegate R, Martin R, Allard M: Benzocaine induced methemoglobinemia after TEE, *Respir Care* 52(11), 2007.
35. Barker SJ, Annabi EH: Life-threatening methemoglobinemia detected by pulse oximetry: a case report, *Anesth Analg* 108(3):898–899, 2009.
36. Macknet M, Norton S, Kimball-Jones P, et al: Continuous noninvasive measurement of hemoglobin via pulse CO-oximetry, *Anesth Analg* 105(6): 2007, S-108.

36a. Macknet MR, Allard M, Applegate RL II, Rook J: The accuracy of noninvasive and continuous total hemoglobin measurement by pulse CO-oximetry in human subjects undergoing hemodilution, *Anesth Analg* 111:1424–1426, 2010.

37. Allard M, Viljoen J: *Casual screening of haemoglobin noninvasively positively affects a colleague's future? A case report.* 14th Annual World Congress of Anesthesiology; March 2008, Capetown, South Africa. Accessed online at http://www.wca2008.com/images/abstractWCA/monitoring.pdf.
38. Pologe JA: Pulse oximetry: technical aspects of machine design, *Int Anesthesiol Clin* 25:137–153, 1987.
39. Kelleher JF, Ruff RH: The penumbra effect: vasomotion-dependent pulse oximeter artifact due to probe malposition, *Anesthesiology* 71:787–791, 1989.
40. Barker SJ, Hyatt J, Shah NK, et al: The effect of sensor malpositioning on pulse oximeter accuracy during hypoxemia, *Anesthesiology* 79:248–254, 1993.
41. Lawson D, Norley I, Korbon G, et al: Blood flow limits and pulse oximeter signal detection, *Anesthesiology* 67:599–603, 1987.
42. Narang VPS: Utility of the pulse oximeter during cardiopulmonary resuscitation, *Anesthesiology* 65:239–240, 1986.
43. Nowak GS, Moorthy SS, McNiece WL: Use of pulse oximetry for assessment of collateral arterial flow, *Anesthesiology* 64:527, 1986.
44. Skeehan TM, Hensley FA Jr: Axillary artery compression and the prone position, *Anesth Analg* 65:518–519, 1986.
45. Barrington KJ, Ryan CA, Finer NN: Pulse oximetry during hemorrhagic hypotension and cardiopulmonary resuscitation in the rabbit, *J Crit Care* 1:242–246, 1986.
46. Freund PR, Overand PT, Cooper J, et al: A prospective study of intraoperative pulse oximetry failure, *J Clin Monit* 7:253–258, 1991.
47. Reich DL, Timcenko A, Bodian CA, et al: Predictors of pulse oximetry data failure, *Anesthesiology* 84:859–864, 1996.

48. Moller JT, et al: Randomized evaluation of pulse oximetry in 20,802 patients, *Anesthesiology* 78:436–453, 1993.
49. Severinghaus JW, Spellman MJ Jr: Pulse oximeter failure thresholds in hypotension and vasoconstriction, *Anesthesiology* 73:532–537, 1990.
50. Graham B, Paulus DA, Caffee HH: Pulse oximetry for vascular monitoring in upper extremity replantation surgery, *J Hand Surg* 11A:687–692, 1986.
51. Lawless ST: Crying wolf: false alarms in a pediatric intensive care unit, *Crit Care Med* 22:981–985, 1994.
52. *Nellcor N-200 pulse oximetry note number 6: C-Lock ECG synchronization principles of operation*, Hayward, California, 1988, Nellcor.
53. Barker SJ, Shah NK: Effects of motion on the performance of pulse oximeters in volunteers, *Anesthesiology* 86:101–108, 1997.
54. Barker SJ: "Motion-resistant" pulse oximetry: a comparison of new and old models, *Anesth Analg* 95:967–972, 2002.
55. Dumas C, Wahr JA, Tremper KK: Clinical evaluation of a prototype motion artifact resistant pulse oximeter in the recovery room, *Anesth Analg* 83(2):269–272, 1996.
56. Kim JM, Arakawa K, Benson KT, et al: Pulse oximetry and circulatory kinetics associated with pulse volume amplitude measured by photoelectric plethysmography, *Anesth Analg* 65:1333–1339, 1986.
57. Bohnhorst B, Peter CS, Poets CF: Pulse oximeters' reliability in detecting hypoxemia and bradycardia: comparison between a conventional and two new-generation oximeters, *Crit Care Med* 28(5):1565–1568, 2000.
58. Malviya S, Reynolds PI, Voepel-Lewis T, et al: False alarms and sensitivity of conventional pulse oximetry versus the Masimo SET technology in the pediatric postanesthesia care unit, *Anesth Analg* 90(6):1336–1340, 2000.
59. Bland JM, Altman DG: Statistical methods for assessing agreement between two methods of clinical measurement, *Lancet* 1:307–310, 1986.
60. Tremper KK, Barker SJ: Pulse oximetry, *Anesthesiology* 70:98–108, 1989.
61. Severinghaus JW, Kelleher JF: Recent developments in pulse oximetry, *Anesthesiology* 76:1018–1038, 1992.
62. Severinghaus JW, Naifeh KH: Accuracy of response of six pulse oximeters to profound hypoxia, *Anesthesiology* 67:551–558, 1987.
63. Kagle DM, Alexander CM, Berko RS, et al: Evaluation of the Ohmeda 3700 pulse oximeter: steady-state and transient response characteristics, *Anesthesiology* 66:376–380, 1987.
64. Severinghaus JW, Naifeh KH, Koh SO: Errors in 14 pulse oximeters during profound hypoxia, *J Clin Monit* 5:72–81, 1989.
65. Barker SJ, Hyatt J: Forehead reflectance pulse oximetry: time response to rapid saturation change, *Anesthesiology* 73(3A):A544, 1990.
66. Barker SJ, Le N, Hyatt J: Failure rates of transmission and reflectance pulse oximetry for various sensor sites, *J Clin Monit* 7:102–103, 1991.
67. Kussmaul A: Über schwielige Mediastino-Peikarditis und den paradoxen Puls, *Berl Klin Wochenschr* 10:433–435, 445-449, 461-464, 1873.
68. Cohn JN, Pinkerton AL, Tristani FE: Mechanism of pulsus paradoxus in clinical shock, *J Clin Investigation* 46(11):1744–1755, 1967.
69. Michard F, Boussat S, Chemla D, et al: Relation between respiratory changes in arterial pulse pressure and fluid responsiveness in septic patients with acute circulatory failure, *Am J Respir Crit Care Med* 162:134–138, 2000.
70. Lopes MR, Oliveira MA, Pereira VO, et al: Goal-directed fluid management based on pulse pressure variation monitoring during high-risk surgery: a pilot randomized controlled trial, *Crit Care* 11: R100, 2007.
71. Michard F: Changes in arterial pressure during mechanical ventilation, *Anesthesiology* 103:419–428, 2005.
72. Partridge BL: Use of pulse oximetry as a non-invasive indicator of intravascular volume status, *J Clin Monitoring* 3:263–268, 1987.
73. Canneson M, Delannoy B, Morand A, et al: Does pleth variability index indicate the respiratory-induced variation in the plethysmogram and arterial pressure waveforms? *Anesth Analg* 106:1189–1194, 2008.
74. Canneson M, Desebbe O, Rosamel P, et al: Pleth variability index to monitor the respiratory variations in the pulse oximeter plethysmographic waveform amplitude and predict fluid responsiveness in the operating theatre, *Br J Anaesth* 101(2):200–206, 2008.
75. Canneson M, Slieker J, Desebbe O, et al: The ability of a novel algorithm for automatic estimation of the respiratory variations in arterial pulse pressure to monitor fluid responsiveness in the operating room, *Anesth Analg* 106:1195–1200, 2008.
76. American Society of Anesthesiologists: Standards for basic intraoperative monitoring, *Anesthesia Patient Safety Newsletter*, 1987; March:3.
77. Eichhorn JH, Cooper JB, Cullen DJ, et al: Standards for patient monitoring during anesthesia at Harvard Medical School, *JAMA* 256:1017–1020, 1986.
78. Coté CJ, Goldstein EA, Coté MA, et al: A single-blind study of pulse oximetry in children, *Anesthesiology* 68:184–188, 1988.
79. Pullerits J, Burrows FA, Roy WL: Arterial desaturation in healthy children during transfer to the recovery room, *Can J Anaesth* 34:470–473, 1987.
80. Tyler IL, Tantisira B, Winter PM, et al: Continuous monitoring of arterial oxygen saturation with pulse oximetry during transfer to the recovery room, *Anesth Analg* 64:1108–1112, 1985.
81. Soliman IE, Patel RI, Ehrenpreis MB, et al: Recovery scores do not correlate with postoperative hypoxemia in children, *Anesth Analg* 67:53–56, 1988.
82. Morris RW, Buschman A, Warren DL, Philip JH, Reamer DB: The prevalence of hypoxemia detected by pulse oximetry during recovery from anesthesia, *J Clin Monit* 4:16–20, 1988.
83. Barker SJ, Tremper KK, Hyatt J, et al: Comparison of three oxygen monitors in detecting endobronchial intubation, *J Clin Monit* 4:240–243, 1988.
84. Murphy KG, Segunda JA, Rockoff MA: Severe burns from a pulse oximeter, *Anesthesiology* 73:350–352, 1990.
85. Keenan RL, Boyan CP: Cardiac arrest due to anesthesia: a study of incidence and causes, *JAMA* 253:2373–2377, 1985.
86. Taylor G, Larson CP Jr, Prestwich R: Unexpected cardiac arrest during anesthesia and surgery: an environmental study, *JAMA* 236:2758–2760, 1976.
87. Chapman KR, Liu FLW, Watson RM, et al: Range of accuracy of two-wavelength oximetry, *Chest* 4:540–542, 1986.
88. Nickerson BG, Sakrison C, Tremper KK: Bias and precision of pulse oximeters and arterial oximeters, *Chest* 93:515–517, 1988.
89. Mihm FG, Halperin BD: Noninvasive detection of profound arterial desaturations using a pulse oximetry device, *Anesthesiology* 62:85–87, 1985.
90. Cecil WT, Thorpe KJ, Fibuch EE, et al: A clinical evaluation of the accuracy of the Nellcor N-100 and the Ohmeda 3700 pulse oximeters, *J Clin Monit* 4:31–36, 1988.
91. Fait CD, Wetzel RC, Dean JM, et al: Pulse oximetry in critically ill children, *J Clin Monit* 1:232–235, 1985.
92. Boxer RA, Gottesfeld I, Singh S, et al: Non-invasive pulse oximetry in children with cyanotic congenital heart disease, *Crit Care Med* 15:1062–1064, 1987.
93. Mok J, Pintar M, Benson L, et al: Evaluation of noninvasive measurements of oxygenation in stable infants, *Crit Care Med* 14:960–963, 1986.
94. Durand M, Ramanathan R: Pulse oximetry for continuous oxygen monitoring in six newborn infants, *J Pediatr* 109:1052–1055, 1986.
95. Yelderman M, New W: Evaluation of pulse oximetry, *Anesthesiology* 59:349–352, 1983.

CHAPTER 12

Blood Pressure Monitoring

Brenton Alexander • Maxime Cannesson • Timothy J. Quill

CHAPTER OUTLINE

OVERVIEW

The frequent measurement of blood pressure during anesthetic administration is a standard practice throughout the world. Because of significant intraoperative blood pressure variance—combined with the presumed value of accurate, frequent, repeatable determinations in predicting certain intraoperative and postoperative problems—the trend in recent years in developed countries has been almost completely toward the use of automatic, digital, electromechanical instrumentation. Many of these devices function quite well and require minimal effort and limited special training. This chapter discusses the most common instrumentation and methods for measuring blood pressure currently in clinical use. This includes principles of operation, perceived advantages and disadvantages, relative accuracy, and factors that may affect operation. It is assumed that the reader is aware of recommended and normal limits for blood pressure and the medical implications of abnormal values.

HISTORY OF BLOOD PRESSURE MEASUREMENT

Nearly every practicing physician is familiar with the originally reported measurement of blood pressure obtained by the Reverend Stephen Hales, who cannulated the femoral artery of a horse and measured the average height of the blood column at approximately 9 feet, corresponding to 200 millimeters of mercury (mm Hg) or 27 kilopascals (kPa). Hales also described respiratory variation and pulsatile pressure, a remarkable achievement in the eighteenth century. Further work was limited until the late nineteenth century, when numerous investigators described noninvasive blood pressure determinations. The auscultatory method of Korotkoff (1905) has been the most common method for blood pressure determination for the past 100 years. However, the oscillometric technique originally described by Roy and Adami in 1890 rapidly gained popularity in the late twentieth century and is the theoretical basis for most automated, noninvasive, blood pressure–measuring equipment manufactured today.

Definitions of Blood Pressure

Accompanying the development of various methods of blood pressure determination was controversy over the actual definition of systolic, diastolic, and mean blood pressures. For invasive methods that produce a pulsatile waveform, the definitions are simple: *systolic pressure* is the maximum instantaneous pressure, *diastolic pressure* is the minimum instantaneous pressure, and *mean pressure* is the area under the waveform-time curve divided by the time interval for one or more beats, a quantity easily determined with simple software.

Blood pressure determinations are highly dependent on the anatomic site being measured.[1] Usually there is an increase in systolic values and a decrease in diastolic values as blood pressure is measured more peripherally in the vascular tree of healthy subjects. Because of the opposite changes of the systolic and diastolic values, mean blood pressure normally remains relatively constant as the measurement site changes. In patients with vascular disease and resultant restricted arterial flow, further errors are introduced that usually produce decreases in systolic, diastolic, and mean flow at more distal locations. Despite these well-known predictable errors, the radial arterial pressure—determined by a small cannula inserted near the wrist, combined with an electronic transducer and digital display system—has become the de facto clinical standard of comparison for human blood pressure determinations. Nearly all published methodology comparisons and so-called accuracy studies use the radial arterial pressure as the reference standard. This is done despite the fact that the choice of the radial artery is more one of safety and convenience than of scientific validity.

Much less affected by arterial system variables is the central aortic root pressure, probably a much more reliable standard, although measurement of aortic root pressure in humans generally involves unacceptable risk.

Instrumentation and Units of Measure

Several different types and models of automated noninvasive blood pressure instrumentation have become available in the United States in recent years, and their use has become ubiquitous in anesthesia over much of the world. Each approach measures different physical quantities, from which values for systolic, diastolic, and mean blood pressure are derived. Noninvasive blood pressure readings never correlate exactly with measured invasive radial arterial blood pressure, irrespective of construction and calibration precision. It is always hoped, however, that the accuracy of any method is such that differences between readings are of little clinical significance. In general, this is true for most commercial oscillometric instruments, although other noninvasive methods do not consistently perform as well in all situations. Reliability of modern automated noninvasive oscillometric equipment has reached the point where it is unnecessary to validate the automated unit with an older method, such as auscultation, because the manual approach is less reliable and more subjective than the automated method and most often represents a step down in accuracy.

The standard unit of measure for blood pressure in the United States is millimeters of mercury (mm Hg), or *torr*, in which 760 mm Hg equals 1 standard atmosphere of pressure at sea level. Elsewhere in the world, the kilopascal (kPa) often is the standard unit of pressure measurement (1 kPa = 7.5 mm Hg). Most commercial digital blood pressure instrumentation provides a readout to within 1 mm Hg, although this implied significance considerably exceeds the actual precision and repeatability of even the best invasive units and certainly does not provide meaningful additional clinical information. The actual precision of the best noninvasive devices is approximately 5 to 10 mm Hg. Calibration accuracy of noninvasive blood pressure devices is most often measured and adjusted by the manufacturer through comparison with radial arterial blood pressure in healthy human subjects. This method obviously involves limitations, not the least of which is using average values without adjustment for anatomic differences, such as body habitus.

As mentioned, radial arterial pressure correlates well with central aortic pressure in healthy subjects,[1] but the two values may disagree by a considerable amount, especially in hypertensive and hyperdynamic patients and in patients with peripheral vasoconstriction or vascular disease.[2] In addition, every noninvasive method measures blood pressure indirectly, by inference from measured physical quantities,[3] such as cuff air-pressure oscillations; the correlation with invasive pressure is never perfect, even under the best of circumstances. This should be kept in mind when interpreting noninvasive blood pressure readings.

Reference Points

If the aortic root is taken as the desired reference point for blood pressure, all measurement techniques must take into account the effect of gravity and the water column hydrostatic pressure that results from a difference of height between the aortic root and the location of the transducer. This amounts to a difference of approximately 7.5 mm Hg for every 10-cm difference in vertical height from the aortic root. The effect is small for a brachial cuff, but it can be large (>50 mm Hg) if, for example, the pressure transducer is accidentally positioned improperly, or if an ankle cuff is used on an individual in a sitting position. Under these circumstances, an accurate pressure can still be obtained, but the operator must add or subtract a fixed amount to the measured blood pressure. This applies to both noninvasive and invasive instruments. Some novel and practical methods have been suggested to accomplish this compensation in everyday clinical situations,[4] but the general rule that 10 cm equals 7.5 mm Hg or 1 kPa always works.

Manual (Riva-Rocci) Measurement Technique

The measurement of blood pressure with an air-inflatable cuff placed on the proximal arm, listening with a stethoscope over the brachial artery for Korotkoff sounds as cuff pressure is slowly decreased, remains the most common and inexpensive method of blood pressure determination. This method was originally described by Scipione Riva-Rocci in the mid-nineteenth century. Five distinct sound phases are heard as pressure decreases from above systolic to below diastolic: in phase I, clear tapping sounds are heard; in phase II, sounds become softer and longer; in phase III, they become crisper and louder; in phase IV, sounds become muffled and softer; and in phase V, sounds completely disappear.[5] Systolic blood pressure is measured as the onset of phase I, and diastolic is measured at the onset of phase V. Mean blood pressure (BP) is not specifically measured, but it often is approximated as follows:

$$\text{Mean BP} = \text{DP} + \tfrac{1}{3}(\text{SP} - \text{DP})$$

where *DP* is diastolic pressure and *SP* is systolic pressure. The advantages of the Riva-Rocci (auscultatory) technique are numerous and include low cost, simplicity, lack of dependence on electricity, and ruggedness. This method suffers from imperfect correlation with invasive measurement of blood pressure because of numerous factors, such as ambient noise, auditory acuity of the clinician, atherosclerotic vascular changes, obesity, and cuff size in relation to the limb.[6] In healthy patients, however, the clinical accuracy is high. Riva-Rocci blood pressure is generally biased low (10 to 30 mm Hg) for systolic blood pressure and high (5 to 25 mm Hg) for diastolic pressure, especially in hypertensive patients.[7] The precision (scatter) is approximately ±20 mm Hg compared with invasive radial arterial pressure.[8] The errors are exacerbated by obesity, edema, and vascular disease. In critically ill hypotensive patients, it is often impossible to obtain a reliable auscultatory blood pressure without resorting to Doppler flow-sensing devices to detect the arterial blood flow. With the increased use of pulse oximetry, systolic pressure can be reliably measured with a much improved sensitivity over manual palpation or Korotkoff sounds by noting the point of occlusion of pulsatile flow in the finger through the observation of the corresponding pulse waveform on the oximeter display.[9] Despite a lack of accuracy and subjectivity compared with automated and invasive methods, manual auscultatory measurement of blood pressure is commonly used for healthy, nonsurgical patients because of the low cost and the unimportance of small errors in the healthy population.

Multiple techniques exist for the physical measurement of cuff pressure throughout deflation. Mercury sphygmomanometers are the more traditional approach, but aneroid and hybrid devices have been consistently increasing in popularity. Actual mercury manometers have mostly disappeared from developed countries because of environmental concerns with liquid mercury. Hybrid devices generally use an electronic pressure gauge that is digitally displayed, replacing the mercury column and circular scale of Bourdon tube mechanical gauges. Hybrid devices usually have the option for the displayed pressure to stop decreasing when significant systolic, diastolic, and mean pressure levels are reached. All pressure techniques are comparable when used properly, although more modern devices are easier to use.

During the 1970s, several automated devices were introduced, such as the Roche Arteriosonde (Roche Diagnostics, Indianapolis, IN), which used the Riva-Rocci technique to measure blood pressure automatically and noninvasively. These devices incorporated either a small microphone or a Doppler transducer built into the cuff, which was placed over the brachial artery, and the cuff was inflated automatically by an air pump. These devices proved to be more technically complicated than oscillometric devices introduced later; they have gradually disappeared from clinical use and are no longer manufactured.

OSCILLOMETRIC BLOOD PRESSURE DEVICES

It is common to observe pulsatile pressure variation in the air pressure gauge during manual measurement of blood pressure using auscultation. Oscillometric cuff blood pressure measurement methods take advantage of this pulsatile variation to allow the extrapolation of arterial blood pressure. The simplest manual technique is to deflate the cuff slowly from a pressure above the expected systolic value. At a pressure roughly corresponding to systolic arterial pressure, the needle of the pressure gauge begins to oscillate slightly (1 to 5 mm Hg) with each cardiac contraction (Fig. 12-1). This value is assumed to be the systolic pressure, and for many years this was the standard method of measuring blood pressure in children, in whom Korotkoff sounds are difficult to hear. An enhancement of this technique was the oscillotonometer, an obsolete mechanical device equipped with two cuffs and a sensitive gauge designed to greatly amplify the observed oscillations and thus increase the sensitivity. The mean pressure is usually assumed to be the cuff pressure that produces the maximum amplitude of oscillations. The diastolic pressure is difficult to measure directly by oscillometric methods, because the oscillations decrease gradually as cuff pressure decreases below

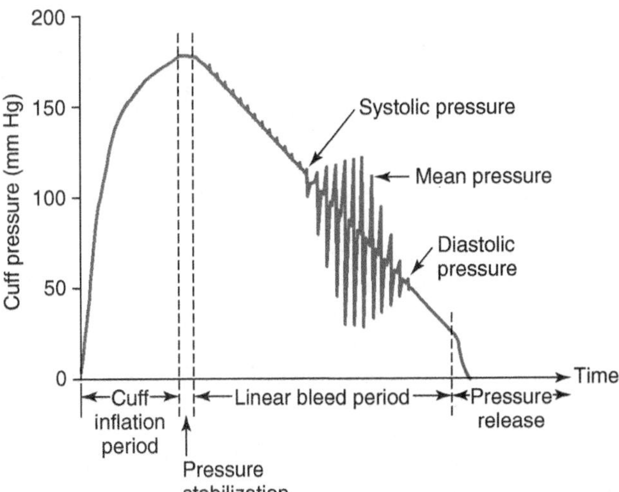

FIGURE 12-1 Observed oscillations in cuff pressure during deflation. The amplitude of oscillations is greatly exaggerated.

the actual diastolic arterial value. The mechanical oscillotonometer lost popularity with the development of automated devices.

Many different electronic oscillometric devices have been developed and commercially introduced and have subsequently become very widely used. Although the specific algorithms used to determine systolic, diastolic, and mean blood pressure values are often proprietary with the manufacturer, it is likely that all of the devices function in a manner similar to the manual oscillometric techniques described above. Cuff pressure is first increased above the expected systolic blood pressure value and then is slowly and gradually decreased, while the pressure oscillations in the cuff are measured electronically. Computation of the diastolic blood pressure is inferred mathematically from the mean value (peak of oscillation strength), the systolic value, and from the characteristics of the "tail" as oscillations decrease at low pressures. Models manufactured since the mid-1980s use high-performance microprocessors and perform remarkably well.[10] They generally incorporate automatic repeated measurement at predetermined time intervals, automatic recording, serial data outputs, and sophisticated alarms.

Automatic oscillometric blood pressure devices offer multiple advantages over manual devices. They eliminate clinician subjectivity and, for a noninvasive monitor, introduce an unprecedented degree of repeatability in regard to subsequent readings. In addition to improved quality and accuracy, automatic devices have been shown to decrease the incidence of "white coat hypertension," the increase in patient blood pressure as a result of being in a medical setting.[11] Larger differences between automatic and auscultatory approaches have been shown to occur more frequently when recorded inconsistencies are apparent in the pressure waveforms.[12] The automated algorithms are presumably optimized to correlate well with invasive blood pressure readings in the average healthy subject. Values have been shown to be algorithm dependent, which indicates a need for a standardized approach.[13] Even so, the precision and bias of well-designed units are generally less than 10 mm Hg.[10]

The oscillometric cuff is the same as the one used for manual auscultatory methods, and problems related to this method remain. In particular, atherosclerosis, edema, obesity, and chronic hypertension introduce errors in systolic (measures too low) and diastolic (measures too high) oscillometric blood pressures when the cuff is used compared with invasive arterial pressure measurements.[14] Using the improper cuff size also introduces significant errors[6]: cuffs that are larger than needed produce erroneously low oscillometric readings, and cuffs that are too small produce higher readings. The proper cuff width has been found to be approximately 46% of arm circumference.[15] Intermittent automated blood pressure monitoring also interferes with ipsilateral intravenous (IV) access and pulse oximetry.

Assuming a properly sized cuff, oscillometric units usually function adequately for obese patients and for children, for whom auscultatory methods fail. Oscillometric cuffs also work well on the calf, ankle, or thigh, a fact often overlooked by the clinician. Finally, the accuracy of an infant cuff used on the adult thumb seems to also be acceptable when brachial or lower extremity cuffs are precluded.[16]

INVASIVE BLOOD PRESSURE MONITORING

Invasive blood pressure monitoring often is the clinical method of choice if large hemodynamic changes are expected or encountered, frequent blood sampling is anticipated, or there is a need for continuous, accurate, beat-to-beat blood pressure determination.[17] The majority of continuous electrocardiograph monitoring units sold in the United States also have the capability to simultaneously measure invasive and noninvasive blood pressure. Besides the obvious advantage of allowing arterial blood sampling, the invasive method provides unsurpassed reliability and accuracy, especially when extremes of blood pressure are expected.

The usual method of invasive blood pressure monitoring consists of the percutaneous insertion of a small-bore (18- to 22-gauge) plastic catheter into a peripheral artery. The catheter is physically connected via high-pressure plastic tubing to an electronic pressure transducer and display unit. The transducer is a sterile, miniature, self-contained assembly that contains the electromechanical components within a clear plastic case. Most transducers incorporate an integral mechanism for providing a continuous, slow flush of sterile solution through the tubing and catheter to prevent clotting. In addition, a mechanism for rapid manual flushing is provided. The entire assembly is designed for single-patient use at a cost of approximately $15 per patient. The use of solid-state, individually calibrated instruments has greatly improved the accuracy over older, partially disposable systems.[18] In general, an absolute accuracy of 5 mm Hg or better throughout the measurement range can be expected. Identical redundant transducer systems typically are used if central venous or pulmonary arterial pressures are simultaneously monitored.

Invasive arterial blood pressure monitoring is not without risk. Potential problems include symptomatic or asymptomatic arterial thrombosis, infection, accidental injection of IV drugs, nerve damage from trauma or hematoma during placement, and exsanguination from accidental disconnection. All these problems have been reported to occur infrequently. Slogoff and colleagues[19] studied arterial cannulation in a large series of surgical patients and concluded that the risks of radial artery cannulation often are exaggerated and that serious morbidity in adults is rare. They also found no evidence to support the long-held beliefs that the shape, size, and material of the catheter and duration of insertion are important predictors of complications. In addition, their study found no objective evidence that noninvasive determination of collateral flow before the catheter is inserted, such as the Allen test, was of any value in predicting morbidity. Furthermore, no evidence suggested that one cannulation site—radial, ulnar, brachial, axillary, femoral, or dorsalis pedis—was safer than another, except perhaps from an infectious disease viewpoint. It is uncertain whether these conclusions can be extended to children and neonates, although the available evidence indicates that arterial cannulation in this population is a reasonably safe procedure.[20]

Arterial cannulation often is painful, and liberal local anesthesia combined with anxiolytic medication is highly recommended for insertion. Although many different insertion techniques have been described—including the guidewire Seldinger technique, transfixion, or direct insertion—most of these methods are successful in trained hands, and there is little reason to suggest that any technique is consistently safer or better than another. Severe hypotension, vascular disease, or previous cannulation can make insertion difficult or impossible. In these cases, direct exposure of the artery via a surgical cutdown may be the only method to cannulate the artery successfully, although infectious complications are much more common with a surgical incision.[21] Also, the use of ultrasound guidance may be useful in these difficult situations.

To minimize possible complications, common sense dictates that arterial catheters should be removed as soon as they are no longer needed.[21] Continuous flushing with heparinized saline at a rate of 5 to 10 mL/h to prevent clotting used to be standard practice. However, because of concerns about heparin-induced thrombocytopenia (HIT, as well as lack of evidence that heparin-containing solutions are superior to plain saline flushing, heparin has been removed from the flush solution. The capability to flush the system automatically has been incorporated into virtually all modern disposable transducer sets. In the intensive care unit (ICU), arterial catheters tend to stop functioning after 1 to 2 weeks because of a combination of arterial inflammation, occlusion, and clot formation. This necessitates removal of the catheter and a change to an alternate site.

Ideally, an invasive blood pressure transducer should be small, reliable, incorporated into the catheter itself, free from nonlinearity and distortion, and inexpensive. Devices approaching this complete ideal are still experimental, but current disposable transducers provide a technology with generally acceptable consistent performance in a reasonably sized package (Fig. 12-2). Many factors influence the accuracy of modern invasive arterial monitoring equipment, not the least of which is the

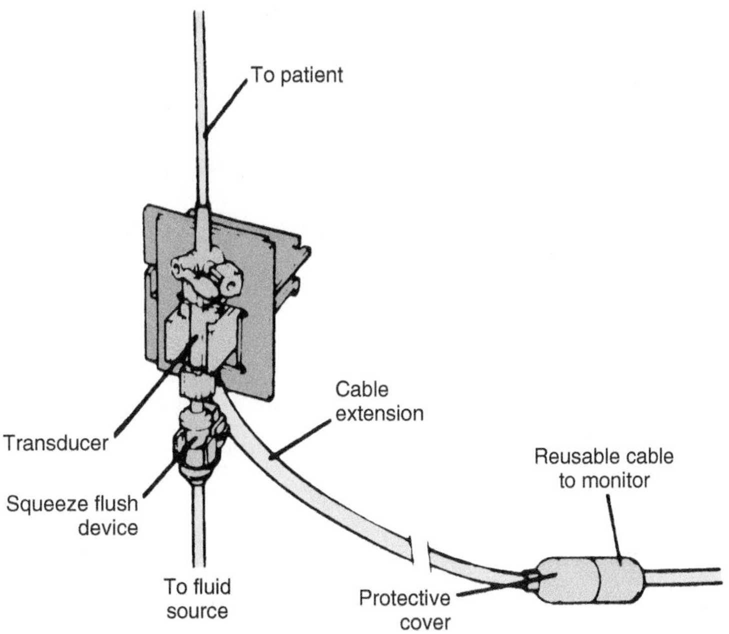

FIGURE 12-2 ■ Typical disposable hemodynamic pressure transducer. (Courtesy Abbott Critical Care Systems, North Chicago, IL.)

ambiguity and disagreement over the exact quantitative definition of blood pressure.[3] Aortic root pressure is the accepted physiologic standard, but safety considerations preclude routine measurement outside the laboratory. Radial arterial pressure reflects aortic pressure well in healthy, young individuals, but this is seldom the condition of patients who require invasive monitoring. As previously mentioned, as the location of the catheter becomes more peripheral, measured systolic pressure tends to increase and diastolic pressure tends to decrease as a result of resonance effects in the arterial tree. Because of the opposing changes of systolic and diastolic blood pressure readings, mean pressure decreases only slightly. Vascular disease and vasoconstriction predictably decrease both systolic and diastolic measurements in proportion to the severity of the condition, and it is fairly common to note an error of 50 mm Hg or more in the cold, severely vasoconstricted patient.[2] In this situation, femoral invasive or brachial noninvasive oscillometric blood pressure readings may more accurately reflect aortic pressure than do radial invasive readings. It should be noted that noninvasive oscillometric blood pressure readings also have been shown to underestimate systolic pressure and overestimate diastolic pressure in first-time stroke patients.[22]

Modern electronic monitors are designed to interface reliably with electromechanical transducer systems without the need for extensive training. A provision for static "zeroing" of the system, eliminating a fixed error, is built into the monitor; after the zeroing procedure is accomplished, the system is ready for operation. As previously mentioned, it is important to position the transducer with the reference point at the approximate level of the aortic root to eliminate the effect of the fluid column height difference. Most monitors display a waveform, preferably with a calibrated scale and a digital numeric display of systolic, diastolic, and mean pressures. Each manufacturer produces an electronic instrument with slightly different, often proprietary, frequency response and filtering algorithms. The various techniques for extracting digital quantities vary from simple peak-and-valley detection to sophisticated algorithms that incorporate digital noise filtering and compensation for artifacts and ringing. Thus it is difficult for two different monitors to read exactly the same numerical blood pressure, although the differences are likely to be clinically insignificant, especially with regard to the mean blood pressure value.

Visualization of the pressure waveform, an important step in assuring the accuracy of digital readings, can be quite useful in qualitatively inferring the inotropic and volume status of the patient. In general, a crisp upstroke implies a more hyperdynamic situation, and a broad peak or plateau of the blood pressure waveform implies adequate diastolic filling and venous volume.[3] Severely hypovolemic patients often demonstrate a sharp upstroke followed by an equally sharp descent nearly to baseline and a secondary, dicrotic wave approximately half the height of the systolic ejection wave. Marked variation of pulse pressure volume (PPV) as a result of the ventilation cycle is often a sign of hypovolemia or tamponade.[23] This can be calculated and displayed in real time using commercially available monitors (Vigileo, LiDCO; Edwards Lifesciences, Irvine, CA) and is increasing in popularity because of the shortage of reliable parameters of fluid status. A marked decrease in the systolic-diastolic difference with a normal mean pressure reading usually indicates a failing catheter or flush system or severe peripheral vasoconstriction.

As blood pressure does not directly correlate well with cardiac output, pulse waveform analysis on invasive arterial pressure waveforms has become a popular approach for minimally invasive cardiac output determinations. This technology has been shown to be reasonably accurate and clinically acceptable, although minimal algorithmic improvements are still necessary.[24] Because of the extreme clinical importance of accurate cardiac output measurement, strong future growth in this field is likely.

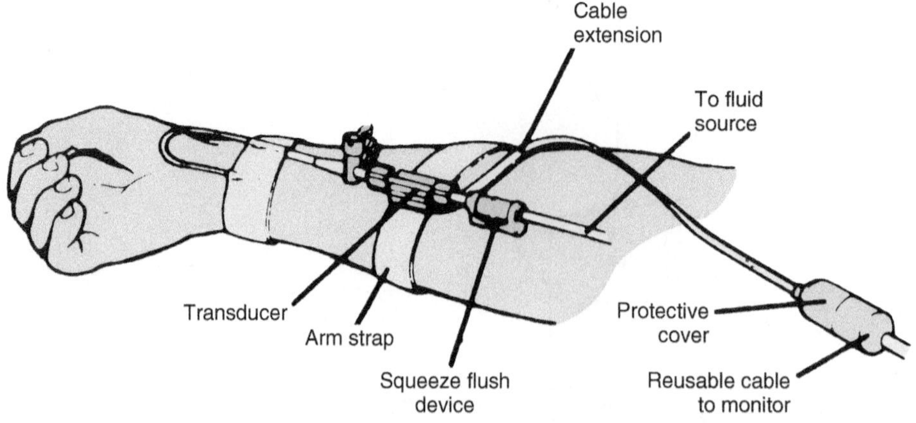

FIGURE 12-3 ■ Recommended setup for invasive, disposable, radial arterial transducer, including short length of connecting tubing.

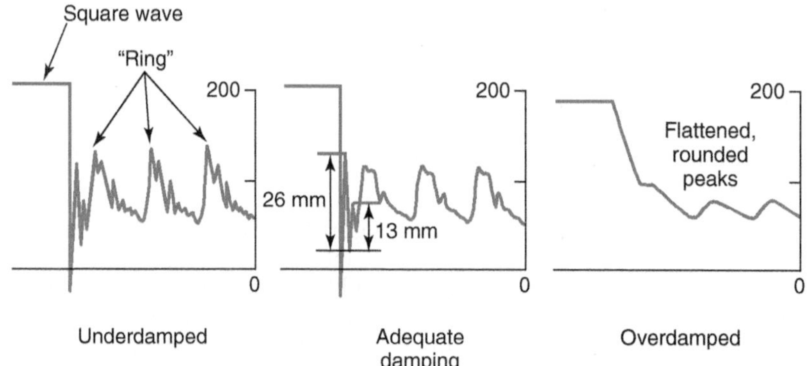

FIGURE 12-4 ■ Effect of damping coefficient on arterial wave morphology. Note the differences in systolic (peak) pressure.

The electromechanical assembly of catheter, transducer, and connecting tubing forms a less than ideal measuring system (Fig. 12-3) with the introduction of resonances and waveform distortion and resultant predictable errors in blood pressure determination.[25] Scaling errors have been all but eliminated with the introduction of disposable, individually calibrated transducers, but older systems require static calibration and comparison with a reference manometer before use.[18] The inherent frequency response of the transducer itself is seldom a limiting factor with modern disposable units, but underdamping and ringing at a characteristic high frequency is the rule.[26] Underdamping increases systolic readings and simultaneously decreases diastolic readings, with little effect on the mean pressure (Fig. 12-4), generally exaggerating the effects of the vascular tree.[1] The fact that the catheter faces into the bloodstream likewise distorts the waveform, produces a pitot-tube effect similar to an airspeed measurement, and exaggerates systolic pressure readings. These errors are especially noticeable in the tachycardic hyperdynamic patient. In practice, resonance errors are usually ignored, in which case mean pressure should be regarded as the value on the basis of which clinical decisions are made. Inexpensive, adjustable, disposable damping devices are available to eliminate the problem of ringing and overshoot and to enable the user to achieve adequate damping (see Fig. 12-4). The use of the shortest possible connecting tubing and careful attention to eliminating air bubbles throughout the system are also essential to ensure accuracy.[26]

In summary, peripheral invasive blood pressure monitoring has become a standard technique in widespread clinical use when continuous, reliable blood pressure monitoring combined with the ability for convenient blood sampling is required. Modern disposable systems enable reasonable accuracy with a minimum of inconvenience. Arterial cannulation in the adult is a reasonably safe procedure to the best of our current knowledge, but it should nevertheless be used only when clinically indicated and appropriate.

CONTINUOUS NONINVASIVE BLOOD PRESSURE MONITORING

Peñaz (Finapres) Technique

The continuous, beat-to-beat measurement of blood pressure is accurately accomplished using an invasive catheter, but this technique involves discomfort and risk for the patient and is not appropriate for use in healthy subjects on a routine basis. Nevertheless, it is desirable to measure blood pressure continuously and noninvasively under many circumstances. This elusive goal was first reached in a practical form and was reported by Peñaz[27] in 1973. The actual measuring element consists of a small air cuff designed to fit around the middle phalanx of the adult finger. The inner surface of the cuff contains a built-in light source that directs an infrared (IR) beam transversely through both digital arteries (Fig. 12-5).

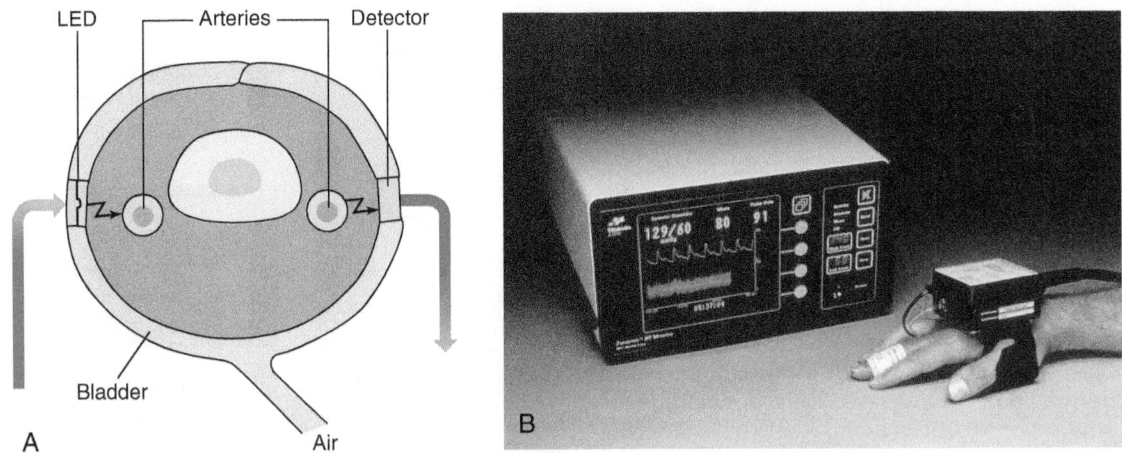

FIGURE 12-5 ■ **A,** The Finapres blood pressure cuff. LED, light-emitting diode. **B,** The finger cuff, transducer, and monitor. (B, Courtesy Finapres Medical Systems, Amsterdam.)

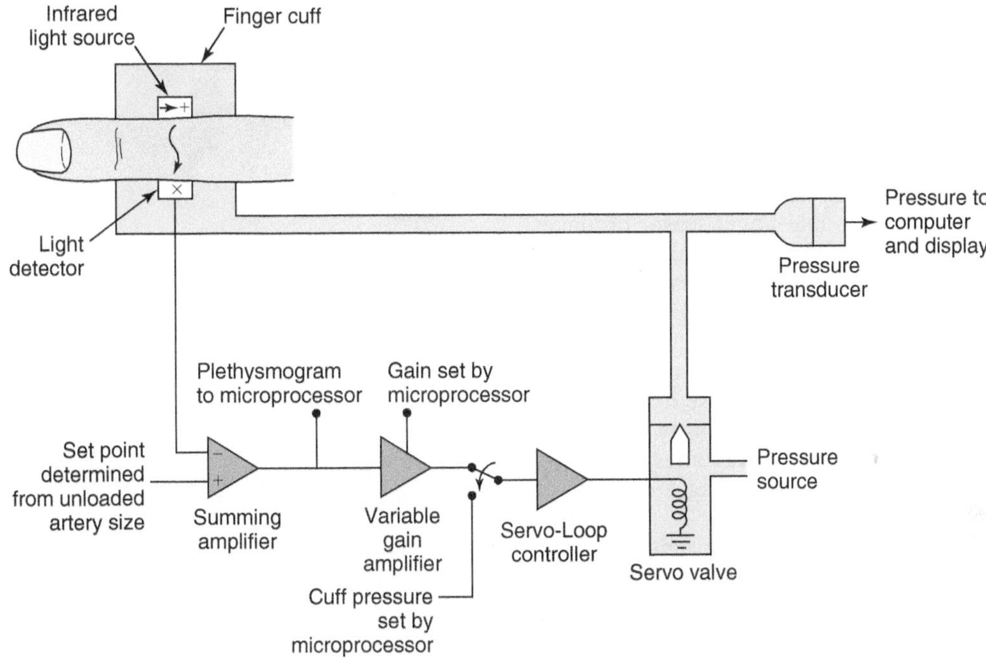

FIGURE 12-6 ■ Basic operation of the Finapres noninvasive blood pressure monitor.

An IR receiver on the opposite side of the finger then generates a signal proportional to the blood volume of the finger. The signal is used as a control signal in a feedback loop that causes rapid inflation or deflation of the cuff. Ideally, the feedback system instantaneously tracks pulsatile changes in the finger and inflates the cuff synchronously to maintain a constant IR light absorbance (Fig. 12-6). This condition, known as *volume clamping*, produces an instantaneous cuff pressure very similar to the instantaneous arterial pressure in the finger. The cuff pressure is then sent to an amplifier and display system similar to that used for invasive pressure measurement. This technology is used in the Finapres blood pressure–monitoring system (Finapres Medical Systems, Amsterdam).[28] Three devices that use this technology are the Nexfin (BMEYE, Amsterdam), the Finometer MIDI (second generation of the Finapres), and CNAP (CNSystems, Graz, Austria).

The Peñaz method has several obvious limitations.[29] Low peripheral perfusion states reduce the useful signal to a point at which oscillation of the feedback system is difficult to prevent, negatively affecting accuracy. When functioning perfectly, the Peñaz method accurately measures the blood pressure in the finger, which may or may not correlate with central arterial pressure. Calibration time has been shown to affect the accuracy compared with intraaortic measurements of blood pressure.[30] In the case of vascular disease or physiologic vasoconstriction, such as in hypothermia, blood pressure in the finger can be very low or even essentially absent, whereas the patient may be centrally hypertensive. Perfusion of the finger during continuous use is marginal, although not apparently to a harmful extent, but fingertip cyanosis often is present.[31] Prolonged use in a conscious patient is sometimes accompanied by reports of pain, although this issue has been improved with most modern devices. One example is the introduction of a "rest period," although the Peñaz device is still probably contraindicated in such conditions as Raynaud disease and sickle cell anemia.

Despite these problems, the Peñaz method is arguably the most successful implementation of beat-to-beat noninvasive blood pressure measurement, and it displays clinical accuracy in healthy subjects similar to that of the best oscillometric devices.[10] The pressure tracings produced by the Finapres method often strikingly resemble those produced by simultaneous invasive radial artery catheters used during comparison studies, including even the dicrotic notch.[28] The Finapres method has also been shown to adequately correlate with arterial blood pressure in determinations of cerebrovascular pressure reactivity.[32] The device has proven useful where measurement of rapid blood pressure transients is desirable without the risk, discomfort, and expense of invasive arterial catheterization. By comparison, even the best oscillometric devices offer a blood pressure reading only approximately every 30 seconds.[33] In addition, confining the transducer system to one finger eliminates interference with IV infusions and pulse oximetry, which is often problematic with oscillometric monitors.

The CNAP Monitor 500 system (CNSystems Medizintechnik AG, Graz, Austria) uses a double-finger sensor to obtain a continuous noninvasive blood pressure measurement (Fig 12-7). This double-finger sensor produces a continuous blood pressure signal that is calibrated to an initial oscillometric value by a special transfer function. The CNAP uses a vascular unloading technique for measuring blood pressure rhythms and pulse waves. Older methods used only a single control loop, which had to manage fast pressure increases and release in the cuff as well as the tracking of blood pressure changes for the stability of the system. The CNAP overcomes the drawbacks of the single-loop system by using a number of interlocking control loops.

The CNAP sensor consists of two semirigid cylinders, one for each finger. Inflatable cuffs, sensors, and electronics are placed inside the semirigid tubes. Three different sizes cover finger diameters from 10 to 30 mm (Fig. 12-8). The device appears to have good correlation with both invasive and oscillometric blood pressure measurements.[34-35]

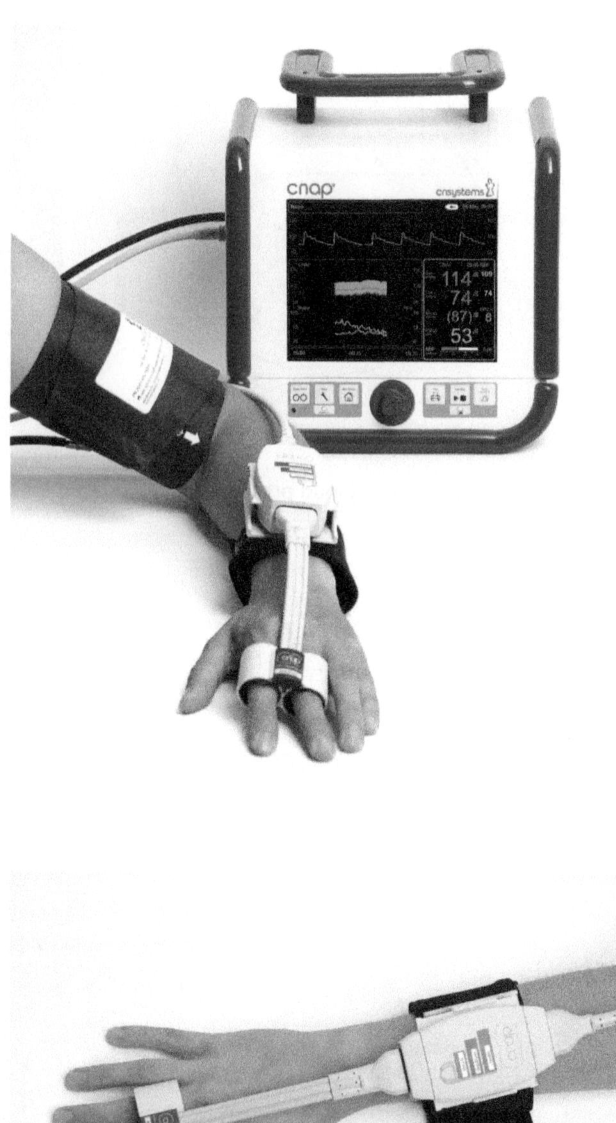

FIGURE 12-7 **A,** The CNAP Monitor 500 with arm and finger blood pressure cuffs. **B,** The CNAP monitor double finger cuff and transducer. (Courtesy CNSystems Medizintechnik AG, Graz, Austria.)

Arterial Tonometry

In this context, *arterial tonometry* (AT) is the external application of a pressure transducer over an artery to discern blood pressure changes from changes in the amplitude of the transduced signal. This method is the oldest proposed method for measurement of beat-to-beat blood pressure, but it has been beset by the lack of a reliable transducer and support system and unacceptable sensitivity to uncompensated changes in dynamic arterial wall tension. Devices using this technology are not common and are considered less clinically useful than oscillometric and invasive measurements.[34] The Vasotrac device (Medwave, Arden Hills, MN) was one of the early tonometers, but it is no longer being produced. It was not a continuous monitor; rather it measured blood pressure three to four times a minute. Studies found reasonable correlation with invasive arterial pressure, but the device was not considered accurate enough for use in liver transplantation.[37-39] The T-Line Tensymeter TL-200 (Tensys Medical, San Diego, CA) is a newer tonometry device that gives continuous blood pressure measurements. A study by Janelle and colleagues[40] found good correlation with simultaneous arterial measurements. AT is more commonly used for the measurement of pulse wave velocity, considered to be the most robust and reproducible measure of arterial stiffness.

Limited development of AT blood pressure devices is still occurring and will no doubt lead to possible future applications. This is due to some unique advantages of AT

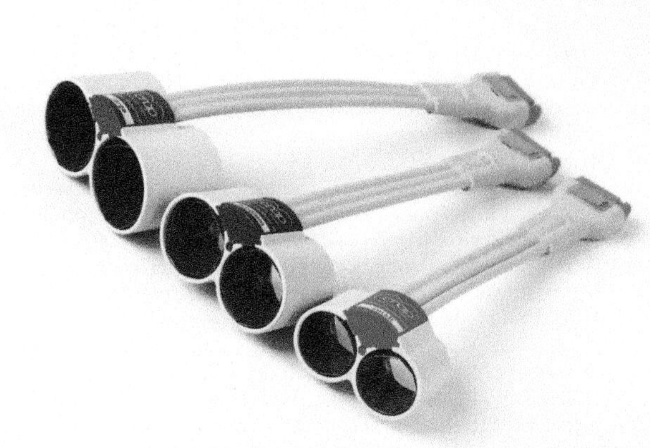

FIGURE 12-8 ■ Three different size cuffs for the CNAP monitor. (Courtesy CNSystems Medizintechnik AG, Graz, Austria.)

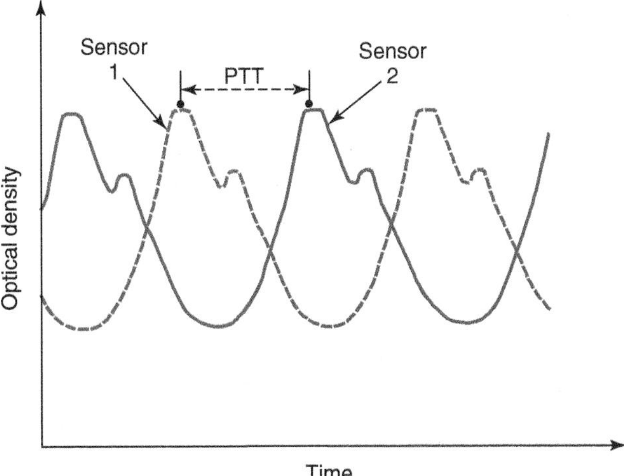

FIGURE 12-9 ■ Definition of pulse transit time (PTT) as measured by two optical sensors. (Courtesy GE Healthcare, Waukesha, WI.)

compared with the Peñaz method for continuous blood pressure recording. AT is theoretically less sensitive than the Peñaz method because of inaccuracies caused by vascular disease and vasoconstriction because the radial artery is so much larger than blood supplies to the finger. Also, discomfort in the awake individual seems to be minimal and cyanosis is not observed. However, future innovations are still needed to improve and expand this technology.

Pulse Transit Time: Photometric Method

The relationship between pulse wave velocity and blood pressure was first described in 1922 by Bramwell and Hill. Pulse transit times (PTTs) are measured by pulse transducers placed at two or more sites on the body. The transducers, located at different distances from the central circulation, measure the delay time between the sites (Fig. 12-9). Alternatively, the time can be calculated as the time delay from the initiation of the cardiac contraction (measure from electrocardiogram) to the photoplethysmograph waveform. PTT has been used in psychiatric studies as a nonspecific index of cardiovascular activity, and it has long been noted that PTT bears a roughly inverse relationship to systolic arterial blood pressure.[41] The relation to diastolic and mean pressure does not seem to be as clear. Calibration is commonly accomplished via a separate oscillometric monitor and brachial cuff placed on the arm. Changes in blood pulse transit time are transformed into blood pressure measurements using a proprietary algorithm.

The accuracy of these devices has not been adequately evaluated in an objective fashion and depends to a large extent on the presumption of a relationship between blood pressure and transit time. Recent preliminary data have shown a strong correlation to invasive blood pressure measurements.[42] This technology theoretically eliminates most of the problems associated with the Peñaz and tonometric methods discussed above. If this methodology continues to demonstrate accurate readings, it will offer a beat-to-beat blood pressure technology only slightly more cumbersome than the now-standard oscillometric unit combined with the similarly standard pulse oximetry.

As mentioned, several methods of noninvasively measuring blood pressure have been developed into practical working devices. Although fast approaching, none of the continuous methods discussed has consistently demonstrated the reliability and ease of use that have been realized by the oscillometric units. In addition, the expense of these alternative technologies has largely limited their use to experimental protocols rather than routine use.

In summary, invasive measurement of blood pressure via a peripherally placed intraarterial cannula remains the method of choice when beat-to-beat blood pressure measurement is required for clinical care. Invasive monitoring is not without risk, but where continuous pressure monitoring and/or frequent blood sampling is required, the morbidity is quite acceptable.

REFERENCES

1. Hamilton WF, Dow P: An experimental study of the standing waves in the pulse propagated through the aorta, *Am J Physiol*(125)48–49, 1939.
2. Pauca AL, Hudspeth AS, Wallenhaupt SL, et al: Radial artery-to-aorta pressure difference after discontinuation of cardiopulmonary bypass, *Anesthesiology* 70(6):935–941, 1989.
3. Bruner JMR: *Handbook of blood pressure monitoring*, Littleton, MA, 1978, PSG Publishing.
4. Pennington LA, Smith C: Leveling when monitoring central blood pressures: an alternative method, *Heart Lung* 9(6):1053–1059, 1980.
5. Pickering TG, Hall JE, Appel LJ, et al: Recommendations for blood pressure measurement in humans and experimental animals. Part 1: Blood pressure measurement in humans: a statement for professionals from the Subcommittee of Professional and Public Education of the American Heart Association Council on High Blood Pressure Research, *Hypertension* 45(1):142–161, 2005.
6. Manning DM, Kuchirka C, Kaminski J: Miscuffing: inappropriate blood pressure cuff application, *Circulation* 68(4):763–766, 1983.
7. Finnie KJ, Watts DG, Armstrong PW: Biases in the measurement of arterial pressure, *Crit Care Med* 12(11):965–968, 1984.
8. Rutten AJ, Ilsley AH, Skowronski GA, Runciman WB: A comparative study of the measurement of mean arterial blood pressure using automatic oscillometers, arterial cannulation and auscultation, *Anaesth Intensive Care* 14(1):58–65, 1986.
9. Talke P, Nichols RJ Jr, Traber DL: Does measurement of systolic blood pressure with a pulse oximeter correlate with conventional methods? *J Clin Monit* 6(1):5–9, 1990.
10. Gorback MS, Quill TJ, Lavine ML: The relative accuracies of two automated noninvasive arterial pressure measurement devices, *J Clin Monit* 7(1):13–22, 1991.

11. Myers MG, Gowin M, Dawes M, et al: Conventional versus automated measurement of blood pressure in primary care patients with systolic hypertension: randomised parallel design controlled trial, *Br Med J* 342:d286, 2011.
12. Amoore JN, Lemesre Y, Murray IC, et al: Automatic blood pressure measurement: the oscillometric waveform shape is a potential contributor to differences between oscillometric and auscultatory pressure measurements, *J Hypertens* 26(1):35–43, 2008.
13. Alpert BS: Oscillometric blood pressure values are algorithm-specific, *Am J Cardiol* 106(10):1524, 2010, author reply 1524–1525.
14. Loubser PG: Comparison of intra-arterial and automated oscillometric blood pressure measurement methods in postoperative hypertensive patients, *Med Instrum* 20(5):255–259, 1986.
15. Marks LA, Groch A: Optimizing cuff width for noninvasive measurement of blood pressure, *Blood Press Monit* 5(3):153–158, 2000.
16. Gorback MS, Quill TJ, Bloch EC, Graubert DA: Oscillometric blood pressure determination from the adult thumb using an infant cuff, *Anesth Analg* 69(5):668–670, 1989.
17. Yocum GT, Gaudet JG, Teverbaugh LA, et al: Neurocognitive performance in hypertensive patients after spine surgery, *Anesthesiology* 110(2):254–261, 2009.
18. Philip JH, Philip BK, Lehr JL: Accuracy of hydrostatic pressure measurement with a disposable dome transducer system, *Med Instrum* 19(6):273–274, 1985.
19. Slogoff S, Keats AS, Arlund C: On the safety of radial artery cannulation, *Anesthesiology* 59(1):42–47, 1983.
20. Selldén H, Nilsson K, Larsson LE, Ekström-Jodal B: Radial arterial catheters in children and neonates: a prospective study, *Crit Care Med* 15(12):1106–1109, 1987.
21. Maki DG, Kluger DM, Crnich CJ: The risk of bloodstream infection in adults with different intravascular devices: a systematic review of 200 published prospective studies, *Mayo Clin Proc* 81(9):1159–1171, 2006.
22. Manios E, Vemmos K, Tsivgoulis G, et al: Comparison of noninvasive oscillometric and intra-arterial blood pressure measurements in hyperacute stroke, *Blood Press Monit* 12(3):149–156, 2007.
23. Cannesson M, Aboy M, Hofer CK, Rehman M: Pulse pressure variation: where are we today? *J Clin Monit Comput* 25(1):45–56, 2011.
24. Della Rocca G, Costa MG, Chiarandini P, et al: Arterial pulse cardiac output agreement with thermodilution in patients in hyperdynamic conditions, *J Cardiothorac Vasc Anesth* 22(5):681–687, 2008.
25. Gardner RM: Direct blood pressure measurement: dynamic response requirements, *Anesthesiology* 54(3):227–236, 1981.
26. Hunziker P: Accuracy and dynamic response of disposable pressure transducer-tubing systems, *Can J Anaesth* 34(4):409–414, 1987.
27. Peñaz J: Photoelectric measurement of blood pressure, volume, and flow in the finger. In Albert A, Vogt W, Hellig W, editors: *Digest of the Tenth International Conference on Medical and Biological Engineering*, Dresden, 104, 1973.
28. Boehmer RD: Continuous, real-time, noninvasive monitor of blood pressure: Peñaz methodology applied to the finger, *J Clin Monit* 3(4):282–287, 1987.
29. Kurki T, Smith NT, Head N, Dec-Silver H, Quinn A: Noninvasive continuous blood pressure measurement from the finger: optimal measurement conditions and factors affecting reliability, *J Clin Monit* 3(1):6–13, 1987.
30. Panerai RB, Sammons EL, Smith SM, et al: Transient drifts between Finapres and continuous intra-aortic measurements of blood pressure, *Blood Press Monit* 12(6):369–376, 2007.
31. Gravenstein JS, Paulus DA, Feldman J, McLaughlin G: Tissue hypoxia distal to a Peñaz finger blood pressure cuff, *J Clin Monit* 1(2):120–125, 1985.
32. Kasprowicz M, Schmidt E, Kim DJ, et al: Evaluation of the cerebrovascular pressure reactivity index using non-invasive Finapres arterial blood pressure, *Physiol Meas* 31(9):1217–1228, 2010.
33. Gorback MS, Quill TJ, Graubert DA: The accuracy of rapid oscillometric blood pressure determination, *Biomed Instrum Technol* 24(5):371–374, 1990.
34. Jagadeesh AM, Singh NG, Mahankali S: A comparison of a continuous noninvasive arterial pressure (CNAP) monitor with an invasive arterial blood pressure monitor in the cardiac surgical ICU, *Ann Cardiac Anaesth* 15:180–184, 2012.
35. Ilies C, Kiskalt H, Siedenhans D, et al: Detection of hypotension during caesarean section with continuous non-invasive arterial pressure device or intermittent oscillometric arterial pressure measurement, *Br J Anaesth* 109:413–419, 2012.
36. Hansen S, Staber M: Oscillometric blood pressure measurement used for calibration of the arterial tonometry method contributes significantly to error, *Eur J Anaesthesiol* 23(9):781–787, 2006.
37. Belani K, Ozaki M, Hynson J, et al: A new noninvasine method to measure blood pressure: results of a multicenter trial, *Anesthesiology* 91:686–692, 1999.
38. Thomas SH, Winsor GR, Pang PS, et al: Use of a radial artery compression device for noninvasive, near-continuous blood pressure monitoring in the ED, *Am J Emerg Med* 22:474–478, 2004.
39. Findlay JY, Gali B, Keegan MT, et al: Vasotrac arterial blood pressure and direct arterial blood pressure monitoring during liver transplantation, *Anesth Analg* 102:690–693, 2006.
40. Janelle GM, Gravenstein N: An accuracy evaluation of the T-Line Tensymeter (continuous noninvasive blood pressure management device) versus conventional invasive radial artery monitoring in surgical patients, *Anesth Analg* 102:484–490, 2006.
41. Lane JD, Greenstadt L, Shapiro D, Rubinstein E: Pulse transit time and blood pressure: an intensive analysis, *Psychophysiology* 20(1):45–49, 1983.
42. Bartsch S, Ostojic D, Schmalgemeier H, et al: Validation of continuous blood pressure measurements by pulse transit time: a comparison with invasive measurements in a cardiac intensive care unit [in German], *Dtsch Med Wochenschr* 135(48):2406–2412, 2010.

CHAPTER 13

ELECTROCARDIOGRAPHIC MONITORING

Jolie Narang • Daniel M. Thys

CHAPTER OUTLINE

ELECTROCARDIOGRAPHY

The intraoperative use of the electrocardiogram (ECG) has developed markedly over the past several decades.[1] Originally, this monitor was primarily used during anesthesia for the detection of arrhythmias in high-risk patients. In recent years, however, it has become a standard perioperative monitor used during the administration of all anesthetics.[2] Beyond its usefulness for the intraoperative recognition of arrhythmias, one of the major indications for ECG monitoring is the intraoperative diagnosis of myocardial ischemia.[3] ECG monitoring for ischemia is inexpensive and noninvasive. Most modern operating room (OR) monitors provide automated ST-segment monitoring, which can be set to alarm if changes are detected.[4]

Normal Electrical Activity

Figure 13-1 shows the segments and intervals of the normal ECG. These elements are explained in the following subsections.

P Wave

Under normal circumstances, the sinoatrial (SA) node has the most rapid rate of spontaneous depolarization and therefore is the dominant cardiac pacemaker. From the SA node, the impulse spreads through the right and left atria. Specialized tracts can conduct the impulse to the atrioventricular (AV) node, but they are not essential. On the ECG, depolarization of the atria is represented by the P wave. The initial depolarization primarily involves the right atrium and predominantly occurs in an anterior, inferior, and leftward direction. Subsequently, it proceeds to the left atrium, which is located in a more posterior position.

PR Interval

Once the wave of depolarization has reached the AV node, a delay is observed. The delay permits contraction of the atria and allows supplemental filling of the ventricular chambers. On the ECG, this delay is represented by the PR interval.

QRS Complex

After passing through the AV node, the electrical impulse is conducted along the ventricular conduction pathways, consisting of the common bundle of His, the left and right bundle branches, the distal bundle branches, and the Purkinje fibers. The QRS complex represents the progress of the depolarization wave through this conduction system. After terminal depolarization, the ECG normally returns to baseline.

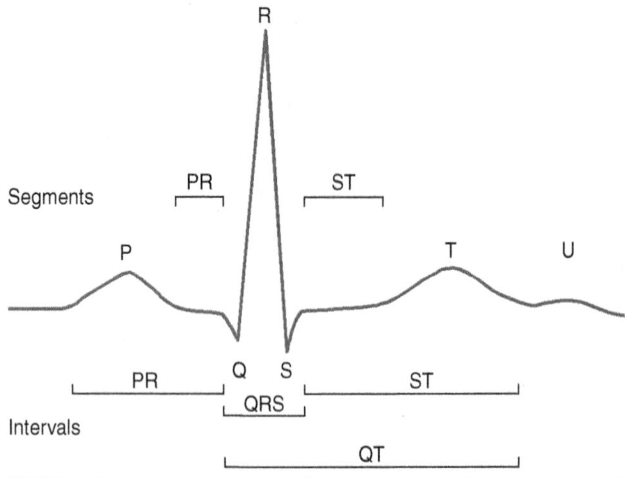

FIGURE 13-1 ▪ Segments and intervals of the normal electrocardiogram.

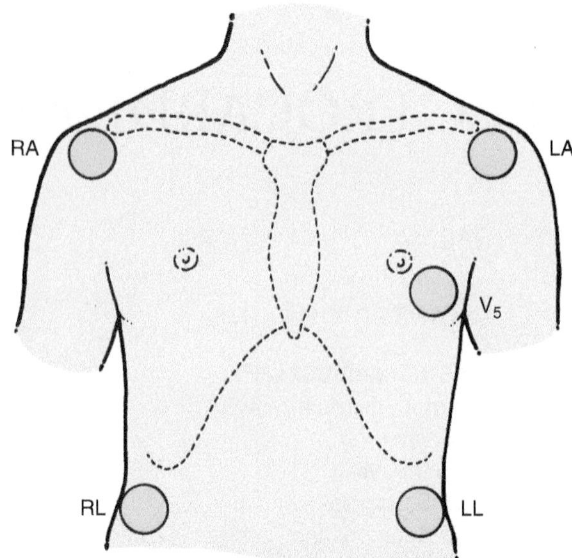

FIGURE 13-2 ▪ Multiple-lead electrocardiographic system consisting of four extremity electrodes: right arm (*RA*), left arm (*LA*), right leg (*RL*), left leg (*LL*), and V_5 leads.

ST Segment and T Wave

Repolarization of the ventricles, which begins at the end of the QRS complex, consists of the ST segment and T wave. Ventricular depolarization occurs along established conducting pathways, but ventricular repolarization is a prolonged process that occurs independently in every cell. The T wave represents the uncanceled potential differences of ventricular repolarization. The junction of the QRS complex and the ST segment is called the *J junction*. The T wave is sometimes followed by a small U wave, the origin of which is unclear. Prominent U waves are characteristic of hypokalemia (as well as hypothermia, hypomagnesemia, and hypocalcemia) and sometimes also observed after cerebrovascular accidents. Very prominent U waves may be seen in patients taking medications such as sotalol or one of the phenothiazines. Negative U waves may appear with positive T waves, an abnormal finding that has been noted in left ventricular hypertrophy and myocardial ischemia.[5]

Lead Systems

Standard Limb and Precordial Leads

The small electric currents produced by the electrical activity of the heart spread throughout the body, which behaves as a volume conductor, allowing the surface ECG to be recorded at any site. The standard leads are bipolar leads because they measure differences in potential between two electrodes. The electrodes are placed on the right arm, the left arm, and the left leg. The leads are formed by the imaginary lines connecting the electrodes, and the polarities correspond to the conventions of Einthoven's triangle. They are labeled leads I, II, and III. By convention, lead I is formed by connecting the right arm and left arm electrodes, with the left arm being positive; lead II is formed by connecting the right arm and left leg, with the left leg being positive; lead III is formed by connecting the left arm and left leg, with the left leg being positive. If the three electrodes of the standard leads are connected through resistances of 5000 ohms each, a common central terminal with zero potential is obtained. When this common electrode is used with another active electrode, the potential difference between the two represents the actual potential. On a standard 12-lead ECG, three unipolar limb leads usually are recorded: aVR, aVL, and aVF. The *a* indicates that the limb leads are augmented and were obtained via Goldberger's modification, in which the resistors are removed from the lead wires and the exploring electrode is disconnected from the central terminal. Goldberger's modification produces larger voltage deflections on the ECG.

Additional information on the heart's electrical activity is obtained when electrodes are placed closer to the heart or around the thorax. In the precordial lead system (Fig. 13-2), the neutral electrode is formed by the standard leads, and an exploring electrode is placed on the chest wall. The ECG normally is recorded with the exploring electrode in one or more of six precordial positions. Each lead is indicated by the letter *V* followed by a subscript numeral from 1 to 6, which indicates the location of the electrode on the chest wall.

Electrocardiogram Monitoring Systems

Three-Electrode System

As the name implies, the three-electrode system uses only three electrodes to record the ECG. In such a system, the ECG is observed along one bipolar lead between two of the electrodes; the third electrode serves as a neutral lead, and a selector switch allows the user to alter the designation of the electrodes. Three ECG leads can be examined in sequence without changing the location of the electrodes. Although the three-electrode system has the advantage of simplicity, its use is limited in the detection of myocardial ischemia because it provides a narrow picture of myocardial electrical activity.

Modified Three-Electrode System

Numerous modifications of the standard bipolar limb lead system have been developed. Some of these are displayed in

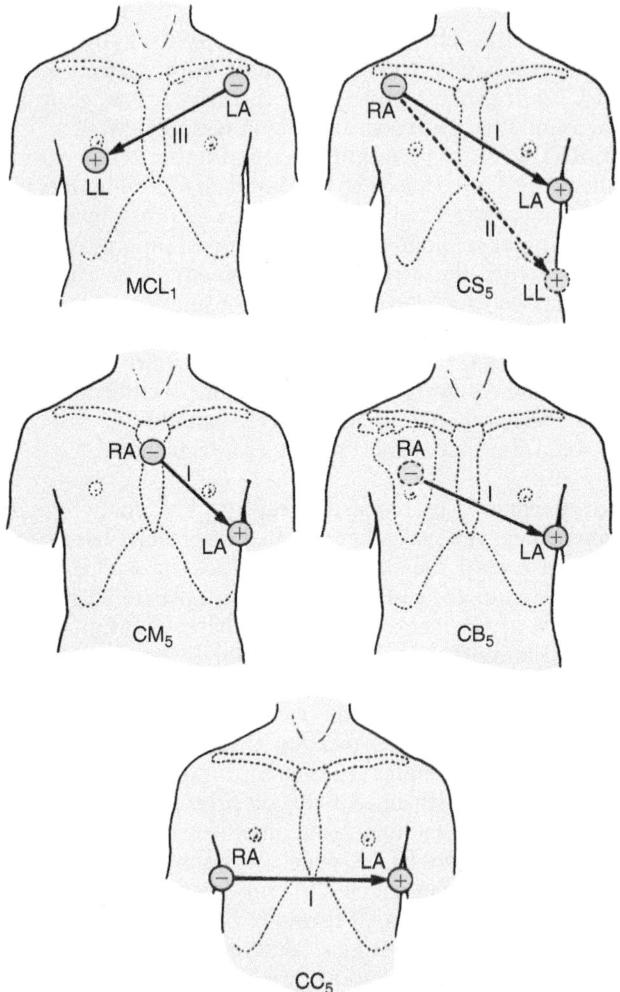

FIGURE 13-3 ■ Modified precordial lead arrangements. *RA,* right arm; *LA,* left arm; *LL,* left leg. (From Thys DM, Kaplan JA, editors: *The ECG in anesthesia and critical care.* New York, 1987, Churchill Livingstone.)

Figure 13-3. They are used in an attempt to maximize P-wave amplitude for the diagnosis of atrial arrhythmias or to increase the sensitivity of the ECG for the detection of anterior myocardial ischemia. In clinical studies, these modified three-electrode systems have been shown to be at least as sensitive as the standard V_5 lead system for the intraoperative diagnosis of ischemia.[6]

Central Subclavicular Lead. The central subclavicular (CS_5) lead (see Fig. 13-3) is particularly well suited for the detection of anterior wall myocardial ischemia. The right arm (RA) electrode is placed under the right clavicle, the left arm (LA) electrode is placed in the V_5 position, and the left leg electrode is in its usual position to serve as a neutral lead. Lead I is selected for detection of anterior wall ischemia, and lead II can be selected either for monitoring inferior wall ischemia or for the detection of arrhythmias. If a unipolar precordial electrode is unavailable, this CS_5 bipolar lead is the best and easiest alternative to a true V_5 lead for monitoring myocardial ischemia.[6]

Central Back Lead. The central back (CB_5) lead is useful for the detection of ischemia and supraventricular arrhythmias, as demonstrated in a study that compared CB_5 and V_5 in patients with closed and open chests.[7] The P wave was 90% larger in lead CB_5 than in lead V_5, and a good association between ventricular deflections of CB_5 and V_5 leads was noted. CB_5 is obtained by placing the RA electrode over the center of the right scapula and placing the LA electrode in the V_5 position. The lead selector switch should be set to lead I. The CB_5 lead may be useful in patients with ischemic heart disease who are susceptible to the development of perioperative arrhythmias.

When modified bipolar limb leads are used, the user should be aware that in certain aspects, they differ significantly from true unipolar precordial leads. The modified precordial leads usually show a greater R-wave amplitude than standard precordial leads, which can result in amplification of the ST-segment response. The criteria for diagnosing myocardial ischemia may therefore need to be adjusted when modified bipolar leads are used. It has been shown during exercise stress testing that normalization of the degree of ST-segment depression to the height of the R wave increases the sensitivity and specificity of the ECG for the recognition of myocardial ischemia.[8] Although similar corrections have not yet been tested during intraoperative monitoring, their possible importance should be kept in mind when intraoperative ECG recordings are examined.

Five-Electrode System

The use of five electrodes permits the recording of the six standard limb leads—I, II, III, aVR, aVL, and aVF—as well as one precordial unipolar lead. In general, the unipolar lead is placed in the V_5 position, along the anterior axillary line in the fifth intercostal space. With the addition of only two electrodes to the ECG system, up to seven different leads can be monitored simultaneously. This allows several areas of the myocardium to be monitored for ischemia, which is helpful in the establishment of a differential diagnosis between atrial and ventricular arrhythmias.

In 1976, Kaplan and King[9] suggested monitoring lead V_5 as the best choice for the detection of intraoperative ischemia. London, and colleagues[10] demonstrated that in high-risk patients undergoing noncardiac surgery, when a single lead was used the greatest sensitivity was obtained with lead V_5 (75%), followed by lead V_4 (61%). Combining leads V_4 and V_5 increased the sensitivity to 90%, whereas the standard combination of leads II and V_5 produced a sensitivity of only 80%. They also suggested that if three leads (II, V_4, and V_5) could be examined simultaneously, the sensitivity would increase to 98%.

Recently, Landesberg and colleagues[11] investigated the usefulness of analyzing data obtained from continuous online 12-lead ECG monitoring for the detection of myocardial ischemia. During 11,132 patient-hours of monitoring, the investigators reported that V_4 was most sensitive to ischemia (83.3%), followed by V_3 and V_5 (75% each). Combining two precordial leads increased the sensitivity for detecting ischemia (97.4% for $V_3 + V_5$ and 92.1% for either $V_4 + V_5$ or $V_3 + V_4$) and infarction (100% for $V_4 + V_5$ or $V_3 + V_5$ and 83.3% for $V_3 + V_4$). They found that the baseline preanesthesia ST segment was above isoelectric in V_1 through V_3 and below isoelectric in V_5 through V_6. Lead V_4 was closest to the isoelectric level on the baseline ECG, rendering it most suitable for ischemia monitoring. The authors recommended that two or more precordial leads were necessary to approach a sensitivity of greater than 95% for the detection of perioperative ischemia and infarction.

However, in an editorial entitled "Multilead Precordial ST-segment Monitoring: 'The Next Generation?'" London[12] concluded that multilead precordial ST-segment monitoring is not practical. It presents a significant logistical problem, particularly if a patient needs to be mobilized quickly. It is also likely to result in a high rate of false-positive responses and artifacts. Instead, London recommended the use of true V_4 or V_5 leads, control of heart rate and pain, and the use of β-blockers as tolerated for all patients at risk (diabetics or patients with left ventricular hypertrophy).

Invasive Electrocardiography

The electrical potentials of the heart can be measured not only from a surface ECG but also from body cavities adjacent to the heart (esophagus or trachea) or from within the heart itself.

Esophageal Electrocardiography. The concept of esophageal ECG is not new, and numerous studies have demonstrated the usefulness of this approach in the diagnosis of complicated arrhythmias. A prominent P wave usually is displayed in the presence of atrial depolarization, and its relationship to the ventricular electrical activity can be examined. The esophageal electrodes are incorporated into an esophageal stethoscope and are welded to conventional ECG wires (Fig. 13-4). To record a bipolar esophageal ECG, the electrodes are connected to the right and left arm terminals, and lead I is selected on the monitor. In one study of 20 cardiac patients, 100% of atrial arrhythmias were correctly diagnosed with the esophageal lead (intracavitary ECG was used as the standard); lead II led to a correct diagnosis in 54% of the cases, and V_5 led to a correct diagnosis in 42% of the cases.[13] In addition, the esophageal ECG may be helpful in the detection of posterior wall ischemia because of its proximity to the posterior aspect of the left ventricle. Jain[14] described the use of esophageal ECG and compared it with surface ECG (SECG) in patients undergoing coronary bypass grafting. He found that the recognition and measurement of all the PQRST waves could be improved and automated by simultaneous use of esophageal ECG and SECG. The P-wave amplitude was greater in esophageal ECG than in SECG, which might facilitate the identification of supraventricular versus ventricular arrhythmias. ST-segment deviation in the unipolar esophageal ECG was not suitable for the routine detection of ischemia because of excessive noise.

To minimize the risk of esophageal burn injury, an electrocautery protection filter capable of filtering radio frequencies greater than 20 kHz should be inserted between the ECG cable and the esophageal lead.

Intracardiac Electrocardiography. For many years, long central venous catheters filled with saline have been used to record the intracardiac ECG (IC-ECG).[15] To best illustrate an IC-ECG, 1) attach a plastic adapter to the hub of the central venous catheter (CVC), whose most distal port is at the low superior vena cava or superior region of the right atrium; 2) instill saline via a syringe needle inserted through the rubber head of the adapter, ensuring by previous aspiration that no blood clots are present and air bubbles are cleared; 3) connect the needle of the syringe with one of the six precordial cables of a standard ECG machine using an alligator clamp; and 4) record a standard ECG, which will show the IC-ECG substituting for the selected V lead. Lead V_1 is used most often, but any of leads V_1 through V_6 can be used.[16]

Chatterjee and colleagues[17] described the use of a modified balloon-tipped flotation catheter for recording intracavitary electrograms. The multipurpose pulmonary artery catheter presently available has all the features of a standard pulmonary artery catheter. In addition, three atrial and two ventricular electrodes have been incorporated into the catheter (Fig. 13-5). These electrodes allow the recording of intracavitary ECGs and the establishment of atrial or AV pacing. The diagnostic capabilities of this catheter are great because atrial, ventricular, and AV nodal arrhythmias and conduction blocks can be demonstrated. The large voltages obtained from the intracardiac electrodes are relatively insensitive to electrocautery interference and

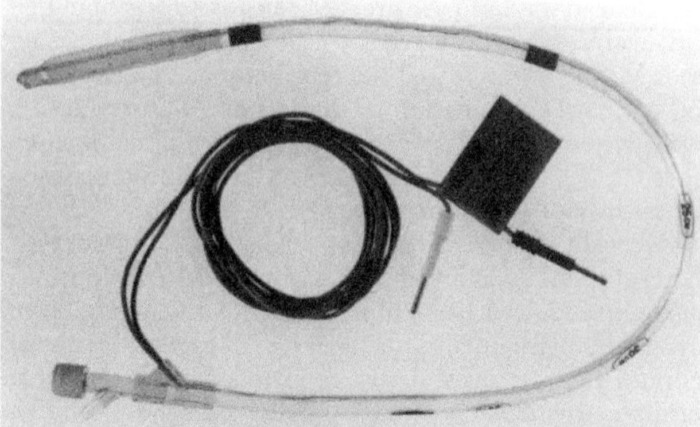

FIGURE 13-4 ■ The cardioesophagoscope. The esophageal leads are embedded in plastic. The electrocardiogram wires are connected to the right arm and left arm leads, and lead I is selected on the monitor.

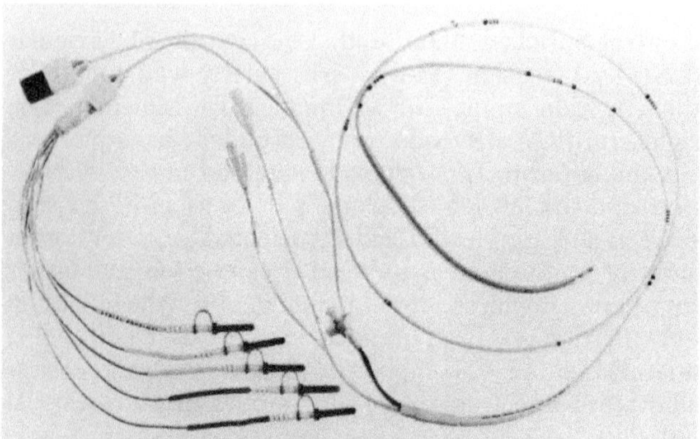

FIGURE 13-5 ■ The multipurpose pacing pulmonary artery catheter. Three atrial and two ventricular electrodes are shown.

are therefore useful for intraaortic balloon pump triggering.[18] Other pulmonary artery catheters have ventricular and atrial ports that allow passage of pacing wires. These catheters also can be used for diagnostic purposes or for therapeutic interventions (pacing).

Benzadon and colleagues[19] compared the amplitude of the P wave obtained by IC-ECG with those of the P waves obtained by esophageal ECG and SECG. They found that IC-ECG and esophageal ECG made it possible to register P waves larger than those registered by SECG but reported no difference between IC-ECG and esophageal ECG.

Tracheal Electrocardiography. Tracheal ECG allows monitoring when it is impractical or impossible to monitor the SECG. The tracheal ECG consists of a standard tracheal tube in which electrodes have been embedded. In a recent report, a tracheal tube was described with two coiled-wire stainless steel electrodes embedded in the tube's cuff (Fig. 13-6).[20] The same safety precautions as for esophageal ECG should be followed for tracheal ECG.

DISPLAY, RECORDING, AND INTERPRETATION

The American Heart Association (AHA) has published instrumentation and practice standards for ECG monitoring in special care units.[21] Because many of the principles enumerated in these standards also are applicable to intraoperative monitoring, they are often referred to in this chapter.

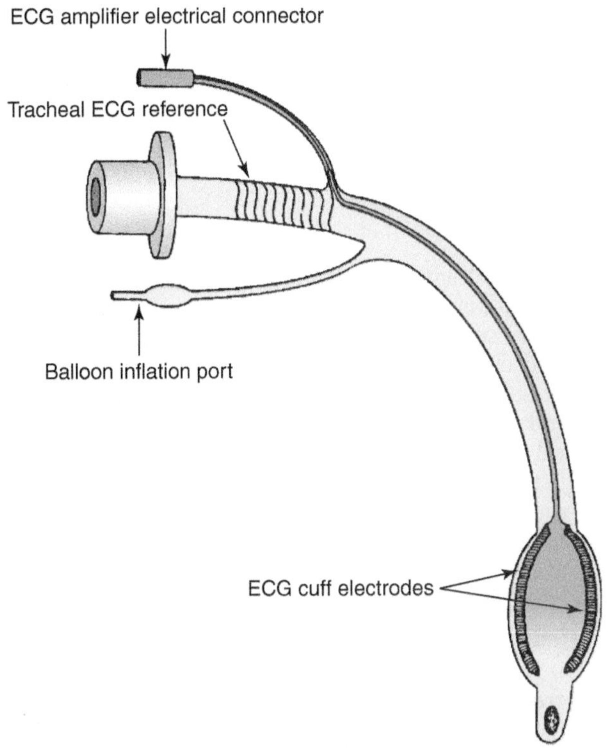

FIGURE 13-6 ■ **Schematic representation of an endotracheal tube with cuff electrodes, spiral reference electrode, and electrocardiograph (*ECG*) amplifier connector.** (From Hayes JK, Peters JL, Smith KW, et al: Monitoring normal and aberrant electrocardiographic activity from an endotracheal tube: comparison of the surface, esophageal, and tracheal electrocardiograms. *J Clin Monit* 1994;10:81-90.)

Basic Requirements

The function of the ECG monitor is to detect, amplify, display, and record the ECG signal. The ECG signal usually is displayed on an oscilloscope, and most monitors now offer nonfade storage oscilloscopes to facilitate wave recognition. All ECG monitors for use in patients with cardiac disease also should have paper recording capabilities. The recorder is needed to make accurate diagnoses of complex arrhythmias and allow careful analysis of all the ECG waveforms. In addition, the recorder allows differentiation of real ECG changes from oscilloscope artifacts. The AHA special report defines a number of requirements that should be met by ECG monitoring equipment (Boxes 13-1 to 13-3).[20]

Oscilloscope Displays

Most modern oscilloscopes are high-resolution monochrome or color monitors similar to those used in computer technology. They frequently allow considerable

BOX 13-1 Electrocardiographic Monitoring Performance Requirements

1. *Protection from overload.* Protection should be adequate (no damage) for 1 V (peak to peak), 60 Hz, applied for 10 seconds to any electrode connection. The device should recover within 8 seconds after a defibrillation shock of at least 5000 V, with a delivered energy of ≥360 J.
2. *Isolated patient connection.* The system should include isolated patient connections to meet standards defined in American National Standards for Safe Current Limits for Electromedical Apparatus.[24]
3. *QRS detection.* Monitors should detect QRS complexes with amplitudes of 0.5-5.0 mV, slopes of 6-300 mV/sec, and durations of 70-140 ms for adult use or 40-120 ms for pediatric use. The system should not respond to signals with an amplitude of ≤0.15 mV or a duration of ≤10 ms.
4. *Accuracy of heart rate meter.* The rate meter should be accurate to within the lesser of ±10% or ±5 beats/min over the range of 30-200 beats/min for adult use or 30-250 beats/min for pediatric use.
5. *Alarm range and accuracy.* Alarm rates should be accurate to within the lesser of ±10% or ±5 beats/min over the range of 30-100 beats/min for the lower limit and 100-200 beats/min (adult) or 100-250 beats/min (pediatric) for the upper limit. Time to alarm after exceeding rate limits should not exceed 10 seconds.
6. *Noise tolerance.* Heart rate meters should remain accurate during application of a 60-Hz signal, 100 mV peak to peak, minimum. Accuracy should not be affected when a triangular wave of 4 mV at 0.1 Hz is superimposed on a train of QRS signals of 0.5-mV amplitude and 100-ms duration.

From Mirvis DM, Berson AS, Goldberger AL, et al: Instrumentation and practice standards for electrocardiographic monitoring in special care units. *Circulation* 1989;79:464-471.

BOX 13-2 Electrocardiographic Monitoring Performance Standards

1. *Input dynamic range.* The device should display, without saturation, differential voltages of ±5 mV at rates up to 320 mV/sec; the output signal's amplitude should not change more than ±10% over the range of direct current offsets of ±300 mV applied to any lead.
2. *Input impedance.* Single-ended input impedance should be 2500 Ω minimum at 10 Hz.
3. *System noise.* Noise from all sources, including manufacturer-recommended patient cables, should be <40 mV peak to peak.
4. *Overall system error.* Input signals with an amplitude limited to ±5 mV and varying at a rate up to 125 mV/sec should be reproduced with an error of less than ±20% or ±100 μV, whichever is greater.
5. *Upper cutoff frequency.* High-frequency cutoff should be at least 40 Hz (−3 dB).
6. *Common mode rejection.* To test common mode rejection, a 60-Hz signal with a 200-pF source capacitance and a 10-V open circuit voltage is applied from power ground to all patient electrode connections attached to a common node and with a parallel combination of a 5100-Ω resistor and 47-nF capacitor imbalance impedance in series with each patient lead (including RL, if supplied). Such a signal should not produce an output signal exceeding 1 mV, peak to peak, with reference to the input over a 60-second period.
7. *Gain selections and accuracy.* Gains of 5 and 10 mm/mV should be provided, with a total allowable gain drift of ±0.66%/min and ±10%/hour.
8. *Pacemaker pulse indication.* The unit should visually indicate on the output display the presence of a minimum pacemaker pulse of 0.2 mV, with reference to the input.
9. *Display during other monitoring function.* At least one electrocardiographic channel should be continuously displayed at all times, including entry and editing of data and procedures, such as thermodilution and cardiac output calculations.

From Mirvis DM, Berson AS, Goldberger AL, et al: Instrumentation and practice standards for electrocardiographic monitoring in special care units. *Circulation* 1989;79:464-471.

flexibility in screen configuration and include waveform positions, colors, and sweep speeds. The norm in modern technology is to display two or three ECG channels simultaneously. These usually consist of two limb leads and one unipolar precordial lead. Average heart rates and optional arrhythmia and ST-segment information are displayed in alphanumeric format in addition to the waveforms.

Standard Electrocardiogram Recordings

The ECG is recorded on special paper marked with a grid of horizontal and vertical lines. Distances between vertical lines represent time intervals, and distances between horizontal lines represent voltages. The lines are 1 mm apart, and every fifth line is heavier than the others. The speed of the paper is standardized to 25 mm/sec; on the horizontal axis, 1 mm equals 0.04 seconds and 0.5 cm equals 0.20 seconds. On the vertical axis, 10 mm represents 1 mV. On every recording, a calibration mark

BOX 13-3 Electrocardiographic Monitoring Disclosure Requirements

1. Electrosurgery and diathermy protection, including disclosure if electrosurgery overload will cause damage
2. Respiration, leads-off sensing, and active noise-suppression methods, including disclosure of waveform type applied directly to the patient for detection
3. T-wave rejection capability, including disclosure of maximum T-wave amplitude for which heart rate indication is within error limits specified above
4. Heart rate averaging algorithm, including disclosure of type of algorithm used and frequency of display update
5. Heart rate meter accuracy and response to irregular rhythm for specified waveforms, including disclosure of meter time to indicate a change of ±40 beats/min from an initial indication of 80 beats/min
6. Time to alarm for tachycardia of specified waveforms
7. Pacemaker pulse rejection capability for specified pacemaker pulses with and without overshoots/undershoots
8. Service procedures and facilities, including name and location of acceptable repair facilities, recommendations for test methods to verify adequate performance, and frequency of recommended preventive maintenance

From Mirvis DM, Berson AS, Goldberger AL, et al: Instrumentation and practice standards for electrocardiographic monitoring in special care units. *Circulation* 1989;79:464-471.

(1 cm = 1 mV) indicates that the ECG is appropriately calibrated. The user should follow the manufacturer's recommended calibration procedures for each monitoring episode. Strip chart recorders that are part of an ECG monitoring system should meet all the standards for time-based accuracy—frequency response, linearity, and so forth—proposed for conventional ECG recording systems.[22,23]

Artifacts

Patient

The electrical signal generated by the heart and monitored by the ECG is very weak, amounting to only 0.5 to 2 mV at the skin surface. To avoid signal loss at the interface of skin and electrode, the skin must be properly prepared. Hair should be removed from the electrode sites with scissors and a razor, and the skin should be cleaned with alcohol and must be free of all dirt. It is best to abrade the skin lightly to remove part of the stratum corneum, which can be a source of high resistance to the measured voltages. To avoid the problem of muscle artifact, electrodes should be placed over bony prominences whenever possible. Muscle movement in the form of shivering can produce significant ECG artifact.

Electrodes and Leads

Loose electrodes and broken leads can produce a variety of artifacts that may simulate arrhythmias, Q waves, or inverted T waves. Pre-gelled, disposable electrodes made of silver metal and silver chloride electrolyte are usually used in the OR. The technical standards for such electrodes have been published by the Association for the

Advancement of Medical Instrumentation (AAMI).[24] It is important that all the electrodes be moist, uniform, and not out of date. Needle electrodes should be avoided because of the risk of thermal injury. Some ECG monitors have built-in cable testers that enable a lead to be tested when the cable's distal (patient) end is connected to test terminals on the monitor. A high resistance causes a large voltage drop, indicating that the lead is faulty. The main source of artifact from ECG leads is loss of the integrity of the lead insulation. This subsequently leads to pickup of other electric fields in the OR, such as the 60-Hz alternating current (AC) from lights and currents from the electrocautery device. Any damaged ECG lead should be discarded for this reason. Movement of leads also can lead to artifact.

Operating Room Environment

Many pieces of equipment in the OR emit electrical fields that can interfere with the ECG. These include the 60-Hz AC power lines for lights, electrosurgical equipment, cardiopulmonary equipment, and defibrillators. Most of this interference can be minimized by proper shielding of the cables and leads, although to date the interference created by the electrosurgical equipment cannot be reliably filtered without distortion of the ECG. Electrocautery, the most important source of interference on the ECG in the OR, frequently obliterates the ECG tracing. Analysis of the electrocautery equipment has identified three component frequencies. Radiofrequency (RF) energy between 800 and 2000 kHz accounts for most of the interference. Also contributing to electrocautery interference are the 60-Hz AC energy and the 0.1- to 10-Hz low-frequency noise from intermittent contact of the electrosurgical unit with the patient's tissues. Preamplifiers can be modified to suppress RF interference, but these filter circuits are still not widely available in the OR.

Other causes of ECG artifacts in the OR environment have been reported. Intraoperative monitoring of somatosensory evoked potentials (SSEPs) has been known to simulate pacemaker spikes.[25] These spikes are caused by the incorporation of a pacer enhancement circuit into certain ECG monitors. The problem can be eliminated by disabling this circuit. Artifactual spikes have been noted to coincide with the drip rate in the drip chamber of a warming unit.[26] The spikes were probably related to the generation of static electricity from water droplets. Use of an automated percutaneous lumbar discectomy nucleotome has been reported to simulate supraventricular tachycardia related to a mechanical interference.[27]

Monitoring System

All ECG monitors use filters to narrow the bandwidth in an attempt to reduce environmental artifacts. The high-frequency filters reduce distortions from muscle movement, 60-Hz electrical current, and electromagnetic interference from other electrical equipment.[28] The low-frequency filters ensure a more stable baseline by reducing respiratory and body movement artifacts as well as those resulting from poor electrode contact. The AHA recommends that a flat frequency response be obtained at a bandwidth of 0.05 to 100 Hz.[12] The high-frequency limit of 100 Hz ensures that tracings are of sufficient fidelity to assess QRS morphology and to accurately evaluate rapid rhythms such as atrial flutter. The low-frequency limit of 0.05 Hz allows accurate representation of slower events, such as P-wave and T-wave morphology and ST-segment excursion.

Most modern ECG monitors allow the operator a choice among several bandwidths. The actual filter frequencies tend to vary from manufacturer to manufacturer. One manufacturer (Hewlett-Packard, Andover, MA) allows a choice between a "diagnostic mode," with a bandwidth of 0.05 to 130 Hz for adults and 0.5 to 130 Hz for neonates, a "monitoring mode" with a bandwidth 0.5 to 40 Hz for adults and 0.5 to 60 Hz for neonates, and a "filter mode" with a bandwidth of 0.05 to 20 Hz.

The importance of bandwidth selection for the detection of perioperative myocardial ischemia has been evaluated by Slogoff and colleagues.[29] They simultaneously used five ECG systems: a Spacelabs Alpha 14 Model Series 3200 Cardule with a bandwidth of 0.05 to 125 Hz and one with a bandwidth of 0.5 to 30 Hz (Spacelabs Healthcare, Issaquah, WA); a Marquette Electronics (now GE Healthcare, Waukesha, WI) MAC II ECG with a bandwidth of 0.05 to 40 Hz and one with a bandwidth of 0.05 to 100 Hz; and a Del Mar Reynolds (now Spacelabs Healthcare) Holter recorder with a bandwidth of 0.1 to 100 Hz. The ST-segment positions with the three systems that used the lower filter limit (0.05 Hz) recommended by the AHA were similar, whereas with the Spacelabs 0.5 to 30 Hz system, they were consistently more negative. The ST-segment displacement on the Holter recorder was consistently less negative and less positive. In at least one automated ST-segment analysis system (Hewlett-Packard), the lower frequency filter (0.05 Hz) is automatically enabled when the ST analyzer is turned on.

INDICATIONS

Diagnosis of Arrhythmias

Arrhythmias are common during surgery, and their causes are numerous. They are most common during tracheal intubation or extubation and arise more frequently in patients with preexisting cardiac disease. The major contributing factors to the development of perioperative arrhythmias are:

1. *Anesthetic agents.* Halogenated hydrocarbons, such as halothane or enflurane, are known to produce arrhythmias, probably by a reentrant mechanism.[30] Halothane has also been shown to sensitize the myocardium to endogenous and exogenous catecholamines. Drugs that block the reuptake of norepinephrine, such as cocaine and ketamine, can facilitate the development of epinephrine-induced arrhythmias.
2. *Abnormal arterial blood gases or electrolytes.* Hyperventilation is known to reduce serum potassium concentration.[31] If the preoperative potassium is

low, it is possible that serum potassium will decrease to the range of 2 mEq/L and thus precipitate severe cardiac arrhythmias.

3. *Tracheal intubation.* This may be the most common cause of arrhythmias during surgery and is commonly associated with hemodynamic alterations.
4. *Reflexes.* Vagal stimulation may produce sinus bradycardia and may allow ventricular escape mechanisms to occur. In vascular surgery, these reflexes may be related to traction on the peritoneum or direct pressure on the vagus nerve during carotid artery surgery. Stimulation of the carotid sinus can also lead to arrhythmias, and the ocular cardiac reflex can be activated during eye surgery, leading to bradyarrhythmias.
5. *Central nervous system stimulation and dysfunction of the autonomic nervous system.*
6. *Preexisting cardiac disease.* Angelini and colleagues[32] have shown that patients with known cardiac disease have a much higher incidence of arrhythmias during anesthesia than patients without known disease.
7. *Central venous cannulation.* The insertion of catheters or wires into the central circulation often causes arrhythmias.

Once an arrhythmia is recognized, it is important to determine whether it produces a hemodynamic disturbance, what type of treatment is required, and how quickly treatment should be instituted. Treatment should be initiated promptly if the arrhythmia leads to marked hemodynamic impairment. In addition, treatment should be instituted if the arrhythmia is a precursor of a more severe arrhythmia (e.g., frequent multifocal premature ventricular complexes [PVCs] with R-on-T phenomenon can lead to ventricular fibrillation), or if the arrhythmia could be detrimental to the patient's underlying cardiac disease (e.g., tachycardia in a patient with mitral stenosis). The standard limb lead II is preferred for the detection of rhythm disturbances, because it usually displays large P waves.

BOX 13-4 Electrocardiographic Criteria for Diagnosis of Ischemia in Anesthetized Patients

- Upsloping ST segment: 2-mm depression, 80 ms after J point
- Horizontal ST segment: 1-mm depression, 60-80 ms after J point
- Downsloping ST segment: 1 mm from PQ junction to top of curve
- ST-segment elevation
- T-wave inversion

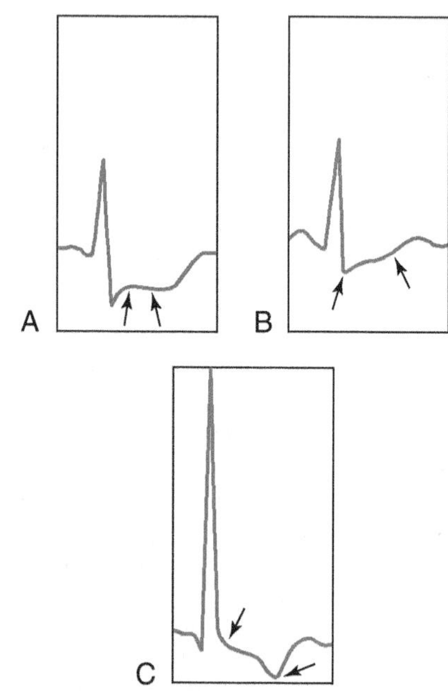

FIGURE 13-7 Examples of ST-segment depression (between arrows). **A,** Horizontal ST segment. **B,** Upsloping ST segment. **C,** Downsloping ST segment.

Diagnosis of Ischemia

Factors that predispose to the development of perioperative ischemia include perioperative events that affect the myocardial oxygen balance and the presence of preexisting coronary artery disease. A number of perioperative clinical studies have found a high incidence of ECG evidence of ischemia (20% to 80%) in patients with coronary artery disease undergoing surgery, both cardiac and noncardiac.[33,34] In the anesthetized patient, the detection of ischemia by ECG becomes even more important because the hallmark symptom of angina is not available.

In recent years, it has also become evident that a significant number of patients have asymptomatic, or silent, ischemia,[35] manifested by characteristic ECG signs of myocardial ischemia in the absence of angina and not necessarily associated with changes in hemodynamics or heart rate. Among patients with chronic, stable angina who have ST-segment depression during exercise, ambulatory ECG monitoring during daily life identifies transient ischemic episodes in approximately 40% to 50% of ambulating patients. In these patients, silent ischemic episodes account for approximately 75% of all ischemic episodes while ambulating.[36] The ECG changes that arise during myocardial ischemia often are characteristic and will be detected with careful ECG monitoring. Although the ECG criteria for ischemia were established in patients undergoing exercise stress testing, they also can be applied to anesthetized patients (Box 13-4).[37] These criteria are 1) horizontal or downsloping ST-segment depression of 0.1 mV (Fig. 13-7, *A* and *C*); 2) slowly upsloping ST-segment depression (Fig. 13-7, *B*) of 0.2 mV, all measured from 60 to 80 ms after the J point; and 3) ST-segment elevation of 0.1 mV in a non–Q-wave lead.

It is commonly believed that monitoring for intraoperative myocardial ischemia is unnecessary in neonates. Whereas ECG lead monitoring for adults is concerned with the detection of ischemia and arrhythmias, neonatal ECG monitoring has focused on arrhythmia recognition alone. Recent studies, however, suggest that the neonatal heart is more susceptible to ischemia than the adult heart. Bell and colleagues[38] have demonstrated the importance of calibrated ECG monitoring in neonates with congenital heart disease.

Although analysis of the ST segment provides sensitive information about myocardial ischemia, it should nonetheless be remembered that in approximately 10% of patients, underlying ECG abnormalities hinder the analysis. Some abnormalities are caused by hypokalemia, administration of digitalis, left bundle branch block, Wolff-Parkinson-White syndrome, or left ventricular hypertrophy with strain. In patients with these problems, other diagnostic modalities, such as transesophageal echocardiography, should be considered.

Diagnosis of Conduction Defects

Conduction defects also can arise during surgery. They can result from the passage of a pulmonary artery catheter through the right ventricle, or they can be a manifestation of myocardial ischemia. Because high-grade conduction defects (second- and third-degree AV blocks) often have deleterious effects on hemodynamic performance, their intraoperative recognition is important.

AUTOMATED RECORDING

A number of anesthesiologists have used Holter monitoring to document the incidence of perioperative arrhythmias and ischemia. In Holter monitoring, ECG information from one or two bipolar leads is recorded by a miniature recorder. Up to 48 hours of ECG signals can be collected. The data are subsequently processed by a playback system, and the ECG signals are analyzed. On most modern systems the playback unit includes a dedicated computer for rapid analysis of the data and automated recognition of arrhythmias. A significant limitation of traditional Holter monitoring in the perioperative period is that recordings usually are analyzed and interpreted retrospectively. A real-time Holter monitor records specific ECG segments for later playback and analyzes the rhythm and ST segment in real time and alerts the user to acute perturbations.[39] The application of Holter monitoring in anesthesiology is, as of yet, primarily limited to the research environment.

Computer-Assisted Electrocardiogram Interpretation

Modern monitoring equipment is highly computerized, and most of the physiologic information is manipulated, analyzed, and stored in a digital format. Therefore an early step in data collection involves the conversion of analog signals (time-variable voltages or amplitudes) into digital format via an analog-to-digital converter. Once in digital format, the physiologic information can be readily subjected to a variety of analyses. In electrocardiography, the most common analyses, besides rate calculations, are related to the recognition of an arrhythmia and the detection of myocardial ischemia.

Arrhythmias

There is little doubt that during prolonged visual observation of the ECG on the oscilloscope, certain arrhythmias will go undetected. This was clearly demonstrated by Romhilt and colleagues,[40] who showed that nurses in coronary care units failed to detect serious ventricular arrhythmias in 84% of their patients. Computers have therefore been designed for the automated detection of arrhythmias in an attempt to increase the detection of abnormal rhythms. Using an early preprocessing algorithm called AZTEC, a computer accurately detected 78% of ventricular ectopic beats. It measured QRS width, offset, amplitude, and area to classify complexes in morphologic families.[41] In a prospective evaluation of such a system, it was found that the computer accurately detected 95.4% of ventricular premature beats but only 82.4% of supraventricular premature beats.[42] Other systems have depended on QRS recognition and cross-correlation with stored QRS complexes.[43] In cross-correlation, each detected QRS complex is compared with a list of previously detected complexes. If a complex does not correlate with a previously stored complex, it is considered to have a new configuration and is added to the list. A number of points of the complex, such as the PR interval and ST segment, are stored as a template for future comparison. Whenever a new complex matches an existing template, it is averaged into that template so that each template represents a running average of all complexes of a particular configuration.[44] Each template is defined as *normal*, *abnormal*, or *questionable* according to previously defined criteria. The AHA has published several parameters that need to be tested to permit a meaningful understanding of a system's values and limitations and to allow a reasonable comparison of systems.[21]

Myocardial Ischemia

Several computer programs for the online detection of ischemia and analysis of ST segments are now commercially available. Most cardiac monitor algorithms are intentionally set for high sensitivity at the expense of specificity.[45] As a result, numerous false alarms occur that must be evaluated by health care professionals so that overtreatment of patients will not occur. Each manufacturer uses a different analysis technique, and not all of the algorithms are in the public domain.

In one system (GE Healthcare, Waukesha, WI), an ST learning phase begins by looking at the first 16 beats, in all leads, for the dominant normal or paced shape. The shapes are correlated via a selected number of points on each of the active, valid lead waveforms. An algorithm looks for leads in the fail or artifact mode to determine the number of valid leads used in the analysis. The algorithm also makes all leads positive to enable the sum of the points on the valid leads to be calculated. This sum is used in determining a peak, or *fiducial point*, which is used as a point of reference on the QRS complex, and a template is formed from selected points around the fiducial point for each ECG lead. As each beat is analyzed, its template is compared to templates of previous beats. If the templates correlate within 75% of a previously stored shape, a match is declared and the template is classified as an *existing shape*. If no match is found, the template becomes a *new shape*. On the seventeenth beat, the dominant QRS shape or paced shape is determined. The algorithm then searches for an additional 16 beats that correlate with the dominant template. With the eighteenth beat, a process called *incremental averaging* is initiated.

Incremental averaging is a method of tracking positive or negative changes occurring on the waveform. These changes are tracked for each of the valid leads. The changes may be either physiologic, such as ST-segment changes as a result of ischemia, or related to artifact caused by high-frequency noise. The changes are tracked by allowing an adjustment of only 0.1 mm, either positive or negative, from the prior shape of each beat. At the 30-second beat, the products of the incrementally averaged templates become the learned ST templates. Until ST is relearned, all changes in the QRS shape are tracked against this learned template. The isoelectric point and ST points are determined during the learning phase and are based on the width of the QRS shape. The isoelectric point is placed 40 ms before the onset of the QRS, and the ST point is placed 60 ms past the offset of the QRS measurement. The isoelectric point provides the point of reference for determining the measurement of the ST segment.

The technique of incremental averaging is well suited to a continuous input with slow changes. However, it links the heart rate to the speed at which changes occur in the template.[46] This system was evaluated intraoperatively in patients undergoing cardiac surgery.[43] The device monitored three selected leads and displayed the absolute values of the ST segment as a line. Upward deflection of the trend line indicated worsening ischemia, whereas a downward trend reflected return of the ST segment toward the isoelectric line. The authors concluded that once the device was clinically accepted, the awareness of ischemic changes increased among the participating anesthesiologists, and therapeutic interventions were instituted more rapidly.

Other systems differ from the above in various ways. In the Hewlett-Packard system, a period of 15 seconds is analyzed first, and the ST displacement is determined on five "good" beats. These displacements are ranked, and the median value is determined. This eliminates the influence of occasional PVCs and ensures that a representative beat is selected. The objective of this procedure is to obtain a representative beat rather than an average template. The measurement point for the ST segment can be selected as the R wave plus 108 ms (default) or the J point plus 60 or 80 ms. ST values and representative complexes are stored at a resolution of 1 minute for the most recent 30-minute trend and at a resolution of 5 minutes for the preceding 7.5-hour trend.

In a third system (Spacelabs Healthcare), a composite ST-segment waveform is developed every 30 seconds and compared with a reference tracing acquired during an initial learning period. The isoelectric and ST-segment points can be manually adjusted to any location on the ECG tracing, or they can be automatically set to predetermined values.

In 1998, Leung and colleagues[47] reported the accuracy of ST trending monitors with that of Holter ECG recorders in detecting ST-segment changes (both analyzed offline) in 94 patients undergoing coronary artery bypass graft surgery. They found the sensitivity of the three ST-trending monitors in detecting ischemia was 75%, 78%, and 60% for Marquette (now GE Healthcare), Hewlett-Packard, and Datex (now GE Healthcare) monitors, respectively. The specificity was 89%, 71%,

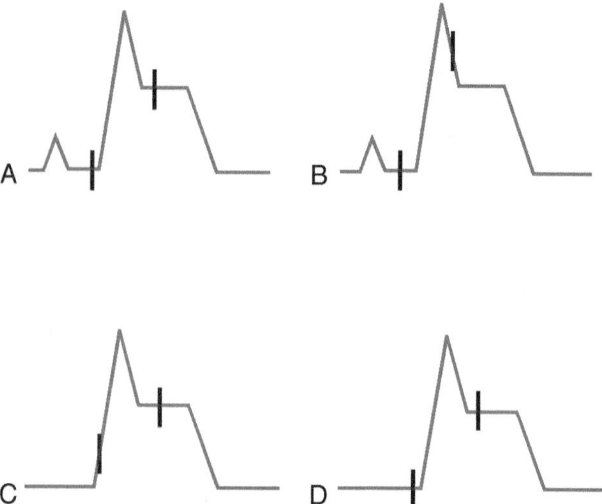

FIGURE 13-8 Schematic representation of isoelectric reference and J-point marker errors in ST-segment elevation templates. The interval between the J point and the isoelectric point is fixed at 115 ms by the algorithm. Two different patterns were noted for each of the two templates. In **B,** the J point is misplaced onto the downstroke of the R wave; in **C,** the isoelectric marker is misplaced onto the upstroke of the R wave. **A** and **D** demonstrate adequate placement of the points. (From London MJ, Ahlstrom LD: Validation testing of the Spacelabs PC2 ST-segment analyzer, *J Cardiothorac Vasc Anesth* 1995;9:684-693.)

and 69% relative to the Holter. Compared with the Hewlett-Packard and Datex monitors, the Marquette monitor had the best agreement with the Holter.

In a case report, Brooker and colleagues[48] described a case in which continuous automated ST-segment analysis (Component Monitoring System, Merlin Software Revision C, Hewlett-Packard) displayed significant and progressive ST-segment depression in three leads. Simultaneous ECG strip-chart recording failed to demonstrate any changes in the ST segments of the three monitored leads. The authors postulated that the erroneous automated interpretation may have been due to an inaccurate location of the measurement points in the ECG tracing.

To better define the role of QRS morphology on automated ST-segment analysis, London and colleagues[49] tested a commercially available ECG monitor (PC2 Bedside Monitor, ECG software version 6.05.16, Spacelabs Healthcare) using an ECG simulator (M311; Fogg System Company, Aurora, CO). Using seven different QRS shapes, they noted subtle errors in placement of the J point for each of the QRS shapes. In two QRS shapes, the isoelectric point was displaced onto the upstroke of an R wave, leading to erroneous ST-segment values (Figs. 13-8 and 13-9). Because each manufacturer uses distinct analysis algorithms, differences in results are expected. London and colleagues suggested that common testing standards be developed. They believe that the factors leading to differences between manufacturers are the location of fiducial points and the number of measurement points being used.

Artifacts mimicking arrhythmias have been reported that can lead to aggressive treatment, which may be unnecessary. Marco and colleagues[50] reported that SSEP monitoring caused an artifact that imitated supraventricular tachycardia; they treated the patient with esmolol before realizing that it was an artifact. According to the

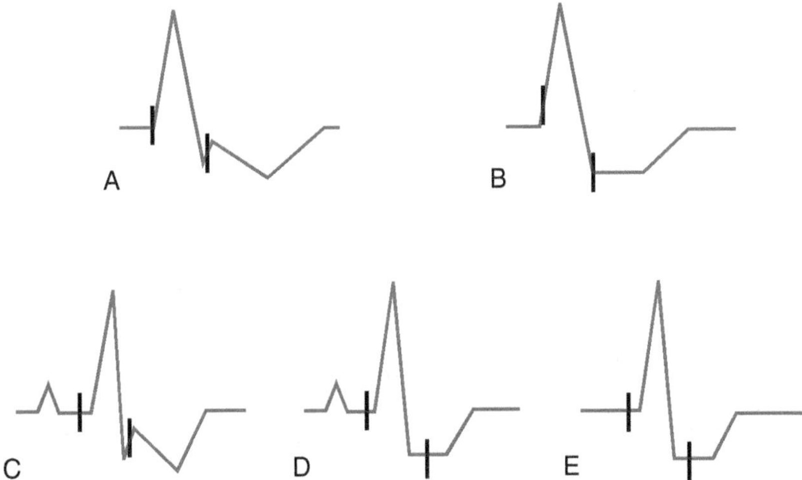

FIGURE 13-9 ▪ Schematic representation of isoelectric and J-point errors noted in ST-segment depression templates. **A** and **B** represent templates with prolonged QRS duration (120 ms), whereas the **C**, **D**, and **E** show those with normal QRS duration (80 ms). (From London MJ, Ahlstrom LD: Validation testing of the Spacelabs PC2 ST-segment analyzer. *J Cardiothorac Vasc Anesth* 1995;9:684-693.)

authors, these artifacts can be explained by partial or complete displacement of the stimulating electrode from the skin or by improper connection between stimulator outputs of the evoked potentials at the different stimulus sites.

Similarly, high-field magnetic resonance imaging (MRI; 1.5 T) in the neurosurgical OR for intraoperative resection control and functional neuronavigational guidance has been reported to cause artifacts.[51] Even MRI-compatible ECG monitoring interferes with electromagnetic fields, so several ECG artifacts can be observed in static and pulsed magnetic fields that can imitate malignant arrhythmias or provoke ST-segment abnormalities. The knowledge of possible and characteristic ECG artifacts during high-field MRI is therefore essential to prevent misinterpretation. When interference makes ECG monitoring difficult, interference-free parameters, such as pulse oximetry or invasive blood pressure curves, can be used for monitoring during intraoperative MRI scans. Others investigators have reported ECG monitoring artifacts inducing pacemaker-driven tachycardia both intraoperatively and in the recovery room.[52,53]

Cleland and colleagues[54] reported ECG pacemaker "pseudo-spikes" from RF interference in a patient in the postanesthesia care unit. The ECG artifact resulted in a misdiagnosis of pacemaker malfunction.

ELECTROCARDIOGRAPHIC MONITORING DURING MAGNETIC RESONANCE IMAGING

Conventional ECG monitoring is not possible during MRI because the lead wires must traverse magnetic fields, which causes distortion of the electrical signal. The need for wires can be eliminated by use of a telemetric ECG.[55] Fiberoptic technology for transmission of ECG signals has become commercially available in MRI-compatible monitoring systems (Veris, Warday Premise, Surrey, UK). The system provides five-lead ECG waveform monitoring and is compatible with 1.5T and 3T MRI systems. Other ECG monitors (Invivo, Gainesville, FL) use wireless technology and 8-hour battery capacity, thus eliminating the need for placement of the ECG monitor in the MRI suite. Digital signal processing and filtering removes MRI-related artifact during all MRI procedures to provide enhanced ECG performance and gating. The proprietary digital cardiac and peripheral gating algorithms ensure the best possible MR image quality.

In addition to ECG signals, capillary blood flow in the earlobe or lip measured by a laser Doppler system can be transmitted using fiberoptics.[56] With either transmission system, ECG artifacts are common with rapid pulse rates from the scanner.

The ECG should be monitored in all patients undergoing regional or general anesthesia. Although it does not provide information on the heart's mechanical function, it allows detection of electrical disturbances that can profoundly affect cardiac function. Today, with the judicious use of selected lead combinations, most arrhythmias and ischemic events can be precisely diagnosed intraoperatively. This diagnostic activity is time consuming, however, and considerable evidence suggests that many intraoperative ECG changes go undetected. There is little doubt that future technologic developments will facilitate the intraoperative recognition of ECG disturbances and lead to better patient outcomes.

REFERENCES

1. Thys DM, Kaplan JA, editors: *The ECG in anesthesia and critical care*, New York, 1987, Churchill Livingstone.
2. American Society of Anesthesiologists: *Standards for basic anesthetic monitoring*, Park Ridge, IL, American Society of Anesthesiologists.
3. Skeehan TM, Thys DM: Monitoring the cardiac surgical patient. In Hensley FA, Martin DE, editors: *The practice of cardiac anesthesia*, Boston, 1990, Little, Brown.
4. Shanewise JS: How to reliably detect ischemia in the intensive care unit and operating room, *Semin Cardiothorac Vasc Anesth* 10:101–109, 2006.
5. Goldberger: *Clinical electrocardiography: a simplified approach*, ed 7, St. Louis, 2006, Mosby, pp 8, 16.
6. Griffin RM, Kaplan JA: Myocardial ischaemia during noncardiac surgery: a comparison of different lead systems using computerized ST-segment analysis, *Anaesthesia* 42:155–159, 1987.
7. Bazaral MG, Norfleet EA: Comparison of CB5 and V5 leads for intraoperative electrocardiographic monitoring, *Anesth Analg* 60:849–853, 1981.

8. Hollenberg M, Mateo G, Massie BM, et al: Influence of the R-wave amplitude on exercise-induced ST depression: need for a "gain factor" correction when interpreting a stress electrocardiogram, *Am J Cardiol* 56:13–17, 1985.
9. Kaplan JA, King SB: The precordial electrocardiographic lead (V5) in patients who have coronary artery disease, *Anesthesiology* 45:570, 1976.
10. London MJ, Hollenberg M, Wong MG, et al: Intraoperative myocardial ischemia: localization by continuous 12 lead electrocardiography, *Anesthesiology* 69:232–241, 1988.
11. Landesberg G, Mosseri M, Wolf Y, et al: Perioperative myocardial ischemia and infarction: identification by continuous 12-lead with on-line ST-segment monitoring, *Anesthesiology* 96(2):259–261, 2002.
12. London MJ: Multilead precordial ST-segment monitoring: "the next generation"? *Anesthesiology* 96(2):259–261, 2002.
13. Kates RA, Zaidan JR, Kaplan JA: Esophageal lead for intraoperative electrocardiographic monitoring, *Anesth Analg* 61:781, 1982.
14. Jain U: Wave recognition and use of the intraoperative unipolar esophageal electrocardiogram, *J Clin Anesth* 9(6):487–492, 1997.
15. Colley PS, Artru AA: ECG-guided placement of Sorenson CVP catheters via arm veins, *Anesth Analg* 63:953–956, 1984.
16. Madias JE: Intracardiac electrocardiographic lead: a historical perspective, *J Electrocardiology* 37:83–88, 2004.
17. Chatterjee K, Swan HJC, Ganz W, et al: Use of a balloon-tipped flotation electrode catheter for cardiac monitoring, *Am J Cardiol* 36:56, 1975.
18. Lichtenthal PR: Multipurpose pulmonary artery catheter, *Ann Thorac Surg* 36:493, 1983.
19. Benzadon MN, Ortega DF, Thierer JM, et al: Comparison of the amplitude of the P-wave from intracardiac electrocardiogram obtained by means of a central venous catheter filled with saline solution to that obtained via esophageal electrocardiogram, *Am J Cardiol* 98(7):978–981, 2006.
20. Hayes JK, Peters JL, Smith KW, et al: Monitoring normal and aberrant electrocadiographic activity from an endotracheal tube: comparison of the surface, esophageal, and tracheal electrocardiograms, *J Clin Monit* 10:81–90, 1994.
21. Mirvis DM, Berson AS, Goldberger AL, et al: Instrumentation and practice standards for electrocardiographic monitoring in special care units, *Circulation* 79:464–471, 1989.
22. Pipberger HV, Arzbaecher RL, Berson AS, et al: Recommendations for standardization of leads and of specifications for instruments in electrocardiography and vectorcardiography. Report of the Committee on Electrocardiography, American Heart Association, *Circulation* 52:11–31, 1975.
23. Sheffield LT, Berson AS, Bragg-Remschel D, et al: Recommendations for standards of instrumentation and practice in the use of ambulatory electrocardiography. The task force of the Committee on Electrocardiography and Cardiac Electrophysiology of the Council on Clinical Cardiology, *Circulation* 71:626A–636A, 1985.
24. Association for the Advancement of Medical Instrumentation (AAMI): *American National Standards for Disposable Electrodes: ANSI/AAMI EC12: 2000(R 2010)*. Arlington, VA, 1984, American National Standards Institute/AAMI.
25. Legatt AD, Frost EAM: ECG artifacts during intraoperative evoked potential monitoring, *Anesthesiology* 70:559–560, 1989.
26. Paulsen AW, Pritchard DG: ECG artifact produced by crystalloid administration through blood/fluid warmer sets, *Anesthesiology* 69:803–804, 1988.
27. Lampert BA, Sundstrom FD: ECG artifacts simulating supraventricular tachycardia during automated percutaneous lumbar discectomy, *Anesth Analg* 67:1096–1098, 1988.
28. Arbeit SR, Rubin IL, Gross H: Dangers in interpreting the electrocardiogram from the oscilloscope monitor, *JAMA* 211:453–456, 1970.
29. Slogoff S, Keats AS, David Y, et al: Incidence of perioperative myocardial ischemia detected by different electrocardiographic systems, *Anesthesiology* 73:1074–1081, 1990.
30. Atlee JL, Rusy BF: Ventricular conduction times and AV nodal conductivity during enflurane anesthesia in dogs, *Anesthesiology* 47:498, 1977.
31. Edwards R, Winnie AP, Ramamurthy S: Acute hypocapneic hypokalemia: an iatrogenic anesthetic complication, *Anesth Analg* 56:786–792, 1977.
32. Angelini L, Feldman MI, Lufschonowski R, et al: Cardiac arrhythmias during and after heart surgery: diagnosis and management, *Prog Cardiovasc Dis* 16:469, 1974.
33. Sonntag H, Larsen R, Hilfiker O, et al: Myocardial blood flow and oxygen consumption during high-dose fentanyl anesthesia in patients with coronary artery disease, *Anesthesiology* 56:416–422, 1982.
34. Coriat P, Harari A, Daloz M, et al: Clinical predictors of intraoperative myocardial ischemia in patients with coronary artery disease undergoing non-cardiac surgery, *Acta Anaesthesiol Scand* 26:287, 1982.
35. Coy KM, Imperi GA, Lambert CR, et al: Silent myocardial ischemia during daily activities in asymptomatic men with positive exercise response, *Am J Cardiol* 59:45–49, 1987.
36. Pepine CJ: Is silent ischemia a treatable risk factor in patients with angina pectoris? *Circulation* 82(Suppl II):135–142, 1990.
37. Chaitman BR, Hanson JS: Comparative sensitivity and specificity of exercise electrocardiographic lead systems, *Am J Cardiol* 47:1335–1349, 1981.
38. Bell C, Rimar S, Barash P: Intraoperative ST segment changes consistent with myocardial ischemia in the neonate: a report of three cases, *Anesthesiology* 71:601–604, 1989.
39. Dodds TM, Delphin E, Stone JG, et al: Detection of perioperative myocardial ischemia using Holter with real-time ST segment analysis, *Anesth Analg* 67:890–893, 1988.
40. Romhilt DW, Bloomfield SS, Chai TC, et al: Unreliability of conventional electrocardiographic monitoring of arrhythmia detection in coronary care units, *Am J Cardiol* 31:457, 1973.
41. Oliver GE, Nolle FM, Wolff GA, et al: Detection of premature ventricular contractions with a clinical system for monitoring electrocardiographic rhythms, *Comput Biomed Res* 4:523, 1971.
42. Shah PM, Arnold JM, Haberen NA, et al: Automatic real-time arrhythmia monitoring in the intensive coronary care unit, *Am J Cardiol* 39:701, 1977.
43. Kotter GS, Kotrly KJ, Kalbfleisch JH, et al: Myocardial ischemia during cardiovascular surgery as detected by an ST-segment trend monitoring system, *J Cardiothorac Vasc Anesth* 1:190–199, 1987.
44. Morganroth J: Ambulatory Holter electrocardiography: choice of technique and clinical uses, *Ann Intern Med* 102:73, 1985.
45. Drew BJ, Robert M, Funk M, et al: Practice Standards for Electrocardiographic Monitoring in Hospital Settings: An American Heart Association Scientific Statement from the Councils on Cardiovascular Nursing, Clinical Cardiology, and Cardiovascular Disease in the Young, *Circulation* 110(17):2721–2746, 2004.
46. London MJ: Monitoring for myocardial ischemia. In Kaplan JA, editor: *Vascular anesthesia*, New York, 1991, Churchill Livingstone.
47. Leung JM, Voskanian A, Bellows WH, Pastor D: Automated electrocardiograph ST-segment trending monitors: accuracy in detecting myocardial ischemia, *Anesth Analg* 87:4–10, 1998.
48. Brooker S, Lowenstein E: Spurious ST segment depression by automated ST segment analysis, *J Clin Monit* 11:186, 1995.
49. London MJ, Ahlstrom LD: Validation testing of the Spacelabs PC2 ST-segment analyzer, *J Cardiothorac Vasc Anesth* 9:684–693, 1995.
50. Marco AP, Rice K: Pseudoarrythmia from evoked potential monitoring, *J Neurosurg Anesthesiol* 13(2):143–145, 2001.
51. Birkholz T, Schmid M, Nimsky C, et al: ECG artifacts during intraoperative high-field MRI scanning, *J Neurosurg Anesthesiol* 16(4):271–276, 2004.
52. Southorn PA, Kamath GS, Vasdev GM, Hayes DL: Monitoring equipment induced tachycardia in patients with minute ventilation rate responsive pacemakers, *Br J Anaesth* 84(4):508–509, 2000.
53. Hu R, Cowie DA: Pacemaker-driven tachycardia induced by electrocardiograph monitoring in the recovery room, *Anaesth Intensive Care* 34(2):266–268, 2006.
54. Cleland MJ, Crosby ET: Electrocardiographic "pacemaker pseudo-spikes" and radio frequency interference, *Can J Anaesth* 44(7):751–756, 1997.
55. Roth JL, Nugent M, Gray JE, et al: Patient monitoring during magnetic resonance imaging, *Anesthesiology* 62:80–83, 1985.
56. Higgins CB, Lanzer P, Stark D, et al: Imaging by nuclear magnetic resonance in patients with chronic ischemic heart disease, *Circulation* 69:523–531, 1984.

CHAPTER 14

TEMPERATURE MONITORING

Bijal R. Parikh • Henry Rosenberg

CHAPTER OUTLINE

OVERVIEW

Body temperature is a critical part of the homeostasis that allows for normal functioning of the human body. Alterations in body temperature can affect a wide array of physiologic processes, from vital chemical reactions catalyzed by enzymes to the optimal functioning of white blood cells and platelets.

Humans maintain body temperature by balancing heat production, primarily by metabolism, with heat loss mainly through a variety of physiologic mechanisms as well as environmental factors. The human body has a complex system in place to regulate body temperature in the awake state. However, during anesthesia many of these temperature-regulating pathways are interrupted or inhibited. This underscores the need for temperature monitoring during anesthesia.

As it relates to anesthesia and the perioperative period, the goal of the anesthesia provider is to minimize deviations in body temperature—unless indicated for specific reasons, such as organ protection—and to determine reasons for any observed deviations in body temperature.

Beginning in the 1960s, a major concern related to body temperature during or immediately following anesthesia was the marked hyperthermia characteristic of the malignant hyperthermia (MH) syndrome. This potentially fatal pharmacogenetic disorder of anesthesia had a marked influence on how the anesthesia community viewed the importance of temperature measurement and regulation.

However, studies conducted more recently have pointed out that even mild hypothermia, as is often noted during anesthesia, carries physiologic risks. Core temperature in the range of 35° C to 36° C triples the incidence of morbid cardiac outcomes, triples the risk of surgical wound infection, and significantly increases blood loss and the need for allogeneic transfusion. In the pediatric population, hypothermia poses additional dangers in terms of acid-base balance and cardiovascular physiology.

This chapter provides an in-depth understanding of perianesthetic thermoregulation in terms of effects of anesthetic agents and techniques, use of monitoring devices, and techniques for maintenance of normothermia. It also provides current recommendations for management of core temperature during surgery and in the recovery period.

THERMOREGULATION

Temperature regulation has three components: 1) an afferent input, 2) a central control, and 3) an efferent response. The afferent component is composed of both heat and cold receptors, which are widely distributed in the body. Heat and warmth receptors travel primarily through unmyelinated C fibers, whereas cold receptors travel along A-δ nerve fibers, although some overlap does occur.[1]

Ascending sensory thermal input is then transmitted to the hypothalamus, the primary thermoregulatory control center of mammals, via the spinal thalamic tracts in the anterior spinal cord.[2] Although most thermal information is integrated by the hypothalamus, some processing and response occurs within the spinal cord itself.[3] For example, patients with high spinal cord transections have better than expected thermoregulation.

Each thermoregulatory response can be characterized by the threshold, gain, and response. The *threshold* is the temperature at which a *response* will occur. The *gain* represents the intensity of that response. The threshold for responses to warmth (sweating and vasodilation) normally exceeds the threshold for the first response to cold (vasoconstriction) by 0.2° C to 0.4° C (Fig. 14-1). Temperatures within this interthreshold range—0.2° C to 0.4° C, the range in between the threshold for response to cold and the threshold for response to warmth—do not trigger any thermoregulatory responses. However, temperatures outside the interthreshold range do trigger a response.[4]

Efferent responses are the activation of effector mechanisms, which either increase metabolic heat production or alter environmental heat loss. The intensity of the response is proportional to the need, or afferent input, and the order in which the responses are used is progressive. Energy-efficient effectors, such as vasoconstriction, are first maximally used before the energy-costly ones, such as shivering, occur. Quantitatively, the most effective responses are behavioral ones: dressing appropriately, moving voluntarily, or adjusting ambient temperature. However, behavioral responses are not relevant for patients under general anesthesia, who are unconscious and often paralyzed.

The major autonomic responses to heat are sweating and active cutaneous vasodilation. Sweating is mediated by postganglionic cholinergic (acetylcholine [ACh]) nerves,[5] and sweat essentially is an ultrafiltrate of plasma. Sweating is the only mechanism by which the body can dissipate heat in an environment in which ambient temperature exceeds core temperature. The body is highly efficient at doing so: 0.58 kcal of heat is dissipated per gram of evaporated sweat.[4] It is also believed that sweat glands release an unidentified substance that mediates cutaneous vasodilation.[6] Cutaneous vasodilation, a unique effector mechanism of humans, diverts blood to the periphery, where heat can be dissipated by the environment more easily and ultimately can lower core temperature.

The major autonomic response to cold is cutaneous vasoconstriction, mediated by α_1-adrenergic receptors and synergistically augmented by hypothermia-induced α_2-adrenergic receptors.[7] Cutaneous vasoconstriction reduces the amount of blood vulnerable to heat loss from the skin surface through convection and radiation. The other major response to cold is shivering, an involuntary muscular activity that increases metabolic heat production by 50% to 100%.[8] Metabolic heat production can be estimated from oxygen consumption or from carbon dioxide production. The response of shivering is absent in the newborn and is probably not fully functional for several years. Infants therefore rely on nonshivering thermogenesis, an important thermoregulatory response that doubles heat production in infants,[9] although it raises temperature only slightly in adults.[10] Nonshivering thermogenesis is mediated by β_3-adrenergic receptors found on brown fat,[11] which contains a unique uncoupling protein that allows the direct transformation of substrate into heat.[12]

EFFECTS OF ANESTHESIA

General anesthesia is associated with an initial decrease in core temperature of approximately 0.5° C to 1.5° C over approximately 30 minutes followed by a slower linear decrease of about 0.3° C per hour until a plateau finally is reached (Fig. 14-2). The initial temperature

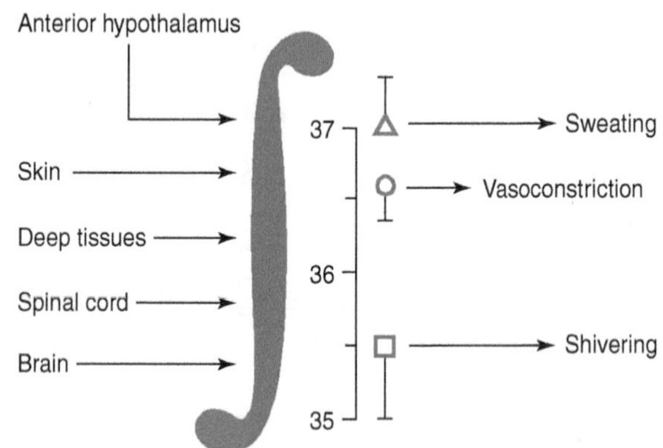

FIGURE 14-1 Thermoregulatory control mechanisms. Mean body temperature is the integrated thermal input from a variety of tissues, including the brain, skin surface, spinal cord, and deep core structures; this input is shown entering the hypothalamus from the left. Temperature thresholds usually are expressed in terms of *core temperature.* A core temperature below the threshold for response to cold provokes vasoconstriction, nonshivering thermogenesis, and shivering. A core temperature exceeding the hyperthermic threshold produces active vasodilation and sweating. No thermoregulatory responses are initiated when the core temperature is between these thresholds; these temperatures identify the *interthreshold range,* which in humans usually is only about 0.2° C. (From Sessler DI: Perioperative hypothermia. *N Engl J Med* 1997;336:1730-1737.)

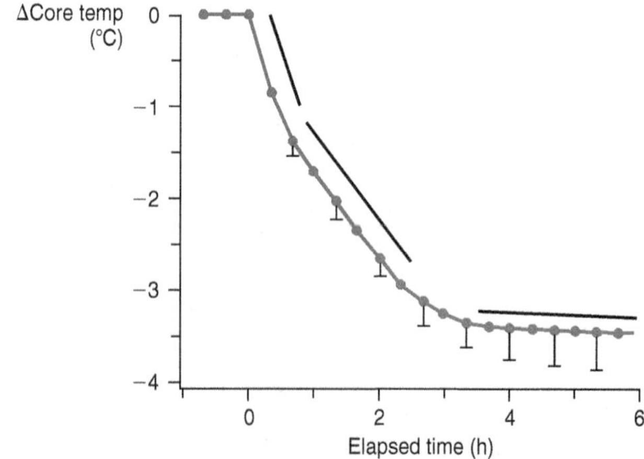

FIGURE 14-2 Hypothermia during general anesthesia develops with a characteristic pattern. An initial rapid decrease in core temperature results from a core-to-peripheral redistribution of body heat. This redistribution is followed by a slow, linear reduction in core temperature that results simply from heat loss exceeding heat production. Finally, core temperature stabilizes and subsequently remains virtually unchanged. This plateau phase may be a passive thermal steady state or may result when sufficient hypothermia triggers thermoregulatory vasoconstriction. Results are presented as mean ± standard deviation.

drop is due in part to increased heat loss during prepping and draping but primarily reflects redistribution of body heat from the core to cooler peripheral tissues with anesthesia-induced vasodilation (Fig. 14-3).[13] The periphery may be 3° C cooler than the core, but body temperature is maintained because of vasoconstriction. With general anesthesia, the vasoconstriction is reduced, leading to mixing of warm core blood with the cooler periphery. The slower linear decrease in temperature occurs as a result of heat loss that exceeds metabolic heat production.[14] General anesthesia completely eliminates any behavioral responses to temperature change. In addition, vasoconstriction is impaired by most anesthetic agents, and muscle relaxants reduce heat production from resting tone in muscles and prevent shivering. Although central regulation of temperature is likely to be depressed, regulation still occurs, albeit at a lower temperature. Sessler and colleagues found that with potent inhaled agents and intravenous (IV) agents, the threshold for the vasoconstrictive response to hypothermia decreases and is dose related (Fig. 14-4) but nevertheless occurs.[15-17]

Major conduction anesthesia has its own implications on body temperature and is almost as severe as general anesthesia.[18,19] There is still an initial drop in core temperature caused by neuraxial blockade–induced vasodilation, resulting in redistribution of perfusion from the core to the periphery.[20] As with general anesthesia, subsequent heat loss exceeds metabolic production owing to a slow linear decline. In contrast to general anesthesia, a plateau may not be reached for two reasons: the vasoconstriction threshold is centrally altered, decreasing the threshold about 0.6° C[21]; more importantly, however, vasoconstriction in the lower extremities is directly inhibited by the nerve block (Fig. 14-5).[22,23] Because the lower extremities represent a major thermal compartment, it is difficult to reach an effective plateau without vasoconstriction in the lower extremities, which would minimize cutaneous heat loss. Both spinal and epidural anesthesia alter the central control of thermoregulation to a similar degree.[21]

The effects of general and regional anesthesia on temperature are additive. The threshold for vasoconstriction during combined regional/general anesthesia is centrally decreased by 1° C more than with general anesthesia alone. Core temperature during regional/general anesthesia continues to decrease throughout the surgery[24]; thus it is especially crucial to monitor temperature during combined regional/general anesthesia.

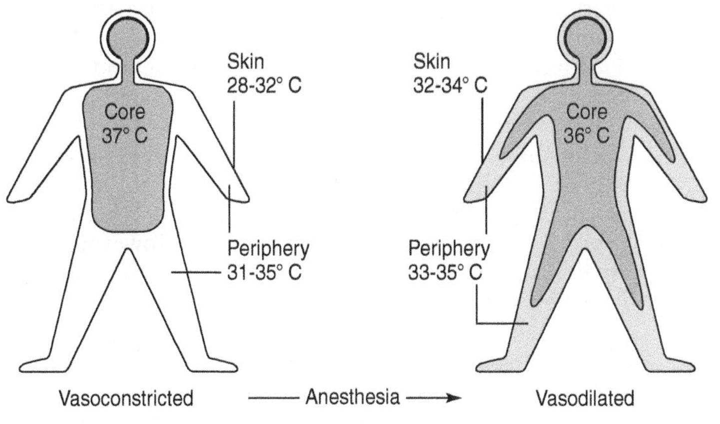

FIGURE 14-3 Internal redistribution of body heat after induction of general anesthesia. Hypothermia after induction of spinal or epidural anesthesia shows similar results, but redistribution is restricted to the legs.

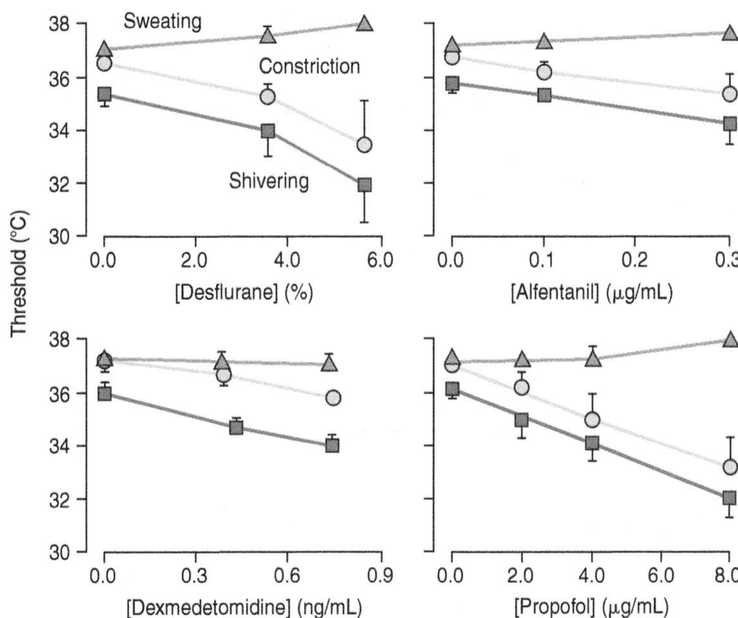

FIGURE 14-4 Changes in thermoregulatory thresholds associated with four anesthetics. The thresholds for sweating (*triangles*), vasoconstriction (*circles*), and shivering (*squares*) are expressed in terms of core temperature at a designated mean skin temperature of 34° C. Doses of desflurane are expressed as percentages of end-tidal expired gas. (From Sessler DI: Perioperative hypothermia. *N Engl J Med* 1997;336:1730-1737.)

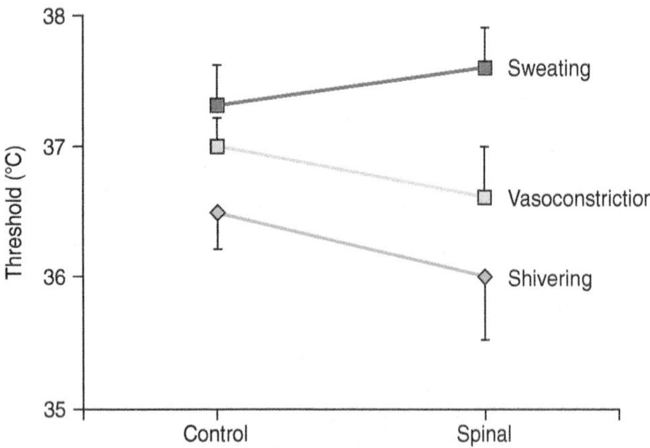

FIGURE 14-5 Spinal anesthesia increased the sweating threshold but reduced the thresholds for vasoconstriction and shivering. Consequently, the interthreshold range increases substantially. The vasoconstriction-to-shivering range, however, remained normal during spinal anesthesia. Results are presented as mean ± standard deviation. (From Kurz A, Sessler DI, Schroeder M, Kurz M: Thermoregulatory response thresholds during spinal anesthesia. *Anesth Analg* 1993;77:721-726.)

MECHANISMS OF INTRAOPERATIVE HEAT LOSS

The four physical processes of heat transfer of interest are *radiation*, *conduction*, *evaporation*, and *convection*. Radiation is the most significant route for intraoperative heat loss, but any one of these processes can overwhelm regulating mechanisms.

Radiant heat transfer likely accounts for the majority of heat loss to the environment.[25] It occurs via infrared radiation and is a function of the body surface area exposed to the environment. Radiant heat transfer is proportional to the fourth power of the absolute temperature difference between the surfaces. Infants have a high surface area/body mass ratio and therefore are especially vulnerable to heat loss by radiation.

Conductive heat transfer occurs from direct contact of body tissues or fluids to a colder material. This may be direct contact between the skin and the operating table or between the intravascular compartment and the infusion of cold fluid. For example, 1 L of crystalloid fluid infused at 21° C to a body temperature of 37° C will decrease mean body temperature by 0.25° C/L, and the infusion of 2 units of cold blood can result in a core temperature decrease of 1° C.[26]

Evaporative heat transfer is attributed to the latent heat of vaporization of water from open body cavities and the respiratory tract. Sweating increases evaporative heat loss but is uncommon during anesthesia. Evaporative heat loss through the skin is usually less than 10% of metabolic heat production.

Convective heat transfer is defined as heat loss as a result of moving fluid (air). This is likely the second most significant route for intraoperative heat loss. Convective heat transfer is proportional to the square root of the air speed and occurs as a result of the ambient air circulation that removes the air warmed by skin and viscera. Clothing or drapes are very effective in decreasing convective heat loss by trapping air near the skin.

EFFECTS OF MILD HYPOTHERMIA

Inadvertent mild hypothermia is a common occurrence during anesthesia. This is due primarily to anesthesia-induced redistribution and partly due to exposure to a cold operating room. The effects of mild hypothermia may be even greater than once thought, and many studies have examined the effects of mild intraoperative hypothermia.

Coagulation is impaired by mild hypothermia; a cold-induced defect in platelet function occurs, and activity of enzymes involved in the coagulation cascade is impaired.[27] Randomized clinical trials have shown that mild hypothermia significantly increases blood loss during hip arthroplasty and increases allogeneic transfusion requirements.[28]

Wound infections are another consequence of mild intraoperative hypothermia.[29] Immune function is directly impaired, and cold-induced vasoconstriction decreases oxygen delivery to the wound site. Mild intraoperative hypothermia (<1° C decrease in core temperature) triples the risk for surgical wound infection in patients undergoing colon surgery. It also delays wound healing and prolongs hospitalization by 20%, even in noninfected patients.[30]

The most serious complication of hypothermia is a threefold increase in morbid myocardial outcomes.[31] This might be due to the elevated blood pressure and heart rate and increased plasma catecholamine levels found in hypothermic patients.

Shivering is uncomfortable for patients and also is potentially harmful because it can increase oxygen requirements by 135% to 468%,[32] although an increase of oxygen consumption above 100% usually is not sustained. This can be especially problematic in the elderly or patients with preexisting cardiac disease who cannot afford acute increases in oxygen demand. However, myocardial infarction is poorly correlated with shivering.[31] Postanesthetic shivering can be effectively treated with meperidine (12.5 to 25 mg IV).

Drug metabolism is decreased by hypothermia. For example, the duration of action for vecuronium is more than doubled by a 2° C reduction in core temperature.[33] During a constant infusion of propofol, the plasma concentration is approximately 30% greater than normal in hypothermic patients.[34] Extra caution should be taken to ensure that residual paralysis and sedation have satisfactorily been reversed or have otherwise worn off.

HYPERTHERMIC STATES

Only a limited number of conditions predispose to intraoperative hyperthermia because anesthesia tends to lower body temperature and blunt the response to interleukins that produce fever.[35] Even patients who are febrile at the onset of anesthesia generally cool down during surgery.

The most common reason for intraoperative hyperthermia is iatrogenic overwarming, particularly in children. The typical scenario is the use of a full-body convective warmer, often accompanied by a warming blanket during surgery on a peripheral body part, such as the hand or the neck. The excess heat is not dissipated because the patient is covered; hence hyperthermia may occur. This condition is best diagnosed based on the clinical condition and the resolution of hyperthermia upon uncovering the patient. Such hyperthermia may be accompanied by mild respiratory acidosis and an increase in carbon dioxide production as a result of an increased metabolic rate secondary to patient warming. In rare cases, a reaction to mismatched blood may be accompanied by intraoperative hyperthermia.

Not to be overlooked is equipment malfunction that may lead to spuriously elevated temperature. An unusual cause of a spuriously elevated body temperature is when a patient's temperature is monitored by a liquid crystal temperature strip on the forehead, and the patient is given a medication that leads to peripheral vasodilation and flushing. In some cases these temperature strips have a built-in 2° C offset to account for the normally cool skin temperature.[36] In that case, when flushing occurs, the temperature strip reads several degrees higher than core temperature.

MH syndrome is the most feared complication of anesthesia accompanied by hyperthermia.[37] This syndrome may be easily diagnosed if muscle rigidity and hypercarbia are noted despite normal minute ventilation. However, a more insidious onset of MH may also occur, marked first by slowly rising, then rapidly rising, end-tidal carbon dioxide ($ETCO_2$). Hyperkalemia and acidosis, both respiratory and metabolic, often are accompanying signs of MH. By the time MH has developed, the syndrome will have been in progress for many minutes.

The treatment must be geared first to discontinuing the triggering anesthetic gases with hyperventilation and immediate parenteral administration of dantrolene, starting with 2.5 mg/kg. Because the syndrome may recrudesce, dantrolene must be continued for at least 36 hours in an intensive care unit (ICU) setting. More information about MH is available from the Malignant Hyperthermia Association of the United States (www.mhaus.org) and in standard anesthesia textbooks.

Of note, MH has *not* been reported to occur later than 40 minutes after discontinuation of anesthesia.[38] In cases of marked hyperthermia in the postanesthesia care unit (PACU), the cause generally is infection. Marked hyperthermia may therefore develop postoperatively in patients undergoing urologic procedures, dental rehabilitation, surgery on body cavities that are "dirty," or drainage of an abscess. In addition, preexisting pneumonia or intraoperative aspiration may lead to postoperative febrile reactions. Rigors sometimes develop at the onset of the fever that are mistaken for the muscle rigidity of MH. Such fevers respond promptly to antipyretics, antibiotics, and surface cooling. However, if there is any doubt as to the cause of the fever, administration of dantrolene is appropriate. A prompt response to dantrolene, however, does not prove that the fever was related to MH.

PERIOPERATIVE TEMPERATURE MANAGEMENT

The importance of temperature regulation within the human body underscores the importance of temperature monitoring during anesthesia. With the normal temperature-regulating pathways being inhibited under anesthesia comes a need for temperature management devices. Because inadvertent mild hypothermia is the most common temperature-related complication, a multitude of patient warming devices are available.

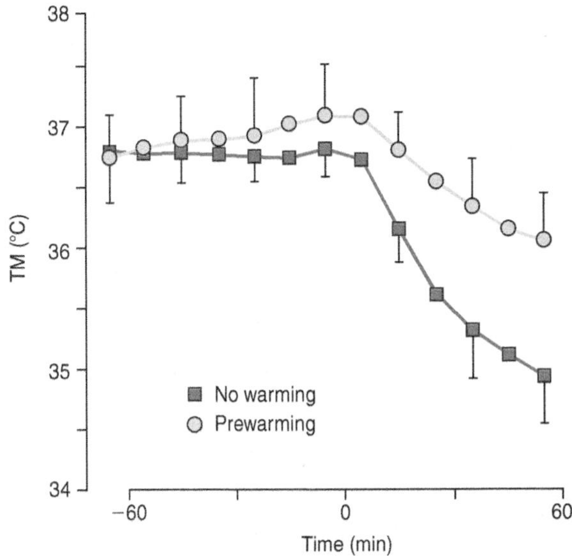

FIGURE 14-6 ■ **The way to prevent redistribution hypothermia is to warm peripheral tissues before induction of anesthesia. During the preinduction period (−120 to 0 min), volunteers were either actively warmed or passively cooled. At induction of anesthesia (time = 0 min), active warming was discontinued, and volunteers were exposed to the ambient environment. During the 60 minutes following induction of anesthesia, core temperature decreased less when volunteers were prewarmed compared with the same volunteers unwarmed.** (From Hynson JM, Sessler DI, Moayeri A, et al: The effects of pre-induction warming on temperature and blood pressure during propofol/nitrous oxide anesthesia. *Anesthesiology* 1993;79:219-228.)

During anesthesia, the initial 0.5° C to 1.5° C reduction in core temperature, reflecting redistribution of blood from the core to cooler peripheral tissues, is difficult to prevent.[39] However, warming the skin surface prior to induction results in less redistribution hypothermia because heat can only flow down a temperature gradient (Fig. 14-6).[40] Active prewarming for as little as 30 minutes likely prevents considerable redistribution.[41] This approach is gaining popularity because it is safe, easy to implement, and inexpensive if the same warming device is used intraoperatively.

Two types of devices attempt to maintain normothermia by affecting respiratory air exchange. One preserves heat by preventing evaporative losses and is often referred to as an *artificial nose*, a passive device that prevents some degree of heat loss but does not compare with active warming devices to maintain normothermia. The other type of device uses heating and humidification of inspiratory airway gases to maintain normothermia. Such devices are inserted in the inspiratory limb of the anesthesia machine, but they are cumbersome and require installation and setup. Because only a small amount of heat is lost through respiratory gases, active heating and humidification only minimally influence core temperature.[42] Most of the heat loss occurs from evaporation rather than gas exchange; devices therefore are only minimally beneficial in preventing heat loss. Furthermore, to avoid airway burns, the temperature of the heated gases must be carefully monitored.

Heat loss from administration of cold IV fluids can become significant when large volumes of fluid are being administered. A number of devices are available that warm the IV fluid pathway to deliver heat. A unit of refrigerated blood or 1 L of crystalloid solution administered at room temperature decreases mean body temperature approximately 0.25° C. When massive transfusion occurs, such as during rapid blood loss from trauma, these devices are helpful in maintaining body temperature.

A variety of devices warm IV fluids. Some, such as the standard Ranger blood/fluid warming system (Fig. 14-7; Arizant Healthcare, Inc., now a part of 3M, Eden Prairie, MN) and the Medi-Temp blood/fluid warming system (Gaymar Industries, Inc., Orchard Park, NY), incorporate a fluid pathway in a cassette device that sits in or fits into a warming dock. Others, such as the Hotline (Smiths Medial, St. Paul, MN), are coaxial systems, in which the administered fluid flows through the inner lumen and is warmed using a counterflow of fluid traveling from a warming device along the outer lumen. Yet another device, the Astotherm Plus (Fig. 14-8; Futuremed America, Granada Hills, CA) warms the fluid pathway by inserting the tubing in a series of grooves in a drum-like device that delivers heat to the fluid as it courses through the tubing. Devices such as the Bair Hugger (Arizant Healthcare) warm the fluid by warm air diverted to an accessory device containing the IV fluid line.

For infusion of large volumes of fluid or blood, it is advisable to warm the patient with both convective and fluid warming devices. According to one study, "the negative thermal balance of infusing 3 L of 21° C crystalloid into a 37° C 70-kg adult patient is 48 kcal. This heat loss represents approximately 1 hour of heat production…and is sufficient to decrease body temperature by 0.75° C or more during general anesthesia."[43] IV fluid warming plus convective warming did lead to better maintenance of normothermia, but the differences between the group with convective warming and the group with convective warming plus fluid warming were small. In any case, the IV fluid will lose significant heat during the infusion unless the length of tubing that contains the heated IV fluid is rather short.

The cost of acquiring the heating device and special tubing must be considered in calculating the value of preventing a small (<0.5° C) drop in body temperature during routine surgery. A detailed analysis of technical and cost considerations may be found in the National Health Service (U.K.) Buying Guide for Intravenous Fluid Warming Devices.[44]

The most basic approach to prevent heat loss during anesthesia is to use cotton blankets kept warm in nearby warming cabinets. This is an easy, low-tech solution and is a quiet method of preventing heat loss. Most blankets are kept in cabinets that can be set from 32° C to 60° C (90° F to 140° F), and a single cotton blanket reduces heat loss by approximately 30% (Fig. 14-9).[45] Adding more layers does not help much for procedures of shorter duration,[46] but for longer procedures adding more cotton blankets does seem to reduce heat loss.[3] Furthermore, the marginal benefit of reflective blankets coated with insulating material must be evaluated in relation to the extra cost. However, such techniques merely prevent heat loss and do not add heat. The forced-air warming device category was created in 1987 by Arizant Healthcare (Fig. 14-10). These devices transfer heat to the patient via convective warming (air-to-surface warming). The disposable warming blankets are placed on the body and connected to forced warm air. Currently, forced air is the most common perioperative warming system used, and about 25 different disposable warming blankets are currently available. The newest blankets, the underbody series, warm patients from below; this allows full-body access to patients, which is ideal for surgeries in which the surgeon needs a greater area of the torso exposed, such as major abdominal and cardiothoracic surgeries. The forced-air warming system is able to maintain normothermia even during major surgery[4] and is superior to the warming provided by circulating-water mattresses.[4,47]

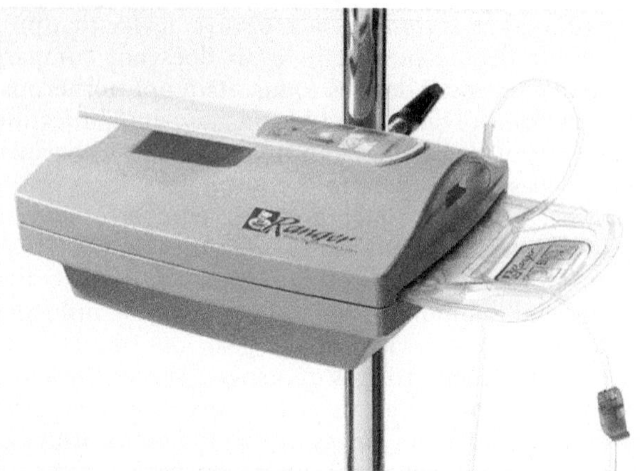

FIGURE 14-7 The Ranger blood-warming device (Arizant Healthcare, Inc. [now part of 3M], Eden Prairie, MN) features a fluid pathway in a cassette that sits in or fits into a warming dock.

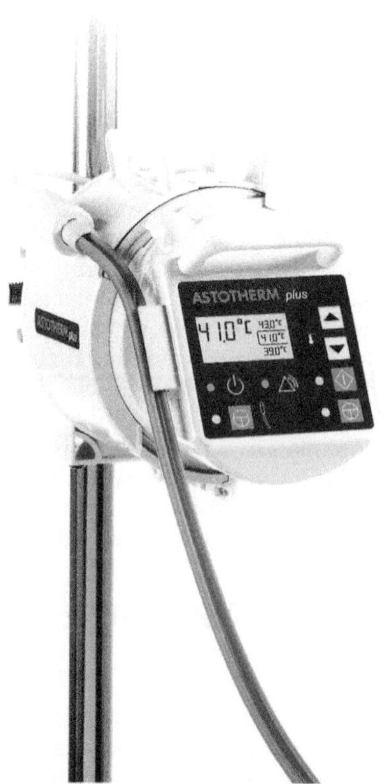

FIGURE 14-8 The Astotherm device (Futuremed America, Granada Hills, CA). The fluid pathway is warmed by inserting the tubing in a series of grooves in a drumlike device that delivers heat to the fluid as it courses through the tubing.

A system introduced by Kimberly-Clark Health Care (Roswell, GA) circulates heated water through thermal pads placed on the patient's body. These disposable, nonslip, hydrogel thermal pads are available in various sizes and conduct heat directly through the skin to safely maintain normothermia while allowing surgical access.[48,49] Use of this warming system has been limited by its high cost.

Conductive fabric warming (CFW) technology, such as the Hot Dog Patient Warming System (Augustine Temperature Monitoring Management, Eden Prairie, MN), is a warming technology consisting of reusable electric blankets and mattresses (Fig. 14-11). The heat is produced by passing low-voltage electric current through fabric coated with a semiconductive polymer. CFW blankets have been shown to be equally effective as forced-air warming (FAW) blankets.[50] The reusable CFW blankets must be wiped clean between uses, but still provide significant savings in the per-patient cost of warming and are ecologically friendly.

Recent evidence shows that CFW prevents the spread of waste heat and waste air that emanate from FAW devices, potentially mitigating sterile field contamination by the waste air. CFW was developed to mitigate the sterile field contamination and orthopedic infection risks now known to be caused by the waste heat and waste air from FAW.[51]

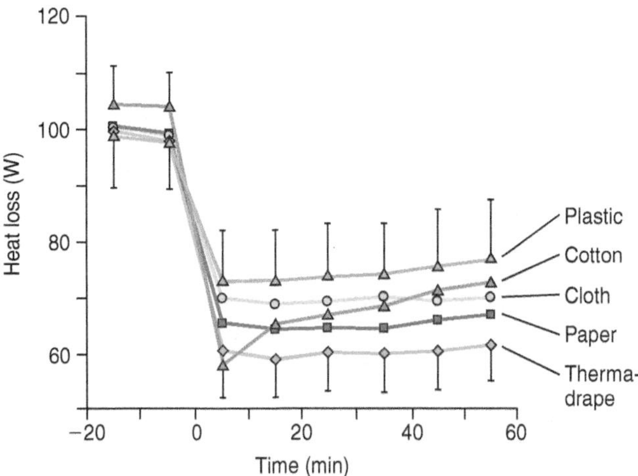

FIGURE 14-9 ▪ Intraoperative heat loss is decreased by passively insulating the patient by a variety of materials. No clinically important differences were noted among the materials, and heat loss in any case can be reduced by 30%. (Data from Sessler DI, et al: Perioperative thermal insulation. *Anesthesiology* 1991;74:875-879.)

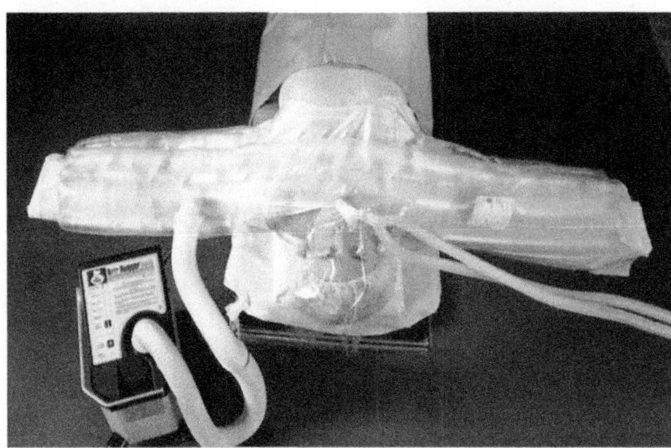

FIGURE 14-10 ▪ Forced-air warming with an upper body blanket (Bair Hugger, Arizant Healthcare, Inc. [now part of 3M], Eden Prairie, MN). Also available are blankets to cover the lower body and one to cover the entire body.

The Insuflow Laproscopic Gas Conditioning Device (Lexion Medical, Austin, TX) delivers gas that has been humidified to 95% relative humidity and warmed to 35° C (95° F), instead of cold and dry carbon dioxide, during insufflation of the peritoneum. This method has not been shown to decrease hypothermia, but interestingly, some authors have reported that the use of heated humidified insufflating gas may reduce postoperative morbidity and pain.[52] However, larger studies are necessary to show the advantages of humidifying insufflating gas.

Recently developed intravascular temperature management devices, such as the Thermogard Temperature Management System (Zoll Medical Corporation, Chelmsford, MA), have proven to be the most effective for rapid manipulation of body temperature. However, intravascular temperature management is also the most invasive method of controlling temperature and usually is reserved for trauma patients, critically ill patients undergoing major surgery, and those undergoing coronary bypass surgery, when manipulation of temperature is necessary. This system consists of a heat-exchanging catheter (Fig. 14-12) inserted into the central venous system via the femoral or subclavian artery or internal jugular vein. The Thermogard system controls the temperature of the saline circulating through the catheter balloon via remote sensing of the patient's temperature. The patient is warmed as venous blood passes over each balloon, exchanging heat without infusing saline into the patient.

Radiant heating with heat lamps is effective primarily in children and is useful during trauma resuscitation, when many providers are crowding around the patient. In addition, warming lights focused on a shivering patient's face and upper torso often reduce shivering; however, warmed hot water bottles should *not* be used because they have been associated with superficial skin burns.

Techniques to cool the patient include uncovering the patient and placing bags of ice on the groin, neck, and axilla; however, it is more effective to lavage various cavities with ice, especially the stomach. This is highly effective in dropping body temperature. Nasogastric and bladder lavage also have been shown to be effective. In addition, some of the convective warmers are sold with the dual capability of delivering cool air. Circulating-water blankets placed over or under the patient also have the capability of passing cold water against the patient's skin. In the case of MH syndrome, it is vital that the hyperthermia and the metabolic changes be treated with the specific treatment drug, dantrolene. Further information is found in the section on hyperthermic states in this chapter.

TRANSDUCERS AND DEVICES FOR MEASURING TEMPERATURE

Mercury Thermometers

The mercury-in-glass thermometer is one of the oldest and simplest devices currently used for clinical thermometry. This is neither the safest nor the fastest method and also is very limited in its access to various remote sites of interest for thermometry in anesthesia. For most purposes,

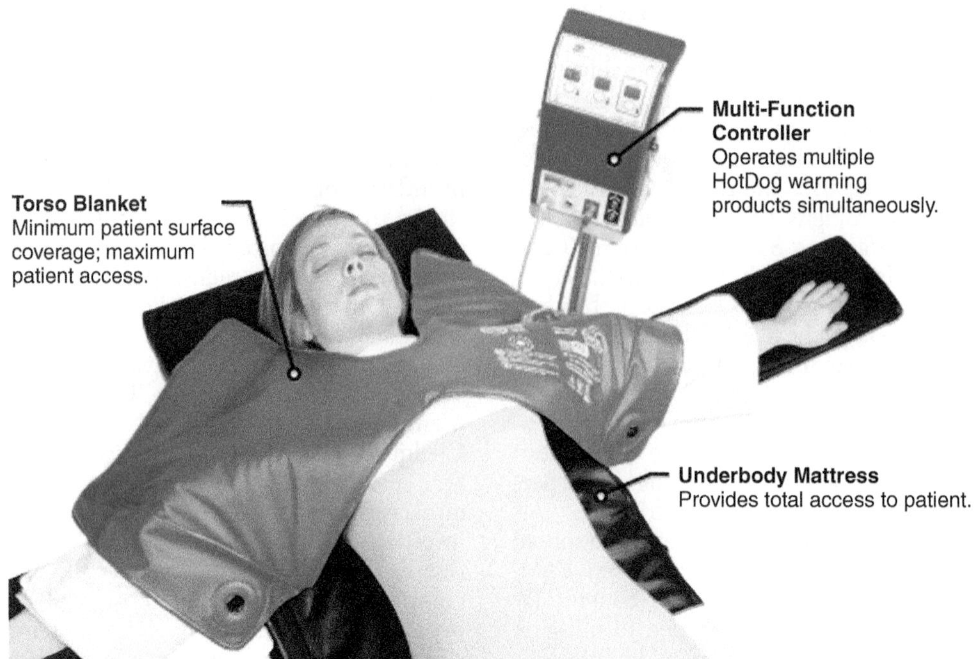

FIGURE 14-11 ■ Hot Dog warming blanket (Augustine Temperature Management, Eden Prairie, MN). An example of an under-body electric warming device along with a torso blanket.

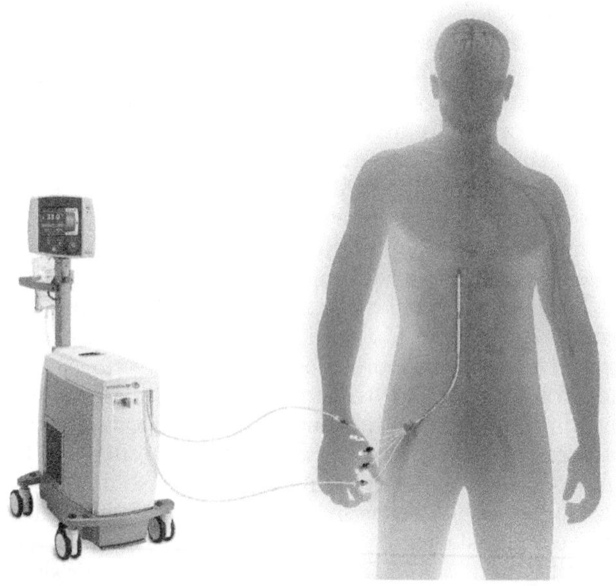

FIGURE 14-12 ■ Intravascular catheter apparatus for delivering heat to patients. The device circulates warmed fluid through a sheath surrounding the catheter.

a telethermometer that consists of a transducer probe connected by a cable to a monitor and a display is an essential arrangement. The most commonly used transducers are thermistors and thermocouples.

Thermistors

Commonly used thermistors are metal-oxide semiconductors.[53] The electrical conductivity of semiconductors depends on thermally excited electrons and "holes" as charge carriers and therefore has a strong temperature dependence dominated by the concentration of charge carriers. A simple battery-powered bridge circuit is shown in Figure 14-13. Thermistor thermometers operate at reasonably low impedances and are relatively immune from interference. Although an outside power source is required, it can be as simple as a single battery cell. Power dissipation rarely is an issue. These transducers are inexpensive and stable, and their readings are reproducible at an accuracy of 0.1° C or 0.2° C. They can be made small enough to fit inside a 25-gauge needle for measurement of muscle temperature. One concern with the circuit in Figure 14-13 is that, although it is battery powered, it is not isolated from ground. If the case is set on a grounded metal surface, microshock or electrosurgical burns at the probe site are possible.[51] Isolated circuits with electrosurgical protection are also available.

Thermocouples

Thermocouples are junctions of two different metals. In a circuit consisting of two such junctions at different temperatures, a small voltage or current is generated from what is known as the *Seeback effect*. The temperature gradient produces a heat flux, carried largely by electrons, in each metal. According to the transport equations, an associated current (or voltage for an open circuit) is induced. Because of differences between metals, voltage gradients in each metal do not precisely cancel, and the voltage difference can be measured with the arrangement shown in Figure 14-14. The second law of thermodynamics is not violated because heat is conducted along the wires from the hot junction to the cold junction.

Thermocouples for clinical thermometry typically use copper-constantan (copper with 40% nickel) junctions. This combination produces a small voltage most

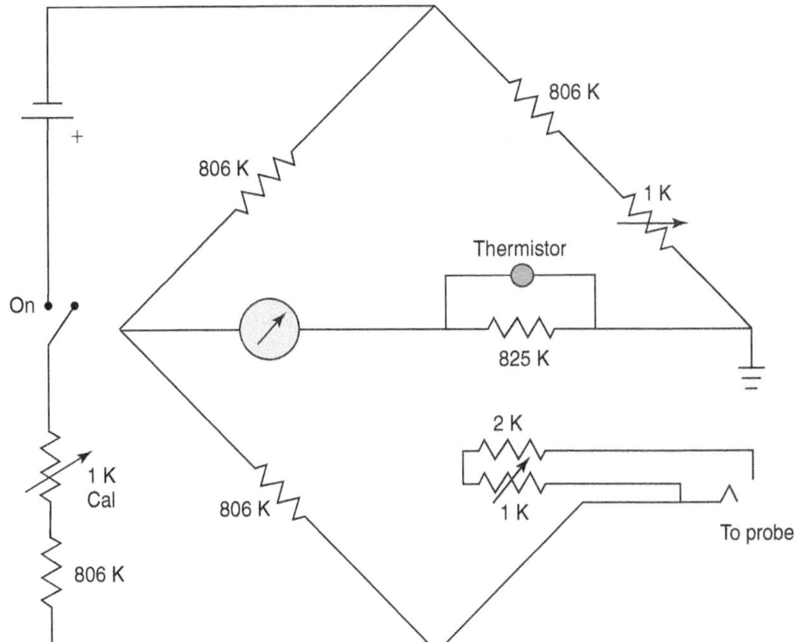

FIGURE 14-13 ■ Circuit for thermistor temperature monitor. This is a simple battery-powered bridge circuit.

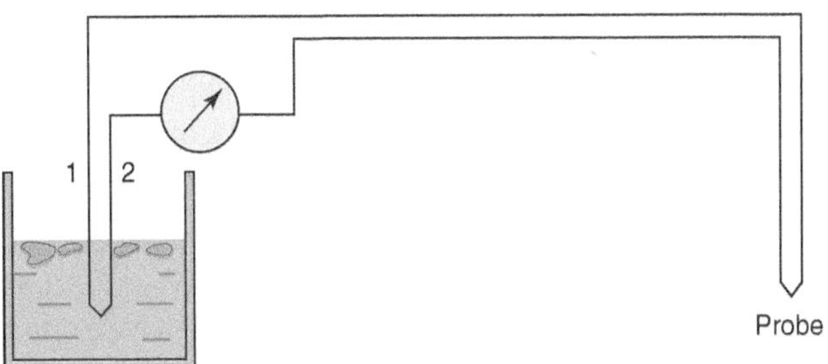

FIGURE 14-14 ■ Circuit for thermocouple thermometer. The probe consists of two different metals (*1* and *2*) that conduct heat differently, which results in the generation of a current that can be measured on the meter (*arrow*).

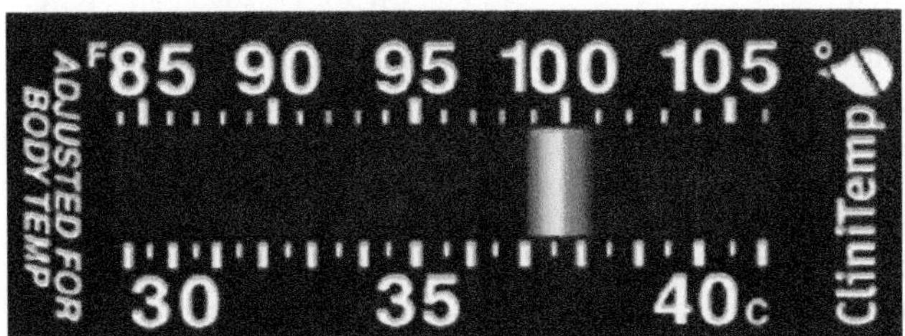

FIGURE 14-15 ■ An example of a skin temperature liquid crystal monitor (Sharn Anesthesia, Inc., Tampa, FL).

easily measured with an amplifier. Although an outside power source is not required, in practice the apparatus is more complicated than the thermistor thermometer. The reference junction can be kept in an ice water bath, in a heated or cooled oven, or even in contact with semiconductor circuits, measuring its temperature and applying an appropriate compensation. Probes are less expensive and also are available in very small sizes. Carefully made junctions are likely to be stable and accurate to 0.1° C.

Liquid Crystal Thermometers

Liquid crystals have complicated structures with large-scale order.[55] Liquid crystal thermometers use cholesteric liquid crystals, which have an ordered layer structure with directional asymmetry in the plane of each layer. The orientation of this asymmetry gradually rotates with each succeeding layer, yielding a periodicity that may be the size of a wavelength of visible light or larger. This structure makes the substance optically active; it rotates the plane of polarized light. The optical properties are highly sensitive to temperature; when liquid crystals are encapsulated in thin films or used with polarizers, the color changes with temperature. Optical changes with phase transitions between various structures also can be used for displaying temperature. These devices are readily applied to measure skin surface temperature. Two forms are available: one displays the actual temperature measured, and the other has a built-in offset so that the temperature displayed estimates core temperature (Figure 14-15).[36] However, under rapidly changing conditions, there is a significant discrepancy between core and skin temperature.[56]

Infrared

The infrared thermometer is a noninvasive device that collects radiation emitted by a warm object. The radiation sensed is converted to a temperature on the basis of an empirical calibration. A small probe covered with a disposable, transparent cover is inserted into the external auditory meatus, where the infrared detector can "see" the tympanic membrane. This method provides a prompt, accurate measure of core temperature.[57] Newer probes have been made for use over the forehead (Fig. 14-16). These infrared devices are placed in the center of the forehead and are scanned along the hairline over the temporal artery. This has become an increasingly popular method for determining temperatures in the PACU because it

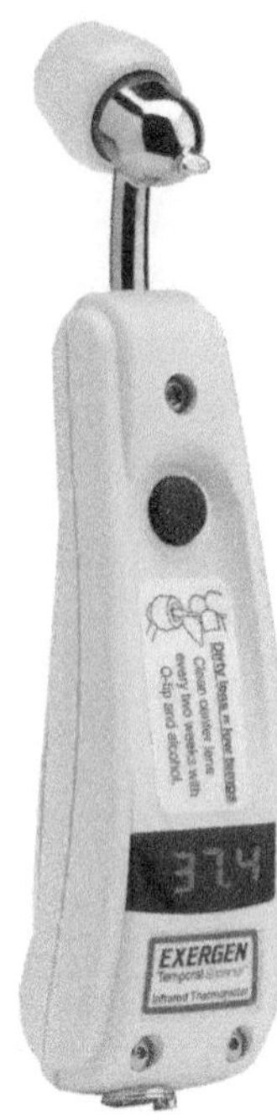

FIGURE 14-16 ■ Temporal Scanner (Exergen, Watertown, MA) infrared forehead temperature-measuring device, which scans the temporal artery.

provides a quick and noninvasive approximation of core temperature.[58] The accuracy of the device was found to be clinically insufficient in one study, but a later updated study found the device to be suitable for clinical use.[59,79]

TEMPERATURE MONITORING SITES

The site for monitoring temperature during anesthesia depends on the surgical procedure, the type of anesthesia used, and the reason for temperature monitoring. When significant changes in body heat are expected, core temperature should be monitored.

The gold standard for measuring core temperature is the temperature of pulmonary arterial blood. The temperature of pulmonary arterial blood correlates well with tympanic membrane temperature, distal esophageal temperature, and nasopharyngeal temperature. When a pulmonary arterial catheter is not otherwise necessary, any of these other sites usually suffices.[60]

The tympanic membrane is close to the carotid artery, and the temperature of the blood supplied to the tympanic membrane approximates that at the hypothalamus.[61] The placement of a temperature probe on or near the tympanic membrane risks perforation and bleeding, especially with heparinization.[62] The external auditory meatus is safer for this purpose but works well only if adequately insulated from the outside temperature.[63]

Nasopharyngeal temperature may reflect the same blood supply as the hypothalamus but is more subject to error from displacement or leakage of respiratory gases and resultant cooling.[64] The insertion of nasopharyngeal temperature probes also can result in epistaxis.[65]

The esophagus is a safe,[66] easily accessible, and accurate site for core temperature measurement during anesthesia. A combination stethoscope and temperature probe is easily passed to a position near the heart; the optimal position for the sensor in adults is 45 cm from the nose.[67] The temperature must be measured in the distal third or quarter of the esophagus to avoid cooling by respiratory gases in the trachea, even though this position may not be optimal for auscultation.

The use of rectal temperature monitoring was more popular in the past, although such readings are affected by heat-producing organisms in bowel, insulation by the feces, and blood returning from the lower limbs. Not only do rectal temperatures not accurately reflect core temperature,[54,68] a small risk of perforation exists with this method. Rectal temperature changes too slowly to follow intraoperatively, and contraindications include obstetrics, gynecologic, and urologic procedures.

Bladder temperature correlates with core temperature well and is easily measured with combination Foley catheter–themistor probe devices.[69] When urine flow is high, correlation between bladder and core temperature increases.[70] During cardiopulmonary bypass, temperature changes too rapidly for the bladder temperature to follow core temperature.[71]

Axillary temperature over the axillary artery with the arm adducted can give a reasonably accurate core temperature and is most reliable in infants and small children.[72] It should not be used on the same side as a blood pressure cuff on the upper arm. Similarly, sublingual temperature, although subject to error, is still useful, and awake patients tolerate the thermometer well.

Although skin temperature contributes to total body heat, it reflects peripheral perfusion rather than core temperature.[73] Total body heat can be calculated via estimates of mean skin temperature measured at multiple sites but is too cumbersome for routine use. Skin temperature, with a 2° C compensation, is a fair estimate of core temperature except in rapidly changing conditions such as malignant hyperthermia.[56,74] Skin temperature is most commonly measured at the forehead because it is easily accessible, has good blood flow, and has very little underlying fat. Readings can be affected by ambient temperature, skin-surface warming devices, and regional vasoconstriction.[74] Skin temperature monitoring also can be used as an indicator of a successful nerve block by observing an increase in temperature. It also can be used in microsurgery to indicate adequate blood flow by seeing an increase in temperature in that area.

Other sites may be of value in special situations. Myocardial temperature is readily measured with a needle probe during cardiopulmonary bypass, and skeletal muscle temperature provides the earliest indication of temperature change with MH.[75]

GUIDELINES FOR TEMPERATURE MONITORING

Although no absolute requirements for routine intraoperative temperature monitoring have been established (except in New Jersey), several guidelines have been proposed by various groups. Sessler,[76] an expert in perioperative temperature monitoring, has published guidelines for temperature monitoring and thermal management that have been published in many major textbooks. The Malignant Hyperthermia Association of the United States endorses these guidelines:

1. Core body temperature should be measured in most patients under general anesthesia for longer than 30 minutes.
2. Temperature also should be measured during regional anesthesia when changes in body temperature are intended, anticipated, or suspected.
3. Unless hypothermia is specifically indicated, efforts should be made to maintain the intraoperative core temperature above 36° C.

This contrasts with the American Society of Anesthesiologists' recommendation that "Every patient receiving anesthesia shall have temperature monitored when clinically significant changes in body temperature are intended, anticipated, or suspected."[77] In our opinion, this recommendation should be modified to reflect the need for continuous monitoring of this physiologic sign.

Other anesthesia societies promulgate the standard followed by the New Jersey State Society of Anesthesiologists that "The body temperature of each patient undergoing general or regional anesthesia shall be continuously monitored." The acceptance of routine intraoperative temperature monitoring is denoted by various quality organizations. The Surgical Care Improvement Project Requirement for Temperature Measurement promulgated by the Centers for Medicare and Medicaid Services to mitigate against the effects of hypothermia is as follows[78]:

All patients, regardless of age, undergoing selected surgical procedures under general or neuraxial anesthesia of greater than or equal to 60 minutes should have at least one body temperature equal to or greater than 96.8° F/36° C recorded within the 30 minutes immediately prior to or the 15 minutes immediately after anesthesia end time.

SUMMARY

There have been significant advances in the understanding of causes and consequences of intraoperative temperature changes in the past 20 years. The effects of even mild hypothermia as well as the consequences of malignant hyperthermia are better appreciated than ever before. This advance in knowledge has resulted in the introduction of a variety of devices and techniques for measuring and maintaining core temperature during the perioperative period. These changes have resulted in improved patient outcome.

REFERENCES

1. Poulos DA: Central processing of cutaneous temperature information, *Fed Proc* 40:2825–2829, 1981.
2. Satinoff E: Neural organization and evolution of thermal regulation in mammals: several hierarchically arranged integrating systems may have evolved to achieve precise thermoregulation, *Science* 201:16–22, 1978.
3. Simon E: Temperature regulation: the spinal cord as a site of extrahypothalamic thermoregulatory functions, *Rev Physiol Biochem Pharmacol* 71:1–76, 1974.
4. Sessler DI: Review article: mild perioperative hypothermia, *N Engl J Med* 336:1730–1737, 1997.
5. Hemingway A, Price WM: The autonomic nervous system and regulation of body temperature, *Anesthesiology* 29:693–701, 1968.
6. Rowell LB: Active neurogenic vasodilation in man. In Vanhoutte P, Leusen I, editors: *Vasodilation*, New York, 1981, Raven, pp 1–17.
7. Flavahan NA: The role of vascular alpha-2 adrenoreceptors as cutaneous thermosensors, *News Physiol Sci* 6:251–255, 1991.
8. Just B, Delva E, Camus Y, Lienhart A: Oxygen uptake during recovery following naloxone, *Anesthesiology* 76:60–64, 1992.
9. Dawkins MJ, Scopes JW: Non-shivering thermogenesis and brown adipose tissue in the human new-born infant, *Nature* 206:201–202, 1965.
10. Jessen K: An assessment of human regulatory nonshivering thermogenesis, *Acta Anaesthesiol Scand* 24:138–143, 1980.
11. Takahashi H, Nakamura S, Shirabase H, et al: Heterogeneous activity on BRI, 35135, a beta 3 adrenoreceptor agonist, in thermogenesis and increased blood flow in brown adipose tissue in anesthetized rats, *Clin Exp Pharmacol Physiol* 21:539–543, 1994.
12. Nedergaard J, Cannon B: The uncoupling protein thermogenin and mitochondrial thermogenesis, *New Comp Biochem* 23:385–420, 1992.
13. Vale RJ: Cooling during vascular surgery, *Br J Anaesth* 44:1334, 1972.
14. Hynson J, Sessler DI: Intraoperative warming therapies: a comparison of three devices, *J Clin Anesth* 4:194–199, 1992.
15. Sessler DI, Olofsson CI, Rubinstein EH: The thermoregulatory threshold of humans during halothane anesthesia, *Anesthesiology* 68:836–842, 1988.
16. Sessler DI, Olofsson CI, Rubinstein EH, et al: The thermoregulatory threshold in humans during nitrous oxide–fentanyl anesthesia, *Anesthesiology* 69:357–364, 1988.
17. Sessler DI: Temperature monitoring. In Miller RD, editor: *Anesthesia*, ed 3., New York, 1990, Churchill Livingstone, pp 1227–1242.
18. Hendolin H, Lansimies E: Skin and central temperatures during continuous epidural analgesia and general anesthesia in patients subjected to open prostatectomy, *Ann Clin Res* 14:181–186, 1982.
19. Sessler DI: Temperature monitoring and management during neuraxial anesthesia, *Anesth Analg* 88:243, 1999.
20. Matsukawa T, Sessler DI, Christensen R, et al: Heat flow and distribution during epidural anesthesia, *Anesthesiology* 83:961–967, 1995.
21. Ozaki M, Kurz A, Sessler DI, et al: Thermoregulatory thresholds during spinal and epidural anesthesia, *Anesthesiology* 81:282–288, 1994.
22. Valley MA, Bourke DL, Hamill MP, Srinivasa NR: Time course of sympathetic blockade during epidural anesthesia: laser Doppler flowmetry studies of regional skin perfusion, *Anesth Analg* 76:289–294, 1993.
23. Modig J, Malmberg P, Karlstrom G: Effect of epidural versus general anesthesia on calf blood flow, *Acta Anaesthesiol Scand* 24:305–309, 1980.
24. Joris H, Ozaki M, Sessler DI, et al: Epidural anesthesia impairs both central and peripheral thermoregulatory control during general anesthesia, *Anesthesiology* 80:268–277, 1994.
25. Hardy JD, Milhorat AT, DuBois EF: Basal metabolism and heat loss of young women at temperatures from 22 degrees C to 35 degrees C, *J Nutr* 21:383–403, 1941.
26. Gentilello LM, Cortes V, Moujaes S, et al: Continuous arteriovenous rewarming: experimental results and thermodynamic model simulation of treatment for hypothermia, *J Trauma* 30:1436–1449, 1990.
27. Michelson AD, MacGregor H, Barnard MR, et al: Reversible inhibition of human platelet activation by hypothermia in vivo and in vitro, *Thromb Haemost* 71:633–640, 1994.
28. Schmied H, Kurz A, Sessler DI, Kozek S, Reiter A: Mild intraoperative hypothermia increases blood loss and allogeneic transufusion requirements during total hip arthroplasty, *Lancet* 347:289–292, 1996.
29. Bremmelgaard A, Raahave D, Beir-Holgersen R, et al: Computer-aided surveillance of surgical infections and identification of risk factors, *J Hosp Infect* 13:1–18, 1989.
30. Kurz A, Sessler DI, Lenhardt RA: Study of wound infections and temperature group: perioperative normothermia to reduce the incidence of surgical-wound infection and shorten hospitalization, *N Engl J Med* 334:1209–1215, 1996.

31. Frank SM, Fleisher LA, Breslow MJ, et al: Perioperative maintenance of normothermia reduces the incidence of morbid cardiac events: a randomized clinical trial, *JAMA* 277:1127–1134, 1997.
32. Bay J, Nunn JF, Prys-Roberts C: Factors influencing arterial PO_2 during recovery from anesthesia, *Br J Anaesth* 40:398–407, 1968.
33. Heier T, Caldwell JE, Sessler DI, Miller RD: Mild intraoperative hypothermia increases duration of action and spontaneous recovery of vecuronium blockade during nitrous oxide– isoflurane anesthesia in humans, *Anesthesiology* 74:815–819, 1991.
34. Leslie K, Sessler DI, Bjorksten AR, Moayeri A: Mild hypothermia alters propofol pharmacokinetics and increases the duration of action of atricurium, *Anesth Analg* 80:1007–1014, 1995.
35. Negishi C, Lenhardt R, Sessler DI, et al: Desflurane reduces the febrile response to administration of interlukin-2, *Anesthesiology* 88(5):12, 1998.
36. Frank SM: Body temperature monitoring, *Anesth Clin North Am* 12:387–407, 1994.
37. Rosenberg H, Brandom BW, Sambuugh N: Malignant hyperthermia and other inherited disorders. In Barash P, Cullen B, Stoelting R, Cahalan M, Stock C, editors: *Clinical anesthesia*, ed 6, Philadelphia, 2009, Lippincott Williams & Wilkins. pp 598–621.
38. Litman RS, Flood CD, Kaplan RF, et al: Postoperative malignant hyperthermia: an analysis of cases from the North American Malignant Hyperthermia Registry, *Anesthesiology* 109(5):825–829, 2008.
39. Matsukawa T, Sessler DI, Sessler AM, et al: Heat flow and distribution during induction of general anesthesia, *Anesthesiology* 82:662–673, 1995.
40. Hynson JM, Sessler DI, Moayeri A, McGuire J, Schroeder M: The effects of pre-induction warming on temperature and blood pressure during propofol/nitrous oxide anesthesia, *Anesthesiology* 79:219–228, 1993.
41. Sessler DI, Schroeder M, Merrifield B, Matsukawa T, Cheng C: Optimal duration and temperature of prewarming, *Anesthesiology* 82:674–681, 1995.
42. Hynson JM, Sessler DI: Intraoperative warming therapies: a comparison of three devices, *J Clin Anesth* 4:194–199, 1992.
43. Smith CE, Desai R, Gorioso V, et al: Preventing hypothermia: convective and intravenous fluid warming versus convective warming alone, *J Clin Anesth* 10:380–385, 1998.
44. National Health Service: *Buying Guide for Intravenous Fluid Warming Devices*, 2010. Available at http://www.wales.nhs.uk/sites3/Documents/443/CEP10013%5B1%5D%20IV%20fluid%20warmers%20BG.pdf.
45. Sessler DI, McGuire J, Sessler AM: Perioperative thermal insulation, *Anesthesiology* 74:875–879, 1991.
46. Sessler DI, Schroeder M: Heat loss in humans covered with cotton hospital blankets, *Anesth Analg* 77:73–77, 1993.
47. Kurz A, Kurz M, Poeschi G, et al: Forced-air warming maintains intraoperative normothermia better than circulating-water mattresses, *Anesth Analg* 77:89–95, 1993.
48. Nesher N, Wolf T, Kushnir I, et al: Novel thermoregulation system for enhancing cardiac function and hemodynamics during coronary artery bypass graft surgery, *Ann Thorac Surg* 72:S1069–S1076, 2001.
49. Stanley TO, Grocott HP, Phillips-Brute B, Landolfo KP, Newman MF: Preliminary evaluation of the Arctic Sun temperature-controlling system during off-pump coronary artery bypass surgery, *Ann Thorac Surg* 75:1140–1144, 2003.
50. Brandt S, Kimberger O, et al: Resistive-polymer versus forced-air warming: comparable efficacy in orthopedic patients, *Anesth Analg* 110:834–838, 2010.
51. Albrecht M, Leaper D, et al: Forced air warming blowers: an evaluation of filtration adequacy and airborne contamination emissions in the operating room, *Am J Infect Control* 39:321–328, 2011.
52. Mouton W, Bessell JR, Millard SH, et al: A randomized control trial assessing the benefit of humidified insufflation gas during laparoscopic surgery, *Surg Endosc* 13:106–108, 1999.
53. Cobboid RSC: *Transducers for biomedical measurements: principles and applications*, New York, 1974, John Wiley & Sons.
54. Parker EO III: Electrosurgical burn at the site of an esophageal temperature probe, *Anesthesiology* 61:93–95, 1984.
55. Fergason JL: Liquid crystals, *Sci Am* 211:76–85, 1964.
56. Larach MG, Gronert GA, Allen GC, et al: Clinical presentation, treatment, and complications of malignant hyperthermia in North America from 1987 to 2006, *Anesth Analg* 110(2):498–507, 2010.
57. Shinozaki T, Deane R, Perkins FM: Infrared tympanic thermometer: evaluation of a new clinical thermometer, *Crit Care Med* 16:148–150, 1988.
58. Al-Mukazeem F, Allen U, Komar L, et al: Comparison of temporal artery, rectal and esophageal core temperatures in sick children: results of a pilot study, *J Pediatr Child Health* 9(7):461–465, 2004.
59. Suleman MI, Doufas AG, Akca O, Ducharme M, Sessler DI: Insufficiency in a new temporal-artery thermometer for adults and pediatric patients, *Anesth Analg* 95:67–71, 2002.
60. Cork RC, Vaughan RW, Humphrey LS: Precision and accuracy of intraoperative temperature monitoring, *Anesth Analg* 62:211–214, 1962.
61. Benzinger TH, Taylor GW: Cranial measurements of internal temperature in man. In Hardy JD, editor: *Temperature: its measurement and control in science and industry*, vol. 3, New York, 1963, Reinhold, pp 111–120.
62. Wallace CT, Marks WE, Adkins WY, et al: Perforation of the tympanic membrane, a complication of tympanic thermometry during anesthesia, *Anesthesiology* 41:290–291, 1974.
63. Keatinge WR, Sloan RE: Measurement of deep body temperature from external auditory canal with servo-controlled heating around ear, *J Physiol* 234:8P–9P, 1973.
64. Siegal MN, Gravenstein N: Use of a heat and moisture exchanger partially improves the correlation between esophageal and core temperature, *Anesthesiology* 69:A284, 1988.
65. Singleton RJ, Ludbrook GL, Webb RK, et al: Physical injuries and environmental safety in anesthesia: an analysis of 2000 incident reports, *Anaesth Intensive Care* 21:659–663, 1993.
66. Riller DM, Rettke SR, Hughes RW, et al: Placement of nasogastric tubes and esophageal stethoscopes in patients with documented esophageal varices, *Anesth Analg* 67:238–285, 1988.
67. Erickson RS: The continuing question of how best to measure body temperature, *Crit Care Med* 27:2307–2310, 1999.
68. Milewski A, Ferguson KL, Terndrup TE: Comparison of pulmonary artery, rectal, and tympanic membrane temperatures in adult intensive care unit patients, *Clin Pediatr* 30(Suppl 4):13–16, 1991.
69. Erickson RS, Kirklin SK: Comparison of ear-based, bladder, oral, and axillary methods for core temperature measurements, *Crit Care Med* 21:1528–1534, 1993.
70. Horrow JC, Rosenberg H: Does urinary catheter temperature reflect core temperature during cardiac surgery? *Anesthesiology* 69:986–989, 1988.
71. Mravinac CM, Dracup K, Clochesy JM: Urinary bladder and rectal temperature monitoring during clinical hypothermia, *Nurs Res* 38, 1989. 73–73.
72. Bissonnette B, Sessler KI, LaFlamme P: Intraoperative temperature monitoring sites in infants and children and the effect of inspired gas warming on esophageal temperature, *Anesth Analg* 69:192–196, 1989.
73. Joly HR, Weil MH: Temperature of the great toe as an indication of the severity of shock, *Circulation* 39:131–138, 1969.
74. Ikeda T, Sessler DI, Marder D, et al: Influence of thermoregulatory vasomotion and ambient temperature variation on the accuracy of core-temperature estimates by cutaneous liquid-crystal thermometers, *Anesthesiology* 86:603–621, 1997.
75. Lucke JN, Hall GM, Lister D: Porcine malignant hyperthermia: metabolic and physiologic changes, *Br J Anaesth* 48:297–302, 1976.
76. Sessler DI: A proposal for new temperature monitoring and thermal management guidelines, *Anesthesiology* 89:1298–1300, 1998.
77. American Society of Anesthesiologists: *Standards, guidelines, statements and other documents*. Available at www.asahq.org/For-Members/Standards-Guidelines-and-Statements.aspx.
78. National Quality Measures Clearinghouse: *Measure summary*. From *Specifications manual for national hospital inpatient quality measures, version 4.1*. Centers for Medicare & Medicaid Services (CMS), The Joint Commission, 2012. Available at http://www.qualitymeasures.ahrq.gov/content.aspx?id=35535.
79. Langham GE, Maheshwari A, Contrera K, et al: Noninvasing temperature monitoring in postanesthesia care units, *Anesthesiology* 111:90–96, 2009.

CHAPTER 15

MONITORING NEUROMUSCULAR BLOCKADE

Sorin J. Brull • David G. Silverman • Mohamed Naguib

CHAPTER OUTLINE

OVERVIEW

In the nearly 70 years since the introduction of curare to clinical anesthesia by Griffith and Johnson,[1] neuromuscular blocking drugs (NMBDs) have emerged as agents that are vital to the care and well-being of patients undergoing anesthesia and surgery. However, there is still uncertainty regarding the best means to administer NMBDs and monitor their effects. Patients vary widely in their response to these drugs,[2,3] necessitating careful titration for induction and maintenance of block and careful assessment of recovery. As a result of this wide interpatient variability, residual block or weakness (residual "curarization") has been documented following a variety of regimens[4-9] despite the intraoperative use of peripheral nerve stimulators.[7,8,10]

NEUROMUSCULAR PHYSIOLOGY

Nerve Conduction

The motor neuron is a single nerve cell whose body is located in the ventral horn of the spinal cord. From here, its axon extends to the muscle fibers that it innervates. When the membrane potential of the motor nerve increases above threshold, an "all-or-none" action potential is generated and translated to the end plate of each muscle fiber by the release of acetylcholine (ACh) across a neuromuscular junction (NMJ). The number of muscle fibers innervated by a single motor neuron, known as the *innervation ratio* of the motor unit, determines the functional intricacy of the particular muscle. For example, where fine movements are required, such as with the extraocular (orbicularis oculi) or digital (lumbrical, interossei) muscles, the same neuron innervates only a few muscle fibers. This low innervation ratio allows very fine control of a single muscle group whose function is modulated by many neurons. In contrast, large muscle groups that do not require fine control over movement, such as the postural muscles of the back, have hundreds of muscle fibers innervated by only one neuron, or a high innervation ratio.[11,12]

Neuromuscular Junction

The NMJ consists of the presynaptic region of the motor neuron, the motor end plate, and the intervening cleft (Fig. 15-1). The region is enclosed by Schwann cells, which separate it from the surrounding tissues and extracellular fluid.[13] The presynaptic terminal is an unmyelinated portion of the axon designed for the synthesis, storage, and release of ACh. The membrane is folded into many closely interposed longitudinal gutters that increase its surface area.[14] Each vesicle appears to contain 5000 to 10,000 molecules of ACh. The ACh contained in a single vesicle often is referred to as a *quantum* of transmitter, which is capable of generating a miniature end plate potential (MEPP). Quanta are continuously released into the synaptic cleft by exocytosis. Excitation of the motor nerve, so-called *motor nerve firing*, causes the synchronized release of multiple quanta, the effects of which summate at the end plate to generate a muscle action potential (MAP).

The postsynaptic membrane, much like the presynaptic membrane, is folded to increase its surface area. The mature postsynaptic end plate contains nicotinic acetylcholine receptors (nAChRs) at a density of 10,000/μm^2, each of which consists of five subunits—two α and one each of β, δ, and ε—arranged in a rosette (Fig. 15-2).[15,16] The recognition site of each of the two α-subunits must be occupied by ACh or an exogenous depolarizing agent (succinylcholine) for the all-or-none opening of a given channel to occur. Each open channel then allows the entry of Na^+ and Ca^{2+} into the cell and allows the exit of K^+. The end plate membrane serves as a resistor, such that the ion flux generates an end plate potential (EPP). Individual EPPs may accumulate and thus summate to

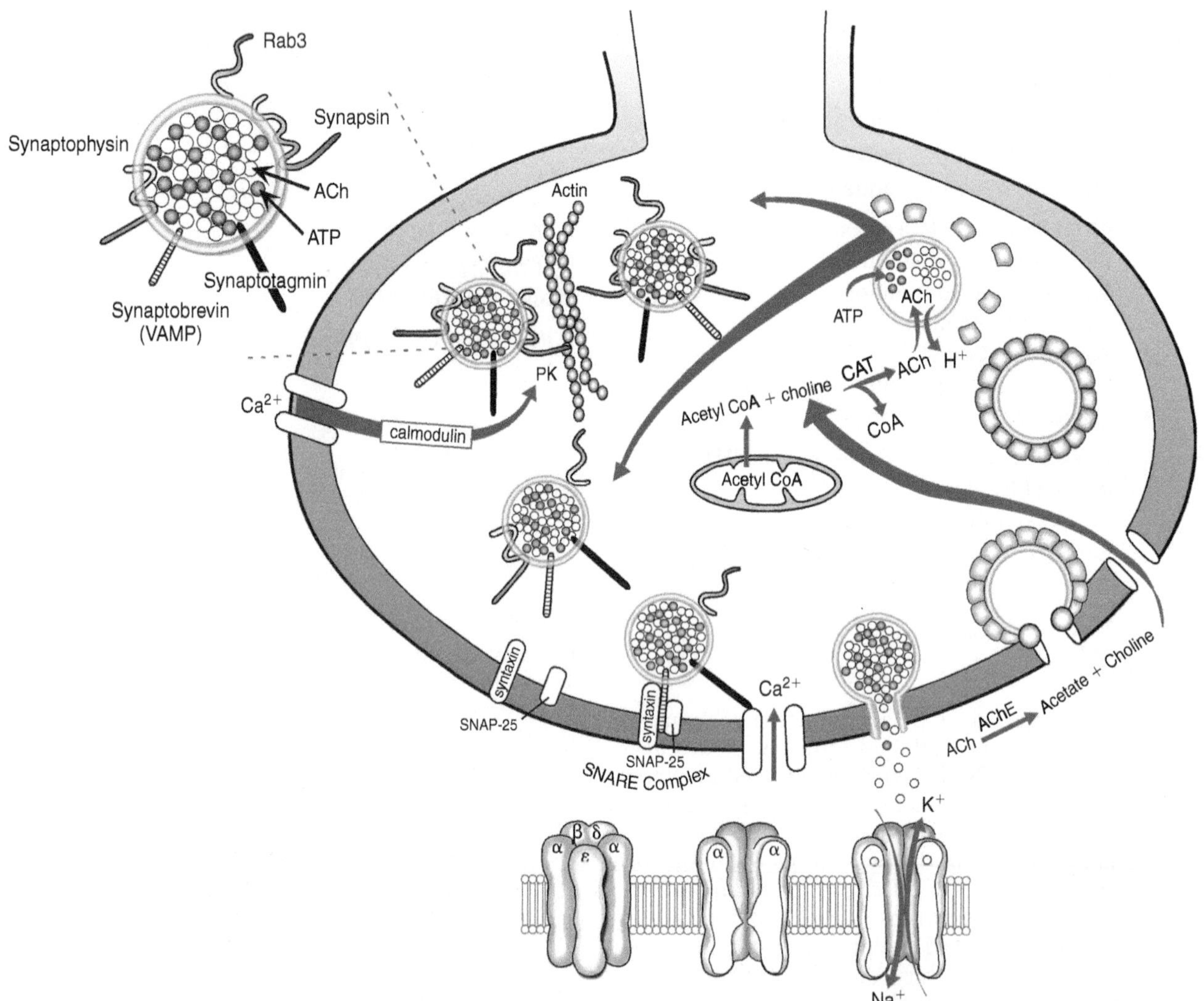

FIGURE 15-1 ■ Neuromuscular junction. The synaptic vesicle exocytosis-endocytosis cycle is shown. After an action potential and Ca^{2+} influx, phosphorylation of synapsin is activated by calcium-calmodulin activated protein kinases I and II. This results in the mobilization of synaptic vesicles (SVs) from the cytomatrix toward the plasma membrane. An essential step for the docking process is the formation of the SNARE complex, which is made of three synaptic proteins. Two of these proteins are from the plasma membrane: synaptosome-associated membrane protein of 25 kd (*SNAP-25*) and syntaxin 1, or HPC1. The third protein is from SVs (synaptobrevin). After fusion of SVs with the presynaptic plasma membrane, acetylcholine (*ACh*) is released into the synaptic cleft. Some of the released acetylcholine molecules bind to the nicotinic acetylcholine receptors on the postsynaptic membrane; the rest is rapidly hydrolyzed by the acetylcholinesterase (*AChE*) present in the synaptic cleft to choline and acetate. Choline is recycled into the terminal by a high-affinity uptake system, making it available for the resynthesis of acetylcholine. Exocytosis is followed by endocytosis in a process dependent on the formation of a clathrin coat and of action of dynamin. After recovery of the SV membrane, the coated vesicle uncoats, and another cycle starts again. CoA, coenzyme A; ATP, adenosine triphosphate; CAT, choline acetyltransferase; PK, protein kinase. (From Naguib M, Flood P, McArdle JJ, Brenner HR: Advances in neurobiology of the neuromuscular junction: implications for the anesthesiologist. *Anesthesiology* 2002;96: 202-231.)

reach threshold. When approximately 250,000 to 500,000 channels (5% to 10%) of a given NMJ are open, the summated EPP typically reaches the threshold required to elicit an MAP.[17] This usually occurs in response to a synchronized release of quanta from the nerve terminal. The end plate response is short-lived because of rapid metabolism of ACh by acetylcholinesterases (AChEs) at the synaptic cleft. At the NMJ, AChE exists in the asymmetric, or A12, form, consisting of three tetramers of catalytic subunits covalently linked to a collagen-like tail.[18] Approximately 50% of the released ACh is hydrolyzed during the time of diffusion across the synaptic cleft before reaching nAChRs. The efficiency of AChE depends on its rapid catalytic activity. In fact, AChE has one of the highest catalytic efficiencies known. It can catalyze ACh hydrolysis (4000 molecules of ACh hydrolyzed per active site per second) at near diffusion-limited rates.

The released ACh binds to α-subunits of the nAChRs. These ligand-gated cation channels allow sodium to enter and depolarize the muscle cell membrane at the NMJ. This depolarization activates voltage-gated sodium channels, which mediate the initiation and propagation of action potentials across the surface of the muscle membrane and into the transverse tubules (T-tubules), which results in the upstroke of the action potential.

There are two types of calcium channels: dihydropyridine receptor (DHPR) in the T-tubules and the ryanodine receptor (RyR1) in the sarcoplasmic reticulum (SR). The DHPRs act as voltage sensors and are activated by membrane depolarization. When the membrane is depolarized, the RyR1 receptors are activated. The DHPR-RyR1 interaction releases large amounts of Ca^{2+} from the SR, causing muscle contraction.[19-21] This process is known as *excitation-contraction coupling*.[22] Repolarization of the muscle membrane is initiated by the closing of the sodium channels and by the opening of the potassium ion channel that conducts an outward K^+ current. The return of the muscle membrane potential to its resting level (approximately −70 to −90 mV) is achieved by allowing Cl^- to enter the cell through voltage-sensitive chloride channels.

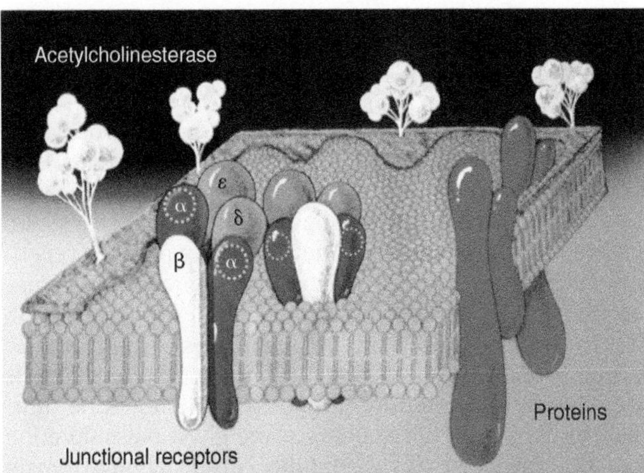

FIGURE 15-2 ■ The postjunctional membrane. The two structures in the center represent receptors. Each member of the pair is made of five subunits—two α and one each of β, δ, and ε—arranged in a circle around a channel. The balloon-like structures at the periphery represent acetylcholinesterase. (From Standaert FG: Neuromuscular physiology. In Miller RD, editor: *Anesthesia*, ed 3. New York, 1990, Churchill Livingstone.)

Neuromuscular Blocking Drugs

Both nondepolarizing and depolarizing relaxants cause flaccid paralysis by their actions at the NMJ. The characteristic patterns of these types of blocks are illustrated in Figure 15-3. Nondepolarizing agents compete with ACh by competitively binding to the α-subunits of the receptor, which have a high affinity for the receptor but exhibit no appreciable agonist activity. Postsynaptic binding prevents the receptor channel from opening. Presynaptic binding opposes the mobilization and release of ACh.[23,24] Studies with nondepolarizing blockers have demonstrated that when twitch height has returned to baseline, significant degrees of fade in the train-of-four (TOF) response may still be present.

It is generally believed that twitch depression results from block of postsynaptic nAChRs, whereas tetanic or TOF fade results from block of presynaptic nAChRs.[23,25] Blockade of the presynaptic nAChRs by neuromuscular blockers prevents ACh from being made available—that is, it prevents its release from presynaptic nerve terminals—to sustain muscle contraction during high-frequency (tetanic or TOF) stimulation. Because the released ACh does not match the demand, fade is observed in response to stimulation.[26] However, there is also strong contrary evidence indicating that fade could be simply a postjunctional (postsynaptic) phenomenon. This latter argument is supported by the fact that the snake α-bungarotoxin, which binds irreversibly to muscle (postjunctional) nAChRs but does not bind to neuronal (prejunctional) nAChRs, does produce fade.[27] Although all nondepolarizing relaxants also bind presynaptically, some drugs such as curare, pancuronium, and rocuronium have an extremely high affinity for these receptors.

Depolarizing blockers bind with high affinity to junctional receptors and act as agonists (i.e., they are similar in structure to ACh) at postsynaptic nAChRs. They cause prolonged membrane depolarization that prevents generation of subsequent action potentials and hence results in neuromuscular block. An MAP can no longer be propagated, and flaccid paralysis ensues. Succinylcholine is the only depolarizing neuromuscular blocker currently in clinical use; it is hydrolyzed in plasma by butyrylcholinesterases (plasma cholinesterases) to succinylmonocholine and choline, such that only 10% of the administered drug reaches the NMJ. Succinylmonocholine is a much weaker neuromuscular blocking agent than succinylcholine and is metabolized much more slowly to succinic acid and choline. Because there is little or no butyrylcholinesterase at the NMJ itself, butyrylcholinesterase influences the onset and duration of action of succinylcholine by controlling the rate at which the drug is hydrolyzed in the plasma before it reaches, and after it leaves, the NMJ. Recovery from succinylcholine-induced blockade occurs as succinylcholine diffuses away from the NMJ, down a concentration gradient as the plasma concentration decreases.

In the case of administration of a depolarizing neuromuscular blocking agent, such as succinylcholine, the muscle response that has been classically described is quite different. Depolarizing block, also called *phase I block*, is often preceded by muscle fasciculation. During partial neuromuscular block, depolarizing block is characterized by 1) a decrease in twitch tension, 2) no fade during repetitive stimulation (tetanic or TOF), and 3) no posttetanic potentiation. However, with prolonged exposure of the NMJ to succinylcholine, or with administration of a single dose in patients with an abnormal genetic variant of butyrylcholinesterase, the characteristics of the neuromuscular block can be changed from those of the classic depolarizing (phase I) block to those of phase II block, characterized by fade during TOF and tetanic stimulation and posttetanic potentiation similar to that induced by nondepolarizing neuromuscular blockers. A recent study, however, demonstrated that posttetanic potentiation and fade in response to TOF and tetanic stimuli are characteristics of neuromuscular block even after a single bolus administration of different doses of succinylcholine.[28] It seems that some characteristics of a phase II block are evident from an initial dose as small as 0.3 mg/kg of succinylcholine.

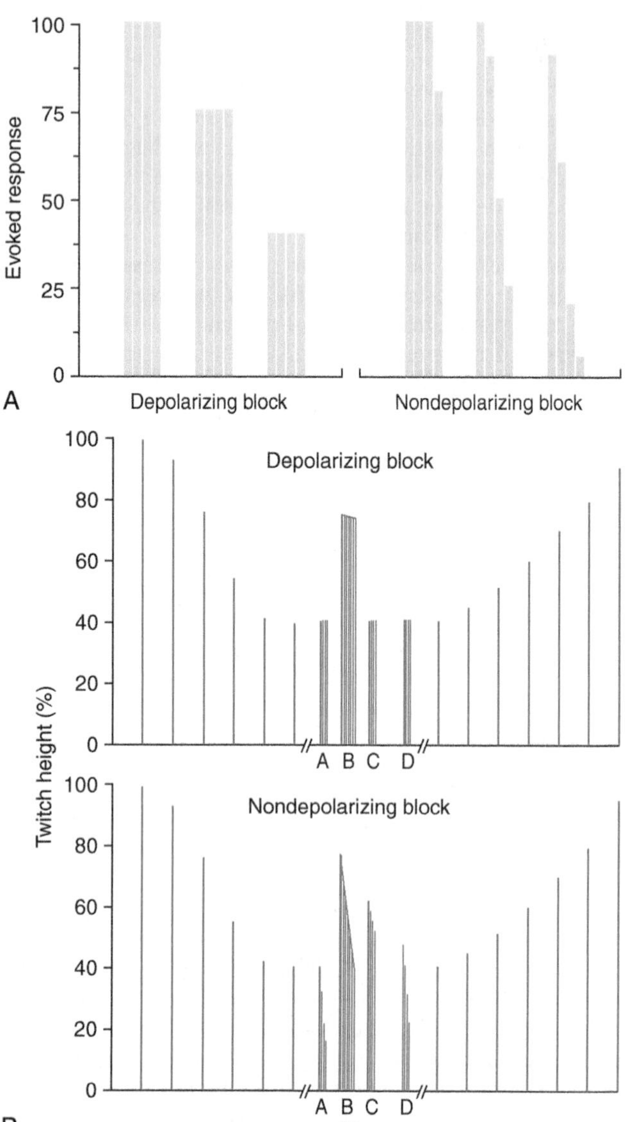

FIGURE 15-3 Characteristics of block. **A,** During depolarizing block, decrease in single-twitch height (T_1) is progressive, but no fade is seen in response to train-of-four (TOF) stimulation. During nondepolarizing block, in addition to the decline in single-twitch amplitude (T_1), there is fade in response to TOF, and the TOF ratio progressively decreases. **B,** During a depolarizing block, there is no fade in either TOF ratio (*A*) or tetanic contraction (*B*), and there is no increase in the amplitude of responses (*C, D*) following a 5-second tetanic stimulation (*B*). In contrast, during a nondepolarizing block, both TOF ratio (*A*) and tetanic contraction (*B*) exhibit fade, and both single-twitch amplitude (T_1) and the TOF ratio (*C, D*) are increased transiently following the 5-second tetanic stimulation (*B*). This posttetanic potentiation, or facilitation period, lasts 1 to 2 minutes (after 50-Hz tetanus), while the responses progressively return to the pretetanic baseline.

In addition to the classic nondepolarizing and depolarizing forms of neuromuscular block, the NMJ also may be inactivated by such phenomena as channel block and desensitization. Channel block entails direct occlusion of the receptor channels. Open-channel block, either use dependent or voltage dependent, involves occlusion of an otherwise open receptor channel, typically by a charged molecule. Closed-channel block involves occlusion independent of channel opening. Desensitization occurs when the receptor and its channel are not responsive to the presence of agonists on both α-subunits. This typically entails a reversible conformational change of variable duration[29,30] as a result of persistent binding of depolarizing agents to the receptor.[31,32] This persistent binding may change the typical (phase I) block of a depolarizing relaxant to one that assumes the characteristics of a nondepolarizing block (phase II). Long-term effects also may be a consequence of inactivation of cellular mechanisms by long, thin molecules such as decamethonium, which may enter the cytoplasm through the open receptors. Barbiturates, potent volatile anesthetics, receptor agonists, cholinesterase inhibitors, local anesthetics, phenothiazines, calcium channel blockers, antibiotics, alcohol, naltrexone, and naloxone all may cause conformational changes of the receptor and/or occlude the channel. All these may enhance or prolong the effects of an existing block from a muscle relaxant.

EXOGENOUS MODES OF NEUROSTIMULATION

In the clinical setting, neurostimulation typically is delivered by a 9-V battery-powered, adjustable direct current (DC) stimulator via subcutaneous needles or surface electrodes. The stimulus should be monophasic (i.e., square wave and unidirectional) because biphasic waves may produce repetitive stimulation. The other critical components of a stimulus are its pulse duration (in milliseconds) and intensity (in milliamperes).[33] Pulse duration must be less than 0.5 ms, so as not to induce repetitive neural firing or direct muscle stimulation. The intensity of the stimulus should be sufficient to depolarize nerve fibers at the given pulse duration (i.e., supramaximal). This stimulus current should remain constant, with the output voltage varying automatically as skin resistance changes over time.[33] Lastly, the stimulator should be able to produce multiple patterns of stimulation, such as single twitch, TOF, tetanic, and so forth. Optimally, a stimulator should have a rheostat for adjusting output current, and lead disconnect, excessive impedance, and low-battery indicators as well as a visual and/or audible stimulus-delivery indicator. The responses to changes in stimulus duration and intensity are illustrated in Table 15-1, which compares mechanomyographic (MMG), electromyographic (EMG), and acceleromyographic (AMG) responses in unblocked, awake volunteers.[34]

When assessing the effect of NMBDs on the response to single stimuli over a period of time, the same number of nerve fibers must be stimulated. For this reason, anesthesiologists traditionally have relied on a supramaximal stimulating current—that is, a current that is 10% to 20% greater than the current needed to stimulate all the efferent fibers in the nerve bundle. Use of a supramaximal current allows current to vary slightly over time without affecting the total number of nerve fibers stimulated. This is readily achieved with needle electrodes, typically at less than 10 mA. Surface electrodes may fail to stimulate all fibers, especially when they are not in close proximity to the nerve, such as with improper electrode placement or in obese patients, even at currents of 50 to 70 mA. It is frequently stated that current intensity determines neural stimulation. In reality, the electrical charge (current [mA] × duration [ms] = microcoulombs [μQ]) is the essential element.

The current output of a stimulator must remain within a narrow range over time and over the range of physiologic resistances. Although delivery of a constant current can be accomplished most effectively with needle electrodes, insertion into the skin may be painful to the awake patient; surface electrodes are most commonly used in the clinical setting.[35] Skin resistance typically is decreased by use of an electrolyte solution, such as silver/silver chloride. However, several minutes are required to allow for it to attain optimal effectiveness. The time for this electrode "curing" may be accelerated by cleansing and degreasing the skin, such as with alcohol or acetone, and by abrading the skin with an abrasive gel (NuPrep; ADInstruments, Colorado Springs, CO; Fig. 15-4).

Although rare, complications associated with the use of nerve stimulators can occur. Needle electrodes may be a source of local irritation, infection, and nerve damage because of intraneural placement.[36,37] They also are more likely to be associated with local tissue burns from electrosurgical units because they provide good contact, with minimal resistance, for exit of high-frequency current over a small area of skin. In general, the use of needle electrodes in clinical practice is not recommended; however, if they are used, caution should be exercised to ensure that the needle is applied adjacent to the nerve, not through it.

TABLE 15-1 Neuromuscular Response to Changes in Stimulus Intensity and Duration in Awake, Unmedicated Volunteers*

Current (mA)	Pulse Width (ms)	MMG (% Response)	EMG (% Response)	AMG (% Response)
20	0.10	0.8	1.0	
	0.15	5.4	1.3	
	0.20	29.7	11.4	12.0
	0.30			29.0
	0.40	67.6	55.8	
40	0.10	13.5	1.5	
	0.15	45.9	20.1	
	0.20	86.5	65.9	54.0
	0.30			79.0
	0.40	97.3	102.6	
50	0.20			80.0
	0.30			101.0
60	0.10	40.5	5.1	
	0.15	81.1	49.0	
	0.20	100.0	100.0	100.0
	0.30			119.0
	0.40	102.7	121.1	
70	0.10	48.6	8.2	
	0.15	102.7	57.5	
	0.20	102.7	106.0	
	0.30			
	0.40	108.1	126.0	

*Values are expressed as percent of the value achieved with a stimulus amplitude of 60 mA and a stimulus duration (pulse width) of 0.2 ms.

AMG, acceleromyograph; *EMG*, electromyograph; *MMG*, mechanomyograph.

Effect of Stimulus Frequency

In the setting of normal, unblocked neuromuscular transmission, increasing the rate of stimulation from single stimuli at 0.1 Hz (one every 10 seconds) to brief tetanic stimulation at 50 Hz results in sustained muscle contractions (tetanus) without fade. At supraphysiologic rates of stimulation (>70 to 200 Hz),[38,39] even normal neuromuscular transmission may fatigue. When a nondepolarizing block is present, such fatigue is noted at slower rates of neurostimulation. This constitutes the basis for assessments of response to tetanic (at 50 Hz) and TOF (at 2 Hz) stimulation.[40,41]

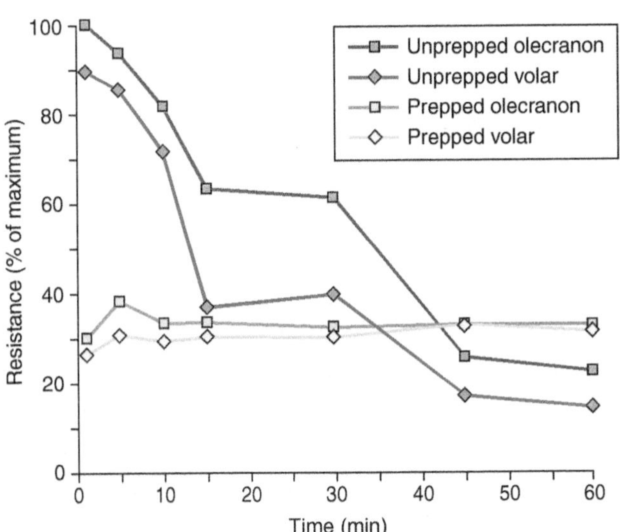

FIGURE 15-4 Effect on skin resistance of cleansing and abrading the skin with abrasive gel. Without prior prepping, resistance at surface electrodes remains elevated for 10 to 30 minutes after electrode application over the olecranon groove and volar forearm. With appropriate skin preparation, skin resistance is lowered by 70%.

The rate of neurostimulation has pronounced effects on assessments of depth of block. In addition to promoting fatigue, frequent stimulation also results in as much as a fivefold to sixfold increase in local blood flow. This may result in more rapid delivery of relaxant to the stimulated muscle,[42,43] especially if neurostimulation is initiated before administration of relaxant.[44] Ali and Savarese[45] reported that the apparent dose requirements for d-tubocurarine at the adductor pollicis muscle decreased by a factor of three as the stimulus frequency increased from 0.1 Hz to 1.0 Hz. Of perhaps even greater clinical significance is the effect of stimulus frequency on the apparent onset of blockade. Increasing the stimulus frequency results in an apparent greater degree of neuromuscular depression at the site of stimulation for both depolarizing[44,46] and nondepolarizing block.[44,45,47,48]

PATTERNS OF STIMULATION

Currently, several patterns of stimulation are used to assess the degree of neuromuscular block. These include single stimuli, tetanic stimulation, TOF, and double-burst stimulation (DBS) (Fig. 15-5). The newer nerve

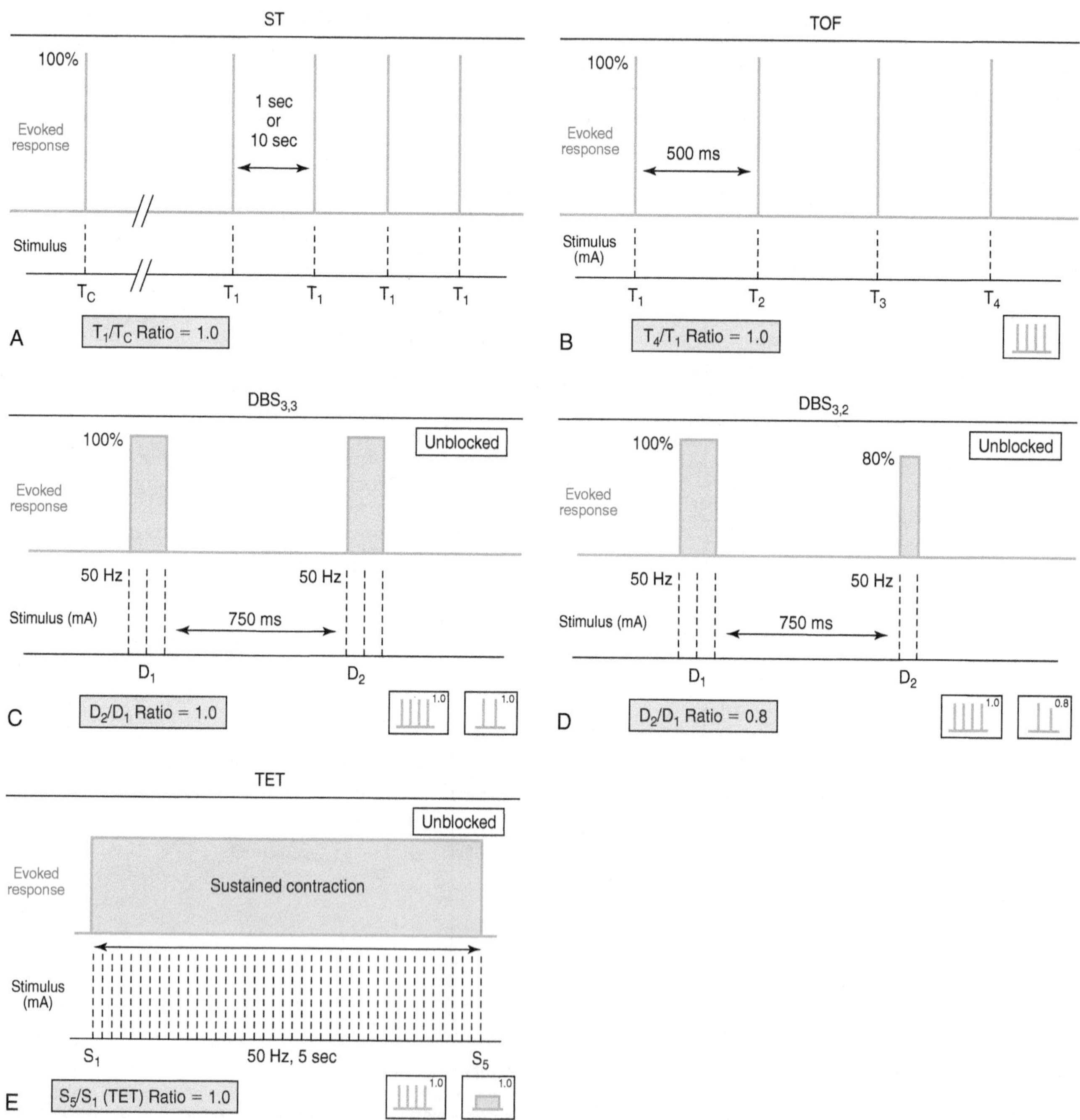

FIGURE 15-5 Comparison of stimulating patterns for single twitch (*ST*) (**A**), train-of-four (*TOF*) (**B**), double burst ($DBS_{3,3}$ and $DBS_{3,2}$) (**C** and **D**), and tetanus (*TET*) at 50 Hz (**E**). The impulses comprising ST, the four twitches of TOF, the two mini-tetanic bursts of DBS, and the 5 seconds of TET are identical in duration (200 μs) and pattern (square wave).

stimulators are capable of functioning in any of these modes as well as in posttetanic count (PTC) mode (Fig. 15-6).

Single Repetitive Stimulation: Single Twitch

This method consists of assessing the response to an individual stimulus or serial stimuli, usually at frequencies between 0.1 Hz (1 stimulus every 10 seconds) and 1.0 Hz (1 stimulus per second). The use of 1.0 Hz should be discouraged for reasons given above. Single-twitch (ST) stimulation is the least precise method of assessing partial neuromuscular blockade under clinical conditions, and it requires measurement of a baseline (no block) ST amplitude for comparison with subsequent responses. In addition, the clinically useful range of block is limited because the response to a single stimulus is not reduced until at least 75% to 80% of the receptors are blocked; the response disappears completely once 90% to 95% of the receptors are blocked.[49] Furthermore, ST monitoring is highly sensitive to variations in stimulating current, temperature, and preload (i.e., resting muscle tension).

As previously noted, it is imperative that the stimulating current remain constant over time to ensure that the same number of nerve fibers reach threshold with each stimulation. By applying a current that is 10% to 20% above the level required to stimulate all fibers of the motor nerve (i.e., supramaximal stimulus), the impact of variables such as temperature, skin resistance, and changes in electrode conductance can be minimized. However, a supramaximal stimulus may not always be delivered when surface electrodes are used. Despite these limitations, the response to ST stimulation is the standard for comparisons of NMBD potency. The effective dose of a muscle relaxant required for 95% depression of the ST height is defined as ED_{95} and is a measure of drug potency.

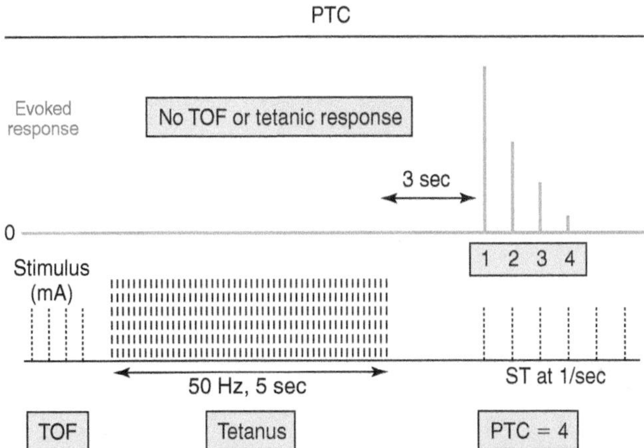

FIGURE 15-6 ■ Posttetanic count (*PTC*): schematic of neuromuscular response. Train-of-four (*TOF*), tetanic, and single-twitch (*ST*) stimuli are represented by *dashed lines* below the zero baseline. Because of a deep degree of block, neither TOF nor tetanic stimulation results in appreciable evoked motor responses (no lines above the zero threshold line). Three seconds after the 5-second tetanic stimulation, there is a brief period of posttetanic potentiation, resulting in the appearance of four ST stimuli that degrade rapidly. In this example, the PTC is 4.

Train-of-Four Stimulation

TOF stimulation consists of four repetitive stimuli at a frequency of 2 Hz. As noted above, even this relatively slow rate of stimulation is associated with fade in the context of nondepolarizing block. TOF is the most commonly used method of neuromuscular assessment in clinical practice. It is far less painful to awake patients than tetanus (a sustained, rapid stimulus) and is not associated with prolonged posttetanic effects at the NMJ. In some cases, it may be more sensitive than tetanus to the presence of residual block.[40] In the context of nondepolarizing block, both TOF and tetanus result in fatigue, which is manifested by fade. However, in contrast to tetanus, TOF does not increase or facilitate neuromuscular responses during and after application.[40,41,50]

Unlike single stimuli, TOF stimulation does not require a prerelaxant baseline for comparison. It assesses the relationship among successive responses, thus serving as its own control. The relationship between the size of the fourth twitch response (T_4) and the first twitch response in the TOF (T_1) is expressed as T_4/T_1, or *fade ratio*. In the absence of nondepolarizing block, the T_4/T_1 ratio is approximately 1.0. In the context of nondepolarizing block, decreases in this ratio depend on such factors as the relaxant used and whether monitoring is performed during onset or recovery. Typically at 70% to 75% receptor occupancy, T_4 will start to decrease selectively. At a T_4/T_1 ratio as low as 0.70, T_1 may still be close to its baseline height. When T_4 is no longer detectable, either visually or mechanomyographically, T_1 is approximately 25% of its baseline size. This corresponds to a block of approximately 80% of the receptors. The third twitch response (T_3) is lost when approximately 85% of receptors are blocked, whereas the second (T_2) is lost when approximately 85% to 90% of receptors are blocked.[51] During the remaining ST monitoring, the height of T_1 is progressively decreased, and T_1 is lost when 90% to 95% of receptors are blocked (Table 15-2).[49,51]

In contrast to ST monitoring, TOF may also allow detection of a phase II block in response to a depolarizing agent. Normally, a depolarizing muscle relaxant causes a progressive decrease in the size of the ST or a symmetrical decrease in the size of all responses of the TOF or response to tetanus. Because no fade is present, the T_4/T_1 ratio is maintained near 1.0 until all twitches disappear. However, when phase II block occurs, the depolarizing relaxant takes on features of a competitive (nondepolarizing) relaxant, and fade develops in response to TOF or tetanic stimulation. This type of block cannot be assessed by ST monitoring.

TOF stimulation provides other advantages as well. The T_4/T_1 ratio is consistent at submaximal and at supramaximal stimulating current intensities, so long as T_1 and T_4 responses are detectable (Fig. 15-7),[52,53] especially at 10 mA or more above the T_4 threshold.[53] Likewise, evidence suggests that although T_1 amplitude increases with both increase in stimulus duration and intensity,[34] the TOF ratio of the evoked responses is independent of stimulus duration, so long as the pulse width is less than 0.5 ms (Fig. 15-8). The consistency of the T_4/T_1 ratio at varying current intensities and at varying stimulus durations facilitates testing of awake patients because discomfort is directly related to the intensity of the stimulating current.[54]

TABLE 15-2 **Approximate Relationships Among Percent Receptor Block and Single Twitch (T_1), Fourth Twitch (T_4), and Train-of-Four Ratio Responses During Nondepolarizing Block**

Total Receptors Blocked (%)	First Twitch (T_1) (% Normal)	Fourth Twitch (T_4) (% Normal)	T_4/T_1
100	0	0	—
90-95	0	0	T_1 lost
85-90	10	0	T_2 lost
	20	0	T_3 lost
80-85	25	0	T_4 lost
	80-90	48-58	0.60-0.70
	95	69-79	0.70-0.75
75	100	75-00	0.75-1.0
	100	100	0.9-1.0
50	100	100	1.0
25	100	100	1.0

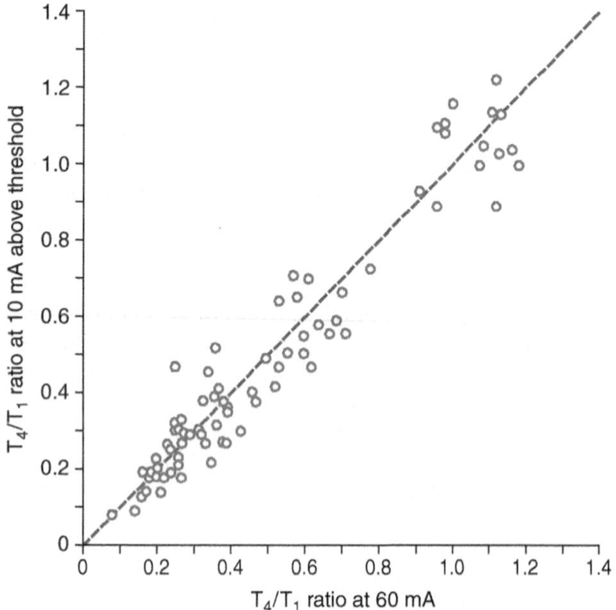

FIGURE 15-7 Comparison of T_4/T_1 ratios at 10 mA above the T_4 threshold with those at 60 mA in patients undergoing general anesthesia and receiving vecuronium infusion. The consistency of fade at these two currents was evidenced by their close correlation (r = 0.94). (From Silverman DG, Connelly NR, O'Connor TZ, et al: Accelographic train-of-four at near-threshold currents. *Anesthesiology* 1992;76:34-38.)

Tetanic Stimulation

Tetanic (TET) stimulation consists of repetitive high-frequency neurostimulation (≥30 Hz). This results in repetitive MAPs and persistent muscle contraction. In the unblocked NMJ, each contraction can be sustained for several seconds at stimulating frequencies as high as 70 to 100 Hz.[38] In clinical practice, a 5-second, 50-Hz TET stimulus is used most often because the evoked muscle tension approximates the tension developed during maximal voluntary effort.[38]

Although normal muscle responds to TET stimulation with summated contractions that overcome elastic forces and produce an augmented response, the TET response fades, or fatigues, in the context of nondepolarizing block (Fig. 15-9).[55,56] Tetanic fade most likely represents a presynaptic inability to mobilize ACh rapidly enough to maintain depolarization despite repetitive nerve firing. It may be attributable to competition by nondepolarizing agents at presynaptic cholinergic receptors involved with Ca^{2+} flux and ACh mobilization.[17] The consequences of the diminished release of ACh are magnified by binding of the nondepolarizing agent to the postsynaptic receptors, thereby decreasing the margin of safety. Evidence also suggests that fade in response to TET stimulation may occur during the use of potent inhaled anesthetics in the absence of nondepolarizing block.[39,57,58]

Another effect of a TET stimulus is the potential alteration of subsequent evoked neuromuscular responses. In the presence of a nondepolarizing NMBD, or phase II block with a depolarizing relaxant, stimulation after tetanus may result in posttetanic facilitation or potentiation. The magnitude of posttetanic effects on evoked twitch size is a function of depth of block.[59] Testing of neuromuscular function within 2 to 5 minutes of a preceding TET stimulation can lead to overestimation of evoked responses, that is, underestimation of depth of block (Fig. 15-10).[59,60] Although this has been shown to be true for T_1, TOF, and DBS, subsequent tetanic fade seems to be relatively

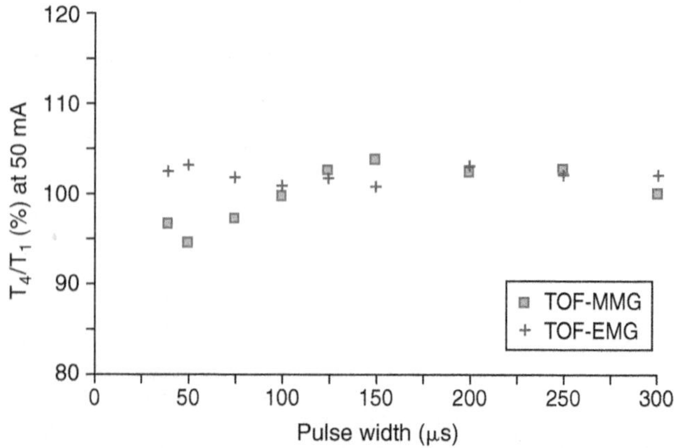

FIGURE 15-8 Consistency of train-of-four (*TOF*) ratio at pulse widths (stimulus duration) ranging from 40 to 300 μs in a healthy volunteer in the absence of neuromuscular blockade. EMG, electromyograph; MMG, mechanomyograph.

immune to the phenomenon.[61] One theory to explain posttetanic facilitation is that the intense tetanic stimulus induces an increase in the mobilization and subsequent release of ACh quanta, which results in an increase in subsequent EPPs.[62] Another theory has suggested that tetanus may have relatively long-term effects on the NMJ by displacing relaxant from the postsynaptic receptor.[63] In either case, posttetanic stimulation during nondepolarizing blockade results in generation of a greater EPP than that obtained before tetanus.

Posttetanic Count

When the use of nondepolarizing NMBDs results in 100% twitch-size depression, the potentiation that occurs following TET stimulation may enable detection of the response to single stimuli.[64,65] The number of twitch responses elicited by serial stimulation at 1 Hz (beginning 3 seconds after a 5-second, 50-Hz tetanus) is inversely related to the depth of block: the greater the number of posttetanic responses, the less the degree of block and the more rapid the ensuing recovery (see Figs. 15-6 and 15-10; Table 15-3). This method of assessment also may be indicated to ensure profound paralysis; that is, ablation of PTC as well as response to twitch and tetanus. It also provides an indication as to when recovery of ST may be anticipated and thus provides a guide for planning reversal of residual block with anticholinesterases.

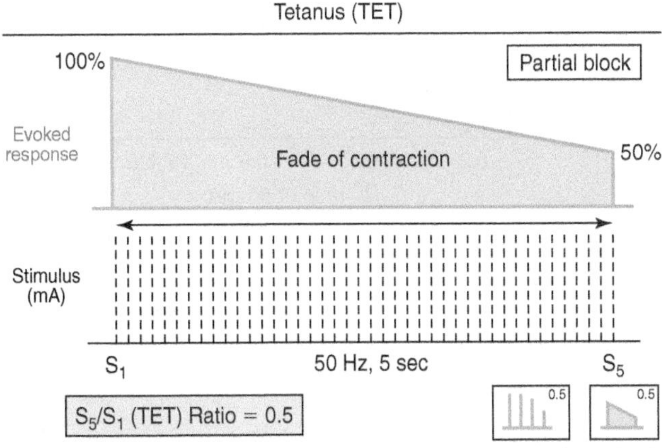

FIGURE 15-9 Tetanic fade. During partial nondepolarizing blockade, the force of muscle contraction at the end of the 5-second tetanic stimulus is lower than the force of contraction at the beginning of stimulation (i.e., contractile fade develops). In the figure, the force of contraction at the end of the 5-second stimulation is half of the force of contraction at the beginning (tetanic fade ratio is 0.5).

Double-Burst Stimulation

Because TOF visual and tactile estimates consistently and significantly underestimate the degree of fade, DBS has been introduced as an alternative means of assessing neuromuscular blockade.[66-68] Although several different combinations of stimuli have been assessed, two patterns are used most commonly. $DBS_{3,3}$ consists of a minitetanic burst of three 0.2 ms impulses at a frequency of 50 Hz, followed 750 ms later by an identical burst. $DBS_{3,2}$ consists of a burst of three impulses at 50 Hz followed 750 ms later by a burst of two such impulses (see Fig. 15-5, *C* and *D*). DBS results in muscle responses of greater magnitude than those elicited by TOF (Fig. 15-11), enabling fade—the percent difference between the last burst and the first—to be more accurately detected visually and tactilely.

When assessed mechanographically, DBS and TOF maintain a close relationship over a wide range in level of block (Fig. 15-12),[69] although TOF and $DBS_{3,3}$ do not correlate well during neuromuscular block recovery.[70] Other DBS patterns have been investigated to decrease fade underestimation bias during the later stages of recovery from neuromuscular blockade ($DBS_{2,2}$: two 0.3-ms stimuli at 50 Hz followed 750 ms later by two 0.2-ms stimuli)[71] and to detect more profound degrees of block ($DBS_{3,3}$ 80/40: three 0.2-ms stimuli at 80 Hz followed 750 ms later by three 0.2-ms stimuli at 40 Hz).[72]

Staircase Phenomenon

Repeated stimulation of a motor nerve may enhance the evoked mechanical response of the corresponding muscle, known as the *staircase phenomenon*.[73,74] This phenomenon does not seem to affect the evoked TOF fade ratio[75] and seems to be equally applicable to AMG and MMG monitoring techniques[76] but not to EMG recordings. This is likely because repetitive stimuli do not increase the size of the compound action potential and therefore do not change the signal height (amplitude) of EMG.[77] This phenomenon affects the degree of twitch stabilization in clinical neuromuscular pharmacodynamic studies but is of limited significance in routine clinical practice. It has been shown that tetanic preconditioning reduces individual variability but does not eliminate it. It also should be noted that the staircase phenomenon is not uniform for all muscles.[78,79]

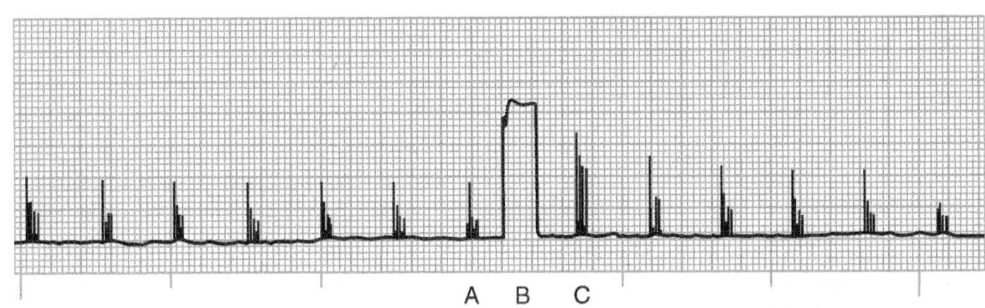

FIGURE 15-10 Effect of tetanic stimulation (5 seconds at 50 Hz) on train-of-four (TOF) monitoring at 12-second intervals during a vecuronium infusion. *A,* Baseline TOF ratio is 0.33. *B,* Following a 5-second tetanic stimulation, T_4 is potentiated to a greater degree than T_1; hence, the T_4/T_1 ratio is increased transiently to as high as 0.70 (*C*) before returning to the pretetanic baseline.

SITES OF STIMULATION AND ASSESSMENT

The primary purpose of intraoperative neuromuscular blockade is to achieve adequate relaxation of the upper airway, vocal cords, and diaphragm to facilitate intubation and surgery. The degree of neuromuscular blockade typically is assessed by stimulating the ulnar nerve and monitoring the response of the adductor pollicis muscle.

Airway Muscles

Although not normally monitored by the clinician, bilateral recurrent laryngeal nerve stimulation may be accomplished by using a negative surface electrode placed over the thyroid cartilage notch and a positive electrode placed on the upper chest or forehead.[80] Diaphragmatic stimulation may be accomplished by needle electrode stimulation of the phrenic nerve at the inferoposterior border of the sternocleidomastoid muscle.[81,82]

Compared with peripheral muscles, the laryngeal and diaphragmatic muscles are less sensitive (more resistant) to nondepolarizing relaxants; that is, the doses required for ED_{95} are approximately 1.5 to 2 times greater than those required for 95% twitch depression of the adductor pollicis.[81,83-85] Hence, coughing, breathing, or vocal cord movement is still possible despite paralysis of the adductor pollicis muscle. Nevertheless, neuromuscular blockade develops faster, lasts a shorter time, and recovers faster at the laryngeal and diaphragmatic muscles (Fig. 15-13).[83,86-91] These observations may seem contradictory because convincing evidence also suggests that, for almost all drugs studied, the half-maximal effective plasma concentration (EC_{50}), a measure of drug potency, is 50% to 100% higher at the diaphragm or larynx than at the adductor pollicis. Fisher and colleagues[92] explain this apparent contradiction by postulating more rapid equilibration (shorter half-time of equilibration between drug concentration in the blood and the effect site [$t_{\{1/2\}}k_{e0}$]) between plasma and the effect compartment at these central muscles. This accelerated rate of equilibrium probably represents little more than differences in regional blood flow. The diaphragmatic muscles likewise evidence decreased sensitivity to depolarizing relaxants[93];

TABLE 15-3 Duration Until Reappearance of First Detectable Twitch Response

Posttetanic Counts*	Atracurium[65] Time (Min)	Pancuronium[64] Time (Min)
1	9	35
2	7	28
4	4	20
6	2	12
8	0-2	6

*Number of responses to single-twitch stimuli at 1 Hz following 50 Hz tetanus for 5 seconds.

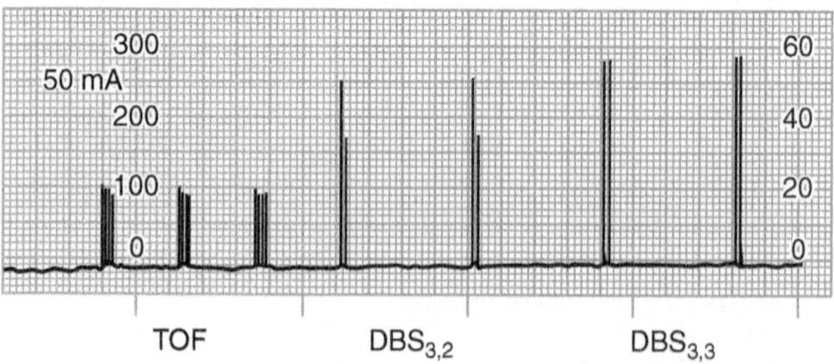

FIGURE 15-11 Evoked responses of train-of four (*TOF*; every 12 seconds), double-burst stimulation (*$DBS_{3,2}$* and *$DBS_{3,3}$*; every 20 seconds) in an unmedicated volunteer. Although the magnitude of the individual responses is greater for DBS, the T_4/T_1 ratio of TOF and the D_2/D_1 ratio of $DBS_{3,3}$ are equivalent. The D_2/D_1 of $DBS_{3,2}$ is lower as a result of its second burst being of shorter duration (two mini-tetanic stimuli) than its first burst (three mini-tetanic stimuli).

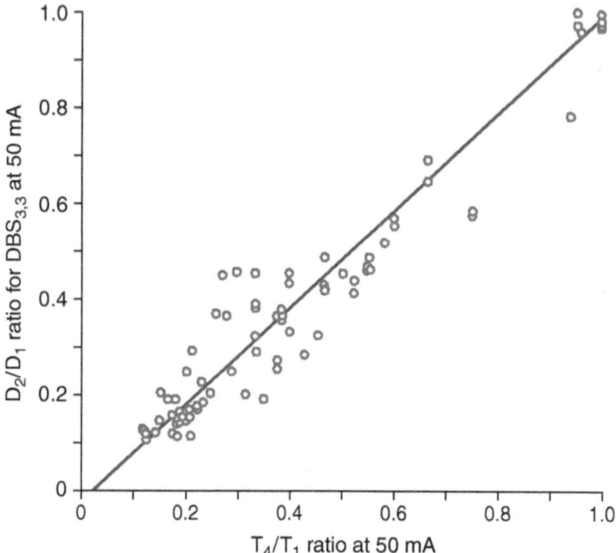

FIGURE 15-12 Correlation of double-burst stimulation (*$DBS_{3,3}$*) and train-of-four in response to 50-mA stimulation (r = 0.98). The straight line represents the line of best fit. Similar consistency was evidenced when train-of-four and $DBS_{3,2}$ were compared. (From Brull SJ, Connelly NR, Silverman DG: Correlation of train-of-four and double-burst stimulation ratios at varying amperages, *Anesth Analg* 1990;71:489-492.)

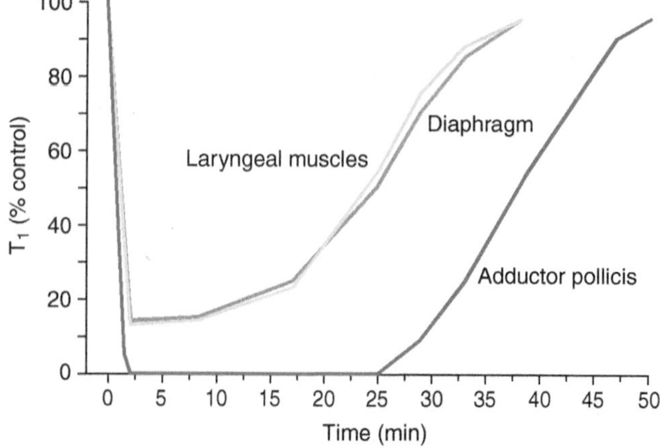

FIGURE 15-13 Relative onset time and duration of action at two central muscle groups (laryngeal muscles and diaphragm) compared with peripheral muscle groups (adductor pollicis muscle) after administration of an intubating dose of nondepolarizing relaxant.

however, neither the laryngeal muscles[86,94] nor the diaphragm[95] show evidence of such sparing in response to succinylcholine.

Muscles of the Extremities

The ulnar nerve primarily innervates the adductor pollicis, abductor digiti quinti, and first dorsal interosseous muscles. One electrode may be placed 1 cm proximal to the wrist on the radial side of the flexor carpi ulnaris, while another is placed proximally, either on the volar forearm or over the olecranon groove; maximal effectiveness is obtained when the negative (depolarizing) electrode is placed distally over the nerve.[34,96-98]

Anesthesiologists typically monitor force of contraction of the adductor pollicis muscle by visual or tactile means or by mechanographic force translation. Because this muscle is on the side of the arm opposite to the site of stimulation, little likelihood of unintentional direct muscle stimulation exists that would falsely suggest incomplete block. Alternatively, the first dorsal interosseous and abductor digiti quinti muscles may be preferable for EMG.[93-95] These muscles are less likely to receive dual innervation, by median as well as ulnar nerves, and the morphology of their EMG response is identified more readily (Table 15-4).[99] However, the abductor digiti quinti (minimi) muscle may be slightly more resistant to block than the adductor pollicis muscle.[68,70] In addition to the wrist and hand, other potential sites of stimulation and assessment on the extremities include the posterior tibial nerve behind the medial malleolus (plantarflexion) and the peroneal and lateral popliteal nerves (dorsiflexion; Table 15-5).

Mainly because of their better perfusion, muscles of the airway have a faster onset of neuromuscular blockade than muscles of the extremities. In light of this more rapid onset, it may be argued that it is not necessary to wait for 95% to 100% adductor pollicis twitch size depression to attain relaxation and intubating conditions.[100] However, monitoring the adductor pollicis at a stimulus frequency of 0.1 Hz provides a desirable safety factor when performing a rapid-sequence induction in settings in which patient movement would be unacceptable.[3,101] In support of this, it was noted that excellent intubating conditions were not observed reliably until 30 seconds after 100% adductor pollicis depression (when stimulating at 0.1 Hz).[101]

Facial Muscles

Monitoring the response of the orbicularis oculi muscle in response to facial nerve stimulation may reflect the level of block at the airway musculature more closely than does monitoring of peripheral muscles.[102-104] However, electrodes placed over the nerve near the tragus of the ear (2 to 3 cm posterior to the lateral border of the orbit) may stimulate the muscle directly and thus may falsely indicate inadequate levels of blockade. In addition, this response is not readily quantified mechanographically.[104] When used to stimulate the facial nerve, surface electrodes should be placed near the stylomastoid foramen, just below and anterior to the mastoid bone.

Other facial muscles have been investigated with regard to their ability to indicate the level of block. The corrugator supercilii muscles can be induced to contract in response to stimulation of the temporal branch of the facial nerve. This stimulation results in a muscular response of the eyelid. For this type of monitoring, the AMG transducer (see below) can be applied to the medial half of the superciliary arch above the eyebrow.[105] Comparison of the corrugator supercilii muscle to the orbicularis oculi muscle

TABLE 15-4 Frequency of Obtaining a Measurable Action Potential at Four Different Hand Muscles in Response to Median and Ulnar Nerve Stimulation

Muscle	Median Nerve (%)	Ulnar Nerve (%)
Adductor pollicis	79	73
Abductor pollicis brevis	93	54
First dorsal interosseous	54	91
Abductor digiti quinti	18	97

Data obtained simultaneously on a four-channel electromyelogram identify the high degree of dual innervation of hand muscles. The adductor pollicis, the muscle most commonly monitored, has a high likelihood of dual innervation; it demonstrated a measurable action potential 79% of the time after median nerve stimulation and 73% of the time after ulnar nerve stimulation.

From Halevy J, Brull SJ, Brooke J, et al: Dual innervation of hand muscles: potential influence on monitoring of neuromuscular blockade [abstract]. *Anesthesiology* 1991;75:A814.

TABLE 15-5 Sites of Neurostimulation in Clinical and Research Settings

Nerve	Site of Stimulation	Movement Observed
Ulnar	Wrist or elbow	Thumb adduction, flexion of fourth and fifth fingers, abduction of fifth finger
Posterior tibial	Posterior to the medial malleolus	Plantarflexion of the big toe
Peroneal	Lateral to the neck of the fibula	Dorsiflexion of the foot
Facial	Near the tragus where the nerve emerges from the stylomastoid foramen, 2 to 3 cm posterior to the orbit	Contraction of orbicularis oculi, orbicularis oris, or corrugator supercilii
Recurrent laryngeal	Notch of thyroid cartilage	Vocal cord adduction
Phrenic	Inferoposterior border of the sternocleido-mastoid muscle	Hemidiaphragm

responses has shown that eye muscles vary in their response to nondepolarizing relaxants. The corrugator supercilii muscles reflect the time course of paralysis and recovery of the laryngeal adductor muscles, whereas the time course of the orbicularis oculi muscles reflects those of peripheral muscles, such as the adductor pollicis.[106]

MONITORING OF NEUROMUSCULAR BLOCKADE AND RECOVERY

Visual and Tactile Assessment of Evoked Responses

In clinical practice, most anesthesiologists rely on visual or tactile means to assess responses to neurostimulation. For visual assessment, the clinician should be positioned 90 degrees to the plane of movement. For tactile assessment, the observer's fingertips should be placed lightly over the distal phalanx of the thumb in the direction of movement. Visual and tactile assessments are limited in that they often underestimate the depth of block; significant degrees of block often may be missed even by experienced observers.[7,9,66,107-109] Precise assessment can be quantified only by EMG (muscle action potential) or MMG (evoked muscle tension). This limitation has been partially overcome by newer means of assessment, such as DBS. Studies have reported that the fade of the sequential bursts of DBS is easier to detect than that between the first and fourth responses of TOF (Table 15-6).[66-68,109,110] In addition, such testing may be performed at least as reliably (Figs. 15-14 and 15-15), as well as more comfortably (Fig. 15-16), using submaximal stimulation (Table 15-7).[52,109-112] Such low-current stimulation affords the clinician the opportunity to confirm a lack of residual blockade in environments where patients are awake and responsive to discomfort, such as in the postanesthesia care unit (PACU) and intensive care unit (ICU).

Electromyography

MAP can be monitored in clinical and laboratory settings by EMG. As illustrated for the muscles of the hand (Fig. 15-17), the EMG recording electrodes are placed over the mid-portion (motor point or innervation zone) of the muscle (abductor pollicis brevis, adductor pollicis, and abductor digiti quinti), and the reference electrode is placed over the muscle's tendinous insertion. The ground electrode is placed away from the recording electrodes and is necessary to provide a common reference. Significant EMG signal data include the latency,

TABLE 15-6 **Ability to Detect Fade by Visual or Tactile Methods at Supramaximal Stimulating Current with Actual TOF Ratio Between 0.40 and 0.70**

	True Positives (Correct Identification of Fade)		
Reference	**TOF (%)**	**$DBS_{3,3}$ (%)**	**$DBS_{3,2}$ (%)**
Engbaeck[67]	—	64	96
Drenck[66]	16	78	—
Viby-Mogensen[107]	36	—	—
Gill[108]	16	69	—
Ueda[68]	—	73	96
Brull[111]	42	67	72

DBS, double-burst stimulation; *TOF*, train-of-four (stimulation).

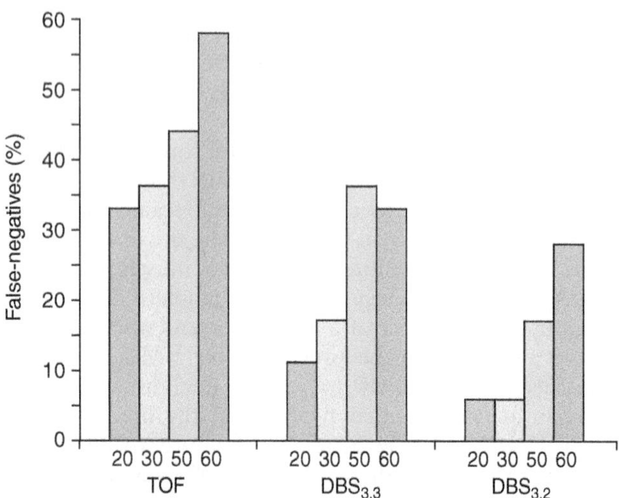

FIGURE 15-14 Failure to identify an actual (mechanographic) train-of-four (*TOF*) ratio below 0.70 by visual inspection using TOF and double-burst stimulation (*$DBS_{3,3}$* and *$DBS_{3,2}$*) at 20, 30, 50, and 60 mA. TOF at 60 mA was associated with the highest incidence of false-negative assessments. (From Brull SJ, Silverman DG: Visual assessment of train-of-four and double burst–induced fade at submaximal stimulating currents. *Anesth Analg* 1991;73:627-632.)

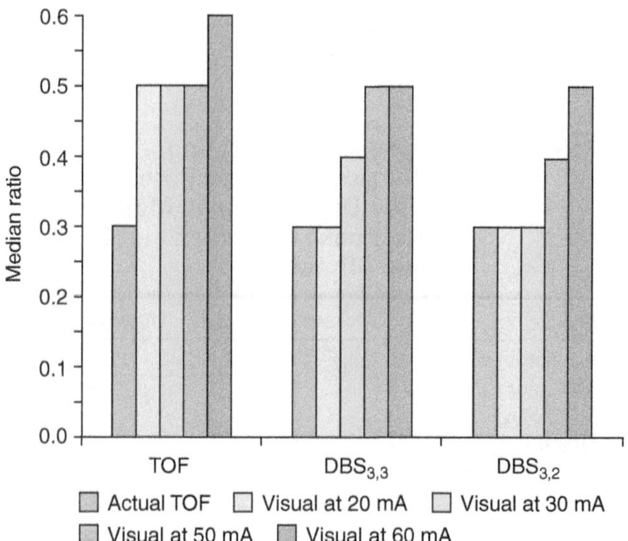

FIGURE 15-15 Degree of overestimation of actual train-of-four (*TOF*) ratio by visual inspection when actual TOF ratio was below 0.70. Quantitative estimation by visual means significantly overestimated the actual ratio (0.3) at all currents for TOF; at currents of 30, 50, and 60 mA for double-burst stimulation (*$DBS_{3,3}$*), and at 50 and 60 mA for $DBS_{3,2}$. (From Brull SJ, Silverman DG: Visual assessment of train-of-four and double burst–induced fade at submaximal stimulating currents. *Anesth Analg* 1991;73:627-632.)

amplitude, duration, and shape of the compound action potential (Fig. 15-18).

The motor latency, expressed in milliseconds, is the time interval between the onset of the stimulus and the initial deflection of the evoked motor response. It includes the nerve conduction time within the motor nerve fiber and the time required for neuromuscular transmission; therefore it reflects the distance from the stimulation site to the muscle group stimulated. Latency also is affected by any influence on nerve transmission velocity: drugs, temperature, nerve injury, and so on. The amplitude of the compound MAP may be measured from the isoelectric line to the peak (baseline-to-peak), from the negative to the positive peaks (peak-to-peak), or as the area under the MAP curve (the root mean squared [rms] value that gives a measure of the power of the signal). It represents the sum of the amplitudes of the individual muscle fibers activated by the stimulus. The duration and morphology of the compound MAP reflect the synchrony and intensity of contraction. For automated analysis of EMG, either analog or digital techniques may be used because they appear to produce results comparable to conventional manual measurement techniques.[113,114]

The EMG most commonly used in the clinical setting until recently was the Relaxograph integrated EMG monitor (Datex, Shrewsbury, MA [now GE Healthcare];

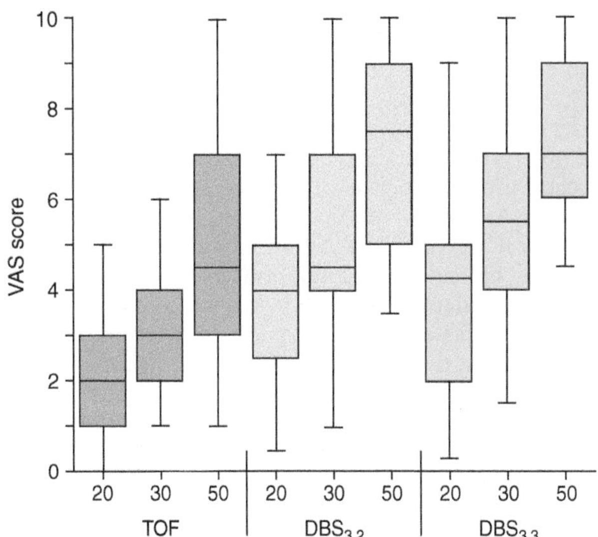

FIGURE 15-16 Effect of train-of-four (*TOF*) and double-burst stimulation (*DBS*) currents at 20, 30, or 50 mA on visual analog scale (*VAS*) pain scores in unpremedicated volunteers. *Shaded areas* represent the 25th to 75th percentiles, *horizontal lines* within shaded areas represent medians, and *extended bars* represent 0 to 100th percentiles. (From Connelly NR, Silverman DG, O'Connor TZ, Brull SJ: Subjective responses to train-of-four and double burst stimulation in awake patients. *Anesth Analg* 1990;70:650-653.)

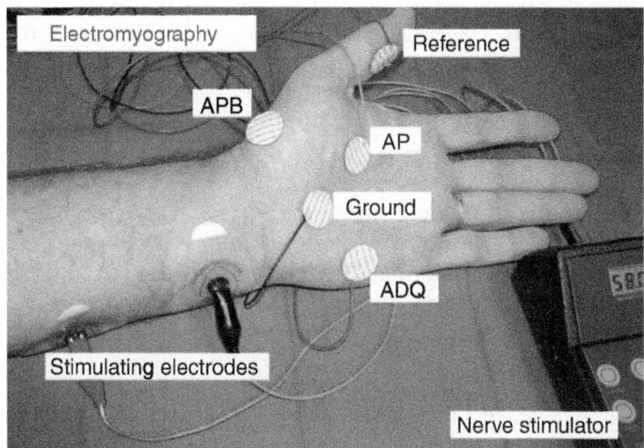

FIGURE 15-17 Electrode placement for electromyographic monitoring of responses to stimulation of the ulnar nerve. ADQ, abductor digiti quinti (minimi) muscle; AP, adductor pollicis muscle; APB, abductor pollicis brevis muscle.

TABLE 15-7 **Consistency of T_4/T_1 Ratios at 20, 30, and 50 mA Stimulating Currents**

T_4/T_1 Classification at 50 mA	20 mA	30 mA	50 mA
≤0.70 (n = 28)	0.500 ± 0.18	0.506 ± 0.17	0.513 ± 0.16
>0.70 to <0.95 (n = 25)	0.915 ± 0.10	0.906 ± 0.08	0.894 ± 0.07
≥0.95 (n = 30)	0.972 ± 0.06	0.972 ± 0.04	0.995 ± 0.02

Data from Brull SJ, Ehrenwerth J, Silverman DG: Stimulation with submaximal current for train-of-four monitoring. *Anesthesiology* 1990;72:629-632.

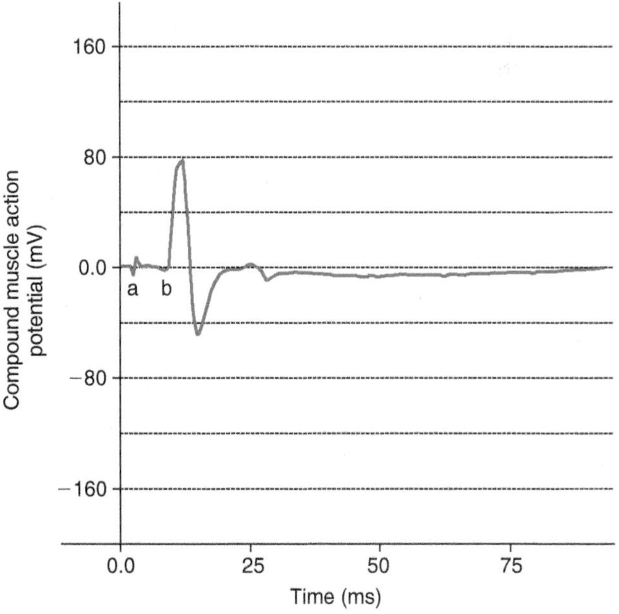

FIGURE 15-18 Electromyographic (EMG) tracing obtained in a healthy volunteer. x-axis, time (in milliseconds); y-axis, compound muscle action potential (MAP, in millivolts); *a,* stimulus artifact; *b,* onset of EMG response. Motor latency is calculated by *b* − *a*. Duration and morphology of the compound MAP are assessed from the first deflection to the time when the MAP returns to the isoelectric line (time epoch).

Fig. 15-19). The Relaxograph is a dedicated EMG instrument that measures the total area of the EMG waveform; that is, the area under the negative and positive deflections: the baseline-to-peak and zero-to-peak amplitudes, latency, and zero cross time. Unfortunately, this monitor is no longer available for purchase, and very few clinical departments still have it in use. Other devices, such as the Excel Plus (Cadwell Laboratories, Kennewick, WA) are multifunctional, so they can evaluate auditory, visual, and somatosensory evoked potentials, conduction velocities, and spectral array. Their multichannel capabilities make these devices well suited for comparisons of responses at multiple sites. However, because of the elaborate and expert setup requirements and the high acquisition costs, these multichannel monitors are rarely used by anesthesiologists in the clinical setting.

Force Translation: Mechanomyography

The adductor pollicis muscle force translation (mechanomyographic) monitor is the device most commonly used to measure evoked muscle response (Fig. 15-20). It consists of a force transducer and a ringed assemblage for appropriate orientation of the thumb. Isometric contraction of the adductor pollicis muscle in response to ulnar nerve stimulation is translated into an electrical signal that can be displayed on an interfaced pressure monitor and also recorded. Currently available force transducers are rarely used clinically and vary considerably in the range of force that they can withstand. Although a transducer with a range of 0 to 5 kg is suitable for most clinical applications in the context of nondepolarizing blockade, tetanic stimulation in the absence of blockade generates a force of 7.1 ± 2.2 kg.[39] This may overload and possibly damage transducers that have not been designed to withstand such forces.[115]

For optimal quantification of thumb adduction in response to ulnar nerve stimulation, and for consistency when evaluating over time, certain practices are important: 1) keep the arm and hand immobilized to attain consistent measurement; 2) orient the ring/thumb complex to align thumb adduction with the axis of the force transducer; 3) abduct the thumb to a constant preload of 200 to 300 g to optimize alignment of actin and myosin filaments; 4) ensure unencumbered movement of the thumb/ring complex; 5) adjust the monitor gain to account for the fact that, depending on the depth of block, the tension developed in response to tetanic stimulation may be three to four times greater than that achieved by a single twitch; 6) place the patient's arm in a position that avoids nerve injury during prolonged immobilization; and 7) place intravenous or intraarterial catheters in, and the blood pressure cuff on, the opposite arm when feasible.

Accelerography (Acceleromyography)

Unfortunately, the adductor pollicis force transducer is relatively cumbersome and must be interfaced with equipment that is not always readily available, especially in the recovery room. This has prompted the introduction of new monitoring techniques, such as accelerography, which uses a miniature transducer (piezoelectric wafer) to measure thumb acceleration (Fig. 15-21). When the mass is constant, changes in force and acceleration are directly proportional because force equals mass × acceleration. As for force transduction, stimulation of the peripheral nerve, most commonly the ulnar nerve, is achieved by indirect stimulation through surface electrodes. Stimulating parameters may be adjusted similarly to those for assessment of force transduction, with the exception that the accelerograph is not suitable for assessing the response to tetanic stimulation. During nondepolarizing block, the accelerograph provides a value for TOF ratio that is virtually identical to that obtained by force transduction.[116,117] However, the T_4/T_1 ratio may be greater than 1.0 in the absence of blockade. This may be attributable to thumb movement or to failure of the unsecured thumb (i.e., without preload) to return to its baseline position after the first of the four contractions of TOF.[118] This monitoring technique is also useful at low stimulating currents, again making it a useful tool for assessing residual blockade in the recovery room.[8] Two

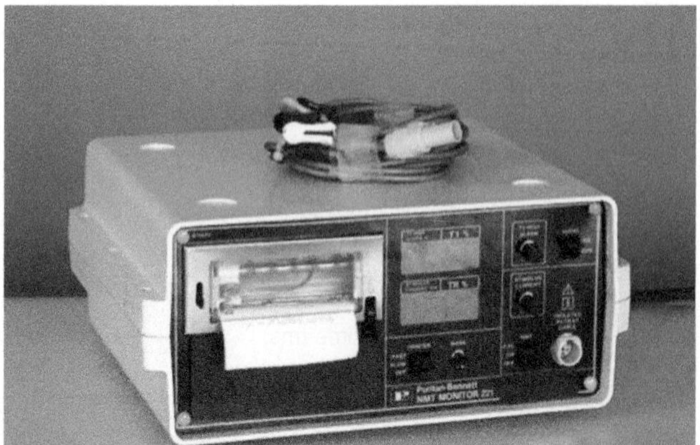

FIGURE 15-19 ■ Datex Relaxograph Neuromuscular Transmission electromyography monitor has an output that shows digital twitch height (T_1%) and train-of-four ratio (T_4%). A sample paper tracing is shown on the left side of the device.

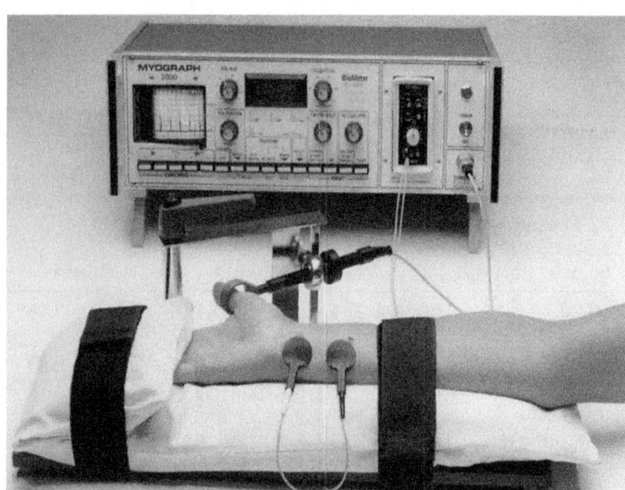

FIGURE 15-20 ■ Mechanomyography with the Biometer Myograph 2000 adductor pollicis force transducer. (Courtesy Biometer International A/S, Odense, Denmark.)

monitors that can measure neuromuscular function using AMG are the highly portable TOF Watch series (TOF-Watch, TOF-Watch S, and TOF-Watch SX; GE Healthcare, Waukesha, WI) and the Infinity Trident NMT SmartPod (Dräger Medical, Telford, PA; Fig. 15-22), a module integrated with the anesthesia workstation.

Kinemyography

The Neuromuscular Transmission Module, E-NMT (GE Healthcare, Waukesha, WI) uses kinemyography (KMG) and is based on a piezoelectric transducer, a strip of piezoelectric polymer applied to molded plastic device placed between the thumb and the index finger (Fig. 15-23). Mechanical movement of the thumb results in a redistribution of the electrical charge on the sensor membrane, a change that can be quantified. The measurement of TOF percent begins by pressing the start-up button. The monitor will start the measurement by automatically setting the stimulus current (maximum 70 mA). The TOF percent is the default mode of analysis because it does not require a reference level (control).

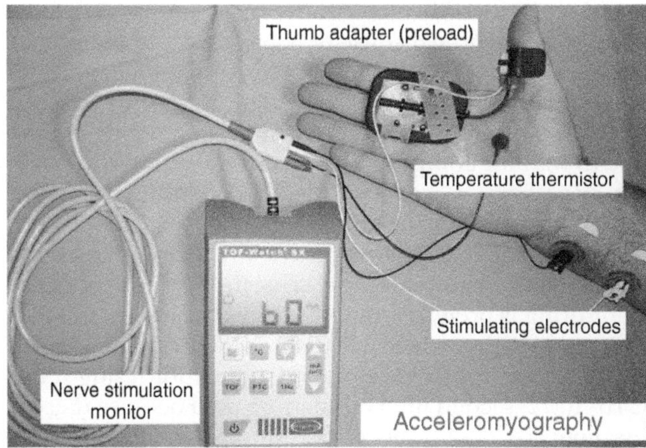

FIGURE 15-21 Acceleromyography with the TOF-Watch SX (GE Healthcare, Waukesha, WI) with interfaced temperature thermistor, piezoelectric crystal attached to thumb adapter, and the two ulnar nerve stimulating electrodes. The thumb adapter is used to maintain constant preload on the thumb and avoid train-of-four ratio measurement error.

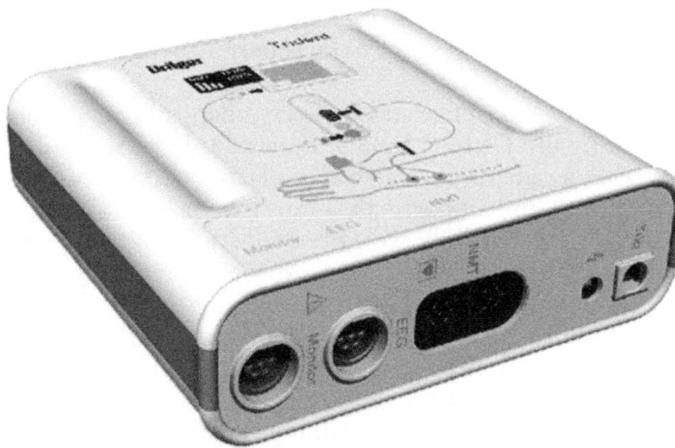

FIGURE 15-22 The Dräger Infinity Trident NMT SmartPod acceleromyography module. (Courtesy Dräger Medical, Telford, PA.)

Phonomyography

Phonomyography (PMG) is based on the fact that muscle contraction evokes low-frequency sounds that can be recorded by special microphones (condenser or piezoelectric) or capacitance accelerometers.[119-121] It has been shown that the peak frequency of a typical signal is at 4 to 5 Hz, and the maximum power occurs over a spectrum of frequencies up to 50 Hz.[122] The advantage of PMG lies in the fact that it can be applied to every muscle site of interest, but the problem that still exists is how to secure the microphone over the muscle of interest. PMG is in its infancy and is not yet available commercially. The agreement between the evoked responses of KMG and PMG with mechanomyography seems to be unacceptable for scientific research but might be acceptable for clinical purposes.[123]

ELECTROMYOGRAPHY VERSUS MECHANOMYOGRAPHY

The EMG and MMG responses do not always agree with one another, nor do changes monitored with one technique necessarily parallel those monitored using the other technique. This may be attributable to the MMG's high sensitivity to factors that affect both muscle contraction and neuromuscular transmission. The EMG tends to be insensitive to mechanical events, but it has been shown to be affected by preload.[124] In addition, the hypothenar muscles, which commonly are monitored for EMG, are less sensitive to nondepolarizing agents than is the adductor pollicis muscle, which is monitored during force transduction.[100] These differences were noted in a study of seven volunteers who received vecuronium.[125] Normal

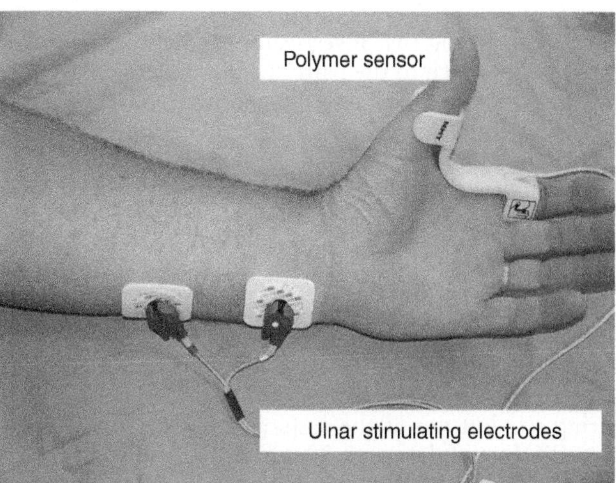

FIGURE 15-23 Kinemyography with the E-NMT Neuromuscular Transmission Module (GE Healthcare, Waukesha, WI). The thumb movement (adduction) in response to ulnar nerve stimulation is detected by bending of the polymer sensor; and the force of muscle contraction is displayed on an interfaced monitor.

vital capacity, inspiratory pressure, and peak expiratory flow rate were achieved at an EMG T_4/T_1 ratio of 0.90. In contrast, the MMG T_4/T_1 ratio associated with normal respiratory tests was only 0.50.

Two other examples may help to elucidate the differences between MMG and EMG monitoring. First, the MMG is affected by dantrolene, whereas the EMG is not; this is due to modulation by dantrolene of the calcium levels responsible for myofibril contraction. Second, the MMG and EMG respond differently to repetitive (tetanic) stimuli. On ST stimulation at a supramaximal current, the muscle does not achieve maximal contraction because of the time required to overcome its elastic properties—a mechanical, not an electrical, feature. Over the time course of a few repetitive stimuli, MMG responses gradually increase to a plateau (asymptote) as elastic forces are overcome. Furthermore, during tetanus, the contractile responses may summate despite a progressive decline in EPPs. These phenomena also explain why, even in the absence of neuromuscular blockade, the MMG—but typically not the EMG—may show amplified response to ST stimulation following tetanus.

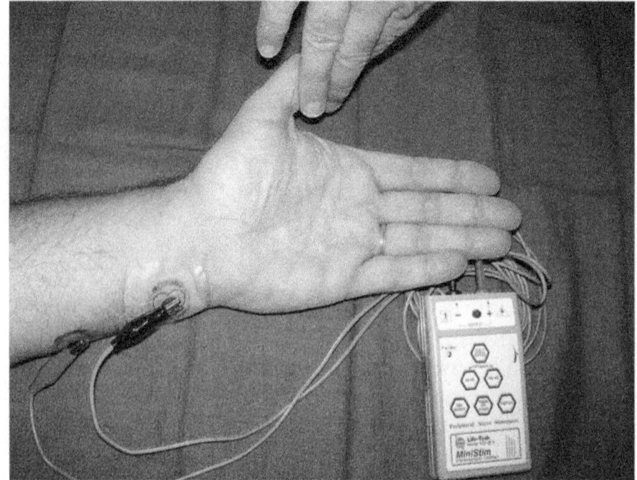

FIGURE 15-24 ■ A nerve stimulator used clinically to assess neuromuscular function subjectively (visually or tactilely). Note the instrument should be termed a "stimulator" and not "monitor," because it only stimulates the nerve; it does not measure the evoked response.

CLINICAL APPLICATIONS

Despite increased understanding of the intricacy of neuromuscular function, consensus is still lacking as how to best monitor blockade during such critical time periods as onset and recovery. Routine clinical care entails a number of compromises. Although assessment of thumb adduction in response to ulnar nerve stimulation is not necessarily indicative of the degree of block at the airway musculature, it is still the most commonly used method of measuring neuromuscular block. Even though mechanographic assessment is more accurate than either visual or tactile assessment, the MMG and EMG monitors are rarely used in routine clinical settings because of cost, lack of availability, and difficulty of use. Instead, nerve stimulators—not monitors, which are frequently misidentified—are used in the clinical setting (Fig. 15-24).

It is disturbing that investigators and clinicians lack a uniform approach to the pattern and rate of neurostimulation; in fact, relatively few use neuromuscular monitors perioperatively. Clearly, rate of stimulation can affect drug delivery and may promote neuromuscular fatigue. Furthermore, the nature of stimulation determines what information may be gained by assessment of thumb adduction.

Onset of neuromuscular paralysis prior to tracheal intubation should be monitored with single stimuli at 0.1 Hz (6/min). Whereas TOF at 10- to 12-second intervals might provide some additional information, it may accelerate apparent onset of blockade at the monitoring site but not at the respiratory or laryngeal muscles. TOF stimulation at 20-second intervals, although not associated with marked acceleration of onset of blockade, may not be frequent enough to effectively monitor the rapid changes typically seen during onset of block. Alternatively, it may be argued that slow stimulation of the ulnar nerve underestimates the rate of onset of blockade at the airway musculature and that it may be less likely to identify minor differences among relaxants. The aforementioned must be viewed in the context of the requirements of the given setting. To document the time at which relaxation is adequate to permit tracheal intubation without coughing or movement, it is preferable to wait for complete ablation of ST at 0.1 Hz. If it is not necessary to ensure "ideal" conditions, a lesser degree of block may be acceptable.

In the patient whose trachea is already intubated, the rate of blockade onset is less critical. Intermittent TOF monitoring is preferred in this setting because it provides information about fade and twitch depression. During maintenance of blockade, nerve stimulation using TOF at 10- to 12-second intervals may be used because there is less concern about the effect of rapid stimulation on delivery of relaxant. At depths of blockade during which there is loss of T_4, the clinician can simply count the number of responses to TOF stimulation. When all four responses to TOF are lost, depth of blockade is assessed by monitoring the PTC. This is particularly helpful to increase the likelihood of vocal cord paralysis during laser surgery; in those cases, PTC should be close to zero. During procedures in which a deep block is desired, such as with middle ear or diaphragm surgery, various DBS patterns have been shown to be superior to TOF and just as reliable as PTC.[72,126,127]

During emergence and recovery, many clinicians rely primarily on TOF or DBS stimulation. When deciding whether extubation of the trachea is indicated, clinicians generally—and incorrectly—consider a T_4/T_1 ratio above 0.70 to be indicative of adequate recovery. However, patients still may be significantly compromised at this degree of recovery.[128,129] Counting the total number of twitches in response to TOF stimulation is helpful at relatively deep levels of blockade, and additional information may be gained by assessing response to tetanic stimulation and examining the degree of posttetanic facilitation. Specifically, if no twitch response is attainable, the response to tetanus or the number of

PTCs provides valuable information about depth of block and degree of spontaneous recovery. However, delivery of a tetanic stimulus may distort the responses to local monitoring for several minutes (1 to 2 minutes after a 5-second, 50-Hz stimulus, and 2 to 3 minutes after a 5-second, 100-Hz stimulation).[60]

In the PACU, clinicians rely on clinical signs and evaluate response to TOF stimulation if residual neuromuscular blockade is suspected. Because many experts agree that significant residual block is common when using intermediate, and especially long-acting, relaxants, it is important to note that many reports have documented the T_4/T_1 of TOF and D_2/D_1 of DBS remain consistent at submaximal currents.[8,52,53,69] Not only does testing with submaximal stimulus currents decrease the discomfort associated with TOF monitoring, it may also improve the quality of visual assessment.[109] If fade is not detectable by visual assessment at low current, it is unlikely to be detected at a higher current. Where there is concern about residual neuromuscular blockade, mechanographic quantification is always preferable to qualitative evaluations.

In all cases, the data generated in response to local neurostimulation should be viewed in the context of clinical signs and symptoms such as head lift and patterns of breathing. Once considered the gold standard indicator of adequate recovery,[130] a T_4/T_1 greater than 0.70 is no longer considered to be a guarantee of airway protection. Likewise, clinical criteria are not definitive, especially in the context of residual anesthetic. A study in awake volunteers noted that even the ability to generate a vital capacity more than 33% of control and to maintain a patent airway without jaw lift did not guarantee effective swallowing and airway protection (Table 15-8).[131] More recently, another study that evaluated the signs and symptoms of awake volunteers during recovery from a TOF ratio in the 50% to 70% range found that "adequate" recovery of neuromuscular function in the outpatient setting requires "return of the TOF ratio to a value greater or equal to 0.90 and ideally to unity."[128] These volunteers were periodically monitored by adductor pollicis EMG, head lift/grip/masseter muscle strength, visual examination, and subjective questioning. Both by subject and observer evaluation, no volunteer was considered "street ready" until well after a T_4/T_1 above 0.85.[128]

Although the benefits of neuromuscular blocking agents are well recognized, the morbidity that may be associated with their use must be considered. Several recent publications have again documented that anesthesiologists across continents vary widely in their use of perioperative monitoring, reversal of residual blockade, understanding of the criteria for adequate reversal, and perceived need for monitoring standards.[132] Recent review articles have documented the need for a unified understanding of the potential complications associated with the perioperative use of muscle relaxants and may provide the needed impetus for a more consistent approach to perioperative neuromuscular monitoring (Box 15-1).[133,134] As recently described, the clinician could use many methods to decrease the incidence of postoperative residual neuromuscular blockade and reduce morbidity.[134] Among these are 1) the avoidance of long-acting neuromuscular blocking agents, unless postoperative mechanical ventilation is planned; 2) recognition that clinical tests to exclude residual neuromuscular blockade are notoriously and consistently unreliable; 3) use of quantitative (not qualitative) perioperative neuromuscular monitors, not just "stimulators," to ensure appropriate dosing of NMBDs and optimal timing of pharmacologic antagonism; and 4) avoidance of overdosing of NMBDs, and the resulting complete loss of evoked responses, unless mandatory for the conduct of surgery.[134] Appropriate dosing of relaxant and reversal drugs and appropriate and careful monitoring of their effects can increase the utility and safety of these valuable agents.

TABLE 15-8 Relationships Among Various Clinical Signs in Healthy Awake Volunteers Receiving Low Doses of Curare to Induce Partial Neuromuscular Block

Parameter	Peak Inspiratory Force (cm H_2O)
Control (no relaxant)	−90
5-second head lift	−53
Effective swallowing	−43
Patent airway without jaw lift	−39
Glottic closure against Valsalva maneuver	−30
Vital capacity >33% of control	−20

Control volunteers could generate a peak inspiratory force of −90 cm H_2O and perform all maneuvers. Following low-dose curare, the ability to maintain an airway (−39 cm H_2O) and swallow effectively (−43 cm H_2O) was not ensured, even when the peak inspiratory force was −30 cm H_2O.

Data from Pavlin EG, Holle RH, Schoene RB: Recovery of airway protection compared with ventilation in humans after paralysis with curare. *Anesthesiology* 1989;70:381-385.

BOX 15-1 Suggested Evidence-Based Practices for Decreasing Residual Paralysis and Improving Patient Outcome

1. Avoidance of Residual Paralysis: General Principles
   a. Use muscle relaxants only when necessary.
   b. Individualize dosing of muscle relaxants based on patient factors, surgical needs, and duration and presence of coexisting diseases.
   c. Avoid long-acting relaxants (e.g., pancuronium).
   d. Avoid reliance on clinical signs of reversal such as head lift, jaw clenching, tidal volume, etc.; such tests are notoriously unreliable.
   e. In patients at risk, rule out residual paralysis by using objective monitors (AMG, MMG, KMG).
   f. Ideally, neuromuscular function should be monitored quantitatively by using objective monitors (AMG, MMG, KMG).
   g. A minimum degree of recovery (TOF count of 4) should be established before pharmacologic reversal with anticholinesterases.
   h. Tactile evaluation of fade and the use of clinical tests of adequacy of reversal do *not* ensure adequate recovery and readiness for tracheal extubation.
2. Pharmacologic Reversal with Anticholinesterases: General Principles
   a. The minimum degree of recovery should be a TOF count of 4 prior to anticholinesterase reversal.
   b. If spontaneous recovery to a minimum TOF ratio above 0.90 assessed objectively (quantitatively) is achieved, neostigmine administration should be avoided. Use of anticholinesterases in fully recovered patients may induce weakness of the airway muscles.
3. Decisions Regarding Pharmacologic Reversal with Anticholinesterases in Clinical Practice
   a. If *no* neuromuscular monitor or peripheral nerve stimulator is available:
      i. Clinical tests of adequacy of reversal are unreliable; always use reversal, and only when spontaneous muscle activity is present. This practice, however, cannot guarantee adequate and safe recovery from neuromuscular blockade and should be discouraged.
   b. If peripheral nerve stimulator is available, but *no* objective means of assessment is available:
      i. If no TOF response is present, delay pharmacologic reversal untill TOF count is 4.
      ii. If TOF count of 4 is present with subjective fade, use reversal.
      iii. If TOF count of 4 is present without subjective fade, consider low-dose reversal (50% of usual dose).
   c. If quantitative monitor *is* available, such as AMG, MMG, KMG, or EMG:
      i. If no TOF response, or if the TOF count is <4, delay reversal.
      ii. If the TOF count is 4, use reversal.
      iii. If TOF ratio is <0.40, use reversal.
      iv. If TOF ratio is between 0.40 and 0.90, consider low-dose reversal (50% of usual dose).
      v. If TOF ratio is >0.90, no reversal is recommended.

AMG, acceleromyograph; *EMG*, electromyograph; *KMG*, kinemyograph; *MMG*, mechanomyograph; *TOF*, train of four.
Data from Murphy GS, Brull SJ: Residual neuromuscular block: lessons unlearned. Part I: Definitions, incidence, and adverse physiologic effects of residual neuromuscular block. *Anesth Analg* 2010;111:120-128; and Brull SJ, Murphy GS: Residual neuromuscular block: lessons unlearned. Part II: Methods to reduce the risk of residual weakness. *Anesth Analg* 2010;111:129-140.

REFERENCES

1. Griffith HR, Johnson G: The use of curare in general anesthesia, *Anesthesiology* 3:418–420, 1942.
2. Katz RL: Neuromuscular effects of d-tubocurarine, edrophonium and neostigmine in man, *Anesthesiology* 28:327–336, 1967.
3. Silverman DG, Swift CA, Dubow HD, O'Connor TZ, Brull SJ: Variability of onset times within and among relaxant regimens, *J Clin Anesth* 4:28–33, 1992.
4. Viby-Mogensen J, Jorgensen BC, Ording H: Residual curarization in the recovery room, *Anesthesiology* 50:539–541, 1979.
5. Lennmarken C, Lofstrom JB: Partial curarization in the postoperative period, *Acta Anaesthesiol Scand* 28:260–262, 1984.
6. Andersen BN, Madsen JV, Schurizek BA, Juhl B: Residual curarisation: a comparative study of atracurium and pancuronium, *Acta Anaesthesiol Scand* 32:79–81, 1988.
7. Bevan DR, Smith CE, Donati F: Postoperative neuromuscular blockade: a comparison between atracurium, vecuronium, and pancuronium, *Anesthesiology* 69:272–276, 1988.
8. Brull SJ, Ehrenwerth J, Connelly NR, Silverman DG: Assessment of residual curarization using low-current stimulation, *Can J Anaesth* 38:164–168, 1991.
9. Beemer GH, Rozental P: Postoperative neuromuscular function, *Anaesth Intensive Care* 14:41–45, 1986.
10. Pedersen T, Viby-Mogensen J, Bang U, et al: Does perioperative tactile evaluation of the train-of-four response influence the frequency of postoperative residual neuromuscular blockade? *Anesthesiology* 73:835–839, 1990.
11. Feinstein B, Lindegard B, Nyman E, Wohlfart G: Morphologic studies of motor units in normal human muscles, *Acta Anat (Basel)* 23:127–142, 1955.
12. Carlsoo S: Motor units and action potentials in masticatory muscles; an electromyographic study of the form and duration of the action potentials and an anatomic study of the size of the motor units, *Acta Morphol Neerl Scand* 2:13–19, 1958.
13. Birks R, Huxley HE, Katz B: The fine structure of the neuromuscular junction of the frog, *J Physiol* 150:134–144, 1960.
14. Israël M, Dunant Y: On the mechanism of acetylcholine release, *Prog Brain Res* 49:125–139, 1979.
15. Peper K, Bradley RJ, Dreyer F: The acetylcholine receptor at the neuromuscular junction, *Physiol Rev* 62:1271–1340, 1982.
16. Salpeter MM, Loring RH: Nicotinic acetylcholine receptors in vertebrate muscle: properties, distribution and neural control, *Prog Neurobiol* 25:297–325, 1985.
17. Wood SJ, Slater CR: Safety factor at the neuromuscular junction, *Prog Neurobiol* 64:393–429, 2001.
18. McMahan UJ, Sanes JR, Marshall LM: Cholinesterase is associated with the basal lamina at the neuromuscular junction, *Nature* 271:172–174, 1978.
19. Rios E, Pizarro G: Voltage sensor of excitation-contraction coupling in skeletal muscle, *Physiol Rev* 71:849–908, 1991.
20. Fill M, Copello JA: Ryanodine receptor calcium release channels, *Physiol Rev* 82:893–922, 2002.
21. MacKrill JJ: Protein-protein interactions in intracellular Ca2+-release channel function, *Biochem J* 337(Pt 3):345–361, 1999.

22. Hoffman EP: Voltage-gated ion channelopathies: inherited disorders caused by abnormal sodium, chloride, and calcium regulation in skeletal muscle, *Annu Rev Med* 46:431–441, 1995.
23. Bowman WC: Prejunctional and postjunctional cholinoceptors at the neuromuscular junction, *Anesth Analg* 59:935–943, 1980.
24. Bowman WC, Marshall IG, Gibb AJ: Is there feedback control of transmitter release at the neuromuscular junction? *Semin Anesth* 3:275–283, 1984.
25. Prior C, Breadon EL, Lindsay KE: Modulation by presynaptic adenosine A1 receptors of nicotinic receptor antagonist–induced neuromuscular block in the mouse, *Eur J Pharmacol* 327:103–108, 1997.
26. Faria M, Oliveira L, Timóteo MA, Lobo MG, Correia-De-Sá P: Blockade of neuronal facilitatory nicotinic receptors containing alpha 3 beta 2 subunits contribute to tetanic fade in the rat isolated diaphragm, *Synapse* 49:77–88, 2003.
27. Chang CC, Hong SJ: Dissociation of the end-plate potential rundown and the tetanic fade from the postsynaptic inhibition of acetylcholine receptor by alpha-neurotoxins, *Exp Neurol* 98:509–517, 1987.
28. Naguib M, Lien CA, Aker J, Eliazo R: Posttetanic potentiation and fade in the response to tetanic and train-of-four stimulation during succinylcholine-induced block, *Anesth Analg* 98:1686–1691, 2004.
29. Standaert FG: Donuts and holes: molecules and muscle relaxants, *Semin Anesth* 3:251–261, 1984.
30. Gage PW, Hamill OP: Effects of anesthetics on ion channels in synapses, *Int Rev Physiol* 25:1–45, 1981.
31. Neubig RR, Boyd ND, Cohen JB: Conformations of Torpedo acetylcholine receptor associated with ion transport and desensitization, *Biochemistry* 21:3460–3467, 1982.
32. Sakmann B, Patlak J, Neher E: Single acetylcholine-activated channels show burst-kinetics in presence of desensitizing concentrations of agonist, *Nature* 286:71–73, 1980.
33. Mortimer JT: Electrical excitation of nerve. In Agnew WF, McCreery DB, editors: *Neural prostheses: fundamental studies*, Englewood Cliffs, NJ, 1990, Prentice Hall, pp 67–84.
34. Brull SJ, Silverman DG: Pulse width, stimulus intensity, electrode placement, and polarity during assessment of neuromuscular block, *Anesthesiology* 83:702–709, 1995.
35. Kopman AF: A safe surface electrode for peripheral-nerve stimulation, *Anesthesiology* 44:343–345, 1976.
36. Gray JA: Letter: nerve stimulators and burns, *Anesthesiology* 42:231–232, 1975.
37. Lippmann M, Fields WA: Burns of the skin caused by a peripheral-nerve stimulator, *Anesthesiology* 40:82–84, 1974.
38. Merton PA: Voluntary strength and fatigue, *J Physiol* 123:553–564, 1954.
39. Stanec A, Heyduk J, Stanec G, Orkin LR: Tetanic fade and post-tetanic tension in the absence of neuromuscular blocking agents in anesthetized man, *Anesth Analg* 57:102–107, 1978.
40. Ali HH, Savarese JJ, Lebowitz PW, Ramsey FM: Twitch, tetanus and train-of-four as indices of recovery from nondepolarizing neuromuscular blockade, *Anesthesiology* 54:294–297, 1981.
41. Lee C, Barnes A, Katz RL: Neuromuscular sensitivity to tubocurarine: a comparison of 10 parameters, *Br J Anaesth* 48:1045–1051, 1976.
42. Goat VA, Yeung ML, Blakeney C, Feldman SA: The effect of blood flow upon the activity of gallamine triethiodide, *Br J Anaesth* 48:69–73, 1976.
43. Saxena PR, Dhasmana KM, Prakash O: A comparison of systemic and regional hemodynamic effects of d-tubocurarine, pancuronium, and vecuronium, *Anesthesiology* 59:102–108, 1983.
44. Curran MJ, Donati F, Bevan DR: Onset and recovery of atracurium and suxamethonium-induced neuromuscular blockade with simultaneous train-of-four and single twitch stimulation, *Br J Anaesth* 59:989–994, 1987.
45. Ali HH, Savarese JJ: Stimulus frequency and dose-response curve to d-tubocurarine in man, *Anesthesiology* 52:36–39, 1980.
46. Connelly NR, Silverman DG, Brull SJ: Temporal correlation of succinylcholine-induced fasciculations to loss of twitch response at different stimulating frequencies, *J Clin Anesth* 4:190–193, 1992.
47. Ali HH, Savarese JJ: Stimulus frequency is essential information, *Anesthesiology* 50:76–77, 1979.
48. Blackman JG: Stimulus frequency and neuromuscular block, *Br J Pharmacol Chemother* 20:5–16, 1963.
49. Waud BE, Waud DR: The margin of safety of neuromuscular transmission in the muscle of the diaphragm, *Anesthesiology* 37:417–422, 1972.
50. Ali HH, Kitz RJ: Evaluation of recovery from nondepolarizing neuromuscular block, using a digital neuromuscular transmission analyzer: preliminary report, *Anesth Analg* 52:740–745, 1973.
51. Lee CM: Train-of-4 quantitation of competitive neuromuscular block, *Anesth Analg* 54:649–653, 1975.
52. Brull SJ, Ehrenwerth J, Silverman DG: Stimulation with submaximal current for train-of-four monitoring, *Anesthesiology* 72:629–632, 1990.
53. Silverman DG, Connelly NR, O'Connor TZ, Garcia R, Brull SJ: Accelographic train-of-four at near-threshold currents, *Anesthesiology* 76:34–38, 1992.
54. Connelly NR, Silverman DG, O'Connor TZ, Brull SJ: Subjective responses to train-of-four and double burst stimulation in awake patients, *Anesth Analg* 70:650–653, 1990.
55. Ali HH, Utting JE, Gray C: Stimulus frequency in the detection of neuromuscular block in humans, *Br J Anaesth* 42:967–978, 1970.
56. Lee C, Katz RL: Fade of neurally evoked compound electromyogram during neuromuscular block by d-tubocurarine, *Anesth Analg* 56:271–275, 1977.
57. Miller RD, Eger EI 2nd, Way WL, Stevens WC, Dolan WM: Comparative neuromuscular effects of Forane and halothane alone and in combination with d-tubocurarine in man, *Anesthesiology* 35:38–42, 1971.
58. Cohen PJ, Heisterkamp DV, Skovsted P: The effect of general anaesthetics on the response to tetanic stimulus in man, *Br J Anaesth* 42:543–547, 1970.
59. Brull SJ, Silverman DG: Tetanus-induced changes in apparent recovery after bolus doses of atracurium or vecuronium, *Anesthesiology* 77:642–645, 1992.
60. Brull SJ, Connelly NR, O'Connor TZ, Silverman DG: Effect of tetanus on subsequent neuromuscular monitoring in patients receiving vecuronium, *Anesthesiology* 74:64–70, 1991.
61. Silverman DG, Brull SJ: The effect of a tetanic stimulus on the response to subsequent tetanic stimulation, *Anesth Analg* 76:1284–1287, 1993.
62. Liley AW, North KA: An electrical investigation of effects of repetitive stimulation on mammalian neuromuscular junction, *J Neurophysiol* 16:509–527, 1953.
63. Feldman SA, Tyrrell MF: A new theory of the termination of action of the muscle relaxants, *Proc R Soc Med* 63:692–695, 1970.
64. Viby-Mogensen J, Howardy-Hansen P, Chraemmer-Jorgensen B, et al: Posttetanic count (PTC): a new method of evaluating an intense nondepolarizing neuromuscular blockade, *Anesthesiology* 55:458–461, 1981.
65. Bonsu AK, Viby-Mogensen J, Fernando PU, et al: Relationship of post-tetanic count and train-of-four response during intense neuromuscular blockade caused by atracurium, *Br J Anaesth* 59:1089–1092, 1987.
66. Drenck NE, Ueda N, Olsen NV, et al: Manual evaluation of residual curarization using double burst stimulation: a comparison with train-of-four, *Anesthesiology* 70:578–581, 1989.
67. Engbaek J, Ostergaard D, Viby-Mogensen J: Double burst stimulation (DBS): a new pattern of nerve stimulation to identify residual neuromuscular block, *Br J Anaesth* 62:274–278, 1989.
68. Ueda N, Viby-Mogensen J, Olsen NV, et al: The best choice of double burst stimulation pattern for manual evaluation of neuromuscular transmission, *J Anesth* 3:94–99, 1989.
69. Brull SJ, Connelly NR, Silverman DG: Correlation of train-of-four and double burst stimulation ratios at varying amperages, *Anesth Analg* 71:489–492, 1990.
70. Kirkegaard-Nielsen H, Helbo-Hansen HS, Severinsen IK, Lindholm P, Bulow K: Double burst monitoring during recovery from atracurium-induced neuromuscular blockade: a comparison with train-of-four, *Int J Clin Monit Comput* 13:209–215, 1996.
71. Saitoh Y, Nakazawa K, Makita K, Tanaka H, Toyooka H: Evaluation of residual neuromuscular blockade using modified double burst stimulation, *Acta Anaesthesiol Scand* 41:741–745, 1997.
72. Kirkegaard-Nielsen H, Helbo-Hansen HS, Severinsen IK, Lindholm P, Bulow K: Response to double-burst appears before response to train-of-four stimulation during recovery from nondepolarizing neuromuscular blockade, *Acta Anaesthesiol Scand* 40:719–723, 1996.

73. Ritchie JM, Wilkie DR: The effect of previous stimulation on the active state of muscle, *J Physiol* 130:488–496, 1955.
74. Krarup C: Enhancement and diminution of mechanical tension evoked by staircase and by tetanus in rat muscle, *J Physiol* 311:355–372, 1981.
75. Kopman AF, Kumar S, Klewicka MM, Neuman GG: The staircase phenomenon: implications for monitoring of neuromuscular transmission, *Anesthesiology* 95:403–407, 2001.
76. Lee GC, Iyengar S, Szenohradszky J, et al: Improving the design of muscle relaxant studies: stabilization period and tetanic recruitment, *Anesthesiology* 86:48–54, 1997.
77. Krarup C: Electrical and mechanical responses in the platysma and in the adductor pollicis muscle: in normal subjects, *J Neurol Neurosurg Psychiatry* 40:234–240, 1977.
78. Van Lunteren E, Vafaie H: Force potentiation in respiratory muscles: comparison of diaphragm and sternohyoid, *Am J Physiol* 264:R1095–R1100, 1993.
79. Deschamps S, Trager G, Mathieu PA, Hemmerling TM: The staircase phenomenon at the corrugator supercilii muscle in comparison with the hand muscles, *Br J Anaesth* 95:372–376, 2005.
80. Donati F, Plaud B, Meistelman C: A method to measure elicited contraction of laryngeal adductor muscles during anesthesia, *Anesthesiology* 74:827–832, 1991.
81. Donati F, Antzaka C, Bevan DR: Potency of pancuronium at the diaphragm and the adductor pollicis muscle in humans, *Anesthesiology* 65:1–5, 1986.
82. Cantineau JP, Porte F, d'Honneur G, Duvaldestin P: Neuromuscular effects of rocuronium on the diaphragm and adductor pollicis muscles in anesthetized patients, *Anesthesiology* 81:585–590, 1994.
83. Donati F, Meistelman C, Plaud B: Vecuronium neuromuscular blockade at the adductor muscles of the larynx and adductor pollicis, *Anesthesiology* 74:833–837, 1991.
84. Debaene B, Guesde R, Clergue F, Lienhart A: Plasma concentration response relationship of pancuronium for the diaphragm and the adductor pollicis in anesthetized man, *Anesthesiology* 73:A887, 1990.
85. Laycock JRD, Donati F, Smith CE, Bevan DR: Potency of atracurium and vecuronium at the diaphragm and the adductor pollicis muscle, *Br J Anaesth* 61:286–291, 1988.
86. Meistelman C, Plaud B, Donati F: Neuromuscular effects of succinylcholine on the vocal cords and adductor pollicis muscles, *Anesth Analg* 73:278–282, 1991.
87. Smith CE, Donati F, Bevan DR: Effects of succinylcholine at the masseter and adductor pollicis muscles in adults, *Anesth Analg* 69:158–162, 1989.
88. Chauvin M, Lebrault C, Duvaldestin P: The neuromuscular blocking effect of vecuronium on the human diaphragm, *Anesth Analg* 66:117–122, 1987.
89. Pansard JL, Chauvin M, Lebrault C, Gauneau P, Duvaldestin P: Effect of an intubating dose of succinylcholine and atracurium on the diaphragm and the adductor pollicis muscle in humans, *Anesthesiology* 67:326–330, 1987.
90. Meistelman C, Plaud B, Donati F: Rocuronium (ORG 9426) neuromuscular blockade at the adductor muscles of the larynx and adductor pollicis in humans, *Can J Anaesth* 39:665–669, 1992.
91. Plaud B, Debaene B, Lequeau F, Meistelman C, Donati F: Mivacurium neuromuscular block at the adductor muscles of the larynx and adductor pollicis in humans, *Anesthesiology* 85:77–81, 1996.
92. Fisher DM, Szenohradszky J, Wright PM, et al: Pharmacodynamic modeling of vecuronium-induced twitch depression: rapid plasma-effect site equilibration explains faster onset at resistant laryngeal muscles than at the adductor pollicis, *Anesthesiology* 86:558–566, 1997.
93. Smith CE, Donati F, Bevan DR: Potency of succinylcholine at the diaphragm and at the adductor pollicis muscle, *Anesth Analg* 67:625–630, 1988.
94. Wright PM, Caldwell JE, Miller RD: Onset and duration of rocuronium and succinylcholine at the adductor pollicis and laryngeal adductor muscles in anesthetized humans, *Anesthesiology* 81:1110–1115, 1994.
95. Dhonneur G, Kirov K, Slavov V, Duvaldestin P: Effects of an intubating dose of succinylcholine and rocuronium on the larynx and diaphragm: an electromyographic study in humans, *Anesthesiology* 90:951–955, 1999.
96. Rosenberg H, Greenhow DE: Peripheral nerve stimulator performance: the influence of output polarity and electrode placement, *Can Anaesth Soc J* 25:424–426, 1978.
97. Berger JJ, Gravenstein JS, Munson ES: Electrode polarity and peripheral nerve stimulation, *Anesthesiology* 56:402–404, 1982.
98. Kalli I: Effect of isometric thumb preload on the evoked compound muscle action potential, *Br J Anaesth* 70:92–93, 1993.
99. Kalli I: Effect of surface electrode position on the compound action potential evoked by ulnar nerve stimulation during isoflurane anaesthesia, *Br J Anaesth* 65:494–499, 1990.
100. Kopman AF: The relationship of evoked electromyographic and mechanical responses following atracurium in humans, *Anesthesiology* 63:208–211, 1985.
101. Hughes R, Payne JP: Clinical assessment of atracurium using the single twitch and tetanic responses of the adductor pollicis muscles, *Br J Anaesth* 55(Suppl 1):47S–52S, 1983.
102. Bencini A, Newton DE: Rate of onset of good intubating conditions, respiratory depression and hand muscle paralysis after vecuronium, *Br J Anaesth* 56:959–965, 1984.
103. Ho LC, Crosby G, Sundaram P, Ronner SF, Ojemann RG: Ulnar train-of-four stimulation in predicting face movement during intracranial facial nerve stimulation, *Anesth Analg* 69:242–244, 1989.
104. Caffrey RR, Warren ML, Becker KE Jr: Neuromuscular blockade monitoring comparing the orbicularis oculi and adductor pollicis muscles, *Anesthesiology* 65:95–97, 1986.
105. Plaud B, Debaene B, Donati F: The corrugator supercilii, not the orbicularis oculi, reflects rocuronium neuromuscular blockade at the laryngeal adductor muscles, *Anesthesiology* 95:96–101, 2001.
106. Ungureanu D, Meistelman C, Frossard J, Donati F: The orbicularis oculi and the adductor pollicis muscles as monitors of atracurium block of laryngeal muscles, *Anesth Analg* 77:775–779, 1993.
107. Viby-Mogensen J, Jensen NH, Engbaek J, et al: Tactile and visual evaluation of the response to train-of-four nerve stimulation, *Anesthesiology* 63:440–443, 1985.
108. Gill SS, Donati F, Bevan DR: Clinical evaluation of double-burst stimulation. Its relationship to train-of-four stimulation, *Anaesthesia* 45:543–548, 1990.
109. Brull SJ, Silverman DG: Visual assessment of train-of-four and double burst-induced fade at submaximal stimulating currents, *Anesth Analg* 73:627–632, 1991.
110. Silverman DG, Brull SJ: Assessment of double-burst monitoring at 10 mA above threshold current, *Can J Anaesth* 40:502–506, 1993.
111. Brull SJ, Silverman DG: Visual and tactile assessment of neuromuscular fade, *Anesth Analg* 77:352–355, 1993.
112. Saitoh Y, Nakazawa K, Makita K, Tanaka H, Toyooka H: Visual evaluation of train-of-four and double burst stimulation, fade at various currents, using a rubber band, *Eur J Anaesthesiol* 14:327–332, 1997.
113. Bergmans J: Computer assisted on line measurement of motor unit potential parameters in human electromyography, *Electromyography* 11:161–181, 1971.
114. Kopec J, Hanusanowa-Petrusewicz I: Application of automatic analysis of electromyograms in clinical diagnosis, *Electroencephalogr Clin Neurophysiol* 36:575–576, 1974.
115. Freund F, Merati J: A source of errors in assessing neuromuscular blockade, *Anesthesiology* 39:540–542, 1973.
116. May O, Kirkegaard-Nielsen H, Werner MU: The acceleration transducer: an assessment of its precision in comparison with a force displacement transducer, *Acta Anaesthesiol Scand* 32:239–243, 1988.
117. Viby-Mogensen J, Jensen E, Werner M, Nielsen HK: Measurement of acceleration: a new method of monitoring neuromuscular function, *Acta Anaesthesiol Scand* 32:45–48, 1988.
118. Brull SJ, Silverman DG: Real time versus slow-motion train-of-four monitoring: a theory to explain the inaccuracy of visual assessment, *Anesth Analg* 80:548–551, 1995.
119. Barry DT, Geiringer SR, Ball RD: Acoustic myography: a noninvasive monitor of motor unit fatigue, *Muscle Nerve* 8:189–194, 1985.
120. Barry DT: Acoustic signals from frog skeletal muscle, *Biophys J* 51:769–773, 1987.
121. Frangioni JV, Kwan-Gett TS, Dobrunz LE, McMahon TA: The mechanism of low-frequency sound production in muscle, *Biophys J* 51:775–783, 1987.
122. Hemmerling TM, Donati F, Beaulieu P, Babin D: Phonomyography of the corrugator supercilii muscle: signal characteristics, best recording site and comparison with acceleromyography, *Br J Anaesth* 88:389–393, 2002.

123. Trager G, Michaud G, Deschamps S, Hemmerling TM: Comparison of phonomyography, kinemyography and mechanomyography for neuromuscular monitoring, *Can J Anaesth* 53:130–135, 2006.
124. Kopman AF: The effect of resting muscle tension on the dose-effect relationship of d-tubocurarine: does preload influence the evoked EMG? *Anesthesiology* 69:1003–1005, 1988.
125. Dupuis JY, Martin R, Tetrault JP: Clinical, electrical and mechanical correlations during recovery from neuromuscular blockade with vecuronium, *Can J Anaesth* 37:192–196, 1990.
126. Braude N, Vyvyan HA, Jordan MJ: Intraoperative assessment of atracurium-induced neuromuscular block using double burst stimulation, *Br J Anaesth* 67:574–578, 1991.
127. Kirkegaard-Nielsen H, Helbo-Hansen HS, Severinsen IK, et al: Comparison of tactile and mechanomyographical assessment of response to double burst and train-of-four stimulation during moderate and profound neuromuscular blockade, *Can J Anaesth* 42:21–27, 1995.
128. Kopman AF, Yee PS, Neuman GG: Relationship of the train-of-four fade ratio to clinical signs and symptoms of residual paralysis in awake volunteers, *Anesthesiology* 86:765–771, 1997.
129. Saitoh Y, Nakazawa K, Toyooka H, Amaha K: Optimal stimulating current for train-of-four stimulation in conscious subjects, *Can J Anaesth* 42:992–995, 1995.
130. Brand JB, Cullen DJ, Wilson NE, Ali HH: Spontaneous recovery from nondepolarizing neuromuscular blockade: correlation between clinical and evoked responses, *Anesth Analg* 56:55–58, 1977.
131. Pavlin EG, Holle RH, Schoene RB: Recovery of airway protection compared with ventilation in humans after paralysis with curare, *Anesthesiology* 70:381–385, 1989.
132. Naguib M, Kopman AF, Lien CA, et al: A survey of current management of neuromuscular block in the United States and Europe, *Anesth Analg* 111:110–119, 2010.
133. Murphy GS, Brull SJ: Residual neuromuscular block: lessons unlearned. Part I: Definitions, incidence, and adverse physiologic effects of residual neuromuscular block, *Anesth Analg* 111:120–128, 2010.
134. Brull SJ, Murphy GS: Residual neuromuscular block: lessons unlearned. Part II: Methods to reduce the risk of residual weakness, *Anesth Analg* 111:129–140, 2010.

PART IV

OTHER EQUIPMENT

CHAPTER 16

AIRWAY EQUIPMENT

William H. Rosenblatt • Tracey Straker

CHAPTER OUTLINE

OVERVIEW

Of all the equipment in the toolbox of the anesthesiologist, airway devices may be the most commonly used as well as the most varied in design and function. The last decade has witnessed a remarkable expansion of the airway armamentarium, necessitating a review of traditional and modern devices. The anesthesia face mask and tracheal tube once comprised the bulk of airway management apparatus; supraglottic airways, video laryngoscopes, and minimally invasive devices have now captured a significant share of both routine and rescue tools. In an attempt to be clinically relevant, this chapter focuses little on historic devices and the forces guiding instrument evolution; that is, the causes, pressure, and findings that led to device development. The exception to this is a historic discussion of the origins of airway management, including tracheal intubation. Although we recognize the importance of historic perspective of all the devices in use today, more authoritative reviews exist.

ANESTHESIA FACE MASK

The anesthesia face mask was invented in 1917. Prior to that, inhalational anesthesia was administered by an open-drop ether technique. The face mask allowed the administration of gases to the patient without instrumentation of the airway. The face mask may be considered the original supraglottic device; it comes in both adult and pediatric sizes. The face mask is held over the patient's face to encompass the patient's nose and mouth. Two fingers are placed over the body of the mask to firmly hold it in place, and three fingers are placed along the bony mandible to complete a tight seal. In edentulous patients, it may be necessary to include the chin of the patient in the mask to compensate for the lack of dentition.

Anesthesia masks are made either of silicone or rubber. In the past, anesthesia masks were opaque, but most modern anesthesia masks are clear to allow the provider to view the patient's lip color, condensation from expiration, secretions, vomitus, and any expelled blood. In some practices, the rubber mask is reusable.

When positioning the mask, the clinician must be careful not to compress the facial nerve and artery, the eyes, or the lips. Face mask fit can be engaged with the help of a head strap (Fig. 16-1) attached to a four-prong ring that encircles the circuit fitting. The head strap is helpful for the clinician with small hands, when the patient is edentulous or has a large face or beard, or to allow providers to have their hands free when the patient is breathing spontaneously.

ORAL AND NASOPHARYNGEAL AIRWAYS

An oral airway prevents the base of tongue and the epiglottis from obstructing the pathway to the larynx. With a few exceptions, oral airways are made from a hard plastic and are inserted into the mouth with their concave surface facing cephalad. Once well within the oral cavity, the airway is rotated 180 degrees so that the preformed concavity comes to its final position following the contour of the tongue. The proximal end of the airway has a flange to prevent the entire device from falling into the mouth; the distal tip sits just above the epiglottis. Because of the position against the base of tongue and posterior pharyngeal wall, oral airways are poorly tolerated in the awake or inadequately anesthetized patient. Nasal airways are made from soft, flexible materials and are tolerated better in awake patients than are oropharyngeal airways (Fig. 16-2). Appropriate nasal airway sizing is determined by measuring the distance from the patient's bony mandible or nostril to the meatus of the ear. Some of the commonly available oral airways include the Berman-Guedel, the split Berman, and the Ovassapian and Williams airways used in fiberoptic laryngoscopy (Fig. 16-3).

Supraglottic Airways

Obstruction of the airway was a poorly understood phenomenon prior to 1874. Opening the mouth with a wooden screw and drawing out the tongue with a forceps or steel-gloved fingers was the height of airway management.[1] Recognition that the base of the tongue falling against the posterior pharyngeal wall accounted for most airway obstruction did not occur until 1880.[2] Credit for the first use of a true supraglottic airway is given to Joseph Thomas Clover (1825–1882), although it is possible that similar devices were used toward the end of the second millennium.[3] Clover used a nasopharyngeal tube for the delivery of chloroform anesthesia. The O'Dwyer tube was introduced in 1884, a device that consisted of a curved metal tube with a conical end that could seal the laryngeal inlet when placed into the oropharynx.[3] Although designed for the treatment of narcotic overdose, it was later modified to be used with volatile anesthetics. Over the next 50 years, several modifications of the basic oropharyngeal airway were described. In the 1930s, Ralph Waters introduced the now familiar flattened-tube oral airway.[4] Guedel modified Waters' concept by fitting his airway within a stiff rubber envelope in an attempt to reduce mucosal trauma.[5]

Tracheal intubation was first described in 1788 as a means of resuscitation of the "apparently dead"[6] but was

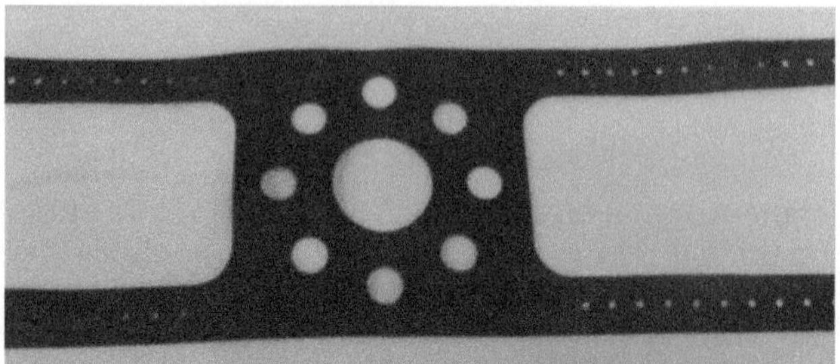

FIGURE 16-1 ■ Mask headstrap.

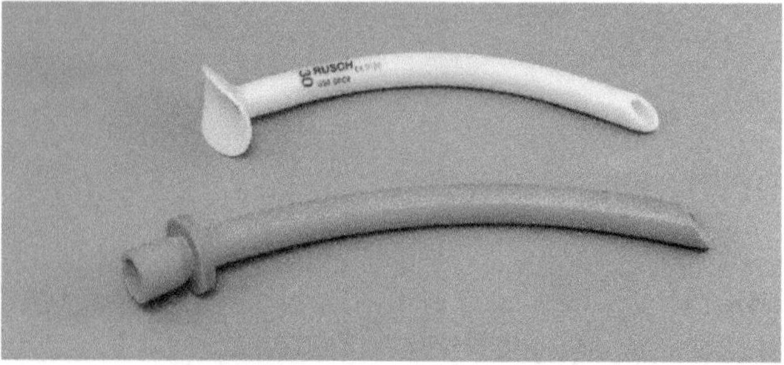

FIGURE 16-2 ■ Nasal airways.

not used for the delivery of anesthesia until almost 100 years later.[7] The forerunner of the modern tracheal tube was designed by the German otolaryngologist, Dr. Franz Kuhn (1866–1929), who developed a flexible metallic tube that resisted kinking and could be shaped to the patient's upper airway anatomy.[8] The tube was inserted using a rigid stylet, and the hypopharynx was sealed with oiled gauze packing. Sir Ivan Magill and Stanley Rowbotham are credited with the initial development of modern tracheal intubation. Performing anesthesia for reconstructive facial surgery during World War I, they developed a two-tube nasal system. One narrow tube of a gum elastic design was passed through the nares and guided into the larynx using a surgical laryngoscope. The other tube was blindly passed into the pharynx to provide for the escape of gases. During use of this "Magill" tube, the exhaust lumen would occasionally pass into the larynx, leading Sir Ivan to describe blind nasal intubation.[9]

Cuffed supralaryngeal airways were initially described in the early part of the twentieth century. The impetus for the development of these devices was threefold. First, the introduction of cyclopropane, an explosive agent, required an airtight circuit for appropriate evacuation. Second, blind and laryngoscope-guided tracheal intubation remained a difficult task. Third, protection of the lower airway from blood and surgical debris in the upper airway was an important concern.[10] The Primrose cuffed oropharyngeal tube, the Shipway airway—which was a Guedel oropharygeal airway fitted with a cuff and circuit connector designed by Sir Ivan Magill—and the Lessinger airway were predecessors of the modern supralaryngeal devices. In 1937 Leech introduced a "pharyngeal bulb gasway" with a noninflatable cuff that fit snugly into the hypopharynx.[11] The use of supralaryngeal airways remained dominant until the introduction of curare in 1942 and the mass training of anesthetists in tracheal intubation in anticipation of and during World War II.[12] Mendelson's description of gastric contents aspiration in obstetric cases (66 of 44,016 patients, with 2 deaths) further pushed the move toward tracheal intubation in most surgical procedures.[13] Within a few years, proficiency in direct laryngoscopy and tracheal intubation became a mark of professionalism.[14] The advent of succinylcholine in 1951 furthered the dominance of tracheal intubation by providing rapid and profound muscle relaxation.

By 1981, two types of airway management prevailed: tracheal intubation and the anesthesia face mask/Guedel airway. Although both were time-tested devices, each had its failings (apart from airway failure in a small number of patients). Tracheal intubation was associated with both dental and soft tissue injury and cardiovascular stimulation, and mask ventilation often required a hands-on-the-airway technique. These difficulties led to the reconsideration of supralaryngeal airways.

Laryngeal Mask Airway

The laryngeal mask airway (LMA) was developed by Dr. Archie Brain in 1982. An exhaustive review of the history of the LMA and its inventor can be found in the text by Joseph Brimacombe.[15] The "classic" LMA (LMA Classic; LMA North America, San Diego, CA) became commercially available in 1988 in England (1992 in the United States). At the time of this writing, the LMA had been used in an estimated 200 million patients. Its components are 100% silicone rubber (no latex), except for a metal spring and a polypropylene component in the inflation valve. It is a reusable device that has a lifespan of 40 uses or cleanings. The mask consists of three components: an inflatable cuff, an airway barrel, and an inflation line (Fig. 16-4). The airway tube is semirigid and semitransparent. Proximally, a standard 15-mm circuit adaptor is permanently fused to the barrel; distally, the barrel is fused to the inflatable cuff. Two flexible aperture bars cross the junction between the barrel and the mask and prevent obstruction by the epiglottis. The aperture bars are flexible enough to allow instrumentation (e.g., intubation) without their removal. The mask is oblong and based on plaster casts of cadavers. The distal aspect is narrow

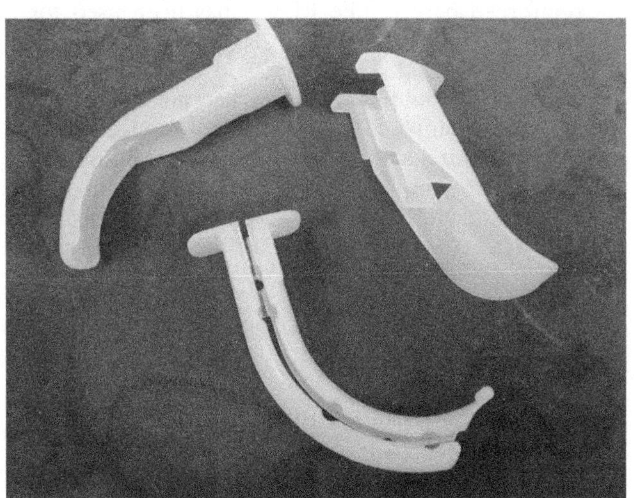

FIGURE 16-3 ■ Williams, Ovassapian, and Split Berman oral airways.

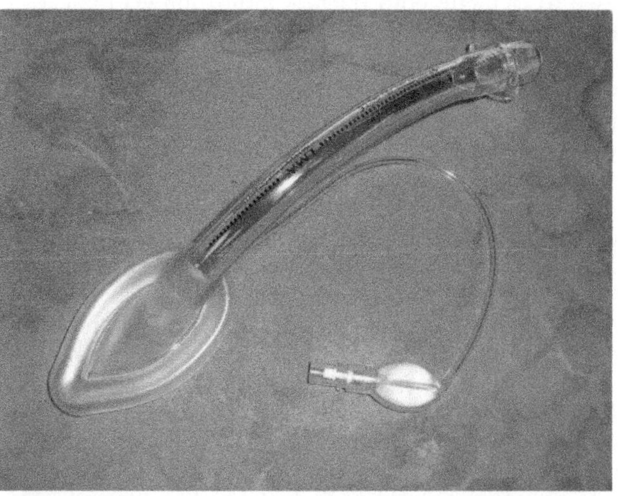

FIGURE 16-4 ■ Single-use version of the classic Laryngeal Mask Airway, the LMA Unique (LMA North America, San Diego, CA).

(over the esophageal inlet), whereas the proximal cuff is broad (upper hypopharynx). With the pilot cuff and syringe tip–activated air valve, the inflation line emerges from the most proximal aspect of the cuff, just behind the barrel-cuff junction.[16] The LMA Classic comes in sizes 1 through 6, with smaller half sizes (1.5 and 2.5); cuff length changes approximately 15% between sizes. The LMA Classic was released in 1998 in a single-use version made of polyvinyl chloride (PVC). Although the LMA Unique has identical dimensions to the LMA Classic, the barrel is more rigid. A rerelease of this device, the LMA Unique in 2000, had a softer barrel and cuff backplate. The LMA has been used in a wide variety of surgical and resuscitative procedures, including spontaneous and controlled ventilation cases,[17] laparoscopy,[18] otolaryngology, and cardiothoracic surgery, in all body positions, in morbidly obese patients, and in other applications.[16] The most feared complication of supraglottic airway (SGA) use, an increased rate of aspiration of gastric contents, has not been realized when the LMA has been used correctly in appropriate patients.[19]

Other versions of the LMA, which were never commercially available, include the nasal LMA, with the barrel and mask assembled in the pharynx; the double-lumen LMA, in which the second lumen is used for instrumentation; the malleable LMA, with a malleable external stylet that allows shaping; the split LMA, to facilitate fiberoptic-aided tracheal intubation; the short-tube LMA, to facilitate through-LMA tracheal intubation; the wide-barrel LMA, to accept a 9-mm tracheal tube; and the gastroscope LMA, to allow passage of an endoscope. Descriptions and citations for these devices can be found in exhaustive reviews by Brimacombe.[15]

A number of accessory devices have been developed by Brain, independent clinicians, and researchers. Two devices have been introduced by Brain to facilitate deflation of the LMA cuff—the *block deflation tool* and the *spring-loaded shoehorn deflation tool.*[20] A wide range of insertion aids include an artificial palate, intralumenal devices, extralumenal devices, and laryngoscope-like blades.[21] Commonly available airway devices have been used to facilitate both tracheal intubation via the classic LMA and its removal after intubation, including the gum elastic bougie, fiberscopes, gastric tubes, and guidewires.[22] Likewise, many different devices have been used to verify the position of the in situ LMA, including light wands, fiberscopes, and the Patil intubation guide (Anesthesia Associates, San Marcos, CA).[22]

Although the LMA shows some resistance to low-power laser strikes, these devices are generally considered non–laser compatible. Details on resistance to a variety of laser sources are available.[23] The metallic spring in the pilot cuff of the LMA Classic and some other LMAs is not MRI compatible; however, no morbidities have been associated with its use, although there have been reports of the spring interfering with the quality of the magnetic resonance image (MRI).[24] An MRI-compatible LMA is available that uses a plastic spring. The metal reinforcement in the LMA Flexible and LMA ProSeal is non–MRI compatible, as is the barrel of the reusable Fastrach and Ctrach LMAs. The silicone cuff of the LMA is permeable to nitrous oxide (N_2O), and intracuff pressure will increase during N_2O anesthesia.[25,26] The LMA contains no natural latex.

Cleaning and sterilization are important steps in the use of any reusable device, and appropriate cleaning improves the safety and longevity of LMA products. Manual cleaning is done with sodium bicarbonate, soapy water, or a mild enzymatic cleaner. Other chemical agents should be avoided, and a soft brush should be used to remove secretions. During cleaning, every attempt should be made to keep the inflation valve dry because water may cause malfunction. After cleaning, the device should be reinspected for soiling or damage. Sterilization is by steam autoclave, and the cuff of all LMAs should be emptied of air immediately before autoclaving (spontaneous reinflation will occur if the device is left for hours prior to sterilization). Immediate spontaneous reinflation may indicate a faulty inflation valve; if this happens, the device should be discarded. Small amounts of gas in the cuff may cause rupture during autoclaving, and autoclave temperature should not exceed 135° C. The duration of the autoclave cycle can be from 3 to 15 minutes depending on the autoclave mechanism. The manufacturer suggests that all reusable LMAs be discarded after 40 uses.

Although a number of LMA modifications have been made, only a handful have found widespread acceptance and commercial success. The following devices are based on the classic LMA but incorporate changes in the barrel or mask design that facilitate usability or improve safety.

The flexible LMA (FLMA; LMA Flexible, LMA North America) was designed to be used in surgical cases where the area in and around the airway must be shared with the surgical team. The barrel of the FLMA is longer and narrower than the classic LMA and is wire reinforced. It may be deflected away from the surgical field without kinking or placing torque on the cuff. When the surgical field includes the head or neck and heavy drapes cover the airway, the drapes can fall on the FLMA barrel with impunity. The FLMA is available in sizes 2 to 6, including a size 2.5. Neither the LMA Classic nor the FLMA is laser resistant, nor are they MRI compatible because of the reinforced barrel. The FLMA has been used for a wide variety of otolaryngeal surgeries, including adenotonsillectomy, uvulopalatoplasty, and dental, intranasal, ear, and eye procedures.[27-29] The narrow barrel of the FLMA is not compressed by a surgical mouth gag, but placement requires cooperation between the anesthesiologist and surgeon. The barrel is placed midline under the grooved blade of the Dingman (or similar) mouth gag. Outward tension is applied on the FLMA barrel as the mouth gag is placed; this maneuver prevents redundancy of the barrel in the pharynx, which occurs as the blade shortens the distance over the tongue. During the mouth gag placement, care must be taken to ensure the FLMA inflation line is not trapped and occluded. The blade of the mouth gag must be appropriately sized; too large a blade can crush the proximal FLMA cuff, and too small a blade can pull the cuff out of position.

The principal concern among clinicians contemplating otolaryngeal procedures with the laryngeal mask has

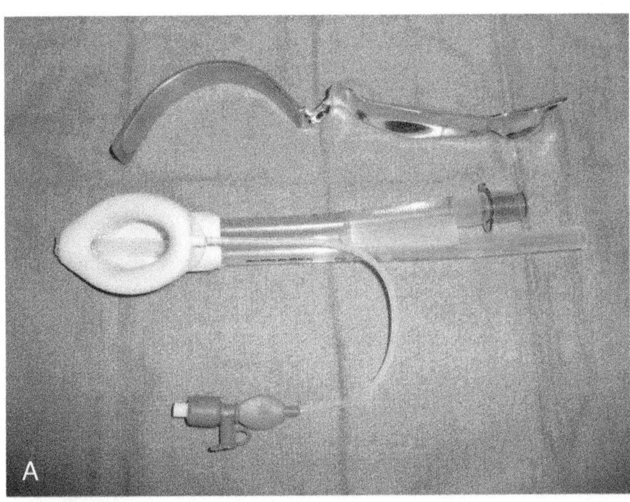

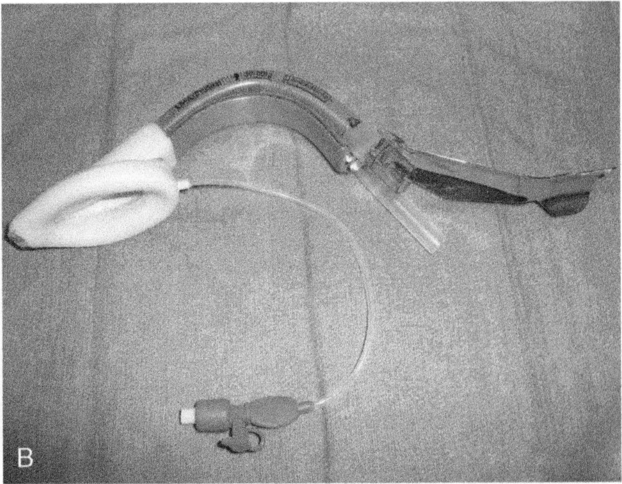

FIGURE 16-5 ■ **A,** ProSeal Larygneal Mask Airway (LMA North America, San Diego, CA). **B,** With insertion handle attached.

been airway protection from surgical blood and debris. Studies have shown superior airway protection compared with the use of a tracheal tube (or nasal mask in dental surgery) by virtue of the supraglottic seal.[30]

The cleaning procedure and life expectancy of the FLMA are identical to those of the LMA Classic. A single-use FLMA is also available.

ProSeal LMA

The ProSeal LMA (PLMA) was introduced in 2001 as an improved version of the LMA Classic. The PLMA is a relatively complex device compared with other laryngeal masks (Fig. 16-5, *A* and *B*). Differences in the ProSeal, compared with the LMA Classic, are listed in Table 16-1.

There are three primary improvements of the PLMA: 1) diagnosis of device position, 2) access to the alimentary track, and 3) higher airway pressures. Although the incidence of complications during LMA anesthesia is similar to that of the tracheal tube, it is believed that poor positioning contributes to most of these events.[19] In one well-described case report, aspiration of gastric contents occurred because of PLMA misplacement. Importantly, the clinician did not perform any confirmatory test to ensure the device's correct position.[31] Several techniques have been described to determine whether the PLMA is correctly inserted (Table 16-2).

Because of the upper esophageal positioning of the PLMA's nonairway lumen, access to the alimentary tract is possible. Gastric emptying may occur that may be passive, via regurgitation, or active, via Salem sump placement. Table 16-3 lists the maximum gastric tube diameter for each PLMA size. Brain suggests that the gastric tube not be left in situ during the maintenance phase of the anesthetic because the lumen of the gastric drain should be left unobstructed (see Table 16-3).

Although the LMA Classic typically achieves a seal pressure of 20 to 25 cm H_2O, some patients, such as the morbidly obese, may require positive airway pressure beyond this.[36] Because of its deep bowl, and possibly the back cuff, the PLMA seals the airway to 40 to 45 cm H_2O or more.[37]

TABLE 16-1 **Unique ProSeal Laryngeal Mask Airway Features***

Gastric drain lumen (secondary lumen)	Diagnostic position testing Passive gastric drain Active gastric emptying (gastric tube) Pressure pop-off valve
No mask aperture bars	Drain tube prevents obstruction by epiglottis
Introducer tool	Creates Fastrach-like insertion
Insertion strap	Fixing of introducer tool Placement of index finger
Wire-reinforced airway tube	Reduces diameter, improves flexibility
Dorsal cuff	Increased seal pressure
Ventral cuff larger in proximal end	Improved seal
Deeper bowl	Improved fit
Integrated bite block	Accessory bite block not required
Hard silicone drain tube rings	Prevents drain tube collapse
Accessory vent (within bowl, under drain tube)	Prevents pooling of secretions

*LMA North America, San Diego, CA.

TABLE 16-2 **Tests to Ensure Proper Positioning of ProSeal Laryngeal Mask Airway***

Test	Observation	Reference
Bite block test	Depth of bite block adequate	32
Suprasternal notch test	Pressing on suprasternal notch moves bubble placed on gastric drain	33
Leak test	No gas leak from drain tube	34
Gastric tube placement	Tube placed into stomach ensures patency	35

*LMA North America, San Diego, CA.

TABLE 16-3 Maximum Gastric Tube Diameters for ProSeal Laryngeal Mask Airways*

Airway Size	OG Tube Size
1½	10 Fr
2	10 Fr
2½	14 Fr
3	16 Fr
4	16 Fr
5	18 Fr

*LMA North America, San Diego, CA.
OG, orogastric.

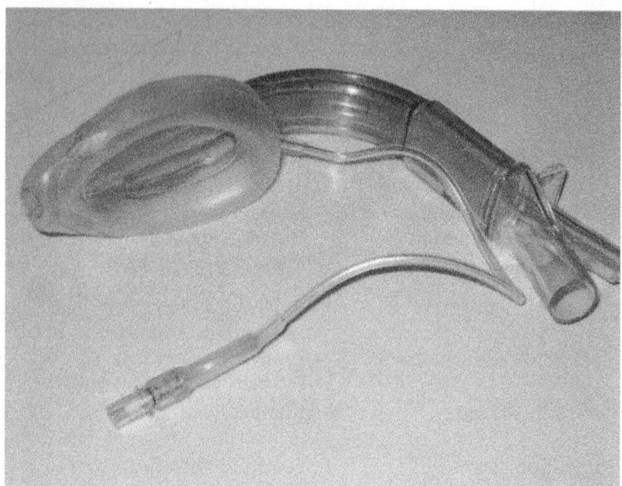

FIGURE 16-6 LMA Supreme (LMA North America, San Diego, CA).

LMA Supreme

The LMA Supreme may first be considered a disposable ProSeal LMA because of a similarly configured drain tube. The LMA Supreme also has a fixed-curve airway tube, like the Fastrach LMA. The LMA Supreme consists of a preformed airway tube, integrated bite block, gastric drain for placement confirmation and gastric decompression, and fixation tabs that help maintain the correct insertion depth. The LMA Supreme is available in adult sizes 3 to 5 (Fig. 16-6).

Fastrach LMA

The Fastrach (LMA North America), or intubating LMA (ILMA), was introduced in 1995 to improve the technique of tracheal intubation through the LMA. Several intubation techniques have been described through the LMA Classic, including blind, retrograde wire-assisted, flexible fiberoptic, light wand, bougie, and tracheal tube exchange catheter placements. Table 16-4 examines the problems with tracheal intubation via the LMA Classic and how the ILMA corrects these problems.

The stainless steel, silicone-coated barrel of the ILMA is anatomically shaped to fit the oral cavity–pharynx-hypopharynx axis, when the head is in the neutral position. This curve was based on the analysis of 60 sagittal MRI sections of patients with normal airways. The barrels of the three available sizes—3, 4, and 5—are identical. The masks vary in the size of the cuff and the placement of the epiglottic lifting bar (ELB). The ELB is a vertically oriented semirigid bar fixed at the proximal end of the bowl aperture and positioned to sit beneath the epiglottis in situ. As a tracheal tube is passed through the barrel, the EBL lifts the epiglottis out of its path to the larynx. A handle at the proximal end of the barrel is used for insertion, repositioning, and removal. A secondary advantage of the handle is that the operator does not need to place fingers into the patient's mouth (Fig. 16-7).

TABLE 16-4 Problems with Tracheal Intubation

LMA Classic	Intubating LMA
22 cm in length, requires long tracheal tube	14 cm in length
Diameter accepts up to size 7.0 tracheal tube	Size 8.0 ID tracheal tube
Obstruction by epiglottis	Lifting bar raises epiglottis away from tracheal tube path
Difficult removal of LMA while leaving the tracheal tube in situ	Removal facilitated by large diameter and short length
Flexible barrel hinders readjustment	Stainless steel barrel
Fingers must be placed in the mouth during placement	Stainless steel handle facilitates insertion

ID, inner diameter; *LMA*, laryngeal mask airway.

The Fastrach is designed to be used with a straight, armored, silicone tracheal tube (Euromedics, Malaysia), although standard or Parker Flex-tip (Parker Medical, Englewood, CO) PVC tracheal tubes have been used.[38] The Fastrach is indicated for routine, elective intubation and for anticipated and unanticipated difficult intubation. Because it was designed to facilitate blind tracheal intubation, the presence of airway secretions, blood, or edema, such as from previous intubation attempts or trauma, has not hindered its usefulness as a ventilating and intubating device after failed rapid-sequence intubation.[38]

Paraesophageal Devices

King Laryngeal Tracheal Tube

The King laryngeal tube (LT; King Systems, Noblesville, IN), is a latex-free, single-use, single-lumen silicone tube that consists of a 130-degree angled airway tube, an average barrel diameter of 1.5 cm, esophageal and oropharyngeal low-pressure cuffs, and two ventilation ports. The distal esophageal tube seals the esophagus and protects against regurgitation, while the proximal oropharyngeal tube sits in the oropharynx and seals both the oral and nasal cavities. During ventilation through the two ventilation ports, the trachea is oxygenated. The King LT is available in sizes 3 to 5 in the United States and in sizes 0 to 2 outside the United States. A double-lumen version of the King LT suction (LTS) also is available. One lumen is available for ventilation, and the other

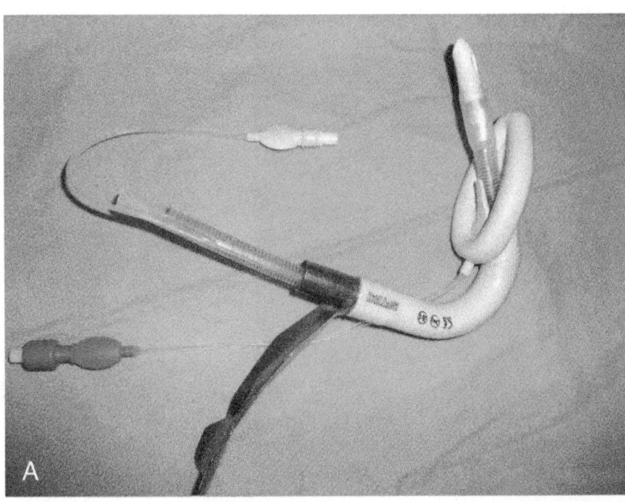

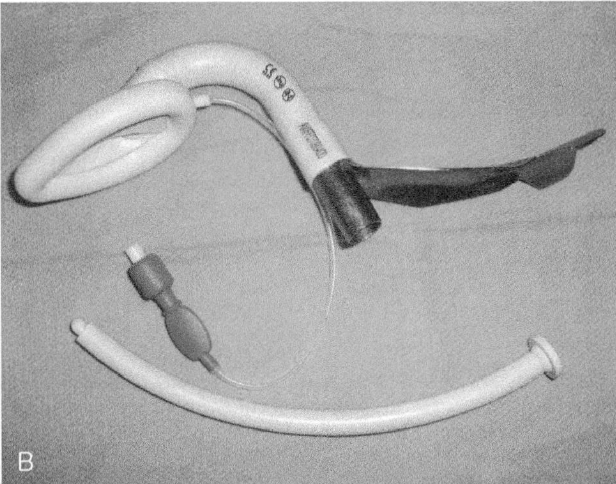

FIGURE 16-7 ▪ **A,** Fastrach (LMA North America, San Diego, CA). **B,** Fastrach with plunger.

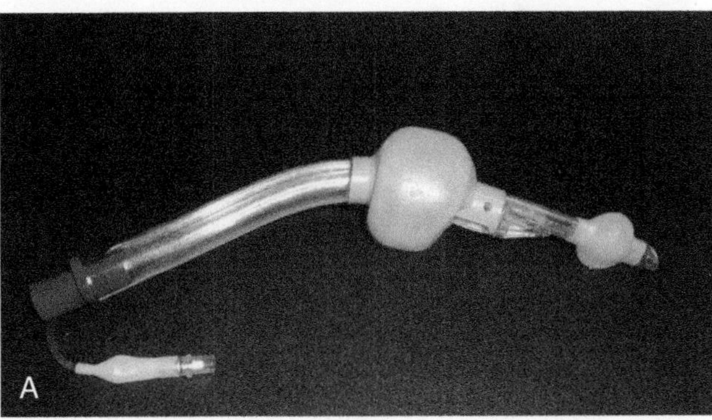

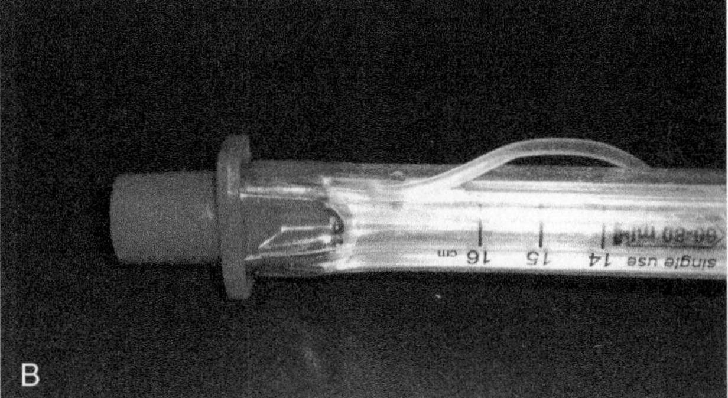

FIGURE 16-8 ▪ **A** and **B,** King laryngeal tube (King Systems, Noblesville, IN).

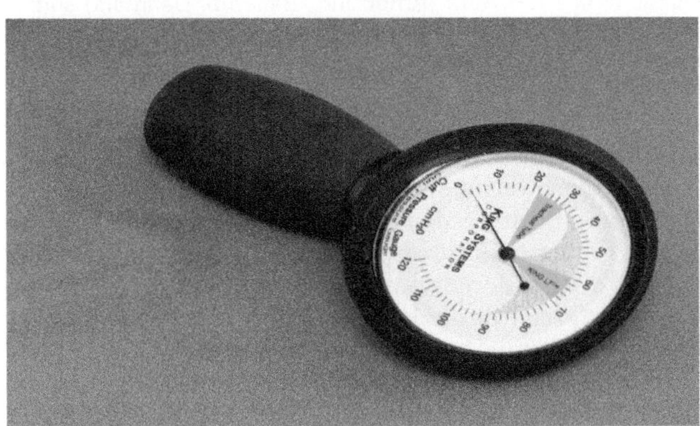

FIGURE 16-9 ▪ Cuff pressure gauge.

lumen is used for decompression of the stomach, suctioning, and placement verification. Both the King LT and King LTS are available in disposable versions (Fig. 16-8).[39] Cuff pressures in supraglottic airways should never exceed 60 cm H_2O. Devices are available to easily measure intra-cuff pressures (Fig. 16-9).

I-Gel

The I-Gel (Intersurgical, Liverpool, NY) is a single-use cuffless supraglottic device made from a thermoplastic elastomer that helps create a seal of the pharyngeal, laryngeal, and perilaryngeal structures. Compression trauma is limited with the use of this material. The I-Gel has a gastric lumen and a built-in bite block along with a buccal cavity stabilizer that aids insertion and eliminates rotation within the oropharynx. The device is available in adult sizes 3 to 5 and accommodates nasogastric tube sizes 12 to 14 (Fig. 16-10).[40]

SLIPA Pharyngeal Liner

The SLIPA streamlined pharyngeal liner (CurveAir Limited, London, UK) is a hollow, cuffless, preformed pharyngeal liner. No cuff is needed for the device to seal the pharynx. The SLIPA was named because it is shaped like a slipper, with a "toe," "bridge," and "heel." During insertion, the jaw is lifted forward "to negotiate the toe of the chamber past the bend in the pharynx at the base of the tongue." The bridge fits into the piriform fossa, sealing the upward outlet at the base of the tongue. The heel anchors the SLIPA into position, sealing off the nasopharynx. The hollow bowl acts as a reservoir for secretions and aids in preventing aspiration as a result of regurgitation. The nonlatex SLIPA is available in six sizes related to patient height and the dimension across the thyroid cartilage. Preformed indentations in the SLIPA help spare the hypoglossal nerve from

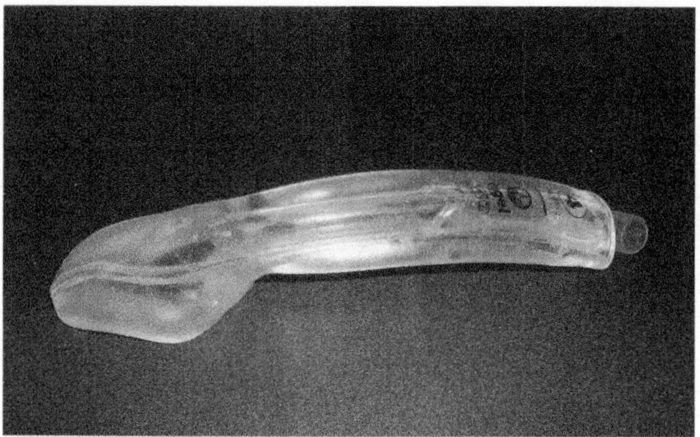

FIGURE 16-10 ■ The I-Gel (Intersurgical, Liverpool, NY) cuffless supraglottic device.

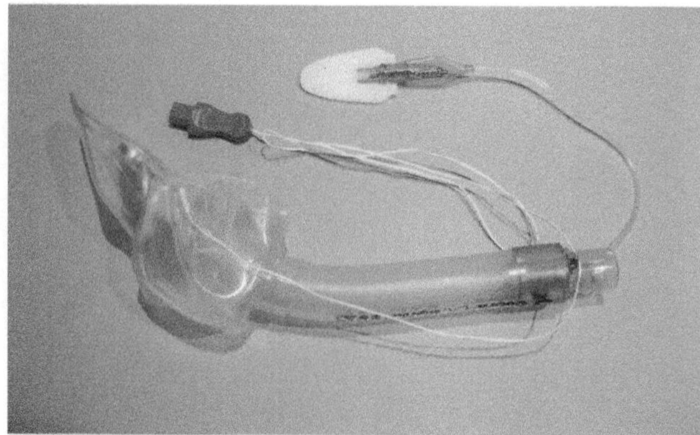

FIGURE 16-12 ■ The Cobra Plus (Engineered Medical Systems, Memphis, TN).

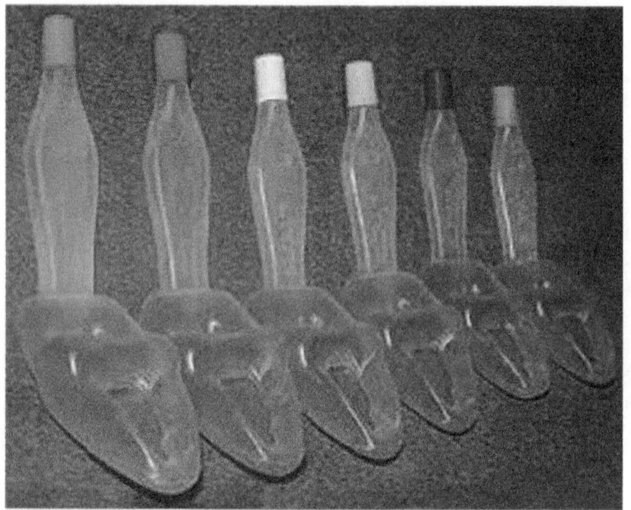

FIGURE 16-11 ■ SLIPA streamlined pharyngeal liners (CurveAir Limited, London, UK).

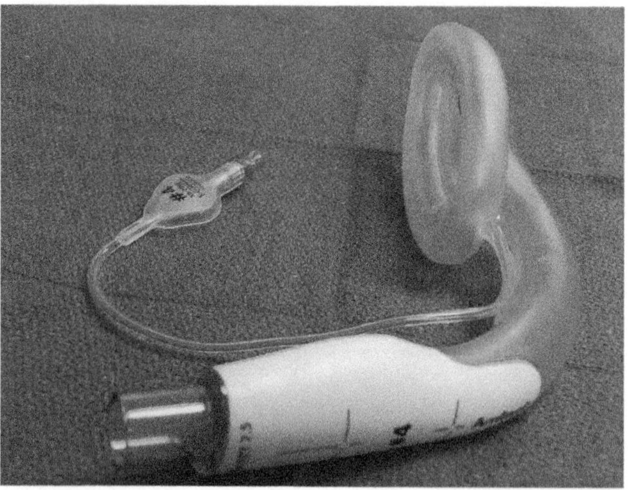

FIGURE 16-13 ■ The Aura (Ambu Inc., Ballerup, Denmark) supraglottic device.

compression, and the stem aids in placement without the need for fingers to be inserted in the mouth. This is a single-use device (Fig. 16-11).[41]

Cobra Plus

The Cobra Plus (Engineered Medical Systems, Memphis, TN) is a single-use, nonlatex supraglottic device designed positioned in the hypopharynx. The device has an airway tube, standard 15-mm connector, and a distal ventilation port surrounded by a slotted port cover that helps prevent the soft tissue and the epiglottis from obstructing the ventilation port. In addition, the Cobra Plus has the ability to monitor the patient's core temperature, has a distal carbon dioxide sampling port, and is available in pediatric sizes. Fiberoptic intubation can be facilitated by this device, which is available in adult and pediatric sizes, ½ to 6 (Fig.16-12).[42]

Aura

The Aura (Ambu Inc., Ballerup, Denmark) is a supraglottic device that has a preformed anatomic curve that simulates human anatomy. This device has no epiglottic bars on the anterior surface of the cuff and has a built-in bite block and an easily removable 15-mm connector that aids in fiberoptic intubation. The Aura comes in reusable and disposable designs, and Ambu recently introduced a wire-reinforced flexible device and devices with straight airway tubes. The Ambu devices are available in sizes 1 to 6, and the reinforced device is available in sizes 2 to 6 (Fig. 16-13).[42]

Obturator and Gastric Tube Airways

Although direct laryngoscopy and tracheal intubation were the standard of airway management in the 1960s, especially in patients who were at risk for gastric content aspiration, concerns regarding out-of-hospital resuscitation were dominant in the emergency medicine literature.[39] Failure of tracheal intubation outside the hospital was common. Recognizing that blind passage of a device into the mouth typically resulted in esophageal intubation, devices that took advantage of this observation flourished. The esophageal obturator airway (EOA) was the first such device.[43] The EOA consisted of a face mask with a blind-ended, cuffed, esophageal obturator, or blocker. Once placed in the esophagus, ventilation could be achieved via perforations in the obturator tube as long as the proximal mask was tightly sealed on the face. Proliferation of EOA use resulted in many criticisms, including reports of accidental tracheal intubations with failure to ventilate, esophageal perforation, gastric insufflations because of cuff failure, and distortion of upper airway anatomy.[11] A modification of the EOA, the esophageal gastric tube airway (EGTA), allowed emptying of the stomach. The concept of the EOA and EGTA was further transformed by Dr. Michael Frass, who substituted a pharyngeal cuff for the poorly fitting face mask of the original devices.

Combitube

The Combitube (Tyco Healthcare [now Covidien], Mansfield, MA) was introduced in 1987 as a substitute for tracheal intubation, especially when trained personnel, proper equipment, or adequate patient access was not available for emergency airway management. The Combitube also has been used for routine anesthetic delivery[44,45] and is available in two sizes: the 37 Fr size is for patients 120 cm to 180 cm in height, and the 41 Fr size is for patients taller than 180 cm. The Combitube is a double-lumen airway composed of a pharyngeal lumen and a tracheoesophageal lumen. The pharyngeal lumen has a standard 15-mm connector at the proximal end (outside the patient) but ends blindly. At the level of the pharynx are multiple perforations that when properly placed are juxtaposed to the laryngeal inlet. The second lumen also has a standard 15-mm connector at the proximal end but terminates with a patent lumen distal to the pharyngeal perforation of the pharyngeal lumen. When properly placed, the distal end of the tracheoesophageal lumen lies within the esophagus. Two cuffs seal the airway; an oropharyngeal balloon lies proximal to the pharyngeal perforations, just posterior to the hard palate. When inflated, the balloon presses ventrocaudally against the tongue and dorsocranially against the soft palate. The distal cuff lies just proximal to the open end of the tracheoesophageal lumen (Fig. 16-14). This configuration allows placement of the distal end of the Combitube into the esophagus (95% of blind placements) or into the trachea. In the esophageal position, which is assumed a priori on first placement, ventilation of the lungs occurs via the pharyngeal perforations; the operator ventilates via the pharyngeal lumen proximally, which is colored blue. In this position, projectile decompression of the stomach via the tracheoesophageal lumen often occurs. Attesting to the ability of the Combitube to decompress the stomach is a "deflation elbow" that can be attached to the esophageal lumen prior to Combitube insertion to prevent soiling.

If tracheal position of the distal Combitube occurs, which can be presumed if ventilation via the pharyngeal lumen is inadequate, the operator switches ventilation to the clear plastic tracheoesophageal lumen. In addition, the Combitube can be inserted with the patient's head in a neutral or extended position; the classic "sniffing" position may impede insertion. In general, the patient's airway reflexes must be obtunded for adequate insertion, which may be performed blindly or with a standard laryngosocope.

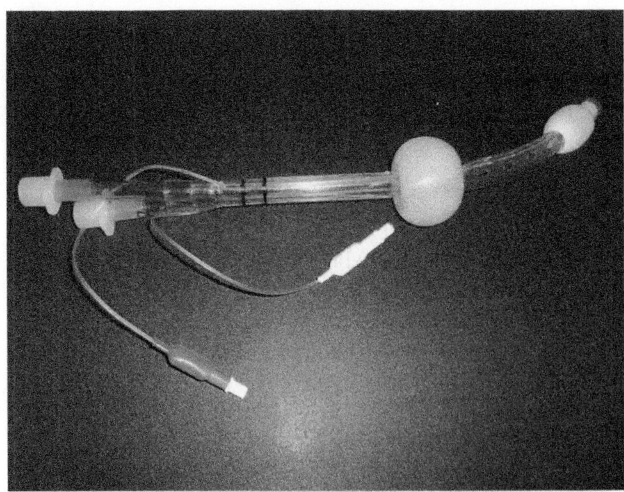

FIGURE 16-14 ■ The Combitube (Covidien, Mansfield, MA).

The Combitube has been left in situ for 8 hours and can be used with mechanical ventilation. Upper limits of achievable airway pressure have been recorded at 50 cm H_2O. The Combitube also may be substituted with a standard tracheal tube by several techniques. The oropharyngeal cuff is deflated, and a laryngocsope or flexible fiberscope is used to achieve tracheal intubation; nasal fiberoptic intubation has also been described with minimal deflation of the pharyngeal cuff, allowing continuous ventilation during the procedure.[44] Once tracheal intubation has been confirmed, the distal cuff is deflated, and the Combitube is removed. If tracheal intubation proves difficult, the pharyngeal cuff is reinflated, and ventilation via the Combitube is resumed.

A similar device released in 2006, the Rusch Easy Tube (Teleflex Medical, Research Triangle Park, NC), also was devised for either tracheal or esophageal intubation, specifically for difficult or emergent intubation. The device consists of a "large-volume pharyngeal nonlatex cuff tapering down from a dual lumen above the pharyngeal cuff to a single lumen at the tip, thereby reducing the potential for trauma to either the trachea or esophagus." The Easy Tube is available in 28 and 41 Fr sizes. The Easy Tube is considerably smaller than the Combitube and affords a better fiberoptic view. The insertion of the Easy Tube is similar to the placement of the Combitube, and the exchange for an endotracheal tube (ETT) can be carried out using techniques described above for the Combitube.[46]

Endotracheal Tubes

The art of endotracheal anesthesia is more than 100 years old. The first orotracheal intubation anesthetic was in 1880 by Glasgow surgeon Sir William Macewen.[47] In 1901 the German physicist Franz Kuhn modified the ETT for an easier intubation.[48]

Several indications exist for ETT intubation. Some important indications for intubation are oxygenation and positive-pressure ventilation, pulmonary toilet, and airway protection. ETTs initially were made of rubber for multiple uses; however, these devices were prone to kinking, and they were unsuitable for patients sensitive to latex. ETTs today are made of many materials, although the most commonly used material is PVC. PVC is inexpensive, and the tubes conform to patient anatomy through thermoplasticity and are more resistant to kinking.[49] ETTs must conform to the American Society for Testing and Materials International (ASTM) standard, which includes specifications for inside and outside diameters, distance markers from the tip, material toxicity, angle and direction of the tip, size and shape of the Murphy eye, and radius of the tube curvature.[50] ETTs may either be cuffed or uncuffed; cuffs provide a seal between the ETT and trachea, thereby protecting the trachea from gastric contents. ETTs in use today have high-volume, low-pressure cuffs that disperse force on the tracheal tissues.

Armored Tubes

Armored tubes, both anode or flexometallic, have a reinforced metal or nylon wire wound in a spiral throughout the shaft of the tube. These tubes are resistant to kinking and compression and often are used in head, neck, and tracheal surgery and in positions in which the neck is flexed. A disadvantage of this tube construction is that once it is kinked or compressed, it does not revert to its original shape; this can result in airway obstruction (Fig. 16-15).[41]

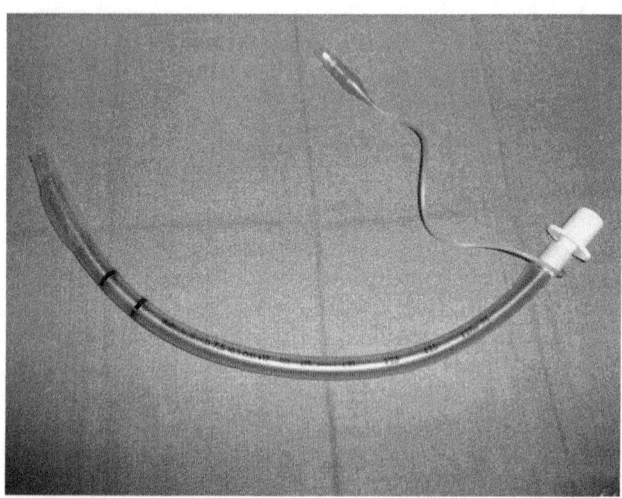

FIGURE 16-15 ■ Anode tube.

Preformed Tubes

Preformed tubes, such as Ring-Adair-Elwyn (RAE) tubes, have a preformed bend and are available for both oral and nasal intubations to prevent the ETT from hindering access to the surgical field. They are predominantly used in oromaxillofacial and nasal procedures (Fig. 16-16).[41]

Parker Flex-Tip Tube

The Parker Flex-Tip ETT (Parker Medical, Highlands Ranch, CO) is designed to facilitate the passage of the tube into the trachea during flexible fiberoptic-aided laryngoscopy. Clefts between the bevel of standard tracheal tubes and the fiberscope may result in entrapment of the right arytenoid cartilage, vocal folds, or other structures. However, the bevel of the Parker Flex-Tip tube decreases the distance between the fiberoptic scope insertion cord and the ETT, thereby increasing the success of first-attempt passage of the ETT.[41]

Hunsaker Mon Jet Tube

The Hunsaker Mon Jet tube (Xiomed, Jacksonville, FL) is designed for elective jet ventilation. The tube consists of a flexible, collapsible cage that positions the distal end of the tube in a midline tracheal position, a 3-mm laser-resistant shaft with a stylet, and a carbon dioxide sampling line. The Hunsaker tube has a Luer-lock top that allows for connection to a jet ventilation device. The carbon dioxide sampling line allows for monitoring of the end-tidal carbon dioxide or airway pressure in an effort to avoid barotrauma. This tube can be used with both carbon dioxide and yttrium-aluminum-garnet (YAG) lasers (Fig. 16-17).[51]

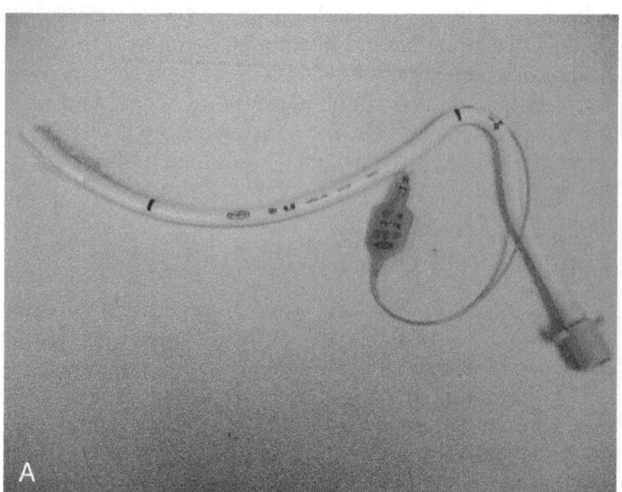

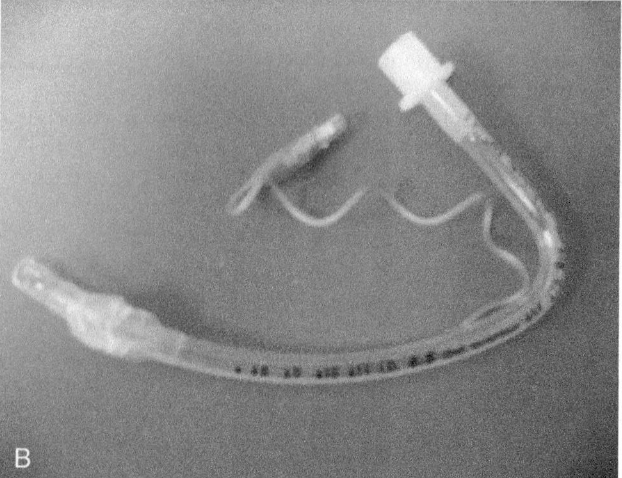

FIGURE 16-16 ■ **A,** Nasal Ring-Adair-Elwyn (RAE) tube. **B,** Oral RAE tube.

LARYNGOSCOPY

Direct Laryngoscopy

Since the 1940s, the most common device used to facilitate tracheal intubation has been the direct laryngoscope (DL). A rapid, easily learned, and highly successful technique, direct laryngoscopy has universal acceptance. The practice of direct laryngoscopy is one of creating a nonanatomic access through a line of sight from the operator to the larynx. With the introduction of anatomically compliant devices (discussed below), the DL is likely to have reduced importance in the future.

All direct laryngoscopes have three basic components: the *handle*, the *blade*, and the *light source*. Although the modern DL in use by the anesthesiologist is based on a right-angle relationship of the handle and blade (with some exceptions), U-type configurations also have been produced and remain popular in otolaryngology. Although fixed-handle blades have been used in the past, most modern systems use a folding latch connector between the two, which also acts as a switch for powering the source of illumination by a variety of mechanisms. Adaptors that can be placed between the handle and blade allow the right angle to be modified to various clinical situations.

The first direct laryngoscopes used external light sources—direct sunlight, head mirrors, and headlamps—to illuminate the larynx.[52] In 1902, Einhorn developed a lightbulb carrier that could be mounted on the blade. In 1907, Jackson developed a blade that used this carrier to provide distal illumination. In 1913, batteries were incorporated into the handle by Janeway. Although the batteries in the handle/lightbulb-on-blade configuration were standard for more than 80 years, the GreenLine DL system (SunMed, Largo, FL) incorporates the entire light-producing mechanism, batteries and light bulb, into the handle. Light transmission to the larynx occurs via a rigid, steel-encased fiberoptic cable. This system offers the advantages of keeping the electrical components in a sealed case and reducing the exposure of the patient to a hot light source.[53]

The DL blade is used to create an axis of visualization of the larynx. The blade spatula compresses the tongue into the mandibular space, while the flange (if present) is used to move the tongue laterally and create a visual lumen. The spatula may be straight, curved, or angular, but the resulting lumen must be a straight line. Flanges have been designed in a variety of cross-sectional shapes that include C, U, and O shapes (the O shape is a completely enclosed tube). The cross-sectional height of the flange is termed the *step*.

The distal end of the blade is referred to as the *tip* and is used to elevate the epiglottis. The tip may be placed either underneath the epiglottis, to lift it directly, or in the vallecula, where stretching of the glossoepiglottic ligament causes elevation. The tip generally is blunt and thickened to reduce trauma.

Although more than 50 DL blades have been designed and marketed, the straight Miller blade and curved Macintosh blade are the predominant ones in clinical use. In lieu of a detailed discussion of each, the unique properties of various blades are highlighted in Box 16-1.

Indirect Laryngoscopy

Advances in the engineering of light-transmitting fibers in the 1950s led to the development of tracheal intubation devices that used indirect imaging of the larynx; a direct line of sight from the operator to the patient larynx was no longer required. Subsequent to this development, the miniaturization of electronics allowed the development of cheaper and more durable devices.

Suspension Laryngoscopy

Suspension laryngoscopy is done with the patient under general anesthesia and consists of a hollow scope used to expose the patient's pharynx and larynx. The laryngoscope is suspended by an external support that allows the surgeon's hand to be free for procedures.

A Dedo scope, a U-shaped scope used during suspension laryngoscopy, is designed to allow examination of the vocal cords at the anterior commissure in patients who have challenging airways. These scopes can be adapted to allow exposure of the airway with microscopes and fiberoptic light sources, tissue removal with lasers, adaptation to video for teaching purposes, and oxygenation and ventilation with a Venturi device. These scopes typically are used by otorhinolaryngologists.[57]

DEVICES

Flexible Fiberoptic Devices

The concept of the fiberscope was first considered in 1954 with the development of glass fiber bundles. Light

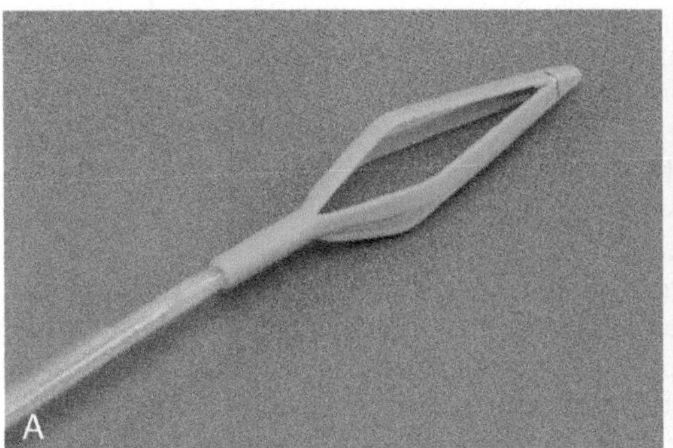

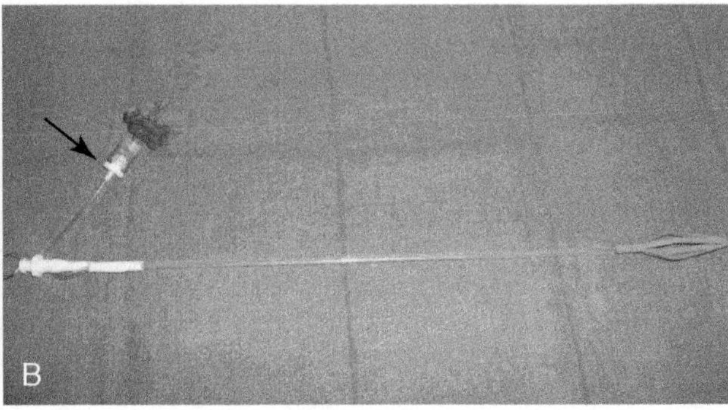

FIGURE 16-17 ■ **A,** The Hunsaker Mon Jet tube cage (Xiomed, Jacksonville, FL). **B,** Hunsaker carbon dioxide sampling port (*arrow*).

BOX 16-1 Unique Design Features and Intended Advantages of Various Laryngoscope Blades

MILLER LARYNGOSCOPE BLADE
- Introduced in 1941. Longer than previous blades. Rounded bottom. Small distal tip. Curve begins two inches from the tip.
- Requires less interincisor space. Used by epiglottic entrapment (direct lift).

MACINTOSH LARYNGOSCOPE BLADE
- Sharply curved blade with large flange. Indirect lifting of the epiglottis by stretching of the glossoepiglottic ligament. Reduced plane of anesthesia required because the posterior surface of the epiglottis, innervated by a branch of the vagus nerve, is not stimulated.

HENDERSON LARYNGOSCOPE BLADE
- Straight blade, large cross-sectional diameter. Used for a paraglossal technique.
- Provides improved view for patients with small oral aperture or enlarged base of tongue.

FLIPPER (RUSCH)
- Hinged tip (70 degrees of movement) is controlled by lever along handle.
- Provides improved view for patients with small oral aperture or enlarged base of tongue.

POLIO LARYNGOSCOPE BLADE
- Blade in line with handle. Developed for the "iron lung" patient.
- Avoids obstructions over the patient's chest (large breasts, morbid obesity, operator hand performing Sellick maneuver).

KESSEL LARYNGOSCOPE BLADE
- Angle of handle/blade is 20 degrees more obtuse than standard Macintosh blade.
- See polio laryngoscope blade.

JELLICO AND HARRIS ADAPTOR
- Adaptor between blade and handle to increase handle/blade angle.
- See polio laryngoscope blade.

PATIL AND STEHLING LARYNGOSCOPE HANDLE (ANESTHESIA ASSOCIATES, INC.)
- Adjustable angle adaptor (180-, 135-, 90-, and 45-degree angles).
- See polio laryngoscope blade.

YENTIS LARYNGOSCOPE BLADE
- Adaptor between blade and handle allows 90-degree pivoting (lateral) position change.

SEWARD LARYNGOSCOPE BLADE (SUNMED MEDICAL)
- 10.5-cm straight blade.
- For patients <5 years.

BRYCE-SMITH LARYNGOSCOPE BLADE
- Short, straight blade with slight 2.5-cm distal curvature. C-shaped cross-section (right side open) with 1.8 cm width (proximal) tapering to 1 cm (distal).
- For newborns to children aged 3 years.

JONES LARYNGOSCOPE BLADE
- Miller-type blade shortened to 6.7 cm. Relatively distal lamp.
- Infant blade, improved illumination.

"FISH-EYE" LARYNGOSCOPE BLADE
- Integrated suction channel on a standard Macintosh blade.
- Continuous suction during intubation attempt.

KHAN LARYNGOSCOPE BLADE
- Integrated suction channel on a standard Miller blade with thumb valve control.
- Intermittent suction during intubation attempts.

DÖRGES EMERGENCY LARYNGOSCOPE BLADE (KARL-STORZ ENDOSCOPY)
- Equivalent in size to a size 2 Macintosh blade with a tapered profile similar to a Miller blade that can be used in adults and in children weighing >10 kg.
- Has 10- and 20-kg markings on the blade to aid in depth of insertion into the oropharynx.

TRUVIEW (TRUPHATEK INTERNATIONAL, NETANYA, ISRAEL)
- Prism mounted on standard Macintosh blade.
- Prism enables a 20-degree refraction around base of tongue.

entering one end of a glass rod undergoes repeated reflections until it emerges from the distal terminus, and small amounts of light are lost with each reflection in the rod. When the glass rod is heated, it may be stretched to a diameter of less than 25 μm. At this diameter, the glass becomes flexible. Reflections of transversing light occur at approximately 10,000 per meter. During transmission down a single fiber, all incoming light is blended to a single, averaged color. Therefore a complex image cannot be transmitted down a single glass fiber; rather, a single colored "pixel" is transmitted. By fusing the terminals of many fibers (e.g., 10,000 to 30,000) and applying an image-magnifying lens, a complex image may be focused onto the objective end of the bundle. The pixelated image is then transmitted to the operator's fused terminus, where a second lens can be used to produce a focused image. The greater the number of fibers and the smaller their size (albeit >8 μm), the higher the resolution of the image. The fiber bundle is fused only at the two termini, maintaining the flexibility of the rest of the bundle. The bundle also must be coherent—that is, the fiber arrangement must be identical at the two termini—if the pixelated image is to be reproduced from one end to the other. Noncoherent fibers, which are less expensive to produce, may be used for applications in which an image is not transmitted, such as with an illuminating source. A second layer of glass, 1 μm

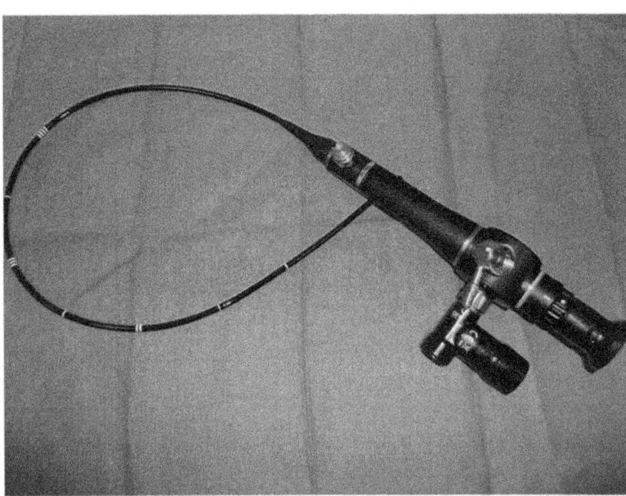

FIGURE 16-18 ■ Fiberoptic scope.

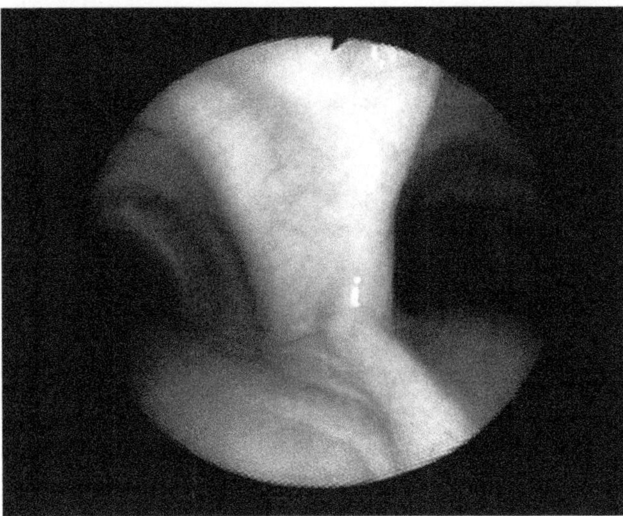

FIGURE 16-19 ■ View down the fiberoptic scope showing the carina and right and left mainstem bronchi. Note that the tracheal rings are anterior and the membranous portion of the trachea is posterior.

thick and with a lower refractive index than the fiber, is fused to the individual fibers; this is termed the *cladding*, and it reduces the amount of light lost with each intrafiber reflection and prevents interfiber light contamination.

The fiber bundle described above comprises the primary functional element of the flexible fiberoptic intubation scope. The remaining elements add functionality. All elements are bound together within a protective, waterproof plastic cover and together are referred to as the *insertion cord* (Fig. 16-18).

Optical Quality

As mentioned, the resolution of the image delivered to the operator at the eyepiece or video screen (Fig. 16-19) depends on the number of fibers as well as the fiber size. The objective (distal insertion cord) has a fixed focus lens. The depth of field is typically 3 to 5 mm. When the tip-bending mechanism is in the neutral position, the field of view is cone shaped. The field of view of the typical fiberscope is 55 to 120 degrees, and the conical field of view may be swung in an arch around the hinged angle.

Light Bundles

As previously mentioned, illumination is provided by noncoherent fiber bundles that travel with the image bundle to bring light to the object. Modern fiberscopes have one or two such bundles. Proximally, the light fibers are supplied with an external light source or battery-powered sources.

Distal Tip–Bending Mechanism

Anterior-posterior bending of the distal tip of the insertion cord is achieved by manipulation of two fine wires embedded in the respective surfaces of the cord. A lever in the handle of the fiberscope is used to tighten or slacken the opposing wires, causing motion of a multifacet joint near the distal end; attempting to bend the tip against force may result in wire damage and inability to direct the tip. Anterior-posterior tip deflection may be purposely asymmetric (i.e., flexion in one direction may be greater than in the opposite direction). The degree of flexion may be up to 180 degrees and depends on the manufacturer and model of the fiberscope.

Working Channel

Most adult intubation fiberscopes house an open lumen that runs the length of the fiberscope from the distal tip to the handle, which also houses the directional controls and proximal optical elements. The working channel of newer fiberscopes has three apertures: one at the distal end of the insertion cord and two on the fiberscope handle. The most proximal aperture, or port, is typically fitted with a valve that allows intermittent application of suction or compressed oxygen. The midport, also on the fiberscope handle, typically has a Luer-lock fitting; syringes for drug or lavage delivery, diaphragm-sealed access ports, biopsy and foreign body retrieval loops, or cleaning brushes may be attached or inserted into this port. Because the working channel is not integral to the primary operation of the fiberscope, it often is eliminated in favor of smaller insertion cord diameters, such as in pediatric models.[54]

Charge-Coupled Devices

Although indirect optical intubation devices have historically used glass fibers to provide image conveyance around anatomic angles, new instruments have incorporated electronic technology to improve image quality and device durability. Charge-coupled device (CCD) technology uses a two-dimensional array of light-sensitive capacitors, which sit at the objective end of the "scope." These light-sensitive silicone semiconductors are buried under multiple layers of polysilicon charge-coupled "gates" that propagate the signal to an interpreting circuit. As photons pass through the gates and strike the semiconductors, a charge is created. The number of photons striking an individual semiconductor is proportional to the intensity of the light. Each semiconductor in the array is electrically isolated from its neighbor and acts as a pixel generator of the final image. In the highest quality imagers, three CCD panels detect the three primary colors, which requires a large area. In most medical and lower cost systems, color is instead detected by the incorporation of a Beyer pattern, which consists of alternating red-green and green-blue filters. These systems can be designed to be significantly more compact than the three-CCD system. Under this scheme, color information for each pixel is determined by interpolation of the signal from its neighboring pixels. For example, a pixel under a red-green filter will determine the correct color information by examining the intensity of light striking its neighboring pixels beneath red-green and green-blue filters.

A CCD system eliminates the need for fragile glass fibers and can give excellent clarity because of the minimal elements between the objective and the chip. At the time of this writing, flexible CCD intubation scopes were four to five times more expensive than a traditional fiberscope.[54]

Rigid Laryngoscopes

Bullard Laryngoscope

The Bullard laryngoscope (Gyrus ACMI, Southborough, MA) is the prototypical anatomically shaped rigid fiberscope. This device consists of a blade 1.3 cm wide and 13.2 cm in length with a fixed anterior curve (3.4 cm radius) meant to replicate the typical adult oral-to-pharyngeal anatomy. To provide indirect imaging around this angle, a fiberoptic bundle is embedded on the posterior surface of the blade, which is 0.64 cm thick. The objective lens is 2.6 cm from the distal end of the blade. Parallel to the embedded image fiber is a 3.7-mm working channel and an illumination fiber bundle. The operator handle with eyepiece and adjustable diopter, standard laryngosocpe handle latch with recessed light bulb, and working channel aperture with Luer-Lock fit a nonmalleable tracheal tube stylet that follows the underside of the blade. The distal 2 cm of the stylet is angled toward the midline. When viewed through the eyepiece, the stylet tip can be seen to direct the path of the tracheal tube as it is extended off the stylet. Three Bullard scope accessories include a hollow tracheal tube stylet, a single-use blade extender, and an external light source cable adaptor. Pediatric and adult sizes are available (Fig. 16-20).

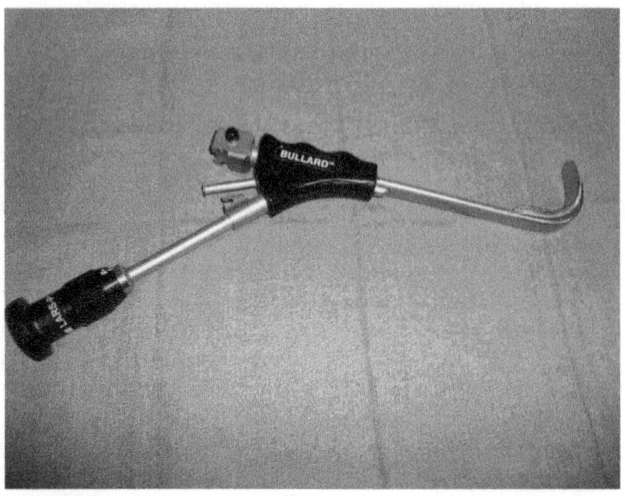

FIGURE 16-20 ■ Bullard-type laryngoscope with blade extender.

WuScope System

The WuScope (Pentax Medical, Tokyo) is similar to the Bullard laryngoscope in that is uses a fixed, shaped blade assembly meant to follow intrinsic patient anatomy. The fiberoptic elements, image and illumination, are provided by a separate, flexible fiberscope (Olympus LF-1, LF-2, or ENF-P3 rhinoscope) that follows a dedicated groove manufactured on the lateral aspect of the blade assembly. A working channel closely parallels the fiberscope groove to provide lens-clearing suction or oxygen insufflation. The WuScope handle is conical and holds the fiberscope handle. The two-blade assembly is attached to the distal handle to produce a channel through which the tracheal tube passes. Optionally, a suction catheter may be passed through the tracheal tube and used as a guide for intubation. Once the glottis is visualized and the tracheal tube has been passed, the blade is disassembled and removed from the mouth. Nasal intubation has been described with the WuScope; the tracheal tube is passed though the nose and into the pharynx, the blade is assembled around the tracheal tube, the glottis is visualized, and the tracheal tube is passed.[55]

Upsher Scope

The Upsher scope and Upsher Ultra scope (Mercury Medical, Clearwater, FL) consist of a C-shaped stainless steel blade encasing fiberoptic bundles, channeled ETT guide, horizontal flange beyond the tube-guided channel, distal lens, and proximal eyepiece. The earlier Upsher scope had an eyepiece that could be focused. The later version, Upsher Ultra, does not have an eyepiece that can be focused, thereby allowing the device to be fully immersible for cleaning.

The device is placed with the patient's head in the neutral position. A small degree of neck flexion may aid in elevating the epiglottis to improve glottic visualization. The Upsher scope can negotiate a 15-mm mouth opening and accommodates size 7.0, 7.5, and 8.0 ETTs. The Upsher Ultra differs from the original scope in that the C-shaped steel blade now has a curvature of almost 90 degrees to more closely approximate the curvature of the base of the tongue and oropharynx. In addition, the Upsher Ultra has a power handle for adaptation to a fiberoptic light source, a snap-on camera that adapts to the eyepiece for remote viewing on a monitor, and the ability to insufflate oxygen down the ETT during intubation, which can be facilitated by passing a bougie down the ETT through the glottis opening and sliding the ETT over the bougie.[56]

Bonfils-Brambrink Endoscope

The Bonfils-Brambrink (infant) endoscopes (Karl-Storz) are optical stylets similar to the Levitan (Clarus Medical, Golden Valley, MN) and Shikani endoscopes. These are rigid-shaft endoscopes with a distal-end fixed deflection. The optical and illuminating elements are encased in a stainless steel shaft, and one model incorporates a working channel. The Bonfils devices also have an adjustable-angle eyepiece to improve ergonomic function. Unlike other optical stylets, the Bonfils-Brambrink endoscopes use a retromolar approach similar to that proposed for the Henderson laryngoscope blade. The endoscope, with a loaded tracheal tube, is guided lateral to the molars. A chin lift or chin-tongue lift maneuver increases the pharyngeal space. Once the pharynx is reached, the scope is rotated until the larynx can be viewed. The tracheal tube is then guided off the stylet and into the larynx under indirect visualization.[58]

Lighted Malleable Stylets

Shikani Optical Stylet

The Shikani optical stylet (Clarus Medical, Minneapolis, MN) is a high-resolution fiberoptic stylet that has a preformed curvature. The metallic casing of the distal scope is malleable and may be shaped by the user. The Shikani has an integrated oxygen port for insufflation and an adjustable tube stop. Made of stainless steel, it is available in adult and pediatric sizes and can be used as an adjunct to direct laryngoscopy or as an independent device. The light source can be a laryngoscope handle or an external cabled light source. A complementary metal oxide semiconductor system is now available (Fig. 16-21).

Levitan

The Levitan (Clarus Medical) is a high-resolution fiberoptic stylet with a malleable distal end. It has an integrated oxygen port, but it does not have an adjustable tube stop. The Levitan also can be used as an adjunct to direct laryngoscopy or as an independent device. It is available only in adult sizes.

Foley Flexible Airway Scope Tool

The Foley flexible airway scope tool (Clarus Medical) is a flexible stylet with a tip that cannot be directed. This device is used as an adjunct to aid tracheal intubation through an intubating laryngeal mask; it can be used for extubation as well. This device also has been adapted for nasal intubation.

Clarus Video Airway System

This system combines a malleable stylet with a 4-inch liquid crystal display (LCD) screen for video assistance. An optional flexible stylet is available.[59]

Alternative Rigid Imaging Devices

CTrach

An early criticism of the LMA Fastrach was the blindness of the tracheal intubation.[60] Although recognized as being a significant advance in the difficult airway armamentarium, especially with its combined faculities of ventilation and intubation, the principle of visualization for verification of glottic intubation was violated.[61] An advanced Fastrach, the CTrach (LMA North America), was introduced in 2005 (Fig. 16-22). The CTrach has a silicone-coated stainless steel barrel and silicone mask identical to that of the Fastrach. Two embedded fiberoptic cables, an image cable and an illumination cable, descend on the lateral aspects of the barrel, from a magnetic latch connector on the proximal barrel, and terminate in the Fastrach-like bowl of the CTrach at a point just distal to the barrel orifice. This objective lens and illumination source position lies directly under the lower third of the epiglottic elevating bar (EEB). To allow illumination and visualization, a window has been cut into the EEB. An LCD display encased in a rechargeable monitor connects with the magnetic latch to give a view of the structures beyond the EEB. The view angle of the CTrach lens is unique among airway devices in that it occurs from a posterior position. Because of this arrangement, the arytenoids, aryepiglottic folds, tracheal tube barrel, and glottic aperture are all often visible during the act of intubation. Contrary to this interesting and useful view is the effect of gravity on secretions, which may pool near the lens. The fiberoptic elements comprise a bundle of 10,000 plastic fibers that gives adequate resolution but is not as clear as many other fiberoptic devices.

The CTrach is inserted in much the same way as the Fastrach. After adequate anesthesia, either general or topical, the barrel handle is held on the chest as the lubricated and completely deflated distal mask tip is placed

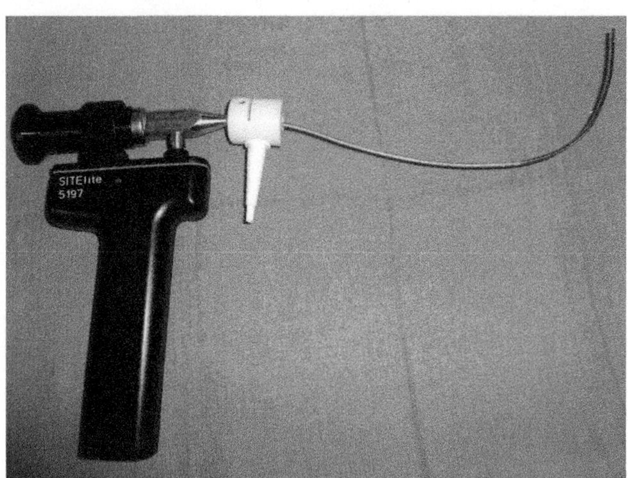

FIGURE 16-21 ■ Shikani optical stylet (Clarus Medical, Minneapolis, MN).

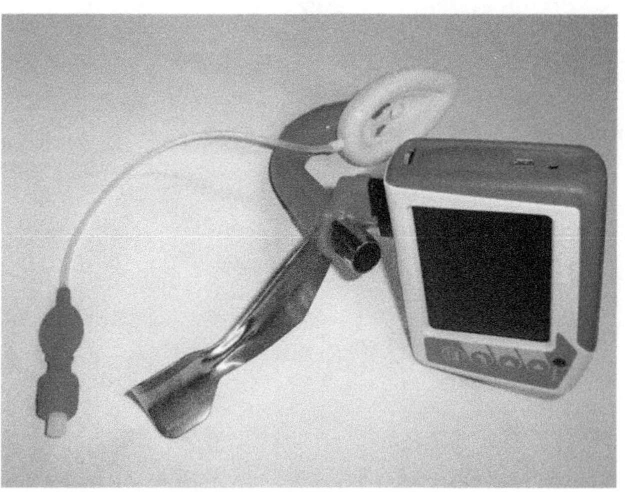

FIGURE 16-22 ■ CTrach (LMA North America, San Diego, CA).

against the hard palate (this initial position prevents monitor attachment). A backward, sweeping, rotational movement introduces the mask into the hypopharynx. Either in mid sweep or after full insertion, the monitor is attached; if placed mid sweep, the passing structures can be appreciated. Next, the mask is inflated, and the glottis should be appreciated at this time. If not, maneuvers common to those used for the Fastrach can be applied, such as Chandy's maneuver (lifting of the mask off the posterior wall) or an up-down maneuver (a 6-cm outward and return "replacement" of the inflated mask).[62] Observation via the monitor during these maneuvers may reveal the location of the laryngeal anatomy.

As with the Fastrach, the CTrach functions adequately as a supraglottic ventilation device. This can be achieved in initial placements regardless of the fiberoptic view.[63] Failure to ventilate adequately and with appropriate airway pressures is most often corrected with the up-down maneuver or Chandy's first maneuver,[62] in which the barrel handle is manipulated to find an ideal optical position.

The imaging capability of the CTrach offers the operator information for diagnosing misplacement during failed Fastrach intubation attempts; a down-folded epiglottis, a distant epiglottis/larynx, and an arytenoid entrapped by the EBB can be seen and corrected with manipulation or CTrach size change.[64] However, failure to obtain an adequate or any image does not preclude adequate ventilation or attempts at intubations.

GlideScope

The GlideScope (Verathon Medical, Bothell, WA; Figs. 16-23 and 16-24) uses an acutely angled blade (60-degree arch) that curves around the base of the tongue. A high-resolution CCD color camera is integrated near the distal tip to give the operator a view of the airway anatomy beyond the curve. Illumination is provided by diodes, eliminating the need for an external light source, and the system also has antifogging capability. Power is provided through a cord emanating from the handle and attached to a portable LCD screen, and both alternating current (AC) and battery-powered units are available. Because of the location of the camera, significant alignment of the oral and pharyngeal axes is unnecessary.[65] The GlideScope has been proven superior to the direct laryngosocpe blade in pediatric and obese patients, those with cervical spine disease, those with a high Cormack and Lehane score (on routine laryngoscopy), patients outside the operating room, as well as where portability is important. Both awake and anesthetized techniques have been used. In one large study, laryngeal view scores of I or II were recorded in 99% of patients, far above what is expected with direct laryngoscopy.[66] Although the laryngeal view may be almost universally achieved, tracheal intubation had a failure rate of 3.7%, despite a grade I or II laryngeal view, in the uncontrolled clinical series.[65] Although the procedure of GlideScope insertion into the airway is familiar to the anesthesiologist, in that it is similar to the procedure of direct laryngoscope placement, ETT placement differs; because of the acute angle of the blade and the fixed shape of the ETT, hand manipulation occurs in an unaccustomed fashion.

Unlike direct laryngoscopy, the GlideScope is inserted in the midline. Airway structures, such as the uvula and epiglottis, should be viewed as the GlideScope moves through the airway. Most investigators recommend that the tip of the blade be placed anterior to the epiglottis, and an ETT with a nonmalleable stylet is recommended. The ETT should be preshaped prior to laryngoscopy: a 60-degree curve can be achieved, similar to that of the GlideScope blade, but operators may find their own ideal contour. Maneuvers that can increase the success of the GlideScope include external laryngeal pressure, sharper angle shaping of the ETT, and placement of an intubating bougie under GlideScope observation and slight withdrawal of the GlideScope blade. A preformed, rigid stylet developed for use with the GlideScope is available, as is a digital video recorder to record intubations, confirm tube placement, and facilitate teaching. Verathon has released a disposable version that uses single-use blades over a CCD baton. Versions that allow video recording and USB drive capability are also available, along with four blade sizes (Table 16-5).[65]

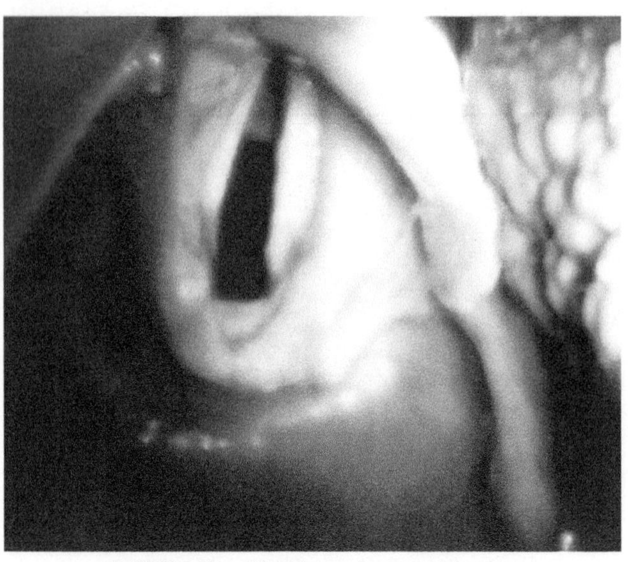

FIGURE 16-23 ■ GlideScope laryngeal image.

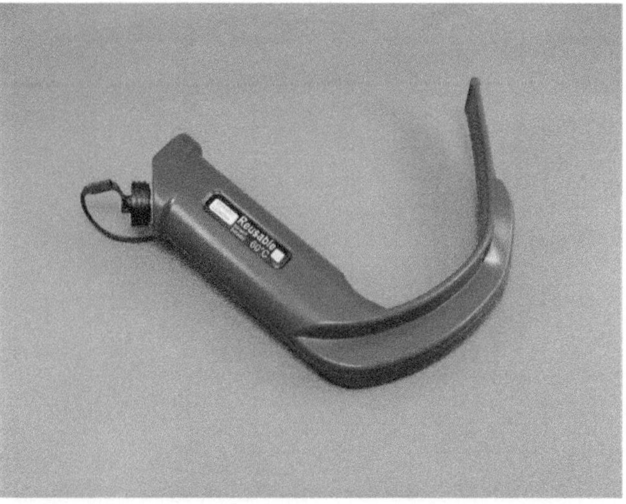

FIGURE 16-24 ■ The GlideScope blade (Verathon Medical, Bothell, WA).

McGrath Laryngoscope

The McGrath laryngoscope (Aircraft Medical, Edinburgh, UK) is a portable rigid glottic imaging device that replicates the look and feel of the direct laryngoscope but with a blade angulation similar to that of the GlideScope. The McGrath Series 5 (Fig. 16-25, *A*) uses a handle and blade configuration reminiscent of the direct laryngoscope but with several additions: a color microcamera is fitted on the distal aspect of a reusable "camera stick," to which a single-use polymer blade is fitted. The handle-to-tip distance is adjustable. The VGA Digital Imaging Sensor transmits the laryngeal image to a flat-panel screen mounted on the handle. The McGrath Mac Scope has a less angulated blade of fixed length (Fig. 16-25, *B*); whereas the Series 5 is an indirect visualization device, the McGrath Mac Scope is meant to allow direct or indirect laryngeal vision techniques. The maximum interdental width of the blade is 14 mm. Although data are limited, several abstracts favorably compare intubation success with the McGrath to the GlideScope.[59]

TABLE 16-5 Verathon Blade Sizes

	Small (mm)	Medium (mm)	Large (mm)	Bariatric (mm)
Blade thickness at level of camera	14.5	14.5	14	14
Camera distance from distal tip	36	52	58	62

Airtraq

The Airtraq (Prodol Meditec, Bilbao, Spain) is a channeled, portable optical device. The optical channel contains prisms, and the guiding channel accommodates the ETT. The device has an in situ antifogging mechanism that activates within 60 seconds, and the internal light source lasts 90 minutes. The Airtraq is inserted midline, and the glottis can be viewed through an eyepiece, adapted to a monitor, or visualized through an optional wireless camera and monitor. The Airtraq is available in both pediatric and adult sizes, and variations of this single-use device include a double-lumen tube and nasotracheal intubation devices (Fig. 16-26).[59]

Tracheal Tube Stylet Devices

As an aid to direct or indirect laryngoscopy, several devices have been introduced for use during tracheal intubation, intubation verification, extubation, and

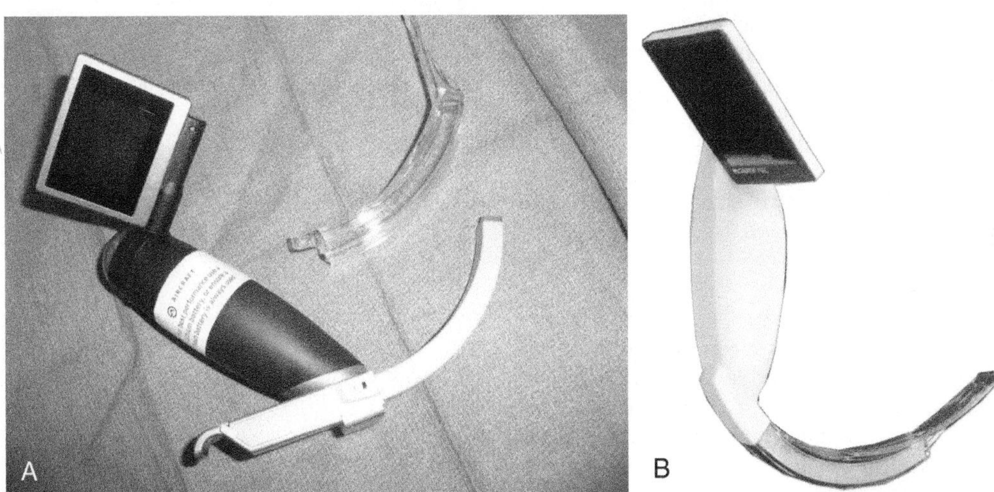

FIGURE 16-25 The McGrath laryngoscope (Aircraft Medical, Edinburgh, UK). **A,** Series 5. **B,** Mac Scope.

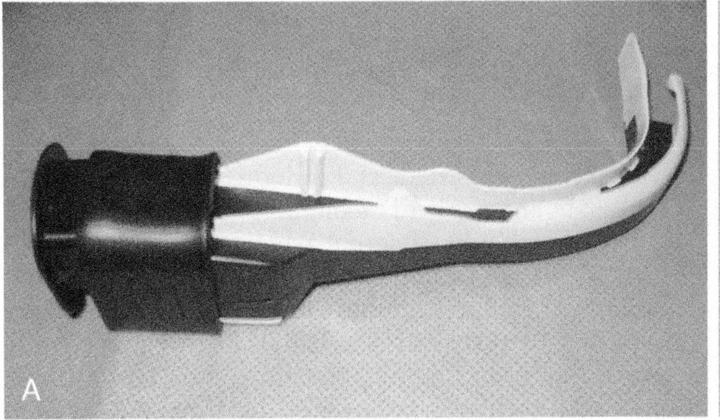

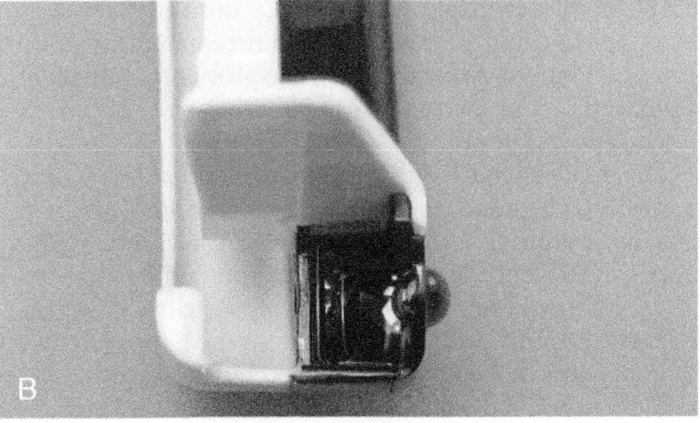

FIGURE 16-26 **A,** The Airtraq, lateral view (Prodol Meditec, Bilbao, Spain). **B,** Distal optical elements.

TABLE 16-6 **Distinctive Features of Sylet Devices**

Device	Features	Principal Application	Manufacturer
Eschmann introducer	Woven polyester base, 15 Fr, 60 cm, angled distal end (35 degrees), reusable	Aid to direct laryngoscopy during poor laryngeal view	Smiths Medical (Kent, UK)
Frova introducer	Angulated distal tip, hollow bore, rapid fit-adaptor compatible[59]; adult, 65 cm for TT tubes >5.5 mm ID; pediatric, 35 cm for TT >3 mm ID	Aid to direct laryngoscopy during poor laryngeal view	Cook Critical Care (Bloomington, IN)
Arndt AEC	Hollow catheter with tapered end; available in 50, 65, and 78 cm lengths with multiple side ports; rapid fit–adaptor compatible	Exchanging LMA for a tracheal tube	Cook Critical Care
Aintree AEC	Large bore (4.7 mm) hollow catheter, will accept fiberoptic bronchoscope; 56 cm	Exchanging LMA for a tracheal tube using a fiberscope	Cook Critical Care
Cook AEC	Firm, long (100 cm) catheter	Exchanging double-lumen tube	Cook Critical Care

AEC, airway exchange catheter; *ID*, inner diameter; *LMA*, laryngeal mask airway; *TT*, tracheal tube.

tracheal tube exchange. Although they differ in design and capabilities, all essentially function as stylets. These devices and their distinctive features are listed in Table 16-6.[59]

Alternative Intubation

air-Q Intubating Laryngeal Mask

The air-Q (Mercury Medical) is an intubating laryngeal airway with a hypercurved airway tube, large mask cavity, and recessed anterior portion. The circuit adaptor is removable, and intubation can be achieved by a large airway tube that is not easily kinked. Intubation is most often described with adjunctive use of a fiberscope. Removal of the air-Q after intubation is facilitated by a removal stylet. The air-Q also has a built-in bite block and is available in adult and pediatric sizes and as reusable and disposable units (Figs. 16-27 and 16-28).[59]

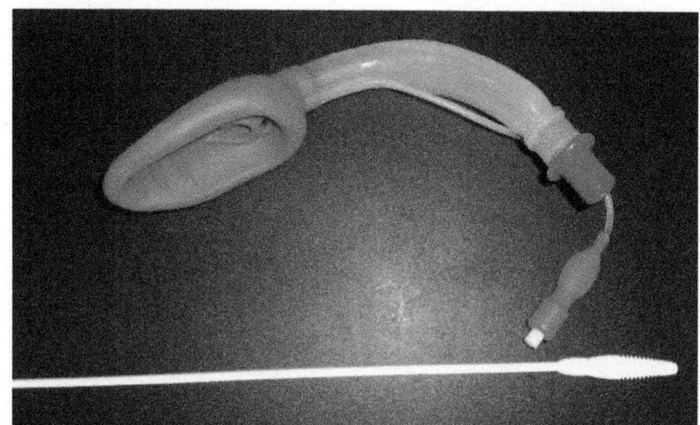

FIGURE 16-27 The air-Q (Mercury Medical) intubating laryngeal airway.

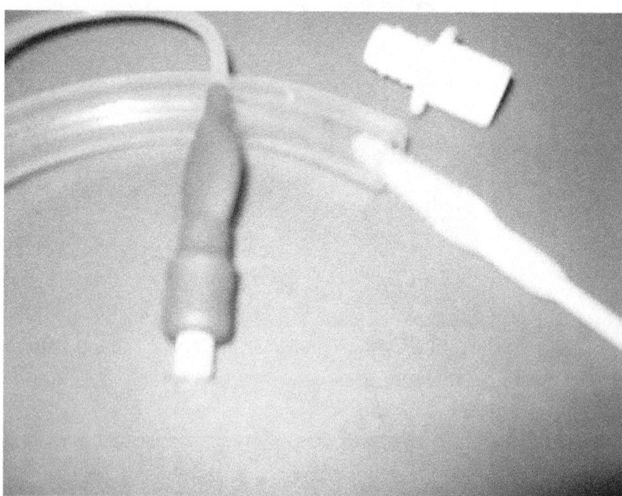

FIGURE 16-28 Intubating laryngeal airway wand and adapter.

Lightwand

Illumination Technique. The first report of the use of transcutaneous illumination, a light source in the airway seen externally, to facilitate tracheal intubation was described in 1959 by Yamamura and colleagues.[67] The transillumination technique relies on the relatively superficial position of the laryngeal tissues in the neck compared with the esophagus. A light source in the larynx produces a well-defined illumination over the neck, typically just below the thyroid prominence; the same light source in the esophagus produces a diffuse glow. The advantage of using a lighted stylet in this manner is that it is independent of visualization of the glottis, a blind technique, and can be successfully used in the "wet" or bloody airway. Several devices are available (Table 16-7).

The disadvantages to this technique are that it is a blind intubation technique facilitated by reducing ambient light: some devices are short (Tube-Stat [Medtronic, Inc., Minneapolis, MN] and Flexilume [Plastic Specialties, Industry, CA] are 25 cm) and may result in inadvertent extubation, and some require two hands to operate the light and place the tube, and the light beam is directed forward (Tube-Stat, fiberoptic lighted intubation stylet [Benson Medical Industries, Markham, Ontario, Canada], fiberoptic lighted stylet [Fiberoptic Medical Products, Allentown, PA]) as opposed to anteriorly (Trachlight; Fig. 16-29).

The Trachlight (Laerdal Medical, Stavanger, Norway), which is no longer manufactured, was specifically marketed for lightwand intubation. It is a reusable device consisting of three parts: a handle with battery pack, a flexible guide with lighted distal tip, and a malleable stylet. The Trachlight is powered by three AAA alkaline batteries. Other features include a locking clamp that

TABLE 16-7 **Available Light Devices**

Device	Manufacturer
Trachlight	Laerdal Medical, Stavanger, Norway (discontinued 2009)
Fiberoptic intubation stylet	Benson Medical Industries, Markham, Ontario, Canada
Flexilume (single use)	Plastic Specialties, Industry, CA
Tube-Stat (single use)	Medtronic, Minneapolis, MN
Fiberoptic lighted stylet	Fiberoptic Medical Products, Allentown, PA

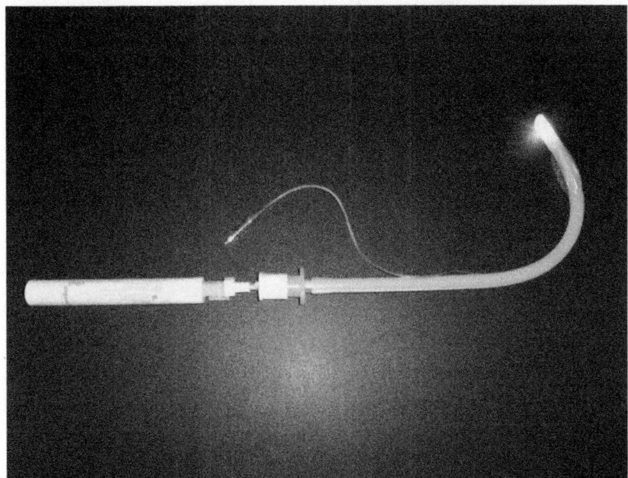

FIGURE 16-29 ■ Lightwand and handle.

holds the tracheal tube in place on the stylet until intubation is complete; a timing device, which causes the light to blink after 30 seconds; and an adjustable handle to accommodate varying tracheal tube lengths. The brightly lit tip will achieve a maximum surface temperature of 60° C, and it projects anteriorly.

MINIMALLY INVASIVE AIRWAY TECHNIQUES

Access to the airway through the cricothyroid membrane, cricotracheal ligament, or intratracheal ligaments increases the clinician's options in both elective airway management and airway rescue. A variety of devices are available.

Cook Retrograde Wire Intubation Kit

Retrograde intubation was described as early as 1960. The technique involves the passage of a catheter or wire via a percutaneous needle through the larynx or trachea and out the upper airway. A tracheal tube can then be threaded over the wire and into the larynx. The catheter or wire is then removed, leaving the tracheal tube in situ.[59] The technique can be awkward if the correct equipment is not immediately available. Kits such as the Cook Retrograde Wire Intubation Kit (Cook Medical, Bloomington, IN) are helpful in this regard. The basic elements of the kit are a 110-cm (0.032-inch) wire and a stainless steel percutaneous needle. This kit also contains a 20-gauge angiocath that may be used instead of the stainless steel needle, a clamp for securing the wire at the puncture site, and a Cook Airway Exchange Catheter (AEC). The Cook AEC can be used to significantly improve the technique, helping overcome two of the most significant procedural difficulties. First, by placing the AEC over the retrograde wire prior to placement of the tracheal tube, the gap that normally occurs between the tracheal tube and the wire is obliterated. This reduces or eliminates hang-up of the tracheal tube on the vocal cords. Second, because the AEC is threaded completely into the larynx and is graduated with centimeter markings, the depth of the tracheal tube passage into the airway can be measured.[59]

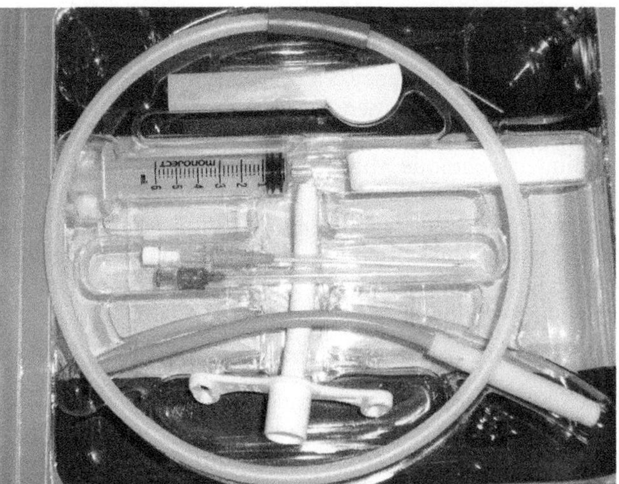

FIGURE 16-30 ■ Melker cricothyrotomy kit (Cook Medical, Bloomington, IN).

Percutaneous Cricothyrotomy

Melker Emergency Cricothyrotomy Catheter Kit

The Melker Emergency Cricothyrotomy catheter set (Cook Medical) is designed for emergency airway access when intubation and ventilation are not possible. The cricothyroid membrane is located with an 18-gauge introducer, and air is aspirated to confirm placement. Next, an Amplatz extra-stiff guidewire is placed, and dilation of the tract follows with a curved dilator. Lastly, a radiopaque airway catheter with a 15-mm adaptor is fed over the guidewire, using a Seldinger-type technique (Fig. 16-30).[59]

Melker Cuffed Emergency Cricothyrotomy Catheter Kit

This kit functions the same as the Melker Emergency Cricothyrotomy Catheter Kit, except the airway catheter has a cuff that allows positive-pressure ventilation in much the same way as an ETT. This cuffed version can be used for short general anesthetic cases. However, the cricothyrotomy does not function as a tracheotomy, and prolonged use of the cricothyrotomy may damage the laryngeal cartilage.[59]

Pertrach Emergency Cricothyrotomy Kit

The Pertrach emergency cricothyrotomy kit (Engineered Medical Systems) is used for cricothyrotomy or tracheotomy in an emergency situation. Rather than using the Seldinger technique, this device uses "splitting needles." Rather than cutting, the splitting needle divides the tissue, which results in less bleeding and scarring. This device is available cuffed or uncuffed in adult and pediatric sizes.[59]

Quicktrach Emergency Cricothyrotomy

The Quicktrach emergency cricothyrotomy device (VBM Medizintechnik, Sulz, Germany) is a preassembled kit used for securing the airway emergently. The device has a built-in stopper to prevent posterior perforation of the trachea. A precision-beveled needle allows insertion into the airway without the use of a scalpel, which results in less bleeding. The Quicktrach is available in pediatric and adult sizes, cuffed and uncuffed.

Ravussin Transtracheal Jet Ventilation Catheter

The Ravussin Transtracheal Jet Ventilation Catheter (VBM Medizintechnik) uses a stainless steel needle that allows easy puncture and kink-free insertion. The needle is covered with a Teflon catheter that is anatomically curved and allows for laser surgery. The catheter has three holes that facilitate centering of the catheter during jet ventilation. A 15-mm adaptor allows positive-pressure ventilation, and a Luer lock aids manual and high-frequency jet ventilation. The catheter is available in three sizes for adults, children, and infants.[59]

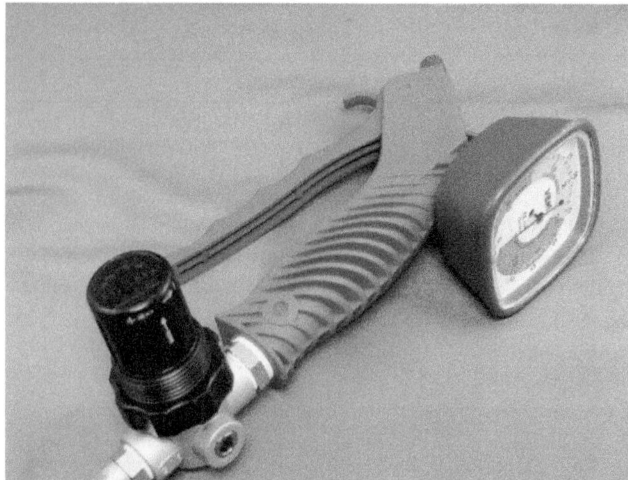

FIGURE 16-31 ■ Manujet III jet ventilator (VBM Medizintechnik, Sulz, Germany).

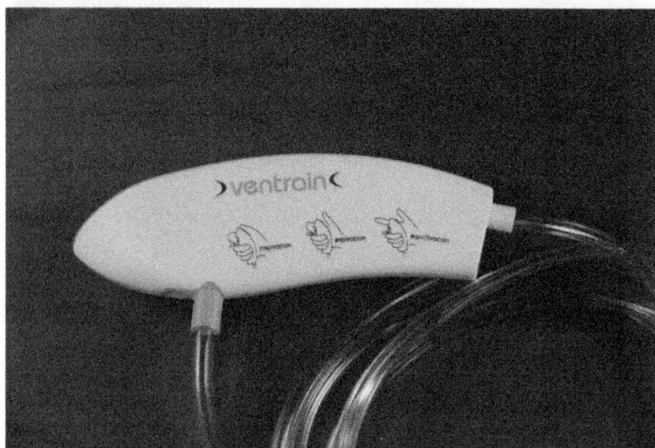

FIGURE 16-32 ■ Ventrain expiratory ventilatory assistance valve (Dolphys Medical, Eindhoven, The Netherlands).

Transtracheal Jet Ventilation

Manujet III Valve

The Manujet III (VBM Medizintechnik) is a hand-held, manually operated jet ventilation valve attached to a 50-psi oxygen source. It includes a 4-mm pressure hose, Luer-lock connecting tubing (for attachment to a jetting needle or jet ETT), Endojet adapter and catheter (for ventilation with an ETT, face mask, or LMA), and pressure regulator. It is indicated for elective airway cases, when the surgeon requests no ETT, or in an urgent "can't ventilate, can't intubate" situation. This device can be used independently with a jetting needle or a Hunsaker Mon Jet ETT. Alternatively, the included Endojet adapter and catheter can be used through an ETT, LMA, or a face mask. This reusable device must be used in an unobstructed airway (Fig. 16-31).[59]

Ventrain

A new concept in jet ventilation is expiratory ventilatory assistance (EVA), in which the Venturi effect is used to assist gas removal during the expiratory phase. The Ventrain (Dolphys Medical, Eindhoven, The Netherlands) device uses EVA. The Ventrain is designed to be used for transtracheal rescue ventilation or electively in laryngeal surgery (Fig. 16-32). EVA may be particularly important in the rescue of a completely obstructed airway, in which the ventilation of gases must occur via a small-bore rescue catheter. Preliminary studies demonstrate that Ventrain ventilation results in superior carbon dioxide removal compared with non-EVA jet ventilation devices.

AincA Manual Jet Ventilator

The AincA manual jet ventilator (Anesthesia Associates) is similar to the Manujet III and has the same indications. The AincA has an on/off thumb control and an internal filter and can be customized to individual specifications (hose lengths, oxygen source connector, and pressure gauge).[59]

Enk Oxygen Flow Modulator

Unlike the above-mentioned devices, the Enk oxygen flow modulator (Cook Medical) is portable, self-contained, and disposable. It is indicated in emergency airway situations when a jet ventilator is not available. The Enk allows manually controlled oxygen flow by

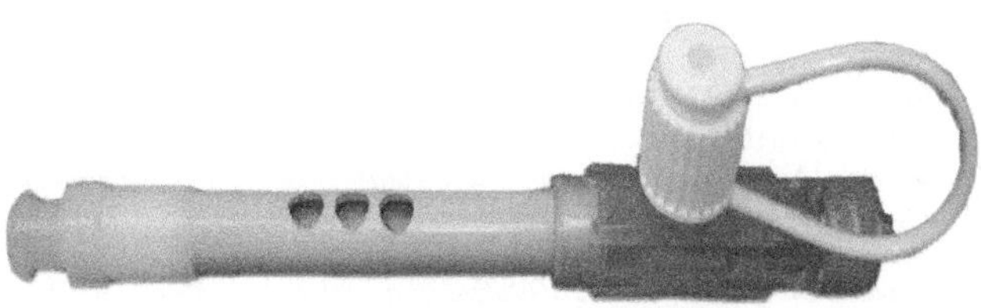

FIGURE 16-33 ENK flow modulator (Cook Medical, Bloomington, IN).

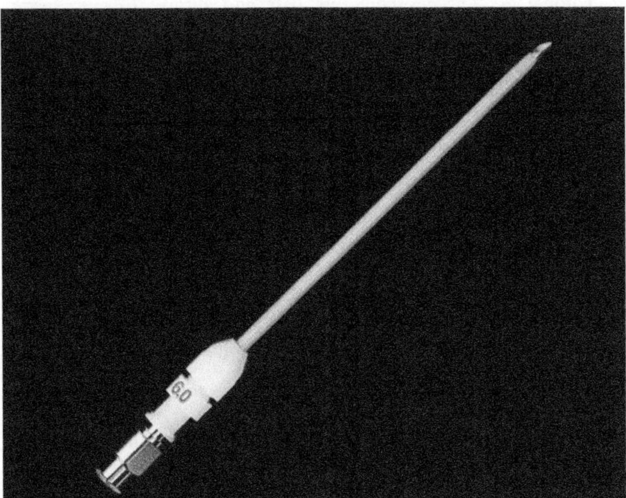

FIGURE 16-34 Cook Transtracheal Jet Ventilation Catheter (Cook Medical, Bloomington, IN).

portholes on the oxygen flow modulator, which are finger occluded to start gas flow. The device can attain nearly 14.7 psi (1 atm) (Fig. 16-33).[59]

Cook Emergency Transtracheal Airway Catheters

These coil-reinforced, nonkinkable catheters are used for emergency access through the cricothyroid membrane when intubation and ventilation are precluded. These 6 Fr catheters have a 2-mm internal diameter and are available in two lengths. They are superior to angiocatheters because flow is not occluded by kinking (Fig. 16-34).[59]

Positioning Pillows

Troop Elevation Pillow

In morbidly obese patients, it is often difficult to stack pillows and blankets to optimize neck extension and potential airway exposure. The Troop device (Mercury Medical) is a sturdy foam pillow designed to place the patient in a head-elevated laryngoscope position. The pillow is for single use only. A head pillow and accompanying arm board pillows also are available.

Pi Pillow Positioning Device

The Pi pillow positioning device (American Eagle Medical, Coram, NY) is a two-part pillow with a base and a removable pad. Both parts together allow comfortable patient positioning. Once general anesthesia is induced, the top pad is removed and the patient's head achieves a "sniffing" position. The Pi pillow comes in single-use and reusable forms and five sizes that range from pediatric to morbidly obese. Once a sniffing position has been achieved, the pillow also facilitates central line placement, Swan Ganz placement, and interscalene blockade. The pillow also facilitates surgical procedures such as thyroidectomy and laryngectomy.

Rapid Airway Management Positioner

The Rapid Airway Management Positioner (RAMP; Airpal, Coopersburg, PA) is an air-assisted patient positioning and lateral patient transfer device. It contains two adjustable air chambers to provide optimal positioning for direct laryngoscopy.

REFERENCES

1. Sykes W: *Essays on the first hundred years of anesthesia*, London, 1982, Churchill Livingstone.
2. Lyman HM: *Artificial anaesthesia and anaesthetics*, New York, 1881, William Wood and Co.
3. Brimacombe J: *Laryngeal mask anesthesia: principles and practice*, ed 2, Philadelphia, 2005, Saunders.
4. Ball C, Westhorpe R: Clearing the airway: the development of the pharyngeal airway, *Anesth Intensive Care* 25:451, 1997.
5. Gudel A: A non-traumatic pharyngeal airway, *JAMA* 100:1862, 1933.
6. Brandt L: The first reported oral intubation of the human trachea, *Anesth Analg* 66:1198–1199, 1987.
7. Sweeny B: Franz Kuhn: his contribution to anaesthesia, *Anaesthesia* 40:1000–1005, 1985.
8. Westhorpe R: Kuhn's endotracheal tube, *Anesth Intensive Care* 19:489, 1991.
9. Magill I: Technique in endotracheal anaesthesia, *Proc R Soc Med* 22:83–88, 1928.
10. Brimacombe J: *Laryngeal mask anesthesia: principles and practice*, ed 2, Philadelphia, 2005, Saunders, p 7.
11. Brimacombe J: *Laryngeal mask anesthesia: principles and practice*, ed 2, Philadelphia, 2005, Saunders, p 6.
12. Griffith HR, Johnson GE: The use of curare in general anesthesia, *Anesthesiology* 3:418–420, 1942.
13. Mendelson C: The aspiration of gastric contents into the lungs during obstetric anesthesia, *Am J Obstet Gynecol* 52:191–204, 1946.
14. IP Latto, Rosen M, editor: *Changing times: changing standards: Difficulties in tracheal intubation*, London, 2000, WB Saunders, pp ix-x.
15. Brimacombe J, editor: *Laryngeal mask anesthesia: principles and practice*, ed 2, Philadelphia, 2005, W.B. Saunders.
16. Brain AI: The laryngeal mask—a new concept in airway management, *Br J Anesth* 55:801–805, 1983.
17. Verghese C, Brimacombe JR: Survey of laryngeal mask airway usage in 11,910 patients: safety and efficacy for conventional and nonconventional usage, *Anesth Analg* 82:129–133, 1996.
18. Maltby JR, Beriault MT, Watson NC, Fick GH: Gastric distension and ventilation during laproscopic cholescystectomy: LMA-Classic vs. tracheal intubation, *Can J Anesth* 47(7):622–626, 2000.
19. Brimacombe JR, Berry A: The incidence of aspiration associated with the laryngeal mask airway: a meta-analysis of published literature, *J Clin Anesth* 47(7):297–305, 2005.
20. Brimacombe J, Brain A, Branagan H, Spry M, Schofield J: Optimal shape of the laryngeal mask cuff: the influence of three deflation techniques, *Anaesthesia* 51:673–676, 1996.
21. Brimacombe J: *Laryngeal mask anesthesia: principles and practice*, ed 2, Philadelphia, 2005, W.B. Saunders, p 47.
22. Brimacombe J: *Laryngeal mask anesthesia: principles and practice*, ed 2, Philadelphia, 2005, W.B. Saunders, p 48.
23. Brimacombe J: *Laryngeal mask anesthesia: principles and practice*, ed 2, Philadelphia, 2005, W.B. Saunders, p 53.

24. Langton JA, Wilson I, Fell D: Use of the laryngeal mask airway during magnetic resonance imaging, *Anaesthesia* 47:532, 1992.
25. Brimacombe J: *Laryngeal mask anesthesia: principles and practice*, ed 2, Philadelphia, 2005, W.B. Saunders, p 57.
26. Reference deleted in proofs.
27. Heath ML, Sinnathamby SW: The reinforced laryngeal mask airway for adenotonsilectomy, *Br J Anaesth* 72:728–729, 1994.
28. Parry M, Glaisyer H, Bailey P: Removal of LMA in children, *Br J Anaesth* 78:337–344, 1997.
29. Williams PJ, Thompsett C, Bailey PM: Comparison of the reinforced laryngeal mask airway and the tracheal tube for nasal surgery, *Anaesthesia* 50:987–989, 1995.
30. Boisson-Bertrand D: Tonsillectomies and the reinforced laryngeal mask. *Can J Anesth* 42:857–861, 1995.
31. Brimacombe J, Keller C: Aspiration of gastric contents during use of a ProSeal LMA secondary to unidentified foldover malposition, *Anesth Analg* 97:1192–1194, 2003.
32. Stix MS, O'Connor CJ Jr: Depth of insertion of the ProSeal laryngeal mask airway, *Br J Anaesth* 90:235–237, 2003.
33. O'Connor CJ, Borromeo CJ, Stix MS: Assessing ProSeal laryngeal mask position: the suprasternal notch test (letter), *Anesth Analg* 94:1374, 2002.
34. Brain AI, Verghese C, Strube PJ: The LMA 'ProSeal'—a laryngeal mask with an oesophageal vent, *Br J Anaesth* 84:650, 2000.
35. Brimacombe J, Keller C, Berry A: Gastric insufflation with the ProSeal laryngeal mask, *Anesth Analg* 92:1614, 2001.
36. Maltby JR, Beriault MT, Watson NC, Liepert D, Fick GH: The LMA ProSeal is an effective alternative to tracheal intubation for laparoscopic cholecystectomy, *Can J Anesth* 49(8):857–862, 2002.
37. Brimacombe J, Keller C, Fukkekrug B, et al: A multicenter study comparing the ProSeal and Classic Laryngeal Mask Airway in anesthetized, nonparalyzed patients, *Anesthesiology* 96(2):289–295, 2002.
38. Rosenblatt WH, Murphy M: The intubating laryngeal mask: use of a new ventilating-intubating device in the emergency department, *Ann Emerg Med* 33:234–238, 1999.
39. Gaitini L, Varda S, Somri M, et al: An evaluation of the laryngeal tube during general anesthesia using mechanical ventilation, *Anesth Analg* 96:1750–1755, 2003.
40. Osborn I, Reinhard PK: *Current concepts and clinical use of the supraglottic airway, anesthesiology news guide to airway management*, ed 2, New York, 2009, McMahon Publishing, p 58.
41. Sinha P, Misra S: Supraglottic airway devices other than Laryngeal Mask Airway and its prototype, *Indian J Anaesth* 49(4):281–292, 2005.
42. Osborn I, Reinhard PK: *Current concepts and clinical use of the supraglottic airway, anesthesiology news guide to airway management*, ed 2, Mumbai, India, 2009, Medknow Publications and Media, p 54.
43. Michael TA, Lambert EH, Mehran A: "Mouth-to-lung airway" for cardiac resuscitation, *Lancet* 2:1329, 1968.
44. Gaitini LA, Vaida SJ, Mostafa S, et al: The Combitube in elective surgery: a report of 200 cases, *Anesthesiology* 94(1):79–82, 2001.
45. Gaitini LA, Vaida SJ, Somri M, Fradis M, Ben-David B: Fiberoptic-guided airway exchange of the esophageal-tracheal Combitube in spontaneously breathing versus mechanically ventilated patients, *Anesth Analg* 88:193–196, 1999.
46. Gaitini L, Vaida S, Somri M, Yanovski B, Toame P: Comparison of the esophageal- tracheal Combitube and Easy Tube in paralyzed anesthetized adult patients [abstract], *Anesthesiology* 101:A517, 2004.
47. James CD: Sir William Macewen and anesthesia, *Anaesthesia* 29:743–753, 1974.
48. Sweeney B: Franz Kuhn: his contribution to anesthesia, *Anaesthesia* 40:1000–1010, 1985.
49. Dorsch JA, Dorsch SE: *Tracheal tubes, understanding anesthesia equipment*, ed 4, Baltimore, 1998, Williams & Wilkins, pp 557–671.
50. American Society for Testing and Materials [ASTM]: *Standard Specification for Cuffed and Uncuffed Tracheal Tubes (ASTM F1242-96)*, West Conshohocken, PA, 1996, ASTM.
51. Davies J, Hillel A, Maronian N, Posner K: The Hunsaker Mon Jet tube with jet ventilation is effective for microlaryngeal surgery, *Can J Anesth* 56(4):284–290, 2009.
52. Cooper R: Laryngoscopy: its past and future, *Can J Anesth* 51(6):R21–R25, 2004.
53. Alberti PW: The history of laryngology: a centennial celebration, *Otolaryngol Head Neck Surg* 114:345–354, 1996.
54. Ovassapian A: *Fiberoptic endoscopy and the difficult airway*, 1996, Raven Press.
55. Rosenblatt W: *Airway management in clinical anesthesia*. In Barash PG, Cullen BF, editors: *Clinical anesthesia*, ed 6, Philadelphia, 2009, Lippincott Williams & Wilkins.
56. Friedrich P, Frass M, Krenn CG, et al: The Upsher scope in routine and difficult airway management: a randomized controlled clinical trial, *Anesth Analg* 85:1373–1381, 1997.
57. DedoScope, Pilling Surgical Instruments, Teleflex Medical, Research Triangle Park, NC.
58. Bein B, Worthmann F, Scholz J, et al: A comparison of the intubating laryngeal mask airway and the Bonfils intubation fiberscope in patients with predicted difficult airways, *Anaesthesia* 59:668–674, 2004.
59. Hagberg CA: Current concepts in the management of the difficult airway, *Anesthesiology New Guide to Airway Management*, 2010, pp 49–71.
60. Ferson DZ, Rosenblatt WH, Johansen MJ, Osborne I, Ovassapian A: Use of the Intubating LMA-Fastrach in 254 patients with difficult-to-manage airways, *Anesthesiology* 95:1175–1181, 2001.
61. Barnes TA, Macdonald D, Nolan J, et al: American Heart Association, International Liaison Committee on Resuscitation: Cardiopulmonary resuscitation and emergency cardiovascular care: airway devices, *Ann Emerg Med* 37(Suppl 4):S145–S151, 2001.
62. Verghese C: Laryngeal mask devices: three maneuvers for any clinical situation, *Anesthesiology News: Guide to Airway Management* 66–67, 2009; May.
63. Goldman AJ, TD, Rosenblatt WH: The Laryngeal Mask Airway CTrach: a multicenter observational series of 230 cases, *J Clin Anesth* 18(4):319–320, 2005.
64. Goldman AJ, Rosenblatt WH: Use of the fibreoptic intubating LMA-CTrach in two patients with difficult airways, *Anaesthesia* 61:601–603, 2006.
65. Cooper RM: Use of a new videolaryngoscope (GlideScope) in the management of a difficult airway, *Can J Anesth* 50(6):611–613, 2003.
66. el-Ganzouri AR, McCarthy RJ, Tuman KJ, Tanck EN, Ivankovich AD: Preoperative airway assessment: predictive value of a multivariate risk index, *Anesth Analg* 82:1197–1204, 1996.
67. Yamamura H, YT, Kamiyana M: Device for blind nasal intubation, *Anesthesiology* 20:221, 1959.

CHAPTER 17

PEDIATRIC ANESTHESIA SYSTEMS AND EQUIPMENT

Simon C. Hillier • William L. McNiece • Stephen F. Dierdorf

CHAPTER OUTLINE

OVERVIEW

The ultimate goal of the anesthesiologist during pediatric surgery is to provide the patient with a safe and smooth anesthetic along with a comfortable and uneventful recovery. A well-considered anesthetic plan for a pediatric patient must include a well-informed choice of appropriate equipment. Which breathing systems are appropriate for the pediatric patient? How do maturational changes in respiratory physiology affect the selection and use of equipment? Does an adult ventilator and breathing system function acceptably for the pediatric patient? Are monitors primarily designed for adults appropriate for pediatric patients? This chapter attempts to answer some of these questions.

A clear understanding of anesthetic equipment is important to the safe delivery of pediatric anesthesia. Approximately 40% of anesthetic incidents were attributed to equipment problems in one 11-year experience, which included both adult and pediatric patients.[1] Standardization of equipment, improved monitoring, and the introduction of new anesthetic drugs have all improved the safety of pediatric anesthesia. Over time, the percentage of pediatric closed claims events attributable to respiratory events or to inadequate monitoring have declined.[2]

PHYSIOLOGY

Work of Breathing Under Anesthesia

Understanding the relevant aspects of pediatric respiratory physiology provides a rationale for the recommendations presented later in this chapter. Several factors may increase the work of breathing under anesthesia (Table 17-1). These factors can be broadly divided into two groups: first is the increased work of breathing that may be imposed by the anesthesia breathing system, including inspiratory and expiratory resistance of breathing circuits, circuit dead space, and rebreathing of carbon dioxide. Second are changes in the mechanics and in the control of breathing induced by general anesthesia. These include decreased total respiratory compliance, decreased lung volume, airway closure, and upper airway obstruction. Thus, during general anesthesia, many factors conspire to increase the demands placed on the respiratory system while simultaneously decreasing the patient's ability to cope with these demands.

TABLE 17-1 **Perioperative Factors that Increase the Work of Breathing**

Anesthetic Breathing System	General Anesthesia
Circuit and tube resistance	Decreased lung volume
Absorber resistance	Decreased respiratory compliance
Valvular resistance	Upper airway obstruction
Apparatus dead space	
Rebreathing of carbon dioxide	

Table 17-2 compares some selected infant and adult respiratory physiologic values. In general, neonates and infants have less respiratory reserve than adults and may demonstrate an unpredictable response to any additional work of breathing through a circuit under general anesthesia. Patients breathing spontaneously with the Mapleson D, E, and F circuits will rebreathe alveolar gas if the fresh gas flow is less than 2.5 to 3 times the predicted minute ventilation.[3] Under normal circumstances, most of these patients will increase their minute ventilation in response and thereby prevent significant hypercarbia. However, even some anesthetized adults are unable to respond to increases in inspired carbon dioxide by hyperventilation and thus become significantly hypercarbic.[4]

Olsson and Lindhal examined the response of spontaneously breathing anesthetized infants[5] (nitrous oxide and 1% to 1.5% halothane) to an increase in inspired carbon dioxide. Patients younger than 6 months did not significantly increase their minute ventilation in response to the added carbon dioxide, whereas patients older than 6 months showed a markedly attenuated response to increased inspired carbon dioxide. When the halothane concentration was reduced to 0.8%, the ventilatory response to carbon dioxide returned in patients younger than 6 months; thus, inhalational anesthesia attenuates the ventilatory response to carbon dioxide in small infants.

General anesthesia also adversely affects infants' ventilatory response to increased respiratory work in the forms of tubular resistance, dead space, and valvular resistance. For a given increase in apparatus dead space, the infant must increase minute ventilation to a proportionately greater degree to maintain normocarbia when compared with the older child.[6] The neonate is prone to respiratory compromise in the face of prolonged increases in

TABLE 17-2 **Comparison of Selected Normal Respiratory Values in Infants and Adults**

Normal Value	Infant	Adult
Weight (kg)	3.0	70
Surface area (m^2)	0.2	1.8
Surface area/weight (m^2/kg)	0.06	0.03
Respiratory frequency (breaths/min)	30-40	10-16
Tidal volume (V_T, mL/kg)	7	7
Dead space (V_D, mL/kg)	2.2	2.2
V_D/V_T	0.3	0.3
Functional residual capacity (mL/kg)	30	30
Specific compliance (mL/cm H_2O/mL)	0.05	0.05
Airways resistance (cm H_2O/L/sec)	25-30	1.6
Work of breathing (J/L)	0.5-0.7	0.5-0.7
Alveolar ventilation (mL/kg/min)	100-150	70
Oxygen consumption (mL/kg/min)	6 to 8	4

respiratory work. The newborn's diaphragmatic muscle is immature, having a smaller proportion of fatigue-resistant high-oxidative muscle fibers.[7] In addition, the infant diaphragm is less able to generate a maximal inspiratory force compared with the adult diaphragm.[8]

PEDIATRIC ANESTHESIA EQUIPMENT

Face Masks

The face mask must be able to provide a good seal to the child's face to facilitate effective positive-pressure ventilation, avoid entrainment of room air, and reduce operating room (OR) pollution. Other desirable face mask features include low dead space, increased patient comfort, and construction with transparent material that allows observation of patient color and the presence of secretions or vomitus (Fig. 17-1); in addition, transparent masks are less threatening to the patient.[9] The ability to ventilate the patient by mask is of the utmost importance, but low dead space is also desirable to avoid retention of carbon dioxide and increased respiratory work. However, in practice, the functional dead space of most face masks is significantly less than the measured dead space because streaming of gas eliminates significant rebreathing.[6,9]

Maintaining an airway with a face mask occasionally can be challenging in children because the anesthesiologist's fingers can cause external compression of the compliant upper airway. Care should be taken to ensure that fingers do not stray from the mandible onto the soft tissues surrounding the airway. Mask anesthesia with spontaneous ventilation should probably not be used for prolonged procedures in small infants because infants are unable to tolerate the increased work of breathing and may respond with apnea or hypoventilation. Inhalational induction of anesthesia may be facilitated by the application of an odorant (e.g., lip gloss) to the inside of the face mask to disguise the smell of the potent volatile agents and the unpleasant plastic odor of the mask and breathing circuit.

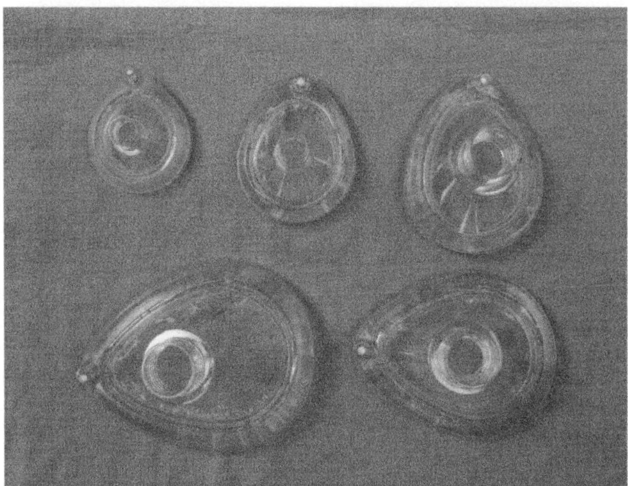

FIGURE 17-1 ■ Transparent anesthesia face masks in various sizes, with syringe-adjustable air cushion.

Tracheal Tubes

Selection of the correct tracheal tube type and size, along with its accurate and secure positioning, is vitally important.

Cuffed Versus Uncuffed Endotracheal Tubes

The decision to use cuffed instead of uncuffed endotracheal tubes (ETTs) in pediatric patients depends on multiple factors. The use of cuffed tubes has historically been discouraged in children younger than 8 to 10 years. Most pediatric anesthesiologists have strong opinions on this matter, and evolving practice patterns are not always evidence driven. Although this topic generates vigorous debate, irrespective of whether a cuffed or uncuffed tube is selected, most experts would agree that safe use of any tube depends on meticulous attention to technical detail.

The vocal cords are the narrowest point of the pediatric airway, but they are more mobile that the cricoid cartilage, which completely surrounds the airway. Although the cricoid often is described as a "ring" of cartilage, the airway at this level has an ellipsoid cross-section.[10-12] Intuitively, it would seem that the ellipsoid cross-sectional configuration of the airway makes it unlikely that a circular, cross-sectional tube can both provide an optimal airway seal and avoid local trauma to some part of the airway circumference, particularly the posterolateral walls of the larynx. However, the subglottic region is lined with loosely bound pseudostratified epithelium. Thus, trauma to this region, such as by intubation with a tube of too large a diameter, readily results in edema that decreases the lumen of the airway and increases resistance to gas flow. During laminar flow, resistance is inversely proportional to the fourth power of the radius. However, flow conditions in the upper airway are likely to be transitional or turbulent.[13] Under these conditions, resistance is inversely proportional to the fifth power of the radius. A 1-mm ring of edema in the newborn will reduce the cross-sectional area of the airway by 75%. Under laminar flow conditions, resistance will increase 16-fold. By comparison, a 1-mm ring of edema in a healthy adult would have a less significant effect on airway resistance.[14]

Avoiding trauma to the vulnerable subglottic region is obviously critical. This applies whether the insult is generated by the shaft of an uncuffed tube or from an ETT cuff. Therefore, an important consideration of pediatric ETTs is their cuff design characteristics. Over time, cuff pressure-volume characteristics have led to the development of less traumatic high-volume low-pressure cuffs. However, recent attempts have been made to eliminate cuff contact with the subglottic region altogether by locating a shorter, ultrathin polyurethane cuff more distally on the shaft of the tube, thus producing a cuff-free subglottic zone.[15] The more distal cuff location has forced the elimination of the Murphy eye. The intent of this design modification is to create a tracheal, rather than a cricoid, cuff seal. The cross-sectional configuration, presence of a nonrigid muscular posterior wall, and U-shaped cartilage make the trachea a more suitable site for cuff placement than the cricoid region. Modern high-volume, low-pressure, ultrathin polyurethane cuffs conform readily to the trachea and provide acceptable seals at lower pressures (<15 cm H_2O).

We prefer to use cuffed ETTs in our practice. However, the use of cuffed tubes is predicated on the availability of tubes of the appropriate design and careful attention to leak pressure. Use of cuffed tubes must be accompanied by careful attention to cuff pressure and may require using a half-size smaller tube to provide space for the uninflated cuff. However, these limitations are offset by several advantages: first, use of a cuffed tube with appropriate inflation provides a reliable airway seal, reduces the risk of aspiration, and limits inspired gas leakage. Second, the improved seal also improves tidal volume measurement and the accuracy of airway gas samples. Third, contamination of the OR ambient atmosphere by anesthetic gas is reduced. Fourth, more consistent ventilation and better carbon dioxide management particularly benefits patients with congenital heart disease or pulmonary hypertension.

TABLE 17-3 **Determination of Endotracheal Tube Size and Depth of Insertion**

Patient Age	Tube Size	Depth
Premature, ≤1000 g	2.5 mm ID	7 cm for a 1-kg infant: +1 cm/kg body weight up to 4 kg
Premature, 1000-2500 g	3.0 mm ID	>4 kg and ≤1 year: 10 cm at the alveolar ridge
<6 years	(Age/3) + 3.75 mm ID	>1 year: (age/2) + 12 cm
>6 years	(Age/4) + 4.5 mm ID	

Tubes 0.5 mm ID larger and smaller than those calculated from these should be immediately available.
ID, inner diameter.

Uncuffed Tubes

The optimal size of an uncuffed tracheal tube is the largest size that will easily pass into the trachea without traumatizing the larynx. To determine the leak pressure after tracheal intubation, the reservoir bag should be slowly inflated; circuit pressure is measured while listening with a stethoscope, either at the mouth or in the sternal notch, for a leak. The optimal leak pressure has not been definitively determined, but the incidence of postextubation stridor seems to increase as the leak pressure increases, particularly to greater than 25 cm H_2O. Most patients' lungs can be adequately ventilated at leak pressures of 15 to 20 cm H_2O. If the patient has lung disease or is undergoing an intrathoracic or high abdominal procedure, a higher leak pressure, such as 25 to 30 cm H_2O, may be necessary to allow adequate ventilation in the face of decreased respiratory compliance. On occasion, an unacceptably large leak will be present with one size of tube but not with a tube 0.5 mm larger in diameter. Under these circumstances, a cuffed tube of the smaller size with the cuff deflated may produce an acceptable leak. Using a tube that is too small with a large leak may lead to difficulty ventilating the lungs and obtaining accurate end-tidal carbon dioxide measurements and, at least in theory, it increases the risk of aspiration. Suction catheters appropriate to all tube sizes must be immediately available to remove secretions from tracheal tubes.

Formulas to predict correct tracheal tube size are based on weight and age (Table 17-3). It is also good practice to also have tubes available sized 0.5 mm above and below the predicted size (Fig. 17-2).

The peak incidence of postextubation stridor is between 1 and 4 years of age.[16] Factors that contribute to the development of postextubation stridor include a tight-fitting tracheal tube (i.e., a leak at >25 cm H_2O),

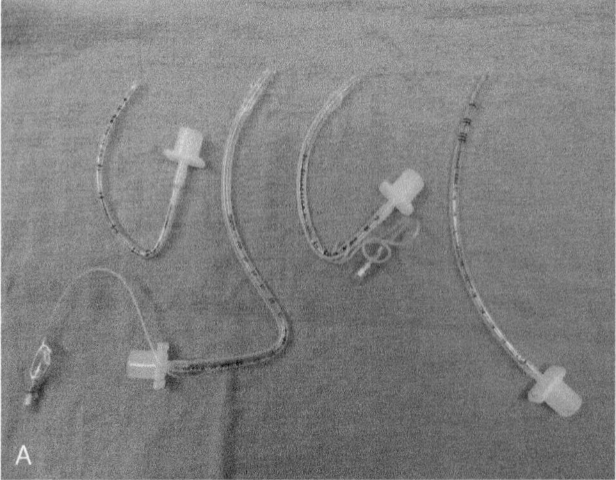

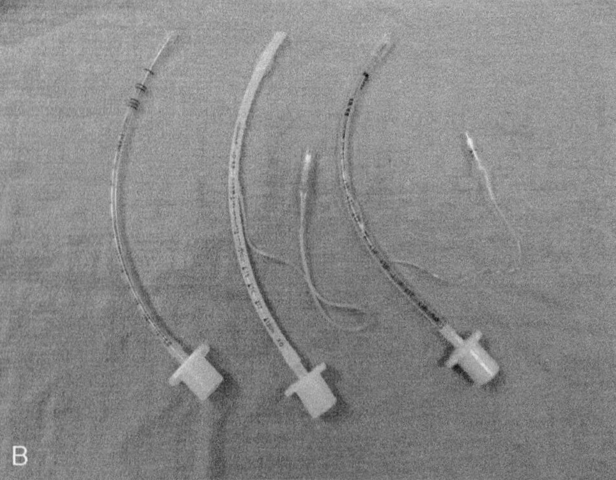

FIGURE 17-2 ■ A selection of preformed and standard pediatric tracheal tubes. **A,** From left to right: uncuffed oral Ring-Adair-Elwyn tube (RAE; Mallinckrodt, St. Louis, MO), cuffed nasal RAE tube, cuffed oral RAE tube, standard oral uncuffed tube. **B,** Cuffed and uncuffed pediatric tracheal tubes.

traumatic or multiple intubations, coughing with the tracheal tube in place during emergence from anesthesia, changing the patient's head position while intubated, intubation lasting more than 1 hour, and operations in the neck region. Although recent upper respiratory tract infection was not initially thought to be a contributing factor, more recent data show that patients younger than 1 year have a 27-fold increased risk of postextubation stridor after upper respiratory tract infection.[17] Patients with Down syndrome may have a narrow subglottic region and are thus prone to postextubation stridor; the clinician should consider using an ETT smaller than that predicted by the patient's age or weight for such patients.

Selecting the Correct Insertion Depth

The term newborn trachea is approximately 4 to 5 cm long. Therefore, the margin of error for a tube located in the mid trachea is approximately 2 cm in either direction. A tube inserted too deeply will result in carinal irritation or endobronchial intubation, whereas too shallow an insertion depth may predispose to accidental extubation. A potential hazard of shallow tube insertion depth is that the cuff may be located in the subglottic, rather than the tracheal, region. To determine the correct insertion depth, gently advance the tube after intubation, while the chest is auscultated bilaterally, to determine the depth at which bronchial intubation occurs. The tube is then carefully withdrawn and secured at the appropriate depth. Of note, when the tube has a Murphy eye, it may be difficult to determine tube position by auscultation because sufficient gas may flow through the eye to produce contralateral breath sounds despite the tube tip being located in a mainstem bronchus.

In small infants, particularly those with lung disease, it is not always easy to determine by auscultation alone at what depth the tube should be secured. When accurate tube position is crucial (e.g., for repair of a tracheoesophageal fistula), a small-diameter flexible fiberoptic bronchoscope may be used to determine the tube location, and 1.8 mm (Olympus PF 18M; Olympus America, Center Valley, PA) and 2.2 mm (Olympus LF-P) outer diameter (OD) flexible fiberoptic bronchoscopes can help in tube positioning. The larger of these bronchoscopes has a directable distal tip. Neither has a suction channel, but both can be passed through a 2.5-mm internal diameter (ID) tracheal tube. If a suitable bronchoscope is unavailable, a chest radiograph may be a reasonable alternative.

Several manufacturers place intubation depth markers on their ETTs. These markers typically are one or more horizontal black bands located near the distal end of the tube. The intent is that when the marker is placed at the vocal cords, the distal tip of the ETT will be located in the mid trachea. Goel and colleagues[18] examined intubation depth markers on several commonly used pediatric ETTs and noted a wide discrepancy in both the number and locations of the markers among manufacturers. Furthermore, a lack of consistency of markers was found among different-sized tubes from the same manufacturer. Thus it is important to be familiar with the location of the intubation depth markers on the tubes most frequently used at an institution. Optimal insertion depth is probably best achieved by using a combination of predictive formulas (see Table 17-3), intubation depth markers, and clinical examination.

Using the Oral RAE Tracheal Tube

The preformed Ring-Adair-Elwyn tube (RAE; Mallinckrodt, St. Louis, MO) (see Fig. 17-2) is often used during ear-nose-throat, plastic, and other head and neck procedures.[19] The RAE tube has several advantages and potential pitfalls: it was originally designed for use during cleft lip and palate surgery at an institution where the surgeon preferred to leave the tube untaped so that its position could be adjusted during the procedure. The designers of the tube intended the distal tip of the tube to lie nearer to the carina than a conventional tube to reduce the likelihood of accidental extubation. Two Murphy eyes, located at the distal end of the tube, are intended to allow continued ventilation should endobronchial migration occur. The acute angle in the RAE tube, the part of the tube most likely to kink, is located outside the mouth and therefore is readily visible.

Although the above design features are useful, several potential hazards have been described. Seemingly appropriate positioning of the acute angle of an RAE tube at the lower lip does not guarantee that the distal tip of the tube is located correctly. The distal tips of 32% of RAE tubes positioned in this way were located at the carina or down a mainstem bronchus.[20] In this situation, the Murphy eyes do not guarantee adequate ventilation during the procedure, but they may allow sufficient gas flow during manual ventilation and chest auscultation to falsely suggest acceptable tube position. It is recommended that a left precordial stethoscope be used to monitor tube position throughout the procedure, particularly during repositioning and mouth-gag insertion, to rapidly detect endobronchial migration. These tubes are labeled by the manufacturer with a suggested patient age range, but these recommendations should be interpreted with caution, as they may advocate a different-sized tube than that predicted by standard formulas for pediatric tracheal tubes.

It should be noted that, although unusual in current practice, occasional patients who require cleft lip and/or palate repair may be smaller than predicted by age, typically as a result of feeding difficulties or coexisting disease. In these patients it can be challenging to select an ETT size that is appropriate in both diameter and length.[21] However, in the majority of patients with cleft lip and palate, standard formulas are acceptable predictors of ETT size and insertion depth.

Another obstacle to correct tube sizing is related to significant differences among manufacturers in the dimensions of oral preformed tubes. For example, when 4.5-mm ID uncuffed tubes from four manufacturers were measured, the distance from the bend to the tube tip ranged between 13.5 and 15 cm.[22]

Problems may occasionally be encountered when performing tracheal suctioning via an RAE tube, and passing a catheter beyond the acute angle in the tube can be

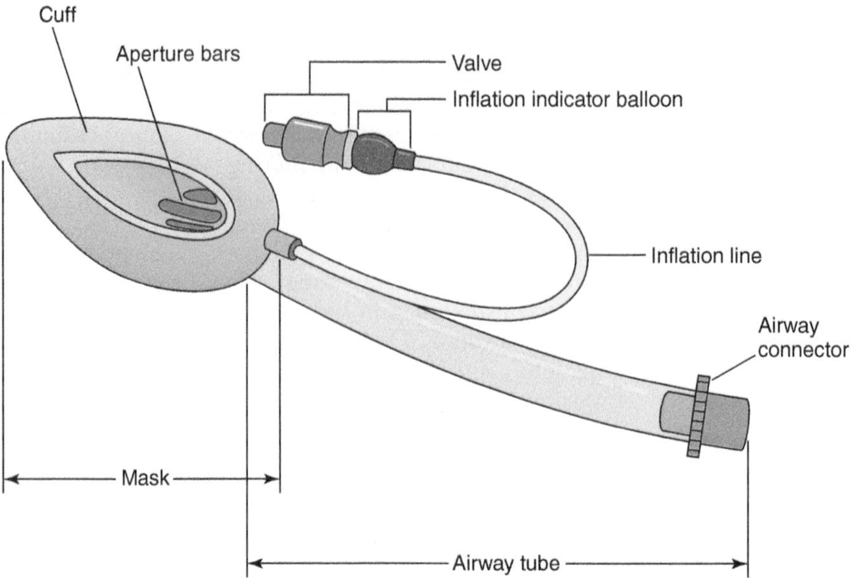

FIGURE 17-3 ■ Parts of the Laryngeal Mask Airway (LMA North America, San Diego, CA). (Courtesy G. Sheplock, MD.)

difficult. Despite these potential problems, and with attention to the details noted above, anesthesiologists have found the RAE tube to be extremely useful during procedures of the head and neck.

SUPRAGLOTTIC AIRWAYS IN PEDIATRIC PATIENTS

The laryngeal mask airway (LMA; LMA North America, San Diego, CA) revolutionized airway management for the practice of anesthesia (Fig. 17-3). The LMA provides a more secure airway than a face mask and pharyngeal airway but is less invasive than a tracheal tube. The success of the original LMA design has been underscored by the large number of supraglottic airway variants that have been developed and marketed by other manfacturers. The creation of a separate category of airway devices, the supraglottic airways, is also indicative of the importance of these devices to airway management. Although originally developed for the management of normal airways, the LMA has proven extremely useful for management of difficult airways.[23,24]

Pediatric patients are especially suited for supraglottic airways, because upper airway obstruction during anesthesia is more likely in children than in adults. Children often require general anesthesia for short surgical or diagnostic procedures, and their small size can place the anesthesiologist at a considerable distance from the patient's head and airway. Prior to the introduction of the LMA, tracheal intubation was often required for such procedures. Compared with tracheal intubation, advantages of the supraglottic airway include less hemodynamic response to insertion and, during emergence, a reduced risk of laryngeal complications such as croup; a decreased incidence of sore throat; and, quite possibly, less nausea and a faster discharge from the postanesthesia care unit (PACU).

Disadvantages of supraglottic airways in children are generally related to malposition of the device, excessive pressure on the oropharyngeal mucosa, hypoventilation, laryngospasm, and aspiration of gastric contents. A light plane of anesthesia may predispose to regurgitation or laryngospasm with a supraglottic airway in place.

Education and the Supraglottic Airway

Airway management during the administration of anesthesia requires precise positioning of the supraglottic airway to maximize ventilatory exchange and minimize the risk of hypoventilation, laryngospasm, and mechanical distortion of the upper airway. Instruction of supraglottic airway use to anesthesiology trainees must be methodical and controlled and must permit adequate experience for the trainee to understand the indications and contraindications for use.[25] Fiberoptic examination of the supraglottic airway after insertion is invaluable for anyone learning to see position variation and how malposition may adversely affect airway function. Experience with different types of supraglottic airways is important for trainees because different institutions use different types.

Insertion Technique

The original insertion technique for LMA insertion has been modified by many users during the past 30 years. Ideal insertion of a supraglottic airway places the airway channel immediately above the glottic inlet, with the distal end resting in the upper esophageal sphincter and the upper border of the device bowl below the hyoid bone. The airway should slide along the hard and soft palates, between the tonsillar pillars, and into the hypopharynx. Insertion techniques for supraglottic airways with cuffs have been described with the cuff completely deflated, partially inflated, and completely inflated (Fig. 17-4). The potential problem with insertion with the cuff inflated is that the epiglottis will fold downward, and the device will be high in the hypopharynx, thereby increasing pressure on the base of the tongue and the lateral

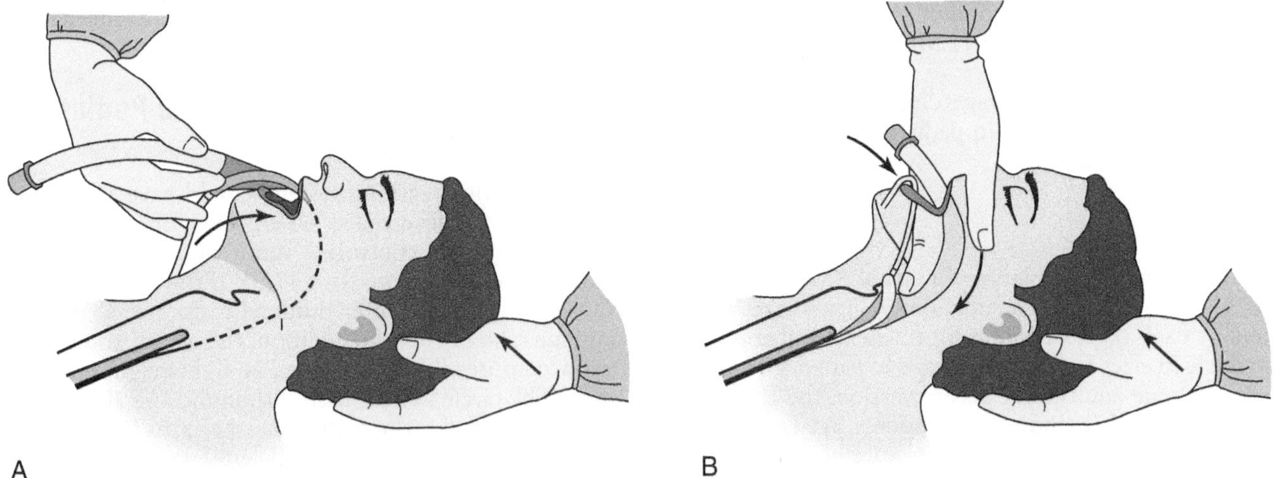

FIGURE 17-4 ■ Insertion of the Laryngeal Mask Airway (LMA; LMA North America, San Diego, CA). **A,** During the initial part of the insertion, it is important that the LMA be directed in a maximally cephalad direction, with the wrist in complete flexion, so that the tip of the LMA follows the curvature of the hard and soft palates. **B,** The LMA is completely inserted when resistance is encountered by the guiding index finger, indicating that the tip of the cuff has reached the inferior recess of the hypopharynx. (Courtesy G. Sheplock, MD.)

oropharyngeal wall. Insertion of a supraglottic airway upside-down and partially inflated, with rotation of the device after it enters the pharynx, has been advocated by many authors.[26,27] Large inflation volumes may cause a greater incidence of sore throat and increase the risk of excessive pressure on the pharyngeal mucosa.

An adequate depth of anesthesia must be attained prior to supraglottic airway insertion. Insertion of the device before attenuation of upper airway reflexes may provoke emesis or regurgitation. Satisfactory anesthesia can be achieved with both intravenous (IV) and inhaled agents.[28,29]

TYPES OF SUPRAGLOTTIC AIRWAYS

Several manufacturers produce supraglottic airways, and product lines continue to evolve (Box 17-1). Many supraglottic airways do not undergo rigorous evaluation prior to clinical introduction, and potential complications do not become known until enough patient uses have been achieved. Consequently, some supraglottic airways have a very short market life. Most institutions now use single-use (disposable) supraglottic airways to minimize the risk of infectious disease transmission and to reduce processing costs.

Some supraglottic airways may be especially suited for a particular procedure, and it is unlikely that one supraglottic airway will fit all needs. Flexible bronchoscopy is easily performed through a supraglottic airway, but bronchoscope manipulation is easier through a silicone airway (e.g., classic reusable LMA).[30] The pediatric anesthesiologist should be facile with several types of supraglottic airways to confront a wide array of patient airways.

Laryngeal Mask Airway

Since its introduction into clinical practice in the late 1980s, several models of the LMA have been developed (Box 17-2). In addition to the LMA Classic, single-use LMAs (LMA Unique), flexible LMAs, intubating LMAs (Fastrach), the ProSeal LMA, and Supreme LMA are currently available. The Fastrach LMA is noted for its ease of insertion and for the fact that it can serve as both a conduit for ventilation and tracheal intubation. The intubating LMA is available only in sizes 3, 4, and 5. All other models are available in smaller sizes. The LMA C Trach is an advanced model of the LMA Fastrach intubating LMA that has imaging capability of the larynx after insertion of the LMA. Although the C Trach has been most frequently used in adults, successful pediatric experience has been reported for children aged 9 to 17 years.[31] The ProSeal LMA and the LMA Supreme are perhaps the most advanced of the LMAs and consist of a more anatomically designed bowl that results in a higher leak pressure without excessive pressure on the

BOX 17-1 Commonly Used Supraglottic Airways

Laryngeal Mask Airway (LMA North America, San Diego, CA)
air-Q (Mercury Medical, Clearwater, FL)
Ambu Airway (Ambu Inc., Ballerup, Denmark)
I-Gel (Intersurgical, Liverpool, NY)

BOX 17-2 Laryngeal Mask Airway Models*

LMA Classic
LMA Unique
LMA Flexible
LMA Fastrach
LMA ProSeal
LMA Supreme

*LMA North America, San Diego, CA.

hypopharynx. A gastric conduit is built into the LMA Supreme and the ProSeal LMA and permits gastric decompression.

The medical literature regarding the LMA is extensive and documents its utility in pediatric patients with normal and difficult airways.

air-Q

The air-Q intubating laryngeal airway (Mercury Medical, Clearwater, FL) is a supraglottic airway that can be used by itself or as a conduit for tracheal intubation. It is available in sizes to fit a wide range of patients from neonates to large adults. One recent version, the ILA-SP, is self-pressurized. A study of 352 patients, aged newborn to 18 years, reported a mean leak pressure of 20.4 cm H_2O, complications in 14 patients, and no cases of regurgitation or aspiration. Successful placement on the first attempt was performed in 95% of the patients.[32] Tracheal intubation via the air-Q can be performed efficiently and effectively with guidance from a flexible fiberscope.[33]

Ambu Airway

There are five models of the Ambu laryngeal airway: the AuraFlex, AuraStraight, AuraOnce, Aura-I, and Aura40 (Ambu Inc., Ballerup, Denmark). The AuraFlex is available in sizes 2 through 6 with a small half size (2.5). All other models are available in sizes 1 through 6 with two small half sizes (1.5 and 2.5). The Aura40 is a curved reusable supraglottic airway, and the AuraOnce is a curved single-use supraglottic airway. Performance of the Ambu laryngeal airway compares favorably with other supraglottic airways, although few published studies have been done in pediatric patients.[34]

I-Gel

The I-Gel (Intersurgical, Liverpool, NY) is a supraglottic airway with a laryngeal cuff composed of a thermoplastic elastomer that produces a perilaryngal seal without an inflatable cuff. The purpose of this design is to provide an adequate laryngeal seal while minimizing the risk of pressure trauma to the hypoharyngeal tissue. A bite block and gastric drain port are also built into the device to permit decompression of the stomach. Reported experience with the I-Gel in children is limited but indicates a high insertion success rate and a mean leak pressure of 25 cm H_2O.[35] There are 7 sizes of the I-Gel that cover patients weighing 2 kg to more than 90 kg.

PEDIATRIC BREATHING SYSTEMS

The preterm infant can be adversely affected by hyperoxia.[36,37] Consequently, no matter what breathing system is used, it is important to control the delivered oxygen concentration, which may be room air. The modern anesthesia machine can be used very successfully for most pediatric cases and has the great advantage of operator familiarity. However, it is very important that the machine have the capability of delivering air.

Fundamental Requirements of the Pediatric Breathing System

The pediatric breathing system should have a low resistance and low dead space, be efficient for use with both spontaneous and controlled ventilation, and be easy to humidify and scavenge (Box 17-3). If the circuit contains valves, they should offer minimal resistance to gas flow and must be reliable. In addition, the circuit should have a low compressible volume and be lightweight and compact. The circle system with carbon dioxide absorbent is commonly used for pediatric anesthesia, as is the Mapleson D and F systems for manual ventilation and in PACU settings.

Mapleson D, E, and F System Development

The Mapleson D, E, and F systems are direct descendants of the original T-piece system introduced in 1937 by Philip Ayre of Newcastle, England.[38] The original Ayre T-piece has been greatly modified over the years and is rarely used today. All have the common feature of containing no valves that direct gas flow toward or away from the patient. The most commonly used configurations are the Mapleson D and F systems (Figs. 17-5 and 17-6). The Mapleson F system is a modification that is generally attributed to Jackson Rees, who added a reservoir bag with an adjustable valve to the expiratory limb.[39] When used with the valve largely open, the movement of the reservoir bag allows monitoring of spontaneous ventilation. With the valve partially closed, manual compression of the bag allows controlled ventilation. The Mapleson D system has an expiratory valve located at the end of the expiratory limb and functions in a manner similar to the Mapleson F circuit. The volume of the expiratory limb should exceed the patient's tidal volume. The Mapleson D and F circuits can be used with mechanical ventilation by removing the reservoir bag and connecting a ventilator.

The absence of valves with the Mapleson systems can result in rebreathing of exhaled gases in a setting of decreased fresh gas flow (FGF). The use of capnometry to determine if there is rebreathing ($PiCO_2$ >0) allows titration of FGF to eliminate rebreathing if desired. In general, an FGF of not less than 2.5 and up to 3 times the minute ventilation will usually eliminate rebreathing

BOX 17-3 Characteristics of an Ideal Pediatric Anesthetic Breathing System

Low dead space
Low resistance
Lightweight and compact
Low compressible volume
Easily humidified
Easily scavenged
Suitability for both controlled and spontaneous ventilation
Economy of fresh gas flow

(Box 17-4).[40] Neonates generally require an FGF of 3 L/min. FGF may need to be increased in the presence of a large tracheal tube leak. Significant FGF will be required in larger children and adults to prevent rebreathing, where peak inspiratory flows may exceed 20 L/min. FGF of this magnitude is both difficult to humidify and expensive. In general, a circle system is more efficient in terms of FGF requirements during anesthesia, particularly in older children and adults.

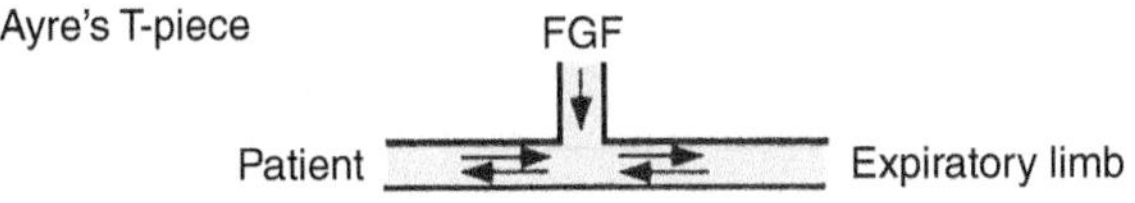

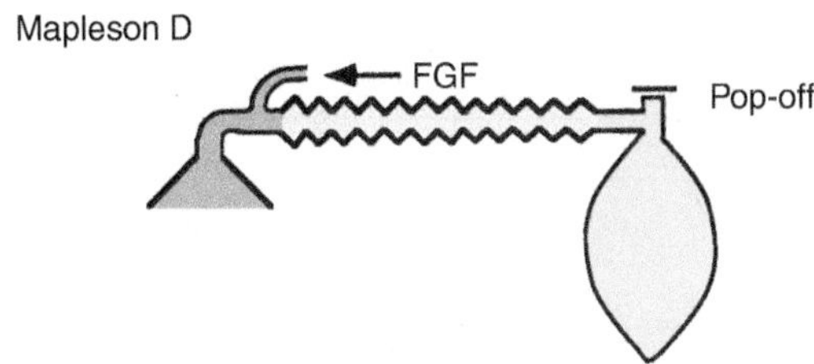

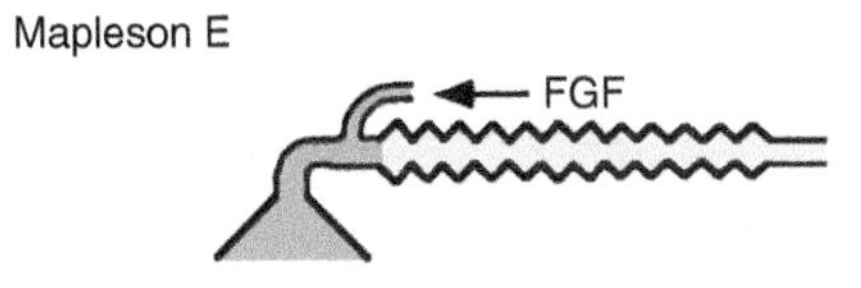

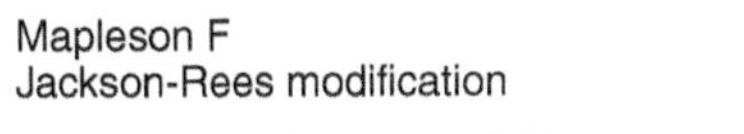

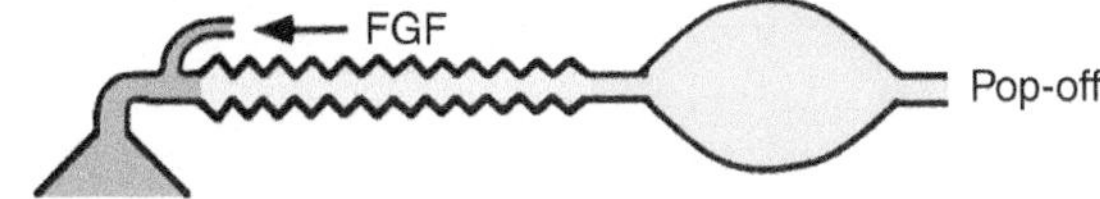

FIGURE 17-5 ■ The Ayre T-piece and its direct descendants, the Mapleson D, E, and F circuits. *FGF,* fresh gas flow.

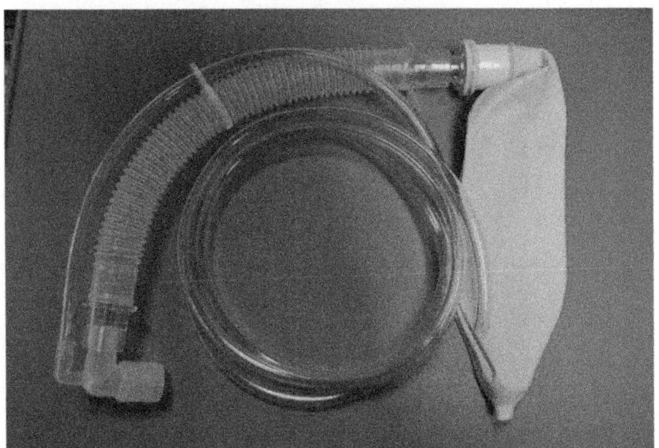

FIGURE 17-6 ■ A portable, disposable Jackson-Rees circuit (Mapleson F) for use to transport an infant or to administer anesthesia. (Courtesy K. Premmer, MD.)

A valved self-inflating breathing bag is appropriate for manual ventilation of larger children and adults when inhaled anesthetic delivery is not being used, particularly during patient transport.

The Bain circuit, described by Bain and Spoerel in 1972, is functionally identical to the Mapleson D system from which it is derived.[41] In the Bain circuit, the FGF is carried in a smaller inner hose, contained within the expiratory limb, attached to the machine using a special adapter (Fig. 17-7). The outer expiratory limb ID is 22 mm and is 7 mm for the inner fresh gas tubing. FGF requirements for the Bain system are similar to those recommended for the Mapleson D and F systems.

Before using the Bain circuit, it is important to verify that the fresh gas inner tube is not fractured or disconnected. In this situation, fresh gas will enter the expiratory limb near the reservoir bag, and a huge dead space will result.[42] Pethick's maneuver has been recommended to test the integrity of the circuit.[43] First, the patient end of the circuit is occluded and the reservoir bag is filled. The patient end is then opened, and a high flow of oxygen is passed through the circuit using the oxygen flush valve. The high gas flow exiting from the patient end of an intact fresh gas hose will cause a reduction in pressure in the expiratory limb because of the Venturi effect, collapsing the reservoir bag. If the inner tube is disrupted, oxygen under pressure will enter the expiratory limb and distend the reservoir bag. This technique has been criticized because small leaks may go undetected, and the test itself may cause circuit disruption. Similarly, if the inner tube is intact but does not extend completely to the end of the expiratory limb, significant dead space will exist that may not be detected. An adapter has been described that tests the integrity of the inner and outer tubing separately (Fig. 17-8).[44] A similar malfunction of a breathing

BOX 17-4 Fresh Gas Flow Requirements to Prevent Rebreathing in a T-Piece System

SPONTANEOUS VENTILATION

Mask Anesthesia

<30 kg body weight:
FGF = 4 × (1000 + [100 × kg body weight])
>30 kg body weight:
FGF = 4 × (2000 + [50 × body weight])

Intubated

<30 kg body weight:
FGF = 3 × (1000 + [100 × kg body weight])
>30 kg body weight:
FGF = 3 × (2000 + [50 × body weight])

CONTROLLED VENTILATION

10-30 kg body weight:
FGF = 1000 mL + 100 mL/kg
>30 kg body weight:
FGF = 2000 mL + 50 mL/kg

From Rose DK, Byrick RJ, Froese AB: Carbon dioxide elimination during spontaneous ventilation with a modified Mapleson D system: studies in a lung model, *Can Anaesth Soc J* 1978;25:353-365.

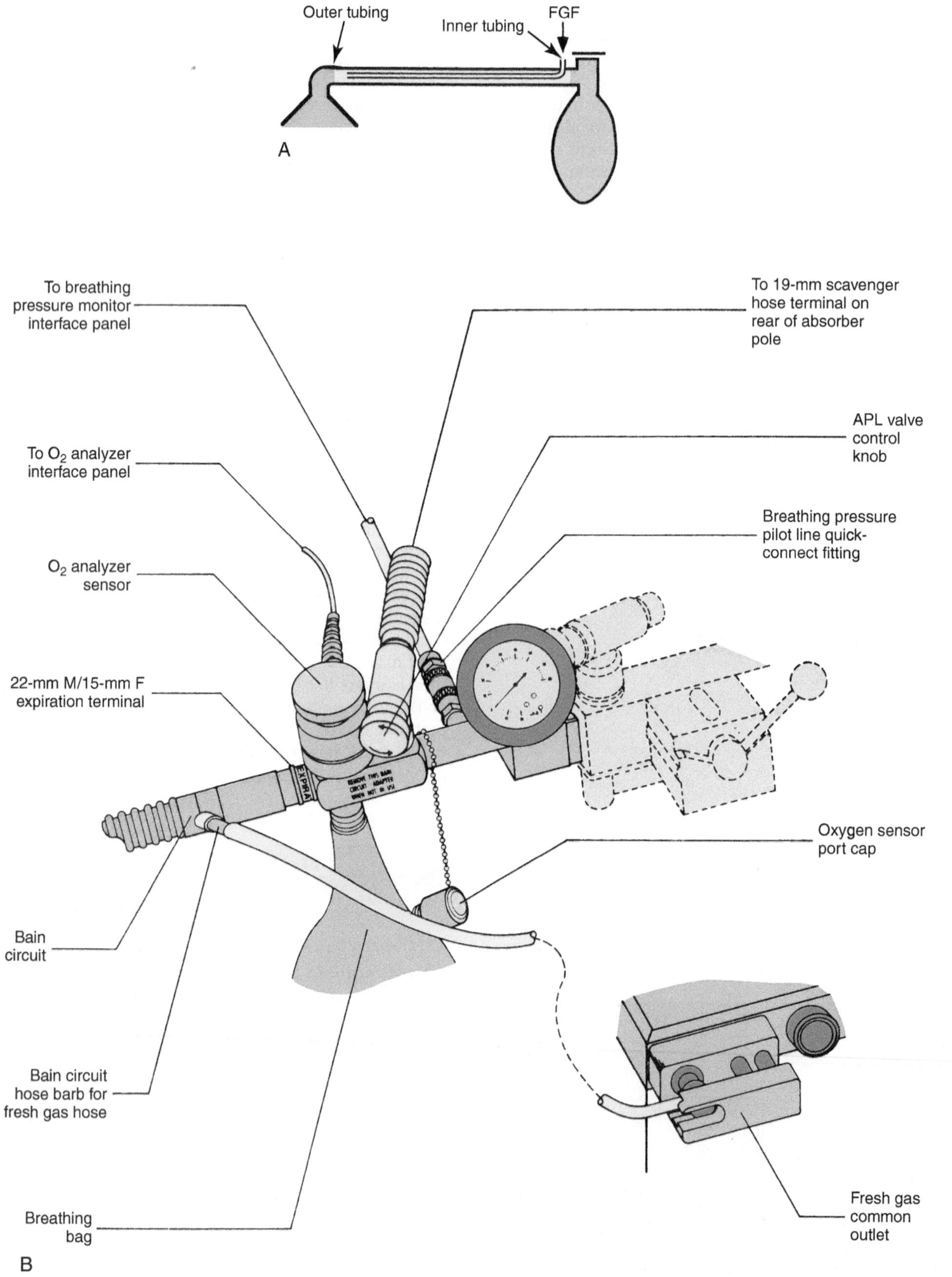

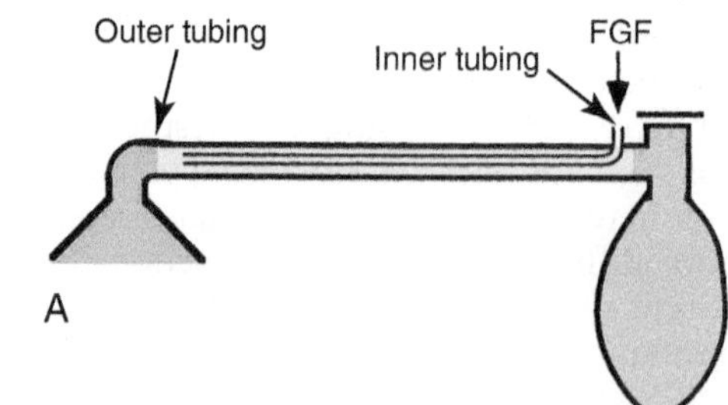

FIGURE 17-7 ■ **A,** The Bain modification of the Mapleson D circuit. **B,** A Bain circuit adapter, which incorporates a bag mount, pressure gauge, adjustable pressure limiting (*APL*) valve, and a 19-mm scavenging connector. (Courtesy Dräger Medical, Telford, PA.)

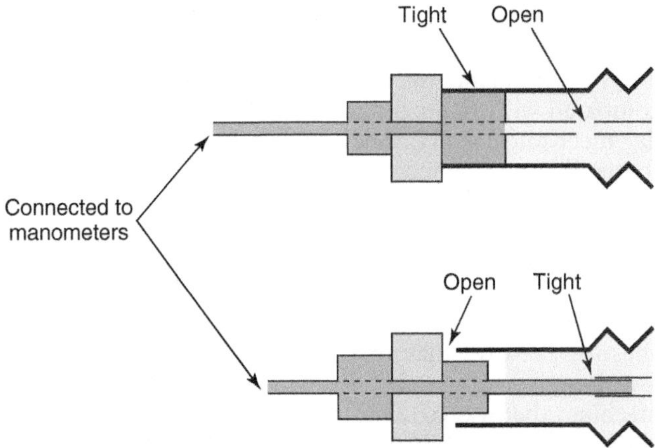

FIGURE 17-8 ▪ Bain circuit test adapter. One end of the device is connected to a manometer and a sphygmomanometer bulb to allow inflation and pressure measurement. The other end is inserted into the patient end of the Bain circuit. The specific calibers and lengths of the components of this device allow it to be inserted in one of two ways. In the top illustration, by occluding the outer lumen of the Bain circuit, the integrity of the entire circuit is determined. If the device is removed, reversed, and reinserted, the inner inspiratory limb can be isolated from the outer expiratory limb, and its integrity may be determined separately. (Modified from Berge JA, Gramstad L, Budd E: Safety testing the Bain circuit: a new test adaptor. *Eur J Anaesthesiol* 1991;8:309.)

system caused by disconnection of the central coaxial tubing can occur with a coaxial circuit used with a circle system.[45]

There has been substantial investigation of the functional characteristics of Mapleson circuits.[46] The near uniform use of capnography during anesthesia has greatly changed the clinical use of these systems and has largely supplanted previous work. Based on the capnogram, FGF can be adjusted as needed to ensure appropriate levels of rebreathing of exhaled gases.

Summary of Mapleson D and F Circuit Properties

The Mapleson D and F circuits are simple, lightweight, and have low resistance and dead space. Some means of humidification is necessary because of the high FGFs required by these circuits. Fresh gases entering the circuit can be passed through a heated humidifier, or a heat and moisture exchanger (HME) can be placed between the circuit and the tracheal tube. Despite the high FGFs required by these circuits, several scavenging systems have been found to be effective for both controlled and spontaneous ventilation.[47] However, in larger patients, the clinician may prefer to use a Mapleson A or circle system during spontaneous ventilation. (Most newborns and small infants will not be breathing spontaneously while anesthetized for prolonged periods.) During spontaneous ventilation in infants and children, it is probably advisable to avoid rebreathing, in view of their unpredictable response to the increased work of breathing. During controlled ventilation, a certain amount of rebreathing is acceptable and may even be advantageous. Capnometry allows the monitoring of inspired carbon dioxide to detect rebreathing and has improved the anesthesiologist's ability to accurately adjust FGFs when using these circuits.

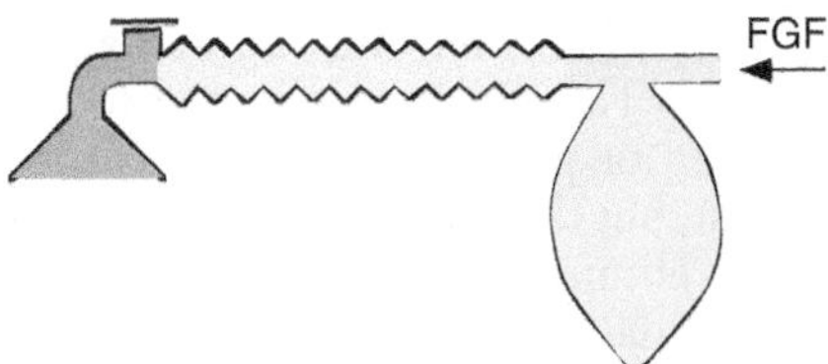

FIGURE 17-9 ▪ The Mapleson A (Magill) circuit. *FGF,* fresh gas flow.

Mapleson A (Magill) Circuit

The Mapleson A (Magill) circuit has the advantage of economy of FGF when used for the spontaneously breathing patient (Fig. 17-9). However, when used for controlled ventilation, this advantage is lost, and a Mapleson D or circle system is a better choice. For anything but the shortest duration of controlled ventilation, there are more appropriate alternatives to this system.

Circle Systems

The circle system is the most commonly used breathing circuit in the United States. Its main advantages are those of economy of anesthetic gas use, decreased environmental pollution, and conservation of heat and moisture. However, early experiences with the use of adult circle systems to anesthetize small children resulted in respiratory compromise in spontaneously breathing patients.[48] High resistances of the valves, tubing, and soda lime and a relatively large apparatus dead space were the factors that led to early recommendations that the circle system not be used for children younger than 6 years.[49] Since that time, developments in circuit design have led to the introduction of circle systems with smaller canister and tubing volumes, decreased compliance, and lower resistance valves and connectors. In contrast to the earlier experiences, recent clinical experience in pediatric patients has been extremely favorable. Compared with the Mapleson D or F circuit, the circle is more economical, offers better heat and moisture conservation, and is easier to scavenge.[3] Although the resistance of circle systems has been found to be slightly higher than or similar to that of a Mapleson D or F system, it does not appear to significantly affect the minute ventilation or blood gas homeostasis of spontaneously breathing infants.[50] To add some clinical perspective, the resistance to breathing of a circle system is significantly less than that of a size 3 or 3.5 mm tracheal tube. Hence, circle circuits appear to be acceptable for short-term spontaneous ventilation for healthy older infants.

Factors that Affect Delivered Tidal Volume

Several factors can make the patient's actual delivered tidal volume differ significantly from that delivered into the circuit by the ventilator. These include compressible volume, tracheal tube leak, and augmentation of tidal volume by FGF. The volume delivered to the patient may be less than or greater than that expected by the anesthesiologist, but the importance of these factors can be reduced or eliminated using available technology. The use of end-tidal capnography provides a continuous monitor of ventilation with or without technology to address compressible volume and augmentation of tidal volume.

Compressible Volume

When a ventilator bellows delivers a tidal volume into a breathing circuit, a portion of that volume will not enter the patient's lungs. This wasted ventilation is partly due to the compressible (compression) volume.[51] The compressible volume is that volume loss attributable to the compliance of the circuit and the compression of the gases within the circuit. The loss of delivered volume as a result of distention of the circuit is a function of the circuit volume, circuit compliance, and peak inflation pressure. Disposable plastic circuits are more distensible than wire-reinforced circuits, and the nondisposable rubber circle system is more distensible than a nondisposable Mapleson D circuit.[3] Breathing circuits can expand both in diameter and length when internally pressurized. The ventilator itself may also contribute to the compressible volume. An adult ventilator bellows usually has a significantly larger compressible volume than a pediatric bellows (4.5 mL/cm H_2O vs. 1 to 2.5 mL/cm H_2O).[52] Volume loss as a result of compression of gases is a separate entity from that resulting from circuit distention and is purely a function of circuit volume and peak inflation pressure. Volume loss because of gas compression is significantly increased by including a humidifier chamber in the circuit.

Endotracheal Tube Leaks

The presence of a leak around the tracheal tube results in volume loss during inhalation and exhalation whenever the airway pressure is greater than the leak pressure of the tracheal tube. Maintaining constant minute ventilation in the presence of a variable tracheal tube leak can be difficult. In this situation, pressure-preset ventilation has some advantages (see also Chapter 6). An alternative approach is to use a cuffed tube, provided that the leak pressure is carefully adjusted and monitored as appropriate.

Tidal Volume Augmentation by Fresh Gas Flow

Depending on the type of anesthetic breathing system in use and its FGF requirements, the tidal volume delivered by a ventilator can be significantly augmented by continuous fresh gas inflow from the anesthesia machine.[53,54] For example, when the FGF is 5 L/min and the inspiratory time is 0.6 seconds, the delivered tidal volume will be augmented by 50 mL (5000 mL/60 sec × 0.6 sec). The practical implication is that alterations in FGF may produce a change in tidal volume that may not be reflected by a change in the ventilator bellows displacement.[55]

The compliance of circle systems can be substantial compared with the compliance of smaller patients. Earlier mechanical ventilators used for the delivery of anesthesia did not compensate for the circuit compliance. In addition, the FGF could affect delivered volumes. Consequently, these earlier ventilators were problematic for use with smaller patients.

More recent anesthesia ventilators address many of the factors that influenced delivered tidal volumes during anesthesia.[56] Investigation of anesthesia ventilators using test lungs demonstrates that more recent anesthesia machines that use ventilators that compensate for circuit compliance and FGF deliver very predictable tidal volumes, even with simulated lung compliances consistent with preterm infants.[57,58] In contrast, older technology that does not compensate for these factors is considerably less accurate in volume delivery.

Compliance compensation and fresh gas decoupling are important advances for anesthesia ventilators. These and other changes, such as improved flow measurement, have eliminated many of the problems earlier generation anesthesia ventilators presented for use with pediatric patients. With these advances, delivered volumes are much more predictable and reliable. Current anesthesia ventilators offer additional forms of supported and controlled ventilation. As with any device, a good understanding of the operation of the ventilators is important for optimal utilization of the capabilities of the machines for clinical application.

Monitoring Ventilation

Adequacy of oxygenation and adequacy of carbon dioxide elimination are the most important endpoints to monitor during controlled ventilation. Tidal volumes, peak inflating pressures, gas delivery patterns, pressure-volume loops, markers of spontaneous respiratory effort, and capnography provide guides to assessing the appropriateness of patient ventilation.

Miscellaneous Aspects of Mechanical Ventilation

Positive End-Expiratory Pressure

During general anesthesia, several factors may decrease the patient's functional residual capacity (FRC; Box 17-5). This drop in FRC can lead to airway closure, ventilation/perfusion (V/Q) mismatch, and hypoxemia.[59] It has been demonstrated that the application of 5 cm H_2O positive end-expiratory pressure (PEEP) can partially restore FRC and increase oxygenation.[60,61] If PEEP is applied, airway pressure should be carefully monitored to allow the detection of excessive airway pressure. Ideally, airway pressure should be monitored as close to the tracheal tube as possible. In practice, airway pressure is usually monitored in the expiratory limb of the circuit. Of note, the application of PEEP may decrease the tidal volume delivered depending on the design of the ventilator.[62] More recent anesthesia

BOX 17-5 Factors that Decrease Functional Residual Capacity in Infants During the Perioperative Period

Decreased intercostal muscle tone
Loss of diaphragmatic muscle tone
Abolition of glottic tone/absence of PEEP
Apnea during induction

PEEP, positive end-expiratory pressure.

ventilators include electronically applied PEEP, which is intended to prevent inaccurate, improper, or unintended PEEP.[56]

Practical Hints for Ventilating Neonates and Infants

Although the healthy newborn has a normal spontaneous respiratory rate of approximately 40 breaths/min, in practice, most healthy newborns who undergo anesthesia are adequately ventilated at somewhat lower respiratory rates, such as 20 to 30 breaths/min.[63]

Some of the factors that determine the adequacy of mechanical ventilation of the neonate have been modeled mathematically.[48] Although these data were derived several decades ago and modern anesthesia systems have since evolved significantly, the authors' conclusions remain pertinent. The anesthesia circuit, ventilator bellows (if present), and humidifiers all have significant compliance. During inspiration a portion of the total flow delivered by the ventilator (Qt) is expended in distending the circuit (Qc), thus the inspiratory flow to the patient (Qp) will be reduced accordingly (Qt = Qc + Qp; Fig. 17-10). This explains in part why very small infants can be ventilated safely with ventilators that have minimum inspiratory flows that greatly exceed those of a spontaneously breathing infant.

The disparity between Qp and Qt is greatest at the start of inspiration, when the circuit pressure is low, and the circuit is most compliant. During the latter portion of the inspiration (after 360 ms), as the circuit becomes pressurized and less compliant, Qp approximates Qt (Qp/Qt = 0.9). Thus, as inspiratory time is prolonged, there may be a disproportionate increase in tidal volume. Conversely, if the inspiratory time is short, Qp will be small in relation to Qt for most of the inspiratory period. To complicate matters, at rapid respiratory rates, shorter inspiratory times (500 ms) may be necessary to allow sufficient time for exhalation. Therefore, when rapid ventilatory rates are used with short inspiratory times, significantly higher inspiratory flows and pressures may be required to ventilate the patient effectively. At lower respiratory rates with longer inspiratory times, a proportionately larger increase in the duration of the later, more effective period of inspiration occurs, and lower inspiratory flows may be sufficient. This may explain the apparently paradoxic deterioration in gas exchange occasionally observed in small infants when they are ventilated at rapid respiratory rates and the inspiratory time is shortened.

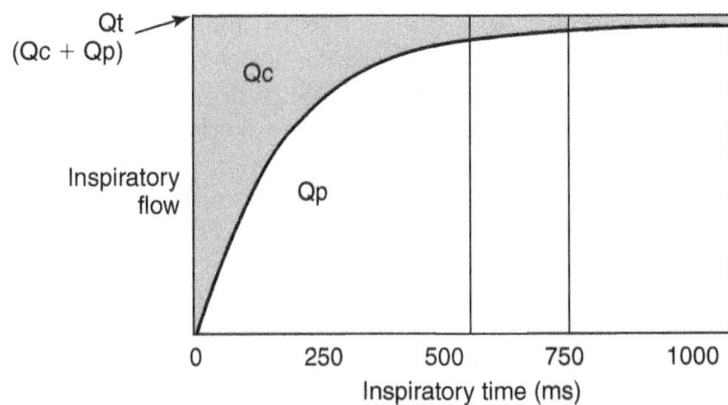

FIGURE 17-10 ■ A schematic of the inspiratory flow pattern during constant flow ventilation. The total flow from the ventilator (*Qt*) is constant throughout inspiration. The proportion of flow spent in distending the anesthesia circuit (*Qc*) is large at the start of inspiration and decreases as inspiration continues. Thus longer inspiratory times may be more effective when the circuit compliance is high compared with that of the patient because the early part of inspiration is spent distending the circuit. *Qp,* inspiratory flow to the patient. (Modified from Epstein MAF, Epstein RA: Airway flow patterns during mechanical ventilation of infants: a mathematical model. *IEEE Trans Biomed Eng* 1979:26:299-306.)

Manual Versus Mechanical Ventilation of Neonates and Infants

In the past it was often recommended that the neonate or small infant be ventilated by hand rather than mechanically.[64] A potential advantage of manual ventilation is that it allows the rapid detection of changes in respiratory compliance by the "educated hand" of the pediatric anesthesiologist. Historically, manual ventilation was used because of the lack of both reliable respiratory monitoring and ventilators suitable for neonates. However, with the advent of pulse oximetry, capnography, routine monitoring of airway pressure, and reliable OR ventilators, the arguments for manual ventilation are now less compelling. Objective data suggest that even experienced pediatric anesthesiologists are unable to consistently detect significant changes in respiratory compliance (e.g., complete occlusion of the tracheal tube).[65] Under ideal circumstances, experienced pediatric anesthesiologists (8 years) could detect complete ETT occlusion 83% of the time versus 64% for their less experienced colleagues (<2 years).[66] Less dramatic changes in compliance and resistance than those that went undetected in these studies would probably produce clinically significant adverse changes in ventilation and oxygenation. Compliant reservoir bags combined with the relatively large compressible volume of many pediatric breathing circuits (compared with the neonate's small tidal volume) will make manual detection of changes in the patient's resistance and compliance unpredictable, particularly when higher FGFs are used (e.g., 6 L/min). Mechanical ventilation produces more consistent ventilation and frees the anesthesiologist's hands to perform other essential tasks. The argument that the large compressible volume of the breathing circuit makes mechanical ventilation unpredictable in the neonate applies equally to manual ventilation of the neonate.[67,68] When using volume-preset mechanical ventilation, the volume delivered to the circuit is constant. Although changes in the patient's compliance may change the tidal volume delivered to the patient, changes in tidal volume should be accompanied by changes in airway pressure, thus enabling the detection of changes in the patient's compliance. Manual ventilation has no advantage over mechanical ventilation for the detection of changes in the patient's compliance, provided that mechanical ventilation is accompanied by continuous measurement of airway pressure, chest excursion, breath sounds, oxygen saturation, and end-tidal carbon dioxide concentration. However, in the case of acute adverse changes in respiratory function, it is still usual to revert to manual ventilation of the patient to confirm adequate lung inflation and allow breath-to-breath adjustment of ventilation.

Summary of Mechanical Ventilation of Infants and Children During Anesthesia

Most *healthy* children can be ventilated adequately with ventilators primarily designed for adults, provided they are used with appropriate respiratory monitoring. These adult devices have the advantage of being familiar to most anesthesiologists, and their operating characteristics are well understood. These devices are safest when used with age-appropriate, low-compliance/low-volume breathing circuits and when capnometry, oximetry, airway pressure, exhaled tidal volume, and auscultation of breath sounds are used to monitor ventilation. Although both pressure-limited ventilation and volume-controlled ventilation can be used safely, the operator should be aware that variable tube leaks, tube obstructions, and changes in pulmonary compliance and resistance may have differing presentations and effects depending on the mode of ventilation. Appropriately sized and adjusted cuffed tracheal tubes, along with anesthesia machines and ventilators that compensate for FGF and circuit compliance, eliminate many of these concerns and provide highly predictable volume ventilation for infants and older pediatric patients. Ventilators specifically designed for neonates, infants, and children are available that can be used in the OR (Fig. 17-11).

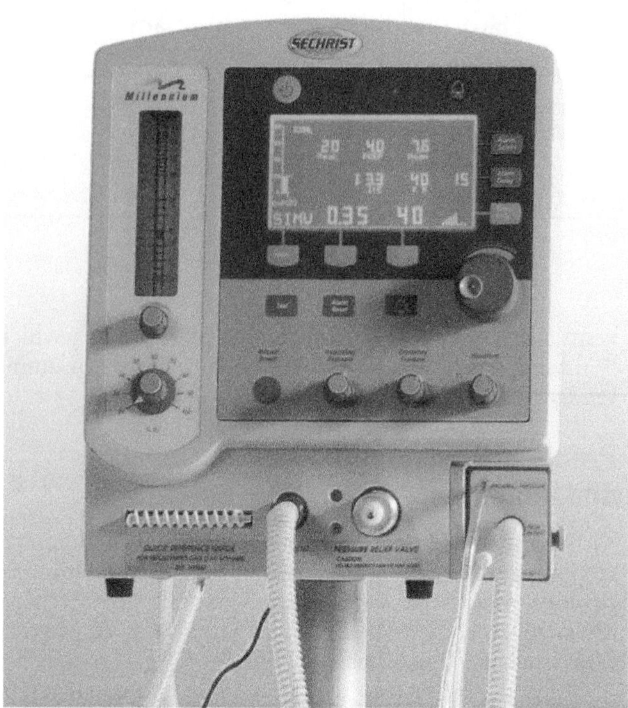

FIGURE 17-11 ■ The Sechrist Millennium neonatal/infant/pediatric ventilator. The ventilator can operate in the SIMV/IMV, Assist-Control, and back-up ventilation continuous positive airway pressure modes. IMV, intermittent mechanical ventilation; SIMV, synchronized intermittent mechanical ventilation. (Courtesy Sechrist Industries, Anaheim, CA.)

High-Frequency Oscillatory Ventilation

Although high-frequency oscillatory ventilation (HFOV) is an established therapy in the neonatal and pediatric intensive care units (ICUs), the perioperative use of HFOV is less well described. As the complexity and number of procedures performed in sicker and smaller neonates increase, anesthesiologists will be even more exposed to patients who require this mode of ventilation. Perhaps the most common scenario is the neonate who is already receiving HFOV prior to patent ductus arteriosus ligation or exploratory laparotomy for necrotizing enterocolitis. However, anesthesiologists may occasionally encounter critically ill neonates who are receiving conventional ventilation, in whom HFOV represents a viable elective option for perioperative ventilation. Importantly, HFOV also represents an invaluable intraoperative rescue strategy that might be considered in certain circumstances.

The most important issues relating to the perioperative use of HFOV include the anesthesiologist's relative unfamiliarity with this technology, the inability to monitor end-tidal carbon dioxide or to deliver volatile agents, and the inability to transport patients while delivering HFOV. Furthermore, it is possible that the neonate who requires HFOV is too sick to transport to the OR. Under these circumstances, the anesthesiologist will be working in the relatively unfamiliar environment of the neonatal intensive care unit (NICU).

On the other hand, although formal data are lacking, it is often the anesthesiologist's experience when HFOV is used during thoracotomy for patent ductus arteriosus ligation that lung retraction appears to be relatively well tolerated, with less interference from ventilation with surgical exposure. Indeed, some anesthesiologists advocate the elective conversion to HFOV prior to this procedure.[69] The use of HFOV has been reported during congenital diaphragmatic hernia repair, necrotizing enterocolitis, excision of pulmonary bullae, and surgery for congenital cystic adenomatoid malformations.[70-72] The assistance of the neonatologist and the respiratory therapist can be helpful in adjusting HFOV settings and troubleshooting. A total IV anesthetic must be used, typically with an opioid-based technique. Because accurate end-tidal carbon dioxide measurement is not possible, transcutaneous or blood gas monitoring of carbon dioxide is needed. If the neonate requires transport prior to surgery and is already on HFOV, it is useful to test his or her ability to tolerate short periods of manual ventilation prior to leaving the NICU.

An in-depth discussion of HFOV weaning and adjustment strategies is beyond the scope of this chapter. However, the basic approach includes adjustment of the fraction of inspired oxygen (FiO_2) and mean airway pressure to optimize oxygenation and manipulation of amplitude, usually referred to as ΔP, and optimizing inspiratory time to achieve the desired carbon dioxide elimination. A commonly monitored parameter of ventilation is the presence of abdominothoracic oscillation. Optimum alveolar recruitment is achieved when lung expansion to 8.5 to 9 ribs is observed on routine chest radiograph.

HUMIDIFICATION

The safe and precise function of the components of a modern anesthesia machine requires a supply of clean, dry anesthetic gases. However, the inhalation of dry, cold gases is suboptimal for the patient, and minimum levels of temperature and humidification have been recommended.[73] The humidification of inspired gases is of particular importance during anesthesia in infants and children (see also Chapter 7). Available approaches include the active humidification of inspired gases, the use of HMEs, and minimizing FGF. Unfortunately, all have limitations in clinical applicability.

Beneficial Effects of Humidification

Beneficial effects of humidification include the reduction of heat and water loss from the respiratory tract, the prevention of airway damage, and the prevention of inspissation of secretions that could cause tracheal tube obstruction.

Reduction of Heat and Water Loss from the Respiratory Tract

During the course of normal breathing, cold, dry atmospheric air is inhaled, warmed to body temperature, and saturated with water vapor by the time it reaches the distal bronchi. Air fully saturated with water vapor at 37° C contains 44 mg/L of water (absolute humidity 44 mg/L, relative humidity 100%). To humidify inhaled gases, heat and water vapor are transferred from the mucosal lining of the airway. Under normal circumstances, most of the heat and water is returned to the respiratory mucosa during exhalation. If the upper airway is bypassed by a tracheal tube, significant heat and water loss will occur from the patient if inspired gases are not humidified. Because of the very low specific heat and thermal capacity of dry gas, it is difficult to provide sufficient energy to the patient to prevent intraoperative hypothermia without causing thermal injury to the airway. A 3-kg infant with a minute ventilation of 500 mL/min will expend 0.0035 kcal/min to raise the temperature of cold, dry inspired gases to body temperature. However, if in addition, another 0.012 kcal/min are required for the heat of vaporization to saturate the dry inspired gases with water vapor at body temperature,[74] the total amount of energy expended will be 0.015 kcal/min. This amounts to approximately 10% to 20% of the total energy expenditure of the infant.

Prevention of Respiratory Tract Mucociliary Dysfunction

The inhalation of dry gases causes ciliary paralysis and decreases mucus flow, thus impeding mucociliary transport.[75] Decreased humidity causes the viscosity of mucus to increase markedly, and greater than 50% relative humidity is required to allow continued flow of mucus.[76] Humidification of inspired gases may reduce the incidence of postoperative pulmonary complications in adults,[77] although similar data in pediatric patients are lacking.

Prevention of Tracheal Tube Obstruction

Given the small internal diameter of pediatric tracheal tubes, even a small amount of inspissated mucus within the lumen of the tube may produce significant airway obstruction. A small premature infant may require a 2.5-mm ID tracheal tube. These small patients have very little respiratory reserve and would be expected to benefit the most from humidification of inspired gases.

Methods of Providing Humidification in Pediatric Systems

Several methods are available to reduce heat and water loss from the airway during anesthesia. Even the tracheal tube itself may act as a low-efficiency passive HME, as the moisture in exhaled gases condenses within the tube and is then added to the inspired gas mixture. In the absence of either active or passive humidification, measurements of humidity at the distal end of the tube demonstrate that the tracheal tube alone will produce an inspired relative humidity of 30% at its distal end.[78] However, this is less than the 50% relative humidity reported to be necessary to allow normal mucus flow.

Humidifiers in common use are either active, adding exogenous heat and water to the breathing system, or passive, conserving and allowing the rebreathing of the patient's endogenous heat and moisture. Alternatively, the use of a circle system with low FGF will generate heat and humidity that can be inhaled by the patient. Each method of humidification has its specific advantages and disadvantages.

Passive Humidification

The simplest method of humidification is passive humidification, using an HME, although HMEs do not add heat or water to the inspired gas other than that exhaled by the patient in the preceding breaths. These devices are placed between the tracheal tube and the breathing system. The HME contains an exchange medium with a large surface area, and its ability to humidify inspired gas is highly dependent on the ambient conditions. When breathing room air (at 20° C with 50% relative humidity and 7 mg H_2O/L absolute humidity), HMEs can produce a relative humidity of almost 100% in the inspired gas; however, when breathing cold, dry anesthetic gases (0 to 20° C, 0% relative humidity), the inspired gas relative humidity may be as low as 60% at 37° C. Improvements in the design of these devices have increased their efficiency.

Concerns about the use of these devices in pediatric anesthesia practice relate to the issues of dead space, resistance, and efficiency. Several HMEs have been developed specifically for use in infants (Fig. 17-12). The characteristics of one such device, the Mini Humid-Vent (Teleflex Medical, Research Triangle Park, NC) have been measured.[79] Although the device has a dead space of 4.2 mL when measured in isolation, when added to the circuit, its dead space decreases to 2.7 mL because of the volume occupied by the circuit and tracheal tube connectors. The dead space is likely to be small in relation to the tidal volume (50 mL) of the pediatric patient, for whom this device is recommended. The resistance of the device at gas flows between 2 and 10 L/min approximates that of a 5.0-mm tracheal tube. At a gas flow of 10 L/min, the pressure drop across a 3.0-mm tracheal tube was increased from 9.6 cm H_2O to 10.4 cm H_2O by the addition of an HME. The resistance to flow across the HME was increased by 10% to 30% when humidified air was compared with dry air.

In contrast, Rodee and colleagues[80] determined that the increased work of breathing imposed by some HMEs is significant. The Mini Humid-Vent was found to increase the work of breathing by up to 60% when dry, and even more when saturated. Investigation of the effect of a ClearTherm HME (ClearTherm Limited, Leicester, UK) found a 43% increase in the work of breathing.[81] Those authors suggest that the HME be removed from the circuit during spontaneous ventilation. Bissonnette and colleagues[82] compared the performance of an HME with that of active humidification in ventilated anesthetized children weighing between 5 and 30 kg and found that although passive humidification was less efficient than active humidification, it was significantly better than no humidification. Although the relative humidity of inspired gases with passive humidification was initially only 50%, after 80 minutes of anesthesia, the relative humidity of the inspired gases had increased to a level (80%) that was not significantly different from that of active humidification (90%). Passive humidification effectively reduced the mean temperature drop that occurred during surgery, from 0.75° C to 0.25° C. An investigation of two other HMEs concluded that the devices conserved airway humidity well but did not achieve desired levels of heat and humidity.[83]

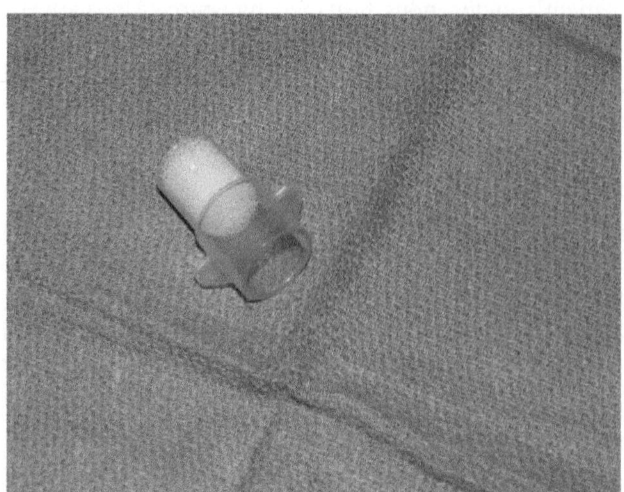

FIGURE 17-12 ■ A low dead space, high-efficiency pediatric heat and moisture exchanger (Breathe Easy; Vital Signs, Totowa, NJ).

HMEs can be effective in reducing heat loss during the perioperative period. Devices are manufactured whose resistance and dead space can be acceptable, especially considering that most infants and children undergoing surgery for an appreciable length of time will be ventilated rather than being allowed to breathe spontaneously. The humidification efficiency of HMEs is predicted to be decreased in the presence of a large leak around the tracheal tube because a variable proportion of the exhaled, heat- and moisture-rich gas will bypass the HME.

Active Humidification

Active humidification prevents energy and water loss from the respiratory tract. The temperature of the inspired gases is continuously monitored to avoid hyperthermia or thermal injury to the respiratory tract. Although active humidification may be more efficient than passive humidification, it is more cumbersome and costly. The presence of the humidifier chamber in the breathing system adds significant compressible volume to the circuit. The potential for circuit disconnection is increased because of the additional connections required for both the humidifier chamber and the temperature-monitoring equipment. Other potential hazards of humidifiers, particularly with ultrasonic nebulization, include overhydration and increased airway resistance. Ultrasonic nebulization adds small droplets (1 to 10 μm diameter) of unheated water to the airway in the form of an aerosol. Molecular humidification, such as with a heated water bath or HME, simply adds molecular water vapor to the airway (see also Chapters 7 and 26).

Active humidification using a heated water system has the advantages of being applicable to patients of all sizes, being highly efficient, and avoiding the problems of dead space and resistance encountered with HMEs. It has the disadvantages of additional compressive volume, higher cost, and increased circuit complexity. Thus active humidification can be used safely during both controlled and spontaneous ventilation.

Minimizing FGF reduces the amount of gas that must be humidified for optimal delivery. Although reducing the amount of FGF improves the level of humidification, the approach is inadequate in infants in the absence of active humidification and/or heat and moisture exchange.[84]

CAPNOGRAPHY AND RESPIRATORY GAS ANALYSIS IN PEDIATRIC PATIENTS

Capnography is vitally important in the monitoring of ventilation during anesthesia (see also Chapter 10). Capnography is also used to confirm tracheal tube placement and to aid in the diagnosis of critical events that occur during anesthesia, including venous air embolism and malignant hyperthermia; however, it is important to be aware of the technical limitations in obtaining accurate capnometric data from small children (Table 17-4). Capnometers can be divided broadly into two groups, *mainstream* (flow-through) devices and *sidestream* (aspirating) devices (see also Chapter 8). Sidestream devices are more commonly used in the OR.

The accuracy of sidestream devices in pediatric patients, defined in this context as the degree to which end-tidal carbon dioxide tensions approximate arterial carbon dioxide tensions, has been investigated by several groups. Several factors appear to be important.

Gas Sampling Site

The site of gas sampling from the breathing circuit appears to be important in patients weighing less than 12 kg.[85] When gas is sampled from the distal end of the tracheal tube with a sampling catheter, the accuracy of measurement was considerably improved over measurements made at the tracheal tube circuit connector (proximal sampling). On the other hand, distal versus proximal sampling may not affect the accuracy of measurement when a nonrebreathing circuit and ventilator with no fresh gas blowby is used, such as a Servo 900C system (Siemens, Munich, Germany).[86] Gas need not be sampled from the distal tip of the tracheal tube but may be sampled with similar accuracy from the point of narrowing of the tracheal tube adapter (Fig. 17-13).[87]

Breathing System

When the Mapleson D circuit is used, end-tidal values are often decreased compared with arterial values. The relatively high FGF required in these circuits dilutes the end-expired carbon dioxide, thereby artifactually lowering the end-tidal CO_2 reading. However, this "dilutional" effect is attenuated when certain ventilators are used, such as the Sechrist Infant Ventilator (Sechrist, Anaheim, CA).[88]

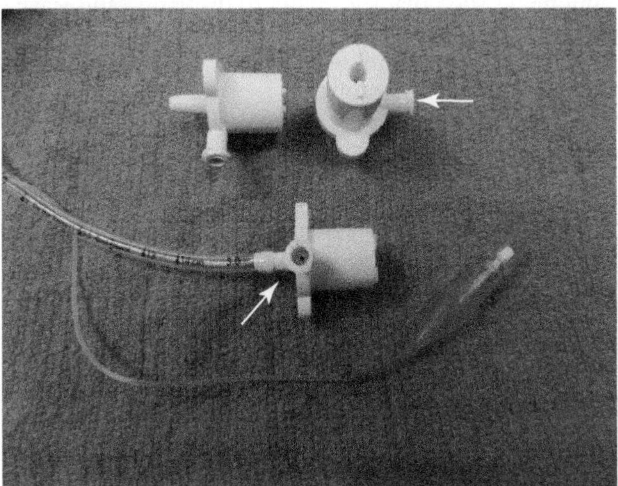

FIGURE 17-13 ■ A low dead space tracheal tube connector with a gas sampling port (*arrows*).

TABLE 17-4 **Techniques to Improve Accuracy of End-Tidal Carbon Dioxide Monitoring in Infants and Children**

Technique	Advantage	Disadvantage
Distal sampling	Decreases dilution by FGF	Requires special sampling port (purchased or made)
Cuffed tube (absence of leak)	Decreases dilution by ambient air in oropharynx	Requires careful management to avoid tracheal injury
Sechrist ventilator*	Uses low FGF (250 mL/min) and simulates a nonrebreathing system by Venturi effect on respiration	Not commonly used in the operating room
Circle system	Valves isolate FGF to minimize dilution of sample	Valves increase work of breathing in infants who are spontaneously ventilating
Low FGF	Decreases dilution of expired sample	May increase rebreathing in a Mapleson D or Bain system
Lower sampling rates	Minimizes dilution by FGF	Decreases accuracy by increasing lag time and reducing response time, especially at rapid respiratory rates and low tidal volumes (does not record true CO_2 peak)
Long I:E ratios (1:3.5)	Prevents rebreathing	Probably not significant
Controlled ventilation	Increases tidal volume relative to FGF	Prevents weaning from mechanical ventilation
Discontinuation of FGF during sampling	Prevents dilution of sample	Interrupts normal ventilation
Mainstream capnometer	Prevents plugging of the sampling catheter with secretions or humidity, decreases response time; minimally affected by FGF	Adds dead space and weight; patient must be tracheally intubated

*Sechrist Industries, Anaheim, CA.

FGF, fresh gas flow; *I:E,* inspiratory/expiratory.

Modified from Dubose R: Pediatric equipment and monitoring. In Bell C, Hughes C, Oh T, editors: *The pediatric anesthesia handbook.* St. Louis, 1991, Mosby–Year Book.

Mainstream Versus Sidestream Analysis

When mainstream capnometers have been compared with sidestream analyzers in children, they were found to be as accurate as distally sampling sidestream analyzers and considerably more accurate than proximally sampling sidestream analyzers.[89] The sampling rate of sidestream capnometers affects their accuracy. High gas sampling rates (>250 mL/min) exaggerate the dilution effect by entraining fresh gas and diluting expired carbon dioxide. On the other hand, low sampling rates (<100 mL/min) can prolong the response time of the capnometer such that the ability to display a valid waveform at rapid respiratory rates is lost.[90] Badgwell and colleagues[91] have examined the effect of ventilation at rapid respiratory rates on the capnographic waveform and demonstrated significant artifactual elevation of the sidestream baseline attributable in part to longitudinal mixing of gas within the sampling line. No artifactual elevation was observed in flow-through capnograph waveform baselines. This study utilized multiplexed mass-spectrometer gas analysis with a sampling line that was approximately 50 m long. The authors predict that artifactual elevation of the baseline waveform would be less when using stand-alone sidestream monitors with shorter sampling lines.

Patient Factors

In general, the accuracy of sidestream measurements is reduced when used with small infants and in the presence of lung disease. With many neonatal lung diseases, measurements of end-tidal carbon dioxide do not accurately reflect arterial carbon dioxide.[92] Also, patients with cyanotic heart disease who have reduced pulmonary blood flow or mixing lesions also tend to have reduced end-tidal carbon dioxide values compared with arterial measurements.[93] Furthermore, for capnometry to be useful even as a monitor of trend in those patients, the arterial/end-tidal carbon dioxide difference must remain constant. Unfortunately, patients with cyanotic heart disease may have variations in shunt fraction, pulmonary blood flow, and dead space/tidal volume ratios during anesthesia and surgery. These variations will produce a variable arterial/end-tidal carbon dioxide difference, thereby reducing the utility of capnometry, even as a monitor of trend.

Although expired carbon dioxide monitoring may not always accurately reflect arterial carbon dioxide tension in children, it does appear to be very useful as a trend monitor in patients without cyanotic heart disease. Capnometry will continue to have a vital role in maintaining the safety of pediatric anesthesia.

MONITORING

Blood Pressure Determination

Periodic blood pressure determination is an essential part of monitoring during anesthesia,[94] and a variety of techniques and equipment are available to achieve this (see also Chapter 12).[95,96] All noninvasive forms of blood pressure determination depend in part on a snugly fitting cuff that contains an air-filled bladder that can be inflated to controlled pressures. The American Heart Association has developed recommendations for indirect blood pressure determination, including those for cuff sizes.[95] The width of the inflatable bladder of the cuff should be 0.4 times the circumference of the extremity, and its length should be at least twice its width to cover at least 80% of the extremity circumference. Cuffs that are too narrow will result in an overestimation of the blood pressure, and cuffs that are too wide will underestimate the blood pressure.[97,98] Given the same degree of mismatch, cuffs that are somewhat too wide will result in less error than cuffs that are too narrow.[99] As a result, a series of blood pressure cuffs of various sizes must be available for the accurate, noninvasive determination of blood pressure in pediatric patients.

Ultrasound Detection of Arterial Flow

Doppler ultrasound detection of arterial flow is a useful method of determining systolic blood pressure even in small infants.[100] One commonly used unit made by Parks Medical Electronics (Aloha, OR) is battery powered and has an ultrasonic detector and an emitter capable of identifying arterial blood flow and converting it into an audible sound; the return of arterial flow with the onset of systole is easily recognized and correlates well with both auscultatory assessment and intraarterial pressure measurement.[100,101]

Ultrasonic blood pressure determination has several advantages: it can be used even in hypovolemic patients, does not require a regular heart rate, and provides a method of beat-to-beat confirmation of cardiac contraction. Once the monitor has been positioned and secured, a blood pressure determination can be obtained rapidly with minimal effort. However, it has two primary limitations: it results in additional room noise and requires operator action to obtain each value.

Automated Noninvasive Systems

Most automated, noninvasive systems that measure blood pressure use an oscillometric method,[102] which uses a rapid inflation of the blood pressure cuff, until the artery is occluded, followed by incremental reductions in cuff pressure. As arterial blood flow resumes, oscillations in the cuff pressure occur, indicating systole. Maximal oscillations appear to correlate with mean arterial pressure, and dampening of the oscillations indicates diastole.

Noninvasive blood pressure devices that use an oscillometric method are available from several manufacturers. The Dinamap unit (Device for Indirect Noninvasive Automated Mean Arterial Pressure, GE Healthcare, Waukesha, WI) was the first commercially available oscillometric device and has been investigated in a variety of clinical settings.[96,102-107] Oscillometric devices provide a safe, easy method of periodic automated blood pressure determination in pediatric patients, including neonates, although accuracy may decrease in severely ill patients. The method does require several heartbeats to determine the blood pressure value. As a result, it cannot be applied when beat-to-beat information is needed, and it may fail when the heart rhythm is irregular.

Whatever method is used to determine the blood pressure, the value must be compared with the expected values for a patient of that age. Various tables of normal values are available in standard texts and other sources.[95,108-111]

Electrocardiographic Monitoring

The electrocardiogram (ECG) is an excellent noninvasive monitor of heart rate and rhythm (see also Chapter 13). Apart from sinus bradycardia and tachycardia, rhythm changes are not common in pediatric patients. Premature atrial and ventricular contractions, junctional rhythms, and respiratory variations are seen on occasion. Rhythm changes in pediatric patients generally relate to some aspect of the ventilatory, metabolic, anesthetic, or surgical management rather than to a primary cardiac event. They can generally be identified using standard limb lead electrode positions, although special leads may be helpful in some instances.[112]

Although the ECG is a very useful monitor of heart rate and rhythm, it can continue to be normal even in the presence of moderate to severe circulatory or ventilatory abnormalities. Indeed, the ECG can appear normal, at least briefly, without systemic perfusion. As a result, additional monitors must be used to supplement the ECG to assess the adequacy of systemic perfusion.

Pediatric ECG monitoring requires equipment capable of processing higher frequency signals.[113] At a minimum, the equipment must be able to identify individual heartbeats and provide accurate rate analysis. Normal values for QRS amplitudes can vary depending on the frequency of sampling in digitized systems because slower sampling frequencies may miss the peak QRS amplitudes.[114]

Although myocardial ischemia is a rare event during uncomplicated pediatric anesthesia, it can occur in some circumstances.[115] Kawasaki disease is an acute exanthematous condition usually seen in infants and children younger than 5 years.[116] The illness is associated with coronary artery aneurysms in 20% to 25% of patients. These aneurysms generally resolve over time, but the lesions may become stenotic. Cardiac ischemia is well recognized in these patients, and appropriate ECG monitoring is indicated perioperatively.[117] Other pediatric clinical situations in which cardiac ischemia may occur include surgery involving the coronary arteries, congenital coronary artery abnormalities, and systemic air embolism.

Pulse Oximetry

Hypoxemia is a major concern during any anesthesia procedure. Its incidence is increased during anesthesia administered to children aged 2 years and younger.[118] Pulse oximetry provides a reliable method to detect hypoxemia prior to the time it is detected clinically (see also Chapter 11).[119] Although pulse oximetry values may change several seconds after the arterial saturation changes,[120] it is sufficiently rapid to detect changes in oxygen saturation as needed in clinical practice.

Pulse oximetry is applicable to all pediatric patients, including neonates.[121,122] The probes must allow the emitter and detector portions of the probe to face each other across some pulsatile bed, and careful attention to probe placement is essential. Oximetry during anesthesia induction and emergence can also be difficult, because the probes may displace or dislodge with the patient's movements. Fetal hemoglobin (HbF) does not affect pulse oximetry but does have an oxyhemoglobin dissociation curve to the left of normal adult hemoglobin.[123] Common sources of inaccurate pulse oximetry values (SpO_2) are summarized in Table 17-5.

Unlike adult patients, hyperoxia is of concern in neonates with immature retinas because elevations in arterial oxygen tension are associated with the development of retinopathy of prematurity. The upper limit of desirable oxygenation varies from infant to infant depending on a variety of factors that include postconceptual age and the clinical stability of the infant. In infants with a patent ductus arteriosus, the pulse oximetry probe should be located at a site that indicates preductal saturation; this value will reflect the oxygenation state of blood supplying the brain and retina.[124] The range of oxygen saturation of concern in hyperoxia occupies the flat portion of the oxyhemoglobin dissociation curve, where large changes in oxygen tension occur with small changes in hemoglobin saturation. Typical safe limits for SpO_2 for the stable preterm infant are 85% to 93%.[123] Preterm infants born at 24 to 27 weeks' gestation have improved survival when managed with SpO_2 of 91% to 95% compared with 85% to 89%.[125] A single best range has not been established.[123] Nonetheless, pulse oximetry is a valuable aid to the anesthesiologist caring for any patient, particularly the neonate, infant, and young child.

Tissue Oximetry

Tissue oximetry offers a noninvasive method to monitor areas of body perfusion.[126,127] It uses near-infrared spectroscopy (NIRS) to assess tissue oxygenation.[128] Both cerebral and somatic monitoring can provide the clinician with important information regarding patient condition,[126,129] and multiple products are available from different manufacturers for this purpose. Technologic approaches to better address the infant patient have been introduced or are in process from multiple manufacturers.[126] NIRS has been used as a routine monitor perioperative status of infants following stage 1 palliation of univentricular congenital heart disease.[130] The role of NIRS in optimizing patient management continues to evolve.[131-132]

Temperature Monitoring and Maintenance

The normal human tightly regulates body temperature within a narrow range using defense mechanisms that prevent both hypothermia and hyperthermia.[133] These defense mechanisms are more effective in adults compared with children, children compared with infants, and less premature infants compared with more premature infants. General anesthesia broadens the range of body temperature that must be reached before homeostatic

TABLE 17-5 **Common Sources of Inaccurate Saturations Obtained by Pulse Oximetry (SpO_2)**

Type of Interference	Cause	Solution
Excessive ambient light	Operating room light	Cover sensor with opaque material, such as a blanket or foil
	Bilirubin lights Bright fluorescent lights Infrared heating lamps Sunlight Xenon surgical lamps	
Optical shunt	Too large a sensor; lets light reach the sensor without passing through a pulsatile bed	Sensor must be completely adherent to skin and must be of the appropriate size
Optical cross-talk	Multiple sensors too close to one another	Cover each sensor with opaque material or use separate sensors (one per extremity)
Movement artifact	Shivering Active child	ECG pulse rate must correlate with that displayed by the oximeter before credence can be given to the oximeter SpO_2 reading Move the probe to a more central location (ear vs. finger) Change the oximeter mode to a longer average time.
Absorption of light by nonhemoglobin sources	Nail polish Intravenous dye Bilirubin	Remove nail polish Verify readings with laboratory CO-oximetry
Electrical interference	Usually caused by electrocautery; can be affected by 60 Hz interference	60-cycle interference may be improved by changing the plug to another outlet Some machines have a built-in mechanism to decrease interference by cautery
Low perfusion	Cold extremities Decreased cardiac output Peripheral vasoconstriction	Warm extremities Use inotropic agents or vasodilators Use a more central location for probe site (tongue or ear)
Active venous bed	Right heart failure Tricuspid regurgitation	Use an oximeter with a visual display of plethysmograph waveform to help interpretation
Altered hemoglobin	Hemoglobin F: oximeter remains in the range of acceptable accuracy Hemoglobin S: possibly accurate if oxygenated; probably very inaccurate in crises Methoglobin: R = 1.0, SpO_2 = 85% Carboxyhemoglobin: Falsely elevated SpO_2	Verify readings of laboratory CO-oximetry

CO, carbon monoxide; ECG, electrocardiograph.
Modified from Dubose R: Pediatric equipment and monitoring. In Bell C, Hughes C, Oh T, editors: *The pediatric anesthesia handbook.* St Louis, 1991, Mosby–Year Book.

mechanisms become active.[134] Mild to moderate degrees of intraoperative hypothermia are common because of factors that include altered temperature homeostasis, cool environments, exposed skin surface, administration of cool fluids, increased evaporative losses, and redistribution of heat.[135] Mild to moderate degrees of hypothermia can adversely affect outcome measures such as shivering, infection, platelet function and bleeding, cardiac events, drug metabolism, and PACU discharge time.[136-138]

The American Society of Anesthesiologists Monitoring Standards state that intraoperative temperature monitoring is indicated whenever a clinically significant change in body temperature is intended, anticipated, or suspected.[94] In combination with the limited ability of the infant and young child to maintain normothermia during anesthesia, this strongly suggests that body temperature should be measured for the majority of young infants and in most pediatric patients undergoing anesthesia.

The approaches generally used to maintain the body temperature of nonanesthetized young infants—clothing, blankets, and heated and humidified enclosures—often cannot be applied in the OR setting. Warmed ORs can be used, but the degree of warmth necessary to maintain body temperature generally makes working conditions uncomfortable, particularly when wearing surgical gowns. Radiant warmers and the use of heated, humidified anesthetic gases can reduce heat loss to a limited degree.

Fluid warmers are useful in maintaining body temperature, particularly during procedures in which large volumes of either room temperature or 4° C blood or blood products are administered.[139] However, at low fluid

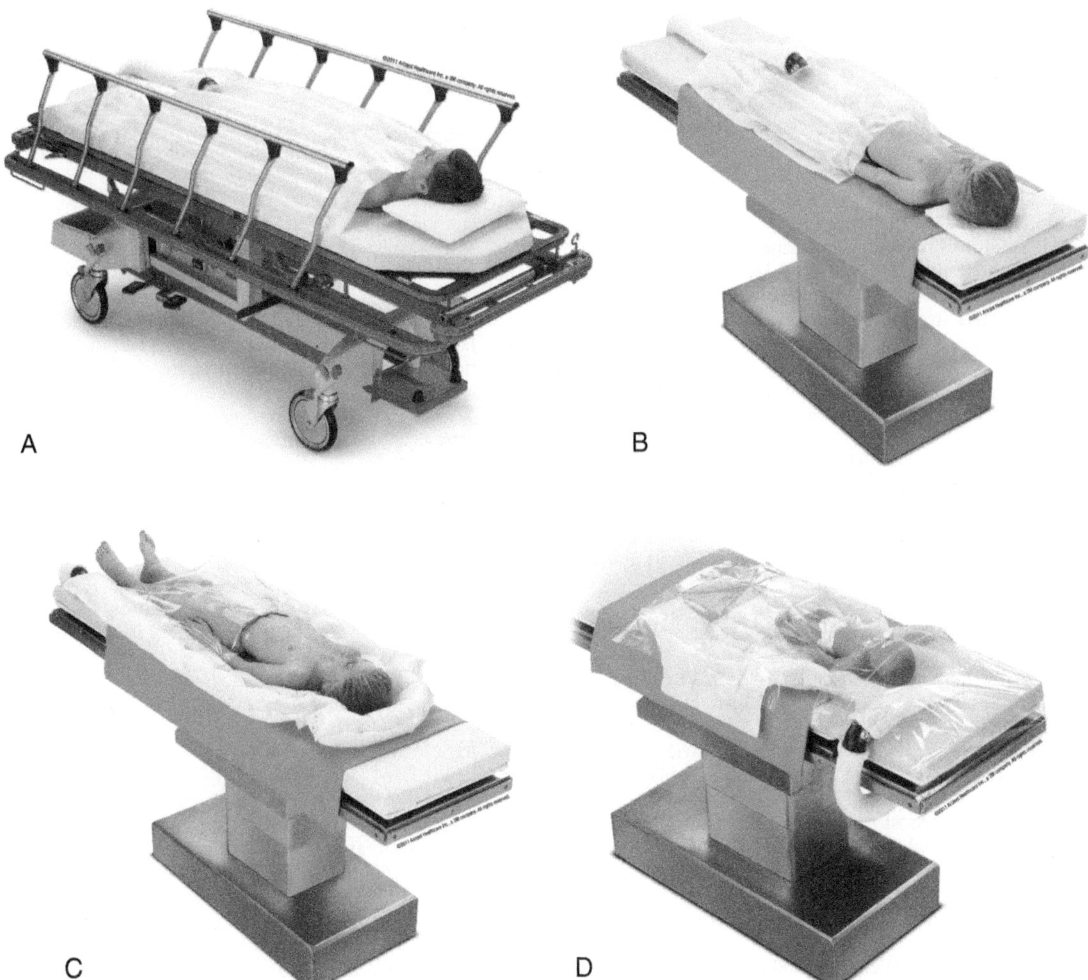

FIGURE 17-14 ■ Examples of forced-air convective warming blankets for pediatric use. **A,** Whole-body blanket. **B,** Lower body blanket. **C,** Child under-body blanket. **D,** Infant underbody body blanket. (Courtesy Arizant Inc. [now 3M], Eden Prairie, MN.)

administration rates, warmed IV fluid tends to cool before reaching the patient. The Hotline fluid warming system (Smiths Medical, St. Paul, MN) uses a water-jacketed administration set able to deliver warm fluid to the end of the administration set at low and high flow rates more effectively than conventional dry warmers. This is advantageous with infants and young children, in whom the absolute rate of fluid administration is low, but the proportionate fluid administration rate to the patient is high.

In contrast to approaches of reducing heat loss, forced-air warmers can effectively add heat to patients. These warmers are manufactured with a variety of air dispersal products, allowing their adaptation for a variety of surgical procedures and patient sizes (Fig. 17-14).[140-142]

ULTRASONOGRAPHY

The term *ultrasound* refers to frequencies above the range of human hearing. For clinical application, frequencies between 2 and 15 MHz are typically used. An inverse relationship exists between the ability to identify smaller structures and the depth of penetration of ultrasound beams. Consequently, two or three probes with different frequencies provide both resolution of small superficial structures and penetration for deeper, larger structures. A good understanding of the basics of ultrasound and ultrasonography and of the appearance of structures with ultrasound are important to utilization of the technique in clinical practice,[143] and ultrasonography is entering the curriculum of many medical schools.[144]

Since 2000, ultrasound equipment has become more portable and less expensive with greater capabilities. It has wide application across specialties in areas of procedural guidance, diagnosis, and screening.[145] In anesthesiology, applications include vascular imaging and access, regional anesthesia, echocardiography, limited trauma examination, and assessment of bladder volume.[146] Appropriate training, education, and experience, including the development of hand skills, is important to the clinical utilization of ultrasonography.[146,147] Ultrasound-guided vascular cannulation and regional anesthesia have become widely adopted in pediatric anesthesia.[148-152]

REFERENCES

1. James RH: 1000 anaesthetic incidents: experience to date, *Anaesthesia* 58:856–863, 2003.
2. Jimenez N, Posner KL, Cheney FW, et al: An update on pediatric anesthesia liability: a closed claims analysis, *Anesth Analg* 104:147–153, 2007.
3. Rasch DK, Bunegin L, Ledbetter J, et al: Comparison of circle absorber and Jackson-Rees systems for paediatric anaesthesia, *Can J Anaesth* 35:25–30, 1988.
4. Byrick RJ: Respiratory compensation during spontaneous ventilation with the Bain circuit, *Can Anaes Soc J* 27:96–105, 1980.
5. Olsson AK, Lindhal SGE: Pulmonary ventilation, CO_2 response and inspiratory drive in spontaneously breathing young infants during halothane anaesthesia, *Acta Anaesthesiol Scand* 30:431–437, 1986.
6. Charlton AJ, Lindhal SGE, Hatch DJ: Ventilatory responses of children to changes in dead space volume, *Br J Anaesth* 57:562–568, 1985.
7. Keens TG, Bryan AC, Levison H, et al: Developmental patterns of muscle fiber types in human ventilatory muscles, *J Appl Physiol* 44:909–913, 1978.
8. Scott CB, Nickerson BG, Sargent CW, et al: Developmental pattern of maximal transdiaphragmatic pressure in infants during crying, *Pediatr Res* 17:707–709, 1983.
9. Fisher DM: Anesthesia equipment for pediatrics. In Gregory GA, editor: *Pediatric anesthesia*, New York, 1990, Churchill Livingstone, p 470.
10. Litman RS, Weissend EE, Shibata D, Westesson PL: Developmental changes of laryngeal dimensions in unparalyzed, sedated children, *Anesth Analg* 98:41–45, 2003.
11. Dalal PG, Murray D, Messner AH, et al: Pediatric laryngeal dimensions: an age-based analysis, *Anesth Analg* 108:1475–1479, 2009.
12. Motoyama EK: The shape of the pediatric larynx: cylindrical or funnel shaped? *Anesth Analg* 108:1379–1381, 2009.
13. Lerman J: Gas flow in the upper airway: turbulent or laminar? *Pediatr Anesth* 19:1241, 2009.
14. Adewale L: Anatomy and assessment of the pediatric airway, *Pediatr Anesth* 19(Suppl 1):1–8, 2009.
15. Dullenkopf A, Gerber AC, Weiss M: Fit and seal characteristics of a new paediatric tracheal tube with high volume–low pressure polyurethane cuff, *Acta Anaesthesiol Scand* 49:232–237, 2005.
16. Koka BV, Jeon IS, Andre JM, et al: Post intubation croup in children, *Anesth Analg* 56:501–505, 1977.
17. Cohen MM, Cameron CB: Should you cancel the operation when a child has an upper respiratory tract infection? *Anesth Analg* 72:282–288, 1991.
18. Goel SA, Lim SL: The intubation depth marker: the confusion of the black line, *Paediatr Anaesth* 13:579–583, 2003.
19. Ring WH, Adair JC, Elwyn RA: A new pediatric endotracheal tube, *Anesth Analg* 54:273–274, 1975.
20. Black AE, Mackersie AM: Accidental bronchial intubation with RAE tubes, *Anaesthesia* 46:42–43, 1991.
21. Kohjitani A, Iwase Y, Sugiyama K: Sizes and depths of endotracheal tubes for cleft lip and palate children undergoing primary cheiloplasty and palatoplasty, *Paediatr Anaesth* 18:845–851, 2008.
22. Sugiyama K, Shimomatsu K, Kohjitani A: Lengths of preformed pediatric orotracheal tubes for children with cleft palate, *Pediatr Anesth* 19:640–641, 2009.
23. Campo SL, Denman WT: The laryngeal mask airway: its role in the difficult airway, *Int Anesthesiol Clin* 38:29–45, 2000.
24. Walker RWM, Ellwood J: The management of difficult intubation in children, *Paediatr Anaesth* 19(Suppl 1):77–87, 2009.
25. Dierdorf SF: Education in the use of the laryngeal mask airway, *Int Anesthesiol Clin* 36:19–28, 1998.
26. Ghai B, Wig J: Comparison of different techniques of laryngeal mask placement, *Curr Opin Anaesthesiol* 22:400–404, 2009.
27. Yun MJ, Hwang JW, Park SH, et al: The 90° rotation technique improves the ease of insertion of the ProSeal laryngeal mask airway in children, *Can J Anesth* 58:379–383, 2011.
28. Kol IO, Egilmez H, Kaygusuz K, et al: Open-label, prospective, randomized comparison of propofol and sevoflurane for laryngeal mask anesthesia for magnetic resonance imaging in pediatric patients, *Clin Ther* 30:175–181, 2008.
29. Park HJ, Lee JR, Kim CS, et al: Remifentanil halves the EC50 of propofol for successful insertion of the laryngeal mask airway and laryngeal tube in pediatric patients, *Anesth Analg* 105:57–61, 2007.
30. Baker PA, Brunette KEJ, Byrnes CA, Thompson J: A prospective randomized trial comparing supraglottic airways for flexible bronchoscopy in children, *Pediatr Anesth* 20:831–838, 2010.
31. Maurtua MA, Finnegan PS, DeBoer G: The use of the CTrach™ laryngeal mask airway in pediatric patients: a retrospective review of 25 cases, *Can J Anaesth* 58:409–410, 2011.
32. Jagannathan N, Sohn LE, Mankoo R, et al: Prospective evaluation of the self-pressurized air-Q intubating laryngeal airway in children, *Pediatr Anesth* 21:673–680, 2011.
33. Jagannathan N, Kozlowski RJ, Sohn LE, et al: A clinical evaluation of the intubating laryngeal airway as a conduit for tracheal intubation in children, *Anesth Analg* 112:176–182, 2011.
34. Theiler LG, Kleine-Brueggeney M, Luepold B, et al: Performance of the pediatric-sized I-Gel compared with the Ambu AuraOnce laryngeal mask in anesthetized and ventilated children, *Anesthesiology* 115:102–110, 2011.
35. Beylacq L, Bordes M, Semjen F, Cros AM: The I-Gel, a single-use supraglottic airway device with a non-inflatable cuff and an esophageal vent: an observational study in children, *Acta Anaesthiol Scand* 53:376–379, 2009.
36. VanderWalt J: Oxygen—elixir of life or Trojan horse? Part 1: oxygen and neonatal resuscitation, *Paediatr Anaesth* 16:1107–1111, 2006.
37. VanderWalt J: Oxygen—elixir of life or Trojan horse? Part 2: oxygen and neonatal anesthesia, *Paediatr Anesth* 16:1205–1212, 2006.
38. Ayre P: Anaesthesia for intracranial operation: a new technique, *Lancet* 1:561–563, 1937.
39. Rees GJ: Anaesthesia in the newborn, *Br Med J* 1:1419, 1950.
40. Rose DK, Byrick RJ, Froese AB: Carbon dioxide elimination during spontaneous ventilation with a modified Mapleson D system: studies in a lung model, *Can Anaesth Soc J* 25:353–365, 1978.
41. Bain JA, Spoerel WE: A streamlined anaesthetic system, *Can Anaesth Soc J* 19:426–435, 1972.
42. Hannallah R, Rosales JK: A hazard connected with the use of the Bain circuit: a case report, *Can Anaesth Soc J* 21:511–513, 1974.
43. Pethick SL: (Letter to the editor), *Can Anaesth Soc J* 22:115, 1975.
44. Berge JA, Gramstad L, Bodd E: Safety testing the Bain circuit: a new test adaptor, *Eur J Anaesthesiol* 8:309–310, 1991.
45. De Armendi AJ, Mayhew JF, Cure JA: Another cause of hypercapnia during induction of anesthesia, *Pediatr Anes* 20:1055, 2010.
46. Hillier SC, McNiece WL: Pediatric anesthesia systems and equipment. In Ehrenwerth J, Eisenkraft JB, editors: *Anesthesia equipment: principles and applications*, St. Louis, 1993, Mosby, pp 537–564.
47. Hatch DJ, Miles R, Wagstaff M: An anaesthetic scavenging system for paediatric and adult use, *Anaesthesia* 35:496–499, 1980.
48. Adriani J, Griggs T: Rebreathing in pediatric anesthesia: recommendations and descriptions of improvements in apparatus, *Anesthesiology* 14:337–347, 1953.
49. Stephen CR, Slater HM: Agents and techniques employed in pediatric anesthesia, *Anesth Analg* 20:254, 1950.
50. Conterato JP, Lindahl SGE, Meyer DM, et al: Assessment of spontaneous ventilation in anesthetized children with use of a pediatric circle or a Jackson-Rees system, *Anesth Analg* 69:484–490, 1989.
51. Coté CJ, Petkau AJ, Ryan JF, et al: Wasted ventilation measured with eight anesthetic circuits with and without inline humidification, *Anesthesiology* 59:442–446, 1983.
52. Binda RE, Cook DR, Fischer CG: Advantages of infant ventilators over adapted adult ventilators in pediatrics, *Anesth Analg* 55:769–772, 1976.
53. Ghani GA: Fresh gas flow affects minute volume during mechanical ventilation. (letter), *Anesth Analg* 63:619, 1984.
54. Scheller MS, Jones BL, Benumof JL: The influence of fresh gas flow and I: E ratio on tidal volume and arterial PCO_2 in mechanically ventilated surgical patients, *J Cardiothorac Anesth* 3:564–567, 1989.
55. Aldrete JA, Castillo RA, Bradley EL: Changes in fresh gas flow affect the tidal volume delivered by anesthesia ventilators [abstract], *Anesth Analg* 65:S4, 1986.

56. Stayer S, Olutoye O: Anesthesia ventilators: better options for children, *Anesthesiol Clin North Am* 23:677–691, 2005.
57. Bachiller PR, McDonough JM, Feldman JM: Do new anesthesia ventilators deliver small tidal volumes accurately during volume-controlled ventilation? *Anesth Analg* 106:1392–1400, 2008.
58. Hjalmarson O, Sandberg K: Abnormal lung function in healthy preterm infants, *Am J Respir Crit Care Med* 165:83–87, 2002.
59. Mansell A, Bryan C, Levison H: Airway closure in children, *J Appl Physiol* 33:711–714, 1972.
60. Katayama M, Motoyama EK: Respiratory mechanics in children under general anesthesia with and without PEEP., *Anesthesiology* 61:A514, 1984, (abstract).
61. Motoyama EK, Brinkmeyer SD, Mutich RL, et al: Reduced FRC in anesthetized children: effects of low PEEP, *Anesthesiology* 57:A418, 1983, (abstract).
62. Mukkada TJ, Khathiwada S, Fernandez J, et al: Effect of positive end expiratory pressure on tidal volume, *Anesthesiology* 69:A269, 1988. (abstract).
63. Epstein MAF, Epstein RA: Airway flow patterns during mechanical ventilation of infants: a mathematical model, *IEEE Trans Biomed Eng* 26:299–306, 1979.
64. Steward DJ: Pediatric anesthetic techniques and procedures. In Steward DJ, editor: *Manual of pediatric anesthesia*, ed 2, New York, 1985, Churchill Livingstone, p 59.
65. Spears RS, Yeh A, Fisher DM, et al: The "educated hand": can anesthesiologists assess changes in neonatal pulmonary compliance manually? *Anesthesiology* 75:693–696, 1991.
66. Schily M, Koumoukelis H, Lerman J, et al: Can pediatric anesthesiologists detect an occluded endotracheal tube in neonates? *Anesth Analg* 93:66–70, 2001.
67. Picca SM: Mechanical versus manual ventilation of the lungs of infants in the operating room [letter], *Anesthesiology* 76:479, 1992.
68. Steward DJ: (Letter), *Anesthesiology* 76:479, 1992.
69. Tobias JD, Burd RS: Anesthetic management and high frequency oscillatory ventilation, *Pediatr Anesth* 11:483–487, 2001.
70. Miguet D, Claris O, Lapillonne A, et al: Preoperative stabilization using high-frequency oscillatory ventilation in the management of congenital diaphragmatic hernia, *Crit Care Med* 22:S77–S82, 1994.
71. Ratzenhofer-Komenda B, Prause G, Offner A, et al: Intraoperative application of high frequency ventilation on thoracic surgery, *Acta Anaesth Scand Supp* 109:149–153, 1996.
72. Aubin P, Vischoff D, Haig M, et al: Management of an infant with diffuse bullous pulmonary lesions using high-frequency oscillatory ventilation, *Can J Anaesth* 46:970–974, 1999.
73. Brock-Utne JG: Humidification in paediatric anaesthesia, *Pediatr Anesth* 10:117–119, 2000.
74. Ryan JF, Vacanti FX: Temperature regulation. In Ryan JF, Todres ID, Coté CJ, editors: *A practice of anesthesia for infants and children*, Orlando, 1986, Grune & Stratton, pp 19–23.
75. Dalham T: Mucous flow and ciliary activity in the trachea of rats and rats exposed to respiratory irritant gases, *Acta Physiol Scand* 123:36, 1956.
76. Forbes AR: Humidification and mucous flow in the intubated trachea, *Br J Anaesth* 45:118, 1973.
77. Chalon J, Patel C, Ali M, et al: Humidity and the anesthetized patient, *Anesthesiology* 50:195–198, 1979.
78. Bissonnette B, Sessler DI, LaFlamme P: Passive and active inspired gas humidification in infants and children, *Anesthesiology* 71:350–354, 1989.
79. Jones BR, Ozaki GT, Benumof JL, et al: Airway resistance caused by a pediatric heat and moisture exchanger, *Anesthesiology* 69:A786, 1988 (abstract).
80. Rodee WD, Banner MJ, Gravenstein N: Variation in imposed work of breathing with heat and moisture exchangers, *Anesth Analg* 72:S226, 1991, (abstract).
81. Bell GT, Martin KM, Beaton S: Work of breathing in anesthetized infants increases when a breathing system filter is used, *Pediatr Anesth* 16:939–943, 2006.
82. Bissonnette B, Sessler DI: Passive or active inspired gas humidification increases thermal steady state temperatures in anesthetized infants, *Anesth Analg* 69:783–787, 1989.
83. Luchetti M, Pigna A, Gentili A, Marraro G: Evaluation of the efficiency of heat and moisture exchangers during paediatric anaesthesia, *Pediatr Anesth* 9:39–45, 1999.
84. Hunter T, Lerman J, Bissonnette B: The temperature and humidity of inspired gases in infants using a pediatric circle system: effects of high- and low-flow anesthesia, *Pediatr Anesth* 15:750–754, 2005.
85. Badgwell JM, McLeod ME, Lerman J, et al: End-tidal pCO_2 measurements sampled at the distal and proximal ends of the endotracheal tube in children, *Anesth Analg* 66:959–964, 1987.
86. Badgwell JM, Heavner JE, May WS, et al: End-tidal pCO_2 monitoring in infants and children ventilated with either a partial-rebreathing or a non-rebreathing circuit, *Anesthesiology* 66:405–410, 1987.
87. Halpern L, Bissonnette B: A new endotracheal tube connector for sampling end-tidal CO_2 in infants, *Anesthesiology* 75:A930, 1991 (abstract).
88. Hillier SC, Badgwell JM, McLeod ME, et al: Accuracy of end-tidal measurements using a sidestream capnometer in infants and children ventilated with the Sechrist infant ventilator, *Can J Anaesth* 37:318–321, 1990.
89. Gravenstein N: Capnometry in infants should not be done at lower sampling flow rates, *J Clin Monit* 5:63–64, 1989.
90. Hillier SC, Lerman J: Mainstream vs. sidestream capnography in anesthetized infants and children, *Anesthesiology* 71:A357, 1989 (abstract).
91. Badgwell JM, Kleinman SE, Heavner JE: Respiratory frequency and artifact affect the capnographic baseline in infants, *Anesth Analg* 77:708–712, 1993.
92. McEvedy BAB, McLeod ME, Mulera M, et al: End-tidal, transcutaneous, and arterial pCO_2 measurements in critically ill neonates: a comparative study, *Anesthesiology* 69:112–116, 1988.
93. Burrows FA: Physiologic dead space, venous admixture, and the arterial to end-tidal carbon dioxide difference in infants and children undergoing cardiac surgery, *Anesthesiology* 70:219–225, 1989.
94. American Society of Anesthesiologists [ASA]: *Standards for basic anesthetic monitoring*, Approved by the ASA House of Delegates on October 21, 1986, as last amended October 20, 2010. Accessed 2012 Feb 11 from http://www.asahq.org/For-Members/Standards-Guidelines-and-Statements.aspx.
95. Pickering TG, Hall JE, Appel LJ, et al: Recommendations for blood pressure measurement in humans and experimental animals. Part 1. Blood pressure measurement in humans: a statement for professionals from the Subcommittee of Professional and Public Education of the American Heart Association Council on High Blood Pressure Research, *Hypertension* 45:142–161, 2005.
96. Roguin A: Scipione Rova-Rocci and the men behind the mercury sphygmomanometer, *Int J Clin Pract* 60:73–79, 2006.
97. Kimble KJ, Darnall RA Jr, Yelderman M, et al: An automated oscillometric technique for estimating mean arterial pressure in critically ill newborns, *Anesthesiology* 54:423–425, 1981.
98. Okahata S, Kamiya T: Influencing factors on indirect measurement of blood pressure in children, *Jpn Circ J* 51:1400–1403, 1987.
99. Geddes LA, Whistler SJ: The error in indirect blood pressure measurement with the incorrect size of cuff, *Am Heart J* 96:4–8, 1978.
100. Gordon LS, Johnson PR Jr, Penido JR, et al: Systolic and diastolic blood pressure measurements by transcutaneous Doppler ultrasound in premature infants in critical care nurseries and at closed-heart surgery, *Anesth Analg* 53:914–918, 1974.
101. Reder RF, Dimich I, Cohen ML, et al: Evaluating indirect blood pressure measurement techniques: a comparison of three systems in infants and children, *Pediatrics* 62:326–330, 1978.
102. Ramsey M: Blood pressure monitoring: automated oscillometric devices, *J Clin Monit* 7:56–67, 1991.
103. Dellagrammaticas HD, Wilson AJ: Clinical evaluation of the Dinamap non-invasive blood pressure monitor in pre-term neonates, *Clin Phys Physiol Meas* 2:271–276, 1979.
104. Friesen RH, Lichtor JL: Indirect measurement of blood pressure in neonates and infants utilizing an automatic noninvasive oscillometric monitor, *Anesth Analg* 60:742–745, 1981.
105. Park MK, Menard SM: Normative oscillometric blood pressure values in the first 5 years in an office setting, *Am J Dis Child* 143:860–864, 1989.
106. Wong SN, Sung RYZ, Leung LCK: Validation of three oscillometric blood pressure devices against auscultatory mercury sphygmomanometer in children, *Blood Press Monit* 11:281–291, 2006.

107. Chiolero A, Paradis G, Lambert M: Accuracy of oscillometric devices in children and adults, *Blood Press* 19:254–259, 2010.
108. The Fourth Report on the Diagnosis, Evaluation, and Treatment of High Blood Pressure in Children and Adolescents. U.S. Department of Health and Human Services. NIH Publication No. 05-5267, revised May 2005.
109. Nielsen PE, Clausen LR, Olsen CA, et al: Blood pressure measurement in childhood and adolescence: international recommendations and normal limits of blood pressure, *Scand J Clin Lab Invest Suppl* 192:7–12, 1989.
110. Kent AL, Kecskes Z, Shadbolt B, et al: Blood pressure in the first year of life in healthy infants born at term, *Pediatr Nephrol* 22:1743–1749, 2007.
111. Nafiu OO, Voepel-Lewis T, Morris M, et al: How do pediatric anesthesiologists define intraoperative hypotension? *Paediatr Anaesth* 19:1048–1053, 2009.
112. Greeley WP, Kates RA, Bushman GA, et al: Intraoperative esophageal electrocardiography for dysrhythmia analysis and therapy in pediatric cardiac surgical patients, *Anesthesiology* 65:669–672, 1986.
113. Weinfurt PT: Electrocardiographic monitoring: an overview, *J Clin Monit* 6:132–138, 1990.
114. Macfarlane PA, Coleman EN, Pomphrey EO, et al: Normal limits of the high-fidelity pediatric ECG, *J Electrocardiol* 22(Supp l): 162–168, 1989.
115. Bell C, Rimar S, Barash P: Intraoperative ST-segment changes consistent with myocardial ischemia in the neonate: a report of three cases, *Anesthesiology* 71:601–604, 1989.
116. Wood LE, Tullor RMR: Kawasaki disease in children, *Heart* 95:787–792, 2009.
117. McNiece WL, Krishna G: Kawasaki disease: a disease with anesthetic implications, *Anesthesiology* 58:269–271, 1983.
118. Coté CJ, Goldstein EA, Coté MA, et al: A single-blind study of pulse oximetry in children, *Anesthesiology* 68:184–188, 1988.
119. Coté CJ, Rolf N, Liu LMP, et al: A single-blind study of combined pulse oximetry and capnography in children, *Anesthesiology* 74:980–987, 1991.
120. Severinghaus JW, Naifeh KH: Accuracy of response of six pulse oximeters to profound hypoxia, *Anesthesiology* 67:551–558, 1987.
121. Deckardt R, Steward DJ: Noninvasive arterial hemoglobin oxygen saturation versus transcutaneous oxygen tension monitoring in the preterm infant, *Crit Care Med* 12:935–939, 1984.
122. Hay WW Jr, Brockway JM, Eyzaguirre M: Neonatal pulse oximetry: accuracy and reliability, *Pediatrics* 83:717–722, 1989.
123. Fouzas S, Priftis KN, Anthracopoulos MB: Pulse oximetry in pediatric practice, *Pediatrics* 128:740–752, 2011.
124. Dimich I, Singh PP, Adell A, et al: Evaluation of oxygen saturation monitoring by pulse oximetry in neonates, *Can J Anaesth* 38:985–988, 1991.
125. SUPPORT Study Group of the Eunice Kennedy Shriver NICHD Neonatal Research Network. Target ranges of oxygen saturation in extremely premature infants, *N Engl J Med* 362:1959–1969, 2010.
126. Mittnacht AJC: Near infrared spectroscopy in children at high risk of low perfusion, *Cur Opinion Anesth* 23:342–347, 2010.
127. Murkin JM, Arango M: Near-infrared spectroscopy as an index of brain and tissue oxygenation, *Br J Anaesth* 103(Suppl 1):i3–i13, 2009.
128. Chakravarti S, Srivastava S, Mittnacht AJ: Near infrared spectroscopy (NIRS) in children, *Sem Cardiothorac Vasc Anesth* 12:70–79, 2008.
129. Owens GE, King K, Gurney JG, Charpie JR: Low renal oximetry correlates with acute kidney injury after infant cardiac surgery, *Pediatr Cardiol* 32:183–188, 2011.
130. Ghanayem NS, Hoffman GM, Mussatto KA, et al: Perioperative monitoring in high-risk infants after stage 1 palliation of univentricular congenital heart disease, *J Thorac Cardiovasc Surg* 140:857–863, 2010.
131. Grocott HP: Avoid hypotension and hypoxia: an old anesthetic adage with renewed relevance from cerebral oximetry monitoring, *Can J Anesth* 58:697–702, 2011.
132. Kasman N, Brady K: Cerebral oximetry for pediatric anesthesia: why do intelligent clinicians disagree? *Paediatr Anaesth* 21:473–478, 2011.
133. Sessler DI: Temperature monitoring and perioperative thermoregulation, *Anesthesiology* 109:318–338, 2008.
134. Sessler DI: Perioperative thermoregulation and heat balance, *Ann N Y Acad Sci* 813:757–777, 1997.
135. Sessler DI: Perioperative heat balance, *Anesthesiology* 92:578–596, 2000.
136. Sessler DI: Complications and treatment of mild hypothermia, *Anesthesiology* 95:531–543, 2001.
137. Kurz A, Sessler DI, Lenhardt R: Perioperative normothermia to reduce the incidence of surgical-wound infection and shorten hospitalization, *N Engl J Med* 334:1209–1215, 1996.
138. Frank SM, Fleisher LA, Breslow MJ, et al: Perioperative maintenance of normothermia reeuces the incidence of morbid cardiac events: a randomized clinical trial, *JAMA* 277:1127–1134, 1997.
139. Presson RG Jr, Bezruczko AP, Hillier SC, McNiece WL: Evaluation of a new fluid warmer effective at low to moderate flow rates, *Anesthesiology* 78:974–980, 1993.
140. Giesbrecht GG, Ducharme MB, McGuire JP: Comparison of forced-air patient warming systems for perioperative use, *Anesthesiology* 80:671–679, 1994.
141. Bräuer A, Quintel M: Forced-air warming: technology, physical background and practical aspects, *Curr Opin Anaesthesiol* 22:769–774, 2009.
142. Bräuer A, Bovenschulte H, Perl T, et al: What determines the efficacy of forced-air warming systems? A manikin evaluation with upper body blankets, *Anesth Analg* 108:192–198, 2009.
143. Marhofer P, Frickey N: Ultrasonographic guidance in pediatric regional anesthesia. Part 1: theoretical background, *Paediatr Anaesth* 16:1008–1018, 2006.
144. Rao S, VanHolsbeek L, Musial JL, et al: A pilot study of comprehensive ultrasound education at the Wayne State University School of Medicine, *J Ultrasound Med* 27:745–749, 2008.
145. Moore CL, Copel JA: Point-of-care ultrasonography, *N Engl J Med* 364:749–757, 2011.
146. Bodenham AR: Ultrasound imaging by anaesthetists: training and accreditation issues, *Br J Anaesth* 96:414–417, 2006.
147. Marhofer P, Willschke H, Kettner S: Imaging techniques for regional nerve blockade and vascular cannulation in children, *Curr Opin Anaesthesiol* 19:293–300, 2006.
148. Verghese ST, McGill WA, Patel RI, et al: Ultrasound-guided internal jugular venous cannulation in infants, *Anesthesiology* 91:71–77, 1999.
149. Maecken T, Grau T: Ultrasound imaging in vascular access, *Crit Care Med* 35(Supp l):S178–S185, 2007.
150. Froehlich CD, Rigby MR, Rosenberg ES, et al: Ultrasound-guided central venous catheter placement decreases complications and decreases placement attempts compared with the landmark technique in patients in a pediatric intensive care unit, *Crit Care Med* 37:1090–1096, 2009.
151. Tsui BCH, Suresh S: Ultrasound imaging for regional anesthesia in infants, children and adolescents: a review of current literature and its application in the practice of extremity and trunk blocks, *Anesthesiology* 112:473–492, 2010.
152. Tsui BCH, Suresh S: Ultrasound imaging for regional anesthesia in infants, children, and adolescents, *Anesthesiology* 12:719–728, 2010.

CHAPTER 18

INFUSION PUMPS

Wilton C. Levine • Kyle A. Vernest

CHAPTER OUTLINE

OVERVIEW

History and Evolution of Infusion Pumps

In 1638, William Harvey, a British physician, first described the circulatory system and found that the heart circulates blood through the body though continuous circulation. Before this, most people believed that blood flowed in arteries and veins like "human breath," essentially just moving back and forth in the body.[1]

This opened the way for Sir Christopher Wren, the famous English architect, to fashion a quill and porcine bladder system (Fig. 18-1, *A*) in 1658 to test the effects of infusing wine, ale, and opium. His work in this area has earned him the distinction of being the "father of modern intravenous (IV) infusion."

Understanding Flow

The rate of flow is described by the following equation:

$$Q = \Delta P/R$$

where Q is the flow, ΔP is the change in pressure, and R is the resistance. To understand the flow, each part should be reviewed. Change in pressure is given by the following formula, known as *Pascal's law:*

$$\Delta P = \rho \times g \times (h_2 - h_1)$$

The change in pressure depends on the density (ρ), which is approximately 1 kg/L for most liquids; the force of gravity (g); and the differences in head height ($h_2 - h_1$). Head height is the primary factor that drives this pressure gradient that generates the flow.

Resistance is a much harder aspect to deal with, because resistance in a pipe can change based on a large multitude of factors in a number of complex relationships. However, if smooth laminar flow is assumed, this simplifies the relationship. Smooth laminar flow, or resistance (R), is given in the following equation:

$$R = \frac{8\eta L}{\pi r^4}$$

In this expression, η is the viscosity of the liquid, *L* is the length of tubing, and *r* is the radius. Thus the radius of the tubing has the greatest effect on resistance (raised to the power of 4). Doubling the radius decreases the resistance 16 times. It should also be noted, however, that viscosity and tube length play a critical role in resistance and thus in the flow rate. These equations can be combined together to form Poiseuille's law for laminar flow in a pipe:

$$Q = \frac{\Delta P}{R} = \frac{\pi \rho g (\Delta h) r^4}{8\eta L}$$

Thus all the factors affecting the rate of flow in a gravity device are illustrated by Poiseuille's law: density (ρ), gravity (g), difference in head height (Δh), tubing radius (r), fluid viscosity (η), and tube length (L). These factors are part of all infusions, and the clinician should remain cognizant of these at all times.

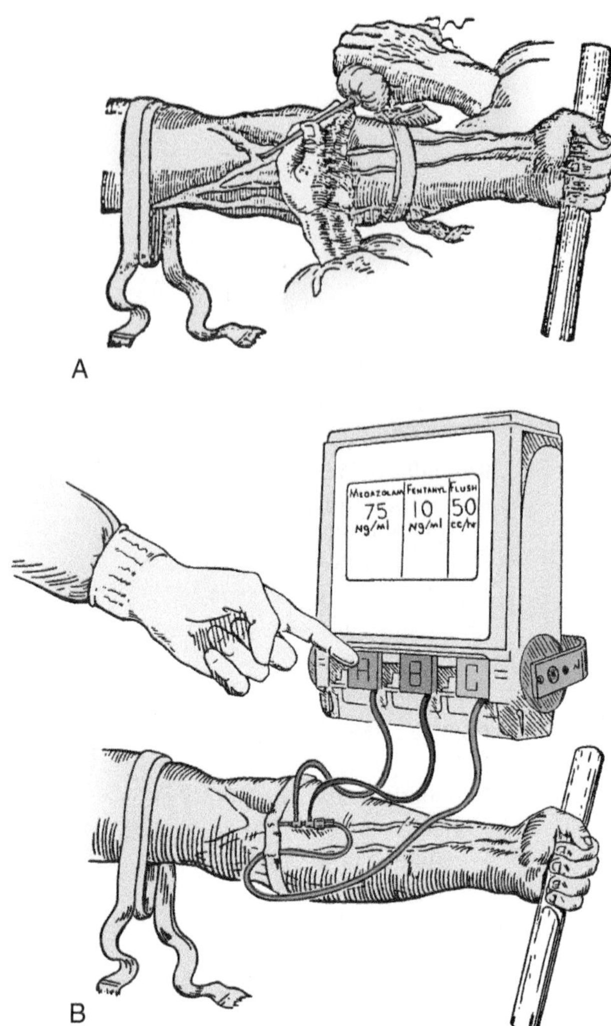

FIGURE 18-1 Intravenous drug delivery: past and future. **A,** A depiction of the first intravenous injection of opium with a quill and bladder. **B,** The future of intravenous drug delivery. Drugs are delivered with the aid of a small, sophisticated infusion pump that permits dosing in terms of plasma drug concentration rather than amount. (From Glass, PSA, Shafer SL, Reves JG: Intravenous drug delivery systems. In Miller RD, Eriksson LI, Fleisher LA, et al, editors: *Miller's anesthesia,* ed 7, London, Churchill Livingstone, 2009.)

INFUSION DEVICES

Nonautomated, Nonregulated Gravity-Induced Flow

The simplest infusion device is a simple IV bag with tubing that has been connected to an IV catheter in a patient. These were the first types of infusions used in the 1900s. It was found that by applying a flow resistor, the flow could be controlled; thus roller clamps were used, and still continue to be used, as a means of modulating flow. By counting the drip rate, the flow rate can be approximated. As such, many infusions were simply set by using the roller clamps and counting drops. However, the flow rate is affected by many factors. Because gravity is the driving force, the height of the IV bag over the infusion location, also known as *head height,* can have a significant role in the rate of an infusion; as the height of the fluid changes, it can change the rate of fluid transfer. Thus the roller clamp would need adjusting for the infusion to maintain a constant flow rate (Fig. 18-2).

Regulated Gravity-Induced Flow

The next step in the progression of infusion devices was the addition of a controller that adjusted the resistance based on the desired flow rate, rather than having a clinician monitor the drip rate (Fig. 18-3).

Mechanism of Operation

Regulated gravity devices primarily operate by using a drip counter. An optical sensor is placed on the drip chamber to count the drops as they fall and thereby block the sensor. The drops have a uniform size based on the temperature, surface tension, and pressure. Because the temperature and pressure remain relatively constant, the viscosity and size of the drip chamber have the greatest role in the flow rate determination.

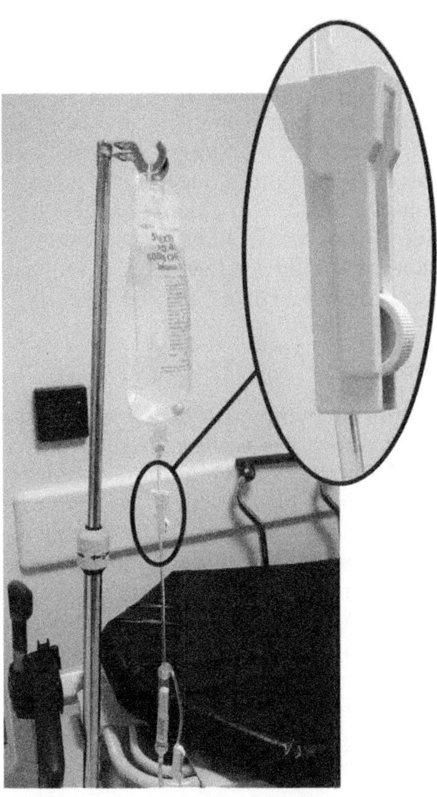

FIGURE 18-2 ■ Roller clamp infusion controller.

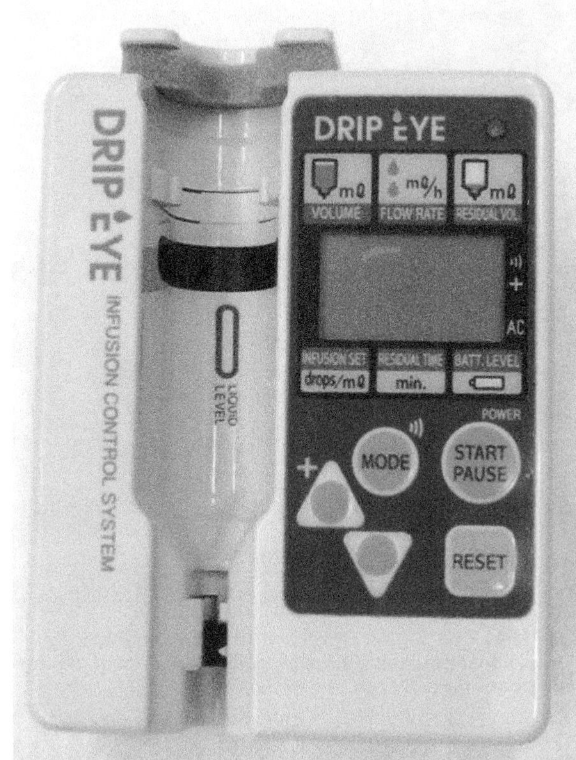

FIGURE 18-3 ■ The Drip-Eye drip counter regulated gravity controller (Parama-Tech Co., Fukuoka, Japan).

Considerations

Advantages

Regulated induced gravity-flow devices, such as drop counters, have several advantages over standard IV systems. First, they can minimize clotting because the controllers have flow sensors that can detect a pressure change that could have resulted from clotting, especially at low flow rates. Second, by the addition of a flow controller, the incidence of rapid infusion dramatically decreases. Last, it can help minimize dry IV lines by monitoring the flow and stopping the infusion before the line runs completely empty. This prevents the infusion of air into the patient's vasculature.

An additional advantage that the regulated gravity devices have is a low driving force, and the device is driven by the pressure at head height. A low driving force decreases the severity of infiltrations. If operating at higher pressures, infiltrations are much harder to detect when the pump is driving with so much pressure.

One of the main attractions of this class of device is its lower cost. Although more expensive than a simple IV bag, it requires less clinician supervision. This allows a single individual to monitor several infusions. In addition, these controllers are substantially less expensive than most positive-pressure infusion pumps and are relatively small.

Drawbacks

Regulated gravity devices have several distinct drawbacks in their operation. Many of these controllers are designed such that they limit the flow when they are closed around the tubing. However, if a device is opened during administration, it can cause free flow of the solution with the potential to give large, unmonitored doses to the patent. In addition, in the programming of drip counters, the *viscosity* of the fluid, or the number of drops per milliliter, must be included in the infusion. This typically requires a look-up chart or similar table, which can be a source of error in programming an infusion. Because different-sized drip chambers are available, the correct chamber size also must be selected when programming the controller. Also, as previously stated, the head height of the device provides the driving force for the infusion; this also has drawbacks with viscous fluids because the flow rate is limited to the force of gravity, and the limited pressure confines infusions to low-pressure target vasculatures (the venous system).

POSITIVE-PRESSURE PUMPS: LARGE VOLUME PUMP

Large volume pumps are one of the most common pumps in a hospital. They are used for many purposes other than drug delivery, such as rapid infusions of fluid and enteric and parenteral feeding. Large volume pumps operate at a wide range of infusions rates but typically are used for infusions between 1 mL/h to 999 mL/h. As previously outlined, positive-pressure pumps can have more severe IV infiltrations, and delays in detection of occlusions at low flow rates may occur as a result of the high pressure generation capability of the pumps.

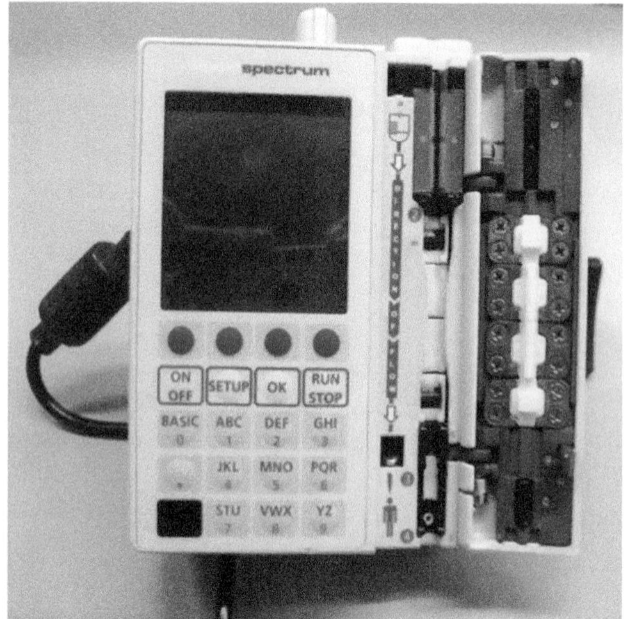

FIGURE 18-4 The Sigma Spectrum (Baxter, Deerfield, IL) large volume, linear peristaltic infusion pump, shown with the mechanism door open.

Positive-pressure pumps do have many advantages over gravity-fed controllers. These pumps can maintain relatively good accuracy at low flow rates compared with the gravity-fed controllers. This is due to the design of their pumping mechanisms; gravity controllers restrict nearly all flow in the tubing at low flow rates. In addition, positive-pressure pumps can reduce the number of minor occlusions with highly viscous solutions and provide faster infusion rates than gravity-fed systems. Moreover, many safety features have been introduced into these pumps, increasing their popularity.

Peristaltic Linear and Rotary Pumps

Mechanism of Action

Linear peristaltic pumps propel fluid by sequentially compressing the fluid-filled tubing using small fingerlike projections in a process similar to peristalsis of food in the gastrointestinal tract (Fig. 18-4). *Rotary peristalsis* propels the fluid by using two or more rotary cams that segment and propel a fixed volume of fluid. This mechanism is infrequently used in infusion pumps because of the increased difficulty in positioning the IV tubing around the cams and possible displacement of the IV tubing during operation. This pump style is more common in large volume pumps, such as rapid infusers and cardiopulmonary bypass pumps (Figs. 18-5 and 18-6).

Peristaltic Pump Considerations

Advantages

Peristaltic infusion pumps have many advantages over both drip counters and manually controlled infusions in addition to having the general advantages of positive-pressure pumps. Peristaltic infusion pumps have improved accuracy in both the rate and volume delivered to the patent over manually controlled infusions. The accuracy of the infusions is comparable to drip counters, and most pumps have ±5% to ±10% accuracy.[2] Although the accuracy is comparable to that of drip counters, one less step is required in the programming of the device, which is one less step in which error can be introduced. In addition, these pumps can handle any volume of liquid and have a broad range of infusion rates, typically from less than 1 mL/h to 999 mL/h.

Disadvantages

Peristaltic infusion pumps also have some drawbacks. One of the largest drawbacks is the pulsatile flow that results when the roller lifts off the tubing; as it completes its cycle, there is a pause in the flow, which decreases the accuracy of the infusion and is a primary reason for decreased accuracy at low flow rates. In addition, because the flexible tubing is constantly massaged, it begins to deform and stretch over time, leading to inaccuracies. These pumps require specialized administration sets, which are often proprietary, to ensure that the tubing is uniform from set to set. Proprietary sets usually cost significantly more than standard IV sets, which increases the cost of every infusion.

Error Curves

The action of the pumping mechanism and variations in the manufacturing of individual administration sets cause short-term fluctuations in the rate accuracy. Two typical performance curves for the pumps often are given (Fig. 18-7):

1. *Start-up curves:* These display the continuous curve of flow rate at a specified flow rate. The overshoot and undershoot of the pump can be seen with this approach. Typically, these are data for the first 2 hours of startup. These curves are significant, because even though the pump screen may display the infusion rate, this rate fluctuates. From these curves the clinician can see exactly how much fluctuation is occurring for that infusion.
2. *Trumpet curves:* These display accuracy over discrete time periods over which fluid delivery is measured. Over a large observational window (30 minutes), short-term fluctuations have little effect on the overall accuracy; this is illustrated in the flat section of the curve. As the observational window shrinks, these errors have increasing significance and result in larger error, forming the open end of the bell of a trumpet-shaped curve, hence the name.

Cassette (Volumetric) Pump

Mechanism

Cassette pump systems work by having a cassette of a measured chamber placed inside the pump. These are often called *volumetric pumps* because they infuse a known volume of fluid with every cycle. The pump operates by a cyclical effect in which the chamber is first filled to the measured volume; a delivery cycle follows in which the

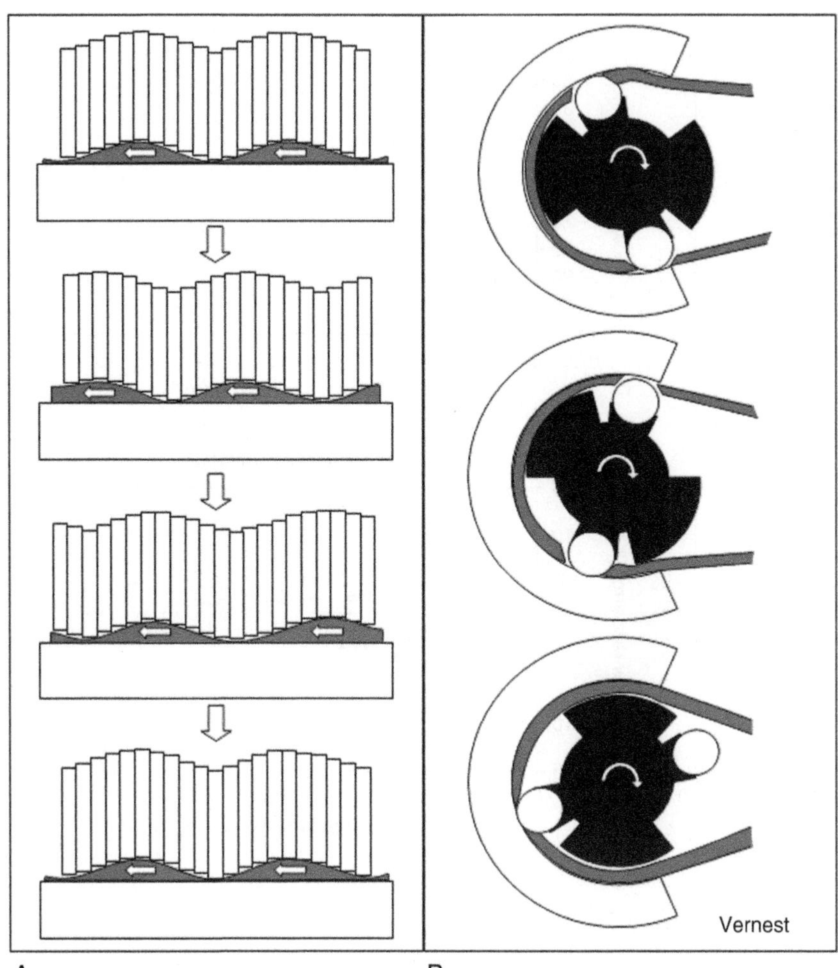

FIGURE 18-5 ■ **A,** A linear peristaltic mechanism: wavelike cyclical movement of fingers propels fluid forward. **B,** A rotary peristaltic mechanism rotates a constant volume of fluid using rotary cams.

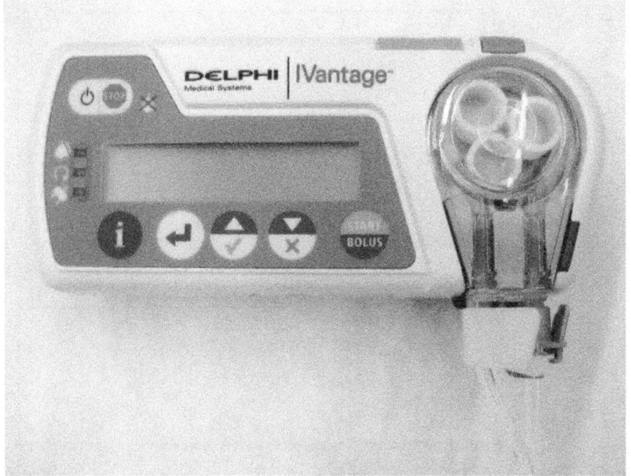

FIGURE 18-6 ■ The Delphi IVantage (Delphi Medical Systems, Longmont, CO) rotary peristaltic pump mechanism.

measured compartment is ejected out of the pump and is infused into the patient (Figs. 18-8 and 18-9).

Cassette Pump Considerations

Advantages. The cassette for the pump is disposable and can be detached from the pump easily, allowing for quick and easy setup from pump to pump. Again, it has one less step in the programming over drip counters because the viscosity of the fluid does not need to be entered. The accuracy of most cassette pumps is typically ±4% to ±10%.[3]

Disadvantages. Although cassette pumps are easy to use once they are primed, they often are difficult to re-prime because of the volumetric balloons and twists in the configuration of the tubing. In addition, each pump uses its own manufacturer's administration set, which often can be a costly ongoing expense. Because of the mechanism of action for cassette pumps, the filling and ejection of chambers, the flow is pulsatile, which can cause greater error at low infusion rates.

Syringe Pump

Mechanism

Syringe pumps (Figs. 18-10 and 18-11) primarily work off a motor-driven lead screw or a gear mechanism to drive the plunger into the syringe barrel. The rate of infusion depends on the speed of the motor that drives the plunger. The flow is characterized as pulsatile continuous flow because the motor often moves in small steps. These pumps achieve an accuracy of approximately ±2% to ±5%, mostly because of stiction, or static friction, and the compliance of the syringe

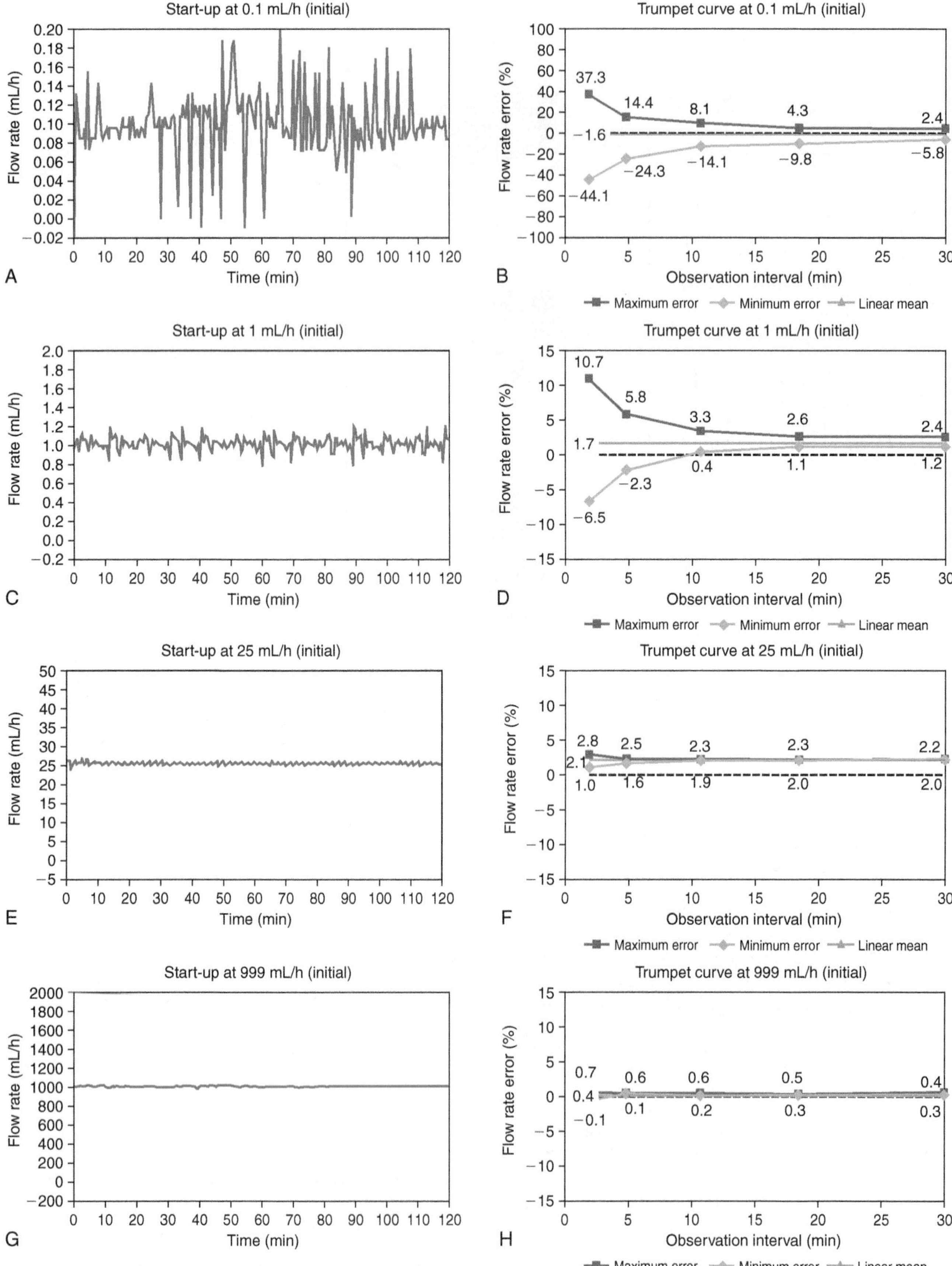

FIGURE 18-7 ■ A standard set of startup and trumpet curves for the Alaris Medley 8100 series (Cardinal Health, Dublin, OH) linear peristaltic infusion pump module.

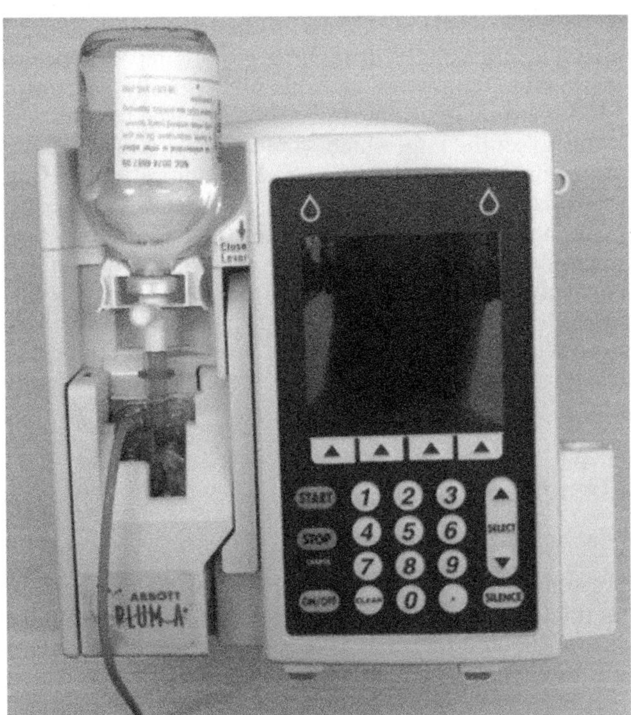

FIGURE 18-8 ■ The Abbott Plum A+ cassette pump (Hospira, Inc., Lake Forest, IL).

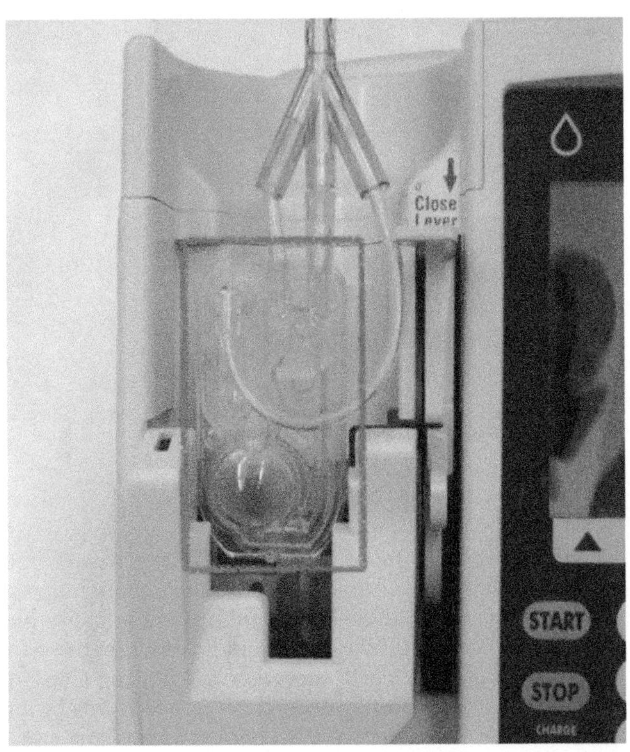

FIGURE 18-9 ■ The Abbot Plum A+ cassette (Hospira, Inc., Lake Forest, IL) removed from the pump.

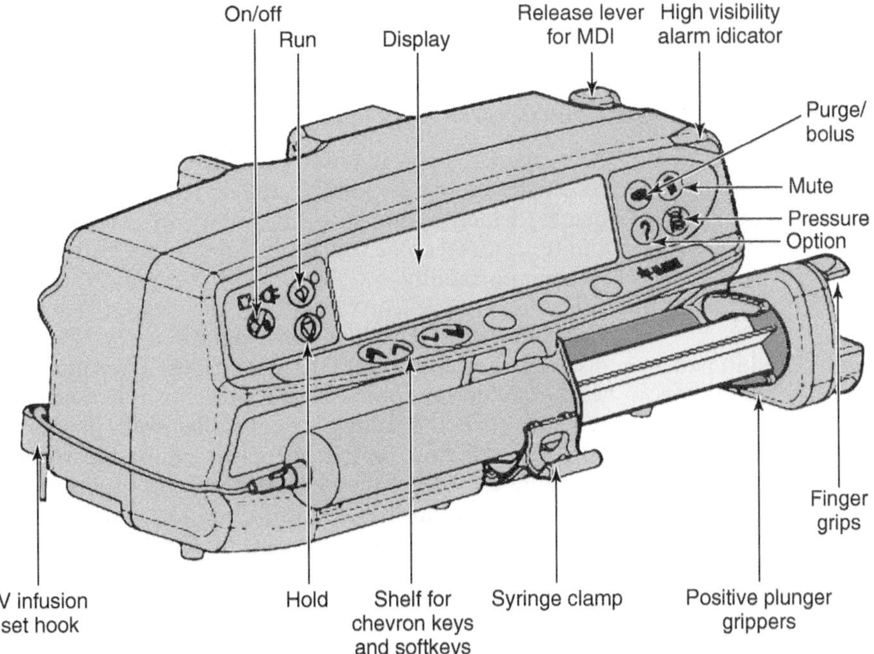

FIGURE 18-10 ■ The Alaris Asena GH syringe pump (Cardinal Health, Dublin, OH).

working against this to start again after it stops (starting and stopping a syringe is not precise because the rubber sticks to the side walls, and force is needed to overcome the static friction). This error is exemplified in the trumpet and start-up curves illustrated in Figure 18-7 (medical device interface).

Considerations for Use

Advantages. Syringe pumps have many attractive features. One of the greatest is the maintenance of precision and accuracy at low flow rates. The accuracy of these pumps is typically ±2% to ±5%. Syringe pumps also are often capable of functioning with different sizes and brands of syringes, including third-party filled syringes, pharmacy-filled syringes, and user-filled syringes. This can potentially reduce costs because clinicians can use a wide variety of syringes and do not need expensive proprietary administration sets; this dramatically reduces the cost per administration.

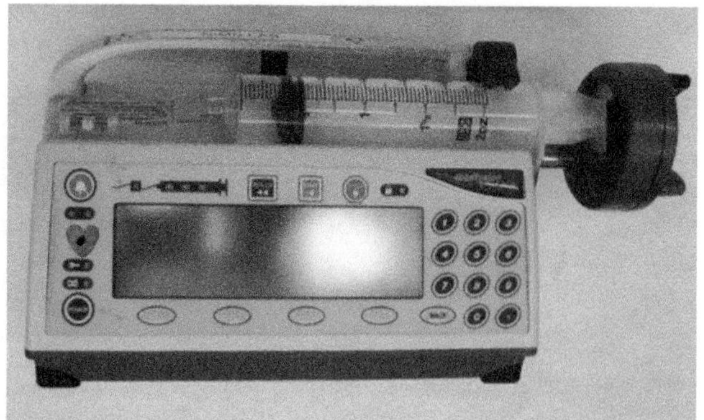

FIGURE 18-11 ■ The Medfusion 3500 syringe "smart" pump (Smiths Medical, St. Paul, MN).

Disadvantages. The major disadvantage of syringe pumps is their limited volume. Most can only handle up to 50-mL syringes; thus syringe pumps are not suitable for large volume infusions. In addition, the time to sound an occlusion alarm increases when using a larger syringe, and eliminating the occlusion results in a bolus proportional to the size of the syringe.[4] Thus it is critical to select the appropriately sized syringe for the infusion rate.

Error Curves. Figure 18-12 illustrates the start-up and trumpet curves for the Alaris Asena Syringe Pump (Cardinal Health, Dublin, OH), which is representative of a typical syringe pump. The effect of stiction can clearly be seen by the imprecise start-up curves and the error in the trumpet curves. However, it can be seen that even with a large 50-mL syringe at a flow rate of 0.1 mL/h, the error and precision are noticeably better than in the linear peristaltic curve shown in Figure 18-7.

Historic Significance

In the past, syringe pumps were primarily used in pediatrics because only a small volume infusion was required. However, many anesthesiology departments have now adopted the syringe pump as their primary pump in the OR. Studies have indicated that excessive fluid balance poses a risk to patients. Reduced forced expiratory volume in 1 minute (FEV_1), renal failure, and positive fluid balances at 24 hours after operation are predictors of prolonged intubation, which increases rates of morbidity and mortality in coronary artery bypass graft (CABG) patients.[5] In addition, a negative fluid balance in the first 3 days of septic shock has been shown to be an independent predictor of survival.[6] It was also shown that a net fluid retention greater than 67 mL/kg/day is a predictor of fatal pulmonary edema in postoperative patients.[7] The volume overload would typically result in furosemide and potassium administration, increased urine output, and hypokalemia, resulting in prolonged mechanical ventilation and intensive care unit (ICU) stays in addition to electrolyte imbalances.

Drugs typically are diluted to improve solubility and safety; by diluting the drug, a margin of safety is added to inaccurate administration. This was typically done with gravity-fed IV infusions, and a clinician used to count the drops to set the rate, which would vary with head height, IV cannula, and flow resistance. In addition, to prevent sclerosis of the vein, drugs are often diluted when inserted into a peripheral vein. Infusion devices provide increased precision in the delivery of fluid; thus, when programmed correctly, less error is associated with the delivery of fluids. When drugs are administered via a central vein, there is no sclerosis of the vein as a result of in vivo dilution of the drug, which takes advantage of the buffering capacity of the blood.

Elastomeric Reservoir

Mechanism

Elastomeric reservoir "pumps" use one of the simplest methods of generating positive pressure: a balloonlike reservoir is used to exert constant pressure on the medication within the balloon. The fluid is passed through a small flow restrictor, and, as specified by Poiseuille's law, the flow (Q) is proportional to the radius to the power of four (r^4); thus the flow rate is the most dependent on the radius of the tubing.

$$Q = \frac{\Delta P}{R} = \frac{(\Delta P)\pi r^4}{8\eta L}$$

Considerations

Advantages. Typically used for outpatients, elastomeric reservoirs are highly portable and do not depend on head height, which allows more flexibility in placement. In addition, they can be hidden in bags or purses to afford discreet portability.

Disadvantages. Although these pumps are portable and discreet, they have several disadvantages. They primarily work only on microbore tubing, which is inherently less accurate than the tubing in controller-style pumps. In addition, the flow rate is not easily adjustable without changing the size of the microbore tubing, and the infusion continues until it is completed. These devices also must be filled at the pharmacy or third-party vendor because of the high pressures required.

Spring-Powered Passive Syringe Pumps

Mechanism

Spring-powered or passive syringe pumps are very similar to the electromechnical syringe pumps, but they use a constant-force spring to apply pressure (Fig. 18-13). The constant-force spring applies pressure to the syringe and forces the fluid out. The flow is then restricted by microbore tubing, which limits the fluid flow to a known level because of Poiseuille's law, as previously demonstrated.

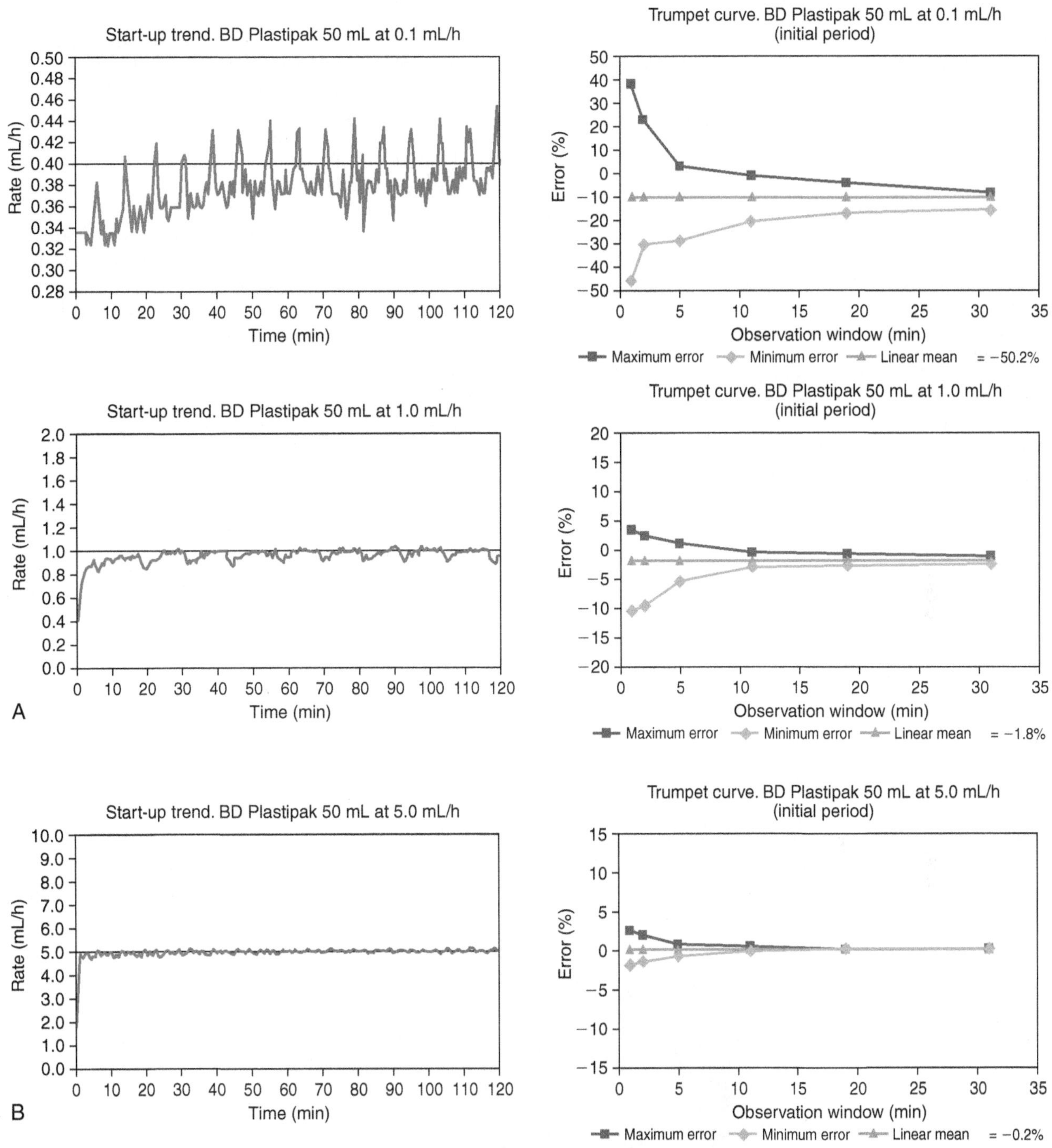

FIGURE 18-12 ■ Start-up and trumpet curves for the Alaris Asena syringe pump (Cardinal Health, Dublin, OH).

Considerations

Advantages. The spring-powered syringe pumps have many advantages; the biggest is probably their low cost. These inexpensive pumps are excellent for the delivery of antibiotics, and they allow an inexpensive but constant means of infusion where high levels of accuracy and precision are not important. Spring-powered syringe pumps can use most syringes and have a high level of interoperability.

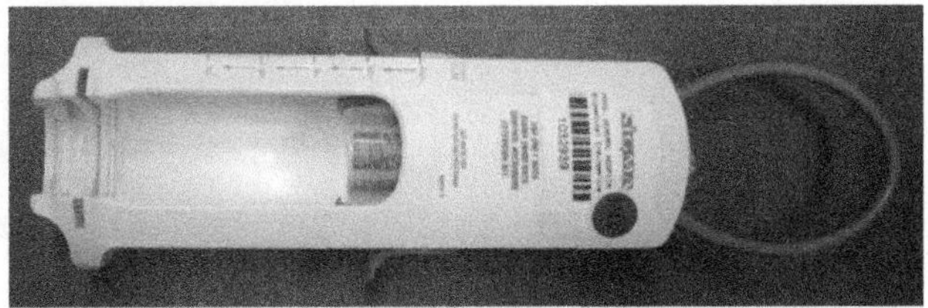

FIGURE 18-13 ■ Sigma Multidoser spring-powered syringe pump (Baxter, Deerfield, IL) without a syringe installed.

Disadvantages. The main disadvantage of spring-powered syringe pumps is lower accuracy compared with controller-style pumps. Also, the flow rate is limited to the flow rate set by the microbore tubing, such that the administration set must be changed to change the flow rate.

PATIENT-CONTROLLED ANALGESIA DEVICES

Patient-controlled analgesia (PCA) pumps were developed as a pain control strategy in the early 1970s. These devices allow patients to self-administer an IV bolus of an analgesic medication by pressing a medication-demand button. Such pumps typically are provided to patients after surgery. They can be programmed to give a baseline infusion of analgesia and then for a patient bolus when pain warrants. This allows the administration of analgesia without nursing intervention and an intramuscular (IM) or IV bolus. Patient-demand boluses are limited in the programming of the device, typically by limiting the number of boluses per unit of time to prevent the user, or anyone else, from overdosing. Nurses and physicians typically have override keys, which allow them to either change the programming or administer additional bolus doses. Typical dosing patterns are illustrated in Figure 18-14.

Portable PCA pumps are becoming increasingly popular. These pumps often are compact and support a locked cartridge of the analgesic agent. Each cartridge typically is prefilled by a pharmacy or third-party vendor, and it allows the analgesic to be locked to the pump to prevent tampering. These pumps typically operate on a linear peristaltic mechanism, drawing the fluid from the contained reservoir. By virtue of the small size and excellent battery life, many portable PCA pumps can be used for long periods, giving users the ability to move around with great ease. Examples are shown in Figures 18-15 and 18-16.

Many syringe pumps support PCA, which allows an increased field of use. Syringe pumps are effective PCA pumps because the flow rate is nearly unchanged no matter what the orientation of the pump.

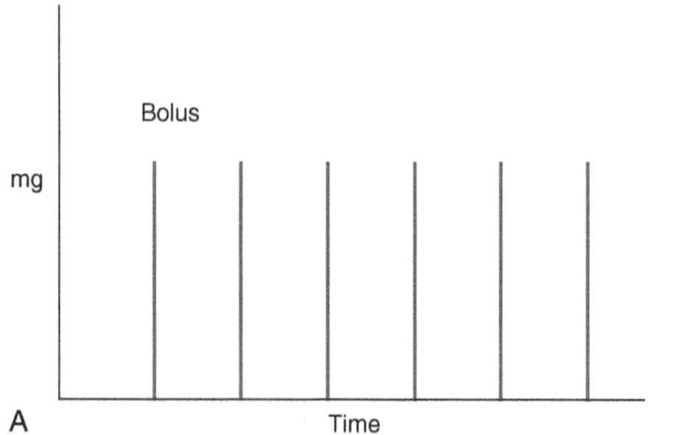

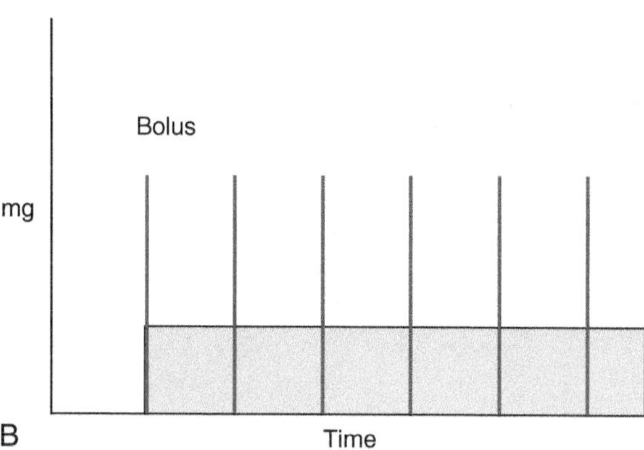

FIGURE 18-14 ■ Common dosing patterns used by patient-controlled analgesia (PCA) pumps. **A,** PCA only. Analgesia is only given when demanded by the user, as denoted by the vertical bolus lines. **B,** PCA and baseline. A baseline infusion (shaded area) is given in addition to user-administrated boluses.

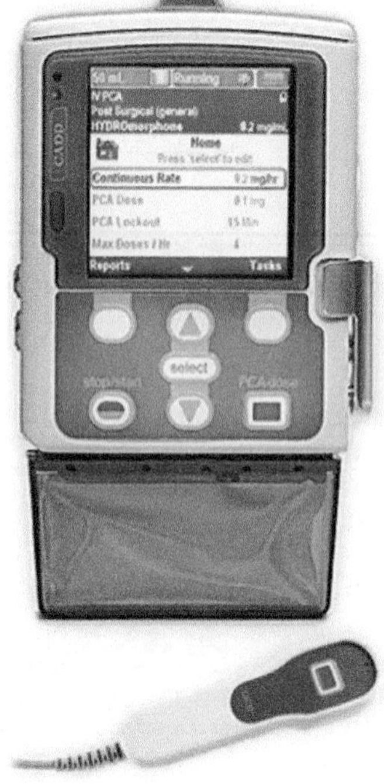

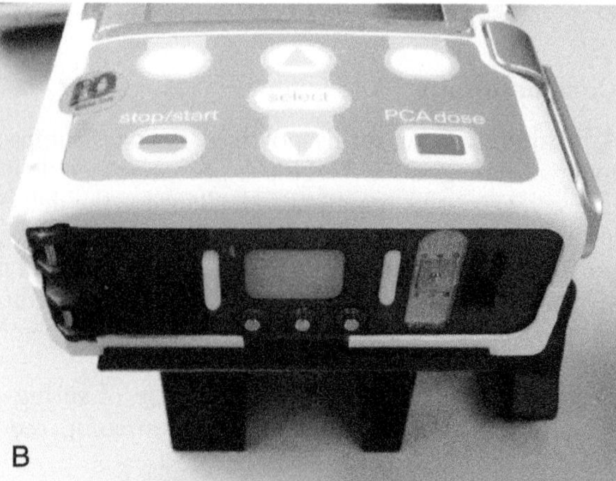

FIGURE 18-15 ■ **A,** CADD-Solis ambulatory infusion pump (Smiths Medical, St. Paul, MN) with external patient-controlled analgesia dose button. **B,** Pump showing the cartridge area.

"Smart" Pumps

Historic Significance

Standard infusion pumps are reliable if regularly maintained and serviced; however, they only deliver medications based on the pump programming. Thus a wrong keystroke can easily cause a 10-fold change in drug delivery. With increased use of syringe pumps to avoid "drowning" patients in fluid, concerns were increasing over potential errors as a result of the much more highly concentrated solutions; a simple keystroke error could change a suitable infusion dose to a deadly one. Pumps therefore needed to be "smarter" to know when a reasonable error was occurring and provide appropriate alarms to the clinicians. The development of pump technology is shown graphically in Figure 18-17.

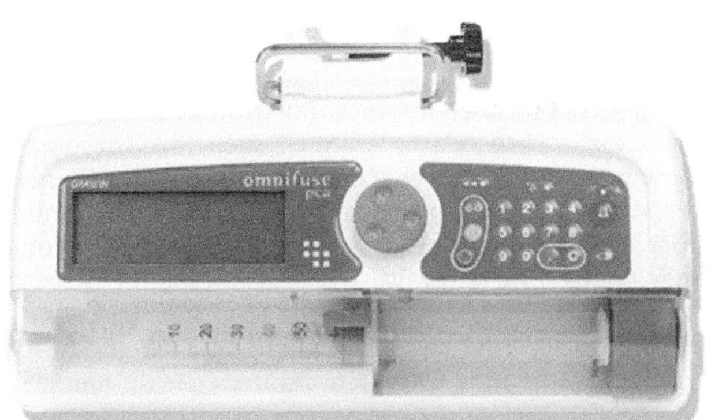

FIGURE 18-16 ■ Graseby Omnifuse patient-controlled analgesia syringe pump (Smiths Medical, St. Paul, MN).

The "Smarts" of Smart Pumps

The solution to this was to have bounds for acceptable dosing limits. From this, the idea of a *hard limit,* an absolute limit that cannot be exceeded, came about. In addition, *soft limits* are added outside the recommended limit that can be overridden if the caregiver accepts the warning. These clinical guidelines are referred to as a *drug library* and typically are defined by the institution based on clinical input. This empowers caregivers with up-to-date best practices, dosing guidance at the bedside, and prompts and alerts during programming that help ensure appropriate settings. In addition, it prevents dosing in wrong *dose rate units*—such as units per hour, rather than mg/kg per minute—and it implements a standard method to warn users of potential overdelivery or underdelivery of drugs with soft and hard limits.

Limitations of Smart Pumps

Smart pump technology is not without limitations. The drug libraries can be bypassed, and the pump can be run like a typical pump, defeating the safeguards. Also, independent double-checks cannot be replaced to ensure that inputs, such as medication or patient weight, are correct; these errors can produce errors in the infusion that are difficult to notice. Lastly, even when alerts are provided to clinicians, most can be overridden, such as soft limits. This can often happen if the drug library is not developed to actual clinical practices that clinicians are following.

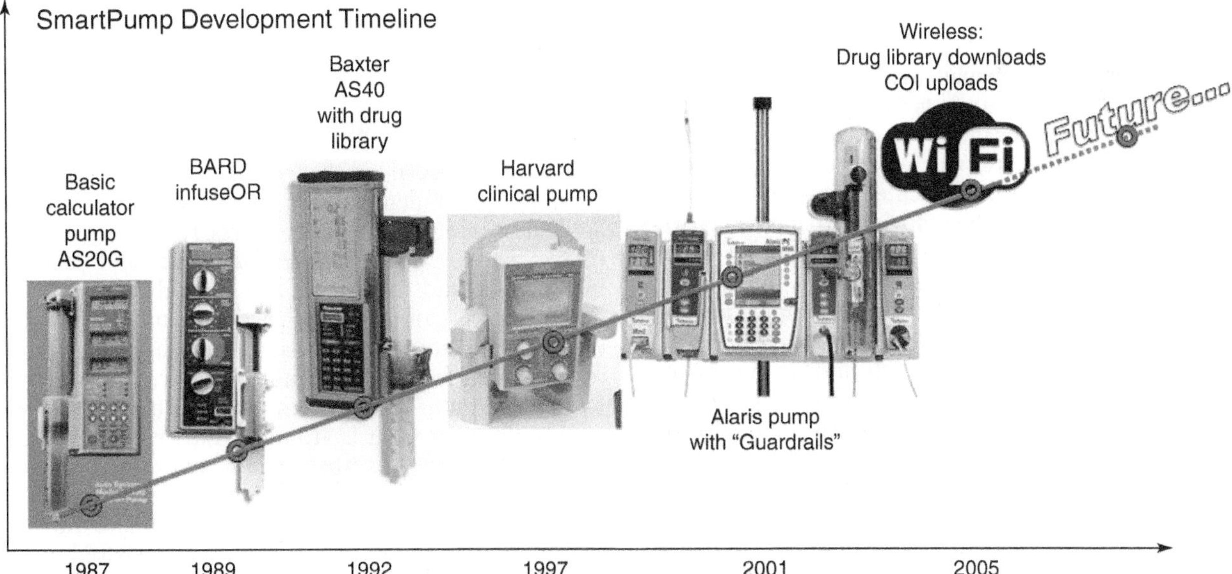

FIGURE 18-17 ■ Smart pump development timeline. **1987:** Baxter AS20G (Baxter, Deerfield, IL), the first calculator pump. It allowed the dose to be programmed directly in mg/kg/min or μg/min rather than mL/h, eliminating the need for conversion tables. **1989:** Bard InfusOR (Bard Medical, Covington, GA), the first "smart" pump, used different magnetic face plates for each drug, which put dosing limits on the rate that a drug could be infused. **1992:** Baxter AS40, the first pump with software drug libraries. This pump was pulled from the market for off-label use of esmolol 3 months after it was introduced. **1997:** Harvard Clinical 2 (Instech Laboratories, Inc., Plymouth Meeting, PA) was the first pump introduced with clinically developed drug libraries. Hospitals were responsible for setting the hard and soft limits on their pumps, removing the liability from the pump manufacturer. **2001:** Alaris was the first manufacturer to hit the mainstream market with drug libraries. They successfully trademarked "Guardrails," became a hard hitter in the pump market, and forced many manufacturers to follow suit in introducing drug libraries. **2005:** Many pumps begin to introduce Wi-Fi to allow the download of drug libraries and upload of quality control information in which an administrator can see how often clinicians exceed soft limits or operate outside the drug libraries. **Future:** remote programming or verification of computerized physician order entry, uploading of current pump information to automated charting systems, automated syringe identification (bar code or radiofrequency identification).

FIGURE 18-18 ■ Bar codes can be verified with many bar code scanning programs available on smart phones in addition to standard bar code scanners. **A,** The simpler bar code on the left contains the number "1." **B,** The MaxiCode on the right contains the nursery rhyme "Mary Had A Little Lamb."

EMERGING TECHNOLOGIES

Making the Five Rights of Medication *Right*

In the delivery of medication, it is important to remember the five rights of medication administration: 1) right patient, 2) right drug, 3) right dose, 4) right route, and 5) right time. Technology is expanding and will continue to develop its role in the area of medication administration. This includes areas such as radiofrequency identification (RFID), bar coding, and various networking methods, including local piconets and larger campus area networks (CANs).

Anesthesia Information Management Systems and Acute Care Documentation

Anesthesia information management systems (AIMS) are part of many hospitals' attempts to automatically record vital signs and other relevant information that is normally part of an anesthesia chart, which is stored electronically. This is part of many hospitals' acute care documentation (ACD) project, which involves moving to paperless charting and record keeping. Currently, these systems document drugs administered by transcribing the information from the pumps. As pumps develop in sophistication, they likely will be able to communicate with AIMS/ACD systems to automatically relay pump information to the electronic chart. However, this will rely on the implementation of other emerging technologies outlined here.

Bar Code Medication Administration

Because many hospitals are moving toward an electronic medication administration record (EMAR), the use of bar coding of medication can be an effective method of providing machine-readable information. This same technology has been implemented into several pumps but has yet to be widely implemented.

The use of bar coding with pumps can provide the pump with contextual awareness. By bar coding items related to infusions—such as provider ID cards, patient ID bracelets, and medications—the pump can use this information to make independent decisions and eliminate entry errors. The most important of these is the bar coded medication, which can be scanned such that the pump knows what drug and concentration is being administered, eliminating the potential to select the wrong drug.

Bar codes have become commonplace on many consumer goods. One kind uses vertical lines and spaces to relay information, check digits, and stop and start points (see Fig. 18-18, *A*). These bar codes have a lower density of information and are often limited to 40 numeric characters.

A second type of bar code, called a MaxiCode (Fig. 18-18, *B*) provides a greater density of information than simple straight-line bar codes. Thus the more data-dense MaxiCode bar codes can provide a great deal of information in text form in a small, compact source, such as drug name, concentration, and date of expiration.

Radiofrequency Identification

RFID uses a special tag that, when triggered, emits a frequency used for identification and tracking; the tag can be applied or built into an object. Most RFIDs are made up of two parts: an *integrated circuit* stores and processes information and modulates and demodulates radiofrequency signals, and a second part contains an *antenna* for receiving and transmitting data. RFID has the potential to take over from bar coding; however, the benefit of RFID is that it uses passive scanning, such that the reader constantly scans what is around it rather than having to present the item to the bar code scanner. In this case, it can know automatically what drug is being infused, who is infusing it, who it is being delivered to, where the pump is, and what additional pumps are nearby. Based on this information, it can then make clinical support decisions. Currently, cost is the limiting factor of RFID, at about $1 per tag; at that cost, it is not feasible to tag all syringes, bags, and other medication containers.

Point-to-Point Networks

Point-to-point networks allow communication between devices over a short distance and in a relatively secure manner, but close proximity is required.

Bluetooth

Bluetooth is a short-distance wireless protocol used to create small networks between portable devices. For medical devices such as infusion pumps, it provides an opportunity to communicate with other devices nearby. This could mean that a pump could communicate with a Bluetooth-enabled computer to upload its infusion data as part of an AIMS/ACD system. In addition, it could communicate with other pumps for that patient to check for drug interactions and perform other patient safety checks, acting as a single unit rather than many individual parts.

ZigBee

ZigBee is a short-distance wireless protocol similar to Bluetooth but simpler and less expensive. It is currently less developed than Bluetooth, yet it holds great promise because of its low energy consumption and secure networking. ZigBee could provide the same options outlined under Bluetooth.

Wi-Fi and Campus Area Networks

Wi-Fi provides the opportunity to access networks wirelessly within a hospital. This can allow pumps to communicate with almost limitless options. Wi-Fi–capable pumps could be integrated into a hospital computerized physician order entry system to ensure that the patient is getting the specified drug. It can also be connected to different databases, such as a patient allergy or drug interactions database. In addition, this method makes it much easier to integrate Wi-Fi technology with an AIMS/ACD system, because the system would communicate with the server as long as it was within the Wi-Fi network.

Target-Controlled Infusion and Closed-Loop Anesthesia

The target-controlled infusion (TCI) method of IV drug administration was first developed in the early 1980s by Schüttler and Schwilden[8] and later improved by Kenny and White[9] in 1990. By understanding the typical pharmacodynamics of opioids and anesthetic drugs, a computer program can predict the level of plasma concentration or effective site concentration for a given patient. By allowing effective site concentration, it allows TCI to specify the central nervous system concentration, the effective location of narcotics. This system can be applied to automatically regulate the level of anesthetic input into the bloodstream, something rather difficult with inhaled anesthetics. Thus total IV anesthesia is the delivery of anesthesia with an IV line, which can be easily controlled by syringe pumps. This method (TCI) works by deriving a computer simulation of a set of pharmacokinetic parameters for a known infusion scheme derived from patient populations for various parameters such as age, weight, and gender. The computer uses these parameters to predict the concentration of the drug at the specified location. The selected model is uploaded to a computer-compatible infusion pump; when activated the system will deliver the required dose to obtain and then maintain the target drug concentration.

With the development of bispectral index monitors to monitor the depth of anesthesia, systems have been developed that regulate the infusion of hypnotic agents. In addition, train-of-four (TOF) often is used to monitor neuromuscular blockade, and it has been suggested that the administration of a paralyzing agent could be automatically administered according to the level of paralysis via TOF. This allows another method for the improvement of TCI and thus close the loop.

The major issue with TCI is the current regulatory challenges that surround these medical devices. At the time of publication, the U.S. Food and Drug Administration (FDA) has not approved any TCI infusion device, thus limiting its clinical applications in the United States. In United States, it is very difficult to get approval for closed-loop drug administration systems because the entire system must be carefully scrutinized; no physician will be present to interpret the results, make decisions, and complete the calculations. This would be done automatically.[10]

Noncontact Flow Sensors

Optical flow sensors have been designed and tested for noncontact flow measuring for use in drug delivery. Current work at the California Institute of Technology has resulted in the development of an optical flow sensor for the monitoring of drug delivery. This miniature flow sensor was developed for flows from 0.8 to 2.9 mL/h with an accuracy better than a 1% coefficient of variation. Although not ready for system integration as of this writing because of a limited range of flows, future models could likely use a larger range.[11]

Noncontact flow sensors could help improve the accuracy of pumps. Because most pumps calculate flow based on mechanism of action—linear peristaltic, rotary peristaltic, or syringe driven—they do not have data on the autual flow rate. By monitoring the flow more accurately, a closed-loop controller could monitor flow rate and achieve better accuracy and precision (Fig. 18-19).

Infusions Based on Drug Infusion Kinetics

Many patients frequently receive life-critical infusions of vasoactive, inotropic, antidysrhythmic, or analgesic drugs via central venous catheters in ICUs and in the operating room (OR), and such infusions also are given to pediatric patients. Several potential dangers are inherent in infusing concentrated drugs at low flow rates, including the delivery of large drug boluses if fluids are given upstream of the concentrated infusion. As such, many concentrated drugs are often piggybacked onto a carrier stream, diluting the concentration of the drug contained within the infusion set and catheter. In a study looking at the characterization of drug-delivery profiles via standard pediatric central venous infusion systems, the authors found that the time to steady-state delivery of a new infusion varied significantly, especially at low flow rates.[12] In addition, research has been done to understand the work of carriers and dead space in drug delivery and how models relate to what is occurring.[13] By understanding the interactions between carriers and drugs, the clinician can better predict the outcome. This can ultimately lead to

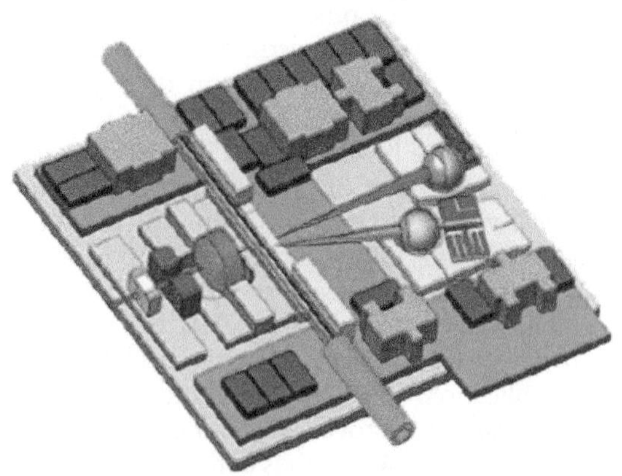

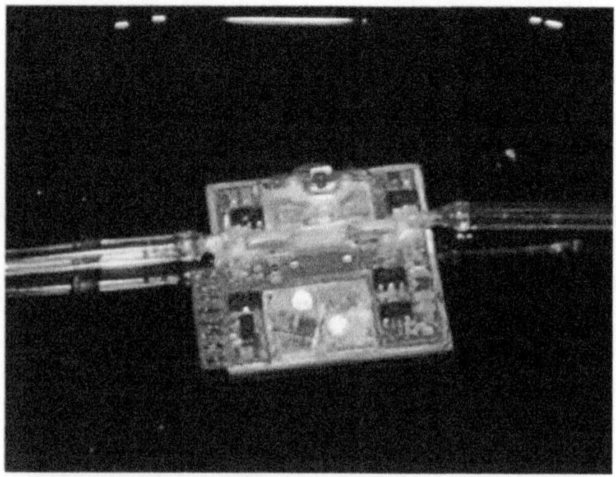

FIGURE 18-19 ■ An example of a noncontact flow sensor.

integrating pumps that consider the drug kinetics that would account for these variances in delivering the correct dose to the patient at the correct time. Thus if the rate of administration was changed, the carrier flow rate could be optimized to deliver that change to the patient sooner. As more research continues into the kinetics of drug infusions, improved mechanisms will likely be built into pumps to increase the precision of the drug administration.[14]

EMERGING NATIONAL RECOMMENDATIONS FOR INFUSION PUMPS

In 2008, two large national meetings were held in Rockville, Maryland. The Institute for Safe Medical Practices (ISMP) Summit on the Use of Smart Infusion Pumps and the Summit on Preventing Harm and Death from IV Medication Errors set out to look at how infusion pumps are used and where development needs to be focused.

The Summit on Preventing Death and Patient Harm from IV Medication Errors was convened by the American Society of Health-System Pharmacists (ASHP), ASHP Research and Education Foundation, Institute for Safe Medication Practices, United States Pharmacopeia, Infusion Nurses Society, The Joint Commission, and the National Patient Safety Foundation. Highlights of their short-term goals included development of national standards for IV drug use to encourage the use of smart pumps, and to ensure that the "smarts" are not turned off. The long-term goals of the conference were very promising. Highlights included encouraging the FDA to require that all drugs bear a single-format bar code that integrates into the system, a resource kit for developing drug and administration guidelines, and establishment of a catalog of best practices in IV medication safety. Many of the steps that the group proposed are a giant step in the right direction; however, much work still needs to focus on developing national and international standards for IV drug administration.

From the ISMP Summit on the Use of Smart Infusion Pumps, the group developed guidelines for safe implementation and use of smart pumps.

CONSIDERATIONS FOR PUMP SELECTION

Cost

Cost is probably one of the biggest factors in selecting new pumps. Obviously, everyone must work within a budget; however, several factors often need to be considered with regard to cost.

Capital Costs

Capital costs for any pump project obviously include the capital purchase price of any pumps, which is the cash required up front to buy the pumps. However, additional capital costs should always be considered. If wireless networks are part of the pump integration, required capital expenditures for the wireless network should be included and consideration given to whether up-front and ongoing costs will be associated with the smart pump systems. Library customization software often is required, as is additional training and staff to support the maintenance of drug libraries and the training of users. In addition, there would be costs incurred to integrate new equipment with other systems.

Operating Costs

In addition to the capital costs of a project, several operating costs typically continue throughout the use of the pumps. Reccurring costs can include the following:

1. *Cost of administration sets* (IV tubing, cassette, or other): proprietary administration sets and cassettes can cost more than $10 each, whereas standard sets typically costs less than $1.
2. *Maintenance plans:* Many pumps come with an optional maintenance plan from the manufacturer to repair any pumps and perform any preventive maintenance required.
3. *Employees:* As pump systems become increasingly complex, more and more employees are needed to support them. Many hospitals now have a hospital pump expert who maintains the drug libraries and helps provide in-service for products.

Size and Weight

The size and weight should always be considered when selecting a new pump. Considerations should be made for extreme cases, such as some cardiac patients, where there may be upward of 12 pumps per patient. Larger and heavier pumps take up more room, making them difficult to position around the patient. Some companies offer a bed-mounted rack system; if selecting this option, be sure that the pump fits on the rack.

User Interface

Quick, easy, and accurate programming must be at the core of pump design. The number of keystrokes or knob turns in the design should be minimized. The human factors involved in the user interface are a key dynamic that many hospitals fail to realize. Not only is it about minimizing the keystrokes, it is also about the minimization of errors that could harm patients. Heuristic and high-fidelity evaluations of the interfaces should take place to evaluate the human factors of the user interface. High-fidelity testing can include videotaping nurses setting a mock infusion; heuristic evaluations often include surveys and visual identification of features. For example, the organization of a keypad should be the same as either a telephone keypad or a computer keypad; changing the organization, such as by moving the zero key, can result in unintentional programming errors due to keystroke errors. Another important consideration is whether the infusion rate can be changed without stopping and restarting the pump. This is particularly important in critically ill patients with rapidly changing physiologic conditions.

Battery

A large part of the size and weight issue is the size of the battery. Pumps should have a large enough battery to run for more than 4 hours at 125 mL/h. A replaceable battery is also a good feature so that the battery can be replaced when it loses the ability hold a charge. Pumps must automatically switch from alternating current (AC) to battery power without losing settings.

Hospital Standardization

It is important to standardize pumps across a facility. This is especially important when integrating with the OR and the emergency department because patents can go nearly anywhere in the hospital on potentially critical medications; switching pumps when moving a patient between departments is a time-consuming and potentially dangerous process because the new pump must be programmed correctly with the infusion.

FINAL THOUGHTS

Ideal Pump Design

What the design of a "perfect" infusion pump would look like is difficult to say because of the many different uses for infusion pumps today. Each pump classification has its own advantages and disadvantages that must be taken into account. One pump cannot really do it all, nor should it. It would not make much sense to have an extremely accurate, very precise infusion pump to administer a general antibiotic, when the requirements for the administration are not that stringent. Similarly, it would not make good sense to have an imprecise infusion pump for a vasoactive medication infusion. As such, there is no real "ideal" design for one pump that can accomplish everything.

A hospital should have at least four types of pumps: 1) a high-volume pump for administration of large volumes of fluids to patients, 2) a syringe pump for life-critical concentrated solutions, 3) a spring-powered syringe pump for the administration of antibiotics and other single-medication doses at low cost, and 4) a PCA pump for the management of acute pain.

The spring-powered syringe pump could likely eventually be replaced by a regular syringe pump; however, most hospitals would not see this as a fiscally responsible decision because of the current high price of syringe pumps and the current low cost of spring-powered syringe pumps. With the remaining three types of automatically regulated pumps a hospital would likely have, a generalization that could be used for all pumps is that clinicians want an inexpensive, quality, easy to use, accurate, and precise pump designed to prevent infusion errors, provide relevant alarms, and integrate with the hospital electronic medical record/physician order entry systems.

Historically, safety has been the major driver for syringe pump development. In the design of future pumps, it is likely that additional safety features and fail-safes will be added to combat the trend of infusion pump recalls as a result of a single failed component. A design style that uses redundant components is not really new; aircraft often have multiple means of calculating position and multiple methods of flight controls, computer servers often have redundant power supplies, and elevators have multiple safeties should a cable break. Similarly, it is likely that infusion pumps will begin using the same design, having multiple means of calculating flow rate and occluding the line to prevent free flow. Redundant designs in these areas could help increase uptime and prevent injury and death.

Integration with other systems and devices will also likely increase the safety of the device because it will allow improved sharing of information. Bidirectional integration with POE will allow orders to be verified—what the clinician is infusing, what was ordered, and the rate at which it was to be delivered—tightening the bounds on what is allowed to be delivered. In addition, the electronic health record system and/or integration with other devices, such as depth-of-sedation monitors and patient vital signs monitors, could provide a more comprehensive view of the patient; alarm algorithms could also be created to alert for specific drug complications. Nevertheless, safety and integration will likely be the two main drivers in the future of infusion pumps because of the constant focus on safety and the increasing demand for connectivity with other medical devices (Table 18-1).

TABLE 18-1 **Infusion Pump Pros and Cons**

Pump Type	Pros	Cons
Regulated gravity-induced flow	Detects clotting, infiltrations, and occlusions Prevents dry IVs Low driving force and decreased severity of infiltrations Low cost Requries less clinical supervision than a gravity IV	No free-flow clamping (currently) Need to know fluid viscosity Needs to be the correct chamber for specific size drip Low pressure, slow infusions Max infusion rate depends on fluid viscosity, head height, and other factors
Peristaltic pumps	Similar accuracy to drip counters Positive pressure can be used to infuse in invasive lines Wide range of infusion rates, up to 999 mL/h Fewer programming errors than drip counters	Pulsatile flow Tubing deforms over time, leading to less precise doses Requires specific tubing set High cost Not accurate for low flow rates
Cassette (volumetric) pumps	Similar accuracy to drip counters and peristaltic pumps Similar function to peristaltic pumps but often easier to load because of the cartridge	More difficult to prime More expensive sets because of the cartridge Pulsatile flow Not accurate for low flow
Syringe pump	Highest accuracy Able to function with many third-party syringes Ability to infuse highly concentrated drugs with accuracy	Limited volume (typically 50 mL) Longer time to determine an occlusion has occurred because of low flow rates
Spring-powered passive syringe pumps	Low cost Can be used with most syringes	Low accuracy Requires special microbore tubing

REFERENCES

1. Millam D: The history of intravenous therapy, *J Intraven Nurs* 19(1):5–14, 1996.
2. Kwan JW: High-technology i.v. infusion devices, *Am J Health Systems Pharm* 48:S36–S51, 1991.
3. ECRI Institute. *Healthcare product comparison system: infusion pumps, general purpose.* Available at www.ecri.org/documents/hpcs_infusion_pumps.pdf.
4. Kim D, Steward D: The effect of syringe size on the performance of an infusion pump, *Paediatr Anesth* 9:335–337, 1999.
5. Cohen AJ, Katz MG, Frenkel G, et al: Morbid results of prolonged intubation after coronary artery bypass surgery, *Chest* 118:1724–1731, 2000.
6. Alsous F, Khamiees M, DeGirolamo A, et al: Negative fluid balance predicts survival in patients with septic shock: a retrospective pilot study, *Chest* 117:1749–1754, 2000.
7. Arieff AI: Fatal postoperative pulmonary edema: pathogenesis and literature review, *Chest* 115:1371–1377, 1999.
8. Schüttler J, Schwilden H, Stoeckel H: Pharmacokinetics as applied to total intravenous anaesthesia, *Anaesthesia* S38:53–56, 1983.
9. Kenny GNC, White M: A portable computerized infusion system for propofol, *Anaesthesia* 45:692–693, 1990.
10. Manberg P, Vozella C, Kelley S: Regulatory challenges facing closed-loop anesthetic drug infusion devices, *Clin Pharmacol Ther* 84(1):166–169, 2008.
11. Catanzaro B, Gillett D, Simmons M, et al: High-accuracy noncontact optical flow sensor for monitoring drug delivery, *Proc SPIE*, 2005. Available at http://proceedings/spiedigitallibrary.org/proceeding/aspx?articleid=858760.
12. Bartels K, Moss DR, Peterfreund RA: Analysis of drug delivery dynamics via a pediactric central venous infusion system: quantification of delays in achieving intended doses, *Anesth Analg* 109:1156–1161, 2009.
13. Lovich MA, Doles J, Peterfreund RA: The impact of carrier flow rate and infusion set dead-volume on the dynamics of intravenous drug delivery, *Anesth Analg* 100:1048–1055, 2005.
15. Summary of proceedings of the 2007 ASHP conference for leaders in health-system pharmacy, *Am J Health Syst Pharm* 65:1270–1271, 2008.

CHAPTER 19

NONINVASIVE TEMPORARY PACEMAKERS AND DEFIBRILLATORS

Ross H. Zoll*

CHAPTER OUTLINE

OVERVIEW

Noninvasive temporary pacemakers and defibrillators are useful devices for treating arrhythmias that may arise during surgery and anesthesia as well as in intensive care or resuscitation settings. Although these are not specifically anesthesia devices, it is important for the anesthesiologist to understand the principles of their function and use.

NONINVASIVE PACING

History

Clinical pacing, first introduced by Paul M. Zoll in 1952, used a device very similar to modern noninvasive pacers.[1-3] However, it was not well accepted because it was a radical innovation in therapy in that it anticipated subsequent developments in monitoring, medical electronics, and intensive care. Although safe and effective,[3] the technique had problems, such as interference with the electrocardiogram (ECG) signal, which made it difficult to determine effectiveness. In addition, the pacing stimulus produced severe pain. Although useful for resuscitation, noninvasive pacing was not satisfactory for long-term pacing therapy.

Implantable pacemakers followed the development of transistors and tissue-compatible stimulating electrodes.[4] Problems of wire breakage, battery life, and circuit reliability were resolved by about 1980. Following the introduction of transvenous pacing,[5] temporary transvenous pacing became popular for resuscitation, prophylaxis, and short-term pacing. However, in certain situations, the transvenous approach has serious disadvantages. Most important, it is not available rapidly enough for resuscitation of an unexpected cardiac arrest, and in such a situation, it is cumbersome and highly unreliable. As an invasive technique, transvenous pacing carries risks such as hemorrhage, infection, tamponade, embolization, and arrhythmias. For prophylaxis, the need for pacing must be weighed against both the expense of the procedure and the risk of complications.

Electrophysiology

As with all excitable tissue, electrical stimulation of cardiac muscle requires forcing decreases in transmembrane potential to activate voltage-dependent ion channels. Subthreshold stimuli have only transient and local effects. Suprathreshold stimuli result in action potentials that propagate throughout the cell membrane and, in the case of cardiac muscle, throughout the contiguous muscle mass. If atrioventricular (AV) conduction is intact, propagation is throughout the heart. Stimuli may be introduced either with transmembrane microelectrodes or by current fields from macroscopic electrodes, such as transvenous or epicardial pacing electrodes or external electrodes on the chest wall. Pacing electrodes in direct contact with tissue, on surface areas of a fraction of a square millimeter, require only 0.1 to 1.0 mA of current for effectiveness. With long-term electrodes, the development of 1-mm thickness or more of scar tissue increases their effective size and may require several milliamperes of current for stimulation. Electrodes on the chest wall are several centimeters distant from the myocardium and typically require 100 times as much threshold current.

*The author was a principal developer of noninvasive temporary pacemakers at Zoll Medical (Redmond, WA).

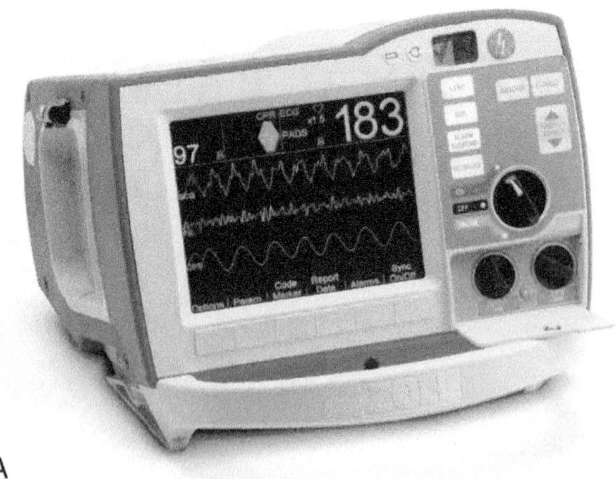

A

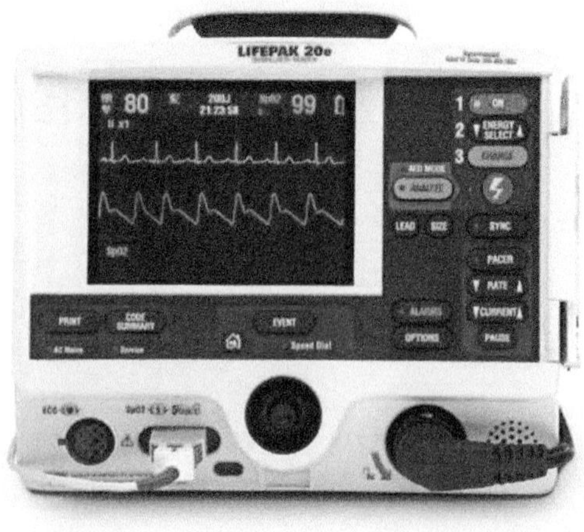

B

FIGURE 19-1 ■ Modern external pacemakers/defibrillators. **A,** Zoll Medical defibrillator (Zoll Medical Corporation, Chelmsford, MA). **B,** Physio-Control Lifepal 20 (Physio-Control, Redmond, WA).

With an external device, unlimited power is available to ensure effectiveness. However, large currents passing through the skin, subcutaneous tissue, and muscle may cause considerable discomfort and even burns. The hemodynamic effects are similar to epicardial or endocardial ventricular pacing.[6,7]

Technology

Improvements in the comfort of noninvasive temporary pacing have contributed greatly to the renewed interest in this technique.[8] The original device of 1952 usually caused unacceptable pain in conscious patients, even following sedation and analgesia. Compared with a typical pacing threshold of 150 mA, a sharp stinging pain was produced at 17 mA. With newer devices, the pacing threshold has been reduced relative to the threshold for discomfort by modifications to the electrodes and stimulus waveforms. Pacing is usually well tolerated for at least a few minutes at currents of 80 mA or more, even without sedation or analgesia.[9] Pacing thresholds vary from 31 mA to more than 100 mA and average about 55 mA. Sedation or analgesia usually improves acceptance by the patient, especially when pacing is required for several minutes.

The modern noninvasive temporary pacemaker system consists of a pacemaker pulse generator incorporated into a portable ECG monitor (most models include a portable defibrillator as well) and disposable self-adherent electrodes for the anterior and posterior chest wall (Fig. 19-1, *A* and *B*). A three-lead ECG monitors effective ventricular capture and is required for the demand ventricular (VVI) pacing mode. The pacemaker has three main controls: the *on/off switch*, the *rate selector*, and the *current amplitude selector*. For operation, the electrodes are applied as in Figure 19-2. A pacing rate (or escape rate in VVI mode) is selected according to clinical criteria, and the pacing current's amplitude is gradually increased until ventricular capture occurs.

Theoretically, there should be an optimum size of electrode. At one extreme, the current field of a point source falls off as the inverse square of the distance from that point. Accordingly, a very small electrode on the chest wall would behave like a point source at a distance from the heart. At the other extreme, a very large electrode will have a uniform current field and will stimulate every muscle in the body, including the heart. A range of sizes and positions for electrodes was tested in a variety of patients to find the optimal size that would be accepted by most patients and for which precise placement was unnecessary (see Fig. 19-2). For the anterior electrode, a diameter of 10 cm was found to be ideal. The posterior electrode is larger and serves as a return path for the current. More recently, computational models have supported the size, position, and impedance determined experimentally.[10] The negative polarity of the stimulus is applied to the anterior electrode for the lowest threshold.

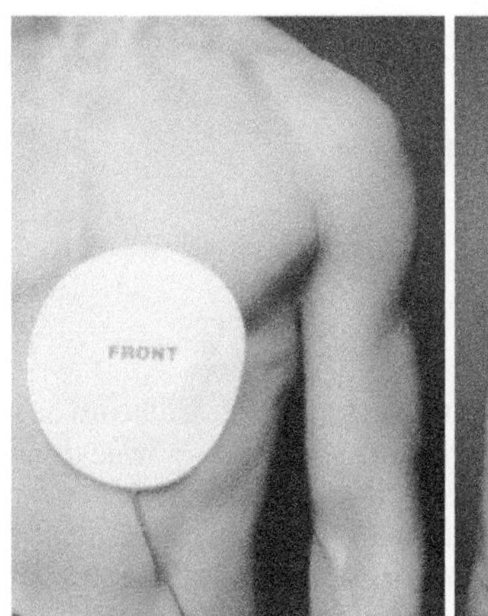

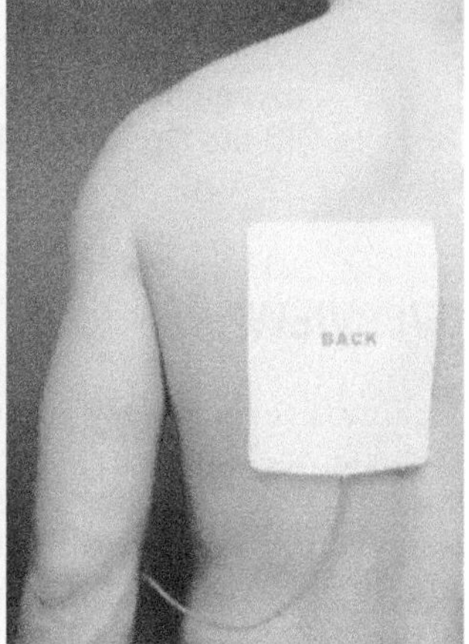

FIGURE 19-2 ■ Nominal positions of electrodes for noninvasive pacing.

An additional step was taken to explore the premise that most of the discomfort from noninvasive pacing was related to current density in the skin and subcutaneous tissues. This component of pain, felt subjectively as a sharp or stinging sensation, is different from pain associated with strong muscle contraction, which also may be uncomfortable. Figure 19-3 shows that the threshold current for skin pain, expressed as current density at the skin,

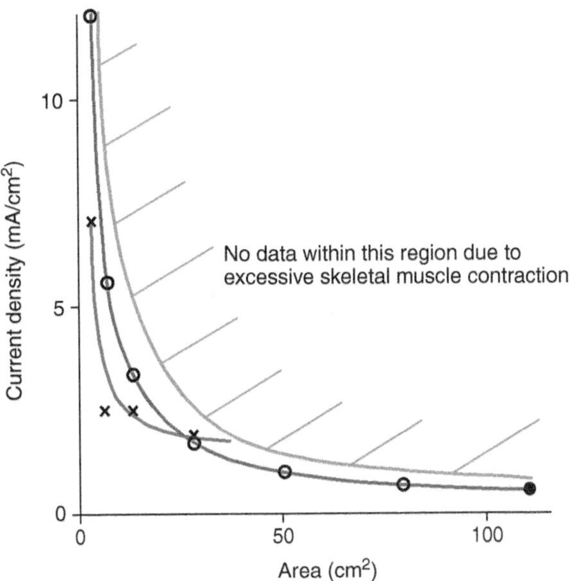

FIGURE 19-3 ■ Relationship of current density at threshold to electrode size for cardiac stimulation. *Circles* show cardiac stimulation; an *x* denotes pain.

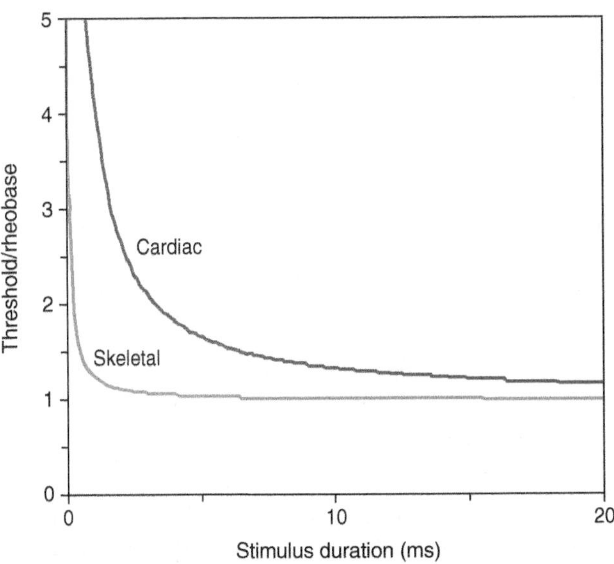

FIGURE 19-4 ■ Strength-duration curves for stimulation of skeletal and cardiac muscle. Rheobase is the minimal strength of an electrical stimulus that is able to cause excitation of tissue.

is independent of electrode area, except for the smallest electrode, where edge effects or coarseness of sensory organs are important. The cardiac stimulation threshold is shown for comparison.

To reduce pain, current density at the skin should be reduced. This can be accomplished by ensuring that the current distribution across the electrode is uniform. Electrodes of relatively high impedance that match skin impedance help reduce edge effects and avoid hot spots if the skin itself is nonuniform.[11] If practical, perspiration or ECG paste should be cleaned from the skin to achieve the most comfortable stimulation. The skin should not be shaved before the electrodes are applied. Because of the high impedance, up to half the energy supplied by the noninvasive external pacemaker may be dissipated in the electrodes. The Zoll NTP (Zoll Medical Corporation, Chelmsford, MA) is designed to supply selected current independent of impedance up to 2000 Ω. However, if the same electrode is to be used for monitoring or defibrillation, a low-impedance medium is necessary.

Electrodes are placed to avoid large muscles yet maintain proximity to the myocardium. The optimum location for the anterior electrode can vary considerably among individuals, and some experimentation may be necessary to achieve greater comfort. Otherwise, the electrode should be placed just to the left of the sternum and mostly below the pectoral muscle. Stimulation directly over the sternum usually is uncomfortable. Precise positioning of the posterior electrode is not necessary.

The noninvasive pacemaker uses the fact that cardiac muscle responds to stimulation somewhat differently than either nerves or skeletal muscle, which respond to stimuli of much shorter duration. Stimuli that are long and uniform in time can reliably pace with less discomfort. Figure 19-4 shows normalized threshold curves for muscle stimulation and for pacing as a function of stimulus duration. Increasing the stimulus duration from 0.5 or 2.0 ms to 40 ms greatly reduces the cardiac stimulation

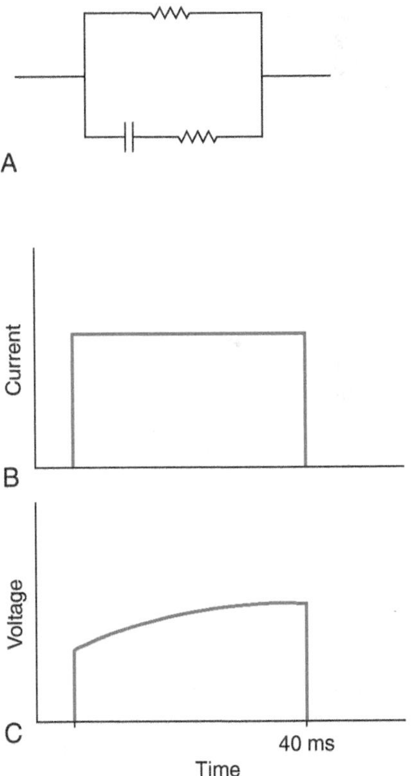

FIGURE 19-5 ■ **A,** Simplified equivalent circuit of tissue and interface. **B,** Controlled-current source waveform. **C,** Resulting voltage waveform (from **B**).

threshold. At 40 ms, threshold amplitude is 5% less than at 20 ms, and discomfort is subjectively halved. Although stimuli of long duration feel different, they are no more intense. Again, the controlled current source design of the Zoll NTP produces a long, constant-amplitude current pulse despite the complex impedance of the tissue and electrodes (Fig. 19-5). The new stimulus does have the disadvantage of increased interference with ECG monitors, and questions of safety have been raised. Noninvasive external pacemakers with shorter stimulus duration and less uniform current amplitude may be more uncomfortable in conscious patients.

Safety

The most serious potential complication of pacing is that of precipitating arrhythmias. Early electrophysiologic studies implicated stimuli of long duration in the production of arrhythmias.[12] However, the original noninvasive pacer used a waveform of 2 to 3 ms and probably never precipitated arrhythmias. By comparison, various permanent and temporary pacers have produced constant voltage or constant current waveforms from 0.2 to 4.5 ms in duration. Demand modes often are used in pacemakers, in part for their hemodynamic benefits, but also because of concern about stimulating during the relative refractory, or "vulnerable," period, when the myocardium is partially repolarized, and a large, suprathreshold stimulus might precipitate ventricular tachycardia or fibrillation. Indeed, when permanent pacing electrodes with small surface areas were introduced to reduce threshold and extend battery life, sudden death occasionally resulted when they were used with older pulse generators that produced higher outputs. Especially when the patient has ischemia or myocardial damage from a recently placed electrode and consequent electrophysiologic inhomogeneity, very large stimuli during the relative refractory period should be avoided. On the other hand, operation of the noninvasive temporary pacer near threshold in the relative refractory period does not produce arrhythmias and is merely ineffective. The maximum output, only four times threshold in the most sensitive patients, is not likely to cause arrhythmias unless the patient's myocardium is so unstable that any extrasystole could degenerate to an arrhythmia. Because the purpose of the device is to produce extrasystole, this risk is unavoidable. Mechanical stimulation from temporary pacing wires occasionally triggers arrhythmias, and this cause is avoided as well. Certain patients who have fibrillated when a temporary wire was passed in the setting of acute myocardial infarction have done well with noninvasive temporary pacing.

The effect of the long-duration stimulus on safety has been studied in dogs.[13,14] A safety factor (i.e., a therapeutic ratio) was defined as the fibrillation threshold divided by the pacing threshold, measured at various stimulus durations. To obtain the worst-case result, the stimulus was intentionally applied during the relative refractory period for fibrillation measurements. Episodes of fibrillation occurred at 5 to 10 times the pacing threshold or higher, and no change was apparent in the safety factor at 40 ms compared with 2 ms.

One significant disadvantage of the long stimulus duration is its interference with ECG monitors. The stimulus artifact is much larger than ECG voltages (1000 times or more) and is within the normal ECG bandwidth. This artifact overloads most monitors, obscuring any real signal. Some monitors include overload recovery circuits and will function normally in this situation. However, the noninvasive temporary pacer is supplied with a rhythm monitor that has preamplifier circuits designed to accommodate the pacing stimulus. The pacemaker circuit inserts a marker on the ECG display to indicate at which point in the cardiac cycle the stimulus occurs. This marker consists of a 40-ms square wave followed by a 40-ms isoelectric period. Following these, the real ECG signal resumes. Part of the QRS response typically is visible as well as the T wave (Fig. 19-6). On occasion, it is necessary to switch leads to obtain a clear tracing. The ECG monitor and pacing output are electrically isolated in accordance with the Association for the Advancement of Medical Instrumentation (AAMI) standards.

Recent Experience

The role of noninvasive external pacing in cardiac arrest situations is under investigation. Fibrillation as a mechanism of arrest is probably more common than asystole, although asystole may follow successful defibrillation. Asystole carries a worse prognosis, in part because it often occurs at a late stage in prolonged arrest. However, some patients are certainly still viable and might be saved with pacing. Some early studies examining the effectiveness of pacing in arrest situations found that pacing held no advantage except in bradycardia. These studies were probably not sufficiently sensitive to discriminate between the situations in which pacing could be effective and those in which the patient was beyond salvage. More recent studies have found pacing to be of benefit in prehospital arrest situations.[15]

Similar to transvenous pacing, noninvasive pacing can be used to interrupt and terminate most supraventricular and ventricular tachycardias using single stimuli, bursts, or overdrive pacing.[16] For tachycardias over 180 beats/min, a special rate generator is needed and is easily added. Often all that is required to interrupt the circus movement in a segment of its AV junctional or ventricular path is a single ectopic ventricular beat.

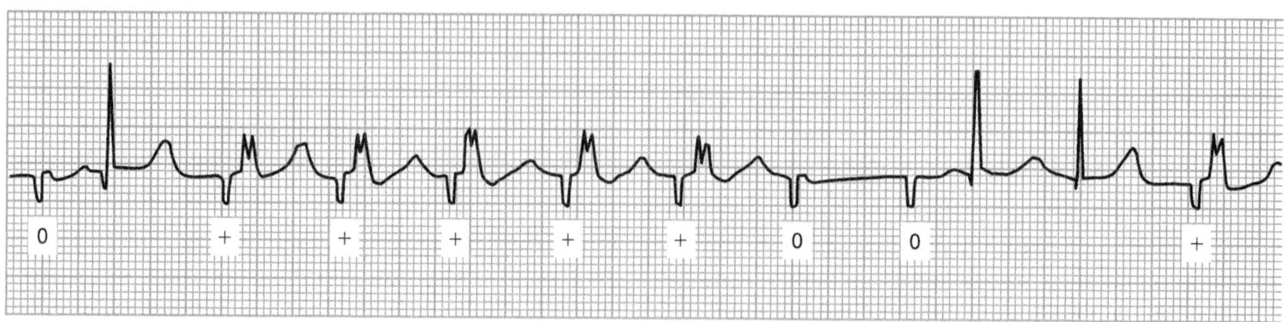

FIGURE 19-6 An electrocardiographic tracing showing effective (+) and ineffective (0, subthreshold) stimulation.

Another potential application of noninvasive pacing is stress testing. As with transvenous pacing, noninvasive temporary pacing at rapid rates simulates exercise stress. This technique does not involve the risks accompanying the insertion of a temporary wire. Stress is alleviated immediately upon cessation of pacing and thus enhances the safety of the procedure. The pacing is interrupted briefly to look for ischemic changes on the ECG. Although rapid noninvasive pacing may be less comfortable than pacing at normal rates, it usually can be performed with analgesia. The effectiveness of the Zoll NTP for stress testing has been confirmed,[17] but extensive experience, and especially correlation to standard protocols, is lacking.

For pediatric use, small electrodes are used for infants and children weighing less than 15 kg. Although pacing thresholds are the same for both children and adults,[18] pediatric pacing rates are likely to be two to three times higher than those for adults. For sick or premature neonates, prolonged use may cause burns if the skin is immature and poorly perfused. However, brief use while securing other means of pacing is safe.

In the Operating Room

Currently, most patients who have significant conduction or sinus node dysfunction have permanent pacemakers. Although bradycardia or asystole unresponsive to atropine or other chronotropic agents is unusual, it has been reported.[19] Temporary pacing frequently is used during the placement of a pulmonary arterial catheter when the patient has preexisting left bundle branch block. Although complete heart block during catheter placement probably occurs in fewer than 1% of cases, it can be disastrous,[20] and noninvasive pacing is ideal for this situation.[21] A temporary transvenous pacemaker requires another site of central access and is not without risk.

Noninvasive pacing is useful for any procedure involving permanent pacemaker systems. It can ensure uninterrupted rhythm during initial implantation of a pacemaker or during revisions or changes of a pulse generator, when mechanical problems occasionally lead to interruption of pacing. The electrodes for the NTP are nearly transparent to radiographs and do not interfere with fluoroscopy.

For patients with permanent pacemakers, the noninvasive pacing guarantees pacing capability during surgery if the system is damaged or reprogrammed by electrocautery. Although uncommon, intraoperative failure of a pacing system occasionally is reported. During surgery, electrocautery usually interferes with the sensing function of the noninvasive pacing, just as it does with permanent pacing systems.

In the event of unexpected arrest, noninvasive pacing can be applied within seconds. When applied promptly, it usually is effective in producing an electrophysiologic response, even if contractility is inadequate. The presence of an electrophysiologic response to pacing stimuli is the appropriate measure of effectiveness, and other pacing modalities produce no additional hemodynamic benefit.

DEFIBRILLATION

History

Defibrillation, introduced into clinical practice by Beck and colleagues in 1947, used electrodes applied directly to the heart.[22] Thoracotomy was advocated as the standard protocol for cardiac arrest. In 1956, Zoll and colleagues[23] introduced closed-chest defibrillation with an alternating current (AC) waveform. Lown[24] and Edmark[25] introduced the direct current (DC) defibrillator in the early 1960s. In the early 1970s, Mirowski and colleagues[26] introduced automatic implantable cardioverter-defibrillators (ICDs) for the treatment of patients with otherwise intractable ventricular arrhythmias. Since that time, there has been renewed interest in other waveforms that might reduce the energy required for defibrillation. Waveforms with improved effectiveness and safety have been discovered and put into practice. Biphasic waveforms with a fixed, opposite polarity component have largely replaced the underdamped oscillator technology.

Technology

The basic principle of defibrillation is to interrupt random and chaotic electrical activity in the heart by using a large stimulus that excites a large and sufficient fraction of the muscle mass at once.[27] However, the detailed mechanism remains extremely controversial. A number of theories and observations have been proposed. One study in dogs found that one small area of fibrillating tissue (approximately 25%) may remain (after treatment) without the fibrillation becoming generalized again; however, two such areas usually lead to clinical failure to defibrillate.[28] It has been observed that the defibrillation threshold may be related to the upper limit of vulnerability for producing fibrillation, although the significance of this is unclear.[29] Much of the myocardium is in the refractory state during fibrillation; therefore a prolongation of recovery may be involved in the defibrillation mechanism.[30] Unlike pacing, which requires an excitement stimulus of only a single cell, a defibrillation shock must excite a considerable portion of the myocardium, even though part of it may be in a relative refractory state, and 1000 times as much current may be required. Cardioversion of atrial or ventricular tachycardia may require much less current, and a pacing stimulus that produces a single extrasystole will occasionally suffice.

On the other hand, too much current can produce damage to the myocardium that may not be thermal in nature. Damage to the cell membrane and contractile structure may lead to depressed function, necrosis, persistent arrest, or single-cell fibrillation.[31] Overdose of current may therefore result in failure to defibrillate. However, there clearly exists a therapeutic window for effective defibrillation. A uniform distribution of current throughout the heart ensures that no part of the heart is overdosed or underdosed, which contributes to the success of defibrillation.

Another factor contributing to success is the defibrillator waveform. The capacitor discharge waveform and, to a lesser extent, the AC waveform are less effective than the truncated exponential (trapezoid) or underdamped harmonic oscillator. Research related to implanted defibrillators has demonstrated new waveforms capable of greater effectiveness with less energy expended as well as greater therapeutic ratio. Biphasic waveforms are in use in Physio-Control (Redmond, WA), Philips Healthcare (Andover, MA), and rectilinear biphasic Zoll Medical devices.

The modern defibrillator works by temporarily storing defibrillation energy in a capacitor. A typical circuit for the underdamped harmonic oscillator waveform is shown in Figure 19-7. The large capacitor is charged to the energy selected by the clinician and then discharged through the paddles. The standard formula for the energy (E) stored by a capacitor (C) at a voltage (V) is as follows:

$$E = \frac{1}{2}CV^2$$

Most of the energy is delivered to the patient, but some is dissipated by parasitic resistance in the inductor. Therefore, by convention, the defibrillator is calibrated in terms of energy delivered into 50 Ω, roughly the average patient's impedance.

The typical underdamped waveform produced is shown in Figure 19-8. For example, a typical old-technology defibrillator (Electrodyne DS95-M [Norwood, MA]) at a setting of 400 J has a capacitor voltage of 7.6 kV corresponding to 450 J stored. At that setting, delivered current into 50 Ω is 66 A, and delivered peak voltage is 3.3 kV. Depending on patient impedance, however, the underdamped negative component may be absent. Evidence suggests that a small negative component reduces defibrillation threshold and increases the therapeutic ratio, perhaps by helping repolarize damaged membranes.

In a biphasic circuit, energy is stored in the capacitor and is discharged through the patient similar to the truncated exponential waveform. However, the current flow is reversed with the H switch circuit; furthermore, the duration of the initial current pulse is adjusted on the fly to deliver a relatively constant energy as selected regardless of impedance, at least in the lower impedance range. This variation in waveform with impedance is shown in Figure 19-9.

The Zoll defibrillator uses a rectilinear biphasic waveform. Because of improved effectiveness, maximum energy into 50 Ω is limited to 200 J. The storage

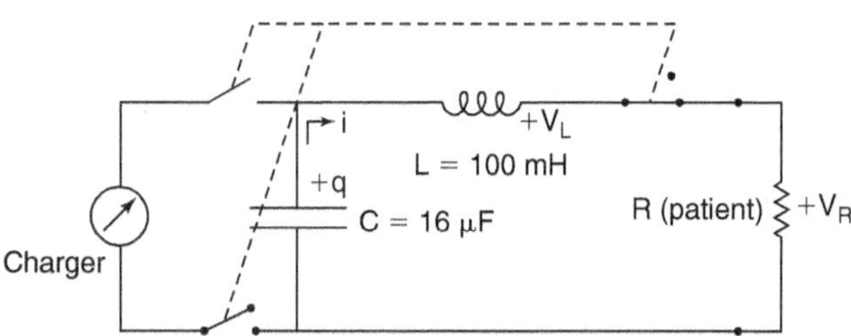

FIGURE 19-7 ■ Typical defibrillator circuit (simplified). Capacitor with a charge of *q*, where capacitance (*C*) is expressed in microfarads (μF); *L*, inductor with inductance expressed in millihenrys (mH); *R*, patient resistance (impedance); *i*, current in circuit; V_L, Voltage across the inductor; V_R, Voltage across the patient.

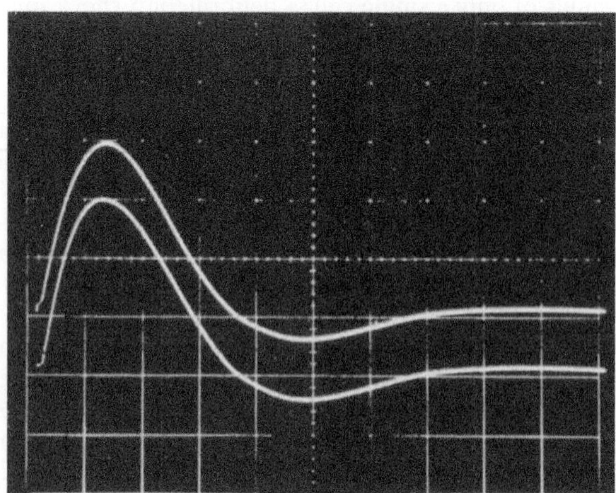

FIGURE 19-8 ■ Defibrillator waveform at a setting of 400 J into a 50 Ω impedance. *Top waveform,* Voltage at 1 kV/division. *Bottom waveform,* Current at 20 A/division. The zero current axis is displaced one division lower to separate the traces. Horizontal scale is 1 ms/division.

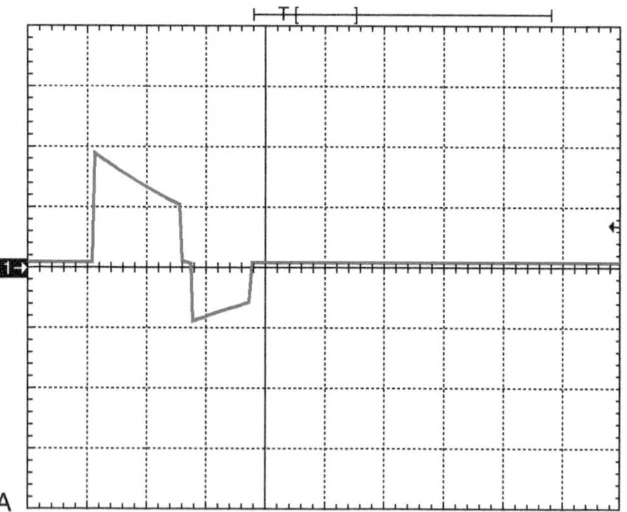

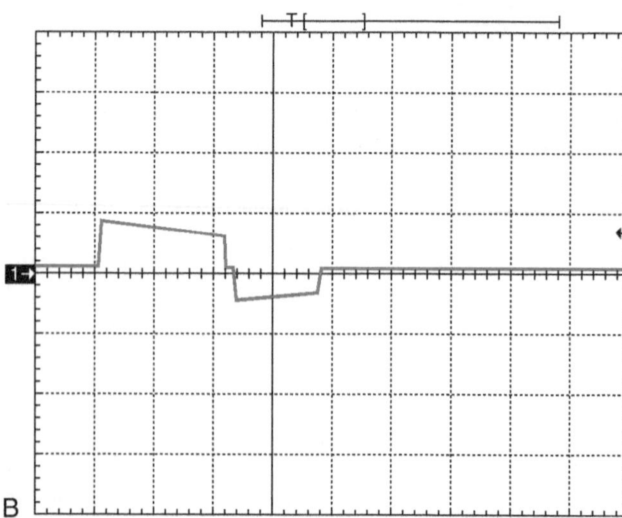

FIGURE 19-9 ■ Biphasic truncated exponential waveform. **A,** Current 20 amp per division vs. 5 ms per division at 50 ohm and 36 J. **B,** At 130 ohm. (From Zelinka M, Buic Z, Zelinka I: Comparison of five different defibrillators using recommended energy protocols. *Resuscitation* 2007; 74:500-507.)

capacitor is charged with up to 2800 V. Before delivering a shock, impedance is tested with an alternating current and a very brief, lower amplitude test shock. Extra resistors are then added into the circuit to adjust the delivered *current* to the appropriate value, relatively independent of patient impedance. They are then switched out, as the capacitor is discharged to maintain a relatively constant current amplitude during the first portion of the discharge. The duration is not adjusted but is kept at the optimum value of 6 ms. It is then switched with the H switch to generate the opposite polarity wave, which is allowed to fall as with the truncated exponential shown in Figure 19-10.

Factors that Affect Success

The primary determinants of success for defibrillation are duration of ventricular fibrillation, and the severity of the hypoxemia, and acidosis. These factors are related to the patient's condition, not to the equipment, and are not discussed further except to the extent that they influence defibrillation studies. Because metabolic state can vary so widely in ventricular fibrillation, the effects on success rates of changes in technique often cannot be discerned. Factors such as weight or paddle location do not seem to affect success rate for ventricular defibrillation in humans. However, these are significant in animal studies of defibrillation and in cardioversion of atrial fibrillation in humans, in whom metabolic factors are more consistent.

Fibrillation is a random and chaotic reentrant arrhythmia. A defibrillation shock at a particular moment finds the myocardium in a unique, unreproducible electrophysiologic state, which is part activated, part refractory, part relative refractory, and perhaps part resting. It is not surprising that the threshold for defibrillation fluctuates with each attempt, even in the same individual. A sigmoid relationship between dose and response exists in the therapeutic range (Figure 19-11). Thresholds vary among individuals for a number of reasons, such as differences in electrophysiologic conditions, geometry, and varying electrical conductivity of the heart and surrounding tissues.

In addition, a number of controllable factors influence the defibrillation threshold, mainly by affecting impedance. Patient impedance can vary widely irrespective of any error in technique. Success in defibrillation correlates better with delivered current than with stored or delivered energy. As with pacemakers, the current flow in the myocardium produces the transmembrane potentials that cause depolarization. Impedance of tissue surrounding the heart and of the electrode interface can vary widely and may absorb a substantial fraction of the delivered energy. Current flow in the myocardium depends almost entirely on delivered current and geometric factors. Peak current can be used as an index of shock strength. Unfortunately, this is practical only for purposes of discussion or research because most defibrillators do not indicate the delivered dose of current. There is some variation in shock duration with impedance, but it is not significant for the underdamped oscillator waveform.

For the defibrillator circuit shown in Figure 19-7, most of the stored energy is delivered to the patient irrespective of the patient impedance. However, delivered energy is the product of current and voltage, summed over time. Variations in patient impedance cause the delivered dose of current to vary widely. For example, at 100 J of stored energy, Figure 19-12 shows the peak current as a function of impedance. Current dose varies by at least a factor of 2 over the domain of common patient impedances. The newer rectilinear biphasic waveform largely corrects for this variation in current dose as well as provides a more effective shape. Clinical studies have confirmed improved effectiveness, especially in cardioversion of atrial fibrillation, when metabolic factors are more consistent.

It has been shown for a wide range of body weights that dose varies with weight (Figure 19-13).[32] Nonetheless, some controversy exists about the dose required for defibrillation of very large, obese humans. No dependence of defibrillation threshold on weight has been demonstrated for adults found in ventricular fibrillation.[33]

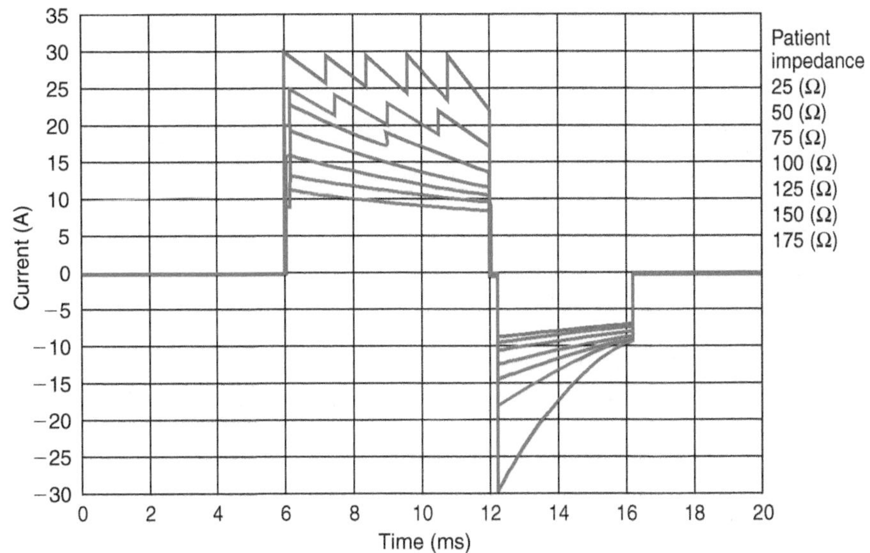

FIGURE 19-10 ■ Rectilinear biphasic waveform. (Courtesy Zoll Medical, Chelmsford, MA.)

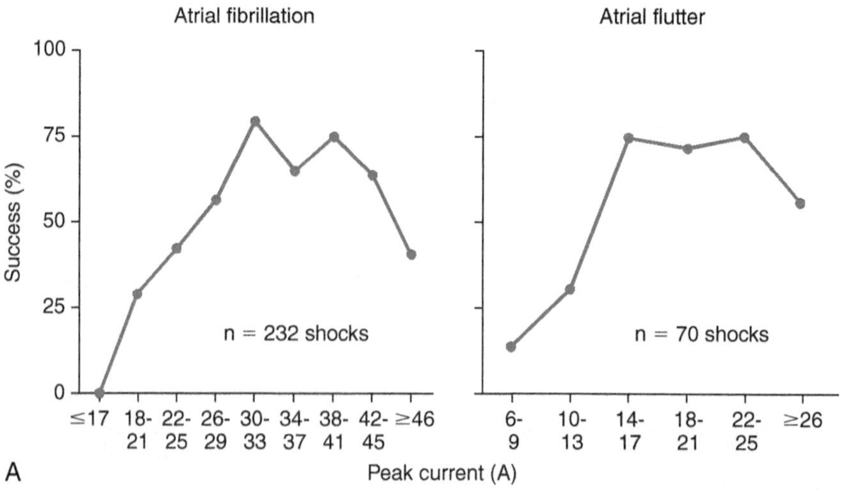

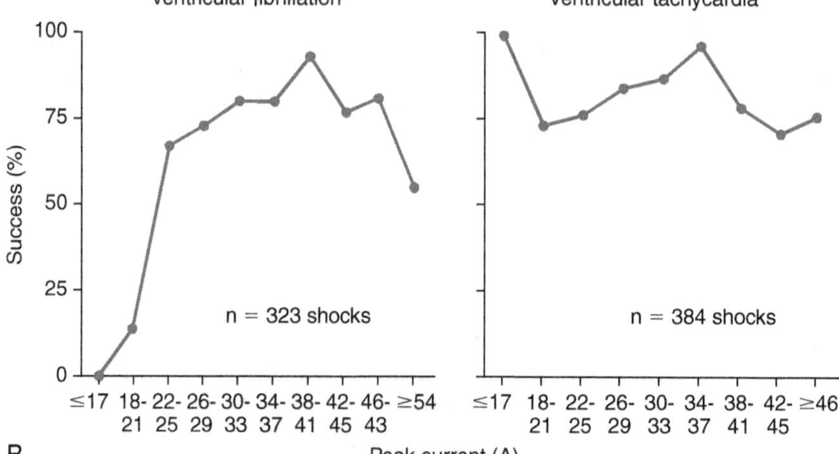

FIGURE 19-11 ■ **Dose vs. response curves for fibrillation and tachycardia in a large population. A, Atrial fibrillation and flutter. B, Ventricular fibrillation and tachycardia.** (From Kerber RE, Martins JB, Kienzle MG, et al: Energy, current, and success in defibrillation and cardioversion: clinical studies using an automated impedance-based method of energy adjustment. *Circulation* 1988;77:1038. Reprinted by permission of the American Heart Association.)

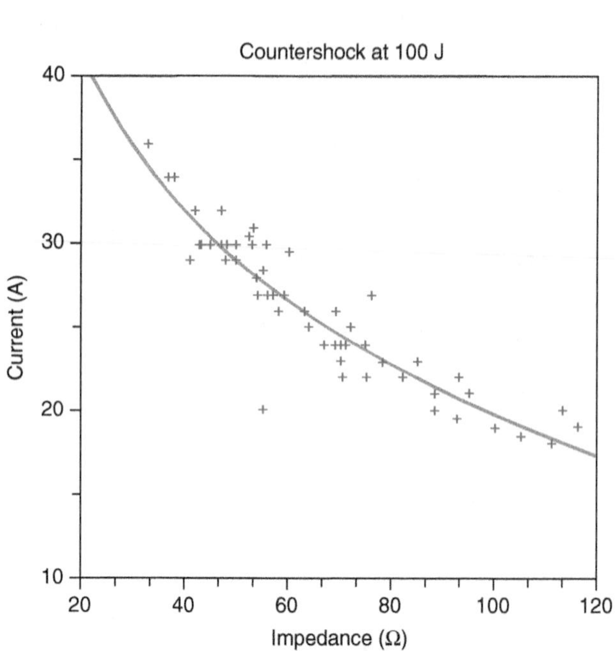

FIGURE 19-12 ■ **Range of patient impedance at 100 J and the resulting variation in peak dose of current.**

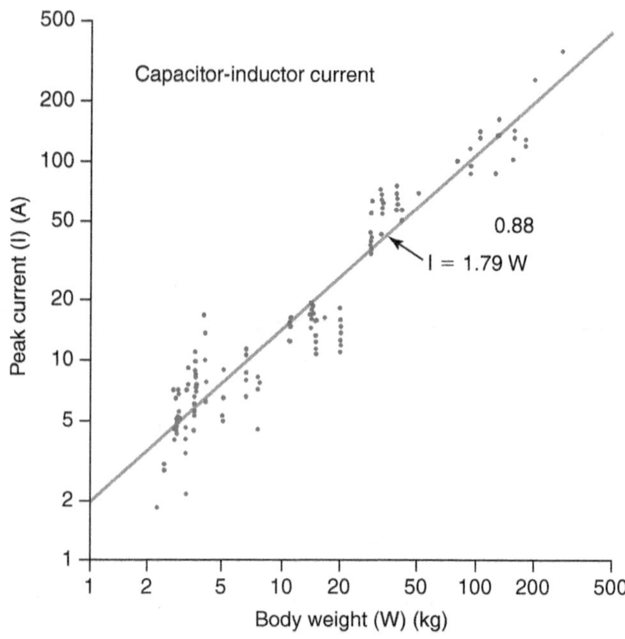

FIGURE 19-13 ■ **Threshold for defibrillation as a function of weight.** (From Geddes LA, Tacker WA, Rosborough JP, et al: Electrical dose for ventricular defibrillation of large and small animals using precordial electrodes. *J Clin Invest* 1974;53:310. Reprinted by permission of the American Society of Clinical Investigation.)

This lack of correlation probably reflects the preponderance of other factors and the relatively narrow range of weights studied.

Shock strength is affected by patient impedance in some defibrillators, which in turn is influenced by numerous factors. Even within the same individual, variations in impedance affect clinical outcome and complicate studies of defibrillation threshold. In general, the body presents a complex (i.e., frequency dependent) and nonlinear impedance. However, for the large currents involved in defibrillation, the frequency dependence is negligible. The nonlinearity is manifest as a much lower resistance at defibrillation currents than at pacing currents and as a continued decrease as shock strength increases. Resistance probably drops 20% to 30% between 50 and 400 J. In addition, a history of previous shocks reduces impedance, perhaps through injury or reflex circulatory changes in the skin and other tissues. Burns are unusual, but erythema under the electrodes is normal and usually fades in a few minutes.

Other factors are important in impedance. The interface material usually contributes insignificantly; however, some gels can add up to 10.5 Ω to the circuit. Paddle pressure typically reduces impedance to 5% to 10% when compared with self-adherent patches without pressure. Geometric changes probably are responsible for this change in impedance. Similarly, there is clearly a small respiratory variation in impedance.

The distribution of current within the body and the heart is affected by size and location of electrodes. The goal is to achieve the most uniform distribution of current possible within the heart. This ensures effective stimulation of all excitable tissue without causing damage by overdosing a portion of the heart. Outcome studies[34] of ventricular fibrillation in humans have shown no difference between anterior and anterior-posterior paddle placement. However, in atrial fibrillation, anterior-posterior placement is more effective.[35] The use of larger electrodes predictably lowers resistance somewhat but also increases current threshold. Any difference in therapeutic ratio would be too subtle to measure in humans. Of note, the presence of myocardial patch electrodes significantly interferes with external defibrillation.[36] In this case, defibrillation thresholds are approximately doubled, emphasizing the importance of current distribution.

These concepts of current and impedance are important. Even though the therapeutic ratio is large, with older defibrillators, the delivered current dose is usually unknown, making overdose easy. The deleterious effects of overdose are evident in animal studies[37] and in studies of single-cell preparations.[31]

Programmed Defibrillators

First-generation automatic pacer-defibrillators[38] have existed since the early 1980s but were not widely used. These instruments were designed to recognize asystole or ventricular arrhythmias requiring defibrillation and to provide the appropriate therapy without the intervention of a physician. Recognition of arrhythmias under adverse conditions of field resuscitation was difficult, and the protocols used for pacing or defibrillation were not the most successful. More recently, new automated external defibrillator devices that recognize ventricular arrhythmias and recommend defibrillation have been approved for use by paramedics, who are not otherwise permitted by local regulation to defibrillate in the field, and by the public.

Newer Electrodes

Traditionally, anterior paddles used for adults are 8 cm in diameter, and a larger 10- to 12-cm paddle is used for posterior placement. One advantage of paddles is that they are applied with force, which reduces impedance. If repeated defibrillation is necessary or if surgical drapes might prevent ready access to the chest, preapplied adhesive electrodes are very convenient. The small increase in impedance is acceptable because more rapid defibrillation can be accomplished.[39] Newer adhesive pad electrodes allow monitoring, pacing, or defibrillation through the same electrodes. One disadvantage is that they may be less comfortable during external pacing. Given the relative rarity of treatable asystole compared with ventricular fibrillation, multifunction electrodes are far more popular. Gelled pads for use with regular paddles offer some convenience compared with paste or gel and avoid arcing or short-circuiting across the chest by leakage of conductive material between the paddles.

Two new related devices that might be encountered are worth mentioning. First, a wearable automatic defibrillator is marketed as a bridge to possible cardioverter-defibrillator implant. Second, an automated cardiopulmonary resuscitation (CPR) device, the Autopulse by Zoll Medical, can provide very consistent and possibly more effective CPR over a prolonged period of resuscitation or transport.

REFERENCES

1. Heller MB, Kaplan RM, Peterson J, et al: Comparison of performance of five transcutaneous pacing devices [abstract], *Ann Emerg Med* 16:166–493, 1987.
2. Zoll PM: Resuscitation of the heart in ventricular standstill by external electric stimulation, *N Engl J Med* 247:768–771, 1952.
3. Abelman WH: Paul Zoll and electrical stimulation of the heart, *Clin Cardiol* 9:131–135, 1986.
4. Zoll PM, Frank HA, Zarsky LN, et al: Long term electric stimulation of the heart for Stokes-Adams disease, *Anesth Analg* 141: 367–376, 1962.
5. Furman S, Robinson G: Use of an intracardiac pacemaker in the correction of total heart block, *Surg Forum* 9:245–248, 1958.
6. Feldman MD, McKay RS, Gervino EV, et al: Noninvasive transthoracic pacing tachycardia stress test: hemodynamic responses [abstract], *Circulation* 72(Suppl III):20, 1985.
7. Feldman MD, Zoll PM, Aroesty JM, et al: Hemodynamic responses to noninvasive external cardiac pacing, *Am J Med* 84:395–400, 1988.
8. Belgard AH, Zoll PM, Zoll RZ: External noninvasive cardiac stimulation, *United States Patent*, 4,349,030, 1982.
9. Falk RH, Zoll PM, Zoll RH: Safety and efficacy of noninvasive cardiac pacing, *N Engl J Med* 309:1166–1168, 1983.
10. Panescu D, Webster JG, Tompkins WJ, Stratbucker RA: Optimisation of transcutaneous cardiac pacing by three-dimensional finite element modelling of the human thorax, *Med Biol Eng Comput* 33(6):769–775, 1995.
11. Williams CR, Geddes LA, Bourland JD, et al: Analysis of the current-density distribution from a tapered, gelled-pad external cardiac pacing electrode, *Med Instrum* 21:329–334, 1987.

12. Wiggers CJ, Wegria R: Ventricular fibrillation due to single, localized induction and condenser shocks applied during the vulnerable phase of ventricular systole, *Am J Physiol* 128:500, 1940.
13. Zoll RH, Zoll PM, Belgard AH: Noninvasive cardiac stimulation. In Feruglio GA, editor: *Cardiac pacing: electrophysiology and pacemaker technology*, Padua, 1983, Piccin Medical Books, pp 593–595.
14. Voorhees WD 3rd, Foster KS, Geddes LA, et al: Safety factor for precordial pacing: minimum current thresholds for pacing and for ventricular fibrillation by vulnerable-period stimulation, *PACE* 7:356–360, 1984.
15. Clinton JE, Zoll PM, Zoll R, et al: Emergency noninvasive external cardiac pacing, *J Emerg Med* 2:155–162, 1985.
16. Estes NA 3rd, Deering TF, Manolis AS, et al: External cardiac programmed stimulation for noninvasive termination of sustained supraventricular and ventricular tachycardia, *Am J Cardiol* 63:177–183, 1989.
17. Feldman MD, Warren SE, Gervino EV, et al: Noninvasive external cardiac pacing for thallium-201 scintigraphy, *Am J Physiol Imaging* 3:172–177, 1988.
18. Beland MJ, Hesslein PS, Finlay CD, et al: *Noninvasive transcutaneous cardiac pacing in children (poster presentation)*, Dallas, 1986, American Heart Association.
19. Kirschenbaum LP, Eisenkraft JB, Mitchell J, et al: Transthoracic pacing for the treatment of severe bradycardia during induction of anesthesia, *J Cardiothorac Anesth* 3:329–332, 1989.
20. Thompson IR, Dalton BC, Lappas DG, et al: Right bundle branch block and complete heart block caused by the Swan-Ganz catheter, *Anesthesiology* 51:359–362, 1979.
21. Buran MJ: Transcutaneous pacing as an alternative to prophylactic transvenous pacemaker insertion [letter], *Crit Care Med* 15: 623–624, 1987.
22. Beck CS, Pritchard WH, Feil HS: Ventricular fibrillation of long duration abolished by electric shock, *JAMA* 135:985–986, 1953.
23. Zoll PM, Linenthal AJ, Gibson W, et al: Termination of ventricular fibrillation in man by externally applied electric countershock, *N Engl J Med* 254:727–732, 1956.
24. Lown B: Cardioversion of arrhythmias, *Br Heart J* 29:469–487, 1964.
25. Edmark KW: Simultaneous voltage and current waveforms generated during internal and external direct-current pulse defibrillation, *Surg Forum* 14:262–264, 1963.
26. Mirowski M, Mower MM, Staewen WS, et al: The development of the transvenous automatic defibrillator, *Arch Intern Med* 129:773–779, 1972.
27. Zipes DP, Fischer J, King RM, et al: Termination of ventricular fibrillation in dogs by depolarizing a critical amount of myocardium, *Am J Cardiol* 36:37–44, 1975.
28. Witkowski FX, Penkoske PA, Plonsey R: Mechanisms of defibrillation in open-chest dogs with unipolar DC-coupled simultaneous activation and shock potential recordings, *Circulation* 82:244–260, 1990.
29. Chen PS, Shibata N, Dixon EG, et al: Comparison of the defibrillation threshold and the upper limit of vulnerability, *Circulation* 73:1022–1028, 1986.
30. Sweeney RJ, Gill RM, Syeinberg MI, et al: Ventricular refractory period extension caused by defibrillation shocks, *Circulation* 82:965–972, 1990.
31. Jones JL, Lepeschkin E, Rush S, et al: Depolarization-induced arrhythmias following high-intensity electric field stimulation of cultured myocardial cells [abstract], *Med Instrum* 12:54, 1978.
32. Geddes LA, Tacker WA, Rosborough JP, et al: Electrical dose for ventricular defibrillation of large and small animals using precordial electrodes, *J Clin Invest* 53:310–319, 1974.
33. Adgey AA, Patton JN, Campbell NP, et al: Ventricular defibrillation: appropriate energy levels, *Circulation* 60:219–223, 1979.
34. Kerber RE, Martins JB, Kelly KJ, et al: Self-adhesive preapplied electrode pads for defibrillation and cardioversion, *J Am Coll Cardiol* 3:815–820, 1984.
35. Zoll RH, Zoll PM, Belgard AH: unpublished data.
36. Lerman BB, Deale OC: Effect of epicardial patch electrodes on transthoracic defibrillation, *Circulation* 81:1409–1414, 1990.
37. Warner ED, Dahl C, Ewy GA: Myocardial injury from transthoracic defibrillator countershock, *Arch Pathol* 99:55–59, 1975.
38. Aronson AL, Haggar B: The automatic defibrillator-pacemaker: clinical rationale and engineering design, *Med Instrum* 20:27–35, 1985.
39. Zoll RH, Zoll PM, Belgard AH: New defibrillation electrodes [abstract], *Med Instrum* 2:56, 1978.

CHAPTER 20

INFECTION PREVENTION: RECOMMENDATIONS FOR PRACTICE

Richard Beers

CHAPTER OUTLINE

OVERVIEW

Patients have a reasonable expectation that anesthesia care will not expose them to infectious disease. Anesthesia professionals, as part of the health care team, have a responsibility to limit the potential for patients to acquire an infection while receiving care. This chapter discusses infection-prevention recommendations and practices as they apply to the anesthesia professional (Box 20-1).

Health care–associated infections (HAIs), formerly termed *nosocomial infections*, are clinically important because they are the most common complication associated with hospital care. In 2002, investigators estimated an incidence of 1.7 million HAIs annually in the United States—1 of every 20 hospitalized patients—leading to 99,000 deaths.[1]

It is important to note that these HAI estimates are extrapolations based on generalizations. Nonetheless, if these 2002 estimates had been accurate, the annual incidence of HAIs would have exceeded that of many reportable diseases, such as hepatitis C and meningococcal meningitis.

Some infections may be inevitable. Harbarth and colleagues[2] estimate that only 20% of all HAIs are likely preventable by using the latest technologies and recommended medical practices. The Study on the Efficacy of Nosocomial Infection Control (SENIC), an investigation conducted from 1971 through 1976, suggested that 6% of nosocomial infections could be prevented by minimal infection control efforts, and that "well-organized and highly effective programs" could forestall 32%.[3]

Nonetheless, some investigators have reported dramatic declines in the incidence of certain HAIs after implementing clinical processes derived from published recommendations. For example, after implementing a "bundle" of five initiatives designed to reduce the chance of infection, Pronovost and colleagues[4] reported a 66% decrease in the rate of bloodstream infections associated with central venous catheters (CVCs). Prior to catheter insertion, the steps these researchers implemented included 1) avoiding the femoral site if possible; 2) performing proper hand hygiene; 3) preparing the skin with chlorhexidine; and 4) using full-barrier precautions prior to catheter insertion. After catheter insertion, the investigators provided ongoing surveillance of the need for the catheter and prompt removal when the central line was no longer essential for clinical care. Other studies have demonstrated that to achieve sustained results, these bundled practices as a whole must be continuously monitored for high compliance.[5] Similar results were achieved using bundled practices to manage hospitalized patients with known or suspected infection with methicillin-resistant *Staphylococcus aureus* (MRSA).[6]

Listed in order of estimated direct socioeconomic costs, the following are the five most prevalent HAIs, comprising more than 80% of those reported: 1) surgical site infection (SSI); 2) *Clostridium difficile*–associated infections (CDIs); 3) central line–associated bloodstream

BOX 20-1 Infection Precautions Glossary

Asepsis: The absence or creation of the absence of potentially pathogenic microorganisms; preventing access by pathogens to any locus of potential infection.

Aseptic technique: Aseptic technique comprises specific, careful practices to minimize contamination by pathogens. It is utilized in the clinical setting to maximize and maintain *asepsis*, the absence of pathogens, to protect the patient from infection, and to prevent the spread of pathogens. For injection safety, this refers to handling, preparation, administration, and storage of medications, solutions, and injection equipment. This applies to all supplies used for injections and infusions, including medication vials, ampoules, syringes, needles, cannulas, fluid containers, intravenous administration tubing, and associated access ports and stopcocks.

Barriers: Equipment such as gloves, gowns, aprons, masks, or protective eyewear, which when worn can reduce the risk of exposure of the health care worker's skin or mucous membranes to potentially infective materials.

Cleaning: The removal, usually with detergents and mechanical action, of all adherent visible soil or debris from the surfaces, crevices, serrations, joints, and lumens of instruments, devices, and equipment by a manual or mechanical process that prepares the items for safe handling and/or further decontamination.

***Clostridium difficile*:** *C. difficile* is a spore-forming, gram-positive anaerobic bacillus that produces endotoxin. It accounts for 15% to 25% of all episodes of antibiotic-associated diarrhea and can cause more serious diseases, such as pseudomembranous enterocolitis and toxic megacolon, both of which can be complicated by perforation, sepsis, and death. *C. difficile* spores are spread from patient to patient by contact transmission. Because alcohol does not kill *C. difficile* spores, use of soap and water is more efficacious than alcohol-based hand rubs. For environmental surface disinfection, consider using an EPA-registered germicide with a sporicidal claim after cleaning in accordance with label instructions; a hypochlorite solution, using household chlorine bleach, may also be appropriately diluted and used.

Common vehicle: Contaminated material, product, or substance that serves as an intermediate means by which an infectious agent is introduced into a susceptible host through a suitable portal of entry.

Contamination: The presence of microorganisms on an item or surface.

Critical device: An item that enters sterile tissue, cavities, or the vascular system. Such items must undergo sterilization prior to reuse.

Decontamination: The use of physical or chemical means to remove, inactivate, or destroy blood-borne pathogens on a surface or item, such that transmission of infectious particles is no longer possible, and the surface or item is rendered safe for handling, use, or disposal.

Disinfection: The use of a chemical or physical process that eliminates virtually all recognized pathogenic microorganisms, but not necessarily all microbial forms (e.g., bacterial endospores), on inanimate objects.

Engineering controls: Controls designed to isolate or remove pathogens from the workplace (e.g., sharps disposal containers, airborne-infection isolation rooms).

Infectious agent: See *Pathogen*.

Hand hygiene: The single most important practice to reduce the transmission of infectious disease in health care settings. Refers to rubbing hands with an alcohol-based product or, if hands are visibly soiled, hand washing with water and plain or antiseptic soap.

Health care–associated infections (HAIs): Infections associated with health care delivery in any setting, including hospitals, long-term care facilities, ambulatory settings, medical and dental offices, and home care.

High-level disinfection: A process that destroys all organisms except high levels of bacterial spores; the process may use a chemical germicide cleared for marketing by the FDA.

Infectious disease: A clinically manifest disease of humans or animals resulting from a transmissible disease caused by the presence and growth of pathogenic biologic agents. Infectious pathogens include viruses, bacteria, fungi, protozoa, parasites, and prions (aberrant proteins).

Injection safety, safe injection practices: A set of measures taken to perform injections in an optimally safe manner for patients, health care personnel, and others. A safe injection does not harm the recipient, does not expose the provider to any avoidable risks, and does not result in waste that is dangerous for the community. Injection safety includes practices intended to prevent transmission of blood-borne pathogens between one patient and another, or between a health care worker and a patient, and to prevent harmful incidents such as needle-stick injuries.

Intermediate-level disinfection: Disinfection that kills mycobacteria, most viruses, and bacteria with a chemical germicide registered as a "tuberculocide" by the EPA.

Low-level disinfection: Disinfection that kills some viruses and bacteria with a chemical germicide registered as a hospital disinfectant by the EPA.

Multidose medication vial: Medication container that holds more than one dose (e.g., insulin preparations, vaccines). Multidose vials used by anesthesia professionals may contain medications such as succinylcholine or neostigmine. When used in an immediate patient care setting, multidose vials should be used as if they are single-dose vials (i.e., for single-patient use only).

Noncritical device: An item that contacts intact skin and requires low-level disinfection.

Pathogen or infectious agent: A biologic, physical, or chemical entity capable of causing disease. Biologic agents may be bacteria, viruses, fungi, protozoa, parasites, or prions.

Personal protective equipment (PPE): Specialized clothing or equipment worn by personnel for protection against a hazard, such as infectious agents.

Portal of entry: The means by which an infectious agent enters the susceptible host.

Reservoir: Place in or on which an infectious agent can survive but may or may not multiply. Health care workers may serve as reservoirs for organisms known to cause health care–associated infections.

Semicritical device: An item that comes in contact with mucous membranes or nonintact skin and requires, at a minimum, high-level disinfection.

Single-dose vial: A single-use vial that contains medication or fluid for single-patient use; the contents do not include preservatives or bacteriostatic agents.

Spaulding scale: A classification system that divides patient care equipment and devices into three classes based on their intended use. Each of the three classes requires a different degree of decontamination: intermediate- or low-level disinfection, high-level disinfection, or sterilization.

Standard precautions: Infection prevention and control practices based on the principle that all blood, body fluids, secretions, excretions (except sweat), nonintact skin, and mucous membranes may contain transmissible infectious agents. Standard precautions apply to all patients, regardless of suspected

Continued

BOX 20-1 Infection Precautions Glossary—cont'd

or confirmed infection status, in any setting in which health care is delivered. Standard precautions include hand hygiene, safe injection practices, and use of barrier protection such as gloves, gowns, masks, eye protection, or face shields, depending on the anticipated exposure. Standard precautions also include the proper handling and cleaning, disinfection, and/or sterilization of reprocessed patient care devices.

Sterilization: The use of a physical or chemical procedure to destroy all microbial life, including highly resistant bacterial endospores.

Surgical site infection: An infection that occurs after surgery in the part of the body where the surgery took place. Surgical site infections can be superficial (skin only) or can involve tissues under the skin, the organs, or implanted material.

Susceptible host: A person or animal who does not possess sufficient resistance to a particular infectious agent to prevent contracting an infection when exposed to the agent.

Transmission: Any mechanism by which a pathogen is spread by a source or reservoir to a person, and the person subsequently develops an infectious disease or evidence of infection.

Work practice controls: Recommended procedures that reduce the likelihood of exposure to blood-borne pathogens by altering the manner in which a task is performed (e.g., prohibiting recapping of needles by a two-handed technique).

EPA, Environmental Protection Agency; FDA, Food and Drug Administration.

infections (CLABSIs); 4) ventilator-associated pneumonia (VAP); and 5) catheter-associated urinary tract infections (CAUTIs).[7] Direct cost estimates do not take into account indirect costs, such as loss of productivity. HAIs are categorized as 1) those associated with a medical *device* (e.g., CLABSI [CVCs]; CAUTI [urinary bladder catheters]); 2) those associated with a medical *procedure* (e.g., VAP [endotracheal intubation and mechanical ventilation]; SSI [surgical procedure]); and, 3) those associated with *antibiotic use*, such as CDIs and infections from multidrug-resistant organisms such as MRSA and vancomycin-resistant *Enterococcus* (VRE).

By following recommended infection-prevention practices, the incidence of infection transmission between patients, between health care personnel and their patients, and from equipment and other inanimate objects to patients can be decreased or eliminated. Timely and effective hand hygiene has frequently been cited as the single most important practice to reduce the transmission of infectious disease in health care settings.[8] After making observations and deductions from clinical practices associated with infectious outcomes, Ignaz Semmelweis, in the mid-1800s, introduced a simple handwashing regimen. The incidence of puerperal sepsis was dramatically reduced when clinicians washed their hands. Since this time, hand hygiene has been a key element of every infection-prevention strategy. Handwashing with soap and water is recommended when hands are visibly soiled or contaminated (Fig. 20-1); hands may be decontaminated with an alcohol-based hand rub when they are not visibly soiled. Gloves do not substitute for or eliminate the need for hand hygiene. Compliance with the hand-hygiene guidelines published by the Centers for Disease Control and Prevention (CDC)[9] and the World Health Organization (WHO)[10] was one of The Joint Commission's National Patient Safety Goals for hospitals in both 2011 and 2012.

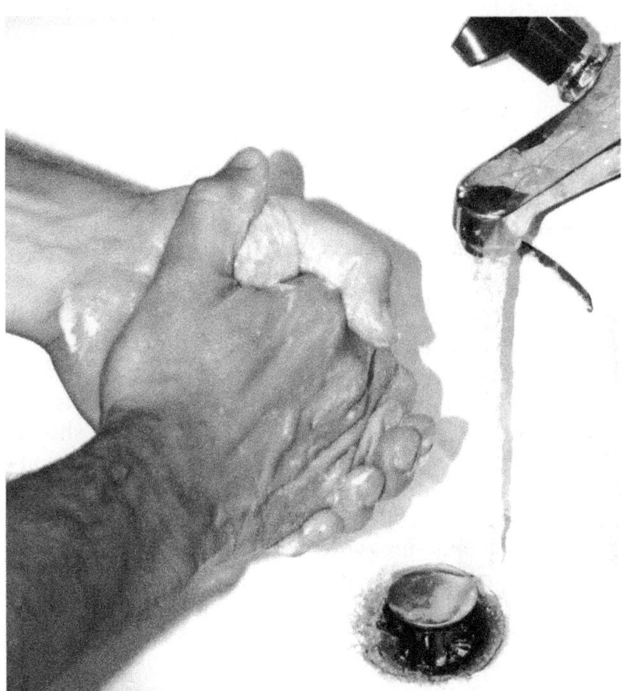

FIGURE 20-1 ■ If hands are visibly soiled, perform hand hygiene by washing vigorously with soap and water for 20 seconds. Wearing gloves does not eliminate the need for hand hygiene.

Injection practices are associated with the use of needles, syringes, medication and fluid containers (ampules, vials, bags, bottles), and infusion supplies (administration sets, ports, connectors, and flush solutions). Recent outbreaks of blood-borne infectious disease have underscored the need for anesthesia professionals to reexamine injection practices. Between 1998 and 2008, there were 33 reported outbreaks associated with the iatrogenic transmission of hepatitis B virus (HBV) and hepatitis C virus (HCV) to patients.[11] These outbreaks were *not* associated with blood-product transfusions or tissue transplantations; each was the result of either reusing a syringe or needle between patients or reusing a syringe or needle to access a medication or fluid container that was subsequently reaccessed and administered to another patient. Delivery of anesthesia care was involved in 7 of the 33 outbreaks. In these 7 outbreaks associated with anesthesia professionals, more than 55,000 patients were identified "at risk," and 144 patients acquired HBV or HCV infections.

Many of the devices, supplies, and equipment used in anesthesia care are labeled "single-use only." After use for one patient, these items should be discarded and not reprocessed for reuse. For equipment and devices labeled as "reusable" by the manufacturer, anesthesia

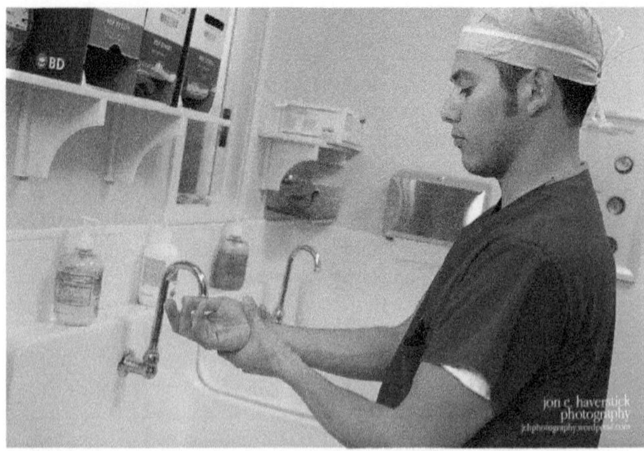

FIGURE 20-2 ■ If hands are not visibly soiled, rub them thoroughly with an alcohol-based gel or foam and let them air dry. Wearing gloves does not substitute for hand hygiene. (Courtesy Jon C. Haverstick Photography, Medcom, Inc., Cypress, CA.)

professionals should be familiar with reprocessing techniques appropriate for anesthesia equipment, including those applicable to the various components of the anesthesia machine.

Anesthesia professionals also should be knowledgeable of how infection prevention recommendations apply to the anesthesia work area, including anesthesia machines, work surfaces, and supply carts. Such knowledge can be extrapolated to other anesthesia care settings: offsite anesthetizing locations, critical care units, obstetric suites, pain management centers, and office-based surgery facilities. In all these settings, anesthesia professionals should be familiar with infection prevention recommendations and practices applicable to all patients (standard precautions) and those that apply to patients known or suspected to have infectious diseases of epidemiologic importance (expanded precautions). Diseases may be epidemiologically important because the infecting pathogen is either highly transmissible (*Mycobacterium tuberculosis*, varicella) or multidrug-resistant, and therefore difficult to treat (MRSA, VRE).

In addition to standard precautions, anesthesia professionals should be familiar with infectious occupational hazards associated with anesthesia care and recommendations intended to limit the potential for acquiring these infections from patients. This discussion will focus on anesthesia work practices, device and facility designs, postexposure prophylaxis, and vaccination.

HAND HYGIENE

Hand hygiene refers to either handwashing with water and plain or antiseptic soap or rubbing hands with an alcohol-based product in the form of a gel, rinse, or foam (Fig. 20-2) followed by air drying. In the absence of visible soiling, approved alcohol-based hand rubs are recommended. Hand hygiene should be performed before and after direct patient contact, before and after wearing gloves, after touching patient care equipment or surfaces in the patient environment, and before and after performing invasive procedures.[9,10]

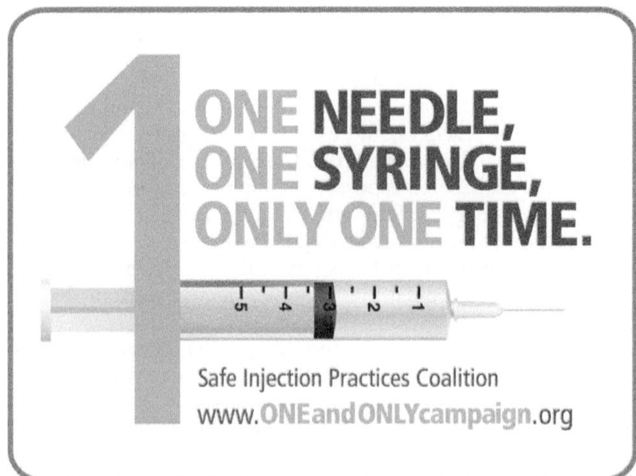

FIGURE 20-3 ■ The Centers for Disease Control and Prevention's "One and Only Campaign" targets the public and health care professionals. It is designed to reinforce the principle that syringes and needles should be used only once and discarded after use. Used needles and/or syringes *should not* be used to reaccess a multidose container of medication or fluid.

STANDARD PRECAUTIONS AND SAFE INJECTION PRACTICES

Because patient examination and medical history cannot reliably identify the presence of infectious disease, the CDC developed standard precautions to apply to *all* patients.[8] Standard precautions require health care personnel to assume that all bodily fluids except sweat are potentially infectious regardless of the diagnosis or perceived risk of the patient. Barrier protection should be used whenever there may be contact with a patient's nonintact skin, mucous membranes, and blood or other bodily fluids; this includes secretions and excretions, regardless of whether they contain visible blood.[8]

Safe injection practices are the application of standard precautions to injection equipment and procedures. Whenever a needle, syringe, medication or fluid container (ampules, vials, bags, bottles), or infusion supply (administration sets and flush solutions) is used, the anesthesia professional must adhere to the principle that *each item is intended for use on a single patient.* A syringe or needle that contacts a patient's blood or body fluids *or any part* of the administration set connected to a patient's vascular (intravenous or arterial) access *should not be reused*, either for another patient *or to reaccess* a fluid or medication container. This is the principle behind the CDC's public health campaign entitled the "One and Only Campaign" to promote the "one needle, one syringe, one time" concept (Fig. 20-3).[12] Safe injection practices also apply to the handling and disposal of injection devices and are designed to protect the anesthesia professional from accidental infection with blood-borne pathogens.

Two unsafe practices by anesthesia professionals have been associated with transmission of blood-borne pathogens: reusing a needle, cannula, or a syringe to administer intravenous (IV) medication to more than one patient and reaccessing a medication vial or flush preparation with

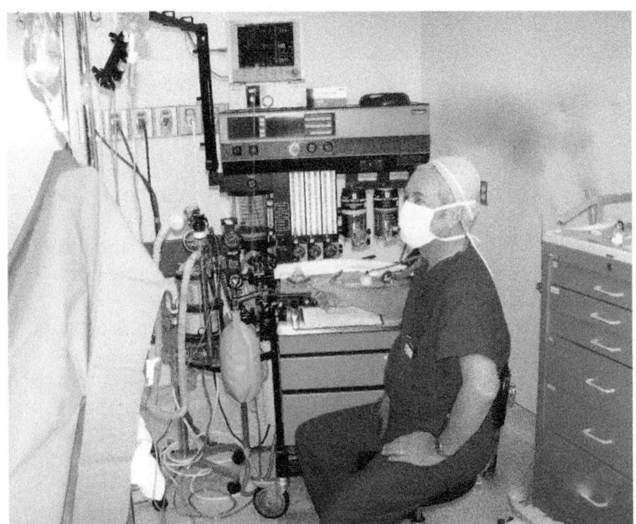

FIGURE 20-4 ■ The "immediate patient care area," as defined by the Centers for Disease Control and Prevention, is a "bedside" area where medications and fluids are sometimes prepared urgently for patients whose medical condition may be changing rapidly, such as within the operating room or delivery room suite or bedside in the critical care, dialysis, or oncology center. Within these locations, stock only single-dose medication and fluid containers if possible. If only multidose containers are available for certain medications and fluids, dispose of these containers *after use on a single patient.* (Courtesy Jon C. Haverstick Photography, Medcom, Inc., Cypress, CA.)

a *used* needle or syringe, then subsequently administering medication or fluid from this contaminated container to another patient. Syringe and/or needle reuse may appear to be a glaring breach of basic infection prevention practices. Unfortunately, it is not universally understood that replacing only the needle on a contaminated syringe is *not* safe; it does not reliably eliminate the potential for transmission of pathogens from the residual syringe contents. Conversely, flushing a contaminated needle with saline and placing it on a new syringe is also not safe. A recent survey of clinicians in U.S. health care settings revealed that a small percentage of health care professionals continue to engage in syringe and needle reuse between patients.[13]

Vials designated for multiple-dose use may be reaccessed to administer residual medication or fluid. If a syringe or needle used for patient care is used again to reaccess a medication or fluid container, contamination occurs, and gross visual inspection is *not* a reliable means of determining its presence. Medication vials labeled for multidose use contain bacteriostatic and/or bactericidal agents; however, these agents *cannot* prevent transmission of infection after contamination from external sources and have *no* antiviral action. Because blood-borne infections have been transmitted through medication or fluid containers contaminated when accessed by used needles and syringes, the CDC recommends that health care professionals refrain from reusing syringes, needles, and cannulas for *any* purpose, even to access a medication or solution container for use for the same patient.

The CDC gives anesthesia work areas and similarly intense bedside areas the term "immediate patient care areas" (Fig. 20-4). In these areas, medications and fluids are sometimes prepared urgently for patients whose medical condition may be rapidly changing, and distracting events may increase the potential for these medications and fluids to become inadvertently contaminated. Within the immediate patient care area, the CDC recommends additional precautions. First, medication and fluid containers should be accessed only by a *clean, sterile* syringe, needle, or cannula. Second, medications and fluids used in these areas should be supplied as single-patient use only (single-dose) containers if possible. Medications in single-use-only containers, regardless of the location in which they are administered, should be discarded after access or when empty; residual medication should *not* be retained for later use. Third, if the manufacturer does not supply a medication in a single-dose container (e.g., neostigmine, succinylcholine), the multidose container should be discarded when empty or at the end of each patient's anesthetic care. The latter procedure provides a second layer of safety to prevent the potential for transmission of blood-borne pathogens.

In accordance with these practices, two techniques *are* acceptable to the CDC to administer aliquots of medication or fluid to the same patient from a container labeled for multidose use. The entire contents of the container may be drawn into a sterile syringe, which may be used for sequential doses for the same patient. Alternatively, sequential doses may be obtained from the medication or fluid container for the same patient using a new, sterile syringe and needle or cannula for each access. The vial should be discarded when empty, or no later than the end of the procedure.

Prefilled syringes provide a well-labeled, ready-to-use medication that is sterile and stable for extended periods, often up to 6 to 8 weeks. The dosage supplied may be tailored to the end user. For example, a clinician may elect to have succinylcholine supplied either as 5 mL of a 20 mg/mL solution, for a total dose of 100 mg, or as 10 mL of a 20 mg/mL solution, for a total dose of 200 mg. Tamper-proof packaging makes it obvious when sterility has been compromised, and no supplies or handling is necessary to prepare the medication. Prefilled syringes are supplied by compounding pharmacies. The anesthesia professional should seek assurance that these sources follow current Good Manufacturing Practices and have a quality control program to test each lot for sterility.

Syringes, needles, medication and fluid containers, the internal surfaces of IV tubing, and any devices in contact with the vascular system or other normally sterile body areas (e.g., epidural, intrathecal, plexus, or peripheral nerve infusion catheters) are required to be *sterile*—that is, free from all bacteria, viruses, fungi, and bacterial spores—before use and maintained as such during use. These include stopcocks and other injection ports for medication injection, fluid infusion, and collection of blood samples and medication vial stoppers. All these represent potential entry sites for pathogens and should be kept free from contamination with a sterile cap and by wiping with 70% isopropyl alcohol during access. Hand hygiene is important before handling injection devices. All the aforementioned items are intended for a single patient and should be discarded after use.

Because of its higher specific gravity compared with IV fluid, blood can travel in a retrograde direction through tubing. A one-way valve does not prevent retrograde blood flow through IV administration tubing. In accordance

BOX 20-2 CDC Safe Injection Practices

The following apply to the use of sterile injection equipment, including syringes, needles, cannulas that may be used in place of needles, medication and fluid containers, and IV delivery systems.

1. Use aseptic technique to avoid contamination of sterile injection equipment.
2. Do not administer medications or other solutions from a syringe to multiple patients, even if the needle or cannula on the syringe is changed.
   - Needles, cannulas, and syringes are sterile, single-use items
   - Do not reuse syringes, needles, or cannulas:
     a. For another patient
     b. To access a medication or solution
3. Use single-dose vials whenever possible.
   - Use single-dose vials, instead of multidose vials, for parenteral medications or other solutions whenever possible.
   - Do not administer medications or other solutions from single-dose containers to multiple patients or combine the remaining contents in the containers for later use.
4. Multidose vials contain more than one dose of medication.
   - If multidose vials must be used:
     a. Each time the multidose container is accessed, use a new sterile syringe and needle or cannula.
     b. Store in accordance with the manufacturer's recommendations and discard if sterility is compromised or questionable.
   - In the immediate patient care area*:
     a. Discard multidose containers when empty or at the end of the case.
5. IV fluid infusion sets and administration and flush systems—including IV bags, tubing, and connectors—are single-use items.
   - Use for one patient only and dispose of appropriately after use.
   - Consider a syringe, needle, or cannula contaminated once it has contacted any part of the system; this includes all tubing, bags, ports, and stopcocks.
   - Do not use bags or bottles of IV solution as a common source of supply for multiple patients.
6. Infection control practices for neuraxial puncture procedures are critical.
   - Wear a surgical mask when inserting a needle, with or without a catheter, into the spinal canal or subdural space (e.g., spinal or epidural anesthesia, diagnostic lumbar puncture, intrathecal injections for imaging studies, or chemotherapy administration).

*The Centers for Disease Control and Prevention (CDC) define "immediate patient care areas" as intense "bedside" settings, where medications and fluids are sometimes prepared urgently for patients whose medical condition may be changing rapidly. In these locations, the potential is higher for medications and fluids to contact body fluids, and health care professionals should exercise more stringent safety practices to prevent transmission of blood-borne pathogens. When possible, medications and fluids used in these settings should be supplied in single-patient-use only (single-dose) containers. Even if labeled for multiple-dose use, medication and fluid containers should be discarded when empty or after use for one patient.

IV, intravenous.

with standard precautions, *all* syringes, needles, cannulas, injection equipment, medication and fluid containers, flush systems, and administration sets that contact a patient's IV access should be discarded at the conclusion of the case *except* those that remain directly connected to the patient.

Multiday infusions should be purchased as premanufactured sterile products or compounded in the hospital pharmacy in accordance with United States Pharmacopoeia (USP) 797 guidelines.[14] Anesthesia work areas do *not* meet these requirements, and medications mixed in this setting should be used or discarded within a period of hours. Infectious risk may be minimized by limiting the number of entries, including top-ups or bag changes, into the sterile infusion sets of continuous systems providing postoperative analgesia, such as epidural or peripheral nerve block infusion systems.

Upon further investigation of the largest outbreaks of blood-borne diseases associated with breaches of injection safety principles,[15] the CDC published "Safe Injection Practices" recommendations (Box 20-2). These recommendations were subsequently adopted by the Healthcare Infection Control Practices Advisory Committee (HICPAC) of the CDC and were incorporated into the 2007 standard precautions.[8] These practices have also been adopted by the American Society of Anesthesiologists (ASA), The Joint Commission, the Association of Professionals in Infection Control and Epidemiology (APIC), the Safe Injection Global Network of the WHO, the Centers for Medicare and Medicaid Services (CMMS), and several state and municipal health departments.

Safe injection practice recommendations also state that the proceduralist who inserts a needle, with or without a subsequent catheter, into the intrathecal or epidural space—such as for spinal or epidural anesthesia and/or analgesia, diagnostic lumbar puncture, myelography, or injection of intrathecal chemotherapeutic agents—should wear a face mask (Fig. 20-5).[8] This recommendation stems from investigations into eight cases of meningitis following lumbar puncture.[15a,15b,15c] Blood and/or cerebrospinal fluid cultures obtained from the affected patients yielded streptococcal species consistent with the oropharyngeal flora of the proceduralist. Aseptic technique had otherwise been followed, and contamination of the equipment and medications had been excluded.

REPROCESSING

Spaulding System

If the manufacturer's instructions indicate that reprocessing is acceptable, the requirements for cleaning, disinfection, and sterilization are based on a classification

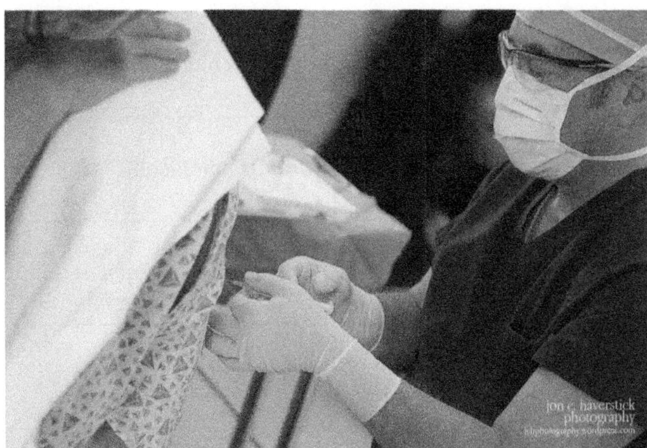

FIGURE 20-5 ■ **Wear a mask when performing a central neuraxial procedure.** (Courtesy Jon C. Haverstick Photography, Medcom Inc., Cypress, CA.)

system developed in the mid to late 1970s known as the *Spaulding scale.* Spaulding and colleagues[16] categorized medical devices based on the risk of infection associated with their clinical use.

Critical Items

These devices—syringes, needles, stopcocks, IV tubing, percutaneous cardiac interventional catheters, surgical instruments, and urethral catheters—either penetrate the skin or are in contact with normally sterile areas such as the bloodstream, tissue planes, neural sheaths, peritoneal or pleural cavity, and urinary bladder. These devices are either disposable or are reprocessed by cleaning followed by sterilization techniques that destroy all endospores, viruses, and vegetative bacteria.

Semicritical Items

Semicritical items contact mucous membranes (e.g., respiratory or alimentary tract) or nonintact skin. These devices—gastrointestinal endoscopes, esophageal echocardiography and temperature probes, laryngoscope blades, endotracheal tubes, laryngeal mask airways, and nasopharyngeal and oropharyngeal airways—require at least cleaning followed by high-level disinfection. Sterilization is not necessary; small numbers of bacterial spores are acceptable.

Noncritical Items

Devices that are in contact with unbroken skin on body surfaces require intermediate- or low-level disinfection; these include stethoscopes, blood pressure cuffs, stretcher side rails, and surfaces within the immediate patient care area.

Limitations

The Spaulding system has limitations, and oversimplification is both its strength and its weakness. First, delicate equipment that requires sterilization under the Spaulding system may be heat sensitive, precluding steam autoclave use. Ethylene oxide gas sterilization may require prolonged turnover and may not be suitable for reprocessing equipment needed for sequential cases. Without evidence of demonstrable differences in outcome, the choice between sterilization and high-level disinfection for reprocessing some of this equipment remains challenging.[17]

Second, at the time the Spalding criteria were established, standard sterilization destroyed all known microorganisms and bacterial spores; however, in the late 1970s, prions were discovered. Prions are "misfolded" proteins that induce normal proteins to also fold abnormally. The word *prion* is derived from the words *protein* and *infection.* These pathogens affect the structure of the brain or other neural tissue; they are associated with currently untreatable and universally fatal transmissible spongiform encephalopathies such as Creutzfeldt-Jakob disease.

"Sterilizing" prions requires denaturation of the infectious protein structure such that the molecule is no longer able to exert its effect on adjacent proteins. Prions contain *no* nucleic acids and are resistant to standard sterilization techniques, including heat, radiation, and formalin. Effective prion decontamination relies on protein hydrolysis or destruction of the protein tertiary structure. First, the item is immersed in a sodium hydroxide (e.g., one normal NaOH) or a sodium hypochlorite (bleach) solution. Second, the item is steam autoclaved at 121° C to 134° C for 1 hour. Guidelines are available for reprocessing of heat-stable surgical instruments that have been used for patients with known or suspected spongiform prion disease.[18] Single-use equipment should be used when possible; it may be necessary to sacrifice some equipment because of the extreme sterilization measures required to prevent prion transmission and the lack of treatment for the progressive and fatal diseases they cause.

Microorganisms can be categorized on a continuum according to their innate resistance to disinfectants. Figure 20-6 illustrates the variation in resistance to disinfectants among general classes of organisms. Resistance to disinfectants is primarily associated with permeability barriers, such as the cell wall or the outer coat of a spore. For example, *Mycobacteria* have impermeable cell walls that act as a barrier to chemical disinfectants; *Mycobacteria* therefore are the most resistant of the vegetative microorganisms. In general, nonenveloped viruses such as poliovirus are more resistant to disinfectants than enveloped viruses (human immunodeficiency virus [HIV], herpesvirus) and vegetative microorganisms except *Mycobacteria.* Resistance to disinfectants *does not* equate with resistance to antibiotics. Antibiotic-resistant bacteria, such as MRSA and VRE, are just as susceptible to sterilization and disinfection as nonresistant bacteria of the same species.

Sterilization

As previously discussed, the Spaulding criteria are designed to determine the appropriate reprocessing technique based on the intended clinical use of the device. Devices that contact normally sterile tissues, potential spaces, or fluid chambers—the bloodstream, tissue planes, neural structures, and urinary bladder—require sterilization. The majority of critical items used in the delivery of anesthesia are single-use items; they are disposed of after use and do not undergo reprocessing.

Most resistant to disinfectants ↑ Least resistant to disinfectants	Pathogen general category	Prototypic organism(s)
	Prions	Creutzfeldt-Jacob Disease
	Bacterial spores	*Clostridium, Bacillus*
	Mycobacteria	*Mycobacterium tuberculosis*
	Small, nonenveloped viruses	Poliovirus, papillomavirus, parvovirus
	Fungi	*Aspergillus*
	Gram-negative bacteria	*Pseudomonas, Escherichia*
	Gram-positive bacteria	*Staphylococcus, Enterococcus*
	Enveloped viruses	Hepatitis B and C viruses and human immunodeficiency virus

FIGURE 20-6 Microorganisms classified according to their sensitivity to disinfectants.

If a hospital chooses to reprocess a single-use device for reuse, the Food and Drug Administration (FDA) holds the hospital to the same standards as it would the original manufacturer of the device. In the anesthesia care setting, reprocessing of disposable devices is not recommended because of the potential for adverse outcomes from device malfunction associated with reprocessing.

Thorough cleaning is an important and essential first step in reprocessing equipment. Cleaning removes soil, debris, and lubricants on the external and internal surfaces of equipment; this residual debris may act as a barrier to prevent disinfectants and sterilants from contacting pathogens.[17] Cleaning involves washing with a detergent or enzymatic agent to remove blood, mucus, and foreign material. Rinsing also is important because residual detergents may inactivate the chemicals used to disinfect or sterilize the items.

Sterilization is the destruction of all forms of microbial life, exclusive of prions, including bacterial spores. Sterilization can be accomplished by either high-temperature steam autoclaving or low-temperature gas (ethylene oxide or ozone) or hydrogen peroxide gas plasma exposure; low-temperature sterilization is also possible by liquid immersion in chemical sterilants. Manufacturers' instructions regarding cleaning of equipment always should be followed to enable sterilization methods to be effective and to avoid damage to the integrity and/or function of the device.

If a device will tolerate high temperatures (typically 134° C; the manufacturer's labeling or documentation will indicate this), it may be processed by steam autoclaving. Steam autoclaving often is the first choice because it is the fastest and most effective method available. At a given temperature, moist heat is more effective than dry heat in penetrating and destroying organisms. When water vaporizes to steam, the change in physical state requires heat energy (the enthalpy of evaporation). Furthermore, the increased pressure effectively increases the steam saturation temperature, or the boiling point of water, within the autoclave. At temperatures of 125° C or higher, saturated steam under pressure readily penetrates and destroys microorganisms, and the amount of time to achieve sterilization is significantly reduced compared with dry heat or boiling at atmospheric pressures. After steam autoclaving, items must be cooled before handling and use.

Ethylene oxide (EtO), an alkylating agent, is a penetrating and reactive gas capable of destroying all known viruses, bacteria, and fungi, including bacterial spores; it is compatible with most materials, even when repeatedly applied. However, it is highly flammable, toxic, and carcinogenic. Gas autoclaving with EtO is useful for items that cannot tolerate exposure to high temperatures and/or water vapor, such as plastic and rubber devices and fiberoptic endoscopes. EtO sterilization requires at least 24 hours for exposure and subsequent aeration; aeration is essential to eliminate residual gas that would otherwise leach out into the tissues and potentially cause chemical burns. EtO sterilizers and aerators need to be installed in separate, well-ventilated areas that have dedicated air-extraction systems to evacuate gas residues to the outside.

Heat-sensitive objects may also be treated with oxidative processes; these include systems that use hydrogen peroxide gas plasma or ozone gas. Hydrogen peroxide plasma sterilization units require no venting (the by-products are water vapor and oxygen); shorter cycle times also are possible, and they avoid the explosive and carcinogenic risks of EtO units. However, they are not compatible with certain cellulose, packaging, dressing, and paper products. Furthermore, the penetrating ability of hydrogen peroxide is not as good as EtO and ozone, so there are limitations on the length and diameter of lumens that can be effectively sterilized and on the volume and complexity of the load.

Ozone is a toxic and unstable gas that has strong oxidizing properties capable of destroying a wide range of pathogens. Ozone is generated within the sterilizer from medical-grade oxygen, so there is no need for handling hazardous chemicals. Waste ozone is destroyed by exposure to a simple catalyst that reverts it back to oxygen. Penetration is excellent, and the cycle time is relatively short (about 270 minutes). However, ozone is immediately hazardous to life and health, so continuous monitoring must be in place to provide a rapid warning in the event of a leak.

Sterilization may also be achieved by exposure to liquid chemical sterilants, such as glutaraldehyde, ortho-phthalaldehyde, or peracetic acid. The FDA maintains a list of liquid chemical sterilants and high-level disinfectants that can be used to reprocess heat-sensitive medical devices; this listing is posted on the Internet.[19] Liquid chemical sterilants reliably produce sterility only if cleaning precedes treatment and strict guidelines are followed regarding the contact time, concentration, temperature, and pH of the sterilant.

Disinfection

Semicritical devices contact mucous membranes or non-intact skin and therefore require high-level disinfection. Such disinfection destroys all viruses, bacteria, and fungi but does not destroy high numbers of bacterial spores (small numbers are acceptable), and it does not destroy prions. Intact mucous membranes, such as those of the lungs and gastrointestinal tract, generally are resistant to infection by common bacterial spores, but they may be susceptible to infection by other pathogens. As with sterilization, meticulous cleaning and rinsing must precede the high-level disinfection process.

Devices that require high-level disinfection include, but are not limited to, laryngoscopes, face masks, laryngeal airways, oral/nasal airways, lightwands, bronchoscopes, endotracheal tubes, transesophageal echocardiography probes, esophageal/rectal temperature probes, and the external anesthesia breathing circuit (distal to the one-way valves). Examples of high-level disinfection techniques include pasteurization and liquid immersion in high-level disinfectants. Depending on the contact time, concentration, temperature, and pH, liquid chemical disinfectants may effectively sterilize a device. For this reason, liquid chemical disinfectants may also be referred to as *liquid chemical sterilants*. Chemical disinfectants and sterilants used to reprocess critical or semicritical medical devices are regulated by FDA.[17] The Environmental Protection Agency (EPA) regulates disinfectants and sterilants used on environmental surfaces.

High-level disinfection of some medical devices may be difficult because of long, narrow lumens and crevices or hinges. More outbreaks involving the spread of infectious disease from patient to patient have been associated with improperly reprocessed endoscopes than with any other medical device.[20,21] Consequently, guidelines have been established for reprocessing these devices.[17,22,23] The challenge is to achieve high-level disinfection without compromising the functionality of the device. Before high-level disinfection, the endoscope must be leak tested. If the device fails leak testing, it cannot undergo cleaning without risking further damage, and the manufacturer should be contacted regarding repair.

High-level disinfection with a liquid chemical generally requires five important steps: 1) cleaning of all surfaces, which includes brushing and flushing internal channels with water and a detergent or enzymatic cleaner; 2) disinfection by immersion and perfusion of all accessible channels (exposure time will vary with the product); 3) rinsing with sterile, filtered, or high-quality potable tap water that meets federal standards; 4) drying by rinsing with alcohol, which may necessitate directing forced air through channels in the device; and 5) storage in a manner that prevents recontamination and promotes drying.

As an important first step, items that require high-level disinfection reprocessing should undergo mechanical cleaning of all surfaces, including internal channels, with a low-sudsing enzymatic detergent as soon as possible after use. This action prevents drying of organic material that may later interfere with the effectiveness of disinfection/sterilization. Organic material retained in the internal channel is a major cause of transmission of infectious disease related to endoscope reprocessing.

After thorough cleaning, endoscopes should undergo a minimum immersion processing of high-level disinfection with a chemical disinfectant. Disinfecting solution should also perfuse the channels within the scope throughout the processing. Glutaraldehyde, hydrogen peroxide, ortho-phthalaldehyde, and peracetic acid with hydrogen peroxide are reliable high-level disinfectants, provided the conditions for their optimal activity are met.

After all surfaces and internal channels of the device have been exposed to chemical disinfectant at the temperature and for the duration recommended, the item should be rinsed thoroughly to remove any residual disinfectant and to reduce the chance of mucous membrane irritation from residual chemicals. After rinsing, the item must be dried both internally and externally. Flushing 70% ethyl alcohol and compressed air through the channel will facilitate drying. The item should be stored (e.g., packaged) in a manner that prevents recontamination and promotes drying (e.g., hung vertically).

Pasteurization is a method of high-level disinfection named after Louis Pasteur, the French chemist who discovered bacteria. After cleaning, a device is submerged in water at 77° C for 30 minutes. The item must then be transferred to a drying cabinet; once dry, it is packaged in plastic bags.

Medications that come in contact with mucous membranes (eye lubricants, topical anesthetics) or those used in conjunction with devices that contact mucosal surfaces (lubricants and topical anesthetics applied to endotracheal tubes) also must be free of pathogens. Contamination cannot always be determined visually; the use of unit-dose packages of these items therefore is recommended.

Noncritical devices contact only intact skin and require intermediate- or low-level disinfection. Noncritical items include blood pressure cuffs, pulse oximeters, stethoscopes, cables, and surfaces of the anesthesia machine and cart. Intermediate-level disinfectants kill vegetative bacteria and fungi, mycobacteria, and most viruses but are not efficient against small, nonenveloped viruses such as human papilloma virus (HPV), and they are ineffective against bacterial spores. The EPA generally classifies intermediate-level disinfectants as tuberculocidals. Low-level disinfectants kill vegetative bacteria and some fungi and viruses but not mycobacteria or spores. The EPA registers these agents as hospital disinfectants. The manufacturers' instructions should be followed regarding concentration and contact time for these products, such as chlorine-based products, phenols, 70% to 90% alcohols, and quaternary ammonium products. Many of these products are supplied as wipes for convenient use (Fig. 20-7).

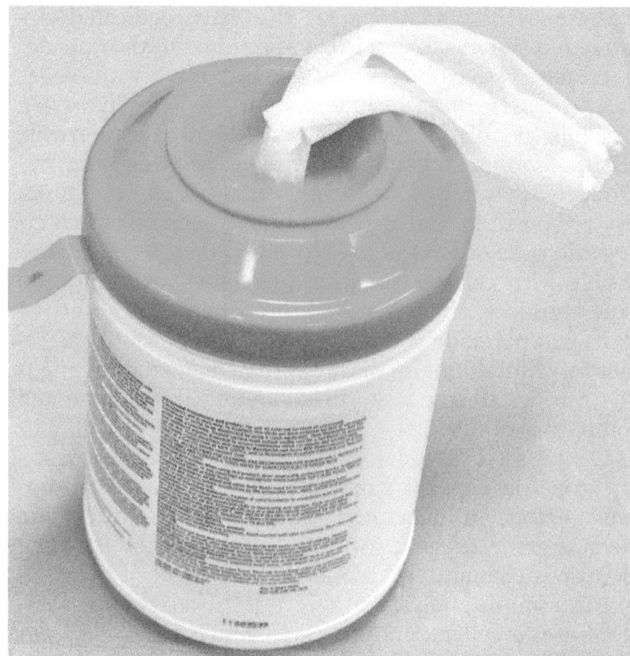

FIGURE 20-7 ■ Intermediate-level disinfectant (tuberculocidal) wipes are used to decontaminate devices that contact intact skin and environmental surfaces within patient care areas.

ANESTHESIA MACHINE AND ANESTHESIA WORK SPACE

The patient breathing circuit that connects to the fixed inspiratory and expiratory ports of the anesthesia machine (Fig. 20-8) and the reservoir bag are in close proximity to the patient and may be contaminated by secretions or exhaled droplets. If reprocessed, items that require high-level disinfection include, but are not limited to, the corrugated plastic tubing with extensions and adapters, the Y-piece and associated straight and elbow connectors, gas sampling ports, and the reservoir bag. It is difficult to clean, disinfect, rinse, dry, and store these items; furthermore, they are available as high-quality, prepackaged, single-patient-use units. For these reasons, anesthesia breathing circuits are not usually reprocessed in the United States. Even when a high-efficiency particulate air (HEPA) filter (Fig. 20-9) is used to protect the internal surface, a breathing circuit should not be reused without appropriate reprocessing because of the potential for contact and droplet contamination of its external surface.[24] There are no reports to date of cross-contamination from reuse of the gas sampling line between patients, and there is little literature to address whether to replace the sampling line between patients.[24a] However, the sampling line may be contaminated by external droplet or contact exposure. It is theoretically possible for fluid and secretions to accumulate on the patient side of the sampling line and then be introduced into a new breathing circuit. Furthermore, gas sampling lines may be labeled "single patient use only." For these reasons, it is recommended that the sampling line be replaced between each patient. The "trap," or the disposable device to which the sampling line connects on the anesthesia machine, does not need replacement between procedures and should only be replaced periodically or if clogged or otherwise malfunctioning. Moisture that accumulates in the anesthesia breathing circuit may be a source of bacterial growth and should periodically be drained from the circuit (away from the patient).[24] There

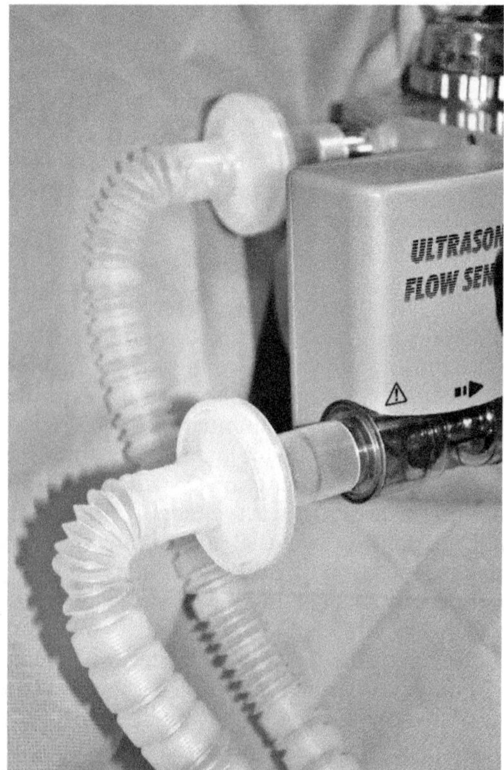

FIGURE 20-8 ■ The expiratory and inspiratory connection ports of the anesthesia machine.

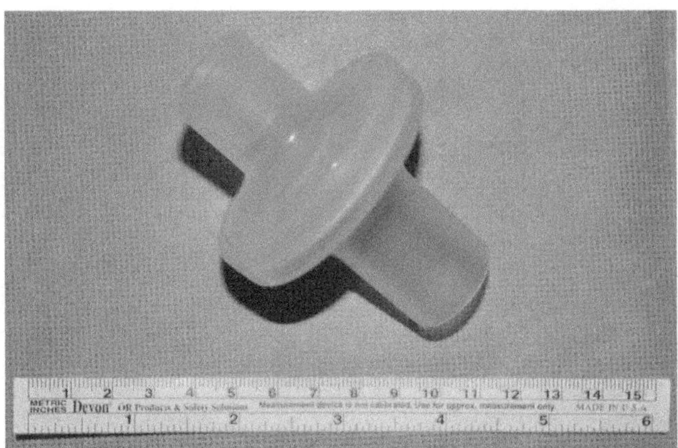

FIGURE 20-9 ■ A high-efficiency particulate air filter used to interconnect into a breathing circuit. The Centers for Disease Control and Prevention recommends a filter capable of trapping at least 95% of particles having a diameter of 0.3 μm, the measurement of the short axis of a tubercle bacterium, or greater. This means that no more than 5% of the particles 3/10 μm in diameter or larger penetrate the filter.

is no recommendation to periodically change the anesthesia breathing circuit during the care for one patient; however, the circuit should be changed when it is visibly soiled or mechanically malfunctioning.[24]

The fixed internal parts of the anesthesia machine that are exposed to respiratory gases—the interior of the unidirectional valves, flow sensors, internal conduits, interior of the ventilator bellows, water traps, nondisposable carbon dioxide absorbent chamber, and oxygen sensor—do not generally harbor or transmit infectious agents among patients.[25] The CDC *does not* recommend routine sterilization or disinfection of the internal components of the anesthesia machine and *does not* recommend obtaining routine bacterial cultures from the anesthesia machine to monitor for contamination.[24]

Similarly, routine sterilization and disinfection are not recommended for nondisposable attachments to the anesthesia machine, such as the scavenging system and fixed suction apparatus (except the suction canister, tubing, and suction tip). Rather, these components are to be cleaned, sterilized, and/or disinfected in accordance with the manufacturer's recommendations. If condensate forms within the tubing that connects the manual ventilation reservoir bag or the ventilator to the internal breathing circuit, it should be drained out, and the tubing should be replaced at the end of the case.[24]

No single reprocessing technique or agent is adequate for all components of and attachments to the anesthesia machine. Most modern anesthesia machines have internal breathing systems that can be disassembled into components, each of which may then be subjected to appropriate reprocessing techniques as specified by the manufacturer. Many of these components are heat stable, enabling sterilization by steam autoclaving (135° C for 8 minutes). Manufacturers have not established time intervals for reprocessing internal anesthesia machine components; rather, a statement is made to reprocess "as necessary," and the determination of the need for and frequency of reprocessing of any particular component is deemed the responsibility of the institution, consistent with established principles of clinical microbiology and infection control. Because some manufacturers suggest performing routine maintenance on anesthesia machines every 6 months, many institutions choose to reprocess internal components following the same schedule.

The Apollo anesthesia machine (Dräger Medical, Telford, PA) has a breathing system that can be disassembled into three parts, each of which can be steam autoclaved.[25] The ventilator bellows and the carbon dioxide absorber canister (if not disposable) can also be steam autoclaved. Other parts, such as the flow sensors, can be disinfected by pasteurization or by wiping with or immersion in a chemical disinfectant. The newer Datex-Ohmeda anesthesia machines (GE Healthcare, Waukesha, WI) can be similarly disassembled into parts, each of which can be subjected to the appropriate reprocessing technique.[26] Most parts can be steam autoclaved; the flow sensors, the oxygen cell, and the scavenging system components are not autoclavable, and appropriate reprocessing techniques for these are described in the manufacturer's manual.

The CDC makes no recommendation for the routine placement of a bacterial filter within the external breathing circuit of an anesthesia machine to protect the internal components exposed to respiratory gases. However, when caring for patients with known or suspected tubercular disease, the CDC *does* recommend placement of a bacterial filter within the external breathing circuit.[27] This is also recommended for viral illnesses such as measles, chickenpox, smallpox, severe acute respiratory syndrome (SARS), and H_1N_1 influenza. These statements seem to contradict the principle of standard precautions; any patient might potentially harbor an airborne-transmissible respiratory pathogen. Respiratory pathogens, including multiple-drug–resistant tubercular bacteria, have been recovered and cultured from the inspiratory limb after nebulization into the expiratory limb of the anesthesia machine circuit.[28] For these reasons, I recommend the routine use of a filter in the external breathing circuit; the CDC recommends a filter capable of trapping at least 95% of particles having a diameter of 0.3 μm, the measurement of the short axis of a tubercle bacterium, or greater. This means that no more than 5% of the particles 0.3 μm in diameter or larger penetrate through the filter. The filter should be placed in the anesthesia circuit, where it will protect both the machine and the ambient air from contamination.[27,29] It should be placed either at the patient end of the Y-piece of the breathing circuit to filter respired gas returning from the patient (Fig. 20-10), or at the expiratory end of the corrugated breathing circuit before entry of gas through the flow sensor or the expiratory one-way valve of the anesthesia machine. Breathing circuit tubing often is supplied with a filter at both of the ends that connect to the anesthesia machine (Fig. 20-11). This is done to avoid the possibility that the filter may be inadvertently attached to the inspiratory port of the anesthesia machine, leaving the expiratory port unprotected. If a filter protects both ends, there is no chance for unfiltered, exhaled gases from the patient to enter the internal breathing circuit of the anesthesia machine. If possible, a filter should also protect the gas sampling port. Sampled gases should be scavenged and not returned to the ambient operating room (OR) air.

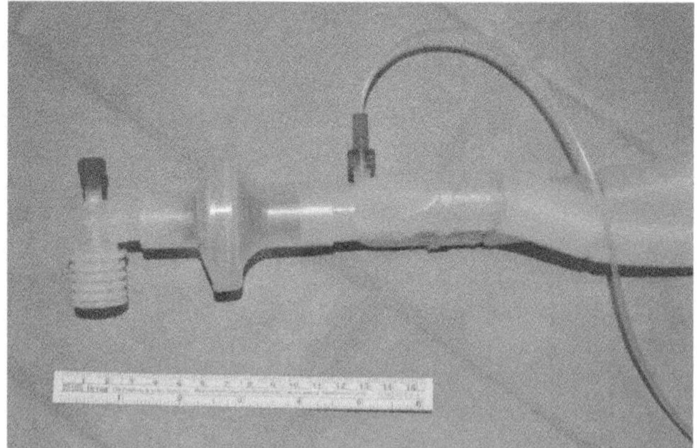

FIGURE 20-10 ■ A filter recommended by the Centers for Disease Control and Prevention may be placed at the patient end of the Y-piece to filter respired gas returning from the patient.

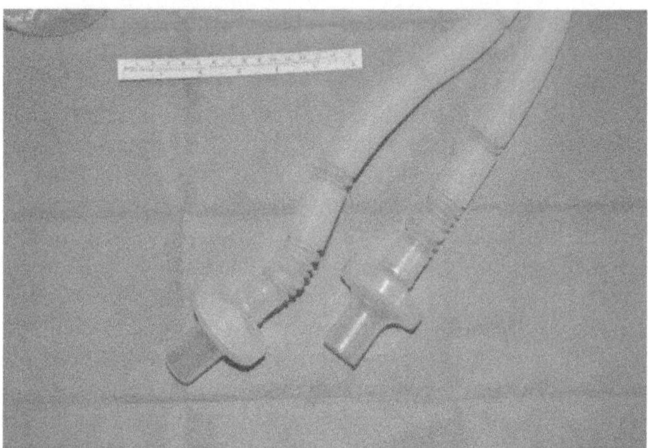

FIGURE 20-11 ■ The Centers for Disease Control and Prevention recommended filter may be placed at the expiratory end of the corrugated breathing circuit before entry of gas through the expiratory port of the anesthesia machine. As shown, the breathing circuit tubing often is supplied with a filter at both of the ends that connect to the anesthesia machine to avoid the chance that the filter may inadvertently be placed on the inspiratory limb of the circuit.

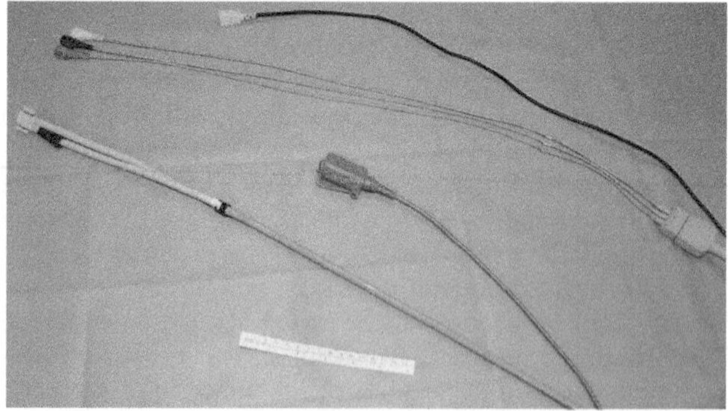

FIGURE 20-12 ■ Cables and leads from noninvasive and invasive patient monitors should be wiped with an intermediate-level disinfectant between cases and at the end of the day.

The anesthesia work space is an area with many opportunities to apply principles of infection prevention. Injection safety and hand hygiene, perhaps the most important practices, have already been discussed. Cables and leads from patient monitors (Fig. 20-12) should be wiped with an intermediate-level disinfectant between cases and at the end of the day. Horizontal surfaces, such as the anesthesia machine and anesthesia cart (Fig. 20-13), and vertical surfaces contacted in the course of anesthesia care—including control knobs, buttons, dials, and handles (Fig. 20-14)—should also be wiped with an intermediate-level disinfectant between cases and at the end of the day. Box 20-3 summarizes the infection prevention recommendations for the anesthesia work area between and during patient cases and for periodic reprocessing of components of and attachments to the anesthesia machine.

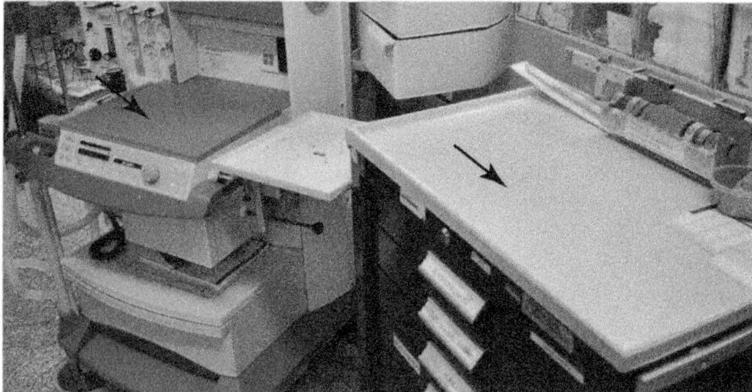

FIGURE 20-13 ■ Horizontal surfaces should be wiped with an intermediate-level disinfectant between cases and at the end of the day (*arrows*).

EXPANDED PRECAUTIONS

Expanded precautions, also known as *transmission-based precautions*, are used in addition to standard precautions for patients with a known or suspected infection or colonization with either a highly transmissible *or* multidrug-resistant pathogen. For the anesthesia professional, knowledge of the management of patients with known or suspected infection with airborne and droplet pathogens is essential.

Airborne transmission occurs when *airborne droplet nuclei*, fine particles less than 5 μm in diameter, disseminate infectious agents. Air currents suspend droplet nuclei and may carry them for long distances. For this reason, diseases spread by airborne droplet nuclei—measles, chickenpox, tuberculosis, smallpox, and severe acute respiratory syndrome (SARS)—are considered highly transmissible.

Patients with known or suspected infection with airborne pathogens require specially designed facilities, equipment, and practices known as *airborne infection isolation precautions*.[30,31] Routine care should be provided in rooms with special air handling and ventilation. Ambient air that contains infectious airborne droplet nuclei is removed from the room, so as not to enter other patient care areas, or it is circulated frequently through filtration capable of removing the infectious particles. Air-cleaning systems that use high-efficiency particulate aerosol (HEPA) filtration or ultraviolet germicidal irradiation (UVGI) technologies can be used in the room or surrounding areas to filter or decontaminate air evacuated from the patient's room.

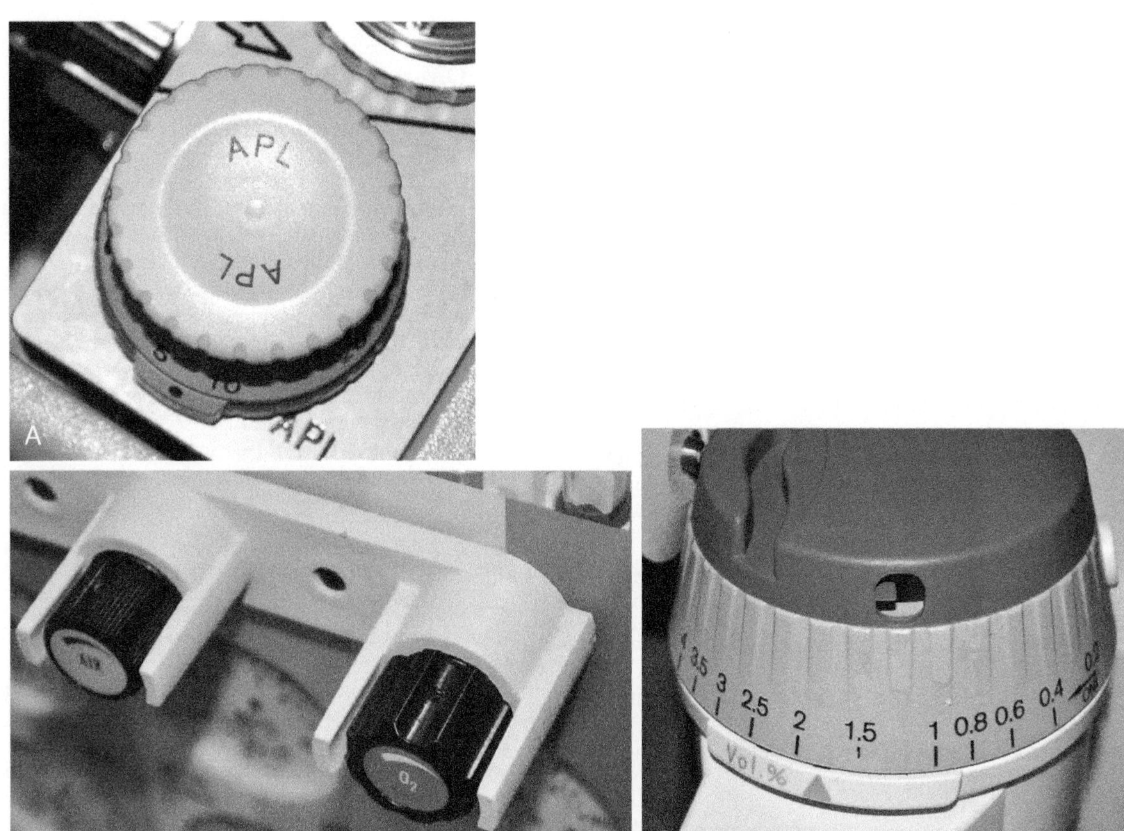

FIGURES 20-14 ■ **A** to **C**, Control knobs, buttons, dials, and handles contacted during the course of patient care should be wiped with an intermediate-level disinfectant between cases and at the end of the day.

During routine care of patients on airborne precautions, health care personnel must wear a properly fitted N95 mask (Fig. 20-15) for protection from infectious droplet nuclei that may be inhaled from the ambient air. The N95 designation indicates that the mask filters out 95% of airborne particles, as certified by the National Institute for Occupational Safety and Health (NIOSH). Barrier protection with gowns, gloves, and eye protection also is required.

Droplets, not droplet nuclei, are generally larger than 5 μm and do not remain suspended in air currents. Droplets travel only a relatively short distance (~3 feet) from the source and infect others by depositing on the conjunctival, nasal, or oral mucosa. Therefore special air handling and ventilation are not required to prevent droplet transmission during routine care. Diseases generally transmitted through droplets include pertussis, viral influenza, and diphtheria.

Certain procedures can be associated with the generation of aerosols that create particles small enough to be considered droplet nuclei; these include bronchoscopy, endotracheal intubation and extubation, open suctioning of airways, and cardiopulmonary resuscitation (CPR). These droplet nuclei may become airborne particles capable of carrying pathogens long distances via air currents. If an anesthesia professional intends to perform an aerosol-generating procedure on a patient or to provide anesthesia care, and the patient has a known or suspected infection with a disease spread by airborne or droplet transmission, the CDC makes several recommendations to protect other patients and their caretakers: consult with the hospital's infection control specialist for these. If possible the procedure should be performed in an airborne infection isolation room, which generates negative pressure inside the room relative to surrounding areas. In contrast, a typical OR is designed to provide positive pressure relative to the outside, with flow-directed, filtered, and temperature- and humidity-controlled incoming air. Therefore an OR does not provide protection for surrounding areas. Infection-control expertise should be sought to guide the management of these patients in an OR setting.[31]

When possible, the procedure should be postponed until the patient is either deemed noninfectious or is determined not to have the disease. When the procedure cannot be postponed, it should first be scheduled at a time when a minimum number of health care personnel and other patients are present in the suite, and when air turnover time between cases is maximized, usually at the end of the day. Second, the number of health care workers within the room during the procedure should be limited, and those present must wear properly fitted N95 respirators along with gowns, gloves, and eye protection. Third, when using a bag-valve-mask device, ventilator, or anesthesia delivery apparatus, a HEPA filter should be placed between the patient's airway device (mask, endotracheal tube, laryngeal mask) and the breathing apparatus to reduce the risk of contaminating the anesthesia machine or discharging infectious particles into the ambient air. Postoperative recovery of a patient with suspected or confirmed disease spread by droplet nuclei should be in an airborne-infection isolation room. Box 20-4 lists the

BOX 20-3 Routine Infection-Prevention Recommendations and Practices to Reduce the Risk of Patient-to-Patient Transmission of Infectious Disease

Between Cases and at the End of the Day

Dispose of:
- Reservoir bag, external breathing tubing, Y-piece, connectors, adaptors, gas sampling ports and gas sampling lines, extensions, heat and moisture barriers and filters, face mask*
- Tubing* connecting the manual breathing reservoir bag and/or ventilator to the anesthesia breathing system, if visibly soiled or moist
- Used and accessed syringes, needles, cannulas, and medication and fluid containers, even if labeled for multidose use
- Used intravenous administration sets and tubing, unless connected directly to a line running into the patient
- Disposable (not reprocessed) airway devices and supplies

Wipe with intermediate-level disinfectant:
- Monitoring cables
- Hand-held portion of equipment such as laryngoscopes and video laryngoscopes
- Horizontal surfaces (e.g., machine and medication cart flat surfaces)
- Knobs, dials, controls, touch screens, and handles contacted during patient care

Special cleaning requirements:
- For initial cleaning prior to reprocessing (sterilization or high-level disinfection), devices such as laryngoscope blades and laryngeal mask airways should be placed in an enzymatic cleanser or detergent recommended by the device manufacturer.
- Endoscopes and other devices with channels may have special cleaning requirements specified by the manufacturer.

During patient cases:
- Follow safe injection practices, including practicing hand hygiene as indicated and using aseptic technique to handle injection supplies and devices.
- Keep injection ports and syringe injection connections sterile by capping and/or wiping with a 70% isopropyl alcohol wipe.
- Maintain physical separation between used and clean injection devices and supplies.
- Use HEPA filtration between either the patient (mask or internal airway device) and the Y-piece *or* between the external breathing tubing and the expiratory entrance port of the anesthesia machine.
- Periodically drain condensate from the anesthesia breathing circuit and from any tubing connecting the ventilator and manual breathing bag to the anesthesia breathing system.
- Replace breathing circuit if it becomes visibly contaminated with secretions.
- Sampled gases should be scavenged and not returned to ambient air; if possible, sampled gases should also be protected by HEPA filtration.

Periodic or "as Necessary" Infection Prevention Recommendations

Anesthesia machine internal components and attachments should be sterilized according to manufacturer recommendations.

For items whose manufacturers deem periodic cleaning and disinfection necessary, consider performing these at the same time as scheduled maintenance.

If a component is not heat sensitive, use steam sterilization (134° C for 8 minutes) after initial cleaning. Components that may be steam autoclaved include the following:
- Disassembled internal breathing system (including the metal valve plate and internal conduits)
- Nondisposable carbon dioxide absorber canisters
- Ventilator bellows, bellows assembly, diaphragm, and piston covers
- Adjustable pressure-limiting valve*

Heat-sensitive components require alternative reprocessing techniques (pasteurization, wiping with or immersion in liquid disinfectants):
- Flow sensors
- Oxygen sensor
- Scavenger system transfer hose and associated connectors
- Scavenger system receiving canister and flow tube

*If any of these items is reusable—breathing bag, tubing, Y-piece, connectors, adaptors, gas sampling ports, extensions, heat and moisture barriers and filters, face mask—it should be subjected to high-level disinfection reprocessing techniques.
HEPA, high-efficiency particulate air.

recommendations for anesthesia professionals caring for patients on airborne or droplet precautions.

PREVENTION OF INFECTIOUS COMPLICATIONS

Device-Related Infectious Complications: Central Venous Catheters

By implementing "bundled" practices shown to reduce infectious complications, the incidence of bloodstream infections associated with CVCs has been reduced. These practices are associated with the planning, placement, ongoing care, and monitoring of CVCs. The "CVC bundle" includes hand hygiene prior to placement, even though sterile gloves are used (hand hygiene is a supplement to barrier protection using gloves); the use of full-barrier precautions (full-length draping of the patient and cap, gown, mask, and sterile gloves for the proceduralist); the use of 70% isopropyl alcohol and 2% chlorhexidine skin prep; avoidance of the femoral site, if possible; and the timely removal of catheters when they are no longer essential for patient care.[32]

Procedure-Associated Infectious Complications: Ventilator-Associated Pneumonia

Ventilator-associated pneumonia (VAP) affects between 9% and 27% of all intubated patients, carries a high

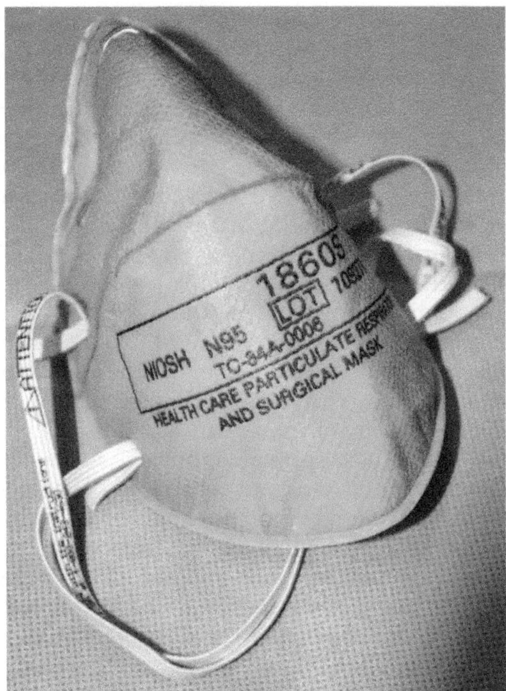

FIGURE 20-15 ▪ An N95 mask. The N95 designation indicates that that the mask filters out 95% of airborne particles, as certified by the National Institute for Occupational Safety and Health. During routine care of patients on airborne precautions, health care personnel should wear a properly fitted N95 mask for protection from infectious droplet nuclei that may be inhaled from the ambient air.

mortality rate, and is among the most common infections acquired by adults in critical care units.[33] In addition to hand hygiene, the measures described here may effectively reduce the incidence of VAP.[33]

If possible, noninvasive respiratory support should be used. Endotracheal intubation increases the risk of hospital-acquired pneumonia from 6-fold to 21-fold. Weaning and sedation protocols may be useful to reduce the duration of intubation and mechanical ventilation.[33,34] Because nasotracheal intubation is associated with a higher incidence of sinusitis, orotracheal intubation is preferred.[34,35] Unless contraindicated, the semirecumbent position (30- to 45-degree elevation of the head of the bed) is independently associated with lower rates of VAP than the supine position,[36] possibly secondary to an increased risk of gastroesophageal reflux and aspiration when supine.[37,38] Endotracheal cuff pressure should be greater than 20 cm H_2O to limit microaspiration, and it should be less than 30 cm H_2O to limit mucosal ischemia.[39] If the expected duration of mechanical ventilation is longer than 3 days, consider endotracheal tubes with subglottic drainage capabilities.[40] Routinely use topical oral antiseptics, such as chlorhexidine, to modulate colonization of the oral bacterial flora.[41,42] The use of sterile water for nebulized medications and drainage of accumulated moisture away from the patient is also recommended. These recommendations are summarized in Box 20-5.

BOX 20-4 Expanded Precautions (Adjuncts to Standard Precautions) for Patients with a Known or Suspected Droplet or Airborne Infection

DROPLET (>5 μm) (E.G., PERTUSSIS, VIRAL INFLUENZA, DIPHTHERIA)*

1. Precautions during routine care (bedside consultation *not* involving the aerosolizing procedures listed below):
   - Wear a mask (N95 not required) when in close proximity (~6 feet) to the patient
2. Precautions during aerosolizing procedures (endotracheal intubation, extubation, airway suctioning, resuscitation):
   - Follow airborne infection isolation precautions for procedures (see below).

AIRBORNE PARTICLES (<5 μm) (E.G., TUBERCULOSIS, MEASLES, VARICELLA ZOSTER (CHICKENPOX), SEVERE ACUTE RESPIRATORY SYNDROME)

1. Airborne infection isolation precautions during routine care:
   - Negative-pressure ventilation *or* special air handling is used to filter or remove ambient air.
   - All personnel must wear a properly fitting N95 mask.
   - When a bag-valve-mask device is used, a HEPA filter should be placed inline to reduce the risk of spread of infectious particles into ventilation equipment and the ambient air.
   - Limit personnel as much as possible.
   - Use barrier precautions such as gloves, gowns, and face shields.
2. Airborne infection isolation precautions for procedures:
   - Follow airborne infection isolation precautions for routine care.
   - If possible, postpone the procedure until the patient is deemed noninfectious.
   - Schedule when minimum personnel and patients are in the vicinity.
   - Schedule when air turnover time to next procedure is maximized, such as at the end of the day.
   - Place an N95 mask on the patient during transport (if the patient is not intubated).
   - Limit health care personnel present to those essential.
   - Plan for recovery of the patient in an airborne-infection isolation room or location with appropriate air handling.

*Droplets often are an order of magnitude larger in diameter than airborne particles.
HEPA, high-efficiency particulate air.

Procedure-Associated Infectious Complications: Surgical Site Infections

Of those patients who have inpatient surgery in the United States, 2% to 5% develop an SSI; when these infections occur, the length of the hospital stay is prolonged an average of 7 to 10 days, and the risk of perioperative death increases 2 to 11 times that of noninfected surgical patients. Anesthesia professionals have a role in the timing of perioperative antibiotic administration, if antibiotics are indicated. Current guidelines recommend the administration of prophylactic antibiotics within

BOX 20-5 List of Recommendations for Ventilator-Associated Pneumonia Prevention Grouped as Priority Modules

PRIORITY MODULE 1: RECOMMENDATIONS FOR ROUTINE CARE OF PATIENTS REQUIRING MECHANICAL VENTILATION

1. Use noninvasive ventilation whenever possible.
2. Use orotracheal, rather than nasotracheal, intubation when possible.
3. Minimize the duration of ventilation, and perform daily assessments of readiness to wean from ventilation.
4. Prevent aspiration by maintaining patients in a semirecumbent position (a 30- to 45-degree elevation of the head of the bed) unless otherwise contraindicated.
5. Use a cuffed endotracheal tube with an endotracheal cuff pressure ≥20 cm H_2O (but <30 cm H_2O) and in-line or subglottic suctioning.
6. Perform regular oral care with an antiseptic solution.

PRIORITY MODULE 2: RECOMMENDATIONS FOR APPROPRIATE CLEANING, DISINFECTION, AND STERILIZATION OF VENTILATOR EQUIPMENT

1. Whenever possible, to reprocess semicritical equipment or devices that are not sensitive to heat and moisture, use steam sterilization by autoclaving or high-level disinfection by wet heat pasteurization (at >70° C) for 30 minutes.
2. Use low-temperature sterilization methods for equipment or devices that are heat or moisture sensitive.
3. After disinfection, proceed with appropriate rinsing, drying, and packaging, taking care not to contaminate the disinfected items in the process.

PRIORITY MODULE 3: RECOMMENDATIONS FOR APPROPRIATE MAINTENANCE OF VENTILATOR CIRCUIT AND ASSOCIATED DEVICES

1. Drain and discard any condensate that collects in the tubing of a mechanical ventilator, taking precautions not to allow condensate to drain toward the patient.
2. Use only sterile fluid for nebulization, and dispense the fluid into the nebulizer aseptically.
3. Use only sterile (not distilled or nonsterile) water to fill reservoirs of devices used for nebulization.

From U.S. Department of Health and Human Services. HHS Action Plan to Prevent Health Care–Associated Infections: Prevention-Prioritized Recommendations. Available at http://www.hhs.gov/ophs/initiatives/hai/prevention.html.

1 hour of incision to maximize tissue concentrations.[43] Because these drugs require up to 1 hour for infusion and have relatively long serum half-lives, vancomycin and fluoroquinolones may be administered up to 2 hours before incision.[43] Perioperative prophylactic antibiotics such as cephalosporins exert bactericidal action only when therapeutic concentrations are maintained within the tissues. Eventually, the antibiotic diffuses back into the circulation and is metabolized by the liver and/or excreted by the kidneys. Periodic redosing is required to sustain the therapeutic effects of preventative antibiotics. When the duration of an operation is expected to exceed the time in which therapeutic levels of the antibiotic can be maintained, the anesthesia professional must determine a redosing time interval based on the approximate serum half-life of the drug, the tissue levels achieved in normal patients by the initial dosage, and the approximate minimum concentration of the antibiotic at which 90% inhibition is achieved, a concentration determined in vitro.[44] For example, the redosing interval for cefazolin is estimated to be 3 to 4 hours. Because the serum half-life of cefazolin is 1.8 hours in normal adults, this represents approximately twice the half-life of the drug.

A randomized, controlled study of 200 patients undergoing colorectal surgery found that those treated with measures to maintain core temperature around 36.5° C, such as with forced-air convection surface warming and fluid warmers, had a significantly lower SSI rate than those provided normal intraoperative thermal care.[45] This and one other study[46] formed the basis for the current recommendation that all perioperative patients undergoing general or neuraxial anesthesia have active warming measures used or a body temperature of 36° C or greater recorded around the time of anesthesia emergence or the end of surgery. Currently, this recommendation is a core SSI prevention strategy of the CDC[47] and has been implemented as part of the Surgical Care Improvement Project (SCIP).[48] A recent retrospective, case-control study using data from the National Surgical Quality Improvement Program (NSQIP) showed no independent association between perioperative normothermia and infectious surgical site complications.[49] However, no randomized, controlled trials refute the link between SSI and perioperative normothermia. Furthermore, perioperative hypothermia may be associated with adverse cardiac events, reduced drug metabolism, and altered coagulation function.[50]

A 1997 retrospective study showed that perioperative hyperglycemia (glucose >200 mg/dL) was associated with a greater risk of SSI in patients undergoing cardiovascular surgery.[51] In addition, good preoperative glucose control (hemoglobin A1c <7%) was associated with fewer infectious complications following major noncardiac surgery.[52] Recent studies have indicated that perioperative patients subjected to "tight control" (blood glucose concentrations between 80 and 120 mg/dL) suffer outcomes equivalent or worse than those managed with conventional glucose control (glucose <180 mg/dL).[53] Maintaining perioperative glucose levels below 180 to 200 mg/dL may be beneficial, but aggressive glucose control requires further study.[54]

MANAGING INFECTIOUS DISEASE RISKS TO ANESTHESIA PROFESSIONALS

For anesthesia professionals, caring for patients who have infectious disease is an unavoidable and often routine occurrence. The key to avoiding infection is to prevent direct exposure to pathogens. Most exposures do not result in infection; nonetheless, significant exposure, such as a needle-stick injury, may lead to anxiety and stress for the affected individual. Strategies to reduce the risk of transmission of disease among anesthesia professionals and their patients include 1) use of barrier precautions, 2) implementation of practices and use of devices that reduce exposure risk, 3) immunization against diseases for which vaccination is effective, and 4) expeditious and appropriate medical attention in the event of an exposure.

Barrier protections are required whenever there may be contact with a patient's nonintact skin, mucous membranes, blood, bodily fluids, secretions, and excretions (except sweat). These measures are the essence of standard precaution and should be routinely used regardless of the diagnosis or perceived risk of the patient and the presence or absence of visible blood.

Hand hygiene is necessary not only to prevent transmission of pathogens to patients but also to protect the anesthesia professional. Hand hygiene should be performed, and gloves should be worn, before contact with a patient's nonintact skin, mucous membranes, or bodily fluids. In most instances, it is not necessary that the gloves be sterile. Gloves should be removed promptly after contact, and hand hygiene should be repeated after glove removal. Anesthesia professionals should use a standard face mask and eye protection or a face shield to protect their mucous membranes during any procedure or patient care activity likely to generate splashes or sprays. A clean gown must be worn to protect the skin and to prevent soiling of clothing. The gown should be appropriate for the activity and the amount of fluid likely to be encountered. Remove a soiled gown as promptly as possible, and perform appropriate hand hygiene. Soiled patient care equipment should be handled in a manner that prevents skin or mucous membrane exposure, contamination of clothing, or transfer of pathogens.

When caring for patients on airborne precautions, anesthesia professionals should protect themselves by wearing a properly fitted N95 face mask and checking to ensure that appropriate air-handling measures have been instituted. Ordinary surgical face masks do not provide protection from airborne pathogens. If the patient is intubated, a HEPA filter should be used during mechanical or manual ventilation to prevent airborne droplet nuclei from contaminating the anesthesia machine or being discharged to the ambient environment. A patient who is not intubated should wear a mask when not enclosed within an airborne-infection isolation room.

Influenza viral infections are generally transmitted through droplets generated during talking, sneezing, and coughing. Droplets are larger than 5 μm in diameter and are generally not propelled more than 3 to 6 feet from their source. However, during procedures such as endotracheal intubation, suctioning of airway secretions, and bronchoscopy, droplets may become aerosolized into finer particles, and these particles are capable of traveling in air currents and traversing ordinary surgical masks. When performing these procedures on patients known or suspected of having infections that require droplet precautions, anesthesia professionals and those in the room should consider wearing N95 masks.[55] If possible, these cases should be performed in an airborne-infection isolation room with only essential personnel present.

Anesthesia professionals are at a relatively high risk for needle-stick injuries compared with health care personnel in other medical and nursing disciplines. Greene and colleagues[56] found that 69% of contaminated percutaneous, hollow-bore needle-stick injuries in anesthesia personnel may have been prevented. The investigators deemed a needle-stick injury preventable when it occurred after the needle had been used for its intended purpose; in such instances, percutaneous puncture may have been avoided by shielding the needle or refraining from recapping or disassembling the device harboring the needle.[56] Tait and colleagues[57] surveyed anesthesiologists and found that 31.8% had had a contaminated needle-stick injury within the previous year; of those who incurred such an injury, only 45% sought appropriate treatment and follow-up. An investigation targeting U.S. surgeons found that almost every surgeon experienced at least one needle-stick injury during his or her training.[58] Unfortunately, health care personnel may not report many of these needle-stick injuries, because they downplay the risk, do not wish to take the necessary time, or fear stigmatization and professional consequences. This is especially dangerous, because timely postexposure prophylaxis is effective to prevent disease after percutaneous exposure to HIV and hepatitis B virus (HBV). Although needle-stick injuries have the potential of transferring bacteria, protozoa, viruses, and prions, from a practical standpoint, the transmission of HIV, HBV, and HCV are of greatest concern.[59]

The greatest risk of transmission of a blood-borne infection with HIV, HBV, or HCV is from a blood-contaminated percutaneous injury with a blood-filled hollow-bore needle. Efforts to reduce the risk of sharps injuries to health care personnel have taken the form of safety-engineered devices and modifications of work practices. Many devices designed to reduce the risk of needle-stick injury are available; these include needleless devices (stopcocks, needleless access ports, and valves), needle products with needle-stick protection safety features (self-sheathing needles, safety IV catheters, and recessed needles), and scalpels with safety-activated blade covers.

Recapping needles with a two-handed technique, in which the needle is directed toward the hand holding the cap, is strongly discouraged because it is one of the most common causes for accidental contaminated needle-stick injury among health care personnel. Puncture-resistant, leak-proof containers for disposal of used needles, syringes, scalpel blades, and other sharp items should be located as close as possible to the immediate area where sharps are used. Convenient access to these containers will facilitate the prompt disposal of contaminated needles without recapping or disassembling them from syringes.

Work practice modifications reduce or eliminate exposure risk by altering how a task is performed. For example, discouraging needle recapping is an effort to modify a work practice. If needle recapping is unavoidable, use of a mechanical device or a one-handed "scoop" technique is recommended; importantly, the sheath is *not* held in the contralateral hand. Unless required by a specific procedure, or no feasible alternative exists, bending sharps is not recommended. Shearing or breaking contaminated needles is not acceptable.

The injury rate from straight suture needles is more than seven times the rate associated with conventional, instrument-held curved suture needles.[60] When suturing, anesthesia professionals should use a curved needle with a needle holder, rather than a straight needle held by hand, and forceps should be used, rather than fingers, to hold tissues when suturing or cutting.[61] Double-gloving offers significantly reduced perforations to the innermost gloves[62] and may decrease the risk of infection by decreasing the inoculum size from some types of needle-stick injuries.[63,64] With regard to dried blood on needles and other inanimate objects, the infectiousness of HIV and HCV decreases within a couple of hours; however, even with desiccation, HBV remains stable and infectious for more than a week.[65]

After a needle-stick injury, the affected area should be rinsed and washed thoroughly with soap and water; the practice to "milk out" more blood is controversial and is not recommended by the CDC.[59] Unless the source is known to be negative for HBV, HCV, and HIV, postexposure prophylactic measures should be initiated. Timeliness is important; if anti-HIV medications are indicated, for optimal effectiveness, they should be taken within hours; delay will result in a significant decline in effectiveness.[59] Because needle-stick injuries do not always occur when employee health offices are open, serious consideration should be given to having postexposure prophylactic medications immediately available to anesthesia professionals at the work site. After phone consultation with appropriate infectious disease personnel, necessary prophylactic medication can then be given without delay. Following preventative medication, if indicated, the needle-stick recipient should then have blood tests drawn to determine his or her baseline serologic status; recipients who have been HBV immunized should have hepatitis B surface antibody titers drawn.[59] Unless already known, the infectious status of the source individual should also be determined.

Following a specific exposure to a blood-borne pathogen, the risk of infection may vary with the pathogen, the type of exposure (e.g., superficial or deep, solid-bore or hollow-bore needle), the amount of blood involved in the exposure, and the amount of virus in the patient's blood at the time of exposure. HBV carries the greatest risk of transmission. After a blood-contaminated percutaneous exposure, if the source patient is hepatitis B surface-antigen (HBsAg) positive and hepatitis B e-antigen (HBeAg) *negative*, the risk of HBV transmission to a nonimmune recipient is between 1% and 6%, and the risk of developing serologic evidence of HBV infection is between 23% and 37%. In comparison, if the source patient is positive for both HBsAg *and* HBeAg, the risk to a nonimmune recipient for acquiring clinical hepatitis is 22% to 31%, and the risk of developing serologic evidence of HBV infection is 37% to 62%. In nonimmunized recipients, appropriate and timely provision (within 24 hours of exposure) of hepatitis B immune globulin and initiation of the HBV vaccination series provides an estimated 75% protection from HBV infection.

The HCV transmission rate has been reported at 1.8%,[59] but newer, larger surveys have shown only a 0.3% to 0.5% transmission rate.[66,67] Immunoglobulin therapy for HCV prevention is not effective and is not recommended. In the absence of a currently available postexposure prophylactic treatment, recommendations for postexposure management for the recipient are early identification of disease. Theoretically, prompt treatment with antiviral agents when HCV ribonucleic acid first becomes detectable might prevent the development of chronic infection.[59]

The average risk of acquiring HIV infection after an accidental percutaneous exposure to blood from a known HIV-infected patient is estimated to be 0.3%.[68] Although the average risk of HIV infection is 0.3%, the risk, although not quantified, exceeds 0.3% for an exposure in which there is a greater volume of blood transferred and/or a higher HIV titer in the blood of the source patient.[69] If the source patient is known or suspected to have HIV infection, antiretroviral medications should be administered as soon as possible. The selection of a drug regimen for HIV postexposure prophylaxis must balance the risk for infection against the potential toxicities of any agent used. Antiretroviral medications used for this indication frequently have side effects such as nausea, fatigue, and rash; drug interactions are common and may be serious. For exposures that pose a negligible risk for transmission, the risk of preventative pharmacologic treatment may outweigh the benefit. HIV postexposure prophylactic regimens change periodically, and the NIOSH blood-borne pathogens page on the CDC website (www.cdc.gov)[70] or another expert should be consulted for the most up-to-date guidelines.

The CDC publishes a list of immunizations strongly recommended for health care personnel.[71] Like any other health care personnel who work with sharps, blood, or bodily fluids, anesthesia professionals should be vaccinated against HBV, unless antibody testing has demonstrated immunity the virus.[59] If the anesthesia professional is an employee, the employer is required to offer the HBV vaccine free of charge. Anesthesia professionals should actively participate in periodic health assessments, vaccinations, and screening programs for tuberculosis and other potentially contagious diseases. Periodic mask fit testing is important to ensure that N95 masks provide sufficient protection from airborne pathogens. If the anesthesia professional contracts an acute illness (e.g., fever, upper respiratory illness, weepy rash), it would be appropriate to refrain from patient-care activities until the illness is resolved or adequately treated. Strategies to reduce the risk of infectious disease transmission from patients to anesthesia professionals are summarized in Box 20-6.

BOX 20-6 Strategies to Reduce the Risk of Infectious Disease Transmission from Patients to Anesthesia Professionals

1. When following standard precautions:
   - Use barriers—gloves, masks, face shields, safety glasses, and waterproof gowns—to limit exposure.
   - Practice timely and appropriate hand hygiene.
2. When caring for patients on *airborne precautions:*
   - Wear a well-fitting N95 mask.
   - Ensure appropriate air-handling measures (negative-pressure rooms, HEPA filtration) are in effect in the patient care location.
   - Use a HEPA filter within the breathing circuit to prevent discharge of airborne infectious particles into the ambient environment.
3. When caring for patients on *droplet precautions:*
   - Wear a mask when working in close proximity (within 3 to 6 feet) of the patient.
   - Use airborne precautions when performing aerosolizing procedures such as endotracheal intubation or suctioning or bronchoscopy.
4. When following principles of *injection safety:*
   - Do not recap or disassemble syringe and needle units prior to disposal.
   - Locate puncture-resistant, leak-proof sharps containers where they can easily be accessed during patient care.
   - Whenever possible and practical, use safety-engineered sharps devices (e.g., self-sheathing needles, safety catheters, scalpels with blade covers), and use needleless systems (e.g., stopcocks, valved access ports) for delivering parenteral medications and fluids and for performing anesthesia procedures.
   - Use a one-handed, scoop technique to recap needles if recapping cannot be avoided.
   - Avoid shearing or breaking needles.
   - Use curved needles and needle holders for suturing (vis-à-vis straight needle) and forceps to hold tissue during suturing.
   - Consider "double gloving" when performing procedures associated with a risk of needle-stick injury.
5. If a sharps injury occurs, wash the wound thoroughly with soap and water as soon as possible after the incident and report promptly to employee health or an infection prevention specialist for evaluation for possible prophylactic oral antiretroviral therapy.
6. Actively participate in periodic health assessments and infectious disease screening programs (e.g., periodic surveillance for tuberculosis infection).
7. Get vaccinations recommended for health care professionals.
8. If you are suffering from a flulike or febrile illness, a severe respiratory infection, a weepy rash, or symptoms or signs of a highly transmissible disease (e.g., herpes zoster), refrain from patient care activities until you are no longer contagious.

HEPA, high-efficiency particulate air.

REFERENCES

1. Klevens RM, Edwards JR, Richards CL, et al: Estimating healthcare-associated infections in U.S. hospitals, *Public Health Rep* 2007(122):160–166, 2002.
2. Harbarth S, Sax H, Gastmeier P: The preventable proportion of nosocomial infections: an overview of published reports, *J Hosp Infect* 54:258–266, 2003.
3. Haley RW, Culver DH, White JW, et al: The efficacy of infection surveillance and control programs in preventing nosocomial infections in U.S. hospitals, *Am J Epidemiol* 121:183–205, 1985.
4. Pronovost P, Needham D, Berenholtz S, et al: An intervention to decrease catheter-related bloodstream infections in the ICU, *N Engl J Med* 355:2725–2732, 2006.
5. Furuya EY, Dick A, Perencevich EN, et al: Central line bundle implementation in US intensive care units and impact on bloodstream infections, *PLoS ONE* 6(1):e15452, 2011.
6. Jain R, Kralovic SM, Evans ME, et al: Veterans Affairs initiative to prevent methicillin-resistant *Staphylococcus aureus* infections, *N Engl J Med* 364:1419–1430, 2011.
7. Scott RD: The direct medical costs of healthcare-associated infections in U.S. hospitals and the benefits of prevention. Centers for Disease Control, Division of Healthcare Quality Promotion, March 2009.
8. Siegel JD, Rhinehart E, Jackson M, Chiarello L, and the Healthcare Infection Control Practices Advisory Committee, 2007. Guideline for isolation precautions: preventing transmission of infectious agents in healthcare settings. Centers for Disease Control and Prevention. Accessed online at http://www.cdc.gov/hicpac/pdf/isolation/Isolation2007.pdf.
9. Centers for Disease Control and Prevention: Guideline for hand hygiene in health-care settings: recommendations of the healthcare infection control practices advisory committee and the HICPAC/SHEA/APIC/IDSA hand hygiene task force, *MMWR Recommendations and Reports* 51(RR-16):1–44, October 25, 2002. Accessed online at http://www.cdc.gov/mmwr/PDF/rr/rr5116.pdf.
10. World Alliance for Patient Safety: *WHO guidelines on hand hygiene in health care: a summary*, 2005, Accessed online at http://www.who.int/patientsafety/events/05/HH_en.pdf.
11. Thompson ND, Perz JF, Moorman AC, Holmberg SD: Nonhospital health care–associated hepatitis B and C virus transmission: United States, 1998-2008, *Ann Intern Med* 150(1):33–39, 2009. Accessed online at http://www.annals.org/cgi/content/short/150/1/33.
12. Centers for Disease Control and Prevention: Injection Safety: May 16, 2008 Division of Healthcare Quality Promotion (DHQP): Accessed online 2011 Aug 6 at http://www.oneandonlycampaign.org.
13. Pugliese G, Gosnell C, Bartley JM, Robinson S: Injection practices among clinicians in United States health care settings, *Am J Infect Control* 38(10):789–798, 2010.
14. USP 797 Guidebook to pharmaceutical compounding—sterile preparations. Accessed 2011 August 6 at http://www.usp.org/products/797Guidebook.
15. Centers for Disease Control and Prevention: Transmission of hepatitis B and C viruses in outpatient settings—New York, Oklahoma, and Nebraska, 2000–2002, *MMWR* 52(38):901–906, 2003. Accessed online at http://www.cdc.gov/mmwr/preview/mmwrhtml/mm5238a1.htm.

15a. Centers for Disease Control and Prevention: Bacterial meningitis after intrapartum spinal anesthesia—New York and Ohio, 2008-2009, *MMWR Morb Mortal Wkly Rep* 59(3):65–69, 2010.

15b. Trautmann M, Lepper PM, Schmitz FJ: Three cases of bacterial meningitis after spinal and epidural anesthesia, *Eur J Clin Microbiol Infect Dis* 21:43–45, 2006.

15c. Hebl JR: The importance and implications of aspectic techniques during regional anesthesia, *Reg Anesth Pain Med* 31(4):311–323.

16. Spaulding EH: Chemical disinfection of medical and surgical materials. In Lawrence C, Block SS, editors: *Disinfection, sterilization, and preservation*, Philadelphia, 1968, Lea & Febiger, pp 517–531.
17. Rutala WA, Weber DJ, the Healthcare Infection Control Practices Advisory Committee: Guideline for disinfection and sterilization in healthcare facilities, Centers for Disease Control and Prevention, 2008. Accessed online at http://www.cdc.gov/hicpac/pdf/guidelines/Disinfection_Nov_2008.pdf.
18. Sutton JM, Dickinson J, Walker JT, Raven ND: Methods to minimize the risks of Creutzfeldt-Jakob disease transmission by surgical procedures: where to set the standard? *Clin Infect Dis* 43:757–764, 2006. Accessed online at http://dx.doi.org/10.1086%2F507030.
19. Food and Drug Administration: *FDA-cleared sterilants and high-level disinfectants with general claims for processing reusable medical and dental devices*, March 2009, Accessed online 2012 Nov 5 at http://www.fda.gov/MedicalDevices/DeviceRegulationandGuidance/ReprocessingofSingleUseDevices/ucm133514.htm.

20. Weber DJ, Rutala WA: Lessons from outbreaks associated with bronchoscopy, *Infect Control Hosp Epidemiol* 22:403–408, 2001.
21. Srinivasan A, Wolfenden LL, Song X, et al: An outbreak of *Pseudomonas aeruginosa* infections associated with flexible bronchoscopes, *N Engl J Med* 348:221–227, 2003.
22. Mehta AC, Prakash UBS, Garland R, et al: Prevention of flexible bronchoscopy-associated infection, *Chest* 128:1742–1755, 2006.
23. Association of Perioperative Registered Nurses: Recommended practices for high-level disinfection, *AORN J* 81:402–412, 2005.
24. Centers for Disease Control and Prevention: Guidelines for preventing health-care associated pneumonia, *MMWR*: 2003 53(RR-03):1–36, 2004. Accessed online at http://www.cdc.gov/ncidod/dhqp/pdf/guidelines/cdcpneumo_guidelines.pdf.

24a. Cross-contamination vis gas sampling lines? *Anesth Patient Saf News*/ Summer:27–29, 2009.

25. Dräger Medical: *Operating Instructions, Apollo SW 4.n. Part Number 9039994* ed 2, Telford, PA, 2008, Dräger Medical, 203–228.
26. Cleaning and sterilization: In *Aisys User Reference Manual*, Chapter 2, Madison, WI, 2008, Datex-Ohmeda, a subsidiary of GE Healthcare.
27. Du Moulin GC, Saubermann AJ: The anesthesia machine and circle system are not likely to be sources of bacterial contamination, *Anesthesiology* 47:353–358, 1977.
28. Langevin PB, Rand KH, Layon AJ: The potential for dissemination of *Mycobacterium tuberculosis* through the anesthesia breathing circuit, *Chest* 115:1107–1114, 1999.
29. Demers RR: Bacterial/viral filtration: let the breather beware! *Chest* 120:1377–1389, 2001.
30. Centers for Disease Control and Prevention: Guidelines for environmental infection control in health-care facilities, *MMWR* 52(RR-10), 2003.
31. Centers for Disease Control and Prevention: Guidelines for preventing the transmission of *Mycobacterium tuberculosis* in healthcare settings, 2005. *MMWR* 54(RR-17):20–21, 2005. Accessed online at http://www.cdc.gov/mmwr/PDF/rr/rr5417.pdf.
32. O'Grady NP, Alexander M, Burns LA, et al, for the Healthcare Infection Control Practices Advisory Committee of the Centers for Disease Control and Prevention: Guidelines for the prevention of intravascular catheter-related infections, 2011. Accessed online at http://www.cdc.gov/hicpac/pdf/guidelines/bsi-guidelines-2011.pdf.
33. Bouza E, Burillo A: Advances in the prevention and management of ventilator-associated pneumonia, *Curr Opin Infect Dis* 22:345–351, 2009.
34. American Thoracic Society and the Infectious Diseases Society of America: Guidelines for the management of adults with hospital-acquired, ventilator-associated, and healthcare-associated pneumonia, *Am J Respir Crit Care Med* 171:388–416, 2005.
35. Coffin SE, Klompas M, Classen D, et al: Strategies to prevent ventilator-associated pneumonia in acute care hospitals, *Infect Control Hosp Epidemiol* 29:S31–S40, 2008.
36. Drakulovic MB, Torres A, Bauer TT, et al: Supine body position as a risk factor for nosocomial pneumonia in mechanically ventilated patients: a randomised trial, *Lancet* 354:1851–1858, 1999.
37. Bassi GL, Zanella A, Cressoni M, et al: Following tracheal intubation, mucus flow is reversed in the semi-recumbent position: possible role in the pathogenesis of ventilator-associated pneumonia, *Crit Care Med* 36:518–525, 2008.
38. Torres A, Serra-Batiles J, Ros E, et al: Pulmonary aspiration of gastric contents in patients receiving mechanical ventilation: the effect of body position, *Ann Intern Med* 116:540–543, 1992.
39. Rello J, Sonora R, Jubert P, et al: Pneumonia in intubated patients; role of respiratory airway care, *Am J Respir Crit Care Med* 154:111–115, 1996.
40. Dezfulian C, Shojania K, Collard HR, et al: Subglottic secretion drainage for preventing ventilator-associated pneumonia; a meta-analysis, *Am J Med* 118:11–18, 2005.
41. DeRiso AJ 2nd, Ladowski JS, Dillon TA, et al: Chlorhexidine gluconate 0.12% oral rinse reduces the incidence of total nosocomial respiratory infection and nonprophylactic systemic antibiotic use in patients undergoing heart surgery, *Chest* 109:1556–1561, 1996.
42. Chan EY, Ruest A, Meade MO, et al: Oral decontamination for prevention of pneumonia in mechanically ventilated adults: systematic review and meta-analysis, *Br Med J* 334:861–862, 2007.
43. Anderson DJ, Kaye KS, Classen D, Arias KM: Strategies to prevent surgical site infections in acute care hospitals, *Infect Control Hosp Epidemiol* 29(S1):S51–S61, 2008.
44. Mangram AJ, Horan TC, Pearson ML, Silver LC, Jarvis WR: Guideline for prevention of surgical site infection, 1999, Hospital Infection Control Practices Advisory Committee, *Infect Control Hosp Epidemiol*, (20):250–278, 1999.
45. Kurz A, Sessler DI, Lenhardt R: Perioperative normothermia to reduce the incidence of surgical wound infection and shorten hospitalization, *N Engl J Med* 334:1209–1215, 1996.
46. Melling AC, Ali B, Scott EM, Leaper DJ: Effects of preoperative warming on the incidence of wound infection after clean surgery: a randomised controlled trial, *Lancet* 358:876–880, 2001.
47. Berrios-Torres SI: Surgical Site Infection (SSI)Toolkit, 2009, CDC. Accessed online at http://www.cdc.gov/HAI/pdfs/toolkits/SSI_toolkit021710SIBT_revised.pdf.
48. Fry DE: Surgical site infections and the Surgical Care Improvement Project (SCIP): evolution of national quality measures, *SurgInfect* 9(6):579–584, 2008.
49. Lehtinen SJ, Onicescu G, Kuhn KM, Cole DJ, Esnaola NF: Normothermia to prevent surgical site infections after gastrointestinal surgery, *Ann Surg* 252:696–704, 2010.
50. Kurz A: Thermal care in the perioperative period, *Best Pract Res Clin Anaesthesiol* 22:39–62, 2008.
51. Zerr KJ, Furnary AP, Grunkemeier GL, Bookin S, et al: Glucose control lowers the risk of wound infection in diabetics after open heart operations, *Ann Thorac Surg* 63(2):356–361, 1997.
52. Dronge AS, Perkal MF, Kancir S, et al: Long-term glycemic control and postoperative infectious complications, *Arch Surg* 141:375–380, 2006.
53. Finfer S, Chittock DR, Su SY, et al: Intensive versus conventional glucose control in critically ill patients, *N Engl J Med* 360:1283–1297, 2009.
54. Murray BW, Huerta S, Dineen S, Anthony T: Surgical site infection in colorectal surgery: a review of the nonpharmacologic tools of prevention, *J Am Coll Surg* 211(6):812–822, 2010.
55. Centers for Disease Control and Prevention: Prevention Strategies for Seasonal Influenza in Healthcare Settings, 2010. Accessed online 2011 Aug 6 at http://www.cdc.gov/flu/professionals/infectioncontrol/healthcaresettings.htm.
56. Greene ES, Berry AJ, Arnold WR, Jagger J: Percutaneous injuries in anesthesia personnel, *Anesth Analg* 83:273–278, 1996.
57. Tait AR, Tuttle DB: Prevention of occupational transmission of human immunodeficiency virus and hepatitis B virus among anesthesiologists: a survey of anesthesiology practice, *Anesth Analg* 79:623–628, 1994.
58. Makary MA, Al-Attar A, Holzmueller CG, et al: Needlestick injuries among surgeons in training, *N Engl J Med* 356(26):2693–2699, 2007.
59. Centers for Disease Control and Prevention: Updated U.S. Public Health Service Guidelines for the management of occupational exposures to HBV, HCV, and HIV and recommendations for post-exposure prophylaxis, *MMWR* 50(RR-11), 2001.
60. Centers for Disease Control and Prevention: Evaluation of blunt suture needles in preventing percutaneous injuries among healthcare workers during gynecologic surgical procedures: New York City, *MMWR* (46):25–29, 1997, March 1993–June 1994.
61. Centers for Disease Control and Prevention: *Workbook for designing, implementing, and evaluating a sharps injury prevention program*, 2008. Accessed online at http://www.cdc.gov/sharpssafety/pdf/sharpsworkbook_2008.pdf.
62. Tanner J, Parkinson H: Double gloving to reduce surgical cross-infection, *Cochrane Database Syst Rev* 3:CD003087, 2006 Jul 19.
63. Bennett NT, Howard RJ: Quantity of blood inoculated in a needlestick injury from suture needles, *J Am Coll Surg* 178: 107–110, 1994.
64. Mast ST, Woolwine JD, Gerberding JL: Efficacy of gloves in reducing blood volumes transferred during simulated needlestick injury, *J Infect Dis* 168:1589–1592, 1993.
65. Bond WW, Favero MS, Petersen NJ, et al: Survival of hepatitis B virus after drying and storage for one week [letter], *Lancet* 1:550–551, 1981.
66. Jagger J, Puro V, De Carli G: Occupational transmission of hepatitis C virus, *JAMA* 288(12):1469–1470, 2002.
67. Chung H, Kudo M, Kumada T, et al: Risk of HCV transmission after needlestick injury, and the efficacy of short-duration interferon administration to prevent HCV transmission to medical personnel, *J Gastroenterol* 38(9):877–879, 2003.

68. Do AN, Ciesielski CA, Metler RP, et al: Occupationally acquired human immunodeficiency virus (HIV) infection: national case surveillance data during 20 years of the HIV epidemic in the United States, *Infect Control Hosp Epidemiol* 24(2):86–96, 2003.
69. Centers for Disease Control and Prevention: Updated U.S. Public Health Service Guidelines for the management of occupational exposures to HIV and recommendations for post-exposure prophylaxis, *MMWR* 54(RR-09):1–17, 2005.
70. Centers for Disease Control and Prevention: National Institute for Occupational Safety and Health: Workplace safety and health topics: diseases and injuries: bloodborne infectious diseases: HIV/AIDS, hepatitis B, hepatitis C, Accessed 2011 Aug 6 at http://www.cdc.gov/niosh/topics/bbp.
71. Centers for Disease Control and Prevention: Guidelines for infection control in dental health-care settings, 2003. Appendix B: immunizations strongly recommended for health care personnel, *MMWR* 52(RR-17):65, 2003.

PART V

COMPUTERS, ALARMS, AND ERGONOMICS

CHAPTER 21

COMPUTING AND THE INTERNET IN CLINICAL PRACTICE

Keith J. Ruskin

CHAPTER OUTLINE

OVERVIEW

Anesthesiologists work in a dynamic environment in which information critical to patient care must be transmitted quickly and accurately. Patients undergoing procedures are often critically ill with rapidly changing vital signs. Treatment plans must be changed rapidly to meet the demands of the surgical procedure and the patient's condition. Health information technology (IT) is critical to patient safety in the perioperative environment. Nearly every new piece of equipment in the operating room (OR) contains one or more microcomputers, making a basic understanding of medical informatics essential for every anesthesiologist. Thus, anesthesiology is an information-intense specialty, and computers play an important role in the OR as well as in other areas of the hospital.

The practice of anesthesia requires the use of computers for data management, quality assurance, automated record keeping, and signal processing. An electronic workflow facilitates direct patient care and can also be used for purposes such as quality assurance and submission of health insurance claims.

One study of 98 Florida hospitals suggests that simply adopting IT may improve patient care. These hospitals' use of clinical, administrative, and strategic applications was associated with a decreased risk-adjusted mortality in percutaneous transluminal coronary angioplasty, gastrointestinal (GI) hemorrhage, and acute myocardial infarction. The authors concluded that adopting the use of health IT improved patient outcome. In this study, use of IT systems was also negatively correlated with unnecessary incidental appendectomy. Interestingly, the adoption of strategic IT applications was associated with decreased risk-adjusted morbidity from laparoscopic cholecystectomy and craniotomy.[1]

Studies such as this one underscore the benefits of adopting IT initiatives as part of anesthetic practice. This chapter discusses the role of medical informatics in anesthesia practice and medical education, and includes a brief discussion of information security.

ANESTHESIA WORKSTATIONS

The latest generation of anesthesia workstations and physiologic monitoring systems offers a wide range of capabilities, from advanced monitoring to ventilator functions comparable to those of an intensive care unit (ICU) ventilator. Current designs may help to improve patient safety by incorporating features such as checklists (e.g., the United States Food and Drug Administration [FDA] anesthesia machine checkout) and double-check systems that prevent unintended changes to ventilator or gas flow settings. Anesthesia workstations can exchange information with electronic health record (EHR) systems, thereby creating an accurate, contemporaneous anesthesia record while also making pertinent history and laboratory results available to the anesthesiologist. Incorporation of these features, most of which rely on systems automation and computers, have been recommended to reduce errors in the OR.[2] Anesthesia workstations also can improve patient safety by requiring compliance with established checkout procedures. The software that drives modern anesthesia workstations allows enforcement of policies and helps prevent use errors. This is an important feature because anesthesiologists are not particularly good at identifying machine faults.[3] For example, the Datex-Ohmeda Aisys and Avance workstations (GE Healthcare, Waukesha, WI) require the user to complete the recommended checkout before the workstation can be used for patient care. (This feature can be bypassed for emergency surgery, and an abbreviated checkout can be done after the first anesthetic of the day.) Interlocks prevent use errors, making it difficult or impossible to deliver a hypoxic mixture or dangerously high peak airway pressures. Advanced workstations require the user to confirm settings, forcing a double-check of the selections. New workstations can also be used to deliver novel anesthetics such as xenon.[4]

The newest generation of anesthesia workstations requires that users receive a significant amount of training before using them for patient care. It is no longer possible to simply turn a knob to increase the gas flow or flip a switch to turn on a ventilator. The new machines use a complicated user interface with a layered series of menus. Usability has become an important design feature, and newer designs offer improved ergonomics. In one study comparing a first-generation workstation with four second-generation workstations, 10 specific qualities were evaluated on a 10-point scale; two design and monitoring criteria, four ventilator criteria, and four maintenance criteria were studied. So-called *second-generation workstations* were found to have an improved user interface and superior readability. They also were easier to set up both at the start of the day and between cases. In particular, the ventilator controls were more intuitive and easier to use.[5]

In modern, integrated anesthesia workstations, the gas machine, ventilator, and physiologic monitor share the same physical space and are designed to work together. These systems offer a variety of new features, including multiple ventilator modes, more precise administration of potent volatile anesthetics, the ability to exchange data, and automated checklists. A sophisticated user interface allows multiple features to be accessed at the touch of a button. Online help systems can allow the clinician to find a particular feature, and newer systems are far more intuitive and easy to use. With these features and careful attention, modern anesthesia workstations can be used to improve patient care.

ANESTHESIA INFORMATION MANAGEMENT SYSTEMS

Anesthesiologists have been among the first to develop technology for keeping EHRs. In one recent study, 44% of all academic anesthesiology practices had adopted anesthesia information management systems (AIMS).[6] This ability to collect, store, and organize large amounts of data makes AIMS ideal for quality assurance and clinical research. Anesthesiologists have been working with medical device manufacturers and standards organizations to create new devices that can communicate with each other and with EHRs.

AIMS can improve patient care because they produce customized, legible anesthesia records while storing high-resolution physiologic data in a database that can be easily searched. This simplifies finding a specific record and facilitates new data analysis techniques, such as data mining, which allows large quantities of data to be searched for subtle associations. This information can be used for quality assurance, to search for and track specific events and their outcomes, and to analyze specific personnel. Nair and colleagues[7] reported that including real-time alerts for prophylactic antibiotic administration increased the rate of timely administration by more than 9%, and they concluded that a decision support system that includes real-time guidance and alerts can improve compliance with guidelines.

Perhaps the most significant difficulty in upgrading anesthesia medical records systems occurs when it is time to completely replace one computerized system with another. Although most systems store information in relational databases, such as the Microsoft SQL Server, it may be very difficult to move large numbers of patient records into a new system. When faced with the complexity of matching up a hundred or more fields from one system with another, at least one hospital decided to simply abandon the previous structured records of more than 100,000 patients. This illustrates how important it is to choose a system that can grow and adapt to a changing practice. It is also important to carefully explore problems related to data migration before choosing a new system.

Despite the obvious advantages of EHRs, their complexity and perceived costs have prevented many providers, particularly those in small hospitals or rural practices, from adopting this technology. AIMS can provide a return on investment by ensuring compliance with Physician Quality and Reporting System guidelines and Center for Medicare and Medicaid Services (CMS) documentation requirements. AIMS have also been shown to increase scheduling efficiency, decrease drug costs, and provide better charge capture and diagnosis and procedure coding.[8]

EDUCATION

The amount of knowledge needed to provide high-quality medical care is rapidly increasing, yet physicians have less time than ever to keep abreast of the literature. Computers can help physicians find critical information quickly and have therefore become commonplace in anesthesia education.

Most books, medical journals, and other educational materials can be accessed electronically, and many physicians now prefer electronic references to printed ones. Journals can be extensively cross-referenced and are no longer restricted to the linear flow of text on a page. Search engines and links from websites make it easier to find information, allowing the average clinician to perform complex literature searches with little or no prior computer experience. Interactive educational materials can quiz the student prior to moving on to new material, and they can use three-dimensional models or video clips to explain a difficult concept. One study suggests that physicians frequently ask clinical questions but may pursue the answers to only slightly more than half. The most common reason cited for abandoning a question was the doubt that an accessible answer existed.[9] In one study, anesthesiologists were given a clinical question and were asked to use PubMed, UpToDate, Ovid, or Google to find the answer. Interestingly, those residents who used Google and UpToDate were more likely than those who used PubMed to find the answer to the question, and searches with Google were faster than those with UpToDate or Ovid.[10]

Portable Devices

Because they are portable, smartphones and tablet computers offer access to journal articles, guidelines, and the patient record without the need to leave the patient. One study of these devices in the emergency medicine department showed that physicians who used them were more likely to correct a patient's diagnosis or treatment.[11] Many clinicians use their handheld computers as their primary source of information, and access to the devices appears to improve clinical decision making, although some physicians are slower to accept mobile computing devices than others. Moreover, transmission of microorganisms by these devices is a concern.[12] Video mobile telephones, which are widely available in Europe and are becoming available in the United States, have been proposed as a possible tool to help bystanders perform CPR. Although early studies on this role have been equivocal, specialized training may enable dispatchers to help bystanders at an accident.[13]

Decision Support

During a life-threatening event, being able to quickly recall a series of actions necessary to manage a rapidly unfolding clinical scenario may improve patient outcome. Critical incident analysis has identified specific nontechnical skills that are vital to the successful resolution of a critical incident in the OR.[14] Traditional anesthesia training does not involve the teaching of crisis resource-management skills. Topics such as situational awareness, resource allocation, team management, and medical decision making must be actively taught and cannot be learned by reading or simply by being present in the OR.[15,16] Yee and colleagues[17] studied the effectiveness of simulator-based crisis resource-management training and found that a single exposure to a simulated critical event improved nontechnical crisis-management skills in anesthesia residents. As a result, many institutions have begun to adopt medical simulation as an integral component of their educational programs.

Simulation

Because of their ability to create a standardized clinical scenario, patient simulators allow trainees to practice and to make mistakes without placing an actual patient at risk (see Chapter 25). The simulation can be stopped, restarted, or reset as needed to facilitate teaching; important points are not lost in the rush to stabilize a sick patient. Because critical events can unfold quickly during surgery, anesthesiologists were among the first physicians to adopt the routine use of full-scale simulation. Simulators have been used to teach medical students and new residents the basic principles of airway management and physiology as well as the fundamentals of anesthetic management of patients. Large commercial simulators make extensive use of computers and a manikin to generate appropriate sounds, movements, and signals for monitors. Small PC-based simulators such as Anesthesia Simulator Consultant (Anesoft, Issaquah, WA) and Gas Man (www.gasmanweb.com) can be run on a desktop computer and are used to teach basic concepts.

COMMUNICATION

Anesthesiologists work in a dynamic environment in which information critical to patient care must be transmitted quickly and accurately. Failures in communication were shown to be the second most prevalent cause of medical errors.[18,19] Rapid transfer of relevant patient information prior to surgery can also improve OR efficiency by reducing the incidence of delays on the day of surgery,[20] and reliable IT tools are critical to patient safety in the perioperative environment.

Modern Communication Devices

Anesthesiologists can choose from a variety of tools to gain access to the information they need. Handheld computers, tablets, and smart phones are ubiquitous, and services such as UpToDate provide evidence-based, peer-reviewed information and guidelines. Online communities and social networking sites can be used to form a "virtual coffee room," where physicians can network with their friends and colleagues.

Cellular telephones, wireless computers, and other communication tools can improve patient care by providing rapid access to vital information from any location. Effective communication has been shown to be a critical component of safety in high-risk environments. Several reviews have postulated that improving communication among health care professionals may improve patient safety. Cellular telephones provide rapid, two-way voice communication and can also be used to exchange pictures and short text messages. Several cellular service providers offer a walkie-talkie mode that allows one user to contact a member of his or her group at the push of a button. The results of at least one study[21] suggest that the use of mobile telephones decreases the incidence of errors.

Computer Interfaces and Networks

Most monitors are now capable of transmitting numbers and waveforms, such as an electrocardiogram (ECG) or blood pressure tracing, to another monitor or to a computer at a remote location, making this critical information immediately available to the clinician. An ideal communication system therefore should include paging, voice communication, and data networking. A portable device capable of displaying this critical information allows a physician to be immediately available in the event of a sudden change in the patient's condition.[22,23] Wi-Fi networks can handle multiple data streams at once, are relatively inexpensive to set up and maintain, and are highly versatile.

The development of widely used data transmission standards has made it possible to connect medical equipment together and to transmit medical information through existing networks to desktop computers, servers, or monitoring stations. The end result is that a core communication infrastructure is likely to be compatible with new devices, and it can be installed using readily available equipment. Wi-Fi networks can also be used to carry voice conversations. *Voice over Internet Protocol* (VoIP) is widely accepted by the general public as an alternative to traditional telephone service, and specialized systems can be installed in the health care environment. These advantages, combined with the low cost and wide availability of Wi-Fi equipment, make this technology well suited for many health care applications. In one study, the staff of a pediatric surgical suite—including anesthesiologists, nurses, and surgeons—were provided with VoIP hands-free communication devices. This technology significantly improved each staff member's ability to communicate, but problems were experienced with voice recognition in a noisy environment, and the system was not reliable in all areas of the OR.[24]

Hospitals in the United States and Europe had implemented policies that prohibit the use of wireless communication devices in patient care areas.[25] Unfortunately, most of these policies were developed in response to anecdotal reports of interference and ignore the potential benefits that cellular telephones can bring to patient care. Modern cellular telephones transmit on specific frequencies dedicated to their use and are designed to minimize spurious, out-of-band transmissions. Several large studies have shown that the risk of using wireless devices at a distance at least 3 feet from a medical device is very low.[26,27]

E-mail

E-mail is an effective tool that permits rapid distribution of information and allows images and other attachments to be exchanged easily. The use of e-mail can enhance the patient-physician relationship by making the physician more accessible, but it raises concerns about both privacy and security. Important messages can be saved for future reference, and e-mail's asynchronous nature allows busy health care professionals to exchange information without having to find one another on the telephone. Physicians and patients routinely use e-mail to communicate with each other. In 2006, 17% of physicians routinely used e-mail to communicate with their patients, and over two thirds of physicians used e-mail to communicate with other physicians.[28] As physicians become increasingly comfortable with IT, it is likely that the number of physicians who use e-mail to communicate will increase. One study by Brooks and Menachemi[28] found that only 1.6% of physicians who used e-mail adhered to published guidelines, which include printing e-mail correspondence and placing it into the patient's chart.[28] Only one third of physicians who used e-mail informed patients about privacy issues.

Many of the problems that arise during e-mail communication are caused by the fact that it is difficult to positively identify the true author of the message. Unencrypted e-mail may be intercepted during transmission or if the mail server at either end of the transaction is compromised. E-mail messages can also be intercepted if either the patient's or physician's computer is lost or stolen, or if an e-mail account is compromised. Many physicians assume that an e-mail correspondent is telling the truth about his or her identity and diagnosis, but it is relatively easy to impersonate another individual by registering an e-mail address similar to that of the intended victim. Eysenbach and Diepgen[29] sent e-mail to the owners of medical websites posing as a fictitious patient with a dermatologic lesion. Although 93% of physicians who responded recommended that the patient see a physician, over half mentioned a specific diagnosis in their response.[29]

As a result of these potential problems, the American Medical Informatics Association has developed guidelines for the use of e-mail by physicians and patients. These guidelines recommend obtaining informed consent prior to using e-mail to communicate, prohibiting the forwarding of e-mail without consent, explaining and using security mechanisms such as encryption, avoiding references to third parties, and informing patients as to who will have access to e-mail communications and whether e-mail will become a part of their medical record. The recommendations also included simple tasks such as double-checking all "To:" fields before sending messages and printing paper copies of messages and replies to place in the patient's chart.[30] Taking these relatively straightforward precautions will enhance the use of e-mail while minimizing security risks. Using secured e-mail programs compliant with the Health Insurance Portability and Accountability Act (HIPAA), such as the Accellion (Palo Alto, CA) plugin for Microsoft Outlook, is also a good option and is now required by law in the United States.

Telephone Consultations

Telephone consultations are now widely used in health care delivery and pose a different set of problems. Telephone calls are widely used by both physicians and patients in the health care setting; unfortunately, this practice can lead to a breach of patient confidentiality. Health care workers rarely if ever ask a caller to prove his or her identity before releasing information.[31] Curious friends, attorneys, or other interested parties may potentially lie about their identities (known as *social engineering*) to gain access to confidential information.[32] Even staff who claim that they can recognize a patient's voice can be fooled. Because of the limited bandwidth of the telephone network, it may be possible for another person to impersonate the patient. To alleviate this problem, Sokol and colleagues[31] have recommended the use of an authentication system that requires the caller to provide a password, making it easy for a patient or authorized representative to be identified.[31]

Social Networking

Social networking sites have fundamentally changed the way many people keep in touch with friends and colleagues. Social media sites such as Facebook and

LinkedIn allow their subscribers share news and pictures with friends and acquaintances. Each service offers a different "feel" and encourages the formation of specific types of communities. In general, LinkedIn is used primarily to maintain professional contacts and is used by recruiters to find candidates for positions in a variety of industries, including medicine. As of this writing, Facebook was the largest service, drawing users with both professional and social interests. Most subscribers use these services as a kind of continuously updated "Family and Friends" newsletter. Others use it to keep in touch with professional colleagues.

Although commercial social networking sites should not be used to discuss specific patients, medical groups have begun to develop their own dedicated sites that allow patients and physicians to interact with each other using instant messaging or community web pages.[33] Social networking sites have become an important method of communication among medical students and residents. In one study, half of medical trainees who responded to a survey participated in at least one social networking site, and only one third made their personally identifiable information private. Use of these sites decreased somewhat as trainees approached graduation.[34]

Patient care issues and any confidential information should not be discussed because of the obvious lack of privacy. Many social networking sites do not provide a way to close an account, meaning a user cannot remove his or her profile once it has been created, although it is, of course, possible to remove nearly all of the information associated with that profile. Information that has been posted may therefore be available online long after its owner had wanted it to be removed. Moreover, the business model of Facebook consists of selling information about its users to advertisers and other organizations. As a result, information that a user might have assumed to be private may be widely available to others. It is important to repeatedly check the privacy policies of social networking sites and the privacy settings of each individual account to make sure that confidential information is not being shared.

SECURITY

Electronic generation, transmission, and storage of health data has transformed patient care by making it easy to acquire, search, manipulate, and distribute large amounts of information. Information in the health record is also used for purposes not directly related to patient care, including insurance qualification, law enforcement, and litigation. Subject to specific safeguards, health information may also be used for clinical research and for projects that improve public health. Patients and health care providers have legitimate concerns about how their information will be protected; therefore systematic collection and storage of this information comes with the responsibility of protecting it from unauthorized use.

A recent survey reported that 75% of American consumers polled were concerned that sensitive health information might leak because of weak data security. Patients expect that their medical records will remain confidential, and government regulations, as well as ethical obligations, require that patients' health information be protected whenever it is aggregated, stored, or transmitted. Most of the requirements for storage and transmission of medical records are covered under HIPAA. These requirements extend beyond health professionals who collect information. Any provider of services to a health care organization that handles "protected health information" is bound by HIPAA to defend the security of medical records.

The electronic medical record contains intimate details about a person's physical and mental health. Unauthorized access to this information can have devastating consequences for both health care providers and their patients. Unintentional release of information about disease processes, medication use, or visits to health care providers can result in stigmatization, difficulty in obtaining credit or employment, or disruption of friendships or family relationships. Most importantly, unintended release of information can result in a breach of trust between patient and physician. Privacy and security of health information are therefore crucial to the widespread adoption of EHRs. A comprehensive information security plan encompasses physical protection of hardware, access control, data authentication, and encryption of sensitive information and should be developed in cooperation with information security professionals.

HIPAA includes specific requirements for privacy and security of electronic medical records systems. The primary impact of the Privacy Rule on the development of preanesthetic evaluation systems was to require user identification and authentication and to log every access to the EHR to allow the patient to have access to a list of all personnel who had accessed the record. Under HIPAA, health care organizations face a series of regulations that dictate how protected health information must be stored, distributed, and used. These regulations apply not only to practitioners who collect the information but also to their business associates. If, for example, a physician in solo practice collects information that is then forwarded to a billing service, that billing service must comply with HIPAA privacy rules. Patients must give consent to the use of protected health information, although HIPAA consents can be interpreted broadly. Compliance with HIPAA regulations will ultimately benefit health care providers by preventing or limiting disclosure or damage to protected health information.

The Health Information Technology for Economic and Clinical Health (HITECH) Act was enacted as part of the American Recovery and Reinvestment act of 2009 and is intended to promote the adoption and meaningful use of health IT. HITECH included $20 billion in funding for health information and extends the privacy and data security regulations enacted as part of HIPAA. HITECH also includes provisions for the development of health information standards and even stronger privacy and security regulations. As interoperable EHRs become commonplace, however, it may ultimately be possible for the health care provider or the patient to determine how confidential information is used.[35]

Although patients have a right to privacy, some elements of the health record must be shared. Obvious examples include prevention of serious threats to health or safety and oversight of the health care system.[36] Health care providers in the United States are required to obtain a patient's written consent prior to disclosure of health information, but most patients do not have a clear idea of where their information will go or how it will be used. Although the individual may request that certain restrictions be placed on the use of his or her information, the health care provider is not obliged to agree to the request.[36]

Attacks on personal computers in the form of viruses, keystroke loggers, and "phishing" are a growing threat and have the potential to interfere with patient care. Hundreds of computer viruses are released every day. Many health care applications rely on the Microsoft Windows operating system. As a result, they are vulnerable to the same kinds of viruses that affect home and office computers. Some experts have suggested that terrorists may specifically target the information infrastructure in hospitals and clinics to increase the number of casualties during an attack. In addition to rendering a computer unreliable, viruses and worms can compromise or destroy health information.

Most computer users are aware of such viruses: small programs are attached to e-mail messages or disguised as useful programs that, once activated, can destroy information or simply slow down the computer, as they send copies of themselves to thousands of other computers. The most common purpose of a virus is to turn the victim's computer into a "zombie" device, allowing it to be controlled over the Internet. Access to groups of zombie computers is bought and sold through underground websites. Such computers can be turned into pornography websites, made to pose as financial websites to collect credit card information, or used to distribute unsolicited commercial e-mail.

Adware and spyware programs are usually installed along with other, marginally useful software, such as a screen saver or file-sharing program. Once installed, these programs monitor computer usage and report back to a central site. They may generate pop-up windows with advertisements or may redirect web searches to a preferred site. They also cause the infected computer to slow down and may make it unstable, causing it to crash and lose valuable information. A keystroke logger is a variant of spyware that is usually distributed as an e-mail attachment, through a malicious website, or as the payload of a virus. This program automatically installs itself and then waits for the victim to log into a bank or credit card site, at which point all identifying information is relayed to the scammers. Keystroke loggers are increasingly common and are usually targeted toward specific banking or credit card sites. Many of these programs are professionally written and are designed by organized crime rings to be nearly invisible to the victim.

Fortunately, a few simple precautions, combined with common sense, can minimize the risk of information theft or damage. All access to websites, especially those of financial institutions, must be protected by a carefully chosen password, which should ideally consist of a series of letters, numerals, and punctuation marks. A good password is easy for its owner to remember but should be difficult for anyone else to guess. Remote access to hospital information systems from home computers, which may not have the latest security updates, should be allowed only when necessary, and these computers should have security software installed by the hospital IT department.

Firewalls determine whether information traveling across a network should be allowed to continue. Software firewalls prevent unauthorized programs from using an Internet connection. Specific programs, such as a web client, are permitted to send information to a location on the Internet. If an unknown program attempts to establish a connection, a software firewall blocks the connection until the user grants access. By limiting the programs that can send information to external computers, software firewalls prevent information from being stolen by spyware or adware. A hardware firewall is a piece of equipment, installed between a home or office network and a cable or DSL modem, that helps to protect against attacks from outside computers. Hardware firewalls guard an entire network against an outside attack but usually permit any computer on the local network to establish an outbound connection. As a result, hardware firewalls do not protect against programs that harvest information.

Hardware and software tools decrease the probability that a computer can be infected by a virus, compromised by a hacker, or turned into a zombie. Antivirus programs marketed by Symantec and McAfee, among others, are an essential tool that should be installed on every computer. It is important to update the programs frequently, because new viruses are released every day. Most of these programs also protect against keystroke loggers and Trojan horses. Ideally, protection of computers on a network should involve a comprehensive approach that includes both hardware and software firewalls, antivirus software, and frequent security analyses.

CONCLUSIONS

Technologically advanced anesthesia workstations and physiologic monitors offer a variety of features that include multiple ventilator modes, more precise administration of potent volatile anesthetics, automated checklists, and the ability to exchange data. A sophisticated user interface allows multiple features to be accessed at the touch of a button, and online help systems allow the clinician to find information on a particular feature. Newer systems are far more intuitive and easier to use, although modern workstations require intensive training before they can be used on patients, and the software and electronics may fail. However, if used carefully, new anesthesia workstations can improve patient care.

Clinical care requires rapid communication among health care providers who function in a highly dynamic environment without fixed workspaces. The increasing requirement for anesthesia services in locations such as interventional radiology or endoscopy suites underscores the need for efficient, reliable telecommunication.

Commonly available tools, such as cellular telephones and Wi-Fi computer networks, can be a simple, cost-effective way to improve patient care, and social networking sites and other "web 2.0" applications offer unprecedented opportunities to network with colleagues.

REFERENCES

1. Menachemi N, Saunders C, Chukmaitov A, Matthews MC, Brooks RG: Hospital adoption of information technologies and improved patient safety: a study of 98 hospitals in Florida, *J Healthc Manag* 52(6):398–409, 2007.
2. Schimpff SC: Improving operating room and perioperative safety: background and specific recommendations, *Surg Innov* 14(2): 127–135, 2007.
3. Larson ER, Nuttall GA, Ogren BD, et al: A prospective study on anesthesia machine fault identification, *Anesth Analg* 104(1): 154–156, 2007.
4. Rawat S, Dingley J: Closed-circuit xenon delivery using a standard anesthesia workstation, *Anesth Analg* 110(1):101–109, 2010.
5. Pouzeratte Y, Sebbane M, Jung B, et al: A prospective study on the user-friendliness of four anaesthesia workstations, *Eur J Anaesthesiol* 25(8):634–641, 2008.
6. Halbeis CBE, Epstin RH, Macario A, Pearl RG, Grunwald Z: Adoption of anesthesia information management systems by academic departments in the United States, *Anesth Analg* 107:1323–1329, 2008.
7. Nair BG, Newman SF, Peterson GN, Wu WY, Schwid HA: Feedback mechanisms including real-time electronic alerts to achieve near 100% timely prophylactic antibiotic administration in surgical cases, *Anesth Analg* 111(5):1293–1300, 2010.
8. Sandberg WS, Sandberg EH, Seim AR, et al: Real-time checking of electronic anesthesia records for documentation errors and automatically text messaging clinicians improves quality of documentation, *Anesth Analg* 106(1):192–201, 2008.
9. Ely JW, Osheroff JA, Chambliss ML, Ebell MH, Rosenbaum ME: Answering physicians' clinical questions: obstacles and potential solutions, *J Am Med Inform Assoc* 12(2):217–224, 2005.
10. Thiele RH, Poiro NC, Scalzo DC, Nemergut EC: Speed, accuracy, and confidence in Google, Ovid, PubMed, and UpToDate: results of a randomised trial, *Postgrad Med J* 86(1018):459–465, 2010.
11. Rudkin SE, Langdorf MI, Macias D, Oman JA, Kazzi AA: Personal digital assistants change management more often than paper texts and foster patient confidence, *Eur J Emerg Med* 13(2):92–96, 2006.
12. Lapinsky SE: Mobile computing in critical care, *J Crit Care* 22(1):41–44, 2007.
13. Bolle SR, Scholl J, Gilbert M: Can video mobile phones improve CPR quality when used for dispatcher assistance during simulated cardiac arrest? *Acta Anaesthesiol Scand* 53(1):116–120, 2009.
14. Blum RH, Raemer DB, Carroll JS, et al: Crisis resource management for an anaesthesia faculty: a new approach to continuing education, *Med Educ* 38:45–55, 2004.
15. Howard SK, Gaba DM, Fish KJ, Yang G, Sarnquist FH: Anesthesia crisis resource management training: teaching anesthesiologists to handle critical incidents, *Aviat Space Environ Med* 63:763–770, 1992.
16. Gaba DM, Fish KJ, Howard SK: *Crisis management in anesthesiology*, New York, 1993, Churchill Livingstone.
17. Yee B, Naik VN, Joo HS, et al: Nontechnical skills in anesthesia crisis management with repeated exposure to simulation-based education, *Anesthesiology* 103:241–248, 2005.
18. Hersh W, Helfand M, Wallace J, et al: A systematic review of the efficacy of telemedicine for making diagnostic and management decisions, *J Telemed Telecare* 8:197–209, 2002.
19. Kluger MT, Bullock MF: Recovery room incidents: a review of 419 reports from the Anaesthetic Incident Monitoring Study (AIMS), *Anaesthesia* 57:1060–1066, 2002.
20. Holt NF, Silverman DG, Prasad R, Dziura J, Ruskin KJ: Preanesthesia clinics, information management, and operating room delays: results of a survey of practicing anesthesiologists, *Anesth Analg* 104(3):615–618, 2007.
21. Soto RG, Chu LF, Goldman JM, Rampil IJ, Ruskin KJ: Communication in critical care environments: mobile telephones improve patient care, *Anesth Analg* 102(2):535–541, 2006.
22. Cermak M: Monitoring and telemedicine support in remote environments and in human space flight, *Br J Anaesth* 97(1):107–114, 2006.
23. Kyriacou E, Pavlopoulos S, Berler A, et al: Multi-purpose HealthCare Telemedicine Systems with mobile communication link support, *Biomed Eng Online* 24:2–7, 2003.
24. Richardson JE, Shah-Hosseini S, Fiadjoe JE, Ash JS, Rehman MA: The effects of a hands-free communication device system in a surgical suite, *J Am Med Inform Assoc* 18(1):70–72, 2011.
25. Klein A, Djaiani G: Mobile phones in the hospital: past, present, and future, *Anaesthesia* 58:353–357, 2003.
26. Iskra S, Thomas BW, McKenzie R, Rowley J, Potential GPRS: 900/180-MHz and WCDMA 1900-MHz interference to medical devices, *IEEE Trans Biomed Eng* 54(10):1858–1866, 2007.
27. Dang BP, Nel PR, Gjevre JA: Mobile communication devices causing interference in invasive and noninvasive ventilators, *J Crit Care* 22(2):137–141, 2007.
28. Brooks RG, Menachemi N: Physicians' use of e-mail with patients: factors influencing electronic communication and adherence to best practices, *J Med Internet Res* 8(1):e2, 2006.
29. Eysenbach G, Diepgen TL: Responses to unsolicited patient e-mail requests for medical advice on the World Wide Web, *JAMA* 280(15):1333–1335, 1998.
30. Kane B, Sands DZ: Guidelines for the clinical use of electronic mail with patients. The AMIA Internet Working Group, Task Force on Guidelines for the Use of Clinic-Patient Electronic Mail, *J Am Med Inform Assoc* 5(1):104–111, 1998.
31. Sokol DK, Car J: Patient confidentiality and telephone consultations: time for a password, *J Med Ethics* 32(12):688–689, 2006.
32. Sokol DK, Car J: Protecting patient confidentiality in telephone consultations in general practice, *Br J Gen Pract* 56:384–385, 2006.
33. Hawn C: Take two aspirin and tweet me in the morning: how Twitter, Facebook, and other social media are reshaping health care, *Health Aff (Millwood)* 28(2):361–368, 2009.
34. Thompson LA, Dawson K, Ferdig R, et al: The intersection of online social networking with medical professionalism, *J Gen Intern Med* 23(7):954–957, 2008.
35. Agrawal R, Johnson C: Securing electronic health records without impeding the flow of information, *Int J Med Inform* 76(5-6): 471–479, 2007.
36. Gostin LO: National health information privacy: regulations under the Health Insurance Portability and Accountability Act, *JAMA* 285(23):3015–3012, 2001.

CHAPTER 22

PERIOPERATIVE INFORMATICS

Paul St. Jacques • James M. Berry

CHAPTER OUTLINE

OVERVIEW

In the twenty-first century, perioperative information systems will not only provide answers to clinical questions in near real-time, they will also anticipate these questions.

JAMES M, BERRY, MD

This vision of technology may soon be realized by the careful development and deployment of medical informatics systems in the perioperative environment. Informatics systems hold the potential to transform operating room (OR) management and produce significant improvements in both efficiency and patient safety. Real-time access to both current patient data and historic patterns make the implementation of quality assurance, practice improvement, and safety initiatives both simple and transparent.[1,2]

Compared with other medical or nonmedical environments, the density and complexity found in the OR make technology implementation much more challenging.[3] The need to frequently move equipment and reconfigure the operating room for different procedures makes even simple connectivity an ongoing challenge. Also, the high-noise environment makes alarm sounds or other audio notification problematic. The numerous, often incompatible electronic devices used produce electrical noise, cross-talk, and other interference. Connecting physically separate devices—such as monitors, towers, input devices, and storage—requires tangles of highly specific, and often poorly shielded, data cables (Fig. 22-1).

DATA

Data Gathering

The foundation of any information system is the ability of the system to gather accurate and timely data. Data may come from a variety of sources, either *primary*, data captured directly from the patient, or *secondary*, preexisting data retrieved from other systems and processed into a more specialized database; perioperative data management systems would be a robust example of such a secondary data system. The importance of integrating this data cannot be underestimated; advanced decision support systems will require not only current data but also past data from the patient's history, comparative data from other patients, and best-practice rules to formulate recommendations for clinicians.

Data Sources

Patient vital signs and ventilatory parameters are fundamental to successful perioperative management, because they serve as objective and quantitative measures of the patient's condition and its evolution over time. Because these data serve as the foundation for most perioperative documentation and clinical decision making in all phases of care—preoperative, intraoperative, and postoperative—they must be readily accessible to all clinicians, including surgical, nursing, and anesthesiology providers. Complicating this processing is the sheer volume of data and the multiple, complex networks from which data are derived. For example, a modern operating suite and the associated critical care units may collect 1 gigabyte, the contents of an encyclopedia, *daily* from vital signs alone.

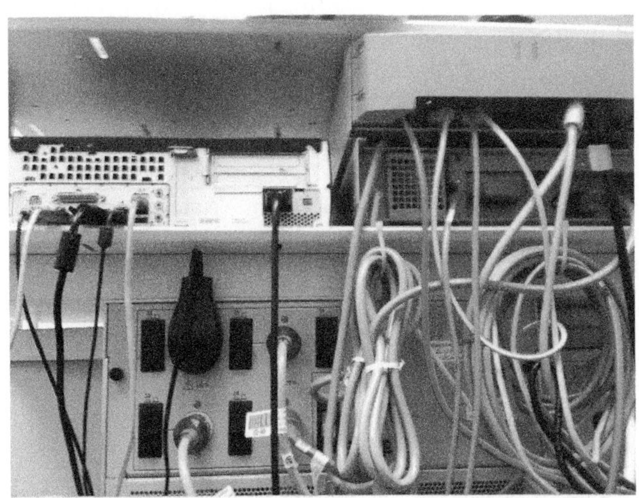

FIGURE 22-1 ■ Example of the multiple interface and power cords on a typical anesthesia workstation.

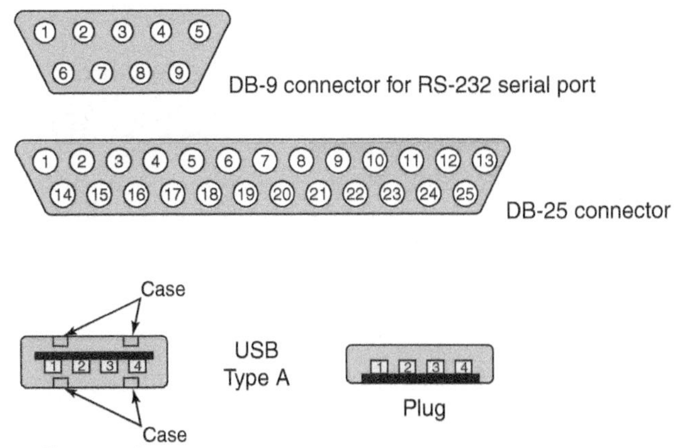

FIGURE 22-2 ■ Port and pin configurations for standard cables and jacks.

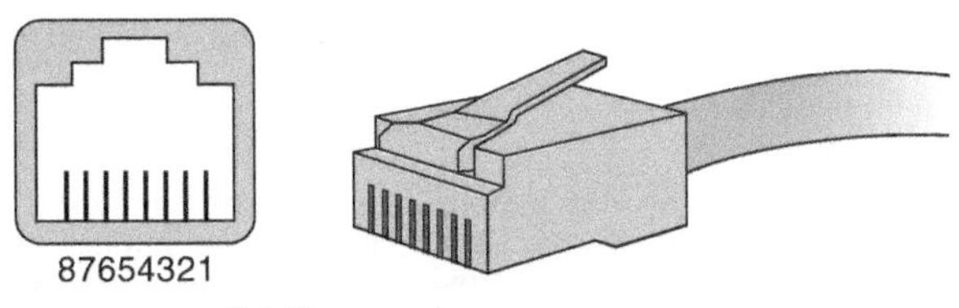

FIGURE 22-3 ■ Standard network cable terminus and jack (RJ-45).

The problem of data volume exists in many professional arenas, not just in medicine,[4] and new software technologies and concepts are helping to resolve this issue. Beyond basic search engines, modern tools such as The Brain (www.thebrain.com) or Wolfram Alpha (www.wolframalpha.com) can analyze a dataset, draw inferences, extract data from other sources, and present artificial intelligence–filtered data to the user. In this way, the computer serves not only as a tool to store and retrieve information but also as a tool to intelligently guide users toward the information they are seeking. Taking a similar approach in medicine, in the future, information systems will be able to examine a constellation of findings in an electronic health record and predict, based on past patterns, likely outcomes and potential morbidity. Additionally, similar algorithms will track numerous care plans and ensure that they are followed to maximize efficacy and minimize morbidity.

Monitor Interfaces

Physiologic monitors come in a variety of designs from a handful of manufacturers. Although they may differ cosmetically and provide similar functionality, data output from monitors is not always standardized. Although RS232 serial output, which uses a 9- or 25-pin connector dating from the 1980s (www.interfacebus.com/RS232_Pinout.html) is still found on some monitor interfaces, RS422 or universal serial bus (USB) output is capable of much higher bandwidth and thus higher data transmission rates (Fig. 22-2).

Also, monitors tend to be both expensive and long lived (10 years typically) in most inpatient environments. This may result in an institution having a mix of physiologic monitors from multiple vendors, with multiple software revisions or hardware generations, many of which may have different physical data interfaces and different interface "languages."

Historically, networked monitors have had proprietary physical connectors that required specialized hard wiring from all the locations in which monitoring occurs. This created a complex network of single-use cabling that would have only one purpose and an investment that would only be viable for a short period of time. Fortunately, most newer generation monitors use not only a standard network cabling infrastructure for hardware connections (RJ-45 Ethernet cabling and jacks; Fig. 22-3) but also are able to transmit data over a standardized Ethernet network.

In this age of health information privacy, a hospital network is required to have significant security measures in place. Virtual local area network (VLAN) or virtual private network (VPN) structures, as well as encryption of wireless traffic, help ensure that network traffic for patient data is segregated and secure. Also, a guaranteed minimum bandwidth available for real-time transmission of critical data and alerts promotes confidence and trust among clinicians that the system is robust, even under stress.[5]

Modern patient monitoring networks typically have intermediate data aggregation points. Data may be stored, transformed, or filtered at these locations. For example, data transmitted from the Philips MP90 bedside physiologic monitors pass through two intermediaries prior to being transmitted to external systems. First, data enter a central station that stores, for 24 hours, all individual data points and waveforms for analysis. Clinicians are able to review, compare, or print data at this central station. The central station may also generate alerts for arrhythmias, hypotension, apnea, and so on to monitoring technicians or nurses. From this hub, data are then transferred to an information server, where the information is both archived and transformed into an externally recognized format for use in other systems (Fig. 22-4).

Physiologic monitoring is but one of a variety of data sources in the perioperative environment. Additional data are required for proper documentation of care and to feed clinical decision-making and decision-support algorithms. Some of these data, such as demographic and

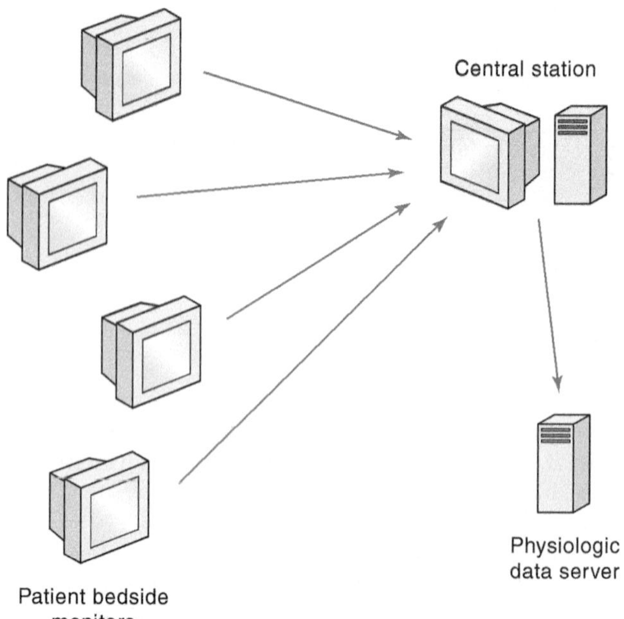

FIGURE 22-4 Data flow from patient bedside monitors to central stations via a secure network. Depending on the manufacturer, data and/or waveforms may be reviewed on the central station. Data are also forwarded to a data server to be stored for real-time retrieval by documentation systems or for off-line analysis.

TABLE 22-1 **Open Systems Interconnection (OSI) Model***

	OSI Model		
	Data Unit	**Layer**	**Function**
Host layers	Data	7. Application	Network process to application
		6. Presentation	Data representation, encryption, and decryption
		5. Session	Interhost communication
	Segments	4. Transport	End-to-end connections and reliability; flow control
Media layers	Packet	3. Network	Path determination and logical addressing
	Frame	2. Data link	Physical addressing
	Bit	1. Physical	Media, signal, and binary transmission

*The OSI model was designed to standardize communications functions. Each layer provides services and data to the layer above while receiving information from the layer below.

laboratory results, are structured in a standard format, but other data are stored as images or in other, nonstructured formats. Demographic databases include patients' nonmedical data: name, date of birth, address, medical record number or other identifiers, diagnoses, and billing information. Wide access to these data is critical to ensure that documentation is timely and accurate, with minimal need for reentry. Rekeying of demographic and identifying data is both time consuming and subject to operator error, and it should be avoided whenever possible. Careful interfacing can bring the previously entered and validated identifying data to the clinician at the point of care.

NETWORKING CONCEPTS AND OPEN SYSTEM INTERCONNECTION

Communicating data across distances requires certain agreements on protocol and format. From the early evolutionary steps of what we now call the Internet, a system of layers of information and protocol developed that may be visualized as parallel systems of information transport, each serving a particular function. In the open system interconnection (OSI) reference model, the most fundamental layer is physical—literally, the wires connecting the computers, servers, and switches. The highest layer is the application, or the way data are presented on a screen (Table 22-1).

Interface Languages

Standardized systems' interface languages ensure the clinician will have easy access to information and save time and effort in formulating treatment plans. For example, the digital imaging and communications in medicine (DICOM) format was developed to ensure interoperability of systems that produce, store, display, process, transmit, or print medical images and structured documents.[6,7] Integration of common data pipelines, using a common language and interface and shared data validation and security, enables images from various modalities—X-ray, ultrasound, medical photography, and electronic documents—to be freely transferred intact among systems and presented to clinicians in widely accepted visual formats. The Health Level 7 (HL7) standard was developed to support the exchange, integration, and retrieval of health information.[8] HL7 provides a communications messaging model at the application level such that systems can communicate and interoperate without manual intervention at each step. Standards such as these enable different manufacturers' products to work together in a clinical environment.[9] From the point of view of the clinician, the underlying standard and processing may be transparent, but the displayed results will not be (Table 22-2).

In addition to traditional sources of patient data, such as monitors and lab systems, modern informatics includes several nontraditional modalities of data collection. Medical imaging and video has become pervasive throughout the practice of medicine, especially in procedural or operative areas.[10] Imaging can be acquired from a variety of sources that include handheld digital cameras, still cameras incorporated into medical devices such as endoscopes, moving video images from surgical instruments (endoscopy, overhead cameras built into lighting fixtures), and other sources. Informatics systems need to be able to capture these images, in real time and only when appropriate, for incorporation into the medical record. Subsequent review of the records for further diagnosis and treatment can then be enhanced with the knowledge provided by having the actual photograph or video loop presented as part of the documentation of the procedure.

TABLE 22-2 **An HL7 Message Format for a Patient Encounter Event***

Code	Description
MSH	Message header
EVN	Event type
PID	Patient identification
ZRB	HIS base registration
ZP2	HIS patient information
PV1	Patient visit
ZV1	HIS patient visit
ZEN	HIS encounter
{ZVP}	HIS patient provider
{DG1}	Diagnosis
ZDX	HIS diagnosis
{PR1}	Procedure
ZPR	HIS procedure
[ZPN]	HIS PHN
{[ZDN]}	HIS dental
[ZDP]	HIS dental op
{[ZIM]}	HIS immunization
{[ZMD]}	HIS medication
{[OBX]}	Health factors
{[OBX]}	Measurements
{[OBX]}	Exams
{[OBX]}	CPT
{[OBX]}	Labs
{[OBX]}	Patient education
{[OBX]}	Skin tests

*Using a standard message structure improves interoperability among devices and decreases provider workload by eliminating the need to reenter data into multiple applications.

CPT, current procedural terminology; HIS, hospital information system; HL7, Health Level 7.

Similar to existing telemedicine applications, such as remote consultations between trauma centers and community hospitals,[11] video feeds have also found utility in management of the perioperative suite.[12] Management can take place at any of several levels. Individual anesthesiologists may provide medical services to patients in a group of two to four ORs in a supervisory role, and charge nurses and anesthesiology coordinators may oversee the flow of patients through entire suites or multiple suites in a large hospital. Video technology, such as that provided through the Vigilance system (Acuitec, Birmingham, AL),[13] provides improved situational awareness of ORs and other perioperative locations from non–point-of-care locations such as OR front desks, offices, preoperative holding rooms, and other OR areas. This system integrates real-time video from ceiling-mounted cameras and presents that video in conjunction with other data derived from information systems to produce a single-screen view of one or more ORs. This view is accessible from a fixed workstation (Fig. 22-5), handheld computer, or even an Internet-connected cellular phone, such as an iPhone (Fig. 22-6).

Additionally, critical voice communications can be facilitated by an informatics system. Voice can either be built in using voice over Internet protocol (VoIP) or information systems that facilitate traditional voice communications by providing phone numbers on the screen or by pages to digital paging systems. Together, these technologies are in the process of revolutionizing real-time voice communication.[14]

Central Storage and Servers

Complex information systems, such as those used in a perioperative setting, generate large datasets. After several years of operation, a large hospital may find itself

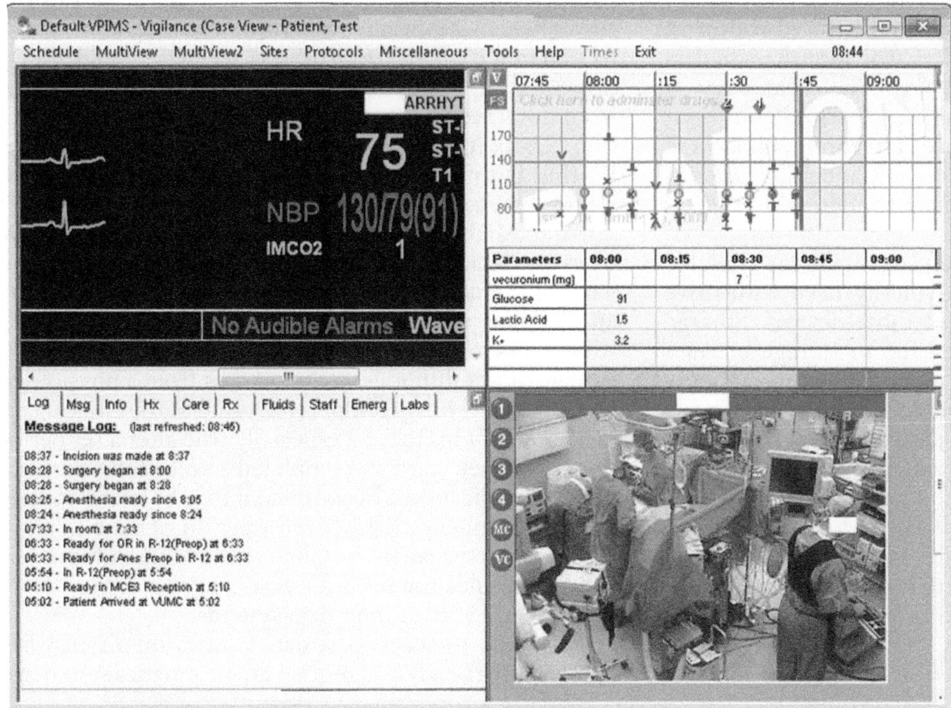

FIGURE 22-5 Data integration to improve situational awareness. Incorporation of video technology into a situational awareness tool that provides a live view into an operating room (OR). In addition to video, users are able to review vital signs trends and waveforms from each OR at any computer workstation location. (Courtesy Acuitec, Birmingham, AL.)

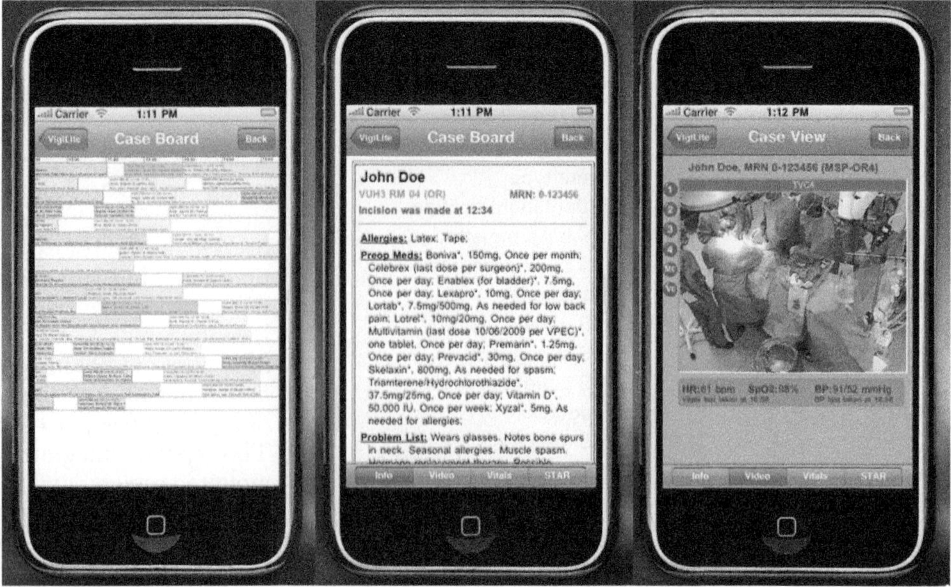

FIGURE 22-6 ■ Handheld situational awareness tools. A handheld version of the situational awareness tool allows users to review data and case progress via a handheld device, such as Apple's iPhone. (Courtesy Acuitec, Birmingham, AL.)

with over a billion data points comprising a database that spans more than one terabyte of data. Compounding the data storage situation is the potential need to keep multiple copies of the database either for back-up or research purposes. In an effort to protect patient privacy, research datasets are often required to be deidentified and stored in such a manner that there can be no linkage from the research dataset to the original data. The U.S. Health Insurance Portability and Accountability Act of 1996 (HIPAA) provides a good standard rule set for data privacy. In addition to removing key patient identifying information, the informatics system may be required to keep a research dataset on a physically separate server to minimize the risk of unintended release of protected patient information. These factors make data storage and security a crucial issue.

Data storage and security are often unseen components of an information system. Data may be stored within an institution or at an external facility that specializes in data management and security. Through the technology of networking, data can flow seamlessly across miles or hundreds of miles of physical distance. The three hallmarks of data storage are 1) *capacity*, 2) *security*, and 3) *availability*. Each of these concepts is important to address, and all are interrelated.

Central storage capacity is fundamentally the available *space* on the physical devices, typically fixed hard-drive storage, and the *configuration* of those devices. Storage can either be on a server dedicated to storage or on a mixed-use server that stores data and also runs applications, called *processes*, which manipulate data or provide the data to applications that use it, called *clients*. This client/server architecture forms the basis of many medical systems (Fig. 22-7).

The storage devices typically used for these implementations are similar to the hard drives found in desktop computers; however, they tend to be faster, of lower individual capacity, and organized into groups, a *redundant array of independent disks*, better known as *RAID arrays*.[15] RAID is a fundamental concept in server storage in which multiple disks are configured in a manner that allows them to work as a team to provide additional capacity and/or redundancy to a stored dataset. For example, a RAID array of three disks may be used to store data such that if any one of the single disks were to fail or "crash," the other two disks could be used to automatically rebuild the data on the third disk once it is physically replaced. Often these disks can be replaced while the server system is running, a process called *hot swapping*.

Lastly, storage systems must come with a plan for data recovery in the event of a disaster, either one internal to the data center, corruption of data from faulty hardware, or in the event of an external attack on the system.[16] Typically this recovery strategy involves a *fail-over plan*, whereby a failing system can have its workload taken up by a secondary server, either automatically or by a manual process usually geographically remote from the primary server, which is typically running and waiting in the wings to step in for a failed primary server. Data should also be protected by a back-up plan, whereby data are archived from the server to a separate location and separate media (Fig. 22-8). Magnetic tape has been a common medium for this, but it is being replaced by other formats, such as removable magnetic or optical disks.

After establishment of the physical devices used to store the data, the next question that must be addressed is what data will be stored on the devices, in what format, and for how long. The answers may vary depending on what types of data are in consideration. For example, storage of a continuous stream of data from a physiologic monitor may or may not provide value to the clinical care of a patient. This may be especially true after a set period of time, when care is completed successfully with no noted complications. In contrast, it may be useful to keep a higher frequency dataset for a period of time to allow for retrospective analysis. Clinicians and institutions will need to balance the need for access to past data with the available capacity of their data systems.

The need to access past data is very important when considering the advantages that an informatics system has

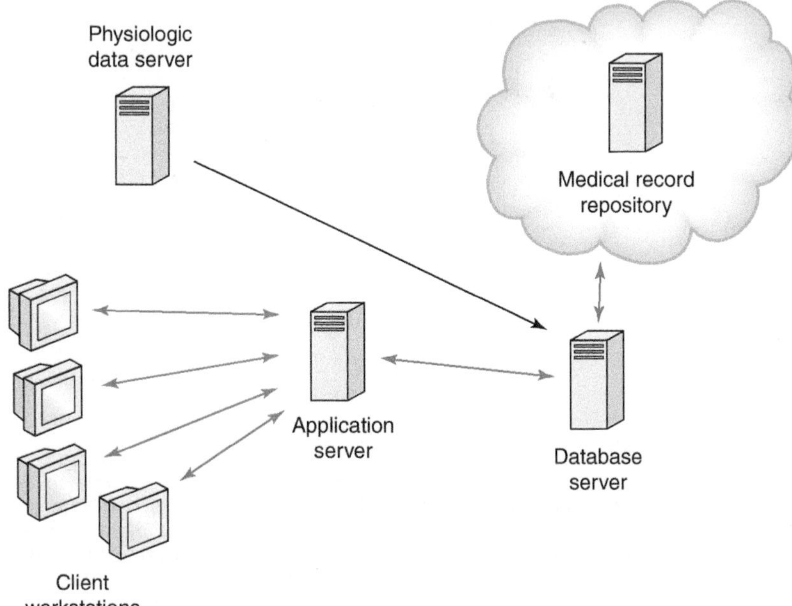

FIGURE 22-7 ■ The relationships of the components of a client server architecture system. Users interact with the system via the client computers, which receive data and application code from an application server and database server. Using this model, applications and data are stored on central servers, enabling any client workstation to access the same revisions of the data and software. Also, security and data integrity are increased, because data are not stored on multiple vulnerable computers but rather on one secure server.

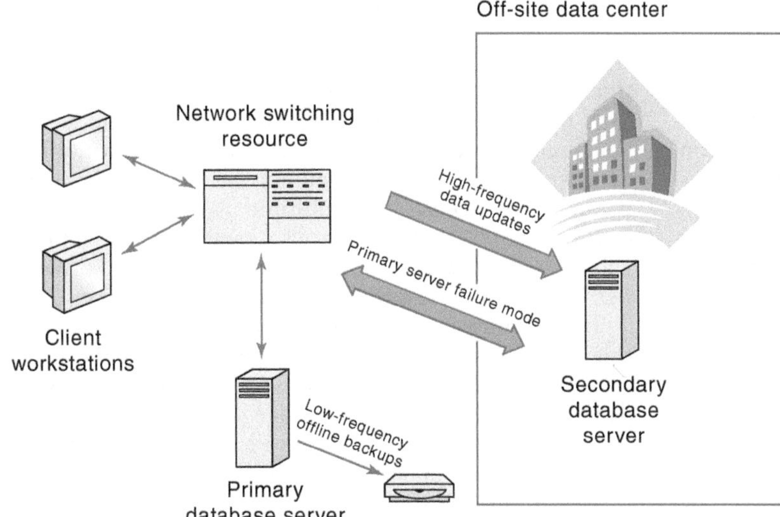

FIGURE 22-8 ■ Disaster recovery. Every software installation should have a defined disaster recovery plan. Typically, a primary server has a mirrored second server of similar capacity. Both servers are kept current in terms of database software and operating systems. The secondary server receives regular updates, for example every 15 minutes, of data that have been entered onto the primary server. In the event of a failure of the primary server, the secondary server can be immediately brought online by rerouting network traffic from the primary server to and from the secondary server. The secondary server is typically housed in a separate facility, so that a single disaster, such as a fire or power outage, will not affect the primary and secondary locations. Off-line backups are made less frequently, daily for example, and are stored on magnetic tape or optical disk. These may be stored in a third location to provide an additional level of data safety.

in serving as a tool for process improvement and research. The ability of a computerized query to search through hundreds of thousands or even millions of patient records is revolutionizing research, compared with hand extraction of data from traditional paper medical charts.

However, storage of these data also comes at a price in terms of data transformation and data cleaning. Raw data entered into a database may be considered "dirty" in that they may be unverified, artifact ridden, or improperly formatted. The field of data warehousing considers these concepts to create a transcribed database that has been subject to computerized processing to clean the data of extraneous values and ensure that the data present are in a final, verified format. Also, data warehousing can ensure patient privacy by following regulations such as those provided by HIPAA and local privacy compliance offices. This is done be either removing patient identifying data or by providing a coded string in the dataset called a *one-way hash* that allows further data to be entered under the same patient record but provides no ability to regenerate the patient identifiers from the hashed information (Fig. 22-9).[17]

The goal of the data processing and deidentification is to create a database that is useful for research: for science, process improvement, or both. A clinical database created for data entry and retrieval is called an *online transaction processing* (OLTP) database.[18] The data processing and deidentification then creates a database suitable for *online analytical processing* (OLAP)[19] from an OLTP original. An OLAP database is specifically configured for rapid execution of complex queries on existing data. Data in an OLAP database are often organized into cubes, often called *hypercubes* or *multidimensional cubes.* Conceptually difficult to visualize, because a typical data table has only rows and columns, a data cube may have numerous different dimensions, each representing a variable. The interrelations of the data are complex, and the data can be analyzed from the point of view of any dimension; but the

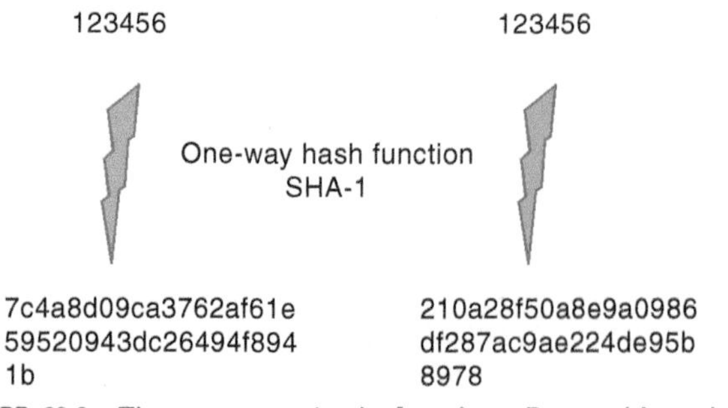

FIGURE 22-9 The one-way hash function. Researching data stored in databases requires maintenance of patient privacy standards. Certain data fields—such as name, Social Security number, and date of birth—must be kept confidential. One method of doing this is to utilize a one-way hash, a mathematical function applied to a string of data to yield a secondary string of data, which is reproducible (the same input string will always yield the same output string) yet cannot easily be reverse engineered (there is virtually no way to return to the original data). Additionally, small changes in the input data result in large variations in the output string.

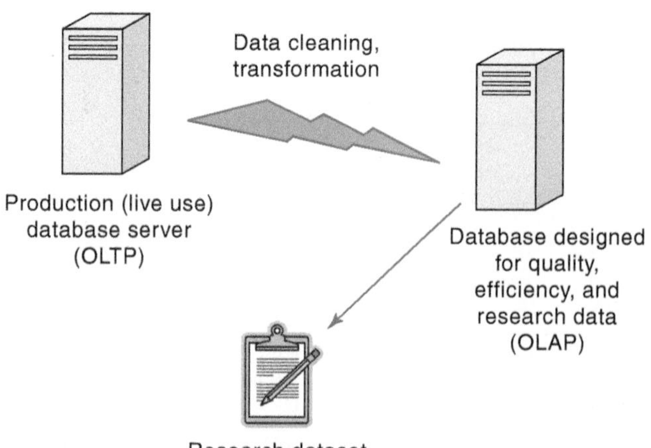

FIGURE 22-10 Data transformation for research. Clinical data are entered into a production database optimized for transaction entry and retrieval. Periodically, data from this database are copied to a database structured to facilitate drawing inferences from the data rather than organizing it for transactions. As the data are copied, computer algorithms are applied to weed out erroneous data and to ensure that all data conform to a common standard. This secondary dataset then serves as the source for data for research and process-improvement questions. OLAP, on-line analytical processing; OLTP on-line transaction processing.

end result is a data structure that can produce answers to complex queries in a fraction of the time of a traditional OLTP database (Fig. 22-10).

Local Versus Central Processing

All data entry or presentation actions rely on some form of data handling. This data handling can occur either on the local computer or on a central computer. Computers or applications that rely on a remote computer to do their basic data handling roles are called *thin clients.* This is in contrast to a *thick client,* or *fat client,* which is designed to do the primary data handling by itself and then forward the results of the computation to the database (Fig. 22-11). Through these types of systems designs, it is possible for applications to be widely accessed and distributed throughout an organization and beyond.[20]

The advantages of a thin-client structure are that thin clients have a significantly decreased requirement for computer resources at the point of care. Because most if not all of the computational needs are handled by the remote computer, the local computer does not need all of the usual components of a full computer. For example, there may be no CD-ROM or hard drive, no modem, and memory may be reduced. The installed computer workstation is therefore less costly initially and has a decreased support requirement and potentially a longer life cycle. Also, because most of the client application may reside on a remote computer, upgrades and distributions of software updates may occur transparently or with minimal intervention.

In contrast, the traditional thick client offers several advantages of functionality but at the cost of more expensive hardware, both at the time of installation and for ongoing maintenance. Thick clients are better able to format data and create a user experience that is richer in graphics and interaction. This is due to the utilization of the local computing resources for central processing unit (CPU)-intensive operations, such as managing on-screen graphics or recording audio or video. In addition, because thick clients do most of the work of the application on the local machine, it places much less of a load on the server, which can therefore be configured to be drastically less expensive than if it were supporting the simultaneous computation needs of the multiple users in a thin client environment. Thick clients also tend to offer a more robust user experience in multiple media and also provide flexibility in the breadth of scope of the applications.

In the interests of data security, robustness, and fault tolerance, it is strongly recommended that applications critical to patient safety be run as thin clients with redundant off-site and encrypted storage of data. This provides the ability to reboot and restore all data in the event of a local hardware problem, by far the most common fault in this environment.

In an enterprise environment, versioning control—that is, the ability of information technology (IT) management to ensure that all computer workstations are running the same version of software—is critical. If different versions of an application are present on different workstations, the results could be that a known bug is allowed to persist longer than it should after the generation of a patch or fix. In the past, this required a team of technicians to attend to each workstation and provide a fix or new installation of software to bring the workstation to the latest revision. However, more recently, sets of Internet-based tools have been developed that allow version control to take place from a central server. This functionality has also been implemented for the initial installation of a software product. Typically, the method involves a user clicking on a web-based link, which initiates an application launcher. The application launcher then checks the current version of the software application against what is present as the most recent version on the server. If the application on the client is not the latest version, the launching application will cause the server to

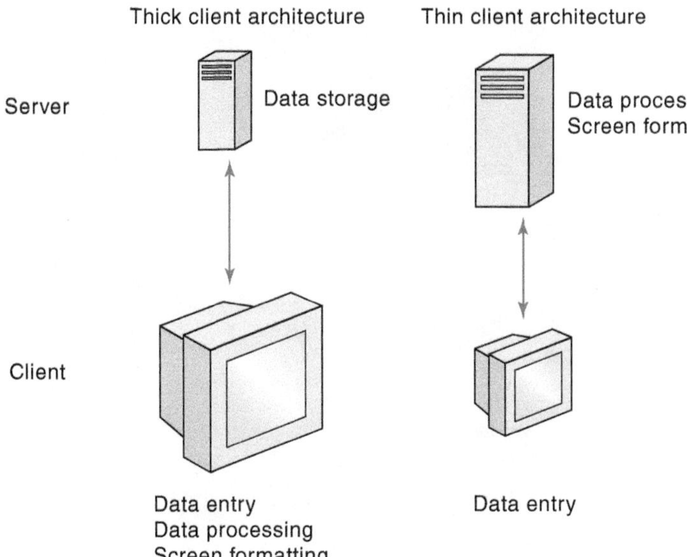

FIGURE 22-11 Client architecture. The difference between "thick" and "thin" client computing is based on the amount of computation that occurs at the user workstation. A thick client system typically has a requirement for a larger workstation, which is responsible for handling data entry, screen formatting, data processing by the application, and data transmission to the server. Under a thin client system, the user workstation is a lower power system that only shuttles data to and from the server. The server therefore has the additional load of data processing, screen formatting, and other functions. In the thin client system, a larger server is generally required, because the server is handling these tasks for all the workstations to which it is connected.

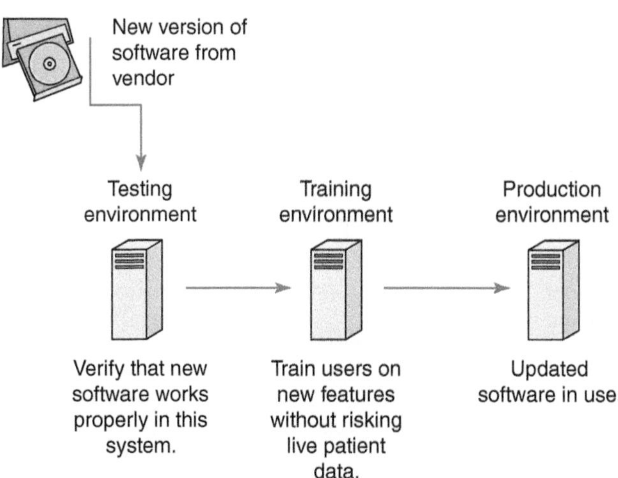

FIGURE 22-12 Software updating process. Different environments offer different functions and protections of the live system against risks from new software updates. A software update is first applied to a testing environment, where support personnel can ensure that no unintended functions have been introduced into the system. Once that verification has taken place, the new software can be loaded into the training environment, where users will be able to explore the new functionality without risking live patient data in an actual clinical encounter. Once training has been completed, the software will be moved to the live production environment.

transfer the updated version to the client before the software launches. This process is virtually seamless to the user and ensures not only that all workstations are running the same version but also that it does so in a manner that does not require a technical call with the associated resources and time necessary to apply a patch (Fig. 22-12).

Presentation

Clinical computer systems are created to provide value to the clinician and patient. Value to the clinician comes in the form of increased work accomplished in the same or less time than without the system. Value to the patient is from less repetition of information, less repeated unnecessary testing, and increased safety from ensuring that known medical history data are available to clinicians in real time at the point of care.

In designing or selecting a system, it is necessary to consider the importance of human factors in interacting with the system. Is the system designed to be user friendly? What does "user friendly" mean? What is the level of general computer competence necessary to operate the software and hardware? Although the competence of the general population continues to grow, and some users have better technical abilities, there is still great variability. Fortunately, the number of clinicians who cannot find the "any" key when instructed to "press any key to continue" is rapidly decreasing. Also, software designers are giving serious consideration to human factors when designing data entry screens and results presentation screens. These screens need to be organized in such a manner—using colors, type fonts, and graphics—to highlight data critical to the current or future process or data that are potentially erroneous or incomplete. Also, the flow of data entry into the system must reflect the work patterns that have been developed over years of clinical experience.

Computerized display technology has undergone revolutionary advancement in the past 10 years. Long gone are the days of heavy, 14-inch cathode ray tube (CRT) displays. Replacing them are light crystal diode (LCD) panels, which offer a larger, sharper image in a more compact and now less expensive form. Additionally, computer equipment is now available that allows for cleaning with antiseptic materials and splash resistance to meet medical and infection-control requirements. This is especially true of keyboards, which have been shown to be vectors of bacterial contamination.[21,22] There are both keyboard overlays and molded-mat keyboards available for use in wet environments.

Limitations in hardware resources (computer workstations) should not limit access to medical information. One solution to the need for point-of-care computing is to install a computer at every point of care. This is a traditional installation schema in which every holding room, postanesthesia care unit (PACU), and OR has a computer workstation. ORs in which both the circulating nurse and anesthesia team are documenting electronically require two or even three workstations if the surgeon has computing needs during the surgery, such as for electronic radiology picture archiving and communications systems (PACS), dictation/note taking or postoperative order set generation with computerized physician order entry (CPOE) systems.

An alternate method of providing computer hardware is to provide each clinician with a portable computer device. Several device manufacturers have entered this arena, but few have been successful. One of the more successful tablet-sized computers is a medical-grade product from Motion Computing (Austin, TX) that includes a built-in bar code scanner and handle for easy portability.

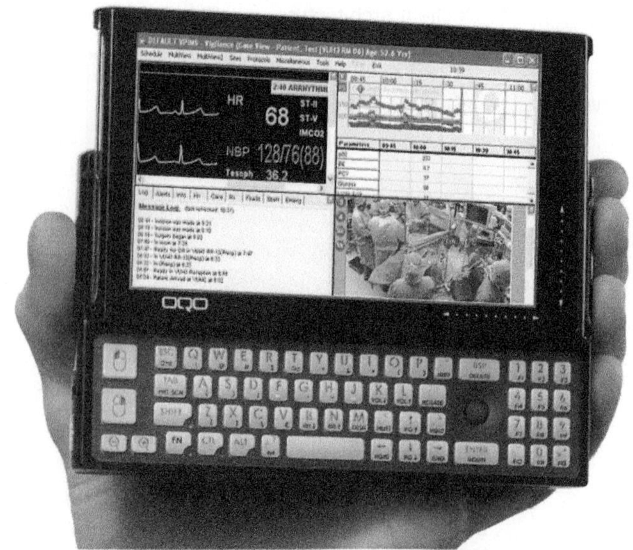

FIGURE 22-13 ■ Mobile computing platform. Handheld or tablet computers allow clinicians to interact with medical record software at the point of care. Small size, light weight, long battery life, and rugged construction are important considerations in selecting a mobile computing device. (Courtesy Acuitec LLC, Birmingham, AL.)

Decision Support

One profound advantage of perioperative information systems is their ability to present the user with decision-support information based on the patient's clinical context. This decision support can be as simple as a reminder that an antibiotic is due at a certain time, or it could be a complex analysis of fluid management based on several parameters. Either way, the autonomously generated data could be presented in several modalities. An on-screen color change can indicate a missing datum, or a pop-up window could present a critical message. Additionally, through short message systems (SMS) such as pagers and the text capabilities of cellular phones, it is possible for an automated system to generate and send a message to a clinician's phone.[23] This may be more of an attention-getter than the screen display, because the phone can be made to provide a sensory alert, such as a vibration or ring tone; whereas a clinician may not be looking at the screen 100% of the time.

In any event, the future holds great promise in this area. Coupled with OLAP processing of existing data, a computer system may be able to one day look at a clinical parameter, compare that parameter to similar patients with similar conditions, and the same surgery at the same point of surgery, and predict a potential pitfall.[24] The clinician can then be notified, and potentially even be provided with additional treatment information, based on previous treatments and outcomes in the OLAP database (Fig. 22-13).

TABLE 22-3 Commercially Available Anesthesia Management Information Systems

Vendor	System Name	Web Site
Acuitec	GasChart	www.acuitec.com
Cerner	SurgiNet	www.cerner.com
Dräger	Innovian Anesthesia	www.draeger.com
Epic	AIMS	www.epic.com
GE Healthcare	Centricity Anesthesia	www.gehealthcare.com
iMDsoft	MetaVision	www.imd-soft.com
Merge Healthcare	Frontiers	www.merge.com
Philips Healthcare	CompuRecord	www.healthcare.philips.com/us
Picis	Anesthesia Manager	www.picis.com
Surgical Information Systems	SIS Anesthesia	www.SISfirst.com

Moving Forward

Transforming an operating suite into an environment that leverages IT is a multistep, multidisciplinary process. Considerations need to be given to hardware, software, users, and support. Each of these categories contains several elements that will need to be addressed. In installing an anesthesiology-based information system, for example, the anesthesia group must be considered in terms of local culture, patient mix, facility needs, and the way the group practices. This analysis can be used to generate a request for proposal (RFP) from vendors. The RFP process may seem tedious, but it pays back significant dividends during the contracting and installation process.

CHOOSING AN ANESTHESIOLOGY INFORMATION SYSTEM VENDOR

A vast array of competing products is available for consideration when making many medical equipment purchasing decisions (Table 22-3).[25] In contrast, when making the decision to install an anesthesiology information management system (AIMS), only a handful of vendors are available from which to choose. Competing systems fit into two distinct categories: enterprise vendors and

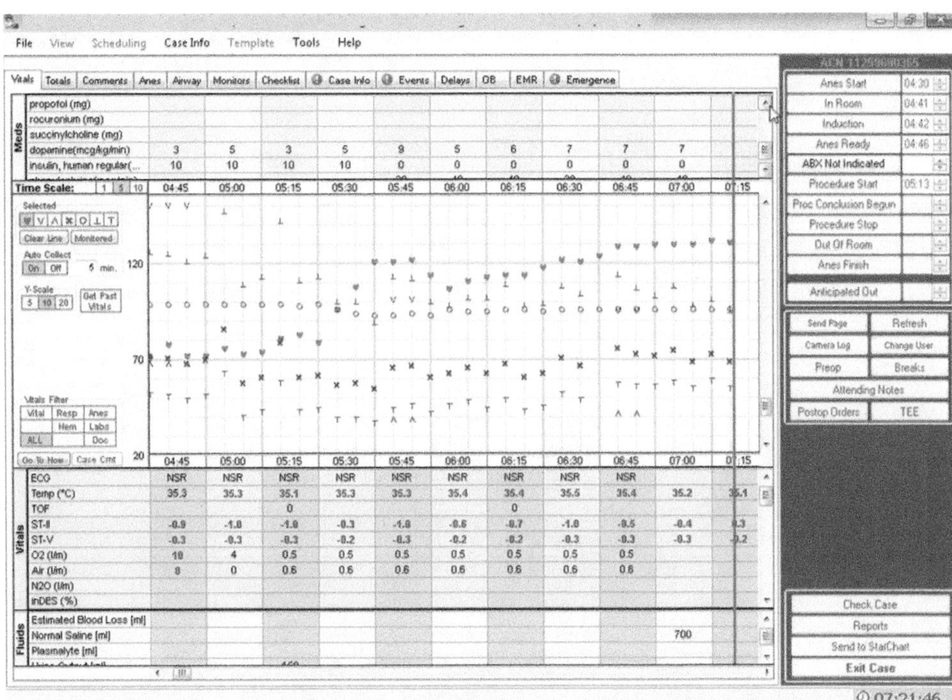

FIGURE 22-14 ■ Sample screen from an anesthesia information management system. (Courtesy Acuitec LLC, Birmingham, AL.)

niche vendors. *Enterprise vendors* often offer an anesthesiology documentation application as part of an overall package purchase by the hospital, along with applications for billing, laboratory, and nursing documentation. In contrast, *niche vendors* focus their product line specifically on the OR environment. Each institution and anesthesiology group needs to decide which model best suits their practice. The advantages claimed by the enterprise vendors are that they offer better integration between the AIMS and other components. In contrast, niche vendors often suggest that their products are better tailored for the OR suite, because expertise in that product line is their sole "best of breed" function, and their businesses are dependent on success in the OR. The look and feel of the user interface varies among vendors. Figures 22-14 to 22-17 show example screens from several vendors. End users should be consulted in determining the optimal solution for each practice.

The process of choosing a vendor may vary depending on the size of the institution and the personnel available to participate in the implementation. Expert guidance will be needed for critical steps in the process, such as needs assessment, product evaluation, implementation, and training.[26] A large anesthesiology group may be able to provide one or more physician champions who can dedicate a significant amount of nonclinical time toward each step of the process. Smaller groups may not be able to absorb a loss in clinical productivity during the selection process and may need to delegate some of these tasks away from clinicians to hospital IT staff or independent consultants.

Financial calculations include costs of the system, initial capital to install and implement the system, and ongoing operation and support expenses; these should be considered early in the process. Once a group or hospital has an estimate of its budget for an implementation, it can better tailor the rest of its processes for system selection and implementation to meet the proposed budget. In many cases, the budget for an implementation may determine which systems or options are suitable for the group to consider, because the initial and operational costs vary widely.

A needs assessment will determine what specifications an AIMS should have. Aspects of the system such as security, compliance, integration, and flexibility all need to be considered. The needs assessment will likely generate an RFP that will be sent to AIMS vendors, who will then respond with a description of how their system matches or does not match the needs outlined in the RFP.

Responses to the RFPs will be reviewed, and qualifying vendors will be selected for demonstrations of their products. Products should be demonstrated on site, and teams from the anesthesiology group and hospital administration should also plan on one or more site visits to other hospitals already using the specific AIMS systems that are being evaluated. These site visits should include time to interact with current users of each proposed system. Through this interaction, the potential user can better understand the problems and achievements of the implementation. They also can benefit from other users' experience with the product and how the vendor responded to software and hardware difficulties.

HARDWARE CONSIDERATIONS FOR AIMS IMPLEMENTATION

Early consideration should be given to hardware installation. Most AIMS have hardware located in a central server area and at the point of care. Point-of-care hardware is located in the OR, PACU, preoperative holding areas, and other places where clinical care is delivered. The central server hardware may be located in a central

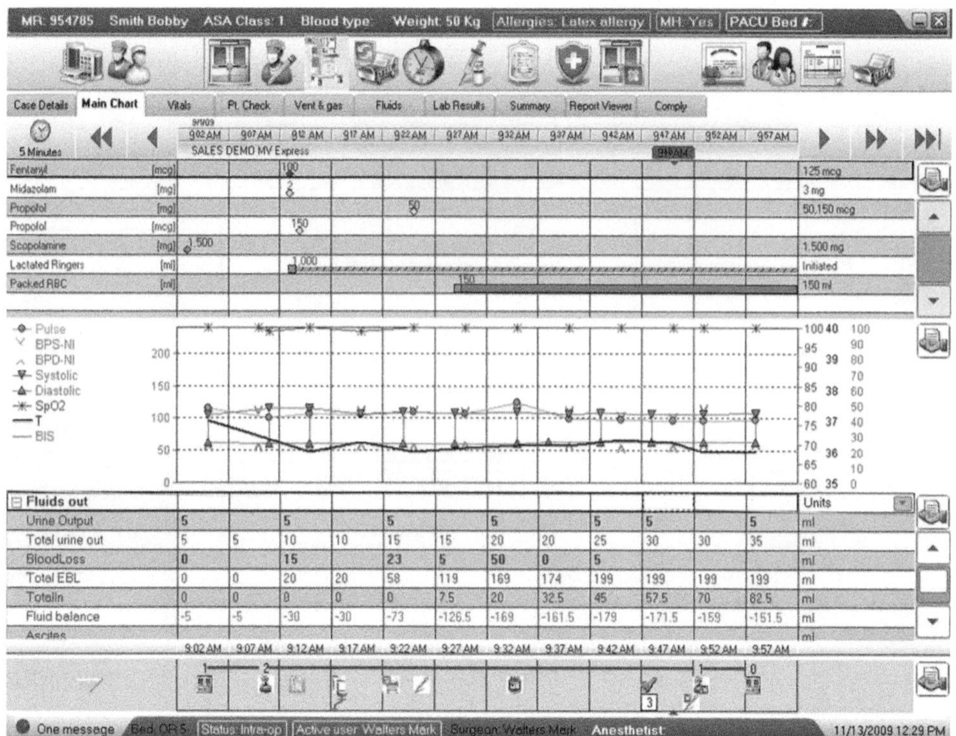

FIGURE 22-15 ■ Sample screen from an anesthesia information management system. (Courtesy iMDsoft, Needham, MA.)

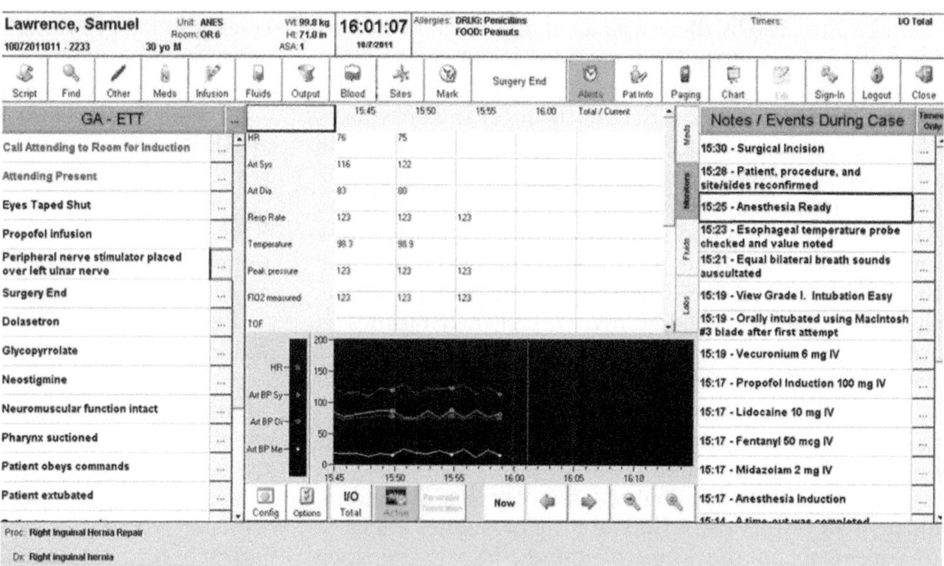

FIGURE 22-16 ■ Sample screen from an anesthesia information management system. (Courtesy General Electric, Cincinnati, OH.)

data closet, hospital data center, or even off site at a separate data center. The future may also introduce AIMS with cloud architecture, using the partial resources of multiple servers in different locations.

Depending on the complexity of the institution and the software being installed, it may be necessary to have different servers, either physical or virtual, for production, training, and testing environments. The production environment is where the actual ongoing "work" takes place; it is where medical data are stored, either entered by the users manually or entered automatically by the monitors. The production environment also produces data for the generation and storage of medical reports, billing data, quality analysis (QA) data, and so on. Typically, production is the most "mission critical" of the environments; as such it should have the greatest level of redundancy and protection from non–production-related factors.

In contrast, the testing environment exists so that new versions of software releases can be tested with other interfacing systems. The testing environment is similar to the production environment in terms of functionality, except that clinicians will not do "work" here, nor will patient information be stored in this location. However, other aspects must be similar to the production environment to ensure that an adequate test can be conducted. Lastly, the

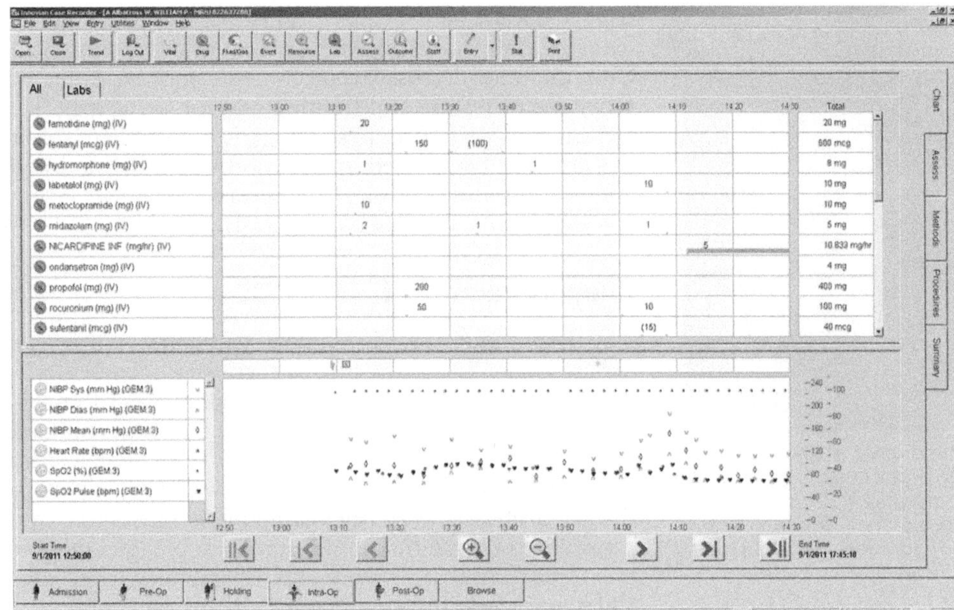

FIGURE 22-17 ■ Sample screen from an anesthesia information management system. (Courtesy Dräger Medical, Telford, PA.)

training environment is typically populated with the latest version of the software, but instead of having actual patient data, as in the production environment, the training environment would be populated with randomly generated patients using artificial names to protect patient privacy. This environment allows users to simulate a patient encounter without risking inputting data to an actual patient chart and without exposing HIPAA-protected patient data to users in training.

At the point-of-care workstation (PC) level, depending on the institution, it may be advisable to use hardware supported by the institution, if it is available. This would be the case if the institution had a standard computer workstation with standard hardware and software components. In this case, support is often available for the hardware, including 24/7 support. Response time is critical, as it is usually not possible to stop an operation or cancel a subsequent case because of a computer workstation being down. In this case, level-of-service (LOS) agreements are necessary, with response times as fast as 1 hr available in some institutions. Even that may not be quick enough, however, and it may be necessary to have spare computer workstations, such as a computer on wheels (COW), that can be rolled into place to substitute for a failed workstation.

The disadvantage to institutional workstations is that they are typically too generic in their configuration. It may not be possible to attach specialized hardware—such as touchscreens, bar code scanners, and so on—unless those items are approved by the institutional team. Also, software restrictions at the operating-system level can prevent legitimate updates from occurring while preventing unauthorized software installations or usage.

In contrast to the institutionally managed standard workstation is the workstation customized for a particular environment. This configuration obviates many of the restrictions of the standardized workstation, in terms of hardware and software, but it comes with its own set of problems to be addressed. One of the primary concerns with this type of workstation is support, especially after-hours support. Several employees may be required to cover call shifts so that one person is available 24/7. Additionally, replacement hardware may need to be kept in a separate inventory, instead of depending on a centralized group to manage the hardware. It is also possible to end up with a patchwork of several different workstations in terms of operability, which may become confusing for less sophisticated users.

Software support is separate from *hardware support.* Although it is possible that the same personnel can support both hardware and software, it is typical, especially in larger institutions, for a separate team to be dedicated to support applications in terms of user training and management of software-related issues. Alternately, vendor support is usually available at a cost, which is either built into the software contract or made available on a term or per-incident basis.

The software support group has two main functions. One is to undertake the training of users on new software packages or on updates to existing packages. Training may be one of the more difficult aspects of perioperative support, because perioperative users have little time on the job to attend training sessions. It is very difficult to have a shift covered, or to do a separate shift, just to attend software training. As a result, the industry relies heavily on self-training tools, such as user manuals and online training modules that use slide-type presentations, usually with narration. In this way, users can learn at a pace that suits them. This is especially useful for minor software updates or for training on specific aspects of existing software. Larger rollouts are more suitable for training centers or learning centers, where a classroom-type presentation can be used to train a large group of users, especially if the training room is set up with computer workstations on which to run trial cases.

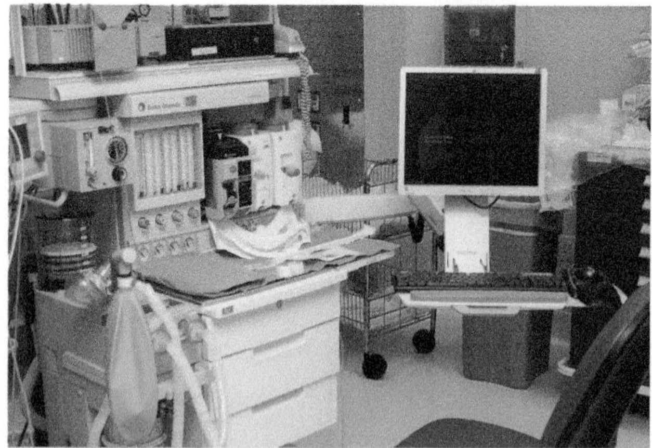

FIGURE 22-18 ■ Computer workstation mounted to an anesthesia machine. The mount allows flexibility in placement of the monitor and keyboard in relation to the machine. The computer's central processing unit is placed on the shelf adjacent to the anesthetic gas analyzer. Alternate configurations place the monitor and keyboard tray to the left of the anesthesia machine.

Hardware Installation

Prior to the successful use of any computerized system, a process of system design and installation must occur. Logistics for the installation may be complex and will require staff to assess physical locations for workstation placement so that computers are available where staff are best able to access them in their normal work processes. For example, in an OR, a computer workstation must be in immediate proximity to the anesthesiologist. Typically this entails mounting the workstation to the anesthesia machine or setting it on a mobile cart adjacent to the anesthesia machine. Several manufacturers—such as Ergotron (St. Paul, MN), GCX (Petaluma, CA), and others—make mounting arms that can be configured to the needs of the individual installation. These mounts are not inexpensive and often require significant effort for assembly and installation (Fig. 22-18).

In addition to mounting the computer workstation where it is needed, both alternating current (AC) electrical power and data networking (RJ-45) must be provided to the workstation. The cost of installing new cabling for the workstation in its new location may exceed the cost of the workstation itself, depending on institutional construction and physical plant requirements. Also, time must be allowed in the installation plan for the completion of these primary cabling and infrastructure tasks. Many institutions have a significant backlog of planned building and infrastructure work, and it may be difficult to obtain prioritization for any particular project.

After installation, all hardware and software must be tested for proper function. Depending on the institution size and number of workstations, this may be a formidable task. Computer hardware must be verified for power, network, monitor, keyboard, and mouse connectors. Software to be installed must be verified, and the workstation must also have the proper network or database access configurations in place. One of the best tests to verify function is by running a test case on the live database. This test case would be erased later or simply flagged to not be processed (billed) or to appear in the database after the testing is done. Larger installations will have multiple database environments for the different functions of testing and training and for the actual, live "production" database. In so doing, it is possible to select the database being used, so that software may be tested and users trained without risking erroneous data being comingled with valid medical records.

Support Personnel

The importance of IT support personnel cannot be underestimated, and the role of these staff members will be of paramount importance during all phases of implementation. Typically, support is divided into several tiers or levels. Tier 1 support is most often a scripted help desk employee available by phone 24/7 to walk users through simple problems with the computer workstation; for example, to ensure that the computer is plugged in, that it is turned on, that network and other cables are secure, and so on. These individuals usually help a wide variety of users over a large area with multiple, different software applications. For more complex problems, hardware and software specialists may be required. If the tier 1 support person is unable to diagnose and resolve a problem, he or she will refer the issue to tier 2 support personnel, usually a hardware or software specialist.

A hardware support specialist would be called in to diagnose and repair or replace malfunctioning computer hardware such as a broken monitor or keyboard or damaged hard drive. Often this is done by swapping out the defective device with an on-hand replacement that is preconfigured and ready for use; this minimizes workstation downtime and the potential effects on patient care or process efficiency. However, it also requires that additional hardware be purchased, maintained, and stored until it is needed. These additional workstations will also need to be maintained with all software updates if they are going to be used in this manner, which creates extra support and storage costs. Despite these costs, it is usually best to budget for at least 3% to 5% more workstations, so that they will be available when the inevitable failure occurs.

If the tier 1 support personnel determine that the hardware is functioning correctly, and the issue is one of user training or software malfunction, the issue may be referred to a tier 2 software support specialist. This staff member serves as an expert on the operation of the software and is available to answer "how do I" questions, to walk users through issues that are not routine, or where the software behavior is counter to what is expected. If the problem is determined to be related to a software bug or malfunction, the software specialist will rely on third-tier support, which is usually the software vendor or developer.

CONCLUSION

Medical informatics is revolutionizing the way medicine is practiced and documented. Informatics holds the potential to provide new levels of patient safety and process efficiency by providing information to clinicians in a just-in-time fashion. Not only is this achieved through medical record retrieval of requested information on demand, it is also accomplished through computerized analysis of existing and incoming data to provide clinicians with live decision-support information with the potential to provide warnings to otherwise unforeseen issues. In the fast-paced operating suite environment, this is of critical importance as adherence to best-practice protocols and reporting compliance with institutional and national standards becomes more prevalent.

Implementing an informatics system in any medical environment is difficult. The constraints of space and density of other technology make the OR a particularly challenging place for the installation of computer resources. However, this can be accomplished successfully with careful planning, budgeting, and accommodation to the requirements of these systems with an understanding that the significant benefit provided is worth many times the cost.

REFERENCES

1. Archer T, Schmiesing C, Macario A: What is quality improvement in the preoperative period? *Int Anesthesiol Clin* 40(2):1–6, 2002.
2. Minear MN, Sutherland J: Medical informatics: a catalyst for operating room transformation, *Semin Laparosc Surg* 10(2):71–78, 2003.
3. St. Jacques PJ, Minear MN: Improving perioperative patient safety through the use of information technology. In Henriksen K, Battles JB, Keyes MA, Grady ML, editors: *Advances in patient safety: new directions and alternative approaches, vol. 4: technology and medication safety*, Rockville MD, 2008, Agency for Healthcare Research and Quality.
4. Hemp P: Death by information overload, *Harv Bus Rev* 87(9):82–89, 2009, 121.
5. Barnes J: *Wired Network Security—Hospital Best Practices.* Available at www.infosecwriters.com/text_resources/pdf/Wired_Security_JBarnes.pdf.
6. Mildenberger P, Eichelberg M, Martin E: Introduction to the DICOM standard, *Eur Radiol* 12(4):920, 2002.
7. Bidgood WD Jr, Horii SC, Prior FW, Van Syckle DE: Understanding and using DICOM, the data interchange standard for biomedical imaging, *J Am Med Inform Assoc* 4(3):199, 1997.
8. Dolin RH, Alschuler L, Beebe C, et al: The HL7 clinical document architecture, *J Am Med Inform Assoc* 8(6):552, 2001.
9. Lyman JA, Scully K, Tropello S, et al: *Mapping from a clinical data warehouse to the HL7 reference information model.* In AMIA, Annual Symposium Proceedings, 2003 [electronic resource], p 920.
10. Satava RM: Emerging technologies for surgery in the 21st century, *Arch Surg* 134(11):1197–1202, 1999.
11. Rogers FB, Ricci M, Caputo M, et al: The use of telemedicine for real-time video consultation between trauma center and community hospital in a rural setting improves early trauma care: preliminary results, *J Trauma* 51(6):1037, 2001.
12. Xiao Y, Schimpff S, Mackenzie C, et al: Video technology to advance safety in the operating room and perioperative environment, *Surg Innov* 14(1):52, 2007.
13. Reference deleted in proofs.
14. Ahuja SR, Ensor R: VoIP: what is it good for? *Queue* 2(6):55, 2004.
15. Patterson DA, Chen P, Gibson G, Katz RH: Introduction to redundant arrays of inexpensive disks (RAID), *COMPCON*112–117, 1989; Spring.
16. Hawkins SM, Yen DC, Chou DC: Disaster recovery planning: a strategy for data security, *Information Management and Computer Security* 8(5):222–229, 2000.
17. Merkie RC: One-way hash functions and DES. *CRYPTO '89 Proceedings on Advanced Cryptology*, New York, Springer Verlag, 1989, pp 428–446.
18. Models D, Design W: Introduction to Data Warehousing and OLAP.
19. Chaudhuri S, Dayal U: An overview of data warehousing and OLAP technology, *ACM Sigmod Record* 26(1):65–74, 1997.
20. Satyanarayanan M: Pervasive computing: vision and challenges, *IEEE Pers Comm* 8(4):10–17, 2001.
21. Schultz M, Gill J, Zubairi S, Huber R, Gordin F: Bacterial contamination of computer keyboards in a teaching hospital, *Infect Control Hosp Epidemiol* 24(4):302–303, 2003.
22. Rutala WA, White MS, Gergen MF, Weber DJ: Bacterial contamination of keyboards: efficacy and functional impact of disinfectants, *Infect Control Hosp Epidemiol* 27(4):372–377, 2006.
23. Spring SF, Sandberg WS, Anupama S, et al: Automated documentation error detection and notification improves anesthesia billing performance, *Anesthesiology* 106(1):157, 2007.
24. Krol M, Reich DL: Development of a decision support system to assist anesthesiologists in the operating room, *J Med Syst* 24(3):141–146, 2000.
25. Ehrenfeld JM: Anesthesia information management systems, *Anesthesiology News* 1–7, 2010; August.
26. Muravchick S, Caldwell JE, Epstein RH, et al: Anesthesia information management system implementation: a practical guide, *Anesth Analg* 107(5):1598–1608, 2008.

CHAPTER 23

Vigilance, Alarms, and Integrated Monitoring Systems

Matthew B. Weinger • James M. Berry

CHAPTER OUTLINE

OVERVIEW

This chapter discusses several areas in which the interface between human and machine—or more accurately, between anesthesiologist and anesthesia equipment—plays a crucial role in patient outcomes. At first glance, the topics may seem unrelated. However, vigilance, alarms, and integrated monitoring systems are, in fact, closely interrelated.

The administration of anesthesia is predominantly a complex monitoring task and, as such, requires sustained vigilance. Unfortunately, humans are not very good at monitoring because we are error prone, and our vigilance is susceptible to degradation by a variety of human, environmental, and equipment factors. Designers of anesthetic equipment therefore have attempted to aid the anesthesiologist by incorporating devices and systems that augment vigilance and clinical performance. Alarms intended to notify the operator of potentially critical situations are effective only if properly designed and implemented. Although many modern anesthesia delivery devices are physically integrated and generally contain systems for gas delivery, monitoring, alarms, and sometimes record keeping, many of the promised benefits of full-scale integration (e.g., "smart" alarms, decision aids) are as of yet unfulfilled.[1] The successful implementation of comprehensive integrated anesthesia workstations will require further technologic advances as well as a more complete understanding of the task of administering anesthesia and the factors that affect performance of the anesthesiologist in this complex human/machine environment. Research to elucidate these "performance-shaping factors" in anesthesia has been under way for a number of years and is beginning to bear fruit. Chapter 24 discusses the role that the field of human factors should play in modern anesthesia practice.

ANESTHESIA MISHAPS

In 1985, as many as 3000 preventable incidences of anesthesia-related death or brain damage were estimated to occur in the United States each year.[2] Although some believe that anesthesia has become safer,[3] many more surgical procedures are now being performed; thus the absolute number of adverse events may not be appreciably decreasing. In addition, patients undergoing surgery today may be older and sicker than they were 10 or 20 years ago, a consequence of population demographics and economically driven changes in the American health care delivery system—a fact that might delay, but will not prevent, the use of surgical therapy. A French group found a 10-fold reduction in anesthesia-related deaths between 1979 and 1999.[4] Finally, studies suggest that the incidence of "potentially serious" clinical events is actually quite common in anesthetized patients, but relatively few evolve into adverse patient outcomes.[5,6]

A number of investigators have suggested that human error is a major contributor to the occurrence of anesthetic mishaps.[2,7-10] For example, clinician errors, such as making an accidental gas flow change or a "syringe swap," accounted for up to 70% of anesthetic mishaps in two early studies.[7,11] In a study by Keenan and Boyan,[2] 75% of intraoperative cardiac arrests were attributed to preventable anesthetic errors; an analysis[12] of incidents under monitored anesthesia care concluded that nearly half of the claims could have been prevented by better monitoring. Holland[13] suggested that inadequate patient observation was a contributing factor in one third of perioperative patient deaths.

In the intensive care unit (ICU), clinical errors often may be associated with failed communication between care providers.[14] On the other hand, as is discussed in detail later in this chapter, the majority of adverse anesthesia incidents are probably the result of systemic factors over which the anesthesia provider has little or no control, such as device designs that predispose to human error.[15]

Even under ideal conditions, performance on complicated tasks is rarely perfect.[16] In complex systems involving both humans and machines, human error is almost always a factor in degraded or faulty performance.[17,18] For example, the percent of accidents that resulted from air crew error was reported to be greater than 50%.[19,20] Accidents usually are caused by the cumulative effect of a number of events rather than one isolated incident.[19,21] Why do highly trained and experienced individuals make errors? What factors influence the occurrence of these errors? What can be done to decrease their incidence or to mitigate their negative outcome? Research has only begun to provide adequate answers to these important questions.

Human Error

Errors are a normal component of human cognitive function and play an important role in learning.[17] Most errors do not result in damaging consequences, but when an error results in an unacceptable outcome, it often is called an *accident*.[22] An error is most likely to deteriorate into a damaging situation when conditions prevent the appropriate corrective responses. Errors committed by anesthesiologists can have catastrophic consequences if not corrected, yet Cooper and colleagues[11] showed that most critical events in anesthetic practice were discovered and corrected before a serious mishap occurred. Therefore it is crucial to understand the determinants of recovery from anesthetic errors; factors such as sleep deprivation, miscommunication, or equipment problems can increase the potential for error as well as preclude effective recovery.

Two types of error are *slips* and *mistakes* (Table 23-1). Both of these can take the form of *errors of omission* (omitting a task step or even an entire task) or *errors of commission* (incorrect performance).[22] *Slips* are most likely to occur during activities for which one is highly trained and that are therefore performed outside active conscious thought. Drug syringe swaps, a commonly described anesthetic critical event,[11,23] are a type of slip. Errors of omission can occur when unexpected distractions interrupt a well-established behavioral sequence. Errors of commission occur when automated schema, or preprogrammed subroutines, are inappropriately called into play by specific stimuli without conscious processing.[17,24] Individuals have a tendency to revert to a high-frequency (well-learned) response in such situations, particularly when under stress. In fact, experts may be more likely than novices to make these kinds of errors.

TABLE 23-1 Types of Human Error

Type of Error	Description
Mistake	Inappropriate intention or action, often the result of a lack of training or knowledge
Slip	Appropriate intention or action at inappropriate time
Mode error	Erroneous classification of the situation
Description error	Ambiguous or incomplete specification of intention
Capture error	Correct schemata at incorrect time, often because of task overlap
Faulty activation	Activation of inappropriate action or failure to activate appropriate action or triggering
Data-driven error	Automatic actions inappropriate for the situation but called into play by ongoing action sequences
Fixation errors	Failure to revise actions with changing conditions, "cognitive lockup"
Confirmation bias*	Tendency to seek confirming data for existing hypotheses
Representational Errors	Faulty mental model of the system and its function or malfunction

*Errors may also occur as a result of a variety of others types of cognitive bias, such as availability, representativeness, similarity, framing, and anchoring.[27,28,368]

In a study of anesthesia residents working a comprehensive anesthesia simulation environment, DeAnda and Gaba[25] documented 132 *unplanned* incidents (i.e., not part of the simulation script but rather created by the subject) during 19 simulations, at a rate of nearly two per case. Human error accounted for 86% of the incidents, whereas equipment failure only accounted for 3%. Of the incidents that resulted from human error, nearly one fourth were the result of so-called *fixation errors*, which occurred when the subject was unable to focus on the most critical problem at hand because of persistent, inappropriate attention or actions directed elsewhere. The overall incidence of human error observed during simulated anesthesia was similar to that suggested by Cooper and colleagues for anesthesiologists in the operating room (OR).[11,26] This study is important because it substantiates the frequent occurrence of error in anesthesia and validates the use of simulation to study the types and causes of critical incidents in anesthesia. Clinical decision making also can be adversely affected by a number of other types of cognitive biases, such as confirmation bias, inappropriate overconfidence, false attribution, the availability and representativeness of heuristics, and anchoring and framing.[27-29]

In contrast to slips and fixation errors, *mistakes* are technical or judgmental errors. Thus mistakes are due to inadequate or incorrect information, poor decision-making skills or inappropriate strategies, inadequate training, lack of experience, or insufficient supervision or backup.

People are more likely to make errors when they are mismatched to the task or the system is not user friendly. Factors that can influence error commission include skill level, attitude, inexperience, stress,[22] poor supervision,[30] task complexity,[22] and inadequate system design (Table 23-2). The topic of human error in anesthesia has been covered in some detail elsewhere.[21,31-33]

At least some of what, on first glance, appears to be human error often can be traced back to poorly designed human/machine interfaces.[34,35] In fact, Norman[36] suggests that "the real culprit in most errors or accidents involving complex systems is, almost always, poor design." Poor operational design can substantially increase the risk of system failure as a result of operator error. Factors related to system-induced error include boredom attributable to overautomation,[37] overreliance on automated devices, and poor team coordination. Good operating practice is essential but not sufficient for minimizing system risk: 1) the design of the system must be fundamentally sound, 2) it must be properly constructed and implemented, 3) the operators must be thoroughly familiar with the system, and 4) ongoing quality control must ensure that system use is appropriate over the full range of possible conditions. This applies to the anesthesia workspace and must be considered when introducing new anesthesia equipment to this unique environment.

VIGILANCE AND MONITORING PERFORMANCE

Vigilance has been equated with "sustained attention."[38] Attention requires alertness, selection of information, and conscious effort; *alertness* indicates the receptivity of the individual to external information (Table 23-3). Mackworth,[39] the father of vigilance research, defined *vigilance* as "a state of readiness to detect and respond to certain specified small changes occurring at random intervals in the environment." Early research was stimulated by the errors of radar operators who performed the task of detecting barely perceivable events at infrequent and aperiodic intervals for extended periods.

The presence of "vigilance" in the official seal of the American Society of Anesthesiologists (ASA) underscores the perceived importance of careful attention to details and detection of subtle signs out of the ordinary. Thus, in a broader sense, *anesthetic vigilance* might be viewed as a state of clinical awareness in which dangerous conditions are anticipated or recognized. *Monitoring*, by definition, is a vigilance task; the administration of anesthesia is a complex monitoring task. The anesthesiologist must continuously evaluate the patient's medical status while assessing the effects of anesthesia and surgical intervention. Memory tasks, decision making, and vigilance are the most vulnerable to compromise under the stressful work conditions often experienced in the OR. Although monitoring during quiescent periods of the maintenance phase of anesthesia appears to closely resemble the classic vigilance tasks studied in the laboratory, anesthesia practice commonly involves more complex situations that

TABLE 23-2 **Typical Causes of Human Error in Anesthesia**

Cause of Error	Representative Example
Human Factors	
Task complexity	Not ventilating when coming off cardiopulmonary bypass
Lack of training or experience	Rapid administration of vancomycin or protamine
Stress	Drug syringe or ampoule swap during critical situation
Ill health	Under the influence of prescribed or recreational substances
Environmental Factors	
Noise/miscommunication	Misheard surgeon, gave wrong antibiotic
Workplace constraints	Circuit disconnect from moving equipment or personnel
Equipment and System Factors	
Poor equipment design	Lightbulb goes out on laryngoscope during a procedure
False and/or noisy alarms	Failure to recognize critical situation after disabling alarms
Mismatch of human/machine functions	Failure to detect ongoing event while manually recording vital signs

TABLE 23-3 **Definitions**

Term	Definition
Perception	To attain awareness or understanding, usually via the senses
Attention	A conscious effort to remain alert and to perceive and select information
Vigilance	A state of readiness to detect and respond to changes in the monitored environment; a state of "sustained attention"
Monitoring	A vigilance task involving the observation of one or several data streams in order to detect specified changes that often occur at random intervals
Vigilance	A state of clinical awareness whereby dangerous conditions are anticipated or recognized
Judgment	The formation of an opinion or evaluation based on available information
Cognition	The act or process of knowing, including both awareness and judgment
Decision making	The act of choosing between alternative diagnoses or possible actions based on judgments
Situation awareness	A coherent mental model or picture of the current state of a complex dynamic system, including an understanding of prior conditions and the implications of ongoing processes to future states

require divided attention, prioritization, and "situation awareness,"[40,41] skills that fall outside the classical definition of vigilance.

A large number of laboratory studies have demonstrated a decline in monitoring performance over time, called the *vigilance decrement*.[42] This performance decline typically is complete within the first 30 minutes of a monitoring session. The vigilance decrement seems to arise primarily as a function of the necessity of attending to a relatively infrequent signal for a prolonged length of time.

Psychologists and engineers have studied vigilance for many years. Investigators in fields outside medicine, most notably aviation, have applied this information to understanding performance on complex monitoring tasks. Studies have identified environmentally induced factors and human/machine interface variables that can impair vigilance and performance in air traffic control,[43] train driving,[44,45] automobile driving,[46] and nuclear power plant control.[47] The armed forces consider the potential impact of such factors at the earliest stages of the design of new weapons systems.[48]

In most complex monitoring tasks, increased task complexity or task duration generally results in impaired performance (Fig. 23-1).[49,50] A major factor in the effect of additional tasks on performance appears to be what personal resources, perceptual or cognitive, are required for each new task, and whether those resources are already taxed. Other factors known to impair vigilance include noise, environmental pollution, fatigue, sleep deprivation, and boredom.[24] Performance also may be impaired if the individual is under stress, is in poor health, or uses drugs. Personality factors, training, and experience also affect performance, and performance on complex monitoring tasks can be strongly affected by environmental or task variables.[51,52]

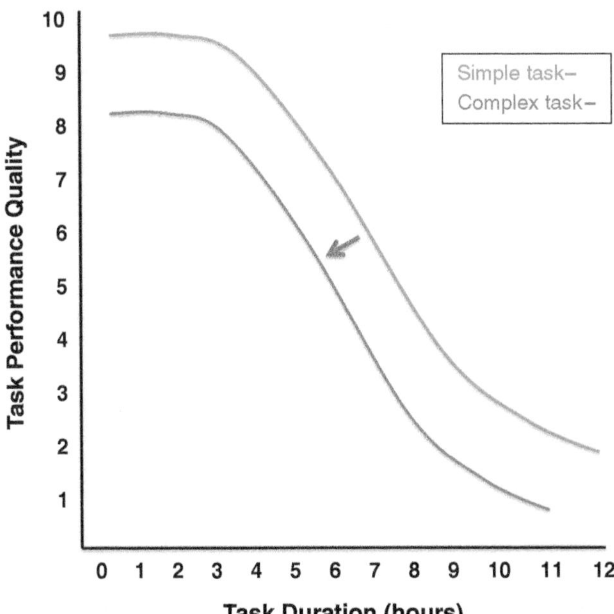

FIGURE 23-1 A curvilinear relationship exists between task performance and task duration in which increasing task duration results in impaired performance. This curve is shifted to the left *(arrow)* as the complexity of the task increases.

Research on Vigilance in Anesthesia

In one of the first ergonomic studies of anesthesia, Drui and colleagues[53] used time-motion analysis to examine how anesthesiologists spent their time in the OR. The practice of anesthesia was divided into a number of discrete activities, and the frequency and sequence of each activity were measured. One principal finding was that anesthesiologists directed their attention away from the patient 42% of the time. Subsequent time-motion studies have corroborated and expanded these early results.[41,54-59]

Subsequent studies have examined the effects of the level of provider experience[59] and of new technologies, such as electronic anesthesia record keeping,[41,58] on the workload and vigilance of residents administering anesthesia. Others have investigated anesthesiologists' vigilance to auditory[60] and visual[59,61,62] alarm cues and to changes in clinical variables[63] in both the laboratory and during actual procedures. For example, Weinger and colleagues[59] demonstrated that novice anesthesia residents were slower to detect the illumination of an alarm light placed within their monitoring array (Fig. 23-2). The response rate was further impaired during periods of high workload, such as during the anesthetic induction.

Well-controlled studies are essential to understand the nature of anesthesia vigilance and monitoring performance. Studies should be designed to use techniques and procedures that have been repeatedly validated by investigators in other fields. Chapter 24 describes in more detail current research in anesthesia related to clinical performance.

Factors that Affect Vigilance

A wide range of factors can affect vigilance and clinical performance in anesthesia (Box 23-1). The following

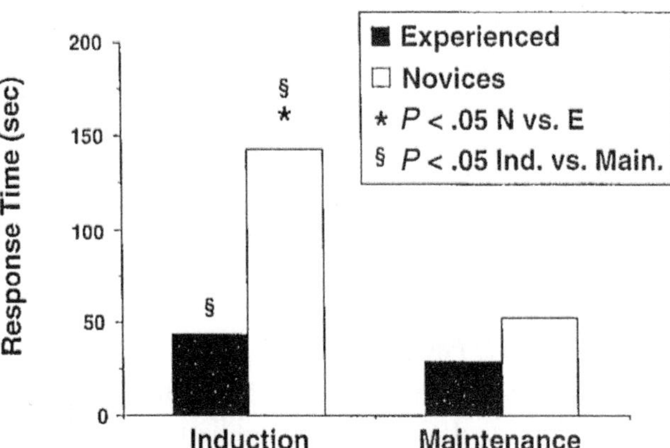

FIGURE 23-2 The mean response time (ordinate, seconds) to a vigilance light is plotted against case segment (abscissa, induction and maintenance). Response latency during induction was significantly delayed compared with the maintenance period ($P < .001$). In addition, novices were significantly slower in their responses ($P < .02$) compared with experienced practitioners, both during induction and over the whole case. (From Weinger MB, Herndon OW, et al: An objective methodology for task analysis and workload assessment in anesthesia providers. *Anesthesiology* 1994; 80:77-92.)

BOX 23-1 Factors Known to Affect Vigilance and Performance

Environmental Factors
- Noise
- Temperature and humidity
- Environmental toxicity
- Ambient lighting
- Workspace constraints

Human Factors
- Human error and cognitive biases
- Fatigue
- Sleep deprivation (acute and chronic)
- Circadian effects and shift work
- Boredom
- Substance use/abuse
- State of health and stress
- Aging
- Training and experience
- Psychosocial factors
- Personality factors

Task and Information Factors
- Primary task load
- Secondary task intrusion
- Interruptions and distractions
- Misinformation
- Alarms and warnings

Interpersonal and Team Communications

System and Equipment Factors
- System-induced errors (e.g., latent errors)
- Equipment failure
- Equipment-induced errors
- Faulty mental models of equipment design/function
- Clumsy automation

Modified from Weinger M, Englund C: Ergonomic and human factors affecting anesthetic vigilance and monitoring performance in the operating room environment. *Anesthesiology* 1990;73:995-1021.

TABLE 23-4 Common Alarms and Other Sounds in the Operating Room

Sound	Decibels
Jet ventilator	120
Monitor alarm sounding (all alarms at highest setting)	91
Humidifier (temperature probe not plugged in)	86
Tourniquet (disconnect alarm)	84
Anesthesia machine (loss of oxygen supply)	84
Anesthesia machine (circuit disconnect)	78
Infusion pump (inclusion alarm)	77
Surgical instruments clanking against each other in a metal basin	75
Monitor alarm sounding (all alarms; at standard setting)	74
Electrocautery unit (return fault)	74
Intercom	72
Tonsil tip suction	70
Pulse oximeter tone (maximum volume)	66
Surgeon's conversation (at patient's ear)	66
"Background" music at patient's ear	65

discussion provides a perspective on how a variety of everyday occurrences in the OR have the potential to significantly impair vigilance, potentially leading to increased risk of critical events and, as a result, anesthetic morbidity or death. The following sections address some of the more important performance-shaping factors organized into environmental, human, and equipment categories.

Environmental Factors

Noise and Music. The noise level in an OR can be quite high. In the early 1970s, Shapiro and Berland[64] measured noise levels associated with specific tasks in the OR during several typical surgical procedures and found that the noise in an OR "frequently exceeds that of a freeway." These findings appear to still be valid; continuous background noise in the modern OR may range from 75 to 90 dB (Table 23-4). High-noise events include mechanical ventilation, suction, music, and conversation. Noise levels up to 118 dB can occur, notably during the operation of high-speed gas-turbine drills; suction tips with trapped tissue yielded up to 96 dB.[65] High noise levels create a positive feedback situation; noisy rooms require louder alarms and louder voices, which contribute to the noise, and so on.[66]

The effects of noise on performance depend on the type of noise and the task being performed.[67,68] In addition, other environmental and human factors can interact with noise to affect task performance.[69] Noise levels similar to those found in ORs detrimentally affect short-term memory tasks[68] and also may mask task-related cues and cause distractions during critical periods.[70] Difficult tasks that require high levels of perceptual and/or information processing are negatively affected by noise.[71] Long-term exposure to high noise levels produces physiologic changes consistent with stress.[72] Exposure to loud noise activates the sympathetic nervous system, a situation that may augment the effects of other performance-shaping factors and result in impaired decision making during critical incidents.[24,69]

There is little doubt that background noise interferes with effective verbal communication.[73] It is critical for the anesthesiologist to be able to hear clearly what other members of the OR team are saying. When multiple tasks are required, the presence of background noise may bias attention toward the dominant task.[74] Although loud noise is clearly disruptive and can impair auditory vigilance—for instance, the ability to hear changes in pulse oximeter tone or to detect and identify alarms—studies have found a beneficial effect on complex task performance in the presence of lower levels of background (white) noise.[75]

Several studies have suggested that the presence of familiar background music could improve vigilance.[76,77] A positive effect of preferred background music on surgeons' mood and laboratory task performance was described.[78] However, the validity of this study's findings were questioned, with no data yet available on the impact of the surgeon's preferred music on the anesthesiologist's monitoring performance.[79] What if the surgeon wanted to listen to country music, for example, and the anesthesiologist did not like that type of music? Swamidoss and colleagues[80] studied the effects of background music on the performance of 30 anesthesia providers using a screen-based computerized anesthesia simulator. They found no significant differences in level of anxiety, time to recognition and correction of critical incidents, or autonomic responses whether subjects listened to their "most enjoyed music," "least enjoyed music," or "no music" at all. However, the number of subjects studied was small, and the applicability of these results to the actual OR environment remains to be examined.

Temperature. Uncomfortable environmental temperatures, a common situation in many ORs, can impair vigilance.[81-83] Although there appears to be significant variability in the effects of temperature on performance depending on the experimental situation (i.e., other environmental, task, and subject variables), as a general rule, temperatures that promote general fatigue decrease performance.[81] Extremely cold temperatures have a deleterious effect on some cognitive tasks, primarily because of the distraction of the cold environment and the associated decrease in manual dexterity.[84] These effects often show up as increased errors and memory deficits.[85] Studies in the industrial workplace suggest that when temperatures fall outside a preferred range (17° to 23° C), workers are more likely to exhibit unsafe behaviors that could lead to occupational injury.[86] Temperatures in some adult ORs can be as low as 7° C, and those in pediatric ORs may approach 30° C. The negative effects of temperature probably are augmented by other factors that enhance fatigue or impair performance.

Environmental Toxicity: Exposure to Vapors. Voluminous literature has been published on the effects of trace anesthetic vapors on anesthesiologist performance. The early studies of Bruce and colleagues[87] reported that exposure to 550 ppm N_2O and 14 ppm halothane led to a significant decrease in performance on complex vigilance tasks. However, their study used as subjects Mormon dental students, who may have been uniquely sensitive to the effects of the anesthetic gases. Smith and Shirley[88] subsequently showed that acute exposure to trace anesthetic gases in amounts commonly seen in an unscavenged OR had no effect on performance in naive volunteers. It thus appears that impaired vigilance related solely to trace anesthetic gases is probably not a problem in the modern, well-scavenged OR. A subsequent, well-controlled crossover study of anesthesiologists showed no differences in either mood or cognitive ability when working in a scavenged OR compared with working in an ICU (i.e., with no trace gases).[89] However, other noxious smells or the need to wear bulky and uncomfortable protective gear could have an adverse impact on clinical performance.[90]

Individual Factors

Fatigue. *Fatigue* is caused by hours of continuous work or work overload,[91] whereas *boredom* is believed to be a function of insufficient work challenge or understimulation. The two, nonetheless, often co-occur. Extreme fatigue results in objectively measurable symptoms of exhaustion and a psychological aversion to further work. There is marked individual variability in the response to factors or situations that can produce fatigue. The continued ability to perform skilled physical or mental tasks in the face of worsening fatigue strongly depends on psychological factors, including motivation. Although some extremely fatigued individuals can be induced to perform,[92] the quality and wisdom of continued work under these circumstances is questionable, certainly so in situations in which human lives may be at stake.

Few fatigue studies have used physicians as subjects. Those that have typically involved sleep loss and, primarily because of poor methodology, raised more questions than they answered. Fatigue and sleep loss often are covariants in studies that examine continuous, long work schedules; in turn, both are modulated by circadian processes. Because the effects of these variables interact,[93] it is difficult to separate the relative contribution of each factor to the performance decrement observed.

Individuals subjected to excessive work, fatigue, or inappropriate shift schedules show degraded performance, impaired learning and thought processes, irritability, memory deficits, and interpersonal dysfunction.[24,94] Fatigued subjects pay less attention to peripherally located instruments and are inconsistent in their response to external stimuli. When coping with task demands, they exhibit less control over their own behavior and tend to select more risky alternatives (shortcuts).[92] If sufficiently motivated, fatigued subjects can attain relatively normal performance on tasks of short duration,[95] but they find it difficult to sustain performance on vigilance or monitoring tasks of long duration.[96,97] Adding sleep loss or shift work accentuates fatigue-induced performance decrements.[98]

Sleep Deprivation. A large body of research supports the contention that sleep deprivation and circadian rhythm disturbances can dramatically impair performance on monitoring tasks.[95,99-103] Although sleep deprivation and fatigue are similar in some of their performance-shaping effects and certainly are interactive, they are different processes. A single night of sleep loss can produce measurable performance decrements, especially on skilled cognitive tasks. Impairment can be seen shortly after task initiation—within 20 to 35 minutes in some situations.[104] However, in most sustained work activities, major decrements usually occur after 4 hours and again after 18 hours.[105] Dawson and Reid[106] showed that the magnitude of cognitive psychomotor impairment after remaining awake for 24 hours was roughly equivalent to that produced by acute inebriation (a blood alcohol level of 0.10%) (Fig. 23-3).

Although wide individual differences exist in the amount of daily sleep required,[107] studies that involve 1 or more days without sleep consistently reveal progressive

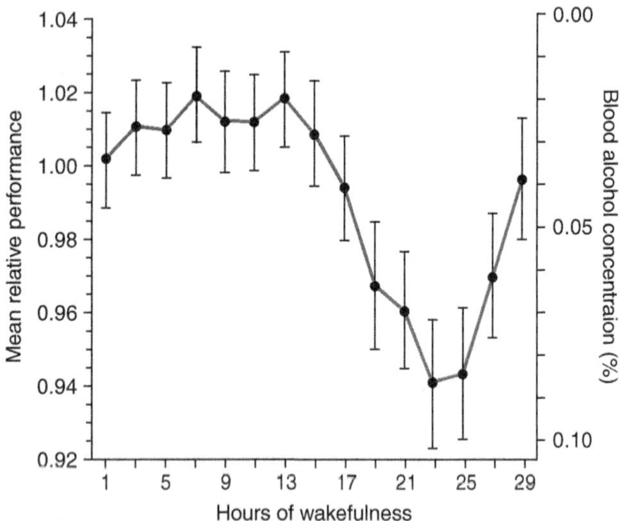

FIGURE 23-3 Mean performance of 40 volunteers on a hand-eye coordination task. *Left, y* axis, expressed as a ratio of baseline performance while remaining awake continuously for over 24 hours, beginning at 8 AM (*x* axis, in hours). In addition, the magnitude of performance impairment on the same test in the same subjects was tested on a different day after consumption of cumulative doses of alcohol at 30-minute intervals until a blood alcohol concentration (BAC) of 0.10% was obtained. The magnitude of cognitive psychomotor impairment after remaining awake for 24 hours was roughly equivalent to that produced by acute inebriation with a BAC of 0.10% (at or above the legal limit for operation of a motor vehicle). (From Dawson D, Reid K: Fatigue, alcohol and performance impairment. *Nature* 1997;388[6639]:235.)

BOX 23-2 Potential Effects of Sleep Deprivation on Vigilance and Performance

Decreases in reaction time
Increases in response variability
Decreases in work rate
Difficulty making choices
Increases in omission errors
Impaired working memory
Failure to appropriately allocate attention
Difficulty setting task priorities
Failure to evaluate potential faulty information

decreases in reaction time and increases in response variability (Box 23-2).[108] Work rate is appreciably slowed, particularly when subjects are required to make choices.[109] In vigilance tasks, omission errors increase, whether or not visual or auditory signals are presented.[110-112] Sleep loss impairs active use of working memory,[108] particularly when the sleep loss precedes learning.[113] Sleep-deprived workers fail to appropriately allocate attention, set task priorities, or sample for sources of potentially faulty information.[114,115] Because many of these skills are essential for optimal anesthesia care, this suggests that sleep loss could be extremely detrimental to clinical performance.

Haslam's early field work[116] indicated that some sleep (2 to 3 hours per day) is better than none at all, at least for soldiers involved in military exercises. For example, in studies of sleep-deprived soldiers, a 2-hour nap was insufficient and a 3-hour nap permitted maintenance of previous levels of already impaired performance; a full 4-hour nap was required before baseline performance was restored.[95,117,118] Taking a short nap (<2 hours) at the circadian low point produces greater cognitive impairment than the same length nap taken at the peak of the circadian cycle.[119,120] In addition, if a sleep-deprived subject is permitted to nap, a period of "sleep inertia" will follow the nap, during which the subject will exhibit a low level of arousal as well as significantly impaired vigilance and performance. Sleep inertia may persist for up to 2 hours.[95]

In one of the first studies of the effects of sleep loss on physician performance, Friedman and colleagues[100] showed that the ability of sleep-deprived medical interns to detect cardiac arrhythmias was significantly compromised compared with well-rested interns. In a well-designed study of 30 first-year medical residents, Hart and colleagues[121] demonstrated mild but significant disturbances in memory, decision making, and motor execution in on-call residents deprived of normal sleep (2.7 ± 2.2 hours slept) compared with those who got a full night's rest (7.9 ± 1.3 hours). Unfortunately, many studies designed to assess the impact of sleep deprivation on the ability of physicians, typically house staff, to perform clinical duties have generally had serious methodologic flaws. One well-regarded study examined 20 interns in critical care units and compared their normal schedules (most worked more than 80-hour weeks) with an intervention period limiting them to 16-hour shifts. During limited work hours, the subjects slept significantly more and had half the attention failures, as defined by electrooculography, than in the control periods.[122] In a similar study, the rate of serious medical errors, as determined by independent observers, was significantly reduced.[123] Percutaneous injuries (needle sticks) were also significantly lower in interns who were not working extended hours.[124] In one examination of complication rates after performing nighttime procedures, no differences were found unless the physician had sleep opportunities of less than 6 hours.[125]

The issue of decreased clinical performance of house officers and other physicians as a result of overwork and sleep deprivation[126,127] gained media attention in the late 1980s.[128] Thereafter, state legislatures, academic institutions, and accrediting bodies implemented restrictions on house staff work schedules; however, there are still no restrictions on the work schedules of fully licensed practicing physicians or nurse anesthetists. As American health care evolves toward capitated managed care, and the financial incentives associated with extended work hours diminish, it will be interesting to see whether more anesthesia providers will voluntarily reduce their work schedules.

Circadian Changes and Shift Work. Periodic, rhythmic fluctuations in bodily processes, including performance and work efficiency, have been well documented.[91,129] More than 50 neurophysiologic and psychological rhythms that potentially influence human performance have been identified.[130] Most studies of rhythmic changes in efficiency have focused on cycles of approximately 1 day, called *circadian processes*. An individual's normal rhythm can be significantly influenced by environmental conditions, illness, time zone changes, and altering shift

BOX 23-3 Potential Problems with Night and Shift Work

Circadian-related fluctuations in performance
Inability to adjust to time changes
Difficulty establishing a normal diurnal rhythm
Sleep deprivation
Exacerbation of other performance-shaping factors
Health problems
Social and interpersonal problems
Increased incidence of on-the-job errors and accidents

schedules. During normal awake times, circadian-related fluctuations in performance can range from 14% to 43% (Box 23-3).[129]

In rapidly changing schedules of regular work hours (e.g., routinely and frequently changing from day shift to night shift), performance rhythm amplitudes show variations as great as 50%.[131] The rate and amount of adjustment to shift changes or extended workdays vary among individuals.[132,133] However, in a study of nurses doing shift work, some individuals were never able to adjust.[134] In general, shift workers exhibit greater sleep, social, and health problems.[135-137] Efficiency of permanent night shift workers is at least 10% less than that of comparable day shift coworkers,[138] and minor accidents[131] and task errors[139] occur most frequently during night shifts and early morning hours. On the other hand, fully acclimated night shift workers have a realigned circadian cycle such that *their* best performance occurs during their normal night shift. Swing shift workers seem to have the most difficulty establishing a normal diurnal rhythm.[99] Because adjustment to shift work takes several days, if shift rotations are required, the rotation should be clockwise—that is, with progressively later shifts—and never less than 2 weeks per shift.[135] The implications for anesthesia is that middle-of-the-night procedures would be optimally performed by anesthesia providers assigned to at least 2 weeks of only night shift duty.

Alterations in the normal circadian rhythms cause changes in arousal as well as in other mental and physical functions. These changes play a major role in the effects on task performance of acute sleep loss, napping, and recovery from disruptions in normal sleep schedule. Phase shifts are introduced by sleep interruption. Some circadian functions are altered, and normal rhythms may be disrupted, even after multiple brief interruptions in an otherwise full night's sleep.[140] The peak and minimal performance times normally expected by the individual are similarly shifted. This can lead to a false sense of competence during "normal working hours" following acute sleep loss. For example, an anesthesiologist who has been working most of the previous night, after recovering from sleep inertia in the early part of the next morning, may feel remarkably awake, perhaps even euphoric. Yet studies have documented degraded performance on complex tasks in such situations (see Fig. 23-3).[119] By mid afternoon, dramatic decreases occur in arousal and the feelings of well-being that accompany parallel performance decrements. That evening, the anesthesiologist will probably have difficulty falling asleep, especially if an afternoon nap was taken. In fact, sleep-wake cycles can be disturbed for up to 36 hours, and the anesthesiologist may remain more error prone during this recovery phase.[118,141]

Performance During Extended Duty Shifts by Anesthesia Personnel. Howard and colleagues[142] have suggested that anesthesia residents are chronically sleep deprived. Using standard sleep study methodology, they demonstrated that undisturbed Stanford anesthesia residents, even if they had not been on call for 2 full days, had daytime sleep latencies comparable to those of patients with narcolepsy. Furthermore, these residents often denied falling asleep during the sleep tests despite objective electroencephalographic (EEG) evidence to the contrary.[143] Post-call anesthesia residents demonstrate significant decrements on laboratory psychomotor vigilance tests.[144]

Cao and colleagues[145] examined the task performance and workload of anesthesia residents performing OR procedures in the middle of the night when on call. Five senior residents performed routine general anesthesia cases at night (between 10 PM and 6 AM) during a 24-hour on-call shift. The same residents were studied again during daytime cases (between 9 AM and 5 PM), which were prospectively matched to the nighttime cases with respect to type and duration of surgery and ASA status. The intraoperative activities of each resident, resolved into 37 task categories, were recorded by a trained observer.[41,59] At night, more time was spent on observation, and each episode lasted longer. During maintenance, residents spent *more* time during the night observing their monitors and *less* time doing manual tasks. Subjective workload was significantly higher at night than during the day. There were no differences, however, in response to a vigilance probe.[145]

These data suggest that in the sleep-deprived state, anesthesia residents perceive a higher workload and are less efficient, suggesting a potential for impaired performance. These results are consistent with the need at night for greater perceptual and cognitive resources to process data and accomplish tasks, although additional experiments will be required to substantiate this hypothesis.

Anesthesia trainees and practitioners may have significant decrements in psychomotor vigilance and reaction times after sleep deprivation.[146] Stanford University anesthesia residents participated in a randomized, controlled crossover study designed to examine the effects on clinical performance of sleep deprivation and fatigue during realistic simulated OR cases.[147] In the "highly fatigued" condition, subjects were kept awake for at least 25 hours prior to a morning experiment. In the comparison well-rested condition, the same resident obtained an extra 2 hours of sleep every night for 1 week before the experiment. The simulated 4-hour routine laparoscopy cases used in the study were designed to accentuate any effects of sleep deprivation. Interestingly, analysis of preliminary data suggest that, through the intraoperative use of a variety of countermeasures, anesthesia residents are able to overcome substantial fatigue and sleep loss to perform almost as well as during routine anesthesia cases. Unfortunately, the effects of sleep deprivation on clinical performance during serious, acute critical events have not yet been examined in either simulated or real cases.

It appears that work schedule can, under some circumstances, be an important factor affecting intraoperative vigilance and performance. Significant individual differences are seen in the response to acute or chronic sleep loss, and each anesthesiologist must be cognizant of his or her own limitations. Individuals must recognize that it is neither unprofessional nor weak to admit sleepiness or fatigue when on the job,[148] and personnel must attempt to either make time to recuperate or seek a clinical replacement.

Breaks. Common sense suggests that relief from a prolonged monitoring task should enhance subsequent performance. Both anecdotal reports and laboratory studies have indicated that people prefer self-paced tasks and will take a break when needed.[105] Short breaks have been shown to alleviate fatigue and increase employee satisfaction and productivity in machine-paced jobs.[104] For worker-controlled sedentary jobs, short breaks or a change in activity increases performance and relieves boredom.[105,149] However, little experimental evidence supports the widely held belief that performance will improve after a break from a prolonged complex monitoring task such as administering anesthesia.

The optimal frequency and duration of breaks is still unknown for most occupations. Warm[40] has recommended that monitoring tasks be limited to sessions of less than 4 hours. Breaks have been required by many union contracts, as well as by legislation in some countries, particularly for occupations in which impaired worker performance could endanger worker or public safety, such as with transportation workers.

In a study of critical incidents associated with intraoperative exchanges of anesthesia personnel, Cooper and colleagues[150,151] identified 90 incidents that occurred during a break. Twenty-eight of these incidents were deemed favorable (the relieving anesthesiologist discovered and corrected a potentially dangerous preexisting situation), and only 10 incidents were considered unfavorable (the relieving anesthesiologist "caused" the critical incident). In some of the remaining incidents, the problem was perpetuated by the relieving anesthesiologist. Unfortunately, because of the possibility of biased reporting, the relative frequency with which relief results in favorable versus unfavorable outcomes cannot be determined from this type of study. On the other hand, of the 1089 total critical incidents studied, Cooper and colleagues did not identify a single relief-related incident that resulted in significant morbidity or mortality. Nevertheless, the detection of problems during a break probably depends on a systematic and comprehensive review of the anesthetic course by the relieving anesthesiologist. Because of this, it has been recommended that specific relief-exchange protocols be developed and strictly adhered to (Box 23-4).[150,151] Several professional organizations are currently developing standardized anesthesia handover protocols and checklists.

BOX 23-4 Recommended Standard Relief Protocol

1. The relieving anesthesiologists must establish familiarity with:
   - Patient's preoperative status
   - Course of the anesthetic
   - Course of the surgical procedure
   - Overall anesthetic plan
   - Arrangement of the equipment, apparatus, drugs, and fluids
2. The two anesthesiologists must communicate relief plans with the surgical team.
3. The original anesthesiologist must not leave the room until the relieving anesthesiologist is in control of the situation and has all of the necessary information to continue with the anesthetic.
4. The original anesthesiologist should not leave the room if the patient is unstable or the anesthetic is not likely to remain in a steady-state condition for at least 5 to 10 minutes.
5. Care must be taken to communicate all special information that is not recorded or may not be readily evident.
6. Under normal circumstances, the relieving anesthesiologists should not appreciably alter the course of preexisting anesthetic management.
7. Before resuming control, the original anesthesiologist should carefully go through these same steps with the relieving anesthesiologist.
8. If the relieving anesthesiologist is to finish the case, special care should be taken to explain the anesthetic plan, including the "to do" list, "to watch for" precautions, and any special issues.

Modified from Cooper JB, Long CD, Newbower RS, Philip JH: Critical incidents associated with intraoperative exchanges of anesthesia personnel. *Anesthesiology* 1982;56:456-461.

Boredom. Boredom is a problem of information "underload," insufficient work challenge, and understimulation.[24,152] Boredom typically results from the need to maintain attention in the absence of relevant task information[152] and may be most likely to occur in semiautomatic tasks that prevent the mind from wandering but are not fully mentally absorbing. Substantial differences exist among individuals as to what types of activities they find boring.[153] Nevertheless, boredom appears to be a major problem in many complex real-life tasks. For example, boredom may be a contributing factor to human error in driving a locomotive[45,154] and in piloting a prolonged routine flight in high-performance and commercial aircraft.[155]

The maintenance phase of most routine anesthetics is a period of very low workload and infrequent task demands.[41,59] This low workload may result in a low arousal state, which can lead to impaired performance. In laboratory experiments, increased effort in the presence of boredom is necessary to suppress distracting stimuli and a generalized feeling of fatigue.[153] The addition of other performance-shaping factors, such as fatigue and sleep deprivation, may augment the negative impact of boredom.[24] Boredom may be minimized by altering the sequence of tasks[156] or by adding tasks to a monotonous job.[157] Dividing attention among several tasks (time sharing) will in some circumstances *improve* monitoring performance.[158,159] Psychological studies suggest that some individuals may be more "boredom prone" but that behavioral interventions can improve these individuals' vigilance.[160]

Observation of experienced anesthesia providers has revealed that, during times of low workload, many add additional tasks to their routine. These secondary tasks include clinically relevant functions, such as rechecking the composition or organization of the anesthesia workspace. Alternatively, it is common to observe anesthesiologists reading, listening to music, attending to personal hygiene, or conversing with their intraoperative colleagues about matters unrelated to patient care. The choice of secondary tasks is probably less important than how those tasks are integrated with the primary tasks of caring for the patient and how easily and quickly the secondary tasks are set aside when anesthesia workload increases.[24,41,161] From a broad perspective, if the anesthesia task environment is optimized to minimize boredom and yet not be as continuously busy as to be stressful, the highest consistent levels of vigilance and performance will be attained.

Reading in the Operating Room. The anesthesia community has discussed the appropriateness of the apparently common practice of the anesthesiologist reading while caring for anesthetized patients.[162,163] Because no objective data exist on the effects of intraoperative reading on patient outcomes, the opinions espoused are largely based on personal beliefs and morals (what is "right").

Most of the time during the administration of an anesthetic, many patient care tasks must be performed, and the diligent anesthesia provider will prioritize and undertake these tasks appropriately. Under this circumstance, if reading occurs, it will only be during "idle time," when no tasks other than general patient monitoring are required. In task analysis studies, the anesthesiologist has been shown to be idle up to 40% of the time during routine cases.[53] This idle time appears to provide a reserve, or spare capacity, that can be called into play during high workload or critical periods, when additional cognitive and physical resources must be rapidly deployed to optimize patient care. Studies suggest that more experienced providers perform tasks more efficiently, report lower workload, and have more spare capacity at a given level of task performance[41,59] than do less experienced providers. It could be speculated that reading during low workload periods could help prevent boredom, sleepiness, and decreased vigilance; however, this hypothesis must be tested in rigorous scientific studies.

Few studies have defined the actual incidence of boredom or of reading in the OR. Some years ago, 57 of 105 anesthesia providers at one institution responded to a questionnaire that included questions on this topic. Almost 90% of those who responded admitted to occasional episodes of "extreme" boredom. To relieve their boredom while in the OR, 29% of the respondents read. Reading was the most common technique to relieve intraoperative boredom; other strategies included "thinking about things," "conversing," and "busying oneself with manual tasks." When asked specifically, "How often do you read while administering anesthesia," 19% of the respondents stated that they read "frequently," 46% said they "sometimes" read, and 33% "rarely" read. Only one respondent claimed that he or she never read in the OR. When they did read, two thirds of the respondents almost always read anesthesia-related material.

Interestingly, despite its common occurrence, 49% of the respondents believed that reading detracted from anesthesia vigilance, 21% believed that reading enhanced vigilance, and 30% were ambivalent. These data are from a Southern California training institution in which intraoperative reading is permitted; it is unclear how these data might generalize to other facilities.

In one institution, trained observers monitored the anesthesia provider in 172 cases and categorized the tasks observed, also noting whether reading was observed. Reading was seen in 35% of cases, almost universally during the maintenance phase. During periods of higher workload, reading was absent, suggesting a "titration" of reading to balance workload.[164]

Laboratory studies suggest that a discrete time-sharing ability can be separated from other vigilance skills[165,166] and that it can be taught. However, anesthesia providers are not given any formal training in time-sharing techniques, although resource allocation and divided attention skills are probably learned on a more informal basis. Tremendous individual variability likely exists in the impact of reading on anesthesia vigilance. For some anesthesia providers, intraoperative vigilance could thus be enhanced by reading during low-workload periods, but in others, the ability to detect acute events may be impaired.

It is also important to be cognizant of the sociopolitical and medicolegal implications of intraoperative reading. Reading will clearly have an adverse impact on performance if it detracts from the anesthesiologist's ability to do the primary tasks of the job, attend to the surgeons' and others' requests, or to respond to new task demands. However, even in the absence of a demonstrable negative impact, reading may simply "look bad" and may give the appearance of inattention and boredom, when it may have the opposite effect. However, in the most recent work on intraoperative reading, no evidence of a change in provider response times to random visual stimuli (as an indicator of vigilance) was demonstrable.[164]

More timely is the issue of distraction from computers, smart phones, or other personal electronics. Although much can be extrapolated from the literature on reading, attention is now turned to the effects that texting and other activities may have on attention.[167] Handheld devices, simultaneously distracting and useful, are becoming ubiquitous. They are also being adapted to "push" information to clinicians as a part of the patient care and monitoring infrastructure.

Stress and Performance. Sources of stress that affect performance can be found in the work environment and may be social and physical[168,169] or related to the tasks involved and their mental load and pacing; individual stressors may be health related or may arise from job matching and personality.[170,171] *Stress* is a broad term. Depending on its type and magnitude, it can result in either degraded or enhanced performance. A subject's performance will be significantly influenced by interaction with the environment and its associated stressors, the work to be performed in this environment, and the level of incentive for performing.

Many personal interactions in the OR can adversely affect performance, such as dealing with the ostensibly difficult surgeon or uncooperative nurse. Other, outside factors can also influence an anesthesiologist's performance, such as financial worries or a recent fight with a spouse. Such domestic stressors have been shown to increase the likelihood of accidents,[172] although being in a bad mood ("induced state negative affect") does not prolong reaction times.[173]

Stressful environmental conditions impair vigilance, especially in situations of conflict.[174] The level of stress can be assessed by measuring either physiologic or psychological parameters. The physiologic correlates of stress generally correspond to sympathetic nervous system activity. Studies have used heart rate,[174-176] skin conductance,[177] respiratory rate,[178] beat-to-beat variability in heart rate,[155,179,180] T-wave peak amplitude on electrocardiogram (ECG),[155] changes in voice characteristics,[155] and catecholamine excretion[181] to assess stress levels during performance of complex tasks. With increasing workload levels during simulated and real flights in high-performance aircraft, pilots who exhibited physiologic signs of stress had more false alarms and exhibited more disorganized task patterns. Thus increased workload or mental stress produces increases in sympathetic nervous system activity that can lead to deleterious physiologic changes.[182,183]

The physiologic response of the anesthesiologist to the stress of giving anesthesia may be a crucial variable, yet it has received little attention. In an early study, Toung and colleagues[184] measured the heart rate of anesthesiologists during anesthetic inductions and found a 60% increase over baseline heart rate in first-year residents at the time of intubation (Fig. 23-4). More experienced clinicians showed less of an increase. Subsequently, these investigators showed that prior medical training, even if not anesthesia related, was associated with a diminished stress response to the

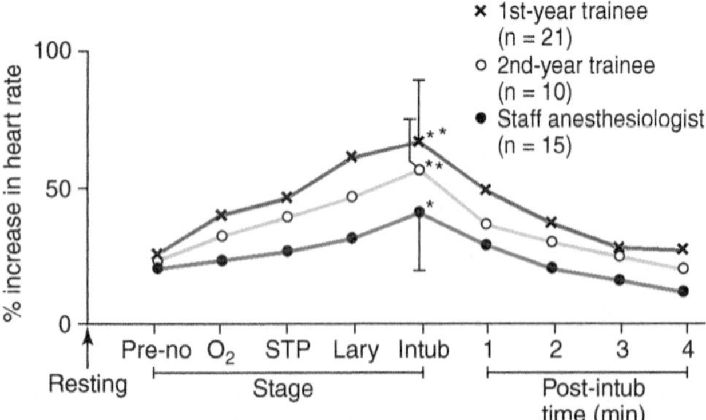

FIGURE 23-4 The heart rate of anesthesiologists increases above baseline during the induction of anesthesia. This increase, a physiologic correlate of stress and workload, is greatest in first-year anesthesia residents and diminishes with increasing experience. (From Toung T, Donham R, Rogers M: The stress of giving anesthesia on the electrocardiogram of anesthesiologists [abstract]. *Anesthesiology* 1984;61:A465.)

administration of anesthesia.[185] Repeated exposures to a specific situation result in diminished endocrine (stress) responses if the subject has learned to cope with the situation.[181] A correlation between clinical workload and the heart rate of anesthesia residents has since been documented,[180] and in another study,[186] the investigators replicated Toung's findings and demonstrated that more emergent procedures generated a greater physiologic stress response. Kain et al[187] documented increases in heart rate and blood pressure of anesthesiologists monitored during their work, especially during induction, although these changes were described as "clinically insignificant." A more recent study of multiple workload measures found consistent increases in heart rates and workload, both self-reported and observed, during anesthetic induction and emergence.[176] The induction-associated tachycardia was greatest in junior trainees. Comparison of teaching and nonteaching cases also produced evidence that clinical teaching increased the workload of the instructor and reduced measures of vigilance.

State of Health. Physicians, like the patients they care for, develop both physical and mental illnesses.[188] The topic of the "impaired" physician has been gaining increasing attention among professional societies, consumer groups, and government regulators. For example, how can these various constituencies be assured that an anesthesiologist infected with HIV does not have neuropsychologic impairment that adversely affects his or her ability to safely administer anesthesia?[189] What should be done with practicing anesthesia providers who are elderly or infirm or those who have been involved in a previous anesthesia mishap? These are complex issues that require more discussion than is possible in this overview.

As individuals age, physiologic and neurologic changes can adversely impact vigilance and task performance.[190-192] Ample "reserve" and years of experience allow most older anesthesiologists to continue to perform at a high level under most circumstances. However, the older practitioner may be more susceptible to the performance-degrading effects of sleep deprivation, fatigue, and stress. In fact, a retrospective analysis by Travis and Beach[193] suggests that older anesthesiologists are proportionally overrepresented in the National Practitioner Data Bank for malpractice claims, although in general, older physicians do not seem to have higher rates of claims.[194,195] Many older anesthesiologists do recognize their limitations and may restrict their practice to routine daytime work. Some also choose to retire rather than continue to work at night.[196]

Anxiety is a major stress factor that can affect job performance. Anxiety adversely affects attention[197] and working memory,[198] and stress-related memory failures probably cause the difficulties in planning and decision making observed in stressed individuals.[91] In addition, the inability to cope with anxiety and stress is likely an important contributing factor in the development of mental illness[198] and substance abuse.

Burnout is a phenomenon first described in the 1970s by Freudenberger[199] and subsequently quantified into components of emotional exhaustion, depersonalization, and reduced sense of personal accomplishment. In a recent study by Hyman and colleagues[200] of perioperative clinicians, they found that residents in anesthesiology had higher burnout scores than attending anesthesiologists or nurses, whereas gender was not predictive of burnout. Riad[201] found that anesthesiologists had significantly higher self-reported components of work-related exhaustion than ophthalmologists or ancillary staff.

Dedication to the "calling" of medicine can produce maladaptive behaviors as well. The phenomenon of *presenteeism*[202,203] refers to the attendance of workers at the workplace when they are ill and not functioning optimally. In health care, it has been described in ill physicians whose attendance at the hospital caused an increased risk of infection in the patients they had been acculturated to try to help.[204,205]

Substance Use and Abuse. Data previously suggested that 1% to 2% of practicing physicians are addicted to drugs, and up to 8% may be classified as alcoholics.[206] However, the rates of substance abuse among physicians are not significantly different than in the general population,[207] although anesthesiologists may be at higher risk for drug abuse than other physicians.[208,209] Whereas the abuse of controlled substances and alcohol is obviously detrimental to job performance, a variety of other, ostensibly more innocuous drugs—such as caffeine, antihistamines, and nicotine—can also affect vigilance.

Small doses of caffeine, such as that found in a typical caffeinated soft drink, can have a positive effect on vigilance and task performance.[210] Yet one study suggested that even among regular coffee drinkers, caffeine ingestion can magnify the physiologic consequences of stress.[211] Antihistamines have been associated with performance decrements on simulated tasks,[212, 213] although nonsedating antihistamines may be without significant performance-degrading effects.[214] Phenothiazines, and perhaps other antiemetics, also can impair performance on complex tasks.[213]

It is well known that alcohol ingestion markedly impairs both vigilance and psychomotor performance.[215-217] In fact, pilot simulator-based training studies have documented significant impairment in performance at blood alcohol levels as low as 20 to 35 mg/dL (0.02% to 0.035%), well below what would be considered legally drunk.[218] Perhaps as important, the effects of a hangover from alcohol can also significantly affect performance,[219] even in the absence of the perception of impairment by the affected individual.[219-221] A study of performance in a laparoscopic simulator by both novices and experienced surgeons showed that hangover effects from the night before persisted until at least 4 PM the following day.[222] The implication of these findings is that individuals should wait *at least 14 hours* after alcohol consumption before performing such complex tasks as flying an aircraft, performing surgery, or administering anesthesia.

Marijuana intoxication impairs performance,[223] and use of the drug has been implicated as a causative factor in several railroad and airline accidents.[224-226] In addition, like alcohol, marijuana intoxication is associated with a hangover condition that may impair performance,[227] even after 24 hours and in the absence of an appreciation by the subjects of their impairment.[228]

Personality. Subjects with different personality types will perform differently on various vigilance tasks.[179] In fact, individual psychological or physiologic differences may be the most important confounding factors in the performance of vigilance tasks.[229] For example, for some tasks, the incidence of error may be better predicted on the basis of individual personality traits, such as emotional stability, than on the nature of the particular task.[230] Individual preferences for particular living, working, and sleeping schedules may have a substantial genetic contribution. Thus working or sleeping at times diametrically opposed to the individual's biologically rooted personality characteristics leads to performance inefficiency and fatigue. Important factors in predicting adjustment to on-call duties may include the person's adaptability to changes in normal sleeping schedule and the ability to overcome drowsiness.[231]

The *disruptive physician* is a term recently applied to a subset of professionals whose behavior is at the extreme end of a normal distribution.[232] As a result of fatigue, anxiety, stress, substance abuse, or any combination of the above, these physicians are at highest risk for patient complaints as well as medical liability claims. Early identification of these at-risk providers is increasingly important because many will respond favorably to counseling and behavior modification.[233]

Training and Experience. Training and experience are clearly important to ensuring a high level of performance on complex tasks. Aviation accident rates directly correlate with flight experience.[20] Individual practice patterns may significantly influence anesthetic morbidity,[234] and one study demonstrated a clear inverse relationship between amount of surgical training and actual complication rates (Fig. 23-5).[235] Although physician experience may not linearly correlate with patient outcomes,[236] additional training and experience may compensate for the

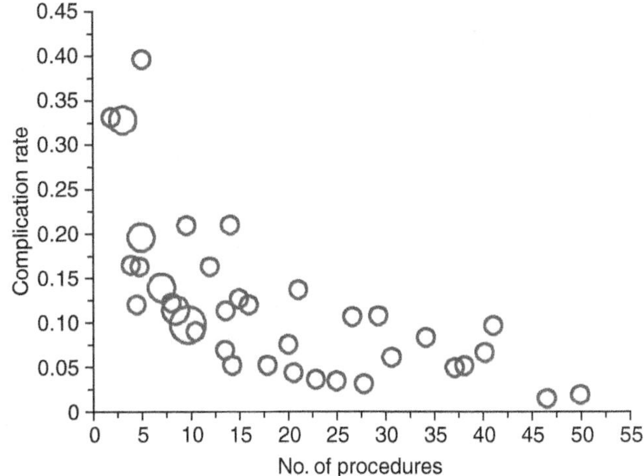

FIGURE 23-5 The correlation is strong between experience and clinical performance in the field of medicine. See and colleagues studied urological surgeons and demonstrated a significant inverse correlation between the number of laparoscopic procedures performed within 12 months of formal training in this surgical technique and the reported rate of complications. (From See WA, Cooper CS, Fisher RJ: Predictors of laparoscopic complications after formal training in laparoscopic surgery. *JAMA* 1993;270:2689-2692.)

negative effects on performance from stress or increased workload.[161] Gaba and DeAnda[237] showed that more experienced residents were better able to correct simulated untoward intraoperative events yet had no faster detection times than residents with 1 year less of training. However, individual differences, perhaps in experience or education, appeared to be much more important than amount of training. Weinger and colleagues[59] showed that during routine anesthesia cases, novice residents exhibited higher workload and decreased vigilance and were less efficient than their more experienced counterparts. Although experience may mitigate some of the adverse effects of other performance-shaping factors, such as fatigue and boredom, it is by no means a complete remedy.

Interpersonal and Team Factors

The anesthesiologist is an integral member of the OR team. In other highly complex tasks involving teamwork, such as commercial aviation, the team has generally been together for a long time and is well practiced. Team communication involves unspoken expectations, traditions, assumptions regarding task distribution and chain-of-command hierarchies, and individual emotional and behavioral components. Alterations in any of these factors can impair effective team function,[238] and unspoken assumptions about goals, duties, and roles may differ among the three main stakeholders in the OR environment.[239] Failures in adequate communication among care providers may contribute significantly to the occurrence of clinical errors in the ICU.[14] Not only were more than a third of all errors reported associated with presumably flawed verbal communication between nurse and physician, errors also seemed to occur more commonly following changes of nursing shifts, suggesting a contribution as well of faulty nurse-nurse communication. Familiar and constant composition of OR teams correlates positively with efficiency and quick turnovers.[240] The added burden of teaching trainees contributes significantly to anesthesiologists' workload and reduces responsiveness to events.[176] These findings suggest that the anesthesiologist who is confronted with a new surgeon, OR nurse, or anesthesia resident should be sensitive to the "new interpersonal environment" and exercise extra vigilance by making a special effort to communicate clearly and unambiguously, particularly in stressful situations. Communication may prove even more difficult when some or all of the team members are subjected to other stressors, such as fatigue or sleep deprivation. In addition, overall OR team performance can be adversely affected by dysfunctional interpersonal interactions among team members.

Workload and Task Characteristics

The specific characteristics of the task itself will interact with other performance-shaping factors. An example of how workload or task requirements can influence performance comes from a study of 12 relatively inexperienced private pilots asked to perform a series of flight maneuvers on a simulator under increasingly difficult conditions until performance failure occurred.[241] Under high-workload conditions, the subjects tended to decompose maneuvers into smaller, more manageable tasks. The subjects also omitted portions of the tasks that were not essential to maintain a minimum level of performance (i.e., safely flying the aircraft). Often the omission of a task component is unintentional, such as a lapse of memory during a routine but important procedure.[242] Task omissions that could have dire consequences in real life become more common in sleep-deprived individuals.

In most complex monitoring tasks, increased task complexity generally impairs performance.[49,50] Human senses can be particularly inaccurate, especially in dynamic situations.[20,243] A major factor in the effect of an additional task on performance appears to be what personal resources (perceptual, cognitive, output modalities) are required for the new task and whether those resources are already taxed.[244] Researchers have proposed a curvilinear relationship among performance, workload, and skill (Fig. 23-6). This relationship appears to apply to the task of administering anesthesia.[24,59]

In a study of pilot performance under various workload conditions, it was shown that with increasing workload, subjects tended to stare longer at the primary (i.e., more important) instruments.[161] In addition to attending less frequently to their secondary instruments (*load shedding*), when pilots did gaze at these instruments, it was for a longer time. The presumption was that with increasing workload, the subjects required more processing time to perceive the information available from each instrument. The performance of more experienced pilots was less strongly influenced by workload. In a comparison of resident performance, Cao et al[145] suggested that the same increased fixation shown by pilots is manifested by residents who were fatigued and relatively task-overloaded. Thus, as task complexity increases in a busy anesthetic case, this same phenomenon may be manifested in poor

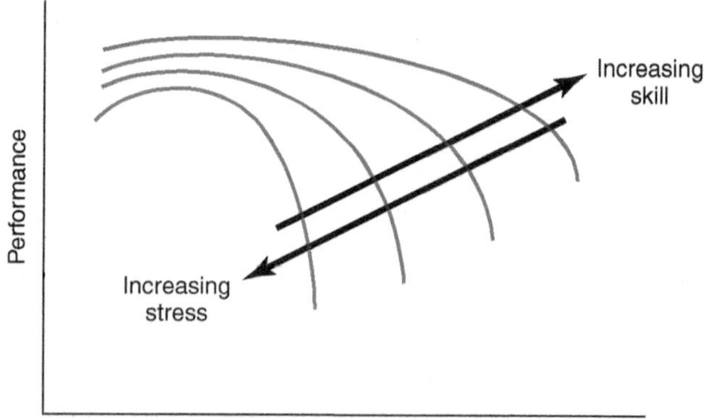

FIGURE 23-6 ■ For most complex tasks, including anesthesia, a curvilinear relationship is apparent between task performance and workload. Performance begins to deteriorate as workload increases. There also may be a less apparent performance decrement at low workload levels, presumably because of boredom or inattention. Increasing skill on the task shifts the performance workload curve upward and to the right; increased stress has the opposite effect. (From Weinger M, Englund C: Ergonomic and human factors affecting anesthetic vigilance and monitoring performance in the operating room environment. *Anesthesiology* 1990;73:995-1021.)

record keeping, sloppy anesthetic routine, or lapses of vigilance. This is supported by task-analysis studies.[41,59] In addition, Lambert and Paget[245] found that intraoperative teaching during "inappropriate" times *markedly detracted* from patient monitoring. Teaching as an independent risk factor was emphasized in one study showing a higher workload, using multiple measures, and a longer alarm response latency in teaching versus nonteaching cases.[176]

Equipment and System Factors

The equipment the anesthesiologist encounters in the OR can be characterized in two ways: those devices primarily for the delivery of substances (gases, drugs, and fluids) and those that permit the clinician to monitor the outcome of substance delivery and the physiologic state of the patient. These two types of equipment increasingly share common attributes (e.g., microprocessor control) along with their associated problems. Although the percentage of anesthesia mishaps primarily as a result of equipment failures appears to be relatively small,[11] the contribution of poor equipment design, maintenance, or performance to user error may be significant. Thus it seems appropriate to wonder about what hidden factors might have contributed to a catastrophe but were not elicited by the "accident" investigation. For example, did distracting alarms contribute to the end result? Or, more importantly, did poor equipment design more or less subtly influence the outcome? One study suggested that the use of transesophageal echocardiograpy during coronary artery bypass graft procedures may, under some circumstances, impair vigilance for other clinical events (Fig. 23-7).[41]

Poor Equipment Design. It has been suggested that almost all human error is due to either inadequate or inappropriate equipment or system design.[36] Equipment problems can manifest in many arenas, including failures of design, device performance, user and service manuals, and maintenance. At least two factors make the design of OR equipment particularly difficult. First, the OR places appreciable physical and environmental stresses on equipment. Second, it is sometimes difficult to elicit from users precise or optimal design requirements for OR equipment. Block and colleagues[246] described the installation of one of the first computerized monitoring systems specifically designed for the OR. Despite doing a careful survey of anesthesiologist users to determine their needs and preferences before designing the system, after the system was built, these users decided that they really wanted something different. This change may not reflect capriciousness as much as it does changing experience and evolving expectations. Nonetheless, it makes the designer's task more difficult. At the very least, in the design and manufacture of new equipment, continuous direct contact between the designer and the user is essential.

Artifact remains a serious problem and can be a function of poor device design. For example, inadequate shielding of ECG cables can lead to motion artifact. If the software cannot handle this artifact, the displayed heart rate will either be absent, or worse yet, incorrect. Computing and displaying incorrect values can be disastrous; the clinician could easily withhold or institute therapy inappropriately or be unable to follow the course of therapy. Substantial improvement has been made in artifact management software over the years. For example, the incidence of pulse oximeter artifact has decreased considerably, such that it is no longer of significant concern to those who use automated anesthesia record-keeping devices.

Poor design can be particularly frustrating because it often is difficult to deal with after the fact. Poor design can be hardware or software related. The former may show up as disorganized, excessive, or inappropriate control mechanisms. Software-related design problems include confusing displays or problems navigating between display screens. Combined hardware and

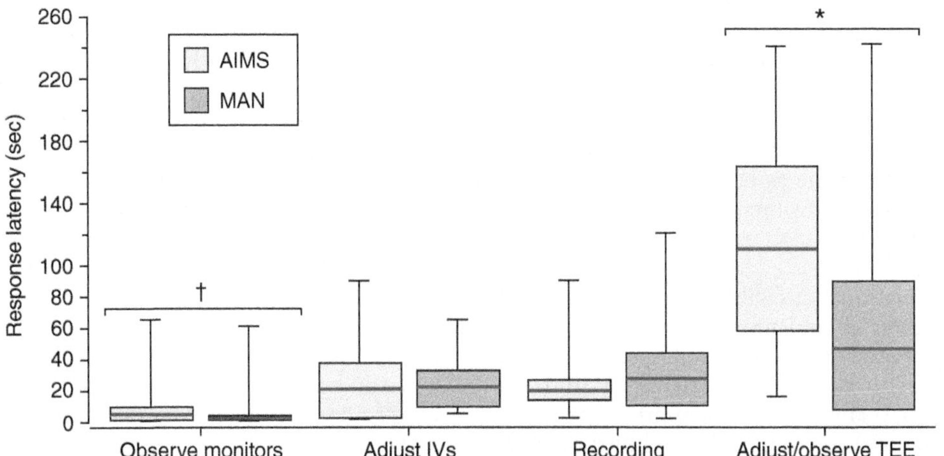

FIGURE 23-7 Intraoperative vigilance, as measured by the response latency to an alarm light positioned within the anesthesia monitoring array, was decreased during use of the transesophageal echocardiography (*TEE*) device compared with the performance of other anesthesia tasks. The minimum and maximum values in each group are shown by the *upper and lower bars*. The rectangle contains 50% of all the data, and the *dark line* depicts the median value in that group. The response latency was significantly slower when observing or adjusting the TEE compared with record keeping, observing monitors, or adjusting intravenous (*IV*) infusions (*$P < .05$). Subjects detected the vigilance light more quickly when observing the monitoring array (†$P < .05$ compared with all three other tasks). *AIMS,* Anesthesia Information Management System; *MAN,* manual charting. (Modified from Weinger MB, Herndon OW, Gaba DM: The effect of electronic record keeping and transesophageal echocardiography on task distribution, workload, and vigilance during cardiac anesthesia. *Anesthesiology* 1997;87:144-155.)

software problems include poor handling of artifact, disruptive display-control relationships, or irrational alarms.

Optimal design of complex microprocessor-based equipment requires a delicate balance between developing a device that is too complicated for the operator to understand versus one that becomes deceptively simple. If there are too many displays, or if the displays are confusing, performance may be suboptimal, and errors can result during crisis situations. The complexity of the Aegis radar display system (Lockheed Martin, Bethesda, MD), and some inherent design flaws, was a major cause of the accidental downing of a commercial airliner by the *USS Vincennes*. On the other hand, well-intended attempts to simplify a device can produce equally poor results. Cook and colleagues[247] describe a humidifier that had been redesigned from a manual device to an automatic one. The clinicians liked the newer device because it was "simpler." Yet research showed that the users did not understand the device's underlying operation. For example, they did not know the procedure necessary to reactivate the device after an alarm, nor did they know that the heating elements were turned off after an alarm. To reset the device after an alarm, users simply turned it off and on again. This device was not intuitive in its design or functionality.

Each individual component of a system may be well thought out, but if the system design as a whole is faulty, the result will be unsatisfactory.[248] Often the design is appropriate for one venue but is transferred to another without taking into account the unique attributes of the new environment. For example, most of the original "integrated" monitors were designed for use in the ICU and provided trend displays using a scale of 6 or more hours. For most anesthetic procedures, the resulting display was far too compressed. The needs of users in the OR can be substantially different than those in the ICU.

The ultimate performance of the equipment is the most important consideration. Poor performance may be related to faults with design, implementation, construction, inappropriate use, or inadequate supporting equipment. Mosenkis[248] suggests that excellent design should allow clinicians to use a device *correctly* the first time they interact with it, preferably without reading the manual, whereas to use that device *well*, practice may be required.[249] He goes on to assert that health care providers use medical devices as they do automobiles: they *expect* that a new device will work more or less the same as equivalent older devices. This cognitive model of how medical devices *should* work can only be supported through user-centered design and by standardization.[250]

The use of simulation may facilitate many of the design goals required for safer and more user-friendly equipment. By testing several designs under almost-real clinical situations, manufacturers will be able to efficiently determine which design, if any, is the most appropriate. Simulation can also be used for training: the clinician will be able to safely and more quickly learn how to use a device, even under the most demanding conditions.

User Manuals/Documentation. The user theoretically depends on the manual for many purposes: becoming acquainted with a device during its initial use, learning its finer points, and troubleshooting. Unfortunately, many manuals and other documentation for medical devices are poorly written, confusing, or incomplete. All too often, the immediately essential or desired information is impossible to find. As a result of these shortcomings, most "user" manuals are simply not used by clinicians. From a practical standpoint, however, most people simply do not bother reading instruction manuals except perhaps to deal with a critical or particularly confusing condition; for example, if they cannot determine how to turn on the device.

On-line real-time help systems can now easily be incorporated into microprocessor-controlled medical devices. For example, an Internet connection can provide ready access to details needed for device operation, troubleshooting, maintenance, or repair. Current implementations typically include text, line drawings, and images. However, digital animations may be a more appropriate method to demonstrate how to calibrate, set up, or troubleshoot a device in real time.

Another consideration is education of anesthesiologists in the use of their equipment, and whether that education is the responsibility of the manufacturer, the hospital, the Food and Drug Administration (FDA), the clinicians themselves, or perhaps some professional society, such as the Anesthesia Patient Safety Foundation (APSF) or the Society for Technology in Anesthesia. Regardless, the technical education of anesthesia providers is sadly deficient at all stages, from the student to the experienced clinician. Until this education problem is addressed, the interaction between the user and complex machines will remain suboptimal, and equipment-induced or system-induced errors will occur that will be inappropriately blamed on the user. Recent efforts by the APSF and the Association for the Advancement of Medical Instrumentation to develop standardized processes for advanced equipment education for clinicians may bear fruit.

Equipment Maintenance. Anesthesia machines in particular require continual maintenance, which must be undertaken by experienced personnel. Maintenance training has traditionally been accomplished at the factory and usually requires several weeks. Optimally, maintenance should either be performed by a representative of the manufacturer or by a well-trained independent maintenance group (see also Chapters 32 and 33).

Maintenance errors often follow the same pattern as other types of errors: a chain of events, each one by itself insufficient to cause a disaster, contributes to the adverse outcome. In one of the most notorious maintenance errors, which occurred decades ago, the OR medical gas lines were switched.[251] A hospital maintenance worker repaired the oxygen hose during the night so he would not disrupt the OR routine. What he initiated in good faith is a classic example of a chain of mishaps. First, an oxygen connector was attached to one end of each of two hoses, and a nitrous oxide connector was attached to the other end. Second, both hoses were black, rather than color coded; third, the maintenance worker carefully and neatly twisted the hoses around each other. In these days before the pulse oximeter, the first patient to be anesthetized with this machine died. The error was soon realized during the procedure on the second patient, whereupon the anesthesia machine was completely disconnected and the patient was ventilated with an independent, portable source of oxygen. The notoriety this case achieved was responsible both for an increased awareness of the possibility of OR gas switches and for the realization that continuous measurement of inspired oxygen is necessary. It has also inspired a generation of studies and simulations to train for proper responses to unexplained hypoxia.[252,253] Sadly enough, gas switches still do occur, but hypoxic mixtures usually are detected by now-mandated oxygen analyzers. One notable exception is the case of a cylinder of carbon dioxide being used in place of a cylinder of nitrous oxide with attendant morbidity from hypercarbia.[254,255]

Equipment Obsolescence. Anesthesia machines are designed to be long lasting and rugged, and manufacturers have largely accomplished this goal. Thus a large number of older machines are still in service, which presents a variety of problems: 1) integral parts wear out and do not function as intended, 2) components do not perform up to today's standards, which can change relatively rapidly, 3) functions available on modern machines are absent, and 4) some components may be dangerous. Examples of dangerous components still found, albeit rarely, on older anesthesia machines in developing countries include the Copper Kettle (Puritan-Bennett; Covidien, Mansfield, MA) and in-circuit vaporizers and vaporizers without an interlock mechanism. Carbon dioxide (CO_2) absorber bypass mechanisms are also still in use in many countries, offering the ability to replace absorbent during a case but also allowing CO_2 accumulation if left on unintentionally. One report detailed the misconnection of an obsolete Bain circuit scavenging outlet to the fresh gas supply.[256]

There will always be out-of-date machines, and it is not cost-effective to replace them all at once. Furthermore, some might argue that an experienced anesthesiologist is safer using customary equipment, instead of a technologically overwhelming "next-generation" workstation. On the other hand, when suddenly confronted with an old piece of equipment during an emergency anesthetic, a less experienced anesthesiologist trained only on modern equipment is placed in a difficult situation that is potentially life-threatening to the patient.

In this era of reduced health care resources and cost consciousness, issues arise when hospitals and anesthesia providers discuss the replacement of old anesthesia machines.[257-259] Older anesthesia machines should be replaced if they do not meet American Society of Testing and Materials (ASTM) standards, are not easily upgradable, or have poor service records (see also Chapter 30 and Box 30-6).[258]

ROLE OF STANDARDS IN ANESTHESIA EQUIPMENT DESIGN

For a number of years, a dedicated group of clinicians, device manufacturers, regulatory agencies, consultants, and other interested parties has been developing voluntary national and international medical device standards to help ensure safe medical practice. One example is the international effort to standardize small-bore connectors to reduce the risk of often-fatal misconnections of gas- and fluid-containing tubing. These standards also help ensure that the devices and their integration will be similar enough to each other to permit clinicians to use different devices from different manufacturers with minimal confusion. The American contributions to medical equipment standards development are sponsored by the nonprofit ASTM, the American National Standards Institute (ANSI), and the Association for the Advancement of Medical Instrumentation (AAMI). The international standards development process includes a joint working group between the International Organization for Standardization (ISO) and the International Electrotechnical Commission (IEC) on integrated monitors, anesthesia workstations, medical device alarms, and connectors.

Standards will continue to be a driving force in the integration of the anesthesia workstation, monitoring systems, and other medical equipment in the clinical work environment. The active involvement of anesthesiologists in the standards-making process is essential to ensure that it results in effective, safe, and easy-to-use devices (see also Chapter 34).

ALARMS

The need to incorporate alarms into monitoring systems stems from several factors. The number of variables to be monitored have increased tremendously; the equipment used to collect and display these variables has become exceedingly sophisticated; and, as discussed, given the complexity of the task and its attendant stress, the anesthesiologist is unlikely to be able to detect all out-of-range variables or conditions without machine assistance. In fact, if displays were easy to comprehend, they presented all the relevant information and no irrelevant information, and all the required clinical information were in one, easy-to-read display, perhaps alarms would be unnecessary.[260] Unfortunately, this situation does not yet exist. In fact, with the increasing sophistication of anesthesia monitors and equipment, the number of alarms has increased almost exponentially.

The objective of any alarm system is to optimize the probability of successfully dealing with the problem at hand.[261] Alarms should serve several functions[260]: 1) assist the anesthesiologist in the detection of adverse or unanticipated conditions, in either the patient or the equipment; 2) aid the fatigued or otherwise nonvigilant anesthesiologist; and 3) assist in situations complicated by stress, workload, lack of training, or other factors that might negatively affect the ability of the anesthesiologist to detect or respond to undesirable conditions.

Once an activated alarm is detected, the next step is to identify the cause. An alarm is of no benefit if it does not also provide the user with sufficient information to correct the alarm condition, either directly or by indicating where to look to get the necessary data. In fact, when the source of an alarm cannot be identified, it is extremely distracting and can exacerbate a potentially difficult clinical situation. Various conditions can cause an alarm condition, including equipment failure, artifact, an unexplained change in one or more of the monitored signals, or an unexpected or undesirable response of the patient to an intervention.[260,262]

An alarm should be more than an indicator of an abnormal condition; it must provide some preliminary information about the condition that triggered activation. However, too much information provided in the initial alarm state can confuse or mislead the operator, especially if the alarm is based on a single variable or if multiple alarms are simultaneously activated. The sounding and subsequent identification of a particular alarm narrows the focus of the user's attention to one aspect of the system. Some alarms, such as a low circuit pressure alarm, are very specific with respect to both the physical location that must be inspected and the fund of knowledge required to correct the problem. In these types of conditions, an experienced user can quickly correct the problem, often with little conscious effort. In contrast, other alarms, such as a high pulmonary arterial diastolic pressure alarm or a low right-hemisphere EEG spectral edge frequency alarm, may require extensive examination of multiple clinical variables and significant contemplation to determine the underlying physiologic condition that activated the alarm state.

The designer of alarm systems must consider the method as well as the consequences of the interruption produced by the alarm.[261] An alarm system should produce a signal as soon as possible after an alarm condition has been detected.[263] It should be easy for the user to identify the source of the alarm, and accurate information about the cause must be provided. The user's attention must then be held long enough to ensure that the problem that caused the alarm has been corrected. Finally, interference from other, less important alarm conditions must be minimized during the response to the original alarm condition.

Human factors principles *must* be applied to the design of alarms. These principles include appropriate selection of physiologic variables that will have alarms, control of alarm limits, reliable detection of out-of-range events, intelligent decisions regarding which states will or will not produce alarms, provision of user-friendly output signals, appropriate application of new technologies (e.g., neural networks, fuzzy logic), and standardization across medical systems (Box 23-5).[264,265] Standardization may best be accomplished through an international multidisciplinary consensus approach such as that used by the ISO/IEC Joint Working Group on Medical Device Alarms.

BOX 23-5 Principles of Good Alarm Design

1. Human factors principles must be applied (see Chapter 24).
2. The physiologic variables to be followed and the alarm limits, along with appropriate user control, must be carefully selected.
3. There must be reliable detection and device intelligence regarding nonalarm states (good "artifact management").
4. Alarms must be prioritized (consider standards such as IEC 60601-1-8).
5. Alarm states must correlate with clinical urgency.
6. The use of different alarm modalities (e.g., audible, visual) and their integration must be considered.
7. The user must be able to silence alarms, at least temporarily.
8. Output signals must be user friendly and must not produce a negative affective response (i.e., "Turn it off!").
9. Designers must consider, on a case-by-case basis, the clinical usefulness of incorporating clinically relevant data into alarms.
10. Alarms should be standardized across all medical devices likely to be used in the same clinical environment.

False Alarms

Although alarms can be useful in terms of improving recognition of critical situations, if improperly designed, they can degrade performance.[264] Intraoperative alarms can give misleading information, and they can be distracting. Alarms may fail to provide adequate notice of a critical situation (a *false negative*), possibly because of intentional inactivation or inappropriate alarm limit adjustment.[266] More commonly, alarms may be activated inappropriately (a *false alarm* or *false positive*), which may be due either to artifact or to an overly sensitive alarm setting.[267] This was a key topic of a 2011 FDA/AAMI Alarms Summit attended by representatives of all relevant stakeholder groups.

False alarms continue to be a significant problem throughout the perioperative period.[268] In one intraoperative study, at least 80% of 731 warnings that occurred during cardiac surgery were of no clinical utility.[269] In another study, 75% of all audio alarms were spurious, and only 3% indicated actual patient risk.[270] In this pediatric study, an alarm sounded every 4.5 minutes, with an average of 10 per procedure. Another study suggests that the implementation of integrated monitors has reduced the incidence of intraoperative false alarms.[271] In that study, only 24% of auditory alarms were spurious, whereas 23% represented a real patient risk. The majority of alarms, both true and false, were observed during induction and emergence; the end-tidal carbon dioxide monitor accounted for 42% of all alarms.

In the recovery room, patient pulse oximeters may sound more often than every 10 minutes, and 75% are false alarms.[272] Apnea alarms were less frequent, about once every 30 minutes, but were more likely to be meaningful; less than one third were false. The ECG alarmed even more infrequently, yet a very high fraction of these alarms were false.

Porciello's survey[273] of critical care unit physicians revealed that many found arrhythmia alarms to be inaccurate, misleading, and disturbing. O'Carroll[274] showed that during a 3-week period in an ICU, only 8 of 1455 alarm soundings indicated potentially life-threatening problems; 45% of the false alarms were from ventilators, and another 35% were from infusion pumps. Lawless[275] concluded that "over 94% of alarm soundings in a pediatric ICU may not be clinically important."

The occurrence of a false alarm requires time and effort to verify the patient's actual condition. This may distract attention away from other tasks or conditions. The false alarm may also lead to an inappropriate action, which will take additional time and also poses a potential risk to patient safety. Anesthesiologists will silence, disable, or ignore alarms that sound falsely or are annoying.[276] Also, many alarm tones are distracting or obnoxious and thereby

TABLE 23-5 **Example of Alarm Hierarchy**

Alarm Priority	Meaning	Desired Response from Operator	Visual Indication	Auditory Indication
High	Emergency, warning	Attend to event	Immediate red; flashing continually repeated	Complex tone, at fast pace
Medium	Caution	Prompt	Flashing yellow	Less complex tone, less frequently repeated
	Alert	Increased vigilance	Continuous yellow	None or simple tone, infrequently repeated
Low	Information, notice	Awareness, confidence	Yellow or cyan	None

elicit a negative affective response ("Make it stop!").[261,277] This is undesirable in an alarm, because not only will it increase stress, but the subject's primary response will be to disable the alarm as promptly as possible, perhaps without adequately investigating the meaning or significance of the alarm state. Some airline pilots believe that all but the most critical aviation alarms should be silenced during high-workload conditions.[278]

Alarm Notification Modality

No crucial alarm condition should be indicated by a single modality. Most experts believe that general information can be presented solely with a visual indication or message, whereas warnings should be indicated by both audible and visual alarm modalities. It is best if both auditory tones and a visual indication occur simultaneously. In a complex environment with many different alarms, a proper mix of alarm notification modalities will prevent confusion and increase subject responsiveness. Visual cues to trend changes also can reduce the "change blindness" seen when monitoring routine visual data.[279]

Consistent with the widespread use of auditory alarms in anesthesia equipment, studies have suggested that for critical information, auditory presentation leads to more rapid and reliable responses than does visual presentation.[280] However, the auditory mode of alarm notification presents several problems. Alarm tones from different devices may sound similar, making identification of the source of the alarm difficult or even stressful. Loeb and colleagues[281] demonstrated that in the absence of other cues, clinicians without distractions could identify the source of alarm tones only 34% of the time. In this study, the authors recorded alarm tones and then played them back to 44 clinicians outside the OR. The recognition of the alarm was greater for alarms heard more frequently, and no relationship was found between the complexity of the alarm tone and the ability to recognize its meaning.

Another problem with auditory alarms is that localization or recognition of specific alarm tones may require normal auditory acuity. Anesthesiologists with hearing deficits may have difficulty determining the source of sounds in the OR. Hearing acuity, especially above 1 kHz, also decreases with age. Yet 50% of all alarm tones in current use have much of their sound energy above 2 kHz. Thus older clinicians may have more difficulty identifying high-frequency alarms.[282] Higher pitched tones are, in general, also more difficult to localize.[283]

The high noise levels in the OR may mask or obscure some alarm tones. Using a Scott Instruments Type 450B sound meter (Maynard, MA), the peak noise level (dB_A) produced by a variety of common alarms was measured in several ORs at the University of California–San Diego Medical Center. Readings were obtained at a distance of 1 foot from the source, and the median maximum value from three successive readings was used. The sound levels of a number of common OR sounds are shown in Table 23-4. It can be shown that frequent alarm activation contributes significantly to the high noise levels reported in the OR.[64,281,282]

Visual alarm lights can be coded by their color, brightness, size, location, and flashing frequency. Flashing lights are more noticeable and are traditionally used for more crucial information. Color codes have been standardized for instrument panels and alarm displays (Table 23-5). Red is used only for emergency or warning signals, yellow indicates caution, and green indicates "power on" or device activation. However, a sizable percentage of the population is color blind; thus crucial alarm information *must* be coded simultaneously by other methods. (Note that color coding is culturally dependent and may be inappropriate for international use.) In addition to lights, visual information can be presented as full or abbreviated text, icons, or other symbols. Coding of these visual messages should be consistent with the protocols used for simple display lights. Alarm tones and visual indications should be different for different levels of alarm priority, and a number of applicable international standards for alarm enunciation have now been consolidated.[284]

Auditory tones can also be coded in several ways in addition to loudness, which is *not* effective because of its disruptive nature. The pattern, pitch, tone, and frequency of an alarm can be modified to provide distinguishing features, so the clinician knows which alarm it is, and other contextual information. A good example of information coding of auditory signals can be found in the frequency modulation of pulse oximeters, in which the pitch of the tone decreases as the patient's oxygen saturation decreases. This modality is implemented differently among manufacturers, leading to the potential for confusion if the ear is "trained" to a certain pitch scale.[285] Some human factors experts have advocated more extensive use of similar "earcons." An example of an immediately understandable alarm sound used in some advanced fighter cockpit designs to indicate low fuel is the sucking noise made by the last bit of sink water going down the drain. More sophisticated types of coding of auditory alarm tones could include melody, as advocated by Block,[286] or actual voice messages. Synthesized voice warning messages may be particularly effective when used sparingly and only for crucial alarms.[287] However, voice messages can be extremely disruptive if they are frequent, present information that is already known ("the car door is open"), or are spurious.

Human factors experts often emphasize the importance of consistency. In the case of auditory alarms, this would suggest that a particular alarm tone should have the same meaning regardless of where it is encountered in a given workspace. In general, within a single clinical care environment such as the OR, no more than 10, but preferably as few as 6, different tones should occur. Several approaches to allocating alarm tones have been proposed.[283] Traditionally, alarm tones have been equipment based, in the sense that each device has a different tone. However, in a truly equipment-based approach, all pulse oximeters would produce identical alarm tones independent of manufacturer. Similarly, ventilators, infusion pumps, monitors, and so on would all have their own unique tones. Alternatively, in a priority-based strategy, taken by many modern integrated monitoring systems, all alarm conditions invoke one of only three tones: *warning*, *caution*, or *notice*. However, this approach makes it more difficult to identify the source and meaning of any given alarm.[288,289]

Another approach to alarm allocation would be based on patient risk; conditions that produce a given magnitude of patient risk would produce a particular tone. The perceived patient risk could be combined with the urgency of required response. The problem with this approach, however, is that patient risk and required response time can vary tremendously depending on individual patient factors and the overall clinical situation. Thus in selected situations, an equipment-generated "low risk/slow response" alarm tone may in fact represent a high risk/rapid response condition, and the anesthesiologist could be lulled into complacency about the importance of the alarm.

A fully integrated OR alarm system should incorporate a combination of patient risk, required response time, and source (which type of equipment and what kind of physiologic variable is generating the alarm) into a coherent prioritized system to optimize appropriate response. When a centralized alarm strategy is used, the system must provide as much information as possible about the source and cause of each alarm condition. The most clinically important alarm must be indicated first, and other, less important alarms should be suppressed during the sounding of the higher priority alarm. In addition, such a system must be flexible enough to permit expansion with new technological and medical advances.

Based on an alarm system for civil aviation in Great Britain, Patterson[290] developed a novel series of general and context-specific alarm tones for use in the medical environment. Patterson's alarm sounds consisted of well-defined, complex sequences of tones that produced distinctive auditory rhythms or signatures. Each tone was composed of at least four harmonics to improve its melodic character. As described by Kerr,[283] three "general" alarm sounds of increasing complexity—advisory, caution, and warning—were proposed. Six "specialized" alarm categories were also described: ventilation, oxygenation, cardiovascular, artificial perfusion, drug administration, and temperature. Each of these had its own unique auditory signature, and for each category, both a caution alarm and a warning alarm were specified. Urgency was indicated by playing the tone more quickly rather than more loudly. Clinicians' estimates of the urgency of particular clinical conditions appeared to be consistent across raters[291] and can thus be used to construct tables of relative clinical risk for alarm conditions.

Use of the Patterson alarm sounds remains controversial. The studies that led to the development of these sounds are more than 30 years old and may not be applicable to the modern OR. This approach requires individual devices to generate several complex tones, adding cost and complexity. More importantly, the OR is a very different workplace than the cockpit of an airplane. In the cockpit, only the flight crew must listen and attend to alarms. In the OR, surgeons, nurses, and awake patients are a captive audience that may find extraneous or excessive sounds disturbing. At a multidisciplinary conference when the Patterson sounds were being debated, the surgeons present were adamant that they were easily distracted by the plethora of auditory alarms in the OR (J. Hedley-White, personal communication, 1996). Although IEC 60601-1-8 specifies Patterson-type alarm tones, developers who implement compliant tones have not been uniformly pleased with the results of either usability testing or customer feedback. In summary, little evidence supports the use of any particular system of alarm tones in the OR environment. Scientific studies must be performed to evaluate the impact of different alarm modes and tones on the anesthesiologist's vigilance and on the performance of the entire OR team.[292]

One unique approach has been investigated in which alarms are transmitted through tactile stimuli through wearable devices.[293] Vibratory stimuli applied to the user's forearm were found to be efficacious and well tolerated. Vigorous research is being conducted to determine both the optimal format and the potential bandwidth of tactile displays and alerts.[294,295]

Alarm Limits

It is generally better to anticipate a critical condition than to respond to it. Thus alarms would be most useful if they were activated *before* the deleterious condition became critical or serious. To prevent patient injury, when setting the values, or limits, at which a particular alarm sounds, five things must be taken into account: 1) the condition of the patient, 2) the rate at which the variable is likely to change (deteriorate), 3) the response time of the measurement system, 4) the response time of the alarm system, and 5) the response (or correction) time of the anesthesiologist.[283] To ensure that alarms sound well before dangerous conditions occur without too frequently being spurious requires considerable intelligence on the part of both the system and the user. Some anesthesia monitoring devices have implemented "alert limits," a kind of prealarm alarm (Fig. 23-8). In theory, systems capable of adjusting alarm thresholds based on each patient's evolving condition could markedly reduce the stress and workload of the user and reduce the incidence

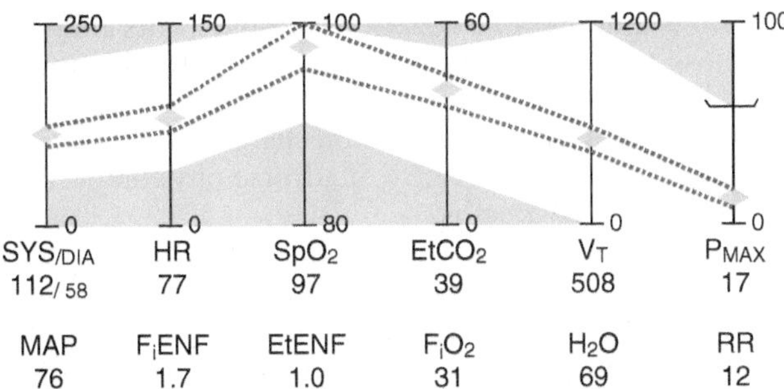

FIGURE 23-8 The use of "alert" limits (*dashed lines*) may provide a more sensitive threshold for detecting adverse trends in patient vital signs. This allows intervention a full "alarm" condition is reached. Such alert zones would be particularly useful if they were modified based on the individual patient's actual ongoing physiologic responses to surgery and anesthesia.

of false alarms. Hence, a major area of interest for alarm designers is the development of automated, intelligent alarm-limit algorithms.

The criteria that determine whether or when a particular alarm sounds is called the *threshold value* or alarm limit. This limit can be set either by the equipment manufacturer or by the user. Except for a few alarm states—such as "wall oxygen disconnect" or "oxygen tank pressure low," whose limits are virtually fixed and rarely if ever need to be changed—other alarm conditions must be adjusted based on the particular clinical situation. The limits that are chosen will, in most situations, determine the incidence of false alarms. Thus it is important to permit the user to easily alter alarm limits. However, if the user must frequently adjust the alarm limits to prevent false or spurious alarms, the alarm will undoubtedly be disabled. Allowing the user to adjust alarm limits to extreme values (e.g., fraction of inspired oxygen [FiO_2] <15%) permits a de facto permanent disabling of the alarm that could potentially result in serious patient injury. Observations of users disabling alarms suggest a problem with the reliability of the underlying parameter and/or deficiencies in alarm design or processing.

Reasonable alarm limits for a particular variable may be determined in several ways.[260] For example, for factory default limits, a consensus of experienced users could be taken; most clinicians would agree that a diastolic blood pressure of greater than 110 mm Hg or less than 40 mm Hg is abnormal. Alternatively, device manufacturers might use previously collected data about a particular physiologic variable, perhaps based on statistical analysis of data from large numbers of similar patients. Either of these approaches would invariably result in alarm limits for some individual patients that are either too restrictive or not restrictive enough. Blum and colleagues[296] examined a rule-based but network-implemented approach to alarm analysis and presentation in the critical care environment. By using median filters and a set of rules, the network was able to reduce false alarms and significantly improve specificity of blood pressure alarms.

A more sophisticated approach would be to design the device so that it dynamically adjusts its alarm limits based on actual ongoing patient values. For example, the system might keep track of the patient's blood pressure over the preceding 30 minutes and then set alarm limits at ±20% of the average of these preceding values. Variable rule-based systems might use the patient's recent history ±1 standard deviation (statistical limits) or rate-of-change limits, rather than absolute numbers, to set limits. One study recently documented a 70% reduction in false alarms using statistical alarm thresholds.[297]

A combination of these approaches was used by plotting blood pressure against the rate of change in blood pressure, both expressed in units of standard deviation. The authors described the advantages as including the detection of "asymmetric" changes, such as alarming with a small decrease in systolic pressure from 90 mm Hg, while ignoring a larger increase.[298] Research on "smart" alarms is now focused on integrating multiple physiologic variables, diagnosing spurious alarm states, and providing additional meaningful information to the user, including suggested responses.

Alarm Fatigue

Numerous reports of patient deaths as a result of alarm deactivation for false alerts has led to regulatory and policy attention to the problem, labeled "alarm fatigue." A meeting jointly convened in 2011 by the AAMI, the FDA, The Joint Commission, and the ECRI Institute reviewed the issues that contribute to this widespread problem. They recommended a cross-disciplinary approach that includes health care professionals, designers, and engineers using a source-path-receiver model to increase the effective signal/noise ratio of alarms.[299] Some of the techniques they suggested include 1) reducing noise levels at the bedside by centralizing alarms; 2) adding sound-absorptive material to reduce background noise and thus enable alarm volumes to be reduced; 3) integrating devices to centralize alarms; 4) using visual alarms, locally or centrally, to limit bedside noise; 5) implementing secondary notification systems (pager or phone); and 6) reducing false-positive alerts through better design and maintenance. In addition, conference attendees supported the increased use of the IEC standard 60601-1-8 for general guidance on alarms[284] and the draft standard IEC 80001-2 concerning integrated alarm systems.

Simple methods are effective in reducing alarm fatigue. Setting alarm limits to individualized, rather than default, parameters reduced false alarms by 43% in one study,[300] but it increased the delay (latency) before alarm sounding and removed 67% of unneeded alarms[301] in another. Recently, Curry and Lynn[302] published an insightful analysis of the relationship between traditional threshold alarms, alarm fatigue, and patterns of unexpected hospital death (PUHD). They identified three patterns of decompensation—heart failure, carbon dioxide narcosis, and sleep apnea—each with distinguishing characteristics. Especially in patients with sleep apnea, repetitive alarms led to alarm fatigue by clinicians and subsequent morbidity. They recommended both multiparameter alarms and further research to identify sentinel patterns of clinical decompensation.

Control of Alarms

If properly designed, visual alarms do not impair critical display information; it should therefore never be necessary to disable them. The system must promptly recognize that the alarm condition has been corrected and must immediately silence the associated alarm tone or indication. Nevertheless, it often is still necessary to silence or disable auditory alarms. In such cases, there must be a visual indication that an auditory alarm has been silenced. High-priority alarm tones should only be able to be temporarily disabled for 45 seconds to 2 minutes.

It is essential that the user be able to test the alarm to ensure that it will produce the expected sound at the appropriate time. Two kinds of tests should be available on any anesthesia workstation: a *power test* and a *limit test.* For the power test, either at power-up or on activation of a "test" switch, all modalities of the alarm should be activated. For the limit test, there should be a way for the user to adjust or modify the device and/or its alarms manually, such that the ability of the alarm to trigger upon reaching the desired limit can be directly tested.

For alarms to perform their function, they must not be disabled. Although every manufacturer allows alarms to be turned off, either temporarily or permanently, this function should rarely, if ever, be used. For this reason, the design of a one-touch control to disable ALL alarms is discouraged. If alarms are both sensitive and specific, the user will feel less burdened and thus be less likely to disable them. Although anecdotes abound of poor outcomes because of disabled alarms, no well-controlled studies have quantitated the risk of deliberate alarm disabling. Incorporating alarm use into routine workflow is as important as designing systems to prevent misuse or nonuse.[303]

Smart Alarms

Appreciable research has been undertaken on "smart" alarms.[304] Theoretically, microprocessor-based smart devices should provide interactive event recognition, reduce the incidence of false alarms, enhance vigilance, and improve data manipulation.[305] Unfortunately, commercially available alarms are not particularly intelligent; part of the problem is that we do not understand the task of administering anesthesia very well. How do anesthesiologists make decisions, and what information is important to those decisions?[306] In addition, any given value of a monitored variable is context specific, so it is difficult for the system to know, for a particular patient and under specific conditions, whether an isolated value is normal or abnormal.

Thus far, investigators have used two approaches in their attempts to develop smart alarms: *rule-based expert systems*[305] and *neural networks.*[307,308] Rule-based expert systems use elaborate "if/then" programs to set contingencies for alarm conditions or limits. Rule-based strategies work relatively well in straightforward and foreseeable situations, such as those that involve the integration of several different devices with known effects on each others' functions. For example, a pulse oximetery monitor could be designed such that if a noninvasive blood pressure cuff is on the same arm as the oximeter probe and the cuff inflates, the SpO_2 alarm would be disabled during the blood pressure reading. Pan and colleagues[309] described a rule-based intelligent monitoring system that incorporated the slope and minimum and maximum values of multiple monitored variables to make specific clinical diagnoses. The system was tested for its ability to diagnose problems of breathing circuit integrity and to assess adequacy of ventilation and oxygenation, and it correctly identified 91% of mechanical malfunctions within 30 seconds and 100% of adverse physiologic conditions within 10 breaths.

In an alternative approach, Beinlich and Gaba[310] used a computerized representation of statistical likelihood (probabilistic) reasoning to aid the clinician in developing clinical diagnoses during critical events. Their prototype system related physiologic variables with potential diseases or problems using objective conditional probability equations; that is, it evaluated the statistical likelihood that a given physiologic state was caused by a particular event. In preliminary testing, their system made the correct diagnosis in only 71% of the test cases presented. Nevertheless, probabilistic techniques have gained favor in some computer-aided diagnostic decision aids.[311]

A neural network is a parallel processor that consists of multiple interconnected nodes.[312] A *node* is a site at which incoming data are processed; the resultant outcome is then presented to subsequent nodes via data flow pathways. The conditions at all adjacent nodes influence the states of the others. In this way, the information passes through the network in a wave, in which all relevant factors, including those that the programmer may not have anticipated, affect the result. The neural network is much more like the human brain than a traditional serial computer; as such, the neural network may be particularly good at tasks that require pattern recognition or associative processing. Theoretically, abnormalities in the state of a complex system, such as the physiologic state of the anesthetized patient, would be particularly amenable to detection by a neural network. The other advantages of a neural network approach are that it can provide information about the interrelationships between and among monitored variables and be robust in diagnosing unanticipated or unusual alarm conditions. A neural network system designed to detect machine/circuit fault conditions was found to be highly effective and permitted more rapid detection of underlying problems than did conventional alarms.[307] Neural networks also may provide important specific diagnostic information during complicated critical events in fully integrated monitoring systems.[307,313] However, neural networks have rarely been incorporated into medical devices, in part because of their inability to deduce or "explain" their results, which poses device validation and regulatory approval obstacles.

Alarm Design

A number of factors must be considered in the design of anesthesia alarm systems (see Box 23-5). Most importantly, human factors principles must be applied.[370] The physiologic variables to be monitored and the alarm limits chosen must be carefully selected; the clinical usefulness of alarms will be enhanced with reliable detection and identification of nonalarm states, or *artifact management.* User-friendly output signals, both auditory and visual, must be provided. Because the anesthesiologist cannot always use visual recognition (e.g., during laryngoscopy), in the face of standardized alarm tones, alternative methods must be incorporated into centralized alarm systems (e.g., tactile alarms) to help the clinician rapidly identify which device is sounding an alarm.

Alarm prioritization remains important, especially in fully integrated systems, and the alarm condition must correlate with the clinical level of urgency. Some organizations advocate industry-wide categorization of alarm priorities (e.g., high, medium, low) as well as standardization across medical devices. However, if standards are too restrictive, innovation or new technology may be impeded. For example, the requirements for alarm sounding used in a personal (earpiece) audio system may be significantly different from those needed for general OR broadcast. Ongoing deliberations of national and international standards organizations are an appropriate forum for consensus on some of these issues. In any case, new alarm designs must undergo rigorous clinical testing, in real or accurately simulated conditions, in conjunction with other alarms and sounds that will be normally present.

INTEGRATED MONITORING SYSTEMS

History and Rationale

In 1902, Harvey Cushing[314] recommended that respiration and heart rate be monitored and recorded whenever anesthesia was administered. A few years later, Cushing introduced the measurement of blood pressure, and it was soon recognized that the anesthetic techniques of the time were associated with labile hemodynamics.

Since Cushing's time, more than two dozen clinical variables have been added to the anesthetic record. Commonly, new variables have been monitored simply because a new device or technique permitted their measurement rather than because a careful scientific study demonstrated that monitoring added significantly to patient safety. In fact, definitive studies, if done at all, usually *followed* the introduction of a new, monitored physiologic variable. In addition, research in anesthesia ergonomics has not kept pace with advances in clinical anesthesia and monitoring technology. As a consequence, for many years, the status quo in anesthesia monitoring was a nonintegrated array of multiple monitors, stacked on top of each other and on top of the anesthesia machine. The location of a particular monitor was usually determined by its size and date of acquisition, with smaller or newer monitors stacked on top of older or larger ones. Each monitor had its own displays, sounds, alarm settings, cables, and methods of operation. The haphazard arrangement and complexity of sights and sounds frequently hindered the acquisition of information on which decision making depended. Setting up, calibrating, attaching to the patient, and monitoring these many devices required additional attention, thereby further decreasing the amount of time spent directly observing or interacting with the patient.

The introduction of integrated monitoring systems in the late 1980s occurred as much for economic reasons as for the compelling ergonomic reasons elucidated above. It became significantly less expensive to produce, and thus to purchase, a single integrated monitor in which one microprocessor controlled multiple previously nonintegrated physiologic monitors. The resulting physical integration nonetheless addressed many of the shortcomings of the older, nonintegrated approach. The first generation of integrated OR monitors, which were hastily modified versions of intensive-care monitors, were heavy and bulky and still wound up on top of the anesthesia machine. Second-generation integrated systems (e.g., Space Labs PC2 or Hewlett-Packard Merlin monitors) were more specifically designed for use in the OR by anesthesiologists. With a few exceptions, enhanced versions of these second-generation systems, which remain physically distinct from the anesthesia machine itself, are still in the vast majority of ORs in the United States. New third-generation systems that integrate physiologic monitoring with all other anesthesia machine functions into an anesthesia workstation are slowly gaining market share (Fig. 23-9).

Although tremendous progress has been made in the physical integration of anesthesia monitors, the true integration of data from all clinical sources is still awkward and incomplete in most OR implementations. Modern anesthesia equipment universally incorporates microprocessor-based intelligent systems, and this provides the ability to both gather and present large amounts of clinical information in new ways. However, as systems become more complicated and automated, they may become more susceptible to both machine and human error.[17,243] Little information exists on how monitored data are actually

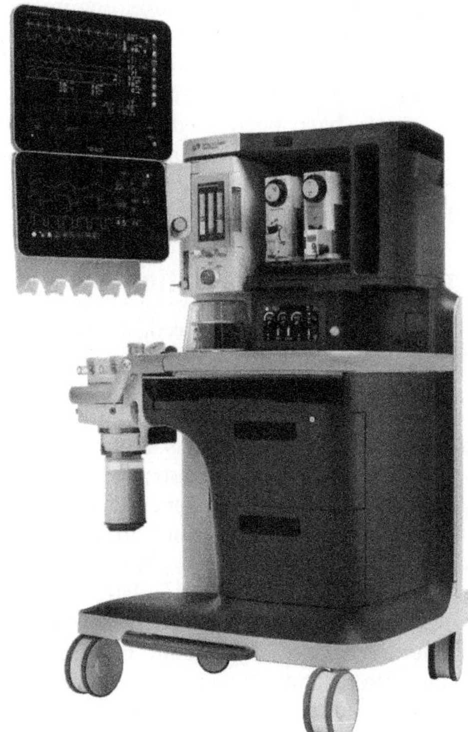

FIGURE 23-9 The Spacelabs Arkon (Spacelabs Healthcare, Issaquah, WA) is an example of a state-of-the-art, fully integrated anesthesia workstation. It seamlessly incorporates a traditional anesthesia machine that includes gas delivery systems, volatile anesthetic delivery systems, and mechanical ventilators with comprehensive physiologic monitoring. Note the use of two data displays; the one on the bottom primarily provides information on gas delivery parameters and anesthesia machine function; the one on the top displays more traditional physiologic cardiovascular and respiratory data. See also Figure 24-16.

TABLE 23-6 **User-Friendliness Scale for the Evaluation and Ranking of Anesthesia Machines and Workstations**

Criteria	Evaluation	Score
Design and Monitoring		
Design	Design, dimensions, and ease of use of the workstation	0 to 10
Screen	Layout and legibility on the monitor	0 to 10
Maintenance		
Self-test	Start-up and self-test of the ventilator	0 to 10
Circuit	Removal and installation of the breathing circuit and absorber of the unit	0 to 10
Absorber	Filling and fitting the absorber	0 to 10
Condensation	Condensation and accumulation of water in the breathing circuit of the unit	0 to 10
Ventilator Use		
Alarms	Setting of alarms (pressure, volume, respiratory rate)	0 to 10
Setting	Setting of ventilation modes	0 to 10
Manual	Manual ventilation with the unit	0 to 10
Switch	Switching from manual to volume-controlled ventilation	0 to 10
	Total Score	0 to 100

The user-friendliness scale evaluated 10 criteria: two criteria of design and monitoring, four of maintenance, and four of ventilation use. Each criterion was evaluated from 0 (poor) to 10 (excellent). The overall score for each tested workstation by a user was calculated on a 100-point basis.

used by clinicians to make decisions.[315,316] The effects of the type of information, display mode, and relationships between them on monitoring performance are still poorly understood. Manufacturers of third-generation workstations are incorporating human factors engineering into their design process. New FDA rules[317] and international standards[250] mandate user-centered design and the consideration of human factors in all medical devices. User-friendliness scales have been used to investigate newer workstations (Table 23-6) with some positive results,[318] and a number of important avenues of research in this area are now under investigation.[63,319-322]

Problem of Physical Integration

The transition from widely scattered, discrete devices to single, integrated systems was slow and painful for several reasons. A large base of installed discrete devices were in use, and the process of replacing them required many years. The integration process itself entails many challenges that relate to physical, electronic, and software issues. Integration implies connection, and unless the same company makes all the components of a monitoring system, there will be incompatibilities—in cabling, in connectors, in signals, and in the software that manipulates and transmits data from one component of the anesthesia workstation to another. The problem of physical and electronic connections was illustrated vividly by reports of overheated pulse oximeter probes when the cable and probe from one manufacturer were connected to another's device.

The software integration process involves *hand shaking*, a digital "meet-and-greet" that sounds easier to arrange than it is, because most companies still have their own unique protocols. For example, one automated anesthetic record-keeping system had to accommodate 75 different protocols to connect to all the available monitors, and one full-time employee in the company did little else but develop handshake protocols. Integrated monitors have vastly simplified the process, especially when the same company or cooperating companies make the workstation, monitors, and record-keeping systems. "Middleware" companies have now appeared that do nothing but facilitate communication among devices and between each device and the hospital information technology (HIT) system. Regardless, as technologic advances lead to new monitoring devices, new devices will continue to be stacked on top of otherwise fully integrated anesthesia workstations. Thus in the absence of comprehensive standards, such as those that allow all consumer stereo components to interface together relatively seamlessly, continued problems related to physical integration of discrete devices can be anticipated. Because of this, a recent attempt to develop an international standard for medical device connection was met with general enthusiasm.

Plug and Play

Bidirectional electronic data communication has been essential to enhancing effectiveness in manufacturing, commerce, banking, and other industries. The ability to interface medical devices with patient care computer systems has been hampered by the lack of an interface standard that meets the unique requirements of the acute patient care setting. One solution was a series of international standards that are collectively called the *Medical Information Bus* (MIB). The MIB promised to be a boon for both manufacturers and users. It would have allowed any two or more pieces of equipment that adhere to the standard to communicate with each other more easily and at a more rapid rate.

The effort to establish the MIB standards began in 1982, when a group of hospitals recognized the problems of medical device interconnection. To meet this challenge, a committee was formed composed of device vendors, computer system vendors, clinical engineers, and clinicians. In 1984, the MIB committee received a sanction from the Institute for Electronic and Electrical

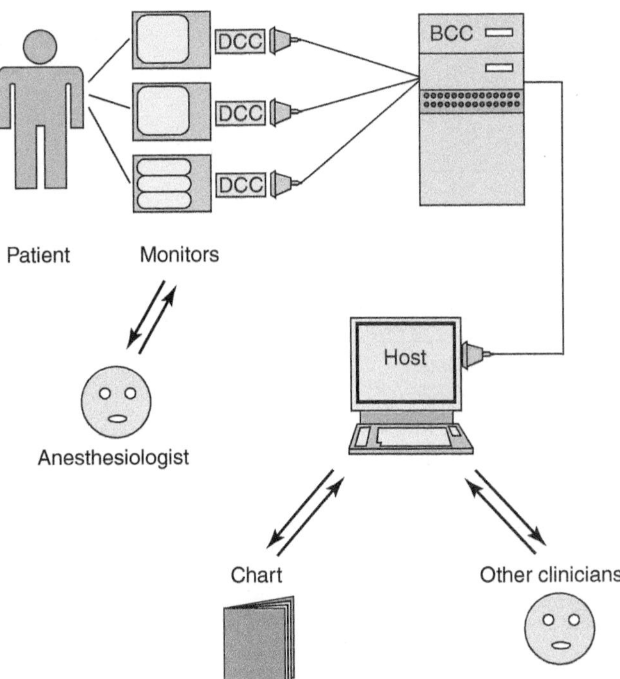

FIGURE 23-10 The medical information bus (MIB) was an attempt at establishing an international standard for hardware and software communication protocols for bidirectional interconnection of medical devices. Not only monitors but computers, record keepers, laboratory equipment, and other devices could easily communicate with one another using the MIB protocol. *DCC,* device communications controller; *BCC,* bedside communications controller. (Modified from Fiegler A, Stead S: The medical information bus. *Biomed Instrum Technol* 1990;24:101-111.)

Engineers (IEEE) to work toward a formal standard (ISO/IEEE 1073). The committee's mission was to develop an international standard for open systems communication in acute health care applications. It was to be modeled after the open systems interconnection (OSI) scheme of "layers" of connectivity.

The MIB was a proposed international standard for bidirectional interconnection of medical devices and computing resources within a medical center or hospital.[323] It specified a local area network (LAN) explicitly designed to provide connection-oriented communication services between medical devices or between medical devices and computers (Fig. 23-10). The LAN was optimized for use in an acute patient care setting. The MIB design goals included 1) to enable host computers to interface with medical devices in a hospital environment in a compatible, vendor-independent fashion; 2) to be highly accurate and reliable; 3) to accommodate the inevitable high frequency of network reconfiguration; 4) to provide a simple user interface, including "plug-and-play" capabilities; and 5) to support a wide range of topologies. Implementation of these objectives was through a family of standards, termed *layers*, that define the overall architecture, electrical characteristics, network characteristics, and software language by which devices will communicate.

The pace of development of the MIB standards was, however, frustratingly slow. By 1996, only two of the seven layers plus the overall framework had been approved. In 2000, the initiative was reborn with the cooperation of European experts as the ISO/IEEE 11073 standard.

TABLE 23-7 Evolution of the Medical Information Bus (IEEE 1073) to the ISO 11073 Standard*

Step	ISO/OSI	Around 2001	Since 2006
7	Application	CEN 13734-Vital	11073-1
6	Presentation	CEN 13735-Intermed	11073-2X
5	Session	CEN 13735-Intermed	11073-2X
4	Transport	IEEE 1073.3X	11073-6X 11073-9X
3	Network	IEE 1073.3x	11073-5x
2	Data link	IEE 1073.3x	11073-3X
1	Physical	IEEE 1073.4x	11073-4x

*The seven-layer open systems interconnection model is also shown for comparison.

IEEE, Institute for Electronic and Electrical Engineers; ISO, International Organization for Standardization; OSI, open systems interconnection.

From Schleifer A: Medical information bus: *Seminar Kommunikationsstandards in der Medizintechnik.* 2010; July:1-12.)

Combining old 1073 standards with evolving European standards resulted in a complete model by 2006 (Table 23-7).[324] Unfortunately, adoption of this standard by industry has not been widespread, with competition from more general computing standards, such as SNMP and XML, as well as from proprietary models offered by large device manufacturers.[325]

One such "standard" is Health Level 7 (HL7), a common language for data interchange at the hospital or enterprise level. Created in 1987, internationally recognized, and now in its third version, HL7 serves as a common language for messaging and data interchange among systems from disparate vendors.[326] A significant new standard, Medical Device Plug and Play (MD PnP), has now been introduced. Beginning in 2004, the MD PnP Interoperability Program introduced the concept of the integrated clinical environment (ICE) as a patient-centric model of interoperability. This culminated in the publication of ASTM standard 2761-2009 describing the new model.[327] The ICE model features the ability to combine clinical information from different devices to enable decision support, distributed control, and closed-loop control. The components of the ICE are shown in Figure 23-11.

Computers in Integrated Monitoring Systems

A major advance in anesthesia equipment was the incorporation of microprocessor-based "intelligent" systems.[328,329] In particular, studies have shown that the precise control of ventilators and measurement of many patient variables can best be performed with microprocessor-based systems.[330] In the 1980s, several institutions developed modular, computer-based anesthesia delivery systems that included the Boston Anesthesia System,[328] the Arizona Program,[331] and the Utah Anesthesia Workstation.[332] These concepts are now being included in new commercial anesthesia workstations.

An understanding of the ergonomic factors that affect the administration of anesthesia will enhance the ability

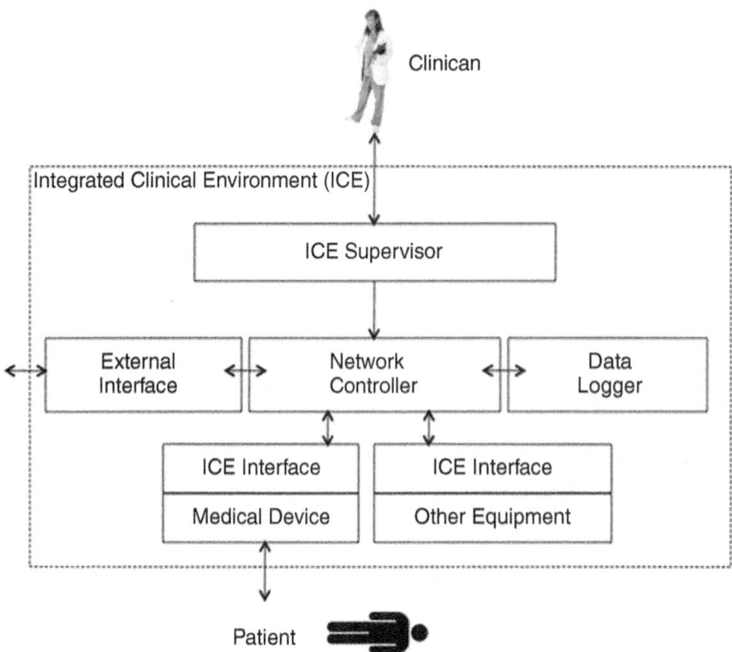

FIGURE 23-11 ■ Functional elements of the integrated clinical environment (ASTM standard F2761-2009).

to effectively implement automated anesthesia tasks, such as drug administration and record keeping; aid in the development of smart alarms; and create novel ways of presenting clinical information. However, if integration and computerization is done poorly, without careful thought and application of human factors design principles (see Chapter 24), poor performance, and the resulting incidence of human error may, in fact, increase.

Data Management in Integrated Displays

One of the major problems in anesthesia monitoring is the need to display a large amount of widely dispersed data in such a way that the human mind can process it efficiently. To pack a lot of information into a small space requires ingenious methods, and many integrated systems currently available do not incorporate appropriate methods to make such compressed data easy to understand. Probably the first attempts to compress clinical information were applied to the EEG and included the compressed spectral array (CSA),[333] the density-modulated spectral array (DSA),[334,335] and aperiodic analysis.[336] These techniques permit the compression of hundreds or thousands of pages of EEG data into just a few pages. More important, the information displayed is much more understandable than the original display. CSA-EEG was included in an early integrated display. The Cerebro Trac (SRD Medical Ltd., Misgav, Israel), an early EEG monitor, was probably the first to use color in a strip-chart format on a monitor screen. The ability to scan both down and across the display allowed the clinician to integrate information easily and to thereby assess cause and effect. An important principle learned from these early integrated displays was that the data must be packed or processed in a way that is intuitive; that is, in a way that corresponds to the "mental model" of the user regarding the source or etiology of the data presented. The compressed analog trend plots found in some modern physiologic displays, such as the one shown in Figure 23-11, can be traced back to these early concepts.

Commercial anesthesia displays have traditionally used time as a variable (i.e., time/effect displays). In contrast, most cockpit displays in aircraft ignore time and simply present the continually changing data, while perhaps also providing an indication of the rate of change. Clinical display designers have explored time-independent display modalities, but few have made it into commercial use. Siegel[337] described a complex polygon-based system for displaying 11 variables in the ICU. The polygon showed one node for each variable, and the distance of the node from the center of the polygon indicated that variable's magnitude. The variables were arranged so that the shape of the polygon could assist the clinician in a quick interpretation of the state of the patient. The Ohmeda CD anesthesia machine (now GE Healthcare, Waukesha, WI) incorporated a similar object display as one of three display options (Fig. 23-12). The Ohmeda polygon contained fewer variables than Siegel's original implementation and, importantly, the Ohmeda CD polygon could be reset at any time to its normal, symmetrical shape. Deneault[338] found that even without training, under simulated conditions, anesthesiologists detected some critical events as well with the polygon system as with a conventional strip-chart (time-based) format. It should be noted, however, that the Ohmeda CD's polygon display was *not* designed to facilitate the use of shape changes to provide specific diagnostic information.

A more rigorous evaluation of the object displays presented on the Ohmeda CD was performed using a partial-task laboratory simulation.[63] The effect of display format on the speed and accuracy of 13 anesthesia residents and five nonmedical volunteers to detect changes in the values of the physiologic variables was measured. Use

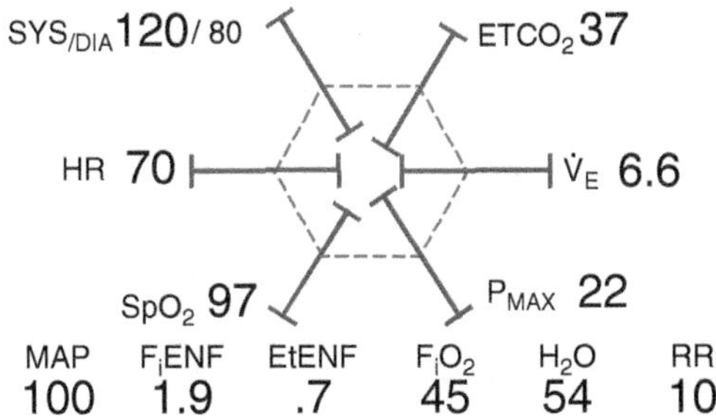

FIGURE 23-12 The polygon display on the Datex-Ohmeda Modulus CD anesthesia machine. The integrated configural display graphically related a number of key physiologic variables. Deformation of the hexagon indicated a deviation from the predefined "normal" physiologic state of the patient. This type of display may be useful for the detection of acute changes in physiologic variables. The use of object displays as an aid to the recognition of evolving clinical conditions in anesthesia is a subject of ongoing research. $ETCO_2$, end-tidal carbon dioxide; EtENF, end-tidal enflurane; FiENF, fraction of inspired enflurane; FiO_2, fraction of inspired oxygen; H_2O, water; HR, heart rate; MAP, mean atrial pressure; P_{MAX}, peak airway presssure; RR, respiratory rate; SpO_2, oxygen saturation; SYS/DIA, systolic/diastolic [pressure]; $\dot{V}_E$, minute ventilation. (Courtesy GE Healthcare, Waukesha, WI.)

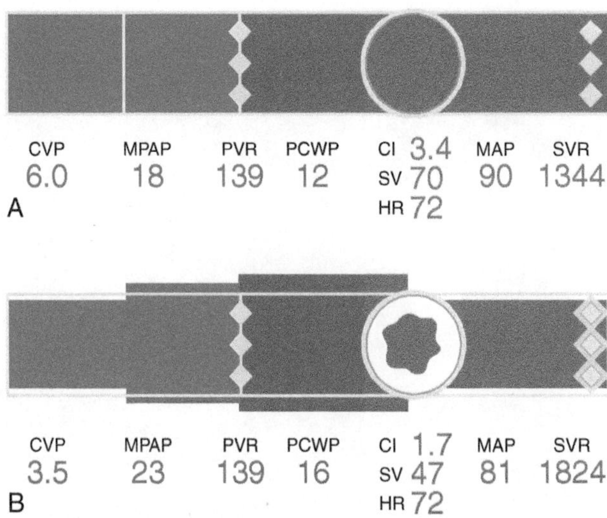

FIGURE 23-13 Advanced physiologic display developed by Westenskow and colleagues at the University of Utah. The display is functionally organized from left to right, depicting normal hemodynamic function (**A**) and the changes with myocardial ischemia (**B**). Advanced display attributes include compressed analog trend plots, alert limits, integrated object display elements in which shape provides additional information (e.g., the product of stroke volume and heart rate is cardiac output), and drug time-concentration plots. CI, cardiac index; CVP, central venous pressure; HR, heart rate; MAP, mean atrial pressure; MPAP, mean pulmonary arterial pressure; PCWP, pulmonary capillary wedge pressure; PVR, pulmonary vascular resistance; SV, stroke volume; SVR, systemic vascular resistance. (From Albert RW, Agutter JA, Syroid ND, et al: A simulation-based evaluation of a graphic cardiovascular display. *Anesth Analg* 2007;105[5]:1303-1311.)

of either the histogram or polygon display format by the anesthesia residents significantly improved detection time and accuracy compared with the numeric display. In contrast, display format did not significantly affect detection time or accuracy in the nonmedical volunteers. The results of this study suggest that graphic displays may enhance the detection of acute changes in patient physiologic status during the administration of anesthesia. More generally, object displays appear to improve detection and recognition of visual patterns, thereby allowing the observer to determine more rapidly the system's overall state. This research also demonstrates the importance of assessing clinical device performance by studying actual intended users.

The results of these clinical studies are consistent with nonclinical display research. In laboratory studies, object displays were superior to bar graph (histogram) displays when the task involved the integration of several individual data values.[339] In contrast, histogram-type displays may provide for faster responses when a change in a single variable must be detected.[340] Object displays appear to be processed "holistically," in which the perception of the whole takes priority over perception of individual parts.[341,342] In process (system) control tasks, especially those involving system uncertainty, graphic displays appear to be superior to numeric displays.[343] The relative disadvantage of numeric displays in these situations may be a consequence of slower serial processing of each individual display element.[344] Thus properly designed object displays may permit more rapid situational assessment and may thereby enhance performance under time stress, particularly when a unique display configuration has specific diagnostic and/or therapeutic implications.[345]

There also appears to be a role for object displays in the clinical diagnosis of complex critical situations.[319,346] For example, Blike's work[347,348] suggests that the use of emergency features, such as graphic features that act as a metaphor for the user's mental model of the underlying system being represented, facilitate the pattern recognition task required to diagnose the etiology of shock. Similarly, two studies from Utah demonstrated that a graphic display of hemodynamic data provided more rapid recognition of adverse events than did "single sensor/single indicator" displays (Fig. 23-13).[349,350]

Advanced displays promise to integrate information seamlessly and to present the data in multiple modalities in hopes of optimizing the use of the available sensory "bandwidth." It is difficult to demonstrate improved outcomes in such a complex environment; therefore studies should focus on response times, perceived workload, and situational awareness.[351]

Design Considerations for Integrated Displays

A large body of literature is available on methods that optimize complex visual displays.[343] Moray[352] enumerates several design priorities for complex display systems. For example, the number of displays and the time required to perceive information should be minimized. The time required to perceive information can be shortened by use of display integration; analog or graphic, rather than digital, visual displays[63,350]; sound and color signatures; highlighting[353]; and poignant visual or audible messages instead of vague, cryptic warnings.[354] Some data suggest that analog displays of information may be easier for the mind to process than digital displays of the same

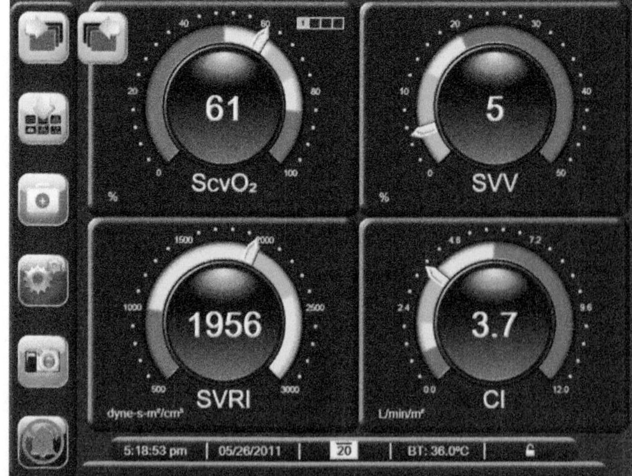

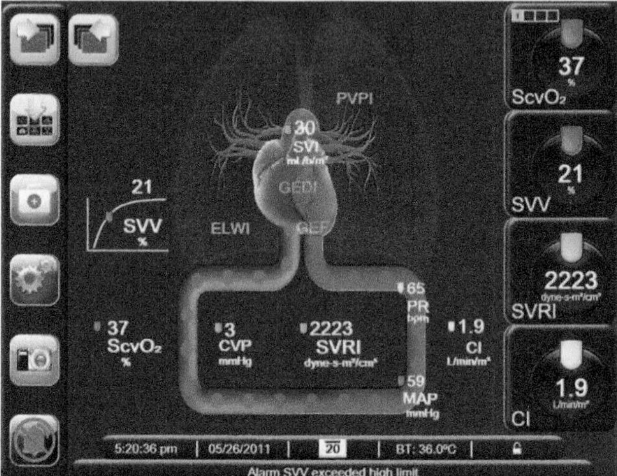

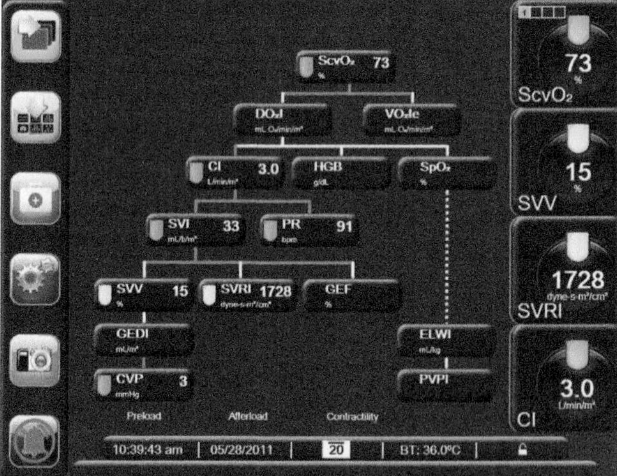

FIGURE 23-14 ■ More advanced displays of physiologic and hemodynamic data use color and shape to call attention to changes as well as to depict relationships among the displayed variables. (Courtesy Edwards Lifesciences, Irvine, CA.)

information, especially in high-workload situations.[63,355] Novel methods of displaying critical information, such as rate-of-change functions,[356] also may improve performance. Integrated displays may be most effective when the displayed variable represents a physiologically relevant interaction of the underlying inputs (e.g., the relationship between heart rate and ejection fraction, as shown in Fig. 23-14).[357] The ultimate integrated display may be the line-drawing face developed by Fukui,[358] in which a few simple lines indicate the patient's status in a format that incorporates everyday experience. However, "logical" designs of displays may not achieve the intended responses and results,[359] and the results also underscore the difficulty of developing a theory of display design.

Modern Integrated Operating Room Monitor

Until recently, logical design concepts were only sporadically applied to anesthesia monitors.[360-362] However, modern anesthesia monitors now incorporate most, if not all, of the important physiologic variables into a single integrated display (Figs. 23-15 to 23-17). These monitors often include ST-segment analysis, cardiac output calculations, respiratory and cardiovascular parameters (Fig. 23-15), real-time on-screen help (Fig. 23-16), and even access to clinical information (Fig. 23-17). Portable monitors are equally sophisticated (Fig. 23-18), and integration of physiologic monitors with electronic anesthesia record keepers continues to increase in popularity (Fig. 23-19; see also Chapter 22). Nonetheless, the design and introduction of newer monitoring devices does not always fully address the needs of the user in the planning and design of displays.[363]

Manufacturers of monitoring equipment have attempted to design their clinical monitors to interface relatively smoothly with existing anesthesia machines (Fig. 23-20). In addition, the software for many modern physiologic monitors runs on off-the-shelf computer hardware, thereby facilitating integration and lowering cost. Finally, most OR monitoring systems are networked together, usually via a nonproprietary architecture. This allows centralized printing and data archiving and facilitates communication with other hospital computers (e.g., to obtain laboratory data) and with other facilities.

Unfortunately, many current devices still have significant shortcomings from an ergonomics standpoint. For example, displays may be crowded and difficult to read, especially during high-workload situations. In the most common menu-driven schemes, crucial waveform and other clinical data may disappear when the user is performing other, secondary tasks such as cardiac output measurement.

At a higher level of integration, all the major anesthesia machine manufacturers have now introduced state-of-the-art integrated anesthesia workstations; these include not only gas and drug delivery systems but also systems that monitor those functions in addition to fully integrated comprehensive clinical monitoring systems (Fig. 23-21). Designers of these third-generation anesthesia workstations appear to have paid more attention to the human–device interface issues.[318] The importance of incorporating human factors into monitors, anesthesia workstations, and other medical devices has been recognized by the federal government. FDA regulations since 1997 have required all manufacturers to incorporate human factors into the design and development of all medical devices.[317]

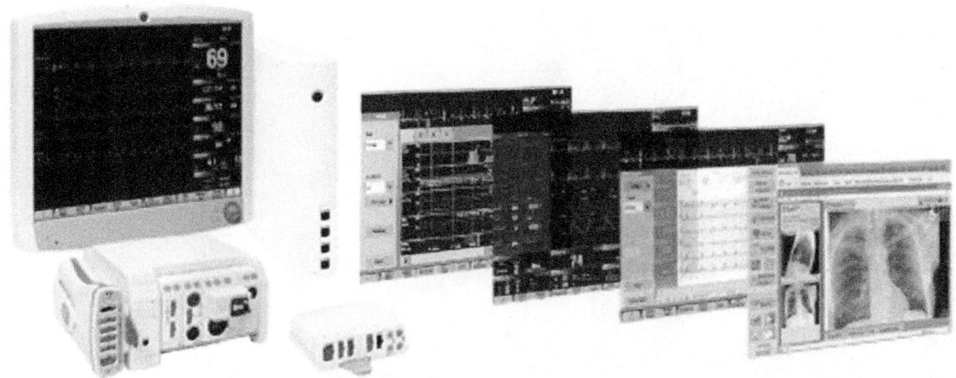

FIGURE 23-15 ■ The Marquette Solar 9500 (GE Healthcare, Waukesha, WI). This integrated physiologic monitor incorporates a full spectrum of cardiovascular and respiratory variables and performs secondary computer processing to display valuable additional clinical information such as ST-segment analysis and cardiac output calculations. Data are presented in multicolor displays in both analog and digital display formats.

Event Setup (Group 4)

Group Name:	Ventil.	Deactivated
Group Type:	Standard	
Notification Type:	None	
Episode Type:	HighRes Trend (4 min): -2 / +2 min	
Trigger Condition:	At Least One Param.	Enhanced ...

HR (Pulse)	*** EXTREME TACHY *** EXTREME BRADY
SpO_2	All ***/** Alarms <Blank>
Resp	All ***/** Alarms <Blank>
$etCO_2$	All ***/** Alarms <Blank>

FIGURE 23-16 ■ Most integrated monitors provide real-time on-screen help. In this example, help is provided for a problem with pacemaker rhythm detection.

Further Issues in Complex Integrated Systems

One advantage of fully computerized systems is that each piece of data can be presented in the context appropriate to the system's current state and the user's immediate needs. Hundreds or thousands of different screens, or menus, are potentially possible, and a hierarchical organization may be inadequate to provide guidance to the user attempting to navigate through the display system.[364] Unfortunately, design guidelines for the relationships between multiple interrelated menus and displays are generally lacking.

With integrated displays, the critical design pitfalls are in the relationships and interactions between displays. Design errors at this level can lead to problems such as having to navigate through too many useless or inefficient displays; getting lost in the display network; tunnel vision or "keyhole" effects, such as restriction to a small subset of displays; and mental overload related to management of the data presented.[364] Woods's comment regarding displays in nuclear power plant control rooms applies equally well to the anesthesia domain[364]: "Given that one of the problems in existing control centers is data overload in rapidly changing circumstances, the shift to more computer-based systems can exacerbate this problem as well as mitigate it." Perhaps paradoxically, the use of rapid prototyping by designers can lead to a proliferation of display screens ("Since we can do it, why not include it?") without adequate consideration of the navigational requirements between displays.

The amount of potentially displayable data is always much larger than the amount of physically available screen space. In complex integrated display systems, the user will have difficulty maintaining a broad overview of system status, especially when required to navigate frequently through multiple displays.[364] One commercially available OR monitor had more than 150 different menu display screens. Additionally, data from modeling of drug concentrations in the patient have been added to the currently existing displays of physiologic data. Research has modeled and simulated the results of these data, which are used in enhancing performance in clinical settings.[365,366] It is therefore important to provide "overview displays" that rapidly present crucial aspects of system status. Wearable head-mounted displays also promise to open up available real estate for presentation of visual information, but their efficacy has yet to be demonstrated.[367]

The ultimate goal of the integrated clinical monitors of the future will be to present only the data the anesthesiologist actually requires at precisely the time required. Information overload must be minimized. Clinical decision making will be enhanced if the relationship between individual physiologic variables is readily apparent. Thus, to accomplish these goals, future displays must use a variety of techniques that include display integration, graphic rather than digital display, sound and color signatures, animation, highlighting, and poignant visual or audible messages. Novel methods of displaying critical information including rate-of-change functions should also be used. A promising approach, validated in the military setting, is the use of sophisticated object displays that contain animated iconic representations that mirror the anesthesiologist's mental model of human physiologic processes (Fig. 23-22, right side of screen).

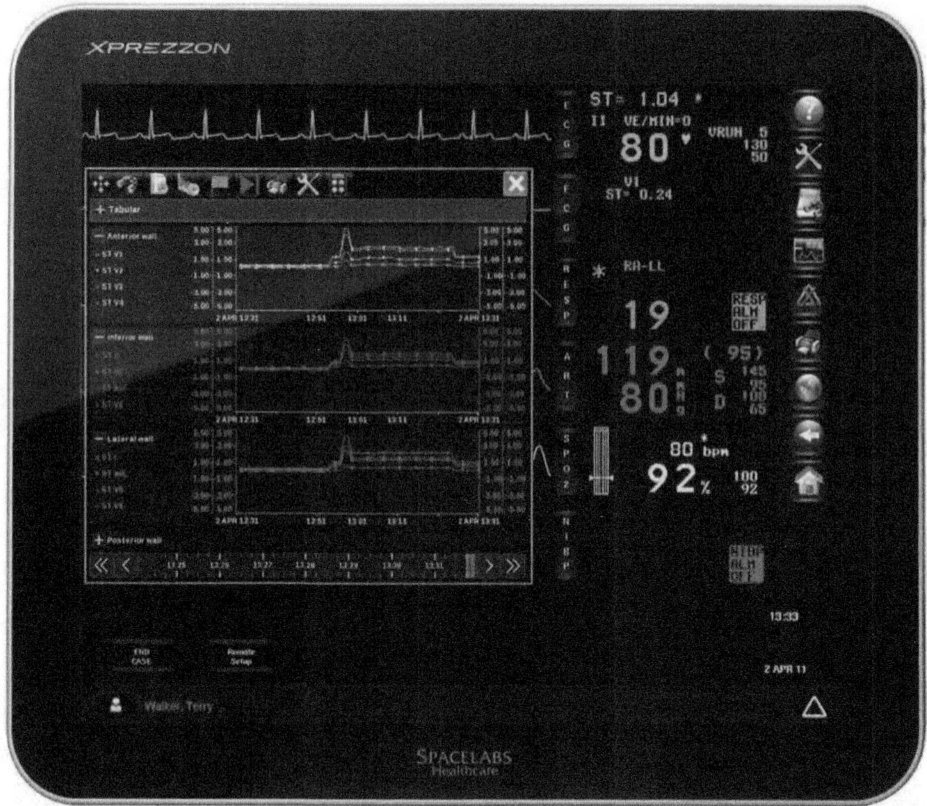

FIGURE 23-17 ■ Many modern operating room monitors incorporate off-the-shelf commercial software and hardware. The use of a commercial computer operating system such as Windows or UNIX facilitates the addition of valuable features by other developers. For example, the Spacelabs PC2 system (Spacelabs Healthcare, Issaquah, WA) can run optional software modules that provide the clinician with valuable clinical information and other reference materials.

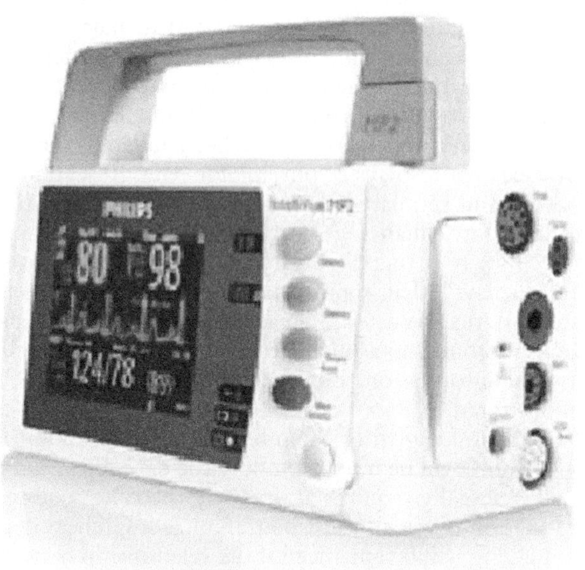

FIGURE 23-18 ■ Sophisticated multiparameter monitors are now available throughout the hospital. In fact, portable monitors such as the Philips MP2 (Philips Healthcare, Andover, MA) are capable of providing high-level display and processing functionality in a relatively lightweight and compact package.

CONCLUSIONS

The administration of anesthesia incorporates a complex monitoring task and, as such, requires vigilance. Human error has been claimed to be a major cause of most anesthetic mishaps. However, poorly designed equipment also contributes to the occurrence of error in anesthesia practice. Human performance is often less than optimal and is particularly susceptible to degradation by a variety of human, environmental, equipment, and system factors. Designers of anesthetic equipment therefore must assist the anesthesiologist by incorporating devices and technologies to augment vigilance and enhance monitoring performance. Alarms intended to notify the user of potential critical situations are effective only when properly designed and implemented.[368]

The completely integrated anesthesia workstation that contains truly intelligent decision support, smart alarms, and closed-loop control systems is still on the horizon. Its successful implementation will require a more complete understanding of the task of administering anesthesia and of the factors that affect performance of the anesthesiologist in this complex task environment.

ACKNOWLEDGMENT

We gratefully acknowledge the contributions, advice, and support of Carl E. Englund, Larry T. Dallen, Holly Forcier, Steve Howard, and David Gaba. Norman Ty Smith was a critical contributor to the previous version of the chapter.

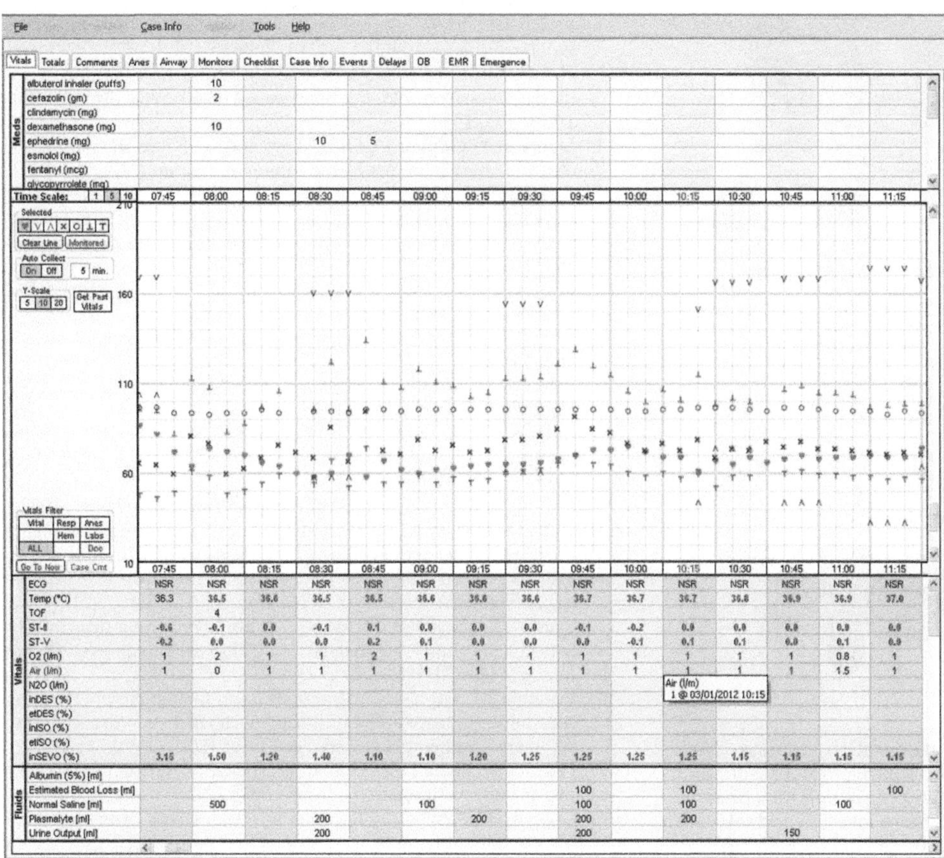

FIGURE 23-19 ■ Electronic anesthesia record-keeping devices, such as this one by Acuitec (Birmingham, AL), may increasingly incorporate traditional physiologic displays, including digital values, analog waveforms, and trend plots.

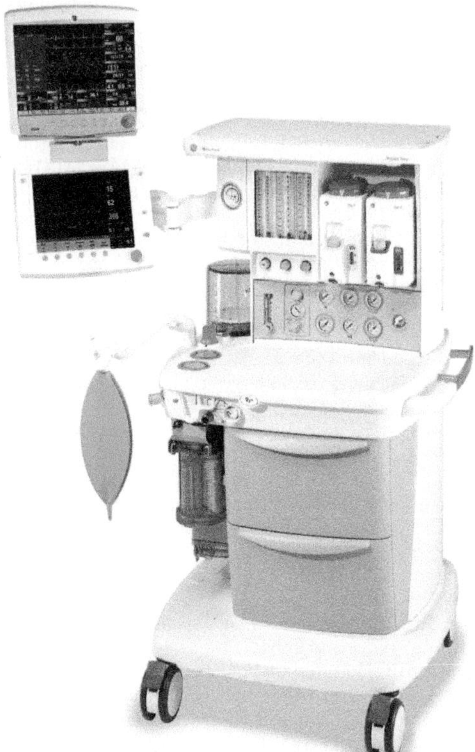

FIGURE 23-20 ■ The Hewlett-Packard (Palo Alto, CA) Merlin system integrated into an Ohmeda Excel anesthesia machine. The collaboration between different manufacturers, such as those that make monitors and those that make anesthesia machines, has resulted in unprecedented interconnectivity to produce well-integrated anesthesia workstations. Many manufacturers now recognize the potential value of the open architecture approach. (Courtesy GE Healthcare, Waukesha, WI.)

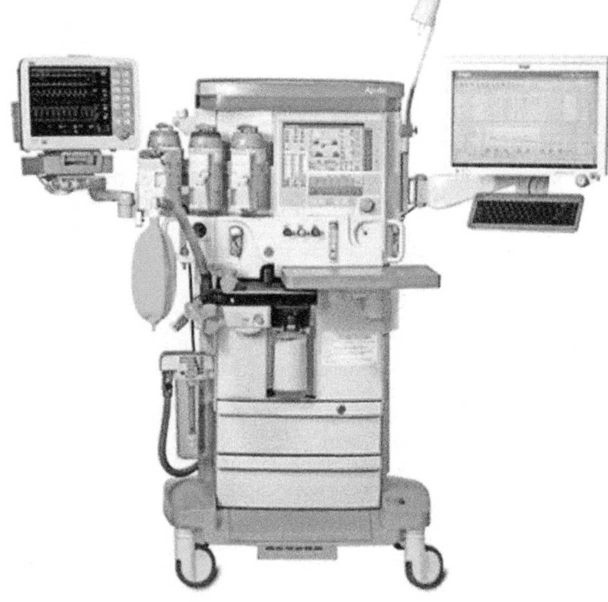

FIGURE 23-21 ■ Dräger Apollo anesthesia workstation. This system takes advantage of the latest technological innovations to fully integrate traditional anesthesia machine functions with physiologic monitoring and electronic record keeping.

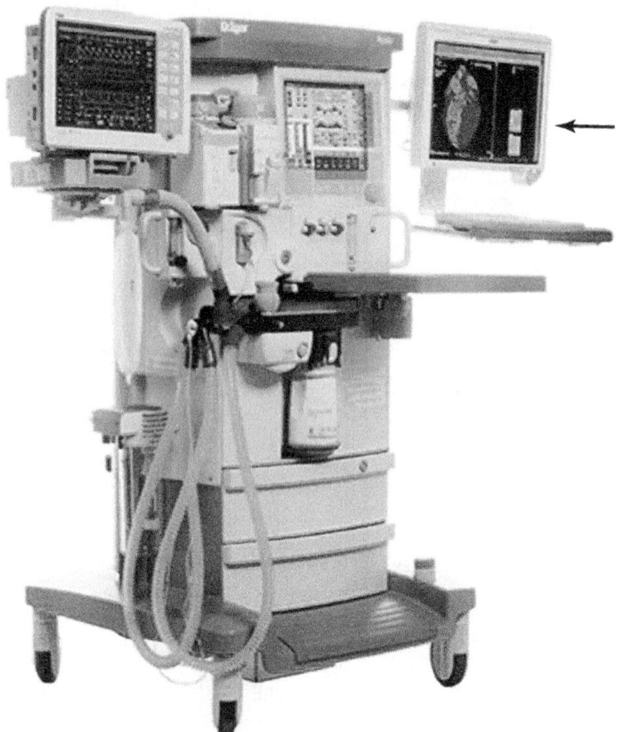

FIGURE 23-22 Integrated anesthesia workstation displays. New technology will take advantage of powerful microprocessors and improved understanding of the human physiologic response to anesthesia to present clinical data in a more intuitive and relevant manner. Note the logical positioning of redundant information. Animation could be used (e.g., a beating heart, *arrow*) to provide increased information content that would obviate the need for waveform displays. Trending of data (not shown) could also be readily incorporated into the display. (Courtesy Dräger Medical, Telford, PA.)

REFERENCES

1. Ansermino JM: Can technology further improve the safety of anesthesia? *Conf Proc IEEE Eng Med Biol Soc* 2008:1026–1027, 2008.
2. Keenan RL, Boyan P: Cardiac arrest due to anesthesia, *JAMA* 253:2373–2377, 1985.
3. Abenstein JP, Warner MA: Anesthesia providers, patient outcomes, and costs, *Anesth Analg* 82:1273–1283, 1996.
4. Lienhart A, Auroy Y, Pequignot F, et al: Survey of anesthesia-related mortality in France, *Anesthesiology* 105(6):1087–1097, 2006.
5. Forrest JB, Cahalan MK, Rehder K, et al: Multicenter study of general anesthesia: II. Results, *Anesthesiology* 72:262–268, 1990.
6. Oken A, Rasmussen MD, Slagle JM, et al: A facilitated survey instrument captures significantly more anesthesia events than does traditional voluntary event reporting, *Anesthesiology* 107(6):909–922, 2007.
7. Craig J, Wilson ME: A survey of anaesthetic misadventures, *Anaesthesia* 36:933–936, 1981.
8. Olsson G, Hallen B: Cardiac arrest during anesthesia: a computer-aided study in 250,543 anesthetics, *Acta Anaesth Scand* 32:653–664, 1988.
9. Utting J, Gray T, Shelley F: Human misadventure in anaesthesia, *Can Anaesth Soc J* 26:73–79, 1979.
10. Williamson JA, Webb RK, Sellen A, Runciman WB, Van der Walt JH: The Australian Incident Monitoring Study. Human failure: an analysis of 2000 incident reports, *Anaesth Intensive Care* 21:678–683, 1993.
11. Cooper JB, Newbower RS, Long CD, McPeek B: Preventable anesthesia mishaps: a study of human factors, *Anesthesiology* 49:399–406, 1978.
12. Bhananker SM, Posner KL, Cheney FW, et al: Injury and liability associated with monitored anesthesia care: a closed claims analysis, *Anesthesiology* 104(2):228–234, 2006.
13. Holland R: Special committee investigating deaths under anesthesia: report on 745 classified cases, 1960-1968, *Med J Austr* 1:573–593, 1970.
14. Donchin Y, Gopher D, Olin M, et al: A look into the nature and causes of human errors in the intensive care unit, *Crit Care Med* 23:294–300, 1995.
15. Runciman WB, Webb RK, Lee R, Holland R: System failure: an analysis of 2000 incident reports, *Anaesth Intensive Care* 21:684–695, 1993.
16. Frankmann JP, Adams JA: Theories of vigilance, *Psychol Bull* 59:257–272, 1962.
17. Allnutt MF: Human factors in accidents, *Br J Anaesth* 59(7):856–864, 1987.
18. Salvendy G: *Handbook of human factors and ergonomics*, ed 3, New York, 2005, John Wiley and Sons.
19. Billings CE, Reynard WD: Human factors in aircraft incidents: results of a 7 year study, *Aviat Space Environ Med* 55:960–965, 1984.
20. Rolfe J: Ergonomics and air safety, *Appl Ergonom* 3:75–81, 1972.
21. Gaba DM, Maxwell M, DeAnda A: Anesthetic mishaps: breaking the chain of accident evolution, *Anesthesiology* 66:670–676, 1987.
22. Sharit J: Human error. In Salvendy G, editor: *Handbook of human factors and ergonomics*. New York, 2006, John Wiley & Sons, pp 708–760.
23. Currie M, Mackay P, Morgan C, et al: The "wrong drug" problem in anaesthesia: an analysis of 2000 incident reports, *Anaesth Intensive Care* 21:596–601, 1993.
24. Weinger M, Englund C: Ergonomic and human factors affecting anesthetic vigilance and monitoring performance in the operating room environment, *Anesthesiology* 73:995–1021, 1990.
25. DeAnda A, Gaba DM: Unplanned incidents during comprehensive anesthesia simulation, *Anesth Analg* 71:77–82, 1990.
26. Cooper JB, Newbower RS, Kitz RJ: An analysis of major errors and equipment failures in anesthesia management: considerations for prevention and detection, *Anesthesiology* 60:34–42, 1984.
27. Reason J: *Human error*, Cambridge, MA, 1990, Cambridge University Press.
28. Tversky A, Kahneman D: Judgment under uncertainty: heuristics and biases, *Science* 185:1124–1131, 1974.
29. Gaba DM, Howard SK, Small SD: Situation awareness in anesthesiology, *Hum Factors* 37, 1995.
30. Cosby KS, Croskerry P: Profiles in patient safety: authority gradients in medical error, *Acad Emerg Med* 11(12):1341–1345, 2004.
31. Gaba DM: Human error in anesthetic mishaps, *Int Anesth Clin* 27:137–147, 1989.
32. Runciman WB, Sellen A, Webb RK, et al: Errors, incidents, and accidents in anaesthetic practice, *Anaesth Intensive Care* 21:506–519, 1993.
33. Arnstein F: Catalogue of human error, *Br J Anaesth* 79:645–656, 1997.
34. Bell TE: The limits of risk analysis, *IEEE Spectrum* 26:51, 1989.
35. Bell TE: Managing risk in large complex systems, *IEEE Spectrum* 26:22–23, 1989.
36. Norman D: *The psychology of everyday things*, New York, 1988, Basic Books.
37. Woods DD, Cook RI, Billings CE: The impact of technology on physician cognition and performance, *J Clin Monit* 11:5–8, 1995.
38. Stroh C: *Vigilance: the problem of sustained attention*, Oxford, UK, 1971, Pergamon Press.
39. Mackworth NH: Some factors affecting vigilance, *Advance Sci* 53:389–393, 1957.
40. Warm J: *Sustained attention in human performance*, New York, 1984, John Wiley and Sons.
41. Weinger MB, Herndon OW, Gaba DM: The effect of electronic record keeping and transesophageal echocardiography on task distribution, workload, and vigilance during cardiac anesthesia, *Anesthesiology* 87:144–155, 1997.
42. See JE, Howe SR, Warm JS, Dember WN: Meta-analysis of the sensitivity decrement in vigilance, *Psychol Bull* 117:230–249, 1995.
43. Singleton W: *The analysis of practical skills*, Lancaster, UK, 1978, MTP Press.
44. Sen R, Ganguli A: An ergonomic analysis of railway locomotive driver functions in India, *J Hum Ergol* 11:187–202, 1982.

45. Kogi K, Ohta T: Incidence of near accidental drowsing in locomotive driving during a period of rotation, *J Hum Ergol* 4:65–76, 1975.
46. Luoma J: Perception and eye movements in simulated traffic situations, *Acta Ophthalmol Suppl* 161:128–134, 1984.
47. Woods D, Wise J, Hanes L: An evaluation of nuclear power plant safety parameter display systems, *Proc Hum Factors Soc* 25:110–114, 1981.
48. Headley D, Hiller J: *MANPRINT guidebook for systems design and assessment 1997*. Accessed online 2012 Feb 14 at http://www.mitre.org/work/sepo/toolkits/risk/taxonomies/files/MANPRINT_Guidebook.DOC.
49. Thackray RI, Bailey JP, Touchstone RM: The effect of increased monitoring load on vigilance performance using a simulated radar display, *Ergonomics* 22:529–539, 1979.
50. Wilkinson RT: Some factors influencing the effect of environmental stressors upon performance, *Psychol Bull* 72:262–270, 1969.
51. Chiles WD: Workload, task, and situational factors as modifiers of complex human performance. In Alluisi EA, Fleishman EE, editors: *Human performance and productivity: stress and performance effectiveness*, Hillsdale, NJ, 1982, Lawrence Erlbaum Associates, pp 32–36.
52. Weinger M: Human factors in anesthesiology. In Carayon P, editor: *Handbook of human factors and ergonomics in health care and patient safety*, Boca Raton, 2012, CRC Press, pp 803–823.
53. Drui AB, Behm RJ, Martin WE: Predesign investigation of the anesthesia operational environment, *Anesth Analg* 52:584–591, 1973.
54. Boquet G, Bushman JA, Davenport HT: The anaesthetic machine: a study of function and design, *Br J Anaesth* 52(1):61–67, 1980.
55. Kennedy PJ, Fiengold F, Wiener EL, Hosek RS: Analysis of tasks and human factors in anesthesia for coronary-artery bypass, *Anesth Analg* 55:374–377, 1976.
56. McDonald J, Dzwonczyk R: A time and motion study of the anaesthetist's intraoperative time, *Br J Anaesth* 61:738–742, 1988.
57. McDonald J, Dzwonczuk R, Gupta B, Dahl M: A second time-study of the anaesthetist's intraoperative period, *Br J Anaesth* 64:582–585, 1990.
58. Allard J, Dzwonczyk DY, Block FE Jr, McDonald JS: Effect of automatic record keeping on vigilance and record keeping time, *Br J Anaesth* 74:619–626, 1995.
59. Weinger MB, Herndon OW, Paulus MP, et al: An Objective methodology for task analysis and workload assessment of anesthesia providers, *Anesthesiology* 80:77–92, 1994.
60. Cooper JO, Cullen BF: Observer reliability in detecting surreptitious random occlusions of the monaural esophageal stethoscope, *J Clin Monit* 6:271–275, 1990.
61. Loeb RG: A measure of intraoperative attention to monitor displays, *Anesth Analg* 76:337–341, 1993.
62. Loeb RG: Monitor surveillance and vigilance of anesthesia residents, *Anesthesiology* 80:527–533, 1994.
63. Gurushanthaiah K, Weinger MB, Englund CE: Visual display format affects the ability of anesthesiologists to detect acute physiologic changes: a laboratory study employing a clinical display simulator, *Anesthesiology* 83:1184–1193, 1995.
64. Shapiro R, Berland T: Noise in the operating room, *N Engl J Med* 287:1236–1238, 1972.
65. Ray CD, Levinson R: Noise pollution in the operating room: a hazard to surgeons, personnel, and patients, *J Spinal Disord* 5(4):485–488, 1992.
66. Hasfeldt D, Laerkner E, Birkelund R: Noise in the operating room: what do we know? A review of the literature, *J Perianesth Nurs* 25(6):380–386, 2010.
67. Broadbent D: Human performance and noise. In Harris CE, editor: *Handbook of noise control*, New York, 1979, McGraw-Hill.
68. Hockey GRJ: Effects of noise on human work efficiency. In May DE, editor: *Handbook of noise assessment*, New York, 1978, Van Nostrand Reinhold, pp 335–372.
69. Jones DM: Noise. In Hockey R, editor: *Stress and fatigue in human performance*, Chichester, England, 1983, John Wiley and Sons, pp 61–95.
70. Poulton E: A new look at the effects of noise: a rejoiner, *Psychol Bull* 85:1068–1079, 1978.
71. Eschenbrenner AJ: Effects of intermittent noise on the performance of a complex psychomotor task, *Hum Factors* 13:59–63, 1971.
72. Andrén L, Hansson L, Björkman M, Jonsson A: Noise as a contributory factor in the development of arterial hypertension, *Acta Med Scand* 207:493–498, 1980.
73. Alapetite A: Impact of noise and other factors on speech recognition in anaesthesia, *Int J Med Inform* 77(1):68–77, 2008.
74. Miles C, Auburn T, Jones D: Effects of loud noise and signal probability on visual vigilance, *Ergonomics* 27:855–862, 1984.
75. Hartley LR, Williams T: Steady state noise and music and vigilance, *Ergonomics* 20:277–285, 1977.
76. Fontaine CW, Schwalm ND: Effects of familiarity of music on vigilant performance, *Percept Motor Skills* 49:71–74, 1979.
77. Wolf R, Weiner F: Effects of four noise conditions on arithmetic performance, *Percept Motor Skills* 35:928–930, 1972.
78. Allen K, Blascovich J: Effects of music on cardiovascular reactivity among surgeons, *JAMA* 272:882–884, 1994.
79. Weinger MB: Cardiovascular reactivity among surgeons: not music to everyone's ears, *JAMA* 273(14):1090–1091, 1995.
80. Swamidoss C, Bell C, Sevarino F, et al: Effects of music on simulated task performance by anesthesiologists [abstract], *Anesth Analg* 84:S215, 1997.
81. Ramsey J: Heat and cold. In Hockey G, editor: *Stress and fatigue in human performance*, Chichester, England, 1983, John Wiley and Sons, pp 33–60.
82. Fine BJ, Kobrick JL: Effect of heat and chemical protective clothing on cognitive performance, *Aviat Space Environ Med* 58:149–154, 1987.
83. Epstein Y, Keren G, Moisseier J, Gasko O, Yachin S: Psychomotor deterioration during exposure to heat, *Aviat Space Environ Med* 51:607–610, 1980.
84. Ellis HD: The effects of cold on the performance of serial choice reaction time and various discrete tasks, *Hum Factors* 24:589–598, 1982.
85. Baddeley A, Cuccuro W, Egstrom G, Weltman G, Willis M: Cognitive efficiency of divers working in cold water, *Hum Factors* 17:446–454, 1975.
86. Ramsey J, Burford C, Beshir M, Jensen R: Effects of workplace thermal conditions on safe work behavior, *J Safety Res* 14:105–114, 1983.
87. Bruce DL, Bach MJ, Arbit J: Trace anesthetic effects on perceptual, cognitive, and motor skills, *Anesthesiology* 40:453–458, 1974.
88. Smith G, Shirley A: A review of the effects of trace concentrations of anaesthetics on performance, *Br J Anaesth* 50:701–712, 1978.
89. Stollery BT, Broadbent DE, Lee WT, et al: Mood and cognitive functions in anaesthetists working in actively scavenged operating theatres, *Br J Anaesth* 61:446–455, 1988.
90. Boucek C, Freeman JA, Bircher NG, Tullock W: Impairment of anesthesia task performance by laser protection goggles, *Anesth Analg* 77:1232–1237, 1993.
91. Hockey GRJ: Changes in operator efficiency as a function of environmental stress, fatigue and circadian rhythms. In Boff KR, Kaufman L, Thomas JE, editors: *Handbook of perception and human performance*, vol II, New York, 1986, John Wiley and Sons, pp 1–49.
92. Holding DH: *Fatigue*. In Hockey R, editor: *Stress and fatigue in human performance*, New York, 1983, John Wiley and Sons, pp 145–168.
93. Dodge R: Circadian rhythms and fatigue: a discrimination of their effects on performance, *Aviat Space Environ Med* 53:1131–1136, 1982.
94. Parker J: The effects of fatigue on physician performance: an underestimated cause of physician impairment and increased patient risk, *Can J Anaesth* 34:489–495, 1987.
95. Englund CE, Ryman DH, Naitoh P, Hodgdon JA: Cognitive performance during successive sustained physical work episodes, *Behav Res Meth Instru Comp* 17:75–85, 1985.
96. Englund CE, Krueger GP: Introduction to special section "Methodological approaches to the study of sustained work/sustained operations." *Behav Res Meth Instru Comp* 17:3–5, 1985.
97. Krueger GP, Englund CE: Methodological approaches to the study of sustained work/sustained operations, *Behav Res Meth Instru Comp* 17:587–591, 1985.
98. Haslam DR: Sleep loss, recovery sleep, and military performance, *Ergonomics* 25:163–178, 1982.
99. Åkerstedt T: Field studies of shiftwork: II. Temporal patterns in psychophysiological activation in workers alternating between night and day work, *Ergonomics* 20:621–631, 1977.

100. Friedman RC, Bigger JT, Kornfield DS: The intern and sleep loss, *N Engl J Med* 285:201–203, 1971.
101. Haslam DR: The military performance of soldiers in sustained operations, *Aviat Space Environ Med* 55:216–221, 1984.
102. Johnson LC, Naitoh P: *The operational consequences of sleep deprivation and sleep deficit (AGARD Report No. AG-192)*, London, 1974, North Atlantic Treaty Organization.
103. Morgan B, Brown B, Alluisi EA: Effects on sustained performance of 48 hours of continuous work and sleep loss, *Hum Factors* 16:406–414, 1974.
104. Krueger GP: Sustained work, fatigue, sleep loss and performance: a review of the issues, *Work Stress* 3:129–141, 1989.
105. Alluisi EA, Morgan BB: Temporal factors in human performance and productivity. In Alluisi E, Fleishman EE, editors: *Human performance and productivity 3: stress and performance effectiveness*, Hillsdale, NJ, 1982, Lawrence Erlbaum Associates, pp 165–247.
106. Dawson D, Reid K: Fatigue, alcohol and performance impairment, *Nature* 388(6639):235, 1997.
107. Webb W: *Sleep: the gentle tyrant*, Englewood Cliffs, NJ, 1975, Prentice-Hall.
108. Williams H, Lubin A, Goodnow J: Impaired performance with acute sleep loss, *Psychol Monogr* 73:1–26, 1959.
109. Wilkinson R: Interaction of lack of sleep with knowledge of results, repeated testing and individual differences, *J Exp Psychol* 62:263–271, 1961.
110. Wilkinson R: Rest pauses in a task affected by lack of sleep, *Ergonomics* 2:373–380, 1959.
111. Wilkinson R: The effect of lack of sleep on visual watchkeeping, *Q J Exp Psychol* 12:36–40, 1960.
112. Williams H, Kearney O, Lubin A: Signal uncertainty and sleep loss, *J Exp Psychol* 69:401–407, 1965.
113. Williams H, Greseking C, Lubin A: Some effects of sleep loss on memory, *Percept Mot Skill* 23:1287–1293, 1966.
114. Hockey GRJ: Changes in attention allocation in a multi-component task under loss of sleep, *Br J Psychol* 61:473–480, 1970.
115. Hockey GRJ: Changes in information selection patterns in multi-source monitoring as a function of induced arousal shifts, *J Exp Psychol* 101:35–42, 1973.
116. Haslam DR: The military performance of soldiers in continuous operations: exercise "Early Call" I and II. In Johnson LC, Tepas DI, Colquhoun W, et al, editors: *The twenty-four hour workday: Symposium on variations in work-sleep schedules*, Cincinnati, 1981, Department of Health and Human Services (NIOSH), pp 81–127.
117. Naitoh P, Angus R: Napping and human functioning during prolonged work. In Dinges DF, Broughton R, editors: *Sleep and alertness: chronobiological behavior and medical aspects of napping*, New York, 1989, Raven Press, pp 221–246.
118. Brown D: Performance maintenance during continuous flight operations: a guide for flight surgeons. U.S, Navy medical publication NAVMED P-6410, 2000.
119. Naitoh P: Circadian cycles and restorative power of naps. In Johnson L, Tepas D, Colquhoun W, Colligan M, editors: *Biological rhythms, sleep, and shiftwork*, New York, 1981, Spectrum, pp 553–580.
120. Dinges DF, Orne MT, Orne EC: Assessing performance upon abrupt awakening from naps during quasi-continuous operations, *Behav Res Meth Instru Comp* 17:37–45, 1985.
121. Hart R, Buchsbaum D, Wade J, Hamer R, Kwentus J: Effect of sleep deprivation on first-year residents' response times, memory, and mood, *J Med Educ* 62:940–942, 1987.
122. Lockley SW, Cronin JW, Evans EE, et al: Effect of reducing interns' weekly work hours on sleep and attentional failures, *N Engl J Med* 351(18):1829–1837, 2004.
123. Landrigan CP, Rothschild JM, Cronin JW, et al: Effect of reducing interns' work hours on serious medical errors in intensive care units, *N Engl J Med* 351(18):1838–1848, 2004.
124. Ayas NT, Barger LK, Cade BE, et al: Extended work duration and the risk of self-reported percutaneous injuries in interns, *JAMA* 296(9):1055–1062, 2006.
125. Rothschild JM, Keohane CA, Rogers S, et al: Risks of complications by attending physicians after performing nighttime procedures, *JAMA* 302(14):1565–1572, 2009.
126. Veasey S, Rosen R, Barzansky B, Rosen I, Owens J: Sleep loss and fatigue in residency training: a reappraisal, *JAMA* 288(9):1116–1124, 2002.
127. Weinger MB, Ancoli-Israel S: Sleep deprivation and clinical performance, *JAMA* 287:955–957, 2002.
128. Lees DE: New York state regulations to be implemented: work hours, resident supervision, anesthesia monitors mandated, *APSF Newslett* 3:18–24, 1988.
129. Englund CE: *Human chronopsychology: an autorhythmic study of circadian periodicity in learning, mood and task performance* [doctoral dissertation], San Diego, 1979, United States International University.
130. Turnbull R: Diurnal cycles and work-rest scheduling in unusual environments, *Hum Factors* 8:385–398, 1966.
131. Folkard S, Monk TH: Shiftwork and performance. In Colquhoun W, Rutenfranz J, editors: *Studies of shiftwork*, London, 1980, Taylor and Francis, pp 263–272.
132. Blake MJ: Relationship between circadian rhythm of body temperature and introversion-extraversion, *Nature* 215:896–897, 1967.
133. Horne JA, Ostberg O: Individual differences in human circadian rhythms, *Biol Psychol* 5:179–190, 1977.
134. Folkard S, Monk TH, Lobban MC: Short and long-term adjustment of circadian rhythms in "permanent" night nurses, *Ergonomics* 21:785–799, 1978.
135. Colquhoun WP, Rutenfranz J: *Studies of shiftwork*, London, 1980, Taylor and Francis.
136. Reinberg A, Vieux N, Andlauer P: *Night and shift work: biological and social aspects*, Oxford, England, 1981, Pergamon Press.
137. Shift work and sleep: optimizing health, safety, and performance, *J Occup Environ Med* 53(Suppl 5):S1–S10, 2011. quiz S11–S12.
138. Colquhoun WP: *Biological rhythms and human performance*, London, 1971, Academic Press.
139. Bjerner B, Swensson A: Shiftwork and rhythm, *Acta Med Scand* 278(Supp):102–107, 1953.
140. Aschoff J, Giedke H, Poppel E, Wever R: The influence of sleep interruption, and of sleep deprivation or circadian rhythms, in human performance. In Colquhoun WE, editor: *Aspects of human efficiency*, Oxford, England, 1972, English Universities Press, pp 135–150.
141. Naitoh P, Englund C, Ryman D: Restorative power of naps in designing continuous work schedules, *J Hum Ergol* 11(Supp):259–278, 1982.
142. Howard SK, Rosekind MR, Katz JD, Berry AJ: Fatigue in anesthesia: implications and strategies for patient and provider safety, *Anesthesiology* 97(5):1281–1294, 2002.
143. Howard SK, Gaba DM, Rosekind MR, Zarcone VP: The risks and implications of excessive daytime sleepiness in resident physicians, *Acad Med* 77(10):1019–1025, 2002.
144. Geer RT, Jobes DR, Gilfor J, Traber K, Dinges D: Reduced psychomotor vigilance in anesthesia residents after 24-hr call [abstract], *Anesthesiology* 83:A1008, 1995.
145. Cao CG, Weinger MB, Slagle J, et al: Differences in day and night shift clinical performance in anesthesiology, *Hum Factors* 50(2):276–290, 2008.
146. Gander P, Millar M, Webster C, Merry A: Sleep loss and performance of anaesthesia trainees and specialists, *Chronobiology Int* 25(6):1077–1091, 2008.
147. Howard SK, Gaba DM, Smith BE, et al: Simulation study of rested versus sleep-deprived anesthesiologists, *Anesthesiology* 98(6):1345–1355, 2003. discussion 5A.
148. Squires B: Fatigue and stress in medical students, interns, and residents: It's time to act! *Can Med Assoc J* 140:18–19, 1989.
149. McCormick EJ, Tiffin J: *Industrial psychology*, Englewood Cliffs, NJ, 1974, Prentice Hall.
150. Cooper JB, Long CD, Newbower RS, Philip JH: Critical incidents associated with intraoperative exchanges of anesthesia personnel, *Anesthesiology* 56:456–461, 1982.
151. Cooper JB: Do short breaks increase or decrease anesthetic risk? *J Clin Anesth* 1:228–231, 1989.
152. Welford A: Fatigue and monotony. In Edholm O, Bacharach A, editors: *The physiology of human survival*, London, 1965, Academic Press, pp 431–462.
153. Davies DR, Shakleton VJ, Parasuraman R: Monotony and boredom. In Hockey GRJ, editor: *Stress and fatigue in human performance*, Chichester, England, 1983, John Wiley and Sons, pp 1–32.

154. Haga S: An experimental study of signal vigilance errors in train driving, *Ergonomics* 27:755–765, 1984.
155. Simonov P, Frolov M, Ivanov E: Psychophysiological monitoring of operator's emotional stress in aviation and astronautics, *Aviat Space Environ Med* 51:46–50, 1980.
156. Wilkinson R, Edwards R: Stable hours and varied work as aids to efficiency, *Psychonomic Sci* 13:205–206, 1968.
157. Froberg JE: Sleep deprivation and prolonged work hours. In Froberg JE, Monk TE, editors: *Hours of work: temporal factors in work scheduling*, Chichester, England, 1985, John Wiley and Sons, pp 67–76.
158. Gould JD, Schaffer A: The effects of divided attention on visual monitoring of multi-channel displays, *Hum Factors* 9:191–202, 1967.
159. Tyler D, Halcomb C: Monitoring performance with a time-shared encoding task, *Percept Motor Skills* 38:382–386, 1974.
160. Sawin DA, Scerbo MW: Effects of instruction type and boredom proneness in vigilance: implications for boredom and workload, *Hum Factors* 37:752–765, 1995.
161. Harris RL, Tole JR, Stephens AT, Ephrath AR: Visual scanning behavior and pilot workload, *Aviat Space Environ Med* 53:1067–1072, 1982.
162. Weinger MB: Lack of outcome data makes reading a personal decision, *J Clin Monit* 12:1–2, 1996.
163. Thomas MA, Weinger MB: Reading in the operating room, *Am J Anesthesiol* 23:81–85, 1996.
164. Slagle JM, Weinger MB: Effects of intraoperative reading on vigilance and workload during anesthesia care in an academic medical center, *Anesthesiology* 110(2):275–283, 2009.
165. Jennings AE, Chiles WD: An investigation of time-sharing ability as a factor in complex performance, *Hum Factors* 19:535–547, 1977.
166. Siering G, Stone L: In search of a time-sharing ability in zero-input tracking analyzer scores, *Aviat Space Environ Med* 57:1194–1197, 1986.
167. Jorm CM, O'Sullivan G: Laptops and smartphones in the operating theatre: how does our knowledge of vigilance, multi-tasking and anaesthetist performance help us in our approach to this new distraction? *Anaesth Intensive Care* 40(1):71–78, 2012.
168. Girodo M: The psychological health and stress of pilots in a labor dispute, *Aviat Space Environ Med* 59:505–510, 1988.
169. Raymond C: Mental stress: "occupational injury" of 80s that even pilots can't rise above, *JAMA* 259:3097–3098, 1988.
170. Dille JR: Mental stress causes accidents, too, *Aviat Space Environ Med* 53:1137, 1982.
171. Smith MJ, Conway FT, Karsh BT: Occupational stress in human computer interaction, *Ind Health* 37(2):157–173, 1999.
172. Bignell V, Fortune J: *Understanding system failures*, Manchester, England, 1984, Manchester University Press, pp 190–204.
173. Clayson PE, Clawson A, Larson MJ: The effects of induced state negative affect on performance monitoring processes, *Soc Cogn Affect Neurosci* 7(6):67–688, 2012.
174. Smith BD, Principato F: Effects of stress and conflict difficulty on arousal and conflict resolution, *Br J Social Psychol* 73:85–93, 1982.
175. Hart SG, Hauser JR: Inflight application of three pilot workload measurement techniques, *Aviat Space Environ Med* 58:402–410, 1987.
176. Weinger MB, Reddy SB, Slagle JM: Multiple measures of anesthesia workload during teaching and nonteaching cases, *Anesth Analg* 98(5):1419–1425, 2004.
177. Barabasz AF: Enhancement of military pilot reliability by hypnosis and psycho-physiological monitoring: preliminary inflight and simulator data, *Aviat Space Environ Med* 56:248–250, 1985.
178. Casali JG, Wierwille WW: On the measurement of pilot perceptual workload: a comparison of assessment techniques addressing sensitivity and intrusion issues, *Ergonomics* 27:1033–1050, 1984.
179. Thackray R, Jones K, Touchstone R: Personality and physiological correlates of performance decrement on a monotonous task requiring sustained attention, *Br J Soc Psychol* 65(3):351–358, 1974.
180. Weinger MB, Shen H, Culp M, Fehrenbacher N, Herndon OW: Real-time workload assessment during anesthesia for outpatient surgery [abstract], *Anesth Analg* 80:S548, 1995.
181. Svensson E, Thanderz M, Sjöberg L, Gillberg M: Military flight experience and sympathoadrenal activity, *Aviat Space Environ Med* 59:411–416, 1988.
182. Rozanski A, Bairey N, Krantz D, et al: Mental stress and the induction of silent myocardial ischemia in patients with coronary artery disease, *N Engl J Med* 318:1005–1012, 1988.
183. Rozanski A, Krantz DS, Bairey CN: Ventricular responses to mental stress testing in patients with coronary artery disease: pathophysiological implications, *Circulation II* 83:137–144, 1991.
184. Toung T, Donham R, Rogers M: The stress of giving anesthesia on the electrocardiogram of anesthesiologists [abstract], *Anesthesiology* 61:A465, 1984.
185. Toung T, Donham R, Rogers M: The effect of previous medical training on the stress of giving anesthesia [abstract], *Anesthesiology* 65:A473, 1986.
186. Dutton RP, Xiao Y, Bernhard W, et al: Measured versus predicted stress during elective and emergency airway management abstract, *Anesthesiology* 87:A444, 1997.
187. Kain ZN, Chan KM, Katz JD, et al: Anesthesiologists and acute perioperative stress: a cohort study, *Anesth Analg* 95(1):177–183, 2002.
188. Bittker TE: Reaching out to the depressed physician, *JAMA* 236:1713–1716, 1976.
189. Shapiro HM, Grant I, Weinger MB: AIDS and the CNS: implications for the anesthesiologist, *Anesthesiology* 80:187–200, 1994.
190. Baracat B, Marquie JC: Age differences in sensitivity, response bias, reaction time on a visual discrimination task, *Exp Aging Res* 18:59–66, 1992.
191. Fozard JL, Vercruyssen M, Reynolds SL, Hancock PA, Quilter RE: Age differences and changes in reaction time: the Baltimore Longitudinal Study, *J Gerontology* 49(4):179–189, 1994.
192. Weale R: *The aging eye*, London, 1963, H K Lewis.
193. Travis KW, Beach ML: Age and professional liability: the National Practitioner Databank [abstract], *Anesthesiology* 87:A983, 1997.
194. Fajardo Dolci G: Malpractice and physician's age, *Gac Med Mex [Article in Spanish]* 147(3):266–269, 2011.
195. Waljee JF, Greenfield LJ, Dimick JB, Birkmeyer JD: Surgeon age and operative mortality in the United States, *Ann Surg* 244(3):353–362, 2006.
196. Katz JD: Factors leading to retirement among anesthesiologists [abstract], *Anesthesiology* 87:A1013, 1997.
197. Eysenck MW: *Attention and arousal: cognition and performance*, Berlin, 1982, Springer-Verlag.
198. Mandler G: Thought processes, consciousness, and stress. In Hamilton V, Warburton DM, editors: *Human stress and cognition: an information-processing approach*, Chichester, England, 1979, John Wiley and Sons, pp 179–201.
199. Freudenberger HJ: The staff burn-out syndrome in alternative institutions, *Psychother Theor Res Pract* 12:73–82, 1975.
200. Hyman SA, Michaels D, Berry JM, et al: Risk of burnout in perioperative clinicians: a survey study and literature review, *Anesthesiology* 114(1):194–204, 2011.
201. Riad W, Mansour A, Moussa A: Anesthesiologists work-related exhaustion: a comparison study with other hospital employees, *Saudi J Anaesth* 5(3):244–247, 2011. Epub 2011 Oct 1.
202. Hemp P: Presenteeism: at work—but out of it, *Harv Bus Rev* 82(10):49–58, 155, 2004. Epub 2004 Nov 24.
203. Dew K, Keefe V, Small K: 'Choosing' to work when sick: workplace presenteeism, *Soc Sci Med* 60(10):2273–2282, 2005.
204. Widera E, Chang A, Chen HL: Presenteeism: a public health hazard, *J Gen Int Med* 25(11):1244–1247, 2010.
205. Landry M, Miller C: Presenteeism: are we hurting the patients we are trying to help? *J Gen Int Med* 25(11):1142–1143, 2010.
206. Colford JM, McPhee SJ: The ravelled sleeve of care: managing the stresses of residency training, *JAMA* 261:889–893, 1989.
207. Hughes PH, Brandenburg N, Baldwin DCJ, et al: Prevalence of substance use among US physicians, *JAMA* 267(17):2333–2339, 1992.
208. Bryson EO, Silverstein JH: Addiction and substance abuse in anesthesiology, *Anesthesiology* 109(5):905–917, 2008.
209. Spiegelman W, Saunders L, Mazze R: Addiction and anesthesiology, *Anesthesiology* 60:335–341, 1984.
210. Leiberman HR, Wurtman RJ, Emde GG, Roberts C, Coviella ILG: The effects of low-dose caffeine on human performance and mood, *Pyschopharmacol* 92:308–312, 1987.
211. Lane JD, Williams RB: Cardiovascular effects of caffeine and stress in regular coffee drinkers, *Psychopharmacol* 24:157–164, 1987.

212. Moskowitz H: Attention tasks as skills performance measures of drug effects, *Br J Clin Pharmac* 18:51S–61S, 1984.
213. Hyman FC, Collins WE, Taylor HL, Domino EF, Nagel RJ: Instrument flight performance under the influence of certain combinations of antiemetic drugs, *Aviat Space Environ Med* 59:533–539, 1988.
214. Gaillard AWK, Gruisen A, deJong R: The influence of antihistamines on human performance, *Eur J Clin Pharmacol* 35:249–253, 1988.
215. Aksnes EG: Effect of small dosages of alcohol upon performance in a Link trainer, *J Aviat Med* 25:680–688, 1954.
216. Collins WE: Performance effects of alcohol intoxication and hangover at ground level and at simulated altitude, *Aviat Space Environ Med* 51:327–335, 1980.
217. Erwin CW, Wiener EL, Linnoila MI, Truscott TR: Alcohol-induced drowsiness and vigilance performance, *J Stud Alcohol* 39:505–516, 1978.
218. Henry PH, Davis TQ, Engelken EJ, Triebwasser JH, Lancaster MC: Alcohol-induced performance decrements assessed by two Link trainer tasks using experienced pilots, *Aerospace Med* 45:1180–1189, 1974.
219. Franck DH: "If you drink, don't drive" motto now applies to hangovers as well, *JAMA* 250:1657–1658, 1983.
220. Seppälä T, Leino T, Linnoila M, Juttunen M, Ylikahri R: Effects of hangover on psychomotor skills related to driving: modification by fructose and glucose, *Acta Pharmacol Toxicol* 38:209–218, 1976.
221. Yesavage J, Leirer V: Hangover effects on aircraft pilots 14 hours after alcohol ingestion: a preliminary report, *Am J Psychiatry* 143:1546–1550, 1986.
222. Gallagher AG, Boyle E, Toner P, et al: Persistent next-day effects of excessive alcohol consumption on laparoscopic surgical performance, *Arch Surg* 146(4):419–426, 2011.
223. Janowksy DS, Meacham MP, Blaine JD, Schoor M, Bozzetti LP: Marijuana effects on simulated flying ability, *Am J Psychiatry* 133:384–388, 1976.
224. Engelberg S: Error by signal operator is called likely cause of Amtrak collision, *New York Times*, 1984.
225. Lewis MF, Ferraro DP: *Flying high: the aeromedical aspects of marihuana*, Springfield, VA, 1973, National Technical Information Service.
226. National Transportation Safety Board [NTSB]: *Central Airlines Flight 27, Newark Airport (March 30, 1983)*, aircraft accident report 84/11, Washington, DC, 1983, NTSB.
227. Yesavage J, Leirer V, Denari M, Hollister L: Carry-over effects of marijuana intoxication on aircraft pilot performance: a preliminary report, *Am J Psychiatry* 142:1325–1329, 1985.
228. Leirer VO, Yesavage JA, Morrow DG: Marijuana carry-over effects on aircraft pilot performance, *Aviat Space Environ Med* 62:221–227, 1991.
229. Ware R, Baker R: The effect of mental set and states of consciousness on vigilance decrement: a systematic exploration. In Mackie R, editor: *Vigilance: theory, operational performance, and physiological correlates*, New York, 1976, Plenum Press, p 607.
230. Verhaegen P, Ryckaert R: Vigilance of train engineers, *Proc Hum Factors Soc* 30:403–407, 1986.
231. Folkard S, Monk TH, Lobban MC: Towards a predictive test of adjustment to shift work, *Ergonomics* 22:79–91, 1979.
232. Brown SD, Goske MJ, Johnson CM: Beyond substance abuse: stress, burnout, and depression as causes of physician impairment and disruptive behavior, *J Am Coll Radiol* 6(7):479–485, 2009.
233. Hickson GB, Entman SS: Physician practice behavior and litigation risk: evidence and opportunity, *Clin Obstet Gynecol* 51(4):688–699, 2008.
234. Slogoff S, Keats A: Does perioperative myocardial ischemia lead to postoperative myocardial infarction? *Anesthesiology* 62:107–114, 1985.
235. See WA, Cooper CS, Fisher RJ: Predictors of laparoscopic complications after formal training in laparoscopic surgery, *JAMA* 270:2689–2692, 1993.
236. Choudhry NK, Fletcher RH, Soumerai SB: Systematic review: the relationship between clinical experience and quality of health care, *Ann Int Med* 142:260–273, 2005.
237. Gaba DM, DeAnda A: The response of anesthesia trainees to simulated critical incidents, *Anesth Analg* 68:444–451, 1989.
238. Kanki BG, Lozito S, Foushee HC: Communication indices of crew coordination, *Aviat Space Environ Med* 60:56–60, 1989.
239. Minnick AF, Donaghey B, Slagle J, Weinger MB: Operating room team members' views of workload, case difficulty, and nonroutine events, *J Healthc Qual*, 2011 Apr 7. [Epub ahead of print].
240. Stepaniak PS, Vrijland WW, de Quelerij M, de Vries G, Heij C: Working with a fixed operating room team on consecutive similar cases and the effect on case duration and turnover time, *Arch Surg* 145(12):1165–1170, 2010.
241. Haskell BE, Reid GB: The subjective perception of workload in low-time private pilots: a preliminary study, *Aviat Space Environ Med* 58:1230–1232, 1987.
242. Bandaret LE, Stokes JW, Francesconi R, Kowal DM, Naitoh P: *Artillery teams in simulated sustained combat: performance and other measures*. NIOSH proceedings: The 24-hour workday (Publication #81-127), Cincinnati, 1981, U.S. Dept of Health and Human Services, pp 581–604.
243. Bergeron HS, Hinton DA: Aircraft automation: the problem of the pilot interface, *Aviat Space Environ Med* 56:144–148, 1985.
244. Wickens C: The structure of attentional resources. In Nickerson R, editor: *Attention and performance VIII*, Hillsdale, NJ, 1980, Lawrence Erlbaum and Assoc, pp 239–257.
245. Lambert TF, Paget NS: Teaching and learning in the operating theatre, *Anaesth Intensive Care* 4:304–307, 1976.
246. Block FEJ, Burton LW, Rafal MD, et al: Two computer-based anesthetic monitors, the Duke automatic monitoring equipment (DAME) system and the MICRODAME, *J Clin Monit* 1:30–51, 1985.
247. Cook RI, Potter SS, Woods DD, McDonald JS: Evaluating the human engineering of microprocessor controlled operating room devices, *J Clin Monit* 7:217–226, 1991.
248. Mosenkis R: Human factors in design. In van Gruting CWD, editor: *Medical devices*, Amsterdam, 1994, Elsevier, pp 41–51.
249. Weinger MB, Wiklund ME, Gardner-Bonneau DJ: *Handbook of human factors in medical device design*, Boca Raton, 2011, CRC Press.
250. International Electrotechinal Commission: *Medical devices: application of usability engineering to medical devices*, Geneva, 2007.
251. Mazze RI: Therapeutic misadventures with O2 delivery systems: the need for continuous in-line O2 monitors, *Anesth Analg* 51:787–792, 1972.
252. Weller J, Merry A, Warman G, Robinson B: Anaesthetists' management of oxygen pipeline failure: room for improvement, *Anaesthesia* 62(2):122–126, 2007.
253. Mudumbai SC, Fanning R, Howard SK, Davies MF, Gaba DM: Use of medical simulation to explore equipment failures and human machine interactions in anesthesia machine pipeline supply crossover, *Anesth Analg* 110(5):1292–1296, 2010.
254. Holland R: Another "wrong gas" incident in Hong Kong, *APSF Newslett* 6:9, 1991.
255. Sato T: Fatal pipeline accidents spur Japanese standards, *APSF Newslett* 6:14, 1991.
256. Hay H: Oxygen delivery failure resulting from interference with a Bain breathing system, *Eur J Anaesth* 17(9):591–593, 2000.
257. Gravenstein JS: In my opinion: to obsolete or not, *J Clin Monit* 13:131–132, 1997.
258. Petty WC: The aging anesthesia machine, *J Clin Monit* 13:129, 1997.
259. Schreiber PJ: Response to question of machine obsolescence, *J Clin Monit* 13:133–136, 1997.
260. Beneken JEW, van der Aa JJ: Alarms and their limits in monitoring, *J Clin Monit* 5:205–210, 1989.
261. Quinn M: A philosophy of alarms. In Gravenstein JS, Newbower RS, Ream AK, Smith NT, editors: *The automated anesthesia record and alarm systems*, Stoneham, MA, 1987, Butterworths, pp 169–173.
262. Hagenouw RR: Should we be alarmed by our alarms? *Curr Opin Anaesth* 20(6):590–594, 2007.
263. Schreiber P, Schreiber J: Structured alarm systems for the operating room, *J Clin Monit* 5:201–204, 1989.
264. Hyman WA, Drinker PA: Design of medical device alarm systems, *Med Instrum* 17:103–106, 1983.
265. Edworthy J, Hellier E: Alarms and human behaviour: implications for medical alarms, *Br J Anaesth* 97(1):12–17, 2006.
266. Campbell RM, Sheikh A, Crosse MM: A study of the incorrect use of ventilator disconnection alarms, *Anaesthesia* 51:369–370, 1996.

267. Takla G, Petre JH, Doyle DJ, Horibe M, Gopakumaran B: The problem of artifacts in patient monitor data during surgery: a clinical and methodological review, *Anesth Analg* 103(5):1196–1204, 2006.
268. Schmid F, Goepfert MS, Kuhnt D, et al: The wolf is crying in the operating room: patient monitor and anesthesia workstation alarming patterns during cardiac surgery, *Anesth Analg* 112(1):78–83, 2011.
269. Meijler A: *Automation in anesthesia: a relief?* Berlin, 1987, Springer-Verlag.
270. Kestin IG, Miller BR, Lockhart CH: Auditory alarms during anesthesia monitoring, *Anesthesiology* 69:106–109, 1988.
271. Block FEJ, Scjaaf C: Auditory alarms during anesthesia monitoring with an integrated monitoring system, *Int J Clin Monit Comput* 13:81–84, 1996.
272. Wiklund L, Hök B, Ståhl K, Jordeby-Jönsson A: Postanesthesia monitoring revisited: frequency of true and false alarms from different monitoring devices, *J Clin Anesth* 6:182–188, 1994.
273. Porciello P: Alarms in coronary care units, *G Ital Cardiol* 10:939–943, 1980.
274. O'Carroll T: Survey of alarms in an intensive therapy unit, *Anaesthesia* 41:742–724, 1986.
275. Lawless ST: Crying wolf: false alarms in a pediatric intensive care unit, *Crit Care Med* 22:981–985, 1994.
276. McIntyre J: Ergonomics: anaesthetists' use of auditory alarms in the operating room, *Int J Clin Monit Comput* 2:47–55, 1985.
277. Stanford L, McIntyre J, Nelson T, Hogan J: Affective responses to commercial and experimental auditory alarm signals for anesthesia delivery and physiological monitoring equipment, *Int J Clin Monit Comp* 5:111–118, 1988.
278. Veitergruber J, Doucek G, Smith W: *Aircraft alerting systems criteria study*, Washington, DC, 1977, Federal Aviation Administration.
279. Tappan JM, Daniels J, Slavin B, et al: Visual cueing with context relevant information for reducing change blindness, *J Clin Monit Comput* 23(4):223–232, 2009.
280. Jones TN, Kirk RE: Monitoring performance on visual and auditory displays, *Percept Mot Skill* 30:235–238, 1970.
281. Loeb RG, Jones BR, Leonard RA, Behrman K: Recognition accuracy of current operating room alarms, *Anesth Analg* 75(4):499–505, 1992.
282. Wallace M, Ashman M: Volume and frequency of anesthetic alarms: are the current alarm systems appropriate for normal human ear aging? *J Clin Monit* 7:134, 1991.
283. Kerr JH: Warning devices, *Br J Anaesth* 57:696–708, 1985.
284. International Electrotechinal Commission: General requirements, tests, and guidance for alarm systems in medical electrical equipment and medical electrical systems. 60601-1-8. Geneva, 2006.
285. Santamore DC, Cleaver TG: The sounds of saturation, *J Clin Monit Comput* 18(2):89–92, 2004.
286. Block FEJ: Evaluation of users' ability to recognize musical alarm tones, *J Clin Monit* 8:285–290, 1992.
287. Hakkinen MT, Williges BH: Synthesized warning messages: effects of an alerting cue in single- and multiple-function voice synthesis systems, *Hum Factors* 26:185–195, 1984.
288. Williams S, Beatty PC: Measuring the performance of audible alarms for anaesthesia, *Physiol Meas* 26(4):571–581, 2005.
289. McNeer RR, Bohorquez J, Ozdamar O, Varon AJ, Barach P: A new paradigm for the design of audible alarms that convey urgency information, *J Clin Monit Comput* 21(6):353–363, 2007.
290. Patterson R: *Guidelines for auditory warning systems on civil aircraft*, London, England, 1982, Civil Aviation Authority, Contract No. 82017.
291. Walsh TC, Beatty PC: Establishing scales of perceived severity for clinical situations during anaesthesia, *Br J Anaesth* 95(3):339–343, 2005.
292. Sanderson PM, Liu D, Jenkins SA: Auditory displays in anesthesiology, *Curr Opin Anaesth* 22(6):788–795, 2009.
293. Ng G, Barralon P, Dumont G, Schwarz SK, Ansermino JM: Optimizing the tactile display of physiological information: vibro-tactile vs. electro-tactile stimulation, and forearm or wrist location, *Conf Proc IEEE Eng Med Biol Soc* 2007:4202–4205, 2007.
294. Jones LA, Sarter NB: Tactile displays: guidance for their design and application, *Hum Factors* 50(1):90–111, 2008.
295. Jones LA: Tactile communication systems optimizing the display of information, *Prog Brain Res* 192:113–128, 2011.
296. Blum JM, Kruger GH, Sanders KL, Gutierrez J, Rosenberg AL: Specificity improvement for network distributed physiologic alarms based on a simple deterministic reactive intelligent agent in the critical care environment, *J Clin Monit Comput* 23(1):21–30, 2009.
297. Connor CW, Gohil B, Harrison MJ: Triggering of systolic arterial pressure alarms using statistics-based versus threshold alarms, *Anaesthesia* 64(2):131–135, 2009.
298. Harrison MJ, Connor CW: Statistics-based alarms from sequential physiological measurements, *Anaesthesia* 62(10):1015–1023, 2007.
299. Logan M: *Clinical alarms*, Herndon, VA, 2011, Association for the Advancement of Medical Instrumentation.
300. Graham KC, Cvach M: Monitor alarm fatigue: standardizing use of physiological monitors and decreasing nuisance alarms, *Am J Crit Care* 19(1):28–34, 2010.
301. Gorges M, Markewitz BA, Westenskow DR: Improving alarm performance in the medical intensive care unit using delays and clinical context, *Anesth Analg* 108(5):1546–1552, 2009.
302. Curry JP, Lynn LA: Threshold monitoring, alarm fatigue, and the patterns of unexpected hospital death, *APSF Newslett* 26(2):32–35, 2011.
303. Svensson MS: Monitoring practice and alarm technology in anaesthesiology, *Health Inform J* 13(1):9–21, 2007.
304. Imhoff M, Kuhls S: Alarm algorithms in critical care monitoring, *Anesth Analg* 102(5):1525–1537, 2006.
305. Watt R, Navabi M, Mylrea K, Hameroff S: Integrated monitoring "smart alarms" can detect critical events and reduce false alarms (abstract), *Anesthesiology* 7(3A):A338, 1989.
306. Kerstholt JH, Passenier PO: Fault management in supervisory control: the effect of false alarms and support, *Ergonomics* 43:1371–1389, 2000.
307. Orr JA, Westenskow DR: A breathing circuit alarm system based on neural networks, *J Clin Monit* 10:101–109, 1994.
308. Mylrea KC, Orr JA, Westenskow DR: Integration of monitoring for intelligent alarms in anesthesia: neural networks—can they help? *J Clin Monit* 9(1):31–37, 1993.
309. Pan P, van der Aa J, Gomez F, et al: Smart anesthesia monitoring system, *Anesthesiology* 73:A450, 1990.
310. Beinlich IA, Gaba DM: The ALARM monitoring system: intelligent decision making under uncertainty, *Anesthesiology* 71:A337, 1989.
311. Heckerman DE, Horvitz EJ, Nathwani BN: Toward normative expert systems: I. The Pathfinder Project, *Meth Inform Med* 31:90–105, 1992.
312. Penny W, Frost D: Neural networks in clinical medicine, *Med Decision Making* 16:386–398, 1996.
313. Factor M, Sittig DF, Cohn AI, et al: A parallel software architecture for building intelligent medical monitors, *Int J Clin Monit Comput* 7(2):117–128, 1990.
314. Cushing H: On the avoidance of shock in major amputations by cocainization of large nerve trunks preliminary to their divisions, with observations on blood pressure changes in surgical cases, *Ann Surg* 36:321–345, 1902.
315. Gravenstein JS, Weinger MB: Why investigate vigilance? *J Clin Monit* 2:145–147, 1986.
316. Philip J, Raemer D: Selecting the optimal anesthesia monitoring array, *Med Instrum* 19:122–126, 1985.
317. FDA: *Human factors implications of the new GMP rule: overall requirements of the new quality system regulation, 2011.* Available at http://www.fda.gov/MedicalDevices/DeviceRegulationandGuidance/HumanFactors/ucm119215.htm.
318. Pouzeratte Y, Sebbane M, Jung B, et al: A prospective study on the user-friendliness of four anaesthesia workstations, *Eur J Anaesthiol* 25(8):634–641, 2008.
319. Michels P, Gravenstein D, Westenskow DR: An integrated graphic data display improves detection and identification of critical events during anesthesia, *J Clin Monit* 13:249–259, 1997.
320. Blike GT, Surgenor SD, Whalen K: A graphical object display improves anesthesiologists' performance on a simulated diagnostic task, *J Clin Monit Comput* 15(1):37–44, 1999.
321. Blike GT, Surgenor SD, Whalen K, Jensen J: Specific elements of a new hemodynamics display improves the performance of anesthesiologists, *J Clin Monit Comput* 16(7):485–491, 2000.

322. Effken J, Loeb R, Johnson K, Johnson S, Reyna V: Using cognitive work analysis to design clinical displays, *Stud Health Technol Inform* 84(Pt 1):127–131, 2001.
323. Fiegler AA, Stead SW: The medical information bus, *Biomed Instru Technol* 101–111, 1990; Mar/Apr.
324. Schleifer A: Medical information bus, *Seminar Kommunikationsstandards in der Medizintechnik.* July 2010, pp 1–12.
325. Gee T: *Is ISO/IEEE 11073 a viable standard?* 2006. Available at http://medicalconnectivity.com/2006/10/03/is-isoieee-11073-aviable-standard.
326. Yuksel M, Dogac A: Interoperability of medical device information and the clinical applications: an HL7 RMIM based on the ISO/IEEE 11073 DIM, *IEEE Eng Med Biol Soc* 15(4):557–566, 2011.
327. American Society for Testing and Materials (ASTM): *Standard F-2761-09, part 1: general requirements and conceptual model,* West Conshohocken, PA, 2009, ASTM International.
328. Cooper JB, Newbower RS: The Boston anesthesia system, *Contemp Anesth Prac* 8:207–219, 1984.
329. Hankeln KB, Michelsen H, Schipulle M, et al: Microprocessor-assisted monitoring system for measuring and processing cardio-respiratory variables: preliminary results of clinical trials, *Crit Care Med* 13:426–431, 1985.
330. Ball GJ: Microprocessors in anesthesia and intensive care, *J Med Eng Technol* 7:303–307, 1983.
331. Jewett WR: The Arizona Program: development of a modular, interactive anesthesia delivery system, *Contemp Anesth Pract* 8:185–206, 1984.
332. Loeb RG, Brunner JX, Westenskow DR, Feldman B, Pace NL: The Utah anesthesia workstation, *Anesthesiology* 70:999–1007, 1989.
333. Bickford RG, Flemming NI, Billinger TW: Compression of EEG data by isometric power spectral plots, *Electroenceph Clin Neurophysiol* 31:632–634, 1971.
334. Fleming RA, Smith NT: An inexpensive device for analyzing and monitoring the electroencephalogram, *Anesthesiology* 50:456–460, 1979.
335. Fleming RA, Smith NT: Density modulation: a technique for the display of three-variable data in patient monitoring, *Anesthesiology* 50:543–546, 1979.
336. Gregory TK, Pettus DC: An electroencephalographic processing algorhythm specifically intended for analysis of cerebral electrical activity, *J Clin Monit* 2:190–197, 1986.
337. Siegel J, Farrell E, Goldwyn R, Friedman H: The surgical implications of physiologic patterns in myocardial infarction shock, *Surgery* 72:126–141, 1972.
338. Deneault LG, Stein KL, Lewis CM, Debbons A, Dewolf A: Comparing geometric objects and conventional displays in patient monitoring, *J Clin Monit* 7:111–113, 1991.
339. Bennett K, Flach JM: Graphical displays: implications for divided attention, focused attention, and problem solving, *Hum Factors* 35(5):513–533, 1992.
340. Carswell CM, Wickens CD: Information integration and the object display: an interaction of task demands and display superiority, *Ergonomics* 30(3):511–527, 1987.
341. Munson RC, Horst RL, editors: *Evidence for global processing of complex visual displays. Proceedings of the Human Factors Society 30th Annual Meeting,* Santa Monica, CA, 1986, Human Factors and Ergonomics Society.
342. Hughes T, MacRae AW: Holistic peripheral processing of a polygon display, *Hum Factors* 36:645–651, 1994.
343. Coury B, Boulette M, Smith R: Effect of uncertainty and diagnosticity on classification of multidimensional data with integral and separable displays of systems status, *Hum Factors* 31:551–569, 1989.
344. Coury BG, Pietras CM: Alphanumeric and graphic displays for dynamic process monitoring and control, *Ergonomics* 32:1373–1389, 1989.
345. Coury BG, Boulette MD: Time stress and the processing of visual displays, *Hum Factors* 34:707–725, 1992.
346. Kruger GH, Tremper KK: Advanced integrated real-time clinical displays, *Anesthesiology Clin* 29(3):487–504, 2011.
347. Blike GT: The boundary information in a gray-scale object display and a color-enhanced variant improve problem recognition compared to an alpha-numeric display [abstract], *Anesthesiology* 87:A458, 1997.
348. Blike GT: The emergent shape features in a gray-scale graphical display improve pattern recognition compared to an alphanumeric display [abstract], *Anesthesiology* 87:A394, 1997.
349. Agutter J, Drews F, Syroid N, et al: Evaluation of graphic cardiovascular display in a high-fidelity simulator, *Anesth Analg* 97(5):1403–1413, 2003.
350. Albert RW, Agutter JA, Syroid ND, et al: A simulation-based evaluation of a graphic cardiovascular display, *Anesth Analg* 105(5):1303–1311, 2007.
351. Sanderson PM, Watson MO, Russell WJ: Advanced patient monitoring displays: tools for continuous informing, *Anesth Analg* 101(1):161–168, 2005.
352. Moray N: The role of attention in the detection of errors and the diagnosis of failures in man-machine systems. In Moray N, editor: *Mental workload: its theory and measurement,* New York, 1979, Plenum Press.
353. Fisher D, Coury B, Tengs T, Duffy S: Minimizing the time to search visual displays: the role of highlighting, *Hum Factors* 31:167–182, 1989.
354. Friedmann K: The effect of adding symbols to written warning labels on user behavior and recall, *Hum Factors* 30:507–515, 1988.
355. Koonce JM, Gold M, Moroze M: Comparison of novice and experienced pilots using analog and digital flight displays, *Aviat Space Environ Med* 57:1181–1184, 1986.
356. Palmer E, Jago S, Baty D, O'Connor S: Perception of horizontal aircraft separation on a cockpit display of traffic information, *Hum Factors* 22:605–620, 1980.
357. Gaba DM: Human performance issues in anesthesia patient safety, *Probl Anesth* 5:329–350, 1991.
358. Fukui J: An expert alarm system. In Gravenstein J, Newbower R, Ream A, Smith N, editors: *The automated anesthesia record and alarm systems,* Stoneham MA, 1987, Butterworths, pp 203–209.
359. Sanderson PM, Haskell I, Flach JM: The complex role of perceptual organization in visual display design theory, *Ergonomics* 35(10):1199–1219, 1992.
360. Calkins JM: Anesthesia equipment: help or hindrance? In Stoelting RK, Barash PG, editors: *Advances in anesthesia,* Chicago, 1985, Gallagher Year Book Medical Publishers, pp 377–406.
361. Thompson P: Safer design of anaesthesia equipment, *Br J Anaesth* 59:913–921, 1987.
362. Waterson C, Calkins J: Development directions for monitoring in anesthesia, *Semin Anesth* 5:225–236, 1986.
363. Daniels JP, Ansermino JM: Introduction of new monitors into clinical anesthesia, *Curr Opin Anaesth* 22(6):775–781, 2009.
364. Woods D, Roth E, Stubler W, Mumaw R: Navigating through large display networks in dynamic control applications, *Proc Human Fac Soc* 34:396–399, 1990.
365. Syroid ND, Agutter J, Drews FA, et al: Development and evaluation of a graphical anesthesia drug display, *Anesthesiology* 96(3):565–575, 2002.
366. Drews FA, Syroid N, Agutter J, Strayer DL, Westenskow DR: Drug delivery as control task: improving performance in a common anesthetic task, *Hum Factors* 48(1):85–94, 2006.
367. Sanderson PM, Watson MO, Russell WJ, et al: Advanced auditory displays and head-mounted displays: advantages and disadvantages for monitoring by the distracted anesthesiologist, *Anesth Analg* 106(6):1787–1797, 2008.
368. Wilcox SB: Alarm design. In Weinger M, Wiklund M, Gardner-Bonneau D, editors: *Handbook of human factors in medical device design,* Boca Raton, 2011, CRC Press, pp 397–423.

CHAPTER 24

ERGONOMICS OF THE ANESTHESIA WORKSPACE

Robert G. Loeb • Matthew B. Weinger • James M. Berry

CHAPTER OUTLINE

HISTORY

Decades ago, accidental delivery of hypoxic gas mixtures was a constant threat during general anesthesia. Many instances of hypoxia were attributed to human error. In some cases, the anesthesiologist mistakenly turned the wrong gas flow control knob or failed to recognize that the oxygen cylinder was empty.[1] In another case, a technician placed the flowmeter tubes in the wrong positions while servicing the anesthesia machine.[2] In each case, these small human errors led to major injury or to death of the patient. With modern anesthesia machines, the risk of accidental hypoxia has been dramatically reduced.[3] In effect, the potential for human error has been reduced by redesigning the equipment. The concept that equipment can be designed for optimal performance by the human user is one of the core principles of ergonomics. This chapter reviews the role of ergonomics in the practice of anesthesia, including the design of the anesthesia workplace.

WHAT IS ERGONOMICS?

Most people have probably thought about ergonomic issues, even if they are not familiar with the term. Accidentally sticking oneself with a hypodermic needle and wondering whether there might be a better way to inject intravenous (IV) drugs is, in effect, thinking about safety, one area of concern in ergonomics. Ergonomics involves optimizing the work environment for the benefit of the user, such as moving the anesthesia machine and elevating the chair to see both the patient and the monitors more easily. Evaluating the ease of use of equipment before purchase is another ergonomic activity.

Ergonomics is a discipline that investigates and applies information about human requirements, characteristics, abilities, and limitations to the design, development, engineering, and testing of equipment, tools, systems, and jobs.[4,5] The objectives of ergonomists are to improve safety, performance, and well-being by optimizing the relationship between people and their work environment. The terms *ergonomics, human factors, human engineering,* and *usability engineering* are often used interchangeably; however, the term *ergonomics* is used exclusively in this chapter.

Scope of Ergonomics

The Software-Hardware-Environment-Liveware (SHEL) model, first introduced by Edwards in 1972,[6] can be used to illustrate the scope of ergonomics (Fig. 24-1). Within this model, all jobs are performed by three classes of resources. The first class is composed of the physical items, or *hardware*. This includes the buildings, equipment, and materials used for the job. The second class, the *software*, consists of the rules, guidelines, policies, procedures, and customs involved in the job. People make up the third class of components, *liveware*. These components act together within a larger context, or *environment*, which is composed of external physical, economic, social, and political factors that affect the job.

Ergonomics is the discipline of designing and testing the human/systems interface with the goal of improving the interactions between the liveware component and the other components. In the broadest terms, ergonomics deals with the study and enhancement of the tools and systems used by humans to interact with the physical world around them.

Ergonomics is both a science and a profession, encompassing both research and application. One goal of ergonomics research is to understand and describe the capabilities and limitations of human performance. Another is to develop principles of interaction between people and machines. Examples of ergonomics research are the investigation of visual perception in relation to a particular task and the measurement and compilation of anthropomorphic data (e.g., what is the distribution in the lengths of the tibia and femur in all men between 18 and 45 years of age). Application involves the use of these data in the development of equipment, systems, and jobs. For example, the selection of color coding for displays is based on an understanding of visual perception, information processing, and decision theory, whereas anthropomorphic data are used in the design of a chair.

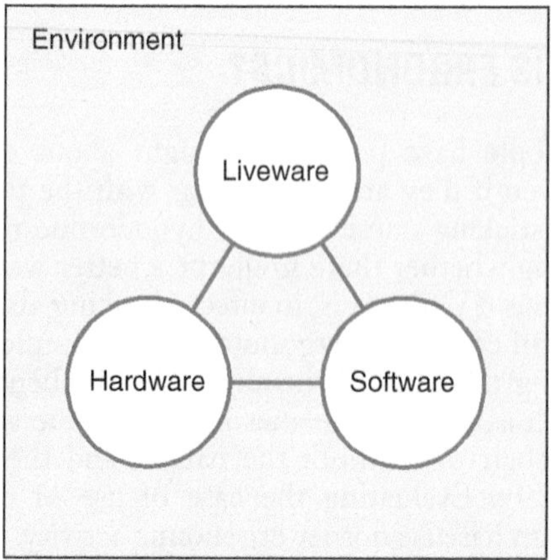

FIGURE 24-1 ■ The software-hardware-environment-liveware (SHEL) model of system resources.

Some aspects of ergonomics focus on the worker and the human-to-human interfaces within the system. This may include task and workload analysis, examination of vigilance and fatigue, and analysis of team interactions. The focus of this chapter is on the interface between the liveware and the hardware, that is, the interface between the human and the machine.

ERGONOMICS RESEARCH IN ANESTHESIOLOGY

The number of ergonomics studies in anesthesiology continues to grow. The focus of these studies has been to identify human/machine interface factors that affect patient safety and the anesthesiologist's job performance.

Task Analysis Studies

Task analysis is a basic ergonomics methodology for evaluating jobs or designing new human/machine systems. Several variants of this methodology are used, such as cognitive task analysis, critical decision method, and time and motion studies, depending on the focus of the problem. Task analysis methods typically involve the structured decomposition of work activities and/or decisions and the classification of these activities as a series of tasks, processes, or classes. At least three interacting components can be identified and described for each task: the task's *goals, constraints,* and *behaviors.*

One of the first formal time and motion studies ever performed was an analysis of surgeons' tasks in the operating room (OR). Frank and Lillian Gilbreth[7] conducted time and motion studies of surgical teams during the early 1900s and concluded that surgeons spent an inordinate amount of time looking for instruments as they picked them off the tray. Their findings led to the current practice of the surgeon requesting instruments from a nurse, who places the instrument in the surgeon's hand.[8]

One of the first time-and-motion studies of anesthesiologists was conducted to identify ways to improve anesthesiologists' job satisfaction. Drui and colleagues[9] filmed eight operations and put the anesthesiologists' activities into 24 categories. They then had anesthesiologists rate each activity's importance, knowledge demand, and skill requirement. They found that filling out the anesthesia record occupied a large proportion of the anesthesiologists' time but was rated as relatively unimportant and easy to perform. They also found that blood pressure and pulse were determined faster when the pressure gauge was located at the head of the OR table instead of on the anesthesia machine. An unexpected finding was that the anesthesiologist's attention was directed away from the patient or surgical field 42% of the time. The authors recommended automating the task of creating an anesthesia record and redesigning the anesthesia machine to increase productivity and decrease the amount of distraction away from the patient and surgical field.

It is interesting that only recently, almost 40 years after Drui's recommendations were published, have electronic anesthesia record-keeping systems and integrated anesthesia workstations attained commercial viability. Kennedy and colleagues[10] recorded three coronary artery bypass procedures on video and coded 13 categories of anesthesiologist activity at 2-second intervals. They found that the two most frequent activities were "observe patient" and "scan entire field" but that attention was directed away from the patient and surgical field 30% of the time. Logging data on the anesthesia record occupied 10% to 15% of the anesthesiologists' time; this activity was tightly linked with observing instrument displays. These authors also recommended automation of the anesthesia record and a more structured arrangement of equipment around the patient and surgical field.

Neither of these studies directly resulted in a redesign of anesthesia equipment. However, in 1976, Fraser Harlake (Orchard Park, NY) produced a prototype line-of-sight anesthesia machine designed by Goodyear and Rendell-Baker.[11] With this machine, the user could see both the patient and the machine controls with minimal eye movement. Although it was never made commercially available, the machine may have nevertheless influenced the design of the Ohio Modulus Wing anesthesia machine (Ohmeda; GE Healthcare, Waukesha, WI). An important feature of the Modulus Wing machine was that the displays and controls had more ergonomic viewing angles and could be positioned closer to the patient.

Boquet and colleagues[12] collected 16 hours of time and motion data during general anesthetic procedures before redesigning an anesthesia system. They recorded and classified 31 manual activities and 26 visual activities. In their study, 40% of the anesthesiologists' visual attention was directed away from the patient or surgical field, and the anesthesiologists were physically idle 72% of the time. The also found that logging data on the anesthesia record occupied 6% of the anesthesiologists' time and was frequently linked to measurement of blood pressure. In addition, the patterns of activity were different during the four quarters of the anesthetic procedure. Based on these observations, the authors proposed a new anesthesia machine design.

More recent studies have confirmed previous findings that anesthesiologists spend significant amounts of time on indirect patient-related tasks and that the distribution of tasks is influenced by the stage of the anesthetic procedure.[13-15] The similarities of the results in these time-and-motion studies are striking, especially because they were conducted over 20 years in a wide variety of clinical settings.

Weinger and colleagues[15] at the University of California–San Diego Medical Center used a combination of task analysis methods to compare the clinical performance of novice and experienced anesthesia care providers. A trained observer used a computer to record, in real time, 28 anesthesia-related tasks during 22 general anesthesia cases. Clinicians also rated their workload at intervals during the case and performed a vigilance task (Fig. 24-2; see also Chapter 23).

Important differences were detected between the novices (residents in their first clinical anesthesia year) and the experts (residents in their third clinical anesthesia year and certified registered nurse anesthetists [CRNAs]). Novices took longer to induce anesthesia, performed fewer tasks per unit of time, and rated their workload as higher (Fig. 24-3). In addition, novices appeared less efficient in their allocation of effort to different tasks. There

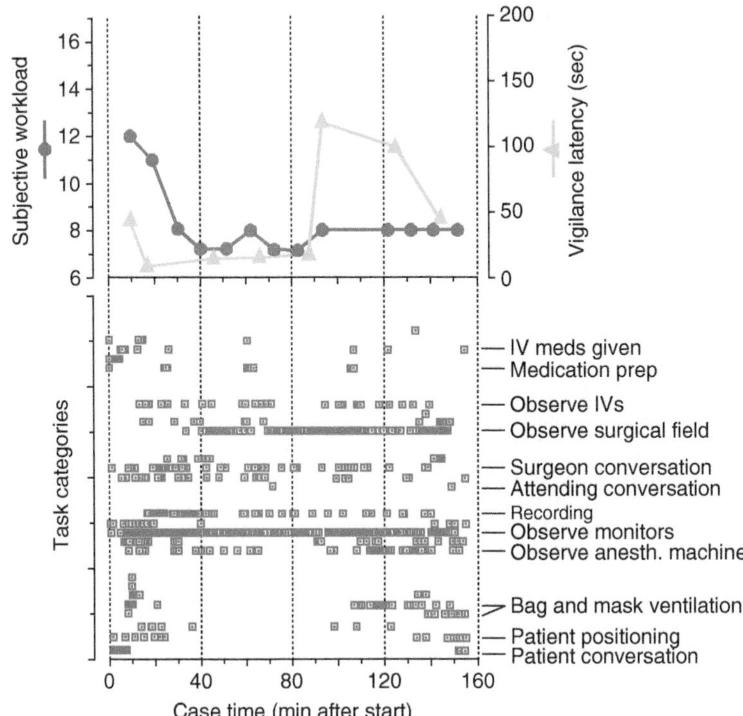

FIGURE 24-2 ■ Task distribution, subjective workload, and vigilance of one senior anesthesia resident during a single, routine, 160-minute general anesthetic procedure. *Top,* Subjective workload score (*circles*) and response latency to a vigilance light (*triangles*) over time. Subjective workload was self-reported on a scale from 6 (no effort) to 20 (maximal effort). Response latency was the time required for the anesthesiologist to recognize the illumination of a small red light located adjacent to the electrocardiograph monitor. *Bottom,* Distribution and pattern of tasks performed. Each data point (*square*) represents a single occurrence of that task category. *IV,* intravenous.

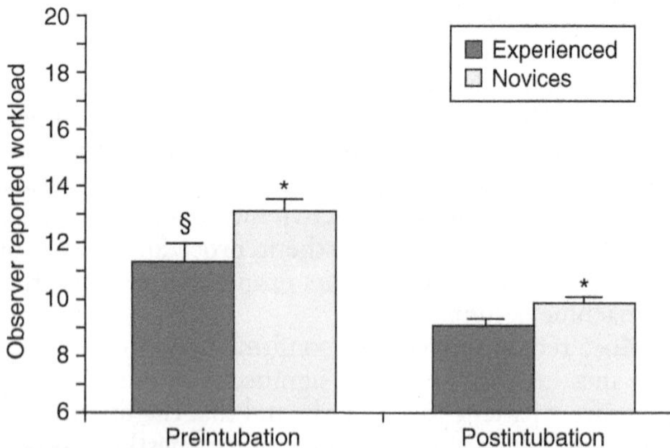

FIGURE 24-3 Workload was higher for novice residents than for experienced practitioners during routine general anesthesia procedures. Subjective workload was scored by an impartial observer, sitting in the operating room, using the 15-point Borg scale (6 = no effort, 20 = maximal effort) throughout a series of procedures performed by novice (2 weeks to 2 months of anesthesia training) or experienced providers (senior residents and certified registered nurse anesthetists). Workload was higher in the novices both before and after intubation (* $P < .05$, novices vs. experienced). In addition, in the experienced providers, but not in the novices, a statistically significant decrease was reported in workload after intubation (§ $P < .05$, preintubation vs. postintubation). Despite a higher reported workload, novices performed fewer tasks per minute and were less vigilant (data not shown). (From Weinger MB, Herndon OW, Zornow MH, et al: An objective methodology for task analysis and workload assessment in anesthesia providers. *Anesthesiology* 1994;80[1]:77-92.)

were, however, many common findings among groups. With few exceptions, task distribution was similar between the novices and experts, although after intubation, experts spent significantly more time observing the surgical field (Fig. 24-4). In both groups, there was a large effect of the stage of the anesthetic on task distribution; during the preintubation period, a more limited set of tasks was performed, and task durations were shorter than during the postintubation phase. Hardly any record-keeping was done by novice or expert practitioners during the preintubation period, but record keeping consumed 15% of their postintubation time.[15]

Workload Studies

Workload assessments are important both for evaluating the cognitive requirements of new workplace designs and equipment and for predicting the worker's cognitive capacity for additional tasks. Workload can have important effects on clinical performance. For example, recovery from critical events may be impaired during high-workload situations. Workload is multidimensional and complex; multiple cognitive, psychological, and physical factors contribute to overall workload, which has been divided into various categories such as *perceptual*, *communicative*, *mediational*, and *motor load*.[16] Specific workload measurement techniques may be more sensitive and/or specific for different types of workload.[17,18] From a

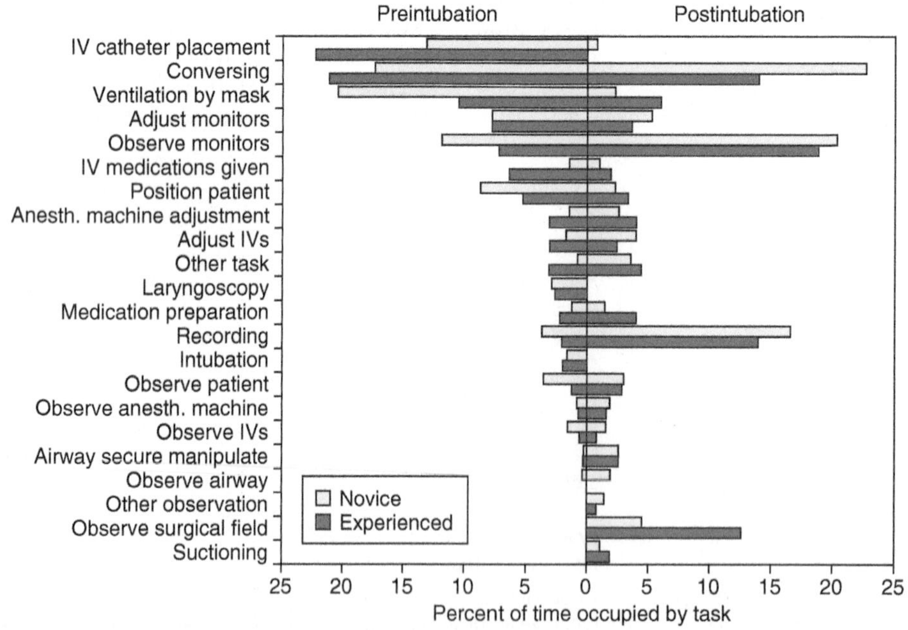

FIGURE 24-4 Distribution of tasks among expert and novice anesthesia providers during general anesthesia. Experienced practitioners (third-year anesthesia residents and experienced certified registered nurse anesthetists) performed 11 procedures under limited supervision by attending anesthesiologists. Novices (anesthesia residents in their first 8 weeks of training) performed 11 procedures under almost constant attending supervision. Each bar represents the percent of time used in one of 22 task categories during the preintubation or postintubation period of the case. For simplicity, five communication tasks are grouped into the "conversing" category, and two mask ventilation tasks are grouped into the "ventilation by mask" category. Both practitioner groups demonstrated dramatic differences in task distribution between the preintubation and postintubation periods. Little record keeping was done by any of the practitioners during the preintubation period, but recording consumed 15% of postintubation time. With few exceptions, task distribution was similar between the novice and experienced providers; after intubation, experts spent significantly more time observing the surgical field, and novices spent more time conversing with the supervising attending. IV, intravenous line. (Data from Weinger MB, Herndon OW, Zornow MH, et al: An objective methodology for task analysis and workload assessment in anesthesia providers. *Anesthesiology* 1994;80[1]:77-92.)

practical standpoint, workload measures can be divided into *psychological*, *procedural* (i.e., task related), and *physiologic* metrics.

Psychological metrics include psychologic tests and survey instruments, either retrospective or prospective. A common example is subjective workload assessment in which either an observer or the subjects themselves rate their workload, or some component of it, on a predefined scale.[19] For example, Weinger and colleagues[14] assessed subjective workload by having an observer and the subject rate the subject's workload every 10 to 15 minutes during general anesthesia cases using an integrated workload scale ranging from 6 (no work) to 20 (extremely hard work). They found a strong correlation between the ratings of the subject and the observer, and subjective workload was significantly higher prior to intubation than during the remainder of the case (Fig. 24-5).

Procedural workload assessment techniques are generally based on alterations in primary or secondary task performance.[20] For example, Gaba and Lee[21] used the ability of anesthesia residents to perform an extra task (paced arithmetic problems) during administration of anesthesia as a measure of the workload of the primary task (administering anesthesia). They found that performance of the secondary task was compromised in 40% of the samples; that is, the problem was skipped, or there was a greater than 30-second excess response time. Workload was highest during the induction and emergence phases of anesthesia. Higher workload occurred during performance of manual tasks, conversations with OR personnel, and interactions with the attending anesthesiologist.

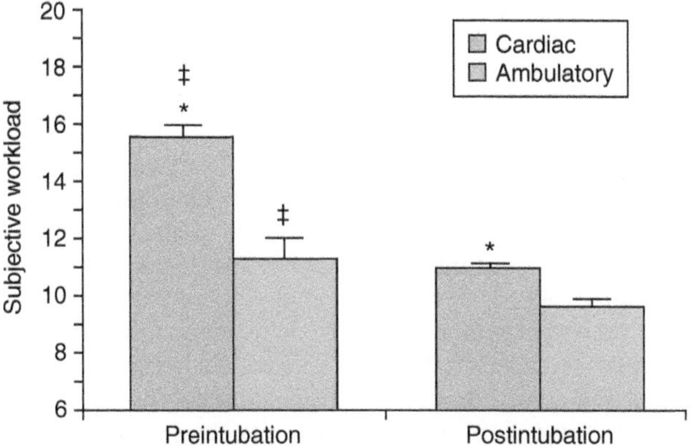

FIGURE 24-5 ■ Workload, as reported by the anesthesia provider, varies with both the type of case and the phase of the anesthetic. Workload reported by experienced anesthesia providers using a Borg scale (6 = no effort to 20 = maximal effort) was higher during induction preintubation than during the maintenance phase postintubation (‡$P < .05$, preintubation vs. postintubation) independent of the type of general anesthetic case performed. In addition, subjective workload during cardiac surgical cases was uniformly greater when compared with routine ambulatory general anesthetics (*$P < .05$, cardiac vs. ambulatory) independent of phase of the case. (Data from Weinger MB, Herndon OW, Gaba DM: The effect of electronic record keeping and transesophageal echocardiography on task distribution, workload, and vigilance during cardiac anesthesia. *Anesthesiology* 1997;87[1]:144-155; and Weinger MB, Herndon OW, Zornow MH, et al: An objective methodology for task analysis and workload assessment in anesthesia providers. *Anesthesiology* 1994;80[1]: 77-92.)

Weinger and colleagues[22] found a correlation between subjective workload and objective workload measured with a different secondary task probe, time to respond to the illumination of a light in the anesthesia monitoring array. Not only was the response time slower during induction than during maintenance, but less experienced anesthesia residents had slower response times compared with more experienced residents, especially during induction. This suggests that less experienced clinicians may have less spare capacity to respond to new task demands, particularly during high-workload conditions. Findings to date suggest that during the course of a typical OR procedure, the anesthesiologist's workload is heavy 20% to 30% of the time and very low 30% to 40% of the time, and the anesthesiologist is physically active but able to respond to additional tasks the remainder of the time.

When workload increases, the sympathetic nervous system is activated, leading to a variety of physiologic changes, many of which can be measured. For example, increased workload is associated with increases in heart rate or respiratory rate, decreases in heart rate variability or galvanic skin response, and changes in pupil size or vocal patterns.[22] In two older reports, Toung and colleagues[23,24] reported that the heart rate of anesthesia providers increased significantly while they were administering anesthesia, and heart rate increased to between 39% and 65% above baseline values at the time of patient intubation, although more experienced individuals manifested less of a heart rate increase.These results have been corroborated by Weinger and colleagues.[25,26] Experienced anesthesia providers showed significant increases in heart rate, above baseline values, during the induction and emergence phases of general anesthesia in healthy outpatients. In addition, their heart rate variability increased throughout the procedure; this is consistent with diminished stress levels as these experienced providers became more comfortable during the course of administration.

Quantitation of the pace and difficulty of the tasks performed in a job may be an alternative type of procedural workload measure. Weinger and colleagues[15] used data from their time-motion study to generate what they called "task density," a continuous measure of the number of tasks performed per unit of time. Although task density correlated well with subjective workload in this study, its value seemed limited by the fact that the demands imposed by different tasks were all weighted equally. *Workload density* has been proposed as a real-time measure that incorporates both task density and a measure of the subjective workload associated with individual clinical tasks (Fig. 24-6).[14] Workload values for common anesthesia tasks were estimated from the results of a questionnaire on which anesthesia providers rated the difficulty of specific tasks (e.g., "observe monitors" or "laryngoscopy") in three different dimensions: 1) *mental workload*, 2) *physical workload*, and 3) *psychological stress*.[26] Factor analysis was used to generate a single index of the perceived workload for each task (i.e., workload factor scores; Table 24-1).[26,27] Workload density was calculated by multiplying the amount of time spent on each task by that task's workload factor score. Workload density correlates with heart rate variability, response latency, and subjective workload.[25]

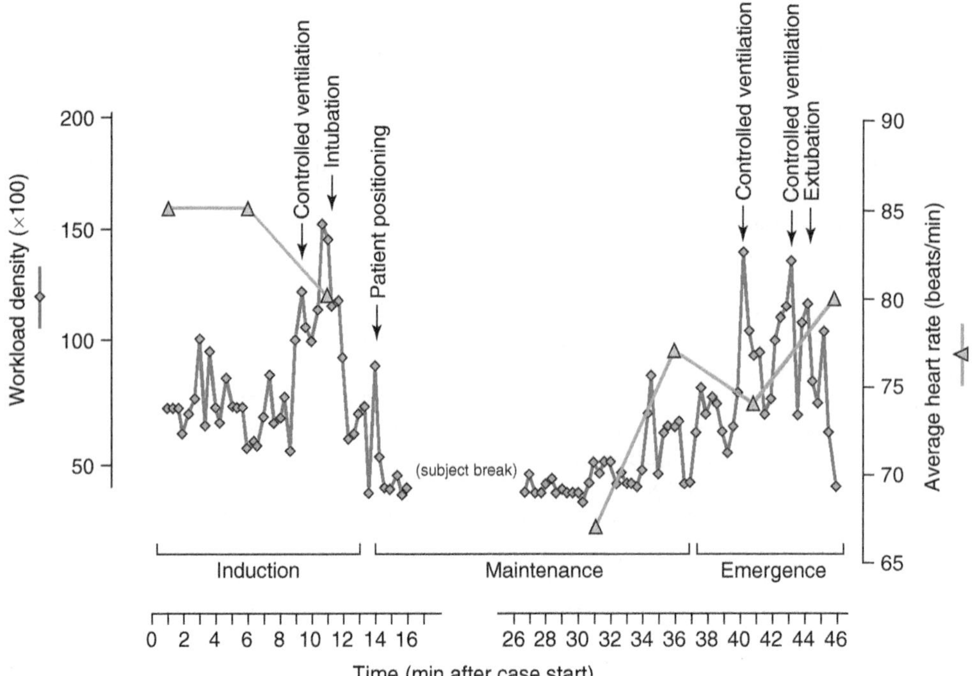

FIGURE 24-6 Workload density (*diamonds*) and average heart rate (*triangles*) for a senior resident during a single, routine, general anesthesia procedure. Workload density is a real-time procedural measure of clinical workload. Note that the subject took a 10-minute break in the middle of the case, during which time data collection was suspended.

Attention Studies

Vigilance has long been considered important to anesthesiologists, as reflected in the word's inclusion on the official seal of the American Society of Anesthesiologists (ASA).[27] Anesthesiologists understand the need to pay attention to details and subtle signs that could easily be overlooked. Vigilance is discussed in some detail in Chapter 23, although several studies pertinent to the above discussion are presented here. Kay and Neal[28] performed one of the earliest studies of anesthesia vigilance, but their experiment had a number of methodological flaws.[29,30] Cooper and Cullen[29] subsequently described a better method for investigating auditory vigilance. They used a computer-controlled device to occlude the stethoscope tubing silently at random intervals during routine general anesthesia cases. Study participants were instructed to press a button to restore function whenever they perceived the absence of stethoscope sounds. The elapsed time between the occlusion of the tubing and the press of the button was automatically recorded. Researchers studied 320 stethoscope occlusions in 32 intubated patients; the interval from occlusion to detection ranged from 2 to 457 seconds with a mean of 34 seconds (Fig. 24-7). They concluded that auditory vigilance during general anesthesia was typically high but not infallible. Manual tasks and conversations interfered with auditory vigilance because the subjects were involved in one of these activities in all instances of response times greater than 5 minutes.

In another study, Loeb[30] evaluated visual vigilance in eight anesthesia residents by displaying numbers at random intervals on an OR monitor during operative procedures. The residents were required to detect an "abnormal" value and asked to respond by pressing a button on the anesthesia machine. During 60 minor operative procedures, the average response time was 61 ± 61 seconds (mean ± standard deviation), and 56% of the detections were made within 60 seconds. Compared with Cooper's study, it appears that response times in the OR are longer for visual than for auditory signals (see Fig. 24-7).

Loeb conducted a second vigilance study to investigate why his subjects took longer to detect changes in monitored data during the induction phase of anesthesia than during the maintenance phase.[31] Residents performed the vigilance task described above, and task analysis data were recorded concurrently by a trained observer. Ten residents were studied during 73 surgical procedures, and performance on the vigilance task correlated with monitor-watching activities. Residents spent less total time watching monitors during induction than during maintenance, and the average duration of monitor observations was shorter. These results, combined with the findings of the above workload studies, suggest that anesthesiologists watch the monitors less during high-workload periods, such as during induction, so they may be less aware of electronically monitored data during that time.

Automation and New Technologies

A recurrent application of task analysis, workload, and attention studies has been to investigate the effect of automation and new technologies on anesthesiologist performance. The impetus for these studies may derive from two opposing schools of thought: one espousing

TABLE 24-1 **Workload Values Associated with Various Anesthesia Tasks**

Task	Value
Procedural	
Laryngoscopy	1.519
Intubation	1.463
Extubation	1.426
Controlled ventilation by mask	1.399
Teaching	1.333
Airway secure/manipulation	1.130
Position patient	1.130
IV catheter placement	0.940
Spontaneous mask ventilation	0.935
Prep for next case	0.909
Adjust TEE	0.841
Other tasks	0.700
Recording (manual)	0.596
Medication preparation	0.519
Tidying up	0.475
Adjust monitors	0.441
IV medications given	0.426
Anesthesia machine adjustment	0.404
Suctioning	0.352
Adjust IVs	0.222
Conversational	
Attending conversation	0.931
Surgeon conversation	0.907
Patient conversation	0.685
Converse with others	0.308
Nurse conversation	0.259
Observational	
Observe TEE	0.672
Observe monitors	0.593
Observe patient	0.574
Observe airway	0.500
Observe anesthesia machine	0.482
Observe surgical field	0.352
Observe IVs/fluids	0.154
Other observation	0.154

Higher values represent greater workload. Workload values were calculated using a factor analysis on data obtained from questionnaires completed by anesthesia providers, who were asked to rate each task on a three-point workload scale (high, medium, or low) based on its associated physical effort, mental effort, and psychological stress. Workload values are used in the calculation of workload density.

IV, intravenous line; TEE, transesophageal echocardiography.

From Weinger MB, Herndon OW, Gaba DM: The effect of electronic record keeping and transesophageal echocardiography on task distribution, workload, and vigilance during cardiac anesthesia. *Anesthesiology* 1997;87(1):144-155; and Keenan RL, Boyan P: Cardiac arrest due to anesthesia. *JAMA* 1985; 253:2373-2377.

technology and the other decrying it. From one side come claims that technology decreases workload, enhances task efficiency, and increases idle time, thereby allowing the anesthesiologist more opportunity to observe and process information from the patient, equipment, and surgical field.[12,32] The other side claims that technology removes the human from the information loop, thereby distancing the anesthesiologist from the patient and decreasing situation awareness.[28,33,34] A more balanced view may be that technology can improve or degrade human performance, depending on how it is implemented. Automation will only prove beneficial if the human was previously overloaded, the automated system is a team player (i.e., responsive, directable, and nonintrusive), and the interface between them supports the human's situation awareness.[35] Systems that do not fulfill these criteria may create new problems and degrade overall system performance.[35,36]

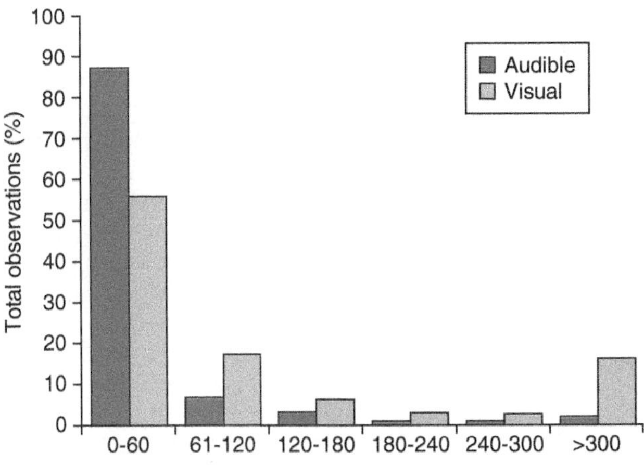

FIGURE 24-7 ■ **Comparison of intraoperative vigilance of anesthesiologists from two different studies. Audible vigilance was assessed as response time to detect occlusion of the esophageal stethoscope. Visual vigilance was measured as response time to detect an abnormal value displayed on a physiologic monitor.** (Modified from Cooper JO, Cullen BF: Observer reliability in detecting surreptitious random occlusions of the monaural esophageal stethoscope. *J Clin Monit* 1990;6:271-275, and Loeb RG: Monitor surveillance and vigilance of anesthesia residents. *Anesthesiology* 1994;80:527-533.)

One study suggests a beneficial effect of automation on anesthesiologist task distribution. McDonald and colleagues[13,37] compared the results of two time-motion studies conducted 5 years apart at the Ohio State University Hospitals. In the newer series, automated blood pressure devices, ventilators, and disconnect alarms were used. With these newer technologies, the time that anesthesiologists spent directly observing or monitoring the patient *increased* from less than 25% to nearly 60% of their total task time. At the same institution, Allard and colleagues[38] examined the effect of an electronic anesthesia record keeper (EARK) on the time spent keeping records and the anesthesia resident's situation awareness. They videotaped 37 general anesthesia procedures in which record keeping was done manually and 29 cases that used a commercial EARK. The intraoperative time of the subjects (33 anesthesia residents and 8 CRNAs) was categorized into 15 predefined activities. Situation awareness was assessed by having the subject turn away from the monitors and recall the value of eight patient variables. No difference was reported between the two groups in the time spent keeping records or the ability to recall clinical data accurately.

Loeb[39] also investigated whether intraoperative vigilance was different when residents kept a manual record than when a human assistant performed the charting. Nine residents were studied during 36 procedures in a within-subjects balanced design. Vigilance was assessed as the subject's response time and detection rate to detect an experimental signal displayed on the physiologic monitor. No overall difference was reported in vigilance between the two record-keeping conditions, but a tendency was observed toward reduced vigilance (i.e., longer response times or lower detection rates) during high-workload periods in the manual record-keeping group.

Weinger and colleagues[14] studied the effects of modern anesthesia technology during the prebypass period of 20 coronary artery bypass graft procedures. In 10 cases record keeping was done manually; in the other 10 cases, a commercially available EARK was used. Transesophageal echocardiography (TEE) was used in all cases. The investigators collected task analysis data (32 task categories, recorded by an observer in real time), subjective workload ratings (10- to 15-minute random intervals), and response latencies to the illumination of a light in the monitoring array. The EARK group spent less time on record keeping between intubation and initiation of bypass and more of their time observing the monitors than did the group keeping manual records. However, no difference was found between the record-keeping groups in subjective workload or rapidity of detecting illumination of the light. Subjects spent nearly 8% of their time observing or adjusting the TEE, and it took an average of 7.4 min to insert the TEE and do a preliminary assessment. Residents were slower to react to the illuminated light while observing or adjusting the TEE than while performing record keeping or other monitor-observation tasks.

In these studies, no demonstrable negative effect was seen of automated record keeping. However, the results from Weinger do demonstrate a high workload imposed by current TEE technology and suggest the potential for impaired vigilance when TEE is used intraoperatively by a solo practitioner.[14]

Critical Incident Studies

A careful analysis of adverse events and "near misses" can lead to productive changes in system structure, equipment design, training procedures, and other interventions to improve safety. Critical incident analysis is an established method for investigating human error that was first used in 1954 to study near misses in aviation.[40] The technique involves structured interviews of people who have either observed or been involved in unsafe acts. Analysis of these interviews often provides evidence of behavior patterns and other recurrent factors that may contribute to accidents.

Cooper and colleagues[41] were the first to apply the critical incident technique to anesthesiology. From 1975 through 1984, they collected descriptions of 1089 critical incidents from 139 anesthesiologists, residents, and nurse anesthetists. The descriptions were obtained through a combination of retrospective interviews and contemporaneous reports. *Critical incidents* were defined as occurrences of "human error or equipment failure that could have led (if not discovered or corrected in time) or did lead to an undesirable outcome, ranging from increased length of hospital stay to death."[41] Their data indicated that human error was responsible for 65% to 70% of the incidents. The 67 incidents that resulted in substantive negative outcomes included 28 technical human errors, 23 judgmental errors, and 13 vigilance errors. A number of recurrent technical human errors were related to the design or organization of equipment. Examples of these included syringe and drug ampoule swaps, gas flow control technical errors, vaporizers unintentionally turned off, drug overdoses (technical), misuses of blood pressure monitors, breathing circuit control technical errors, and wrong IV lines used. On the basis of their findings, the authors recommended a standardized system of syringe labels and redesign of the breathing circuit to prevent disconnections.

A detailed description of one of their critical incidents, gas flow control technical error, illustrates the importance of evaluating equipment designs prior to implementation. At one of the hospitals where the studies were conducted, all the anesthesia machines had been modified. On each machine, the oxygen flow control knob had been replaced with a large, square knob in an attempt to distinguish it from the nitrous oxide knob. However, rather than preventing gas flow control errors, the knob was found to be a contributing factor: half the accidental decreases in oxygen flow occurred when the knob was bumped by an object placed on the desktop surface of the anesthesia machine. This example highlights the importance of field testing new device designs by intended users.

Subsequent critical incident studies[42-45] have been performed using contemporaneous reporting strategies. In each, human error has been a predominant cause of mishaps, and the patterns of incident types and associated factors have been similar. Kumar and colleagues[44] demonstrated that critical incidents decreased when an anesthesia equipment checklist was used, old anesthesia machines were replaced, and incidents were discussed at department conferences. They recommended critical incident surveillance as a method of identifying specific problems and ensuring quality control.

Since 1989, the Australian Patient Safety Foundation has supported an ongoing multiinstitutional collection of anesthesia critical incidents.[45] Anesthesiologists from 90 participating hospitals and practices in Australia and New Zealand anonymously report unexpected incidents using a structured format. Each report is entered into a computerized database after it has been reviewed and classified using standard keywords. In 1993, an exhaustive analysis of the first 2000 incidents was published.[46] Human error was believed to be involved in 83% of the incidents; only 9% of the incidents involved equipment failure. Equipment design improvement was suggested as an appropriate corrective strategy in 17% of the reports. System failure was a contributory factor in 26% of the incidents and, based on the results, the authors recommended 111 system improvements to increase patient safety.[46]

Reporting bias is a recognized shortcoming of the critical incident methodology. Many incidents are never reported, and those that are may be incomplete or inaccurate for a number of reasons.[47] In studies of adverse drug reporting, only a very small fraction of the total number of events are voluntarily reported.[48] Both the number and accuracy of adverse event reports can be enhanced by scanning automatically collected data for predefined criteria, such as out-of-bounds physiologic parameters.[49] A continuing problem, however, is the collection of adverse events that become apparent only in the postoperative period. Until comprehensive computerized medical records are widely available, painstaking follow-up will remain a cornerstone of accurate adverse event collection and analysis.[50,51]

Gaba and DeAnda[52] used a comprehensive anesthesia simulator to investigate factors of accident evolution and techniques used by clinicians to recognize and recover from critical events. The simulator recreated the OR environment with real monitors and equipment, and a patient mannequin was used (see Chapter 25). In an initial study of behavior of residents in response to planned critical incidents, these researchers noted problems and errors that arose in addition to the planned events. They documented 132 unplanned events during 19 simulated cases; 87 events were attributed to human error, and only 4 were equipment failures.[53] However, many of the human failures involved errors in the use of equipment; for example, failure to switch the ventilator power back on after hand-ventilating the patient and neglecting to turn up the oxygen flow during preoxygenation. This study indicated that errors occur commonly, that many errors involve interactions with equipment, and that most errors are detected and corrected before they become hazardous to the patient. These findings also apply to experienced clinicians, who averaged five unplanned incidents during each simulated case.[54] Again, many of the experienced practitioners' errors involved interactions with equipment.

MacKenzie and colleagues[55,56] took an alternative approach to the study of clinical decision making in anesthesia. Similar to the intraoperative task analysis studies described above, MacKenzie's group assessed performance during actual trauma cases at the Maryland Shock Trauma Center and developed a sophisticated audio-video and physiologic data-capture methodology that allows off-line analysis.[57] They described four components of task complexity that appear to have a significant impact on teamwork during emergency resuscitation after trauma: 1) multiple concurrent tasks, 2) uncertainty, 3) changing plans, and 4) high workload.[55] Their work suggests that video analysis methodology can be a powerful tool in the evaluation of factors leading to deficiencies in airway management.[56,58]

ERGONOMICS GUIDELINES

The successful development of ergonomically sound equipment and systems requires that ergonomics principles and guidelines be adhered to throughout the entire design cycle, beginning in the predesign phase. A number of ergonomics handbooks and guidelines have been published for equipment designers in fields outside medicine.[59] In the late 1980s, the Association for the Advancement of Medical Instrumentation (AAMI), the professional organization for American clinical/hospital engineers, began a national standards-making process to develop guidance for medical device manufacturers to improve the human factors of their products. The result, "Human Factors Engineering Guidelines and Preferred Practices for the Design of Medical Devices,"[60] was largely an adaptation of human factors design guidance from other industries (especially for the design of military products). In the early 1990s, the AAMI Human Factors Committee decided to revise this document substantially. The group first developed a process-oriented standard on a structured approach to user interface design for all medical devices. This national standard, ANSI/AAMI HE-74-2001, described design approaches relevant to all aspects of the design of devices, including labeling, documentation, and learning tools. More importantly, the standard and the Committee's deliberations drove greater interest in human factors in the national and even international medical device industry and its regulators. For example, HE-74 was the foundation for the international collateral standard 60106-1-6 on medical device usability from the International Electrotechnical Commission (IEC), which only applied to medical devices requiring electricity to operate. This international standard was subsequently replaced by standard 62366, Medical Devices—Application of Usability Engineering to Medical Devices,[61] a joint standard by the IEC and the International Organization for Standardization (ISO) that applies to *all* medical devices. The content of HE-74 is provided in Appendix G of standard 62366. At the time of this writing, standard 62366 is undergoing another revision expected to be completed in 2015.

Although these standards specify the process of designing medical device user interfaces, they do not provide any guidance on the *design elements* of a good medical device user interface. Thus, the AAMI HF Committee spent 5 years creating a companion standard, HE-75 (Factors Engineering—Design of Medical Devices),[62] which is intended to provide comprehensive human factors design principles for medical devices. In parallel with this effort, a number of the HF Committee members published a handbook intended to amplify HE-75 with greater topical detail, figures, and case studies.[63] The Food and Drug Administration (FDA) is responsible for federal oversight of medical devices and has become increasingly interested in ensuring that medical device manufacturers use human factors design principles and adhere to standardized good manufacturing practices (GMP). The FDA recently published guidelines on this subject,[64] which also are available on the Internet.

Principles of Good Device Design

User requirements must be emphasized during the design of equipment and devices. The goal is to produce devices that are easily maintained, have an effective user interface, and are tailored to the user's abilities.[4] This is best accomplished during the early phases of system and equipment design, when the ergonomics and engineering specialists can work together with end users to produce a safe, reliable, and usable product.[65] Norman eloquently presents this principle of user-centered system design in *The Psychology of Everyday Things*.[66] This book can be recommended for all engineers, programmers, and designers responsible for the development of new medical devices. Some of the key aspects of user-interface design that Norman emphasizes are to 1) make things visible, 2) provide good mapping, 3) create appropriate constraints, 4) simplify tasks, and 5) design for error.

Make Things Visible

A well-designed interface between human and machine conveys to the user the purpose, operational modes, and controlling actions for the device. If the design of the device or system is based on a good conceptual model, its purpose will be readily apparent to the user. Most devices have several operational modes, and the user must be able to determine rapidly and accurately whether the system is in the desired mode and when the mode changes. With most devices, a number of user actions are possible at any given time; with complex systems, the allowable commands often depend on the current operational mode. The user should be able to tell what actions are possible at any given instant and what the consequences of those actions will be. *Feedback* must be provided after each user action that should be readily understandable, and it should match the user's intentions.

The user's understanding of the function and operation of a device is paramount to the effectiveness of the system. The function and operation of many common devices is learned through cultural experience. People also expect certain objects to always function in a particular manner: knobs are for turning, buttons are for pushing, and so on. With other devices, the function can and often should be implied by the device itself. That is, the purpose and operation of a particular control or display should by design be as intuitive as possible for the user; for example, the sturdy horizontal handle on the side of the anesthesia machine is for pulling the device from one location to another. Such intuitive operation may be difficult to attain with complex, microprocessor-controlled multifunction devices. However, when the design requires the user to memorize specialized knowledge to operate the system (e.g., "To see the systolic blood pressure trend plot, I must push a particular sequence of soft buttons in a specific order"), the need for training increases, and the chance of system-induced user error increases, especially under stressful, unusual, or high-workload conditions.

Provide Good Mapping

Mapping is the relationship between an action and a response and may be natural or artificial. *Natural mappings* are intuitive; *artificial mappings* must be learned. Artificial mappings that have been learned so well that the relationship between action and effect is recognized at a subconscious or automatic level are called *conventional mappings*. On an anesthesia machine, squeezing the bag to inflate the lungs is a natural mapping. Turning the oxygen flow control knob counterclockwise to increase gas flow is an artificial mapping. However, because this design follows the conventional mapping of valves, users typically do not have difficulty adjusting the flow of oxygen on the anesthesia machine. Unfortunately, for many medical machines and systems, methods for activating alternate modes of action, adjusting alarm limits, or manipulating data are via artificial, unique, and nonstandard mappings.

Any device has three different stages of mapping: 1) between intentions and the required action; 2) between actions and the resulting effects, and 3) between the information provided about the system and the actual state of the system. Inappropriate mapping at any stage leads to delayed learning and poor user performance. If natural or well-known artificial mappings are not used, the designer should seek preexisting standards or perform tests to ascertain optimal mappings, which should be consistent within a single device or system.

Create Appropriate Constraints

Constraints are limitations on the user's available options or actions and can be physical, semantic, cultural, or logical. The provision of a control that can be oriented only in specific ways is a physical constraint (e.g., a switch can only be either on or off). With a semantic constraint, the meaning of a particular situation controls the set of possible actions.[66] For example, the sounding of an alarm is meant to indicate the need to take some kind of action.

Cultural constraints are a set of allowable actions in social situations: signs, labels, and messages are meant to be read. Natural mappings typically work by logical constraints. When a series of indicator lights are arranged in a row, each with a switch underneath, the logical constraint dictates that the switch underneath a particular indicator light controls, or is associated with, that light. Devices, particularly their human interface components, should contain constraints that facilitate simple, logical, and intuitive operation.

Design for Error

Human performance is prone to error. *Slips*, or actions that do not go as planned, are a common form of human error arising from interactions with devices.[67] Accidentally pushing the wrong button is an example of a slip (see Chapter 23). It is the device designer's responsibility to anticipate user errors and minimize the risk that these inevitable errors will produce ill effects. Actions with potentially undesirable consequences should be reversible and the device should perhaps require additional user acknowledgment prior to completing the action. The designer also can implement a *forcing function*, a type of constraint that prevents performance of an action that is clearly undesirable. An example of a forcing function is the oxygen/nitrous oxide interlock mechanism that prevents the delivery of a hypoxic gas mixture.

These principles of good design are not limited to the interface between user and machine.[4] A well-designed device is also easy to clean, maintain, and repair, and its documentation is organized and understandable. However, many currently available commercial devices violate these basic design principles. In an ergonomics evaluation of a microprocessor-controlled respiratory gas humidifier, Potter and colleagues[68] found that the device had hidden modes of operation, ambiguous alarm messages, inconsistent control actions, and complex resetting sequences. One clinically used respiratory gas analyzer issues arcane alarm messages and has multiple display formats that are difficult to access. Another gas analyzer has a hidden calibration mode that renders it unusable if the sampling tubing is not attached when the unit is initially powered up. We have noted that at least two brands of limb tourniquet controllers have no indicator that the cuff is inflated, although this impression is mistakenly given by a display of "cuff pressure" and a running timer on the front panel.

Crisis situations tend to generate "use errors" that may not occur during less stressful times. For example, during simulated crisis situations, many subjects forgot to coordinate the setting of the bag/ventilator selector switch on the anesthesia machine breathing circuit when switching between controlled and spontaneous ventilation.[69] At least some of what, on first glance, appears to be human error often can be traced back to poorly designed interfaces between human and machine.[70] Devices often are used inefficiently or incorrectly as a consequence of poor design.[68] When the device acts in unexpected ways, the user develops erroneous or inconsistent mental models of its operation.[71] This problem can be exacerbated when the user has not received adequate instruction before using the device.

Visual Displays

Humans rely heavily on the visual sensory channel for communicating or obtaining information. The cathode ray tube (CRT), printed page, vehicle instrument panel, and line drawing are all examples of visual displays. An early application of ergonomics was the design of instrument displays for military applications.[72,73] Research continues on developing and improving visual displays for such diverse areas as the airplane cockpit (Fig. 24-8), the nuclear power plant control room, and the office computerized workstation.[74,75] Although a complete description of this work is outside the scope of this chapter, a number of guidelines that have resulted from these studies are presented. Much of the specific information presented stems directly from the general considerations already discussed.

Properties of Visual Displays

Three criteria are fundamental to the performance of a display: visibility, legibility, and readability.[8] *Visibility* refers to the degree to which the individual characters or symbols on a display are detectable against the background, and it depends on display features such as symbol size and background color. Visiblity is also influenced by environmental factors, such as ambient light levels, and by the limitations of human perception, such as color blindness and deficiencies of refractive index. *Legibility* pertains to the degree to which displayed numerals, characters, and symbols can be differentiated from one another. It is primarily influenced by features of the individual symbols, including size, simplicity of form, and stroke width. *Readability* is a quality that makes possible the quick and unambiguous interpretation of the information intended to be conveyed. For text displays, this is a function of semantics and letter spacing; for symbol displays, simplicity and organization are important.

The preferred size of display components depends on the viewing distance, ambient illumination, and the importance of the information. The perceived size of a display element is a function of the viewing angle. Numerals and letters on a display should be large enough to be easily legible.[8] For visual search tasks, larger characters are required.[76] Tightly packed letters are preferable when text must be read and comprehended quickly, probably because fewer eye fixations are required.[8]

Displays of Magnitude

Displays of magnitude can be either numeric or graphic. Digital displays, such as a digital watch or the odometer of a newer car, are numeric. Analog displays, such as the capnogram or the dial of a pressure gauge, are graphic. Dials are classified as either *moving pointer* on a fixed scale or *moving scale* with fixed pointers. Each type of display has advantages for particular tasks. Numeric displays require less space and are preferable when a precise numeric value is required, because they minimize errors and reading time. However, numeric displays are difficult to read if the value is changing rapidly. For instance, pilots are better at performing basic flight maneuvers in a simulator with analog displays than in one with digital displays.[77] Moving pointers are preferable as indicators of control settings, because they provide the simplest relationship to the control motion. When qualitative information is sufficient—for example, for detecting the

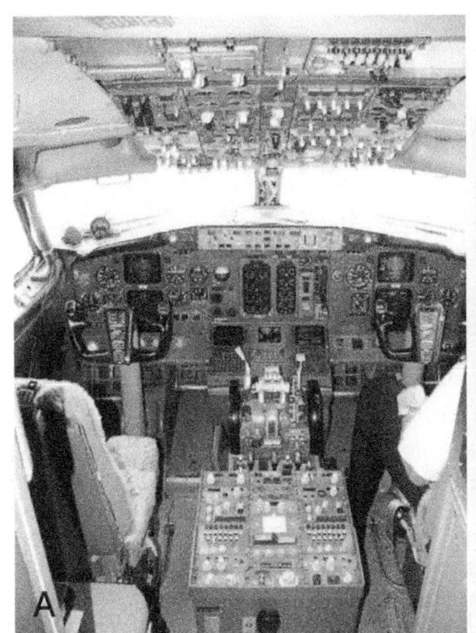

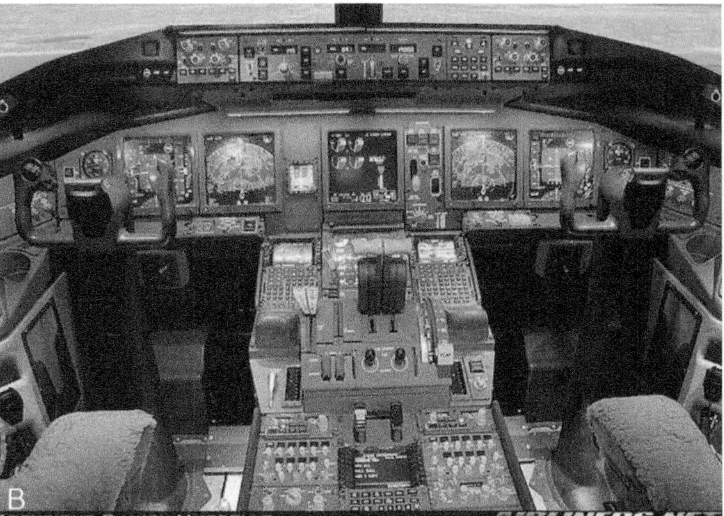

FIGURE 24-8 n Evolution of cockpit displays. **A,** Analog gauges of the Boeing 737. **B,** Computerized screens of the Boeing 777. (B, Photo copyright Daniel Murzello, used with permission. Accessed at www.airliners.net.)

direction or rate of change of a value—a graphic display or moving pointer dial is preferred.[76] Reading a dial to extract quantitative information takes significantly longer (>400 ms) than does a qualitative reading to affirm that the pointer is in the right general location (125 to 200 ms).[78] Graphic displays of recent data are especially useful for trend detection and tracking. When markers are not present for each value, people are able to interpolate, but the time required to obtain the reading is prolonged.[8] All characters should be in a vertical orientation because it takes longer to read a dial when the characters are rotated.[79]

Grouping of Displays

Displays should be grouped for optimal performance. Perceptual studies[76] support the grouping of important displays within the central 30 degrees of the visual field. The normal visual field extends up to about 30 degrees vertically and about 80 degrees horizontally. Three areas of attention have been described based on response time to visual stimuli: the stationary field, the eye field, and the head field.[80] The *stationary field* occupies the central 30 degrees and is the area of foveal vision. Within this field, multiple displays can be viewed simultaneously without eye movements. The visual field between 30 and 80 degrees is the *eye field*—the area of peripheral vision. Even when foveal vision is fixed on a display, information can still be extracted from the periphery. Peripheral vision is especially sensitive to motion and can act reflexively to guide the eye to the target information. Targets within the eye field can be brought into foveal view by eye movements; head movements are not required. The *head field* lies outside the central 80 degrees, and displays in this area are outside the peripheral visual field. To view displays in this area, the head must be moved under conscious control.

The relative importance of particular displays can be deduced from the frequency of readings during task analysis studies.[81] Similarly, link analysis[14,82] can identify recurrent sequences of display readings. Optimally, important displays should be located in the most convenient positions, and displays that are commonly viewed in sequence should be arranged adjacent to each other. To perform a task, a number of displays often are interpreted concurrently. When multiple channels of information must be mentally integrated, performance is often improved when the information is grouped. In contrast, when information from multiple channels must be kept distinct—for example, during focused attention on a single channel—grouped presentation may be deleterious.[83] Most grouping methods are based on Gestalt theory, which describes the ways in which people identify boundaries and groups. The generally accepted Gestalt laws of grouping include *proximity, similarity, closure, continuity, common region,* and *connectedness.*[84] These concepts are illustrated in Figure 24-9.

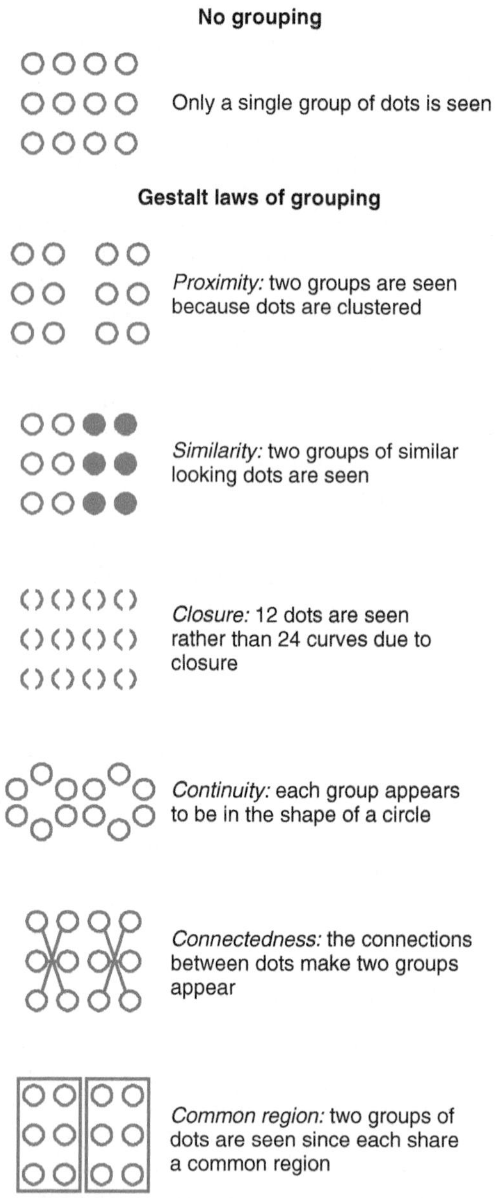

No grouping

Only a single group of dots is seen

Gestalt laws of grouping

Proximity: two groups are seen because dots are clustered

Similarity: two groups of similar looking dots are seen

Closure: 12 dots are seen rather than 24 curves due to closure

Continuity: each group appears to be in the shape of a circle

Connectedness: the connections between dots make two groups appear

Common region: two groups of dots are seen since each share a common region

FIGURE 24-9 ■ Laws of grouping from Gestalt theory.

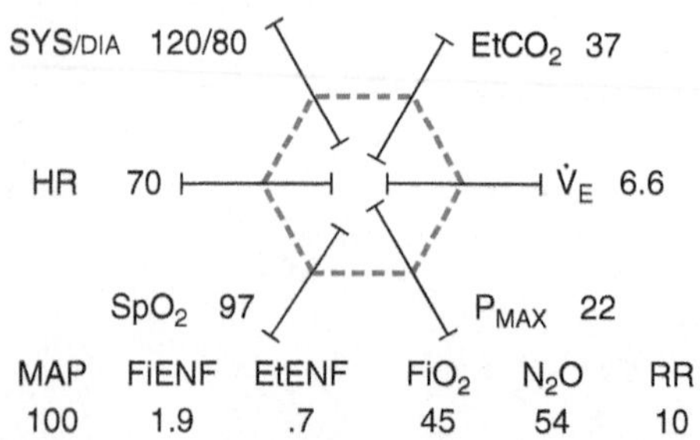

FIGURE 24-10 ■ The polygon display from the Ohmeda Modulus CD machine (GE Healthcare, Waukesha, WI). $ETCO_2$, end-tidal carbon dioxide; EtENF, end-tidal enflurane; FiENF, fraction of inspired enflurane; FiO_2, fraction of inspired oxygen; HR, heart rate; MAP, mean arterial pressure; N_2O, fraction of inspired nitrous oxide; P_{MAX}, peak airway presssure; RR, respiratory rate; SpO_2, pulse oximeter saturation; SYS/DIA, systolic/diastolic [pressure]; $\dot{V}_E$, exhaled minute ventilation.

Object Displays

Dials and numeric displays are typically read sequentially, and clustering of displays can encourage parallel processing. However, placing displays close together in space does not guarantee parallel input of information and may interfere with focused attention on a particular display. One way of ensuring some parallel processing is with object displays, in which multiple data elements are represented as attributes of a single object. When a single object is viewed, its multiple attributes—such as color, shape, and size—are perceived in parallel.

In some nuclear reactor control rooms, object (polygon) displays of safety parameter data have replaced banks of separate instrument dials.[85] In these displays, eight values are represented by eight spokes that form the axes of an octagon. A similar type of polygon display was incorporated into the Ohmeda Modulus CD anesthesia machine (GE Healthcare, Fig. 24-10). In a laboratory study, the Ohmeda polygon display was superior to a numeric display in a simulated detection task.[86] Anesthesia residents detected changes in the values of physiologic variables more quickly and accurately with the polygon display than with a numeric display. However, performance with the polygon display was not much better than that with a histogram display of the same information. The applicability of these findings to the use of graphic displays in the OR during real procedures remains to be determined.

Although object displays might seem implicitly superior to multiple dials, early studies have demonstrated some disadvantages to this approach. Petersen and colleagues[87] compared object displays with multiple bar graph displays in a task of monitoring for changes in the state of a system. They found that the object display was superior when subjects had to detect whether *any* parameter was out of tolerance, but that multiple bar graphs were better for detecting the number and identities of the out-of-bound parameters.[88] Wickens and Andre[89] performed an experiment in which subjects viewed either a bar graph display or an object display of three values for 1.5 seconds. The subject was then asked either to make a judgment on the basis of an integration of the values or to recall a single value. Performance was better on the integration task with the object display, but single values were more accurately recalled with the bar graph display. These findings are consistent with many others that support the principle of *proximity compatibility*, which states that combined displays are best suited to tasks that require information integration, whereas tasks that require independent information processing will benefit from more separate displays.[90,91] The generalizability of this principle has been questioned by Sanderson and colleagues,[92] who asserted that object displays are superior only when a simple geometric feature of the object directly correlates with the goal parameter of the task. For instance, to support judgments about systemic vascular resistance (SVR), an object display of cardiac output and blood pressure might be used instead of two individual bar graph displays. The combined display would be expected to be superior only if a simple geometric feature of the object, such as area, correlated with the goal parameter, in this case SVR.

Cole[93] has evaluated an object display of respiratory data for use in the intensive care unit (ICU). His display consists of two adjacent rectangles: the left one depicts the state of the ventilator, and the right one depicts the state of the patient; the height of each rectangle is proportional to tidal volume; the width is proportional to respiratory rate; and the color is proportional to inspired oxygen concentration. An emergent feature of the rectangles is that their area is proportional to minute volume. Respiratory therapists learned this representational scheme in less than 5 minutes and were able to judge patient status twice as quickly with a flow sheet containing these objects than with a flow sheet containing numbers.

Blike[94] developed a complex object display of hemodynamic data for use during cardiovascular surgery (Fig. 24-11). Using anesthesia residents as subjects, he demonstrated the potential utility of this display format. The residents recognized and diagnosed abnormal hemodynamic states—anaphylactic shock, bradycardia, hypovolemic shock, cardiogenic shock, and pulmonary embolism—25% to 30% faster with the object display than with an alphanumeric display. Even though the residents voiced a negative initial opinion of the display because of its complexity, their performance plateaued after 8 to 12 presentations, suggesting a relatively rapid learning curve.

These studies demonstrate the potential advantages of using object displays to present large sets of physiologic data. Most of these novel displays, however, have been evaluated only under simulated conditions that do not accurately represent real clinical situations. Additional testing of these novel displays must be performed in real or simulated clinical settings before their routine use can be recommended.

Display Coding

Coding methods can be used to highlight targets of visual search tasks and to provide similarities for grouping. Common coding methods for display elements include color, alphanumeric symbols, geometric shapes, size, brightness, location, and flash rate. In a comparison of coding methods, Hitt[95] coded objects on a map with color, numerals, letters, and geometric shapes. Performance was then assessed on tasks of identification, counting, location, comparison, and verification. Color and numeric codes were superior in most tasks. Color is the most effective coding method for search tasks, in which the subject must locate and count items in variable positions on a display. Search times can decrease by as much as 70% with color coding.[96] In a study of color coding to organize instruments on a simulated aircraft display,[88] common color coding of relevant instruments was found to facilitate integration of information, and distinct color coding improved the ability to focus attention on each instrument. Subjects commonly respond to color codes faster than to shape or alphanumeric codes. This may be because color is perceived earlier than other types of visual coding in the sequence of information processing. Another reason that color coding may be advantageous is that short-term memory is better for colors than for shapes or numbers.[88] Color coding may be most effective when the display is unformatted, the symbol density is high, or the operator must search for specified information. Color is less useful for identification tasks in which letters and numbers are preferable. Untrained subjects can reliably discriminate only five to nine colors[8]; however, with training, 24 colors can be reliably discriminated. Color coding is more effective when the chosen colors are consistent with prevailing conventions or accepted standards. In the general population, red indicates danger, and green indicates safety. To U.S. anesthesiologists, but not necessarily to others, green indicates oxygen, blue indicates nitrous oxide, and yellow indicates air.

One disadvantage of color coding is that it cannot be discriminated by the color-vision impaired. Colored lenses, such as those in the protective goggles worn during laser surgery, also impair color perception and may interfere with anesthesia tasks.[97] Redundant coding must therefore always be used when selection of the wrong object could have adverse consequences. Alternative or multiple coding methods should be considered when more than six codes must be discriminated on a single display. A number of studies suggest that irrelevant color coding can interfere with cognitive processing of visual information,[88,98] and the overuse of color for coding purposes also increases the visual clutter of a display.

Tools have been developed for the controlled study of the optimal properties of displays. For example, Berguer and colleagues[99] have used a virtual display design program to rapidly prototype and evaluate medical monitor displays for efficiency and ease of use.

Auditory Displays

Situations in which the auditory modality is preferable to the visual modality are listed in Table 24-2. A primary advantage of the human auditory system is that it can simultaneously detect signals from multiple locations. This makes auditory displays particularly useful for displaying alarms and warnings that require immediate

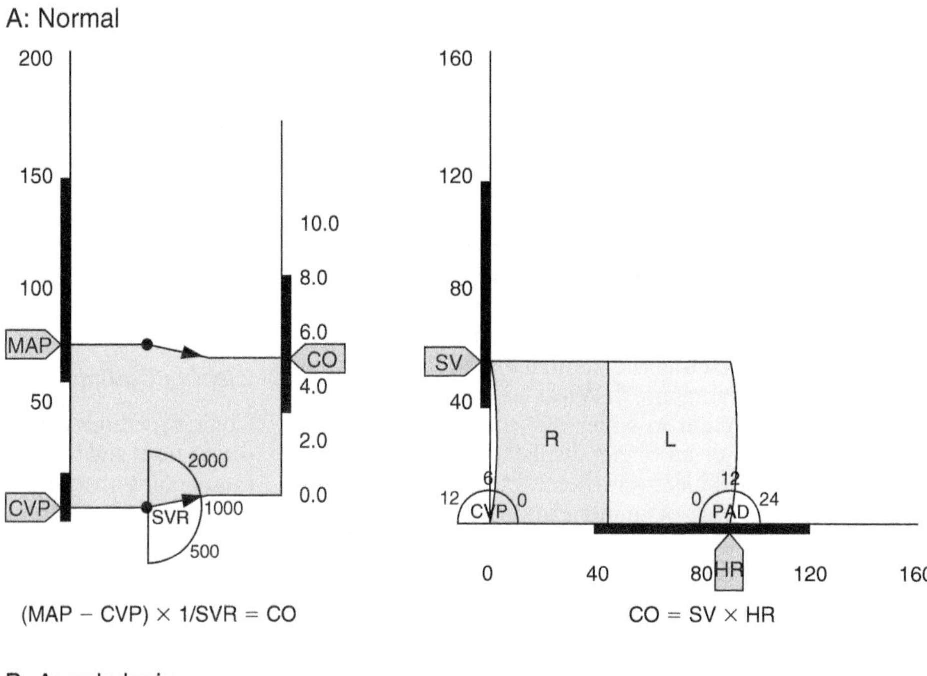

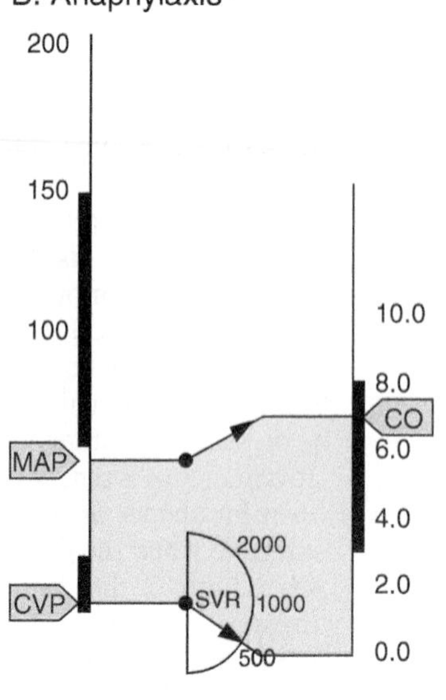

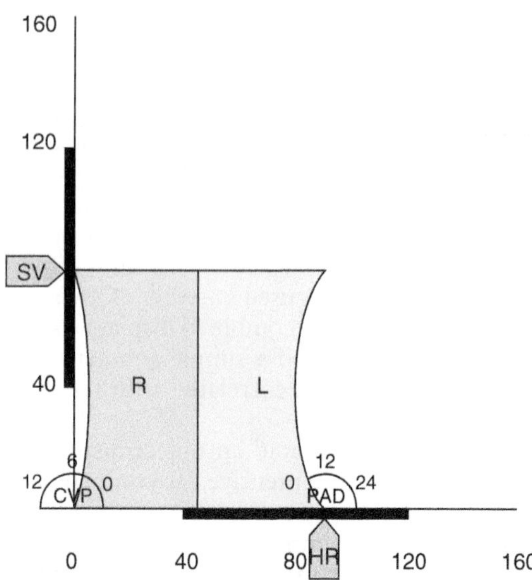

FIGURE 24-11 ■ An experimental object display of hemodynamic data. Six variables—mean arterial blood pressure (*MAP*), heart rate (*HR*), central venous pressure (*CVP*), pulmonary artery diastolic pressure (*PAD*), cardiac output (*CO*), and systemic vascular resistance (*SVR*)—are functionally mapped onto two objects. The graph on the *left* depicts functional relationships among MAP, CVP, SVR, and CO. The graph on the *right* depicts relationships among stroke volume (*SV*), HR, CO, CVP, and PAD; (*R,* right side of heart; *L,* left side of heart). The display is designed to support recognition of critical hypotension and differentiation of five hypotensive states: *anaphylaxis, bradycardia, hypovolemia, ischemia,* and *pulmonary embolus.* **A,** Display under normal conditions. **B,** How the object display might look during anaphylaxis (high CO, low SVR, low CVP, and low PAD). (Courtesy George Blike, MD, Dartmouth University, Hanover, NH.)

response (alarms are discussed in Chapter 23). Signals that must be monitored continuously can be presented on auditory displays because humans can process visual and auditory signals simultaneously.[100]

Auditory displays also should take advantage of learned or natural relationships. For instance, the pitch should increase as the value increases. In general, the same signal should designate the same information in all situations. Because the number of recognizable auditory signals may be limited, auditory displays should not provide more information than is necessary. Complex messages may best be transmitted in two stages. The first stage should be an alerting signal to identify the general category of information. The second stage may then transmit more specific information. Auditory displays must be carefully designed to prevent masking of the signal by the noise of the environment.[100] Extremely loud or abrupt-onset signals should be avoided because they tend to startle the operator. Continuous signals can also be disruptive, and perceptual adaptation may limit their effectiveness. A number of methods may be used to improve the signal/noise ratio.[101] Auditory displays should also take into account the perceptual limitations of the user; for instance, 66% of 188 anesthesiologists had abnormal audiograms, a rate higher than that for the general population.[102]

TABLE 24-2 **Selection Criteria for Auditory vs. Visual Presentation of Information**

Auditory presentation is appropriate when:	Visual presentation is appropriate when:
The message is simple.	The message is complex.
The message is short.	The message is long.
The message will not be referred to later.	The message will be referred to later.
The message deals with events in time.	The message deals with a location in space.
The message must be responded to immediately.	The visual system of the person is overburdened.
The message does not call for immediate action.	The auditory system of the person is overburdened.
The receiving location is too bright.	The receiving location is too noisy.
The person moves about continually to perform the job.	The person performs the job from one position.

Modified from Deathridge BH: Auditory and other sensory forms of information processing. In Van Cott HP, Kinkade RG, editors: *Human engineering guide to equipment design.* Washington, DC, 1972, American Institutes for Research.

Manual Controls

Just as the equipment transmits information to the user through displays, the user transmits information to the device via controls. Different types of controls are preferable for different kinds of tasks. Switches or buttons are used to transmit binary, or on/off, information. Continuous information is usually conveyed with knobs, cranks, wheels, levers, or pedals. Keyboards are frequently used to enter numeric or alphabetic information, and cursor position on computer displays may be controlled with a mouse, joystick, trackball, touch screen, or light pen.

The control's design influences the speed and error rate of user actions. Factors such as control type, control "feel" or resistance, control feedback (visual, audible, and tactile), control placement, and keyboard layout are all important considerations for the equipment designer.

Compatibility of Controls

The degree to which relationships between a stimulus and a response are consistent with human expectations is paramount in the design of controls. When control function conforms to expectations, learning is faster, reaction time is decreased, fewer errors are made, and user satisfaction is enhanced. Although four types of compatibility have been described,[8] spatial and movement compatibility are especially important in the design of controls.

Spatial compatibility deals with the physical arrangement of controls and their associated displays. In general, for optimal performance, each control should be located directly below its corresponding display. When controls are located above the related display, the user's hand may block the view of the display while adjusting the control. When the controls are grouped apart from the displays, controls and their corresponding displays should be arranged in corresponding patterns (Fig. 24-12). Controls should also be arranged to conform with the physical layout of the system; for instance, the throttles on a jet correspond left to right with the spatial relationship of the engines. *Spatial conformity* also refers to the physical similarity between controls and displays. Thus a round dial is a more appropriate display for a knob, and a linear display is more appropriate for a slide control.

Movement compatibility relates to expectations that people have regarding the relationship between control or

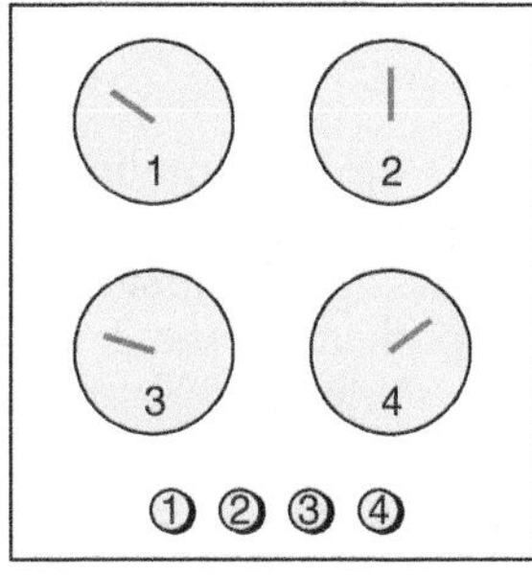

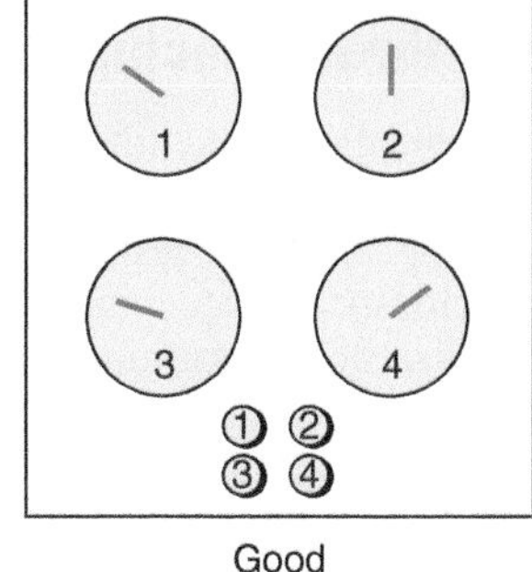

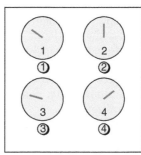

Better

FIGURE 24-12 Acording to the laws of spatial compatibility, controls should be positioned directly below their corresponding displays whenever possible.

TABLE 24-3 **Control Movement Conventions in the United States**

Function	Direction of Control Movement
On	Clockwise, up, right, forward
Off	Counterclockwise, down, left, backward
Increase	Clockwise, up, right, forward
Decrease	Counterclockwise, down, left, backward
Open valve	Counterclockwise
Close valve	Clockwise

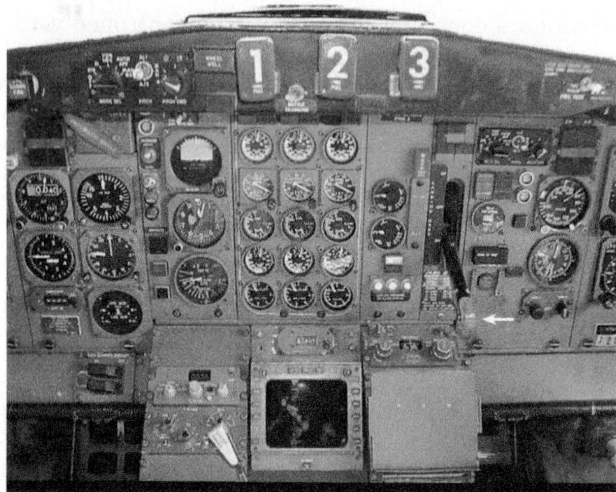

FIGURE 24-13 Cockpit of a Boeing 727. The lever with a wheel on the end that controls the landing gear is shown (*arrow*). Note the three red switches labeled 1-2-3, which control the fire extinguishers for the three engines. (Photo copyright by Mike Olson, used with permission. Accessed at www.airliners.com.)

display movements and system responses. People's expectations regarding movement relationships often are based on population or cultural stereotypes. For example, moving a light switch up generally turns a light *on* in the United States, but the same action turns a light *off* in the United Kingdom and Australia.[103] It therefore is imperative that the designer consider the population that will be using the device. Some guidelines for direction of control movements are listed in Table 24-3.

Coding of Controls

Mistaking one critical control for another has led to serious accidents in aviation (i.e., confusing the landing gear and flap controls), ground transportation (i.e., mistaking the accelerator for the brake pedal), and medicine (i.e., flowmeter control errors, syringe swaps). Unambiguous identification of controls can decrease the incidence of such errors. Primary coding methods for controls include type, shape, texture, size, location, color, and labels. As with coding of display elements, the success of the coding method depends on detectability, discriminability, compatibility, meaningfulness, and standardization.

Shape is an effective method for coding of controls. It provides tactile feedback to the user, which is especially useful when the user does not routinely observe the operation of the control. On most keyboards, special keys are of different shapes, and the F and J keys often are identified by raised dots. The Federal Aviation Administration[104] requires unique, standardized shapes for cockpit controls. Besides being easily distinguishable, some of these knobs have symbolic meaning; for example, the landing gear control resembles a wheel (Fig. 24-13), and the flap control is shaped like a wing.

Surface texture is another useful coding dimension. The textured rims of the dime, quarter, and half dollar provide a common example. Smooth, knurled, and fluted knobs can be reliably discriminated, even by the gloved hand.[105] Color coding of controls can be effective if a small number of coding categories exist and if the colors are meaningful, and color can also be used to associate a control with a display. One disadvantage of color coding, however, is that the user must look at the control during use.

The most common way of identifying controls is with labels. The advantage of labels is that large numbers of meaningful codes can be developed. Disadvantages include the time required to read the label, the effects of lighting conditions and label position on legibility, and the possibility of reading errors in stressful situations and with high workloads. Additional coding methods are therefore indicated when poor lighting or stressful conditions are present and when controls are cluttered or positioned out of the line of sight. Text labels are not appropriate for equipment sold in an international market; graphic or iconic labels are better. International standards organizations have attempted to develop universal icons for medical equipment; however, this endeavor has been hampered by the difficulty of developing icons that have clear meaning across multiple languages and cultures.[106]

ERGONOMICS IN DESIGN

The number of monitors and devices in the typical OR has increased rapidly in past decades, with each year bringing another complicated device that is promoted as being "necessary" for quality care. Such additions include pulse oximetery, capnometry, processed and bispectral electroencephalography (EEG), and multiplane TEE, among others. As each device was introduced, it was necessary to find shelf or floor space for it and an available electrical outlet. Ergonomic problems in the OR still include poor physical layout of displays and controls, cluttered workspaces, and information overload. These cannot be solved at the level of the individual monitors. Integration is one solution, and it must occur on two levels: physical and functional (see Chapter 23).[107]

Anesthesia Machine

The anesthesia machine arguably has the best ergonomic design of any complex piece of equipment in the OR. This is primarily a result of many years of refinement and the widespread acceptance of comprehensive standards, such as those promulgated by the American National Standards Institute (ANSI) and the American Society for Testing and Materials, now known as ASTM International.[108] Equipment users and representatives from anesthesia machine manufacturers serve on the committees that draft these standards. Medical device standards are also based on user experiences, adverse events reported to the FDA, published literature, input from formal organizations, including the American Society of Anesthesiologists (ASA), ECRI Institute, and the Association for the Advancement in Medical Instrumentation (AAMI) as well as relevant experience from other fields (e.g., human engineering).[61]

This section reviews the ergonomic design features of the anesthesia machine with reference to the requirements and rationale of selected specifications from the current (2005) ASTM standard.[108] This standard covers the design of continuous-flow anesthesia machines for human use. The anesthesia machine includes the gas piping and flow control systems between the pressurized gas sources and the common gas outlet, vaporizers, and integrated oxygen concentration and ventilation monitors. Specifications for breathing circuits, ventilators, and such optional devices as humidifiers and positive end-expiratory pressure (PEEP) valves may be found in other standards documents. In light of the ongoing evolution of integrated, microprocessor-controlled anesthesia delivery and monitoring systems, the standards include specifications for data communication and integration of components into a unified anesthesia workstation. These standards take into account several important aspects of the anesthesia work environment: 1) that the operator may be positioned away from the machine; 2) that the anesthesiologist may stand or sit; and 3) that care is sometimes provided in remote locations, such as the radiology suite, where the ambient lighting is poor. This is exemplified by the general specification concerning placement and legibility of controls and displays[108]:

> 2.13.19 *legible*—displayed qualitative or quantitative information, values, functions, and/or markings shall be discernible or identifiable to an OPERATOR with 6-6 (20/20) vision, corrected if necessary, from a distance of 1 m at a light level of 215 lux, when viewing the information, markings, and so on perpendicular to and including 15 degrees above, below, left, and right of the normal line of sight of the OPERATOR.

Another general requirement is that the manufacturer attach a preuse checkout procedure to the anesthesia machine. This is important because the details of operation of anesthesia machines may differ, and clinicians cannot reliably detect faults in anesthesia machines, especially when faults are concealed and do not render the machine inoperative.[109] Cooper[41] identified "failure to perform a preuse check" as an important factor in critical events. Preoperative "preparation and check of equipment, drugs, fluids, and gas supplies" is considered an important part of the anesthesia provider's responsibility.[110]

Gas Systems

A major intention of the specifications regarding anesthesia machine gas piping systems is the deterrence of cross-connections, which can occur when the anesthesia machine is accidentally connected to the wrong cylinder or hospital central gas supply outlet. To prevent this, the ASTM standard requires that anesthesia machines be equipped with pin index safety system and diameter index safety system fittings: the *pin index system* is designed to prevent the attachment of a cylinder of one gas to the hanger yoke of another; the *diameter index system* is designed to prevent crossovers when equipment or flexible hoses are attached to a central pipeline system. Each hanger yoke and pipeline inlet must be permanently marked with the name or chemical symbol of the gas it accommodates, and color coding of each inlet is recommended. Cross-connections also can arise during construction or maintenance of the anesthesia machine or central piping system.[111,112] To reduce the chance that these hidden crossovers will be made by service personnel, the ASTM standard requires that piping be labeled with the gas content at each junction, or where the piping joins the component, and the National Fire Protection Association (NFPA)[113] requires labels on all medical gas piping at 20-foot intervals. Fatalities have resulted from cross-connections in countries where such standards have not been adopted.[114]

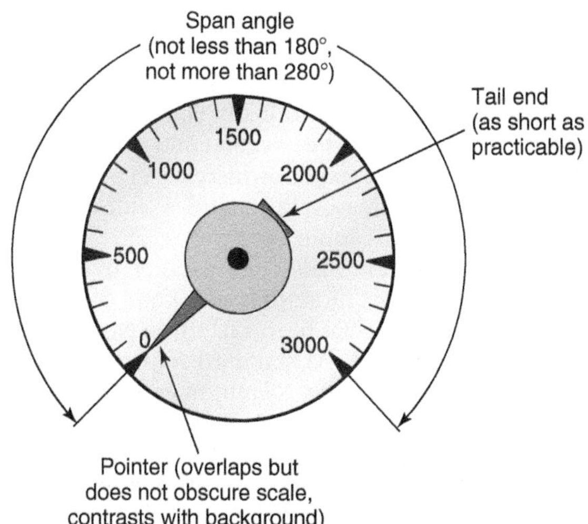

FIGURE 24-14 Recommended pressure gauge features. (From *Minimum performance and safety requirements for components and systems of continuous-flow anesthesia machines for human use, Z79.8-1979,* New York, 1979, American National Standards Institute.)

A poorly designed analog pressure gauge may give the illusion that a gas cylinder is full when it is actually empty.[115] To prevent this, the ASTM standard specifies design criteria for anesthesia machine pressure gauges (Fig. 24-14). The pointer must be designed so that the indicator end is immediately distinguishable from the tail end, and circular pressure gauges must have the lowest pressure reading located in a standard position, between the 6 and 9 o'clock positions. Each gauge must be clearly labeled with the name or chemical symbol of the gas it monitors. Most manufacturers also code the gauge by color. In the United States, the color standards[116] for oxygen, nitrous oxide, and air are green, blue, and yellow, respectively; those for helium, nitrogen, and carbon dioxide are brown, black, and gray, respectively.

Flow Control Systems

The three classes of primary gas controls on an anesthesia machine are 1) the flow controls, 2) the oxygen flush control, and 3) the vaporizer controls (discussed later). Each flow control is associated with a flow indicator, or flowmeter. Together these components form a flow control system. The ASTM standard includes a number of ergonomic design specifications to discourage the unintentional or unrecognized delivery of a hypoxic gas mixture. Flow control knobs are coded by label and color, and the oxygen knob is additionally coded by shape and location. By convention, the oxygen control is located on the right side of the group of flowmeters. A counterclockwise turn always increases flow, and a clockwise turn decreases it.[11,117] This same convention also applies to vaporizer concentration dials. The parallel arrangement of flowmeters, in which more than one knob controls the flow rate of a single gas, has been a factor in patient deaths (Fig. 24-15).[111] The ASTM standard requires that each gas delivered to the machine's common gas outlet be controlled by no more than one knob, and a single flowmeter tube for each gas is recommended. The Thorpe flowmeter, which is commonly used on anesthesia machines, is calibrated for a single gas; thus the standard specifies that flowmeters are not interchangeable.

The above discussion demonstrates that equipment can be designed to decrease the likelihood of user error. Designs also can incorporate constraints to prevent dangerous human errors. All current anesthesia machines in the United States have flow control systems that prevent the administration of hypoxic mixtures of oxygen and nitrous oxide, although the ASTM standard does not require this.

A limitation of the traditional mechanical proportioning systems (i.e., the Ohmeda Link-25 and Dräger ORMC [Dräger North America, Telford, PA]) is that the ratio of only two gases, generally oxygen and nitrous oxide, can be controlled. Hypoxic mixtures can still be delivered when three or more gases are dispensed together. However, the delivery of hypoxic mixtures can reliably be prevented with electronic flow control systems.[118] Such systems are available in some modern anesthesia machines.

Vaporizers

Inhaled anesthetic agents are potent drugs that may cause death as a result of overdosage.[119] Underdosage of these agents can result in an undesirable cardiovascular response to surgical stimulation as well as intraoperative patient awareness.[120] The ASTM standard specifies a number of ergonomic requirements that reduce user errors: 1) the vaporizer must be equipped with a clearly visible liquid-level indicator to prevent underdosage because of a lack of liquid agent; 2) to prevent delivery of liquid anesthetic into the breathing circuit, the vaporizer must be constructed so that overfilling is impossible; 3) to prevent an incorrect agent from being added to a single-agent vaporizer, each should be fitted with an agent-specific keyed filling device.[11] Vaporizers are discussed in more depth in Chapter 3.

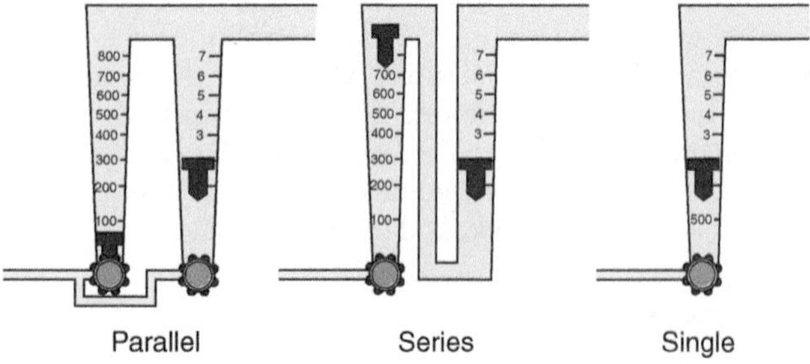

FIGURE 24-15 Arrangements of flowmeters. Serious mishaps have resulted with the parallel arrangement when the low-flow control knob was mistaken for the high-flow knob. The series arrangement is less dangerous, but one flowmeter may still be mistaken for the other. (From Loeb RG: Preventing anesthesia machine-induced hypoxemia. *Wellcome Trends in Anesthesiology* 1990;8:2-10.)

Most manufacturers color code their vaporizers for specific inhaled agents: color codes for desflurane, enflurane, halothane, isoflurane, and sevoflurane are blue, orange, red, purple, and yellow, respectively. All new anesthesia machines produced for human use in the United States have a vaporizer interlock mechanism that prevents the simultaneous administration of a volatile agent from more than one vaporizer. Vaporizers also are securely mounted on the machine to prevent tipping, which can lead to overdosage. Desflurane is a volatile anesthetic with a low boiling point and a high minimum alveolar concentration (MAC); thus it requires use of a special heated, pressurized vaporizer (see Chapter 3) that necessitates use of a special one-way filling system to prevent backflow and vapor spray. Similarly, the traditional glass window sight cannot be used because accidental breakage would result in a pressurized spray of desflurane into the OR.

Automation and Modern Anesthesia Machines

The technology of anesthesia machines is changing rapidly (see Chapter 23). Until recently, the flowmeters, vaporizers, and pressure regulators were all mechanical devices; electronics were added only for monitoring purposes. However, several anesthesia machines with electronic flowmeters and vaporizers are now commercially available for use in the United States, and standards are being updated for this generation of machines.[108]

For decades, research has shown the viability of automatic control of the delivery of inhaled anesthetics,[121,122] IV anesthetics,[123,124] neuromuscular blockers,[125] and ventilation.[126] Yet commercial systems are only now becoming available. Automation can enhance system performance, increase safety, and decrease human workload.[127] However, inappropriate or excessive automation may result in low-workload conditions, leading to boredom and inattention.[128] Poor design of automation processes in which the human operator was not "in the loop" have led to catastrophic accidents.[4]

Electronic anesthesia machines provide manufacturers with the opportunity to redesign the ergonomics of the workstation. This redesign may or may not be a positive step forward. Some manufacturers have chosen to design electronic gas flow controls to operate in the opposite direction of the current manual controls; that is, turning the knob clockwise increases the flow, instead of decreasing it, as it would in a conventional machine. Many anesthesiologists would state that this is not an example of a positive design. The Arkon anesthesia machine by Spacelabs (Spacelabs Healthcare, Issaquah, WA) (Fig. 24-16) offers some innovative ideas to help the anesthesiologist better interact with the workstation. For example, the gas flowmeters have a color bar that increases in size as the flow is increased. It also has a spinning red bobbin at the top to simulate a traditional flowmeter. The gauges for the tank and wall supply pressures are easy to read and interpret, and innovative use of lighting lets the anesthesiologist know that a function has changed from baseline. For instance, if the carbon dioxide absorber is out of the circuit, a red light is illuminated in that spot. Similarly, if the alternate fresh gas flow outlet is selected, it is lit with a green light. In addition, when a vaporizer is turned on, that vaporizer is lit. Finally, a pull-out writing table is provided so the clinician can stand to do charting.

As automation is introduced into the anesthesia workplace, additional training will be required to prevent experienced clinicians from continuing to practice the "old way" with new devices that provide different data or require different control strategies.[129] For example, older clinicians adjusted their behavior to avoid hyperventilating patients with a new anesthesia ventilator that compensates for gas compression within the breathing circuit. Conversely, with overdependence on automation, clinicians may fail to understand the underlying complexity of the system and the methods for resuming control when the technology fails. The burden of retraining must be shared by the device manufacturers, the clinicians, and the health care system in which the equipment is installed.

Intravenous Administration Systems

The ergonomic problems of IV administration systems are all too familiar to the anesthesia practitioner. Tangled

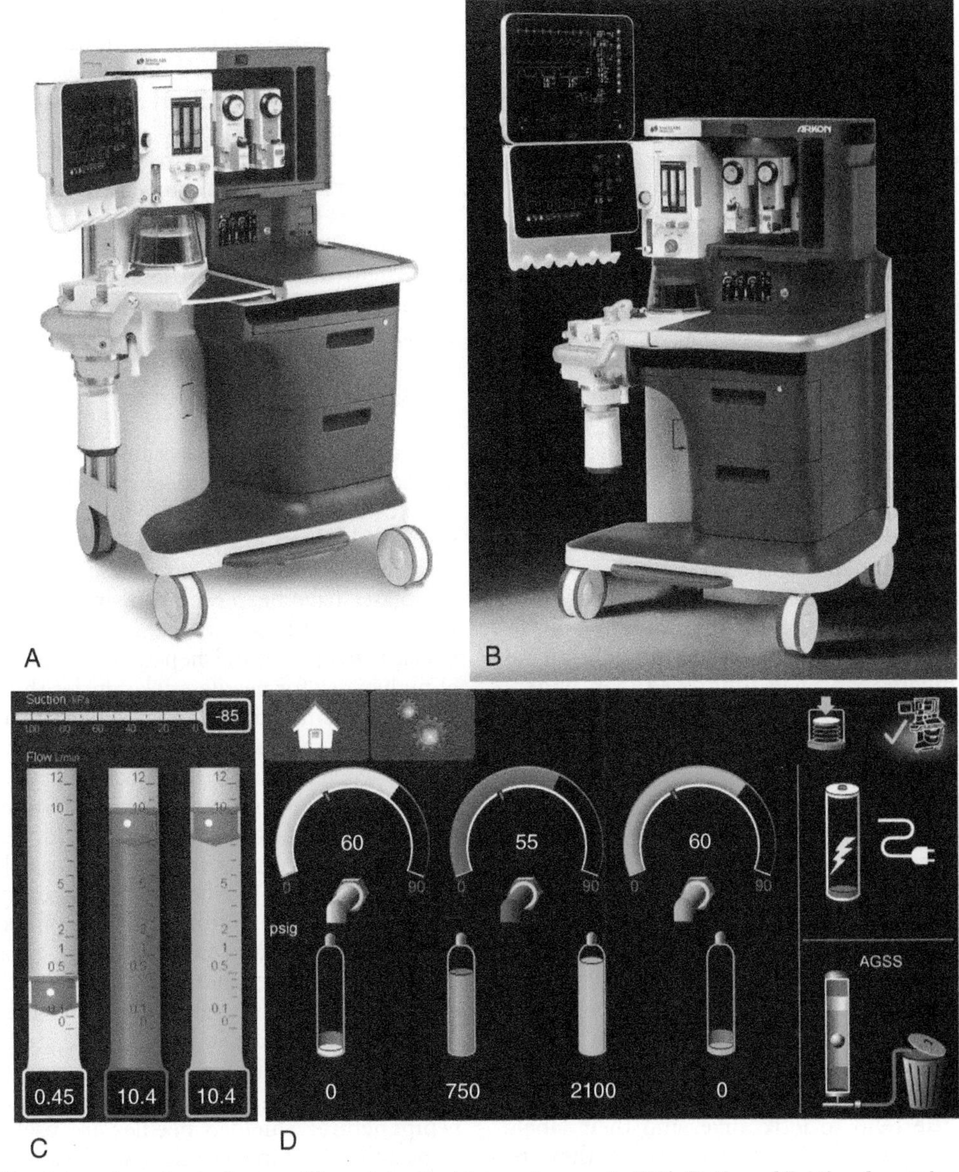

FIGURE 24-16 ■ **A,** The Arkon Anesthesia System (Spacelabs Healthcare, Issaquah, WA). **B,** Use of lighting for various functions; a red light is illuminated when the CO_2 absorber is out of the circuit. The green light next to the absorber indicates that the alternate fresh gas flow outlet is in use. The blue lights show that the ventilator is being used, the vaporizer has been turned on, or that the auxiliary oxygen flowmeter is in use. **C,** The gas flow controls have knobs that control a computer graphic display. Each gas has a red bobbin at the top that spins to simulate a traditional flowmeter. As the knob is turned counterclockwise, the flow increases, and a color-coded bar is filled in below the bobbin. **D,** The dashboard display. Wall supply pressures are clearly displayed. Below these are the reserve tank pressures and a graphic display of how much gas is in each tank. For example, the oxygen cylinder on the left is full, and the one on the right is empty. Other items displayed are whether the anesthesia gas scavenging system (*AGGS*) has sufficient vacuum, the charge of the backup battery and whether it is plugged in to charge, and whether a preuse check has been done (check mark next to the machine icon). The *green arrow* above the bellows icon shows that the ventilator driving gas is O_2 (the arrow would be yellow if air was being used as the driving gas).

lines, inaccessible injection ports, and misidentified tubing are common, especially after a patient has been transported to or from the OR. Most of the complications that arise are never documented; however, multiple cases have been reported of accidental injections of IV medications into arterial or epidural catheters.[130,131] Although no national standard addresses these issues, institutions, departments, and individual clinicians should adopt procedures to minimize problems.

We recommend that different types of tubing be used for IV, intraarterial, and epidural systems. Tubing and injection ports should be clearly labeled; color-coded tubing and stopcocks are commercially available. Tubing used for epidural infusions and arterial pressure monitoring should not have injection ports.[132] Transport racks may help keep tubing organized while the patient is moved; alternatively, superfluous tubing can be converted to heparin locks to prevent tangling during transport. The use of smaller, more user-friendly infusion devices specifically designed for administration of drugs, rather than fluids, may reduce the incidence of medication errors, particularly during the transport of critically ill patients who require multiple drug infusions. Cook and colleagues[133] described four cases of drug administration error that resulted from a poorly designed user interface and inappropriate use of a fluid infusion controller. We advocate that clinicians always use infusion pumps, rather than infusion controllers, when administering vasoactive drugs or anesthetic agents in the perioperative period.

Medication Errors

Drug errors that result in the administration of the wrong drug or wrong dose are among the most frequent errors reported in critical incident studies of anesthesiologists.[42-44,134,135] These errors frequently result in a physiologic change in the patient.[134] A series of studies from the Harvard-affiliated hospitals improved our understanding of the nature and causes of medication errors. These investigations of *all* adverse drug events throughout the entire hospital demonstrate that medication errors are common, often preventable, rarely reported, and result in potentially substantial health care costs.[136,137] Importantly, Leape and colleagues[138] found that system deficiencies, such as failure to disseminate knowledge about drugs to those who use them and failure to provide drug and patient information at the time it is needed, were a contributing factor in *more than three fourths* of the detected adverse drug events. In addition, a number of ergonomic deficiencies contribute to the problem. Labels on vials and ampoules often are illegible, especially when they are printed directly on the glass. Prefilled syringes for emergency use tend to look alike, and their labels often become hidden within the syringe barrel as they are used. Similarities in packaging—vial shape, proprietary drug name, lettering style, and company logo—serve to code the medication by manufacturer rather than by drug type.[139]

The tendency of hospitals to decrease costs by changing drug vendors more frequently may exacerbate this problem. Standards to address some of these problems have been published by the ASTM[140,141] that require the name and concentration of the drug and the volume of the container to be legible at 20 inches in dim hospital lighting. For prefilled emergency syringes, the label must be legible at 5 feet, even after the contents are dispensed. The United States Pharmacopoeia (USP) and the FDA are federally mandated to have jurisdiction over the packaging and labeling of all drugs used by anesthesiologists in the United States. These organizations have begun to show interest in improving the current environment.

Evidence suggests that the risk of drug errors increases following intraoperative exchanges of personnel.[142] The incidence of these errors may be increased as a result of syringes being either unlabeled or labeled incompletely or unconventionally. A label containing the name and concentration of the drug should be affixed to the syringe at the time it is filled; the concentration is especially important when a nonstandard dilution is used. Colored, preprinted labels have been available for some time. A national standard for syringe labels specifies legibility and color codes: induction agents are yellow, muscle relaxants are fluorescent red, and narcotics are blue (Fig. 24-17).[143] Special formats are reserved for succinylcholine, epinephrine, and antagonist agents. Nevertheless, the contribution of human error to these incidents should not be discounted; the anesthesiologist is ultimately responsible for ensuring the identity of a medication prior to administering it.

Needle-Stick Injuries

The danger of needle-stick injuries to health care workers has received a great deal of attention. This is largely due to the epidemic of human immunodeficiency virus (HIV), although only 57 cases of occupationally contracted HIV had been documented as of 2001, and no new cases have been reported since 1999.[144] In contrast, up to 300 health care workers die each year from occupationally acquired viral hepatitis.[145] Anesthesiologists are at higher risk for needle-stick injuries than are other physicians. Needle-sticks most frequently occur during or after needle disposal, rather than while using the needle, and between 20% and 40% occur during recapping.[146]

Improvements in the design of IV administration systems can appreciably reduce the risk of needle-stick injuries. Devices are now commercially available that allow safer recapping of needles, provide protection of the needle during use, or eliminate the use of needles during IV therapy. Items that provide safer recapping include resheathing devices that hold the cap during insertion of the needle and retractable sheaths that extend over the needle from behind after use. These are especially useful when the needle must be exposed during use, such as during catheter placement, intramuscular injection, and venipuncture. Shielded needles are useful for IV injections and IV tubing/needle assemblies. Here, the needle is protected at all times within a plastic cylinder designed to fit over an injection port. A disadvantage of these devices is that without an adapter, they cannot be used to withdraw medications from vials. The elimination of needles from IV therapy has been accomplished, such as by using IV tubing with Luer ports rather than standard latex Y-ports or flashbulbs.[147] Luer ports with integrated antireflux valves are particularly useful during anesthesia

Drug class	Label color	Example
Induction agent	Yellow	Propofol mg/ml
Benzodiazepine	Orange	Midazolam mg/ml
Neuromuscular blocker	Fluorescent red	Vecuronium mg/ml Succinylcholine mg/ml
Relaxant antagonist	Fluorescent red with white stripes	Neostigmine mg/ml
Narcotic	Blue	Morphine mg/ml
Narcotic antagonist	Blue with white stripes	Naloxone mg/ml
Major tranquilizer	Salmon	Droperidol mg/ml
Vasopressor	Violet	Ephedrine mg/ml Epinephrine mg/ml
Hypotensive agent	Violet with white stripes	Nitroprusside mg/ml
Local anesthetic	Gray	Lidocaine mg/ml
Anticholinergic agent	Green	Atropine mg/ml

FIGURE 24-17 Standard color codes for user-applied syringe drug labels.

because they allow intermittent injections to be administered with one hand. One company manufactures a needleless system with special prepierced injection ports accessed with a blunt plastic cannula. A device is also available to permit needle-free drug aspiration from multiple-dose vials. Single-dose glass ampoules still generally require the use of a blunt needle.

Operating Room Environment

Work environment has a pervasive influence on people's ability to perform their jobs. Diverse factors such as the loudness of the ventilation system, the size of a doorway, or the glare from a light fixture can hamper the ability to perform specific tasks. The OR is a workplace for surgeons, anesthesiologists, nurses, technicians, orderlies, and radiographers. Ideally, it should be designed to support the wide variety of tasks performed by each of these individuals. This section briefly reviews some of the implications of OR design on the tasks performed by anesthesiologists. The topic of noise is discussed in Chapter 23.

Ambient Lighting

Most of the clinical information that the anesthesiologist gathers is collected visually. The impact of illumination on task performance has received much attention from ergonomics and lighting specialists.[8] Illumination requirements depend on the characteristics of a given task, such as visibility and speed. In general, the more difficult the psychomotor task, the greater the level of illumination required for optimal performance. For example, the suggested level of illumination for the surgical field is very high (10,000 to 20,000 lux), whereas monitoring in the anesthesia workspace may require only the levels suggested for performance of visual tasks of medium contrast or small size (500 to 1000 lux).[148] Studies have indicated that brighter illumination is more satisfying and may improve performance,[8] decrease reaction time,[149] and increase social interaction.[150]

Other factors such as color, glare, shadows, and heat production must also be considered in the design of OR lighting. The spectral distributions of available light sources differ markedly, and these differences can affect people's ability to discriminate colors. Anesthesiologists must discriminate colors when evaluating the patient for cyanosis or jaundice and when using color-coded equipment. Therefore, minimizing color distortion by use of lights with a high color-rendering index must be a priority. Overhead lighting must also be diffused to decrease the glare and shadows that interfere with the anesthesiologist's ability to see monitor displays or to perform invasive procedures.[22]

Facility Layout

The layout of the physical facility plays a role in user efficiency and satisfaction with the workplace. Factors to be considered with regard to space management for surgical facilities include the total quantity of space required, allocation of space for specific purposes, layout of the ORs, traffic patterns, and accessibility of ancillary and support services.[148] All these factors have a direct impact on the anesthesiologist's job.

The layout of the facility is especially important during the turnover time between surgical cases. A well-planned facility encourages a smooth flow of people and materials. For instance, in an ambulatory surgical facility, patients should proceed in an orderly fashion from the reception area through the changing and preoperative holding areas to the OR. At the conclusion of the procedure, the patient should be transported to the recovery room without crossing paths with preoperative patients. The preoperative holding area and recovery room should be in the immediate vicinity of the ORs, so that the anesthesiologist does not need to change clothes and can be immediately available if required.[151] At the Shock Trauma Center in Baltimore, the trauma patient is directly transported by elevator from the helicopter landing pad on the roof to the triage unit. Immediately adjacent to the triage unit are the ORs and a computerized tomography (CT) scanner facility. This provides an opportunity for the anesthesiologist to be involved in the initial resuscitation. Also, secondary resuscitation is not impaired during radiologic diagnostic procedures.

Efficiency is enhanced when the distances that must be traversed are minimized. If the anesthesiologist must leave the OR to procure drugs or equipment between cases, turnover times will be prolonged. One approach to this problem is to provide centrally located OR satellite pharmacies and anesthesia workrooms.[152] Alternatively, controlled substances can be dispensed in a pack to be worn on the anesthesiologist's body,[153] and carts within the room can be restocked with supplies by an anesthesia assistant.

Insufficient storage space is a common problem in many ORs. This can lead to cluttered hallways, which can be a hazard to patients during transport and to personnel. Cluttered hallways also present a real danger in the event of a fire, and they violate NFPA fire code regulations. ORs should be designed with immediately adjacent space that is set aside for OR personnel to have meals, conferences, breaks, and to perform administrative duties. At every stage of the OR design process, it is critical that all potential users have the opportunity to be involved and provide input.[154]

SUMMARY

The anesthesiologist performs a complex job in a poorly designed workplace, and ergonomic "malpractice" remains pervasive. These problems cannot be addressed at just one level.[155] Research must continue to investigate the tasks of anesthesiologists and the equipment-related factors that influence their performance. Standard design specifications, coauthored by equipment producers and users, must continue to be developed. Equipment manufacturers must strengthen their commitment to ergonomics throughout the design phase. Anesthesiologists, as individuals and as a group, must demand better ergonomics in their equipment and should refuse to purchase devices with suboptimal designs. Finally, multidisciplinary groups that include anesthesiologists, surgeons, nurses, ergonomics specialists, biomedical engineers, and architects must be assembled to address problems at a systems level. Solutions will be found only when there is a comprehensive approach to improve the ergonomics of the anesthesia workspace.

REFERENCES

1. Weller J, Merry A, Warman G, Robinson B: Anaesthetists' management of oxygen pipeline failure: room for improvement, *Anaesthesia* 62(2):122–1226, 2007.
2. Epstein RM, Rackow H, Lee AS, Papper EM: Prevention of accidental breathing of anoxic gas mixtures during anesthesia, *Anesthesiology* 23:1–4, 1962.
3. Mudumbai SC, Fanning R, Howard SK, Davies MF, Gaba DM: Use of medical simulation to explore equipment failures and human-machine interactions in anesthesia machine pipeline supply crossover, *Anesth Analg* 110(5):1292–1296, 2010.
4. Weinger MB, Wiklund M, Gardner-Bonneau D, editors: *Human factors in medical device design: a handbook for designers*, Boca Raton, 2011, CRC Press/Taylor & Francis.
5. Carayon P, editor: *Handbook of human factors and ergonomics in health care and patient safety*, Boca Raton, 2012, CRC Press.
6. Edwards E, editor: *Man and machine: systems for safety. British Airline Pilots Associations Technical Symposium*, London, 1972, British Airline Pilots Associations.
7. Gilbreth FB: Motion study in surgery, *Can J Med Surg* 40:22–31, 1916.
8. Sanders MS, McCormick EJ: *Human factors in engineering and design*, ed 7, New York, 1992, McGraw-Hill, pp xiii, 790.
9. Drui AB, Behm RJ, Martin WE: Predesign investigation of the anesthesia operational environment, *Anesth Analg* 52(4):584–591, 1973.
10. Kennedy PJ, Feingold A, Wiener EL, Hosek RS: Analysis of tasks and human factors in anesthesia for coronary-artery bypass, *Anesth Analg* 55(3):374–377, 1976.
11. Rendell-Baker L: Problems with anesthetic gas machines and their solutions, *Int Anesthesiol Clin* 20(3):1–82, 1982.
12. Boquet G, Bushman JA, Davenport HT: The anaesthetic machine: a study of function and design, *Br J Anaesth* 52(1):61–67, 1980.
13. McDonald JS, Dzwonczyk R, Gupta B, Dahl M: A second timestudy of the anaesthetist's intraoperative period, *Br J Anaesth* 64(5):582–585, 1990.
14. Weinger MB, Herndon OW, Gaba DM: The effect of electronic record keeping and transesophageal echocardiography on task distribution, workload, and vigilance during cardiac anesthesia, *Anesthesiology* 87(1):144–155, 1997, discussion 29A-30A.
15. Weinger MB, Herndon OW, Zornow MH, et al: An objective methodology for task analysis and workload assessment in anesthesia providers, *Anesthesiology* 80(1):77–92, 1994.
16. Wierwille WW, Rahimi M, Casali JG: Evaluation of 16 measures of mental workload using a simulated flight task emphasizing mediational activity, *Hum Factors* 27(5):489–502, 1985.
17. Hicks TG, Wierwille WW: Comparison of five mental workload assessment procedures in a moving-base driving simulator, *Hum Factors* 21(2):129–143, 1979.
18. Reid G, Nygren T: The subjective workload assessment technique: a scaling procedure for measuring mental workload. In Hancock P, Meshkati N, editors: *Human mental workload*, Amsterdam/New York, 1988, Elsevier Science, pp xvi, 382.
19. Hill SG, Iavecchia HP, Byers JC, et al: Comparison of four subjective workload rating scales, *Hum Factors* 34(4):429–439, 1992.
20. Salas E, Maurino D, editors: *Human factors in aviation*, ed 2, Burlington, MA, 2010, Academic Press.
21. Gaba DM, Lee T: Measuring the workload of the anesthesiologist, *Anesth Analg* 71(4):354–361, 1990.
22. Weinger MB, Englund CE: Ergonomic and human factors affecting anesthetic vigilance and monitoring performance in the operating room environment, *Anesthesiology* 73(5):995–1021, 1990.
23. Toung T, Donham R, Rogers M: The stress of giving anesthesia on the electrocardiogram of anesthesiologists (abstract), *Anesthesiology* 61:A465, 1984.
24. Toung T, Donham R, Rogers M: The effect of previous medical training on the stress of giving anesthesia (abstract), *Anesthesiology* 65:A473, 1986.

25. Weinger MB, Reddy S, Slagle JS: Multiple measures of anesthesia workload during teaching and non-teaching cases, *Anesth Analg* 98(5):1419–1425, 2004.
26. Vredenburgh AG, Weinger MB, Williams KJ, et al: Developing a technique to measure anesthesiologists' real-time workload, *Proc IIEA/HFES Cong* 44:4241–4244, 2000.
27. Weinger MB, Vredenburgh AG, Schumann CM, et al: Quantitative description of the workload associated with airway management procedures, *J Clin Anesth* 12:273–282, 2000.
28. Kay J, Neal M: Effect of automatic blood pressure devices on vigilance of anesthesia residents, *J Clin Monit* 2:148–150, 1986.
29. Cooper JO, Cullen BF: Observer reliability in detecting surreptitious random occlusions of the monaural esophageal stethoscope, *J Clin Monit* 6:271–275, 1990.
30. Loeb RG: A measure of intraoperative attention to monitor displays, *Anesth Analg* 76:337–341, 1993.
31. Loeb RG: Monitor surveillance and vigilance of anesthesia residents, *Anesthesiology* 80:527–533, 1994.
32. Drui AB, Behm RJ, Martin WE: Predesign investigation of the anesthesia operational environment, *Anesth Analg* 52:584–591, 1973.
33. Noel KR: Controversy in automated record keeping [letter], *J Clin Monit* 7:280, 1991.
34. Noel T: Computerized anesthesia record may be dangerous [letter], *Anesthesiology* 64:300, 1986.
35. Woods DD, Cook RI, Billings CE: The impact of technology on physician cognition and performance, *J Clin Monit* 11:5–8, 1995.
36. Cook RI, Woods DD, Howie MB, Horrow JC, Gaba DM: Case 2-1992: unintentional delivery of vasoactive drugs with an electromechanical infusion device, *J Cardiothoracic Vasc Anesth* 6:238–244, 1992.
37. McDonald J, Dzwonczyk R: A time and motion study of the anaesthetist's intraoperative time, *Br J Anaesth* 61:738–742, 1988.
38. Allard J, Dzwonczyk DY, Block FE Jr, McDonald JS: Effect of automatic record keeping on vigilance and record keeping time, *Br J Anaesth* 74:619–626, 1995.
39. Loeb RG: Manual record keeping is not necessary for anesthesia vigilance, *J Clin Monit* 11:9–13, 1995.
40. Flanagan JC: The critical incident technique, *Psych Bull* 51(4):327–358, 1954.
41. Cooper JB, Newbower RS, Long CD, McPeek B: Preventable anesthesia mishaps: a study of human factors, *Anesthesiology* 49(6):399–406, 1978.
42. Cooper JB, Newbower RS, Long CD, McPeek B: Preventable anesthesia mishaps: a study of human factors. *Qual Saf Health Care* 11(3):277–282, 2002.
43. Craig J, Wilson ME: A survey of anaesthetic misadventures, *Anaesthesia* 36(10):933–936, 1981.
44. Kumar V, Barcellos WA, Mehta MP, Carter JG: An analysis of critical incidents in a teaching department for quality assurance: a survey of mishaps during anaesthesia, *Anaesthesia* 43(10):879–883, 1988.
45. Webb RK, Currie M, Morgan CA, et al: The Australian Incident Monitoring Study: an analysis of 2000 incident reports, *Anaesth Intensive Care* 21(5):520–528, 1993.
46. Runciman WB, Sellen A, Webb RK, et al: The Australian Incident Monitoring Study: errors, incidents and accidents in anaesthetic practice, *Anaesth Intensive Care* 21(5):506–519, 1993.
47. Runciman WB: Complete retrograde dysmnesia, *J Clin Monit* 11(1):3–4, 1995.
48. Sanborn KV, Castro J, Kuroda M, Thys DM: Detection of intraoperative incidents by electronic scanning of computerized anesthesia records: comparison with voluntary reporting, *Anesthesiology* 85:977–987, 1996.
49. Cullen DJ, Bates DW, Small SD, et al: The incident reporting system does not detect adverse drug events: a problem for quality improvement, *Jt Comm J Qual Improv* 21:541–548, 1995.
50. Mahajan RP: Critical incident reporting and learning, *Br J Anaesth* 105(1):69–75, 2010.
51. Bolsin SN, Colson M, Patrick A, Creati B, Bent P: Critical incident reporting and learning, *Br J Anaesth* 105(5):698, 2010.
52. Gaba DM, DeAnda A: A comprehensive anesthesia simulation environment: recreating the operating room for research and teaching, *Anesthesiology* 69:387–394, 1988.
53. DeAnda A, Gaba DM: Unplanned incidents during comprehensive anesthesia simulation, *Anesth Analg* 71:77–82, 1990.
54. DeAnda A, Gaba DM: Role of experience in the response to simulated critical incidents, *Anesth Analg* 72(3):308–315, 1991.
55. Mackenzie CF, Jefferies NJ, Hunter WA, Bernhard WN, Xiao Y: Comparison of self-reporting of deficiencies in airway management with video analyses of actual performance. LOTAS Group. Level One Trauma Anesthesia Simulation, *Hum Factors* 38(4):623–635, 1996.
56. Xiao Y, Hunter WA, Mackenzie CF, Jefferies NJ, Horst RL: Task complexity in emergency medical care and its implications for team coordination. LOTAS Group. Level One Trauma Anesthesia Simulation, *Hum Factors* 38(4):636–645, 1996.
57. Mackenzie CF, Hu PF, Horst RL: An audio-video system for automated data acquisition in the clinical environment. LOTAS Group, *J Clin Monit* 11(5):335–341, 1995.
58. Mackenzie CF, Martin P, Xiao Y: Video analysis of prolonged uncorrected esophageal intubation. Level One Trauma Anesthesia Simulation Group, *Anesthesiology* 84(6):1494–1503, 1996.
59. Brown CM: *Human-computer interaction design guidelines*. Exeter, UK, 1999, Intellect, pp 236.
60. Association for the Advancement of Medical Instrumentation (AAMI): Human factors engineering guidelines and preferred practices for the design of medical devices (ANSI/AAMI HE-48-21993). Arlington, VA, 2001, AAMI.
61. International Electrotechnical Commission (IEC): *Medical devices—application of usability engineering to medical devices* (IEC/ISO 62366:2007), Geneva, 2007, IEC.
62. Association for the Advancement of Medical Instrumentation (AAMI): *Human factors engineering—Design of medical devices* (ANSI/AAMI HE-75-2009). Arlington, VA, 2009, AAMI.
63. Weinger MB, Wiklund M, Gardner-Bonneau D, editors: *Handbook of human factors in medical device design*. Boca Raton, FL, 2011, CRC Press.
64. FDA: Human Factors Implications of the New GMP Rule Overall Requirements of the New Quality System Regulation. Available at http://www.fda.gov/MedicalDevices/DeviceRegulationandGuidance/HumanFactors/ucm119215.htm.
65. Bock FM 4th: Considering human factors in the initial analysis and design of a medical computer system, *J Med Syst* 6(1):61–76, 1982.
66. Norman D: *The psychology of everyday things*, New York, 1988, Basic Books.
67. Gaba DM: Human error in anesthetic mishaps, *Int Anesth Clin* 27:137–147, 1989.
68. Potter SS, Cook R, Woods D: The role of human factors guidelines in designing usable systems: a case study of opeating room equipment, *Proc Hum Factors Soc* 34:391–395, 1990.
69. Howard SK, Gaba DM, Fish KJ, Yang G, Sarnquist FH: Anesthesia crisis resource management training: teaching anesthesiologists to handle critical incidents, *Aviat Space Environ Med* 63(9):763–770, 1992.
70. Bell TE: The limits of risk analysis, *IEEE Spectrum* 26:51, 1989.
71. Cook RI, Potter SS, Woods DD, McDonald JS: Evaluating the human engineering of microprocessor controlled operating room devices, *J Clin Monit* 7:217–226, 1991.
72. Elkin EH: *Effects of scale shape, exposure time, and display-response complexity on scale reading efficiency: Aero Medical Laboratory*, Air Research and Development Command, U.S. Air Force, 1959, Wright Air Development Center.
73. Fitts PM, Jones RE: *Psychological aspects of instruments display*, Washington, DC, 1947, Department of Commerce.
74. Stokes AF, Wickens CD: Aviation displays. In Wiener EL, Nagel DC, editors: *Human factors in aviation*, San Diego, 1988, Academic Press.
75. Ivergard T: *Handbook of control room design and ergonomics*, New York, 1989, Taylor & Francis.
76. Bennett K, Nagy A, Flach J: Visual displays. In Salvendy G, editor: *Handbook of human factors and ergonomics*, Hoboken, NJ, 2006, John Wiley, pp 1191–1221.
77. Koonce JM, Gold M, Moroze M: Comparison of novice and experienced pilots using analog and digital flight displays, *Aviat Space Environ Med* 57(12 Pt 1):1181–1184, 1986.
78. Allen RW, Clement WF, Jex HR: *NASA CR-1569*, Moffett Field, CA, 1970, National Aeronautics and Space Administration.
79. Diffrient N: *Humanscale 4/5/6*, Boston, 1981, MIT Press.
80. Sanders AF: Some aspects of the selective process in the functional visual field, *Ergonomics* 13(1):101–117, 1970.

81. Harris RL, Tole JR, Stephens AT, Ephrath AR: Visual scanning behavior and pilot workload, *Aviat Space Environ Med* 53:1067–1072, 1982.
82. Shepherd A, Stammers R: Task analysis. In Wilson JR, editor: *Evaluation of human work*, ed 3, Boca Raton, FL, 2005, CRC Press, pp 129–157.
83. Barnett B, Wickens C: Display proximity in multicue information integration: the benefits of boxes, *Hum Factors* 30:15–24, 1988.
84. Rock I, Palmer S: The legacy of Gestalt psychology, *Scientific American* 263(6):84–90, 1990.
85. Schaefer W, Little J, Cooper K, Easter J: inventors; Westinghouse Electric, Pittsburgh, PA (assignee): *Generating an integrated graphic display of the safety status of a complex process plant*, U.S. Patent 4,675,147, 1987.
86. Gurushanthaiah K, Weinger MB, Englund CE: Visual display format affects the ability of anesthesiologists to detect acute physiologic changes: a laboratory study employing a clinical display simulator, *Anesthesiology* 83(6):1184–1193, 1995.
87. Petersen RJ, Banks WW, Gertman DI: *Performance-based evaluation of graphic displays for nuclear power plant control rooms*, Gaithersburg, MD, 1982, Proceedings of the 1982 Conference on Human Factors in Computing Systems. Association for Computer Machinery, pp 182–189.
88. Stokes AF, Wickens CD, Kite K: *Display technology: human factors concepts*, 1990, Society of Automotive Engineers.
89. Wickens CD, Andre AD: Proximity compatibility and information display: effects of color, space, and objectness on information integration, *Hum Factors* 32:61–78, 1990.
90. Reference deleted in proofs.
91. Caroux L, Le Bigot L, Vibert N: Maximizing players' anticipation by applying the proximity-compatibility principle to the design of video games, *Hum Factors* 53(2):103–117, 2011.
92. Sanderson PM, Flach JM, Buttigieg MA, Casey EJ: Object displays do not always support better integrated task performance, *Hum Factors* 31(2):183–198, 1989.
93. Cole WG, Stewart JG: Human performance evaluation of a metaphor graphic display for respiratory data, *Meth Inform Med* 33:390–396, 1994.
94. Blike GT, Surgenor SD, Whalen K: A graphical object display improves anesthesiologists' performance on a simulated diagnostic task, *J Clin Monit Comput* 15(1):37–44, 1999.
95. Hitt WD: An evaluation of five different abstract coding methods—experiment IV1, *Hum Factors* 3(2):120–130, 1961.
96. Christ R: Review and analysis of color-coding research for visual displays, *Hum Factors* 17:542–570, 1975.
97. Boucek C, Freeman JA, Bircher NG, Tullock W: Impairment of anesthesia task performance by laser protection goggles, *Anesth Analg* 77(6):1232–1237, 1993.
98. Macdonald WA, Cole BL: Evaluating the role of colour in a flight information cockpit display, *Ergonomics* 31(1):13–37, 1988.
99. Berguer R, Loeb RG, Smith WD: Use of the virtual instrumentation laboratory for the assessment of human factors in surgery and anesthesia: studies in health technology and informatics, *Stud Health Technol Inform* 39:187–194, 1997.
100. Sanderson PM, Liu D, Jenkins SA: Auditory displays in anesthesiology, *Curr Opin Anaesthesiol* 22(6):788–795, 2009.
101. Wilcox SB: Alarm design. In Weinger M, Wiklund M, Gardner-Bonneau D, editors: *Handbook of human factors in medical device design*, Boca Raton, 2011, CRC Press, pp 397–423.
102. Wallace MS, Ashman MN, Matjasko MJ: Hearing acuity of anesthesiologists and alarm detection, *Anesthesiology* 81:13–28, 1994.
103. O'Hare D, Roscoe SN: *Flightdeck performance: the human factor*, Ames, IA, 1990, Iowa State University Press.
104. United States Code of Federal Regulations, 14CFR 25.781, Federal Aviation Administration, 1990.
105. Westhorpe RN: Ergonomics and monitoring, *Anaesth Intensive Care* 16(1):71–75, 1988.
106. Forcier H, Weinger MB: An evaluation of proposed graphical symbols for medical devices, *Anesthesiology* 79:625–627, 1993.
107. Waterson C, Calkins J: Development directions for monitoring in anesthesia, *Semin Anesth* 5:225–236, 1986.
108. American Society of Testing and Materials: *Standard Specification for Particular Requirements for Anesthesia Workstations and Their Components*, 2005.
109. Buffington CW, Ramanathan S, Turndorf H: Detection of anesthesia machine faults, *Anesth Analg* 63:79–82, 1984.
110. Recommendations for Pre-Anesthesia Checkout Procedures American Society of Anesthesiologists. Available at http://asahq.org/For-Members/Clinical-Information/~/media/For%20Members/Standards%20and%20Guidelines/FINALCheckoutDesignguidelines.ashx.
111. Mazze RI: Therapeutic misadventures with O2 delivery systems: the need for continuous in-line O2 monitors, *Anesth Analg* 51:787–792, 1972.
112. Ward CS: The prevention of accidents associated with anaesthetic apparatus, *Br J Anaesth* 40(9):692–701, 1968.
113. NFPA-99: *Health Care Facilities Code: Gas and Vacuum Systems*, Quincy, MA, 2012, National Fire Protection Association.
114. Sato T: Fatal pipeline accidents spur Japanese standards, *APSF Newslett* 6:14, 1991.
115. Blum LL: Equipment design and "human" limitations, *Anesthesiology* 35:101–102, 1971.
116. Compressed Gas Association: *Standard color-marking of compressed gas cylinders intended for medical use in the United States*, New York, 2004.
117. Katz D: Increasing the safety of anesthesia machines. I. Further modification of the Draeger machine. II. Considerations for the standardization of certain basic components, *Anesth Analg* 48(2):242–245, 1969.
118. Loeb RG, Brunner JX, Westenskow DR, Feldman B, Pace NL: The Utah anesthesia workstation, *Anesthesiology* 70:999–1007, 1989.
119. Keenan RL, Boyan P: Cardiac arrest due to anesthesia, *JAMA* 253:2373–2377, 1985.
120. Guerra F: Awareness and recall, *Int Anesth Clin* 24(4):75–99, 1986.
121. Smith NT, Quinn ML, Flick J, et al: Automatic control in anesthesia: a comparison in performance between the anesthetist and the machine, *Anesth Analg* 63(8):715–722, 1984.
122. Westenskow DR, Wallroth CF: Closed-loop control for anesthesia breathing systems, *J Clin Monit* 6(3):249–256, 1990.
123. Kern FH, Ungerleider RM, Jacobs JR, et al: Computerized continuous infusion of intravenous anesthetic drugs during pediatric cardiac surgery, *Anesth Analg* 72(4):487–492, 1991.
124. Leslie K, Clavisi O, Hargrove J: Target-controlled infusion versus manually-controlled infusion of propofol for general anaesthesia or sedation in adults, *Anesth Analg* 107(6):2089, 2008.
125. Jaklitsch RR, Westenskow DR, Pace NL, Streisand JB, East KA: A comparison of computer-controlled versus manual administration of vecuronium in humans, *J Clin Monit* 3(4):269–276, 1987.
126. Lampard DG, Coles JR, Brown WA: Electronic digital computer control of ventilation and anaesthesia, *Anaesth Intensive Care* 1(5):382–392, 1973.
127. Tsang P, Johnson W: Cognitive demands in automation, *Aviat Space Environ Med* 60:130–135, 1989.
128. Wiener E: Controlled flight into terrain accidents: system-induced errors, *Hum Factors* 19:171–181, 1977.
129. Cook RI, Woods DD: Adapting to new technology in the operating room, *Hum Factors* 38:593–613, 1996.
130. Dror A, Henriksen E: Accidental epidural magnesium sulfate injection, *Anesth Analg* 66(10):1020–1021, 1987.
131. Holley HS, Cuthrell L: Intraarterial injection of propofol, *Anesthesiology* 73(1):183–184, 1990.
132. Fromme G, Atchinson S: Safety of continuous epidural infusions, *Anesthesiology* 66(1):94–95, 1987.
133. Cook RI, Woods DD, Howie MB, Horrow JC, Gaba DM: Case 2–1992: unintentional delivery of vasoactive drugs with an electromechanical infusion device, *J Cardiothorac Vasc Anesth* 6(2):238-244, 1992.
134. Currie M, Mackay P, Morgan C, et al: The Australian Incident Monitoring Study. The "wrong drug" problem in anaesthesia: an analysis of 2000 incident reports, *Anaesth Intensive Care* 21(5):596–601, 1993.
135. Chopra V, Bovill JG, Spierdijk J: Accidents, near accidents and complications during anaesthesia: a retrospective analysis of a 10-year period in a teaching hospital, *Anaesthesia* 45(1):3–6, 1990.
136. Cullen DJ, Bates DW, Small SD, et al: The incident reporting system does not detect adverse drug events: a problem for quality improvement, *Jt Comm J Qual Improv* 21(10):541–548, 1995.
137. Bates DW, Cullen DJ, Laird N, et al: Incidence of adverse drug events and potential adverse drug events: implications for prevention. ADE Prevention Study Group, *JAMA* 274(1):29–34, 1995.

138. Leape LL, Bates DW, Cullen DJ, et al: Systems analysis of adverse drug events. ADE Prevention Study Group, *JAMA* 274(1):35–43, 1995.
139. Murphy JL Jr: Endrate or amidate, *Anesth Analg* 73(2):237, 1991.
140. ASTM: Standard specification for identification and configuration of prefilled syringes and delivery systems for drugs (excluding pharmacy bulk packages), *Philadelphia, PA*, 2009, ASTM.
141. ASTM: Standard specification for labels for small-volume (100 mL or less) parenteral drug containers, *Philadelphia, PA*, 2007, ASTM.
142. Cooper JB, Long CD, Newbower RS, Philip JH: Critical incidents associated with intraoperative exchanges of anesthesia personnel, *Anesthesiology* 56(6):456–461, 1982.
143. ASTM: Standard specification for user applied drug labels in anesthesiology, *Philadelphia, PA*, 2011, ASTM.
144. Centers for Disease Control and Prevention: *Occupational HIV transmission and prevention among healthcare workers, 2001*. Available at http://www.cdc.gov/hiv/resources/factsheets/PDF/hcw.pdf.
145. Tomkins SE, Elford J, Nichols T, et al: Occupational transmission of hepatitis C in healthcare workers and factors associated with seroconversion: UK surveillance data, *J Viral Hepat* 19(3):199–204, 2012.
146. Anderson DC, Blower AL, Packer JM, Ganguli LA: Preventing needlestick injuries, *Br Med J* 302(6779):769–770, 1991.
147. Kempen PM: Eliminating needle stick injuries, *Can J Anesth* 36(3 Pt 1):361–362, 1989.
148. Hejna WF, Gutmann CM: *Management of surgical facilities*, Rockville, MD, 1984, Aspen Systems, pp xv, 345.
149. Zahn J, Haines R: The influence of central search task luminance upon peripheral visual detection time, *Psychonomic Sci* 24:271–273, 1971.
150. Sanders M, Gustanski J, Lawton M: Effect of ambient illumination on noise level of groups, *J Applied Psychol* 59(4):527–528, 1974.
151. Burn JM: Facility design for outpatient surgery and anesthesia, *Int Anesth Clin* 20(1):135–151, 1982.
152. Ziter CA, Dennis BW, Shoup LK: Justification of an operating-room satellite pharmacy, *Am J Hosp Pharm* 46(7):1353–1361, 1989.
153. Partridge BL, Weinger MB, Sanford TJ: Preventing unauthorized access to narcotics in the operating room, *Anesth Analg* 71(5):566–567, 1990.
154. Ehrenwerth J, editor: *Operating room design manual*, Park Ridge, IL, 1999, American Society of Anesthesiologists.
155. Gaba DM, Maxwell M, DeAnda A: Anesthetic mishaps: breaking the chain of accident evolution, *Anesthesiology* 66(5):670–676, 1987.

CHAPTER 25

Simulation Equipment, Techniques, and Applications

Ken B. Johnson • Elizabeth M. Thackeray

CHAPTER OUTLINE

OVERVIEW

Simulation has become an integral part of teaching and evaluation in anesthesia. Because a mannequin is used in simulation, it provides an opportunity for anesthesia practitioners to try out their skills in managing adverse events without consequence to actual patients. They can demonstrate their deployable knowledge, communication skills, and psychomotor dexterity to uncover weaknesses in response to potentially life-threatening events. Simulation provides a means to train for difficult, unusual, or infrequent adverse events. Simulation in anesthesia seeks to recreate real experiences with simulated ones that replicate important aspects of a real clinical environment in an interactive fashion.[1] In its finest form, simulation seeks to immerse participants in a task-oriented experience in which they suspend disbelief and behave much as they would in a real-world clinical scenario.

It is not surprising that anesthesiologists have played a critical role in the development of this technology. In anesthesia, simulation has evolved from using relatively simple, mannequin-based equipment to assess skills in airway management and cardiac lifesaving to using sophisticated environments that allow participants to fully immerse themselves in a simulated perioperative arena and manage adverse events in a realistic manner. Researchers have published a growing number of original manuscripts, reviews, and technical reports in anesthesia and simulation journals to investigate how simulation is used to train and evaluate clinician performance.

Over the past 25 years, advances in simulation have significantly improved education in anesthesia. Simulation centers across the world are growing in number and offer numerous training opportunities to anesthesia care providers. At some institutions, fully trained anesthesiologists participate in periodic simulation training and receive a discount on malpractice insurance.[2] Selected entities that provide board certification currently or will soon require simulation training prior to board certification[3] or as a component of board recertification.[4]

TABLE 25-1 **Definitions Used in Simulation**

Term	Definition
Simulation in anesthesia	Re-creation of a clinical environment in anesthesia for training and evaluation purposes.
Simulator	Equipment used to mimic objects or persons encountered in a clinical environment; simulators used in anesthesia include full-body mannequins, part-task trainers, virtual reality equipment, and computer screen–based simulators.
Part task trainer	Equipment that allows anesthesia care providers to practice psychomotor and decision-making skills; examples of part task trainers include torso and neck body parts that contain imitation blood vessels and tissue on which to practice ultrasound-guided placement of central lines and also head, neck, and chest simulators to practice airway management and other functions.
Computer or screen simulators	Software programs that recreate environments that allow clinicians to practice diagnostic, therapeutic, and decision-making skills; examples include software used to train and evaluate skills in advanced cardiac life support, crises in critical care, pediatric emergencies, and others.
Computer-based anesthetic drug simulators	Software programs that provide graphic illustrations of anesthetic drug behavior; these programs provide predictions of plasma and effect-site concentrations and interactions between different anesthetic drug classes (i.e., the synergistic interaction between opioids and potent inhaled agents).
Virtual reality	Fully immersive simulation environment in which participants interact with a virtual world using computer-based simulation; virtual reality systems in anesthesia are primarily investigational.
Anesthesia crisis resource management	A training technique designed to improve communication and information-sharing among clinicians, especially when managing an adverse event.[60]
Haptic feedback	Technology that provides participants a sense of touch through vibrations, forces, and/or motions; these mechanical simulations may be used to create simulated physiologic phenomenon, such as a radial pulse in a mannequin, or to create the feel of objects that only exist in a simulated virtual world.
Fidelity	The extent to which a simulated environment re-creates a real clinical setting; the four types are *environmental, equipment, physical,* and *psychologic.* Each form of fidelity contributes to the overall *simulation fidelity.*[17] Examples of simulation fidelity in anesthesia include how well 1) simulated hemodynamics respond to blood loss, resuscitation, or pharmacologic agents; 2) simulated difficult airway and compromised respiratory function mimic these findings in a real patient; or 3) interactions among operating room personnel during an adverse event reflect actual behaviors encountered in the operating room.
Reliability	Consistency among experts asked to evaluate a participant's performance in managing a simulated adverse event, often referred to as *interrater reliability,* or consistency in a participant's performance over a series of simulation exercises.[61] This term is used in simulation-based research.
Validity	The ability of an evaluation tool used to assess performance, such as a checklist, to detect differences between participants with low and high skill levels.[61] Types of validity include face, content, construct, and predictive. *Face validity* is how well the evaluation tool looks like it is going to measure what it is intended to measure. *Content validity* refers to whether an evaluation tool covers the content it is trying to measure. *Construct validity* refers to how well the theory behind an assessment tool, such as a checklist used to assess participants' management of an unanticipated airway, translates into actual action (i.e., successful intubation). *Predictive validity* is the accuracy an evaluation tool has in predicting the success of a particular behavior or action. The various types of validity are used in simulation-based research.
Standardized patient	An actor who re-creates a patient; they are used to train and assess clinicians in their performance of routine assessments (e.g., preoperative anesthesia evaluation) or to interact with patients during a challenging clinical scenario (e.g., myocardial infarction in the postanesthesia care unit). Technologies developed to support this line of activity include Internet-based software applications that assist in the development of patient cases, checklists to assess clinician performance, video recording of patient encounters, and standardized reports.

The purpose of this chapter is to provide an overview of existing simulation equipment used in anesthesia education. This overview will include a discussion of components, advantages, and limitations of each type of simulator and will also briefly discuss advances in simulation technologies, innovations in teaching techniques, and core concepts in simulation training. With the implementation of simulation-based education, numerous terms have been developed to describe simulation systems and how they are used. A brief review of selected key terms and phrases that will be used throughout the chapter is presented in Table 25-1.

HIGH-FIDELITY HUMAN PATIENT SIMULATORS

High-fidelity human patient simulators in general consist of a full-body mannequin, a control computer, and a display to present vital signs (Fig. 25-1). Examples of commercially available high-fidelity human patient simulators are presented in Table 25-2. They are designed to be run by an operator independent of the simulation instructor, and they come equipped with patient profiles and a variety of clinical scenarios. Sample scenarios are presented in Box 25-1. High-fidelity human patient simulators are

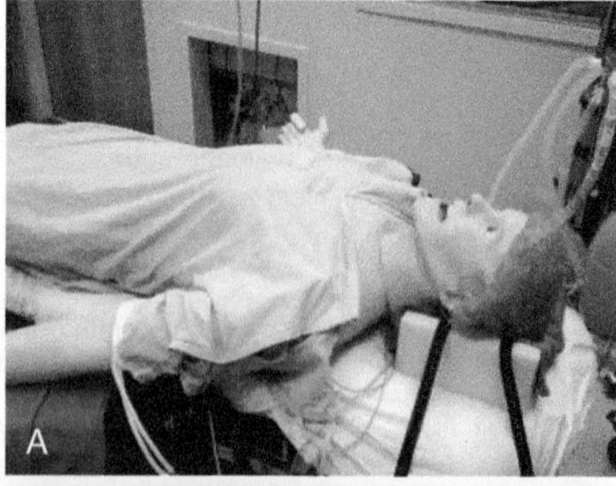

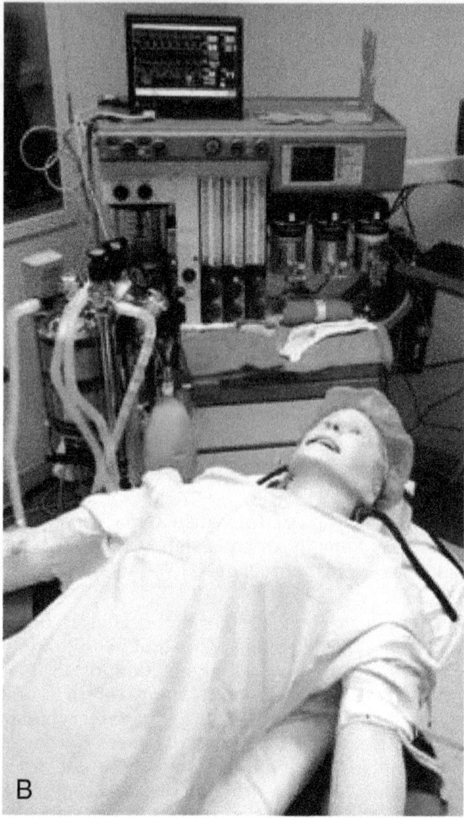

FIGURE 25-1 ■ A high-fidelity human patient simulator (SimMan 3G; Laerdal Medical, Stavanger, Norway). The simulator system consists of a full-body mannequin (**A** and **B**), a control computer (not shown), and a vital sign display (**B**).

a composite of multiple simulation systems of anatomic structure, organ function, and physical appearance. Organ systems include a lung simulator, cardiovascular simulator, airway simulator, and drug simulator and may include an obstetric simulator and neurologic simulator, among others. Each organ-system simulator may have configurable anatomic structures, such as an airway; computer-generated outputs, such as oxygen saturation; or both. Each can be configured to mimic selected disease states, such as a pneumothorax with unilateral chest excursion and breath sounds, and responses to therapeutic interventions, such as restoration of bilateral chest excursion and breath sounds. Components of organ-system simulators commonly found in most high-fidelity human patient simulators are presented in Table 25-3.

TABLE 25-2 **Commercially Available High-Fidelity Human Patient Simulators**

Company	Type of Simulator
Laerdal Medical, Stavanger, Norway	Adult, infant, and neonatal
CAE Healthcare, Montreal, Canada (METI Learning)	Advanced adult, adult prehospital or nursing, 6-year-old child, 3- to 6-month-old infant
Gaumard, Miami, FL	Adult, adult obstetric, 5-year-old, newborn, premature neonatal

BOX 25-1 Sample Scenarios Available in High-Fidelity Human Patient Simulators

Anaphylaxis
Bronchospasm
Congestive heart failure with severe hypotension
Laryngospasm
Hyperkalemia
Malignant arrhythmias
Malignant hyperthermia
Massive hemorrhagic shock
Myocardial ischemia
Subdural hematoma
Tension pneumothorax
Unanticipated difficult airway with hypoxia
Unstable ventricular arrhythmias

Simulation of Pulmonary Function

Simulation of pulmonary function is sophisticated in high-fidelity full-body simulators. Mannequins are equipped with speakers within the chest wall that provide a variety of lung sounds during chest auscultation. One challenge is that during auscultation, breath sounds can be difficult to hear with background noise from the simulator. Recent upgrades provide a means to pause background noise within the mannequin during auscultation to allow for more accurate assessment of breath sounds.

Mannequins produce chest wall movements that coincide with respiratory function. Chest wall excursion can be configured to match findings consistent with endobronchial intubation, pneumothorax, or severe bronchospasm. Mannequins can accommodate needle decompression of a pneumothorax and chest tube placement. Needle decompression provides a rush of air when placed at the midclavicular line of the second intercostal space. Simulation manufacturers recommend the use of a 22-gauge or smaller needle; this is in contrast to the recommended larger, 14- or 16-gauge needle used to treat a tension pneumothorax in a live patient.[5] In some models, construction of the mannequin chest wall out of one continuous piece of material makes unilateral chest excursion difficult to appreciate.

Simulation of one-lung isolation is also possible, but limitations exist. Just beyond the carina, the mainstem bronchi terminate at an apparatus that simulates lung function. When performing fiberoptic bronchoscopy, to confirm placement of a double-lumen tube or an endobronchial blocker, there is little room to advance these

TABLE 25-3 **Selected Features of High-Fidelity Human Patient Simulators**

Organ System	Features
Airway	
Anatomy	Anatomic oral and nasopharygeal airway and glottic opening
	Teeth (both soft and breakaway)
	Mobile cervical spine
	Articulated mandible
Outputs	Inspiratory and expiratory stridor sounds
Configurations	Decreased neck extension
	Difficult intubation with tongue and pharyngeal swelling
	Trismus
	Laryngospasm
Procedures	Manual ventilation with face mask
	Oral and nasopharyngeal suctioning
	Oral or nasotracheal intubation
	Oral and nasopharyngeal airway placement
	Endobronchial intubation
	Esophageal intubation
	Laryngeal mask airway placement
	Combitube placement
	Fiberoptic or lighted stylet intubation
	Tracheostomy
	Cricothyroidotomy
	Retrograde guidewire intubation
	Transtracheal jet ventilation
	Manual ventilation with face mask
Sensors	Jaw thrust
	Depth of endotracheal tube
	Cervical motion monitoring
Pulmonary System	
Anatomy	Tracheobronchial tree
Outputs	Breath sounds synchronized with chest rise, both anterior and posterior
	End-tidal CO_2
	Inspiratory/expiratory O_2
	Tidal volumes
	SpO_2
	Cyanosis
	Gas exchange
Configurations	Adjustable pulmonary mechanics (respiratory rate, tidal volume, airway resistance, lung compliance, etc.)
	Lung sounds: wheezes, rales, absent, unilateral
	Unilateral chest rise
	Flail chest
	Tension pneumothorax or hemothorax
Procedures	Manual or mechanical ventilation
	Bilateral needle decompression
	Bilateral chest tube placement
Sensors	Ventilation
Cardiovascular System	
Anatomy	Arterial pulses
Outputs	ECG, five leads
	Heart sounds synchronized with ECG
	Noninvasive blood pressure via Korotkoff sounds
	Palpable pulses; pulse intensity synchronized with ECG and blood pressure
	Simulated arterial, pulmonary artery, pulmonary capillary wedge, and central venous pressures
	Simulated cardiac output
	Bleeding ports (simulated hemorrhage)
Configurations	Range of heart sounds and intensities
	Adjustable cardiac parameters (heart rate, blood pressure, contractility, afterload, etc.)
	Jugular vein distention
	Extremity hemorrhage and moulage sites
Procedures	Defibrillation, pacing, and cardioversion
	Chest compressions
	Interosseus access (sternal and tibial)
	IV access; bilateral peripheral (dorsal vein and antecubital fossa)
	Central (femoral and jugular) IV lines
	Bilateral thigh autoinjection sites for medication administration
	Pericardiocentesis
	Treatment of hemorrhage: pressure points, tourniquets, surgical clamps
Sensors	Touch-activated recording of pulse assessment
Gastrointestinal System	
Anatomy	Esophagus
Output	Bowel sounds
Genitourinary System	
Anatomy	Interchangeable male or female genitalia
Output	Urine output (normal, none, polyuria)
Procedures	Bladder catheter placement
Central Nervous System	
Anatomy	Eyes, eyelids, and pupils
Voice	
Output	Verbal responses: prerecorded response, real-time responses from operator
	Intracranial pressure
	Convulsions
	Light-reactive pupils
	Secretions: tears, mouth, nose, ears, forehead
Configurations	Eyelid blinking frequency
	Eyelid status: open, partially open, closed
	Pupil size: constricted, normal, dilated, unilateral changes
	Pupil response: normal or sluggish
Procedures	Ventriculostomy

ECG, electrocardiogram; IV, intravenous.

devices much past the carina; it is therefore difficult to achieve an adequate seal within the mainstem bronchus.

Conventional ventilator equipment can be used to mechanically ventilate a mannequin. Measured airway pressures and tidal volumes can be deceiving with some models. In a recent work by Liu and colleagues,[6] they explored the response of the SimMan (Laerdal Medical, Stavanger, Norway) and the Human Patient Simulator (HPS) and Emergency Care Simulator (ECS) (METI; CAE Healthcare, Montreal, Canada) to mechanical ventilation. Their aim was to compare tidal volume and airway pressure values using conventional ventilator settings, and they found that these were appropriate in the HPS but not in the other models. With the SimMan and the ECS, the tidal volumes were lower than expected, and airway pressures were higher than expected. This output makes clinical interpretation difficult. With normal ventilator settings, participants may mistakenly assume findings consistent with bronchospasm. These types of model misspecifications and/or mechanical limitations of the pulmonary simulator require an astute simulator operator who can override simulator output to improve simulation realism.

Simulators provide equipment to mimic gas exchange. Most systems simulate gas exchange and present carbon dioxide and oxygen levels on a simulator-driven physiologic display. In more advanced models, exhaled carbon dioxide levels are generated and can be detected with conventional monitors. In the HPS system, in addition to expired carbon dioxide, inhaled oxygen content and anesthetic gas concentrations are also detected. One limitation in all but one of these systems is apparent during spontaneous ventilation. When simulating an intubated spontaneously breathing patient, the reservoir bag in an anesthesia circuit does not move. A simulated capnograph is available, but no airway flow is present. Only the HPS system provides exhaled carbon dioxide and airway flow during spontaneous ventilation (i.e., the reservoir bag moves). Depending on the scenario, without these features, simulated spontaneous ventilation can be difficult to mimic with high fidelity. Another gas-exchange feature provides a visual representation of cyanosis using a blue light contained within the oral cavity. The blue light is activated once oxygen saturations fall below 90%.

Simulation of Cardiovascular Function

Similar to pulmonary function, models of cardiac function are sophisticated in high-fidelity full-body simulators. Peripheral pulses—radial, brachial, femoral, popliteal, pedal, and carotid—can be modeled, with possible peripheral pulse options that include weak, absent, normal, and bounding. Pulse intensity variations can be linked to changes in blood pressure, such as hypotension and a weak pulse. Cardiovascular simulators generate a variety of heart sounds—normal, muffled, systolic, and diastolic murmurs—and electrocardiograph (ECG) signals that cover a wide range of arrhythmias. They also respond to several interventions, including defibrillation, pacing, chest compressions, volume resuscitation, and, with some systems, pericardiocentesis.

Cardiovascular models are used to simulate right- and left-sided cardiac pressures and estimates of cardiac output. Arterial blood pressures can be represented as noninvasive (blood pressure cuff) or invasive (arterial line) measurements. Pulmonary artery pressures, central venous pressures, and pulmonary capillary wedge pressures are also available, assuming a pulmonary artery catheter is in place. More sophisticated simulators can detect the inflation of a pulmonary artery catheter balloon using electromechanical sensors, and they present the physiologic display estimates of the pulmonary capillary wedge pressure. Manipulation of these parameters can be used to characterize cardiac function in terms of preload, contractility, afterload, and heart rhythm across a variety of cardiovascular states such as hypovolemia, congestive heart failure, pulmonary embolism, sepsis, and so on. These states can either be operator controlled in real time or scripted to mimic a selected cardiovascular state along with responses to resuscitative interventions.

Simulation of Drug Administration

Early high-fidelity full-body simulators used bar code technology and flowmeters for intravenous (IV) drug identification and dosing data. Drug delivery can also be manually recorded by the simulator operator. Newer systems use proximity chips for drug recognition. Proximity chips are small (1.5 × 0.75 inches) and are attached to the syringe. For drugs to be detected, the syringe must be attached at an IV port near a proximity-chip sensor under the skin; in the SimMan 3G, the radiofrequency antenna is in the right arm. With proximity chips, the drug amount is estimated with a flowmeter contained within the simulator. The flowmeters, however, do require periodic calibration.

The response to drug administration can be either model driven or script controlled.[7,8] Model-driven simulators, including the HPS,[8] allow participants and operators to interact with simulated patients in a fashion similar to that of a clinician interacting with real patients. Although useful, model-driven simulators are more expensive,[9] incomplete,[10] and can have inaccurate predictions of drug behavior.[11,12] Responses can be unpredictable when combined with other physiologic models (e.g., hemorrhagic hypotension)[6,13] and may lead to unexpected simulator behavior.

For example, if a participant were to administer a 2.5 mg/kg induction dose of propofol, the simulator would detect the drug name (propofol) and dose (2.5 mg/kg). Without additional input, pharmacologic and physiologic models in the simulator estimate an appropriate response: eyes closing, minor decrease in blood pressure, minor increase in heart rate, and temporary apnea. Programmed responses to IV anesthetics and vasoactive agents based on pharmacokinetic and pharmacodynamic (PK/PD) models are primarily limited to changes in cardiopulmonary function and level of consciousness. The models make predictions of the onset and duration of drug effects and can account for differences in covariates, such as age, weight, and blood volume, in their pharmacokinetic models. They do not, however, account for multiple drug interactions on anesthetic effects (i.e., interactions between sedatives and opioids on analgesia). Simulator operators may have to compensate for modeling limitations by manually overriding responses to drugs in real time; in some cases, the override of undesirable responses is not feasible in a timely manner.

In selected simulation control software, the operator is able to modify both pharmacokinetic and pharmacodynamic models before conduction of a simulation session as appropriate. Tooley and colleagues[12] found the response to IV epinephrine in the METI pediatric simulator to be clinically unrealistic. Unrealistic responses included excessive tachycardia and development of fatal arrhythmias. They modified the time course and magnitude of hemodynamic effects based on feedback from a cohort of pediatric anesthesiologists to fine-tune the response to epinephrine. They emphasized the need for a simulator's response to commonly used IV resuscitation drugs to be consistent with clinician experience in order to maintain a high degree of simulation realism and educational value.

By contrast to model-driven responses, in most simulation systems, the response to a drug is under operator control. For example with script-controlled simulators, such as the SimMan 3G, operators specify the vital signs and simulated patient disposition. With the administration of propofol, an operator would manually close the mannequin's eyes, reduce the blood pressure, increase the heart rate, and halt spontaneous ventilation instead of only entering the dosing information. The advantage of this design is that operators have complete control over what participants see and experience on the monitors and mannequin, but the corresponding disadvantage is that script-controlled simulators require more work and expertise to operate.

Overall, providing participants the opportunity to administer drugs adds fidelity to simulations in anesthesia. Participant tasks associated with drug selection, dosing considerations, and managing drug delivery systems (gravity-driven and syringe pumps) during time-sensitive adverse events improve simulation realism.

Proximity chips can be used to detect actions of participants other than drug administration, such as placement of an oxygen mask on the patient, palpation of the pulse, and depth of intubation. However, a similar proximity chip must be placed on the oxygen mask, so the ability of the simulator to detect and log participant actions must be balanced against interference with the reality of the simulator.

Physiologic Monitors

Pulmonary and cardiovascular simulators generate data for presentation on a vital sign monitor. Some systems require the use of a simulator-specific monitor, but others are configured to emit vital sign signals that conventional physiologic monitors can detect. This is an important feature to consider if simulation goals or research activities require the use of a specific physiologic monitor. For example, anesthesiologists may want to train with the physiologic monitor they are familiar with. Scenario realism may be improved by having participants decide to attach monitor sensors and obtain vital signs, such as during induction of a poorly compliant pediatric patient, who will not allow monitors to be placed before induction.

The importance of this level of fidelity may become important only in high-stakes assessments (i.e., evaluations of clinical competency as part of board certification) and is perhaps not essential in more routine training applications.[14] To the casual observer, full-body simulators may provide impressive clinical realism, but if participants have difficulty interpreting clinically unrealistic responses, simulated adverse events will have limited construct validity.[15]

All the simulators are mobile with the exception of the HPS system. "Mobile" means that they do not require fixed resources to function. The HPS system requires the mannequin to be in close proximity to a computer tower with extensive connections between the mannequin and the tower. Mobile units, however, require only power and proximity to a laptop computer with a wireless connection to function, a feature that provides flexibility in how and where simulations are conducted.

Importance of Orientation

Given the sophistication of current high-fidelity full-body simulations, it is important to conduct an orientation to the simulator before participants using it. This is especially important if the simulator is to be used in an evaluation process. To achieve a high degree of realism, a thorough review of the simulator functionality and its limitations is warranted to avoid participants needlessly pursuing an incorrectly perceived aberrant clinical finding from a simulation artifact. Orientation may include listening to breath and heart sounds, examining the airway, observing chest rise, palpating pulses, hearing the mannequin speak, administering IV drugs, obtaining IV access, and so on. If not addressed prior to initiating a simulation session, participants may focus on simulation artifacts and limitations instead of exploring the limitations of their clinical expertise.

Models of Organ Function and Drug Behavior

Many of the simulation systems integrated into full-body patient simulators use a hybrid of mathematical and mechanical models to characterize organ function and drug behavior. Hybrid models are used in simulating pulmonary and cardiovascular function, whereas mathematical models are primarily used to describe drug behavior.

Some of the models come from published work, but others are built by simulator manufacturers. In some instances, model interactions are not well defined; for example, no body of literature describes how cardiovascular models are modified by the presence of vasoactive agents or IV anesthetics known to suppress cardiovascular function. To improve simulation realism, manufacturers have created programmed responses but often make available to simulator operators the capability to modify model-driven responses or revise the parameters to improve model behavior.

Importance of Integration

Unique to high-fidelity patient simulators is the ability to integrate control of multiple organ simulators to create realistic patient presentations. For example, alterations in the size of the tongue and pharynx, cervical spine range of motion, and vocal cords can be used to block visualization of the glottic opening and/or prevent tracheal intubation. Combined control of airway and pulmonary systems can be used to mimic adverse airway and respiratory events such as can't intubate/can't ventilate, can't intubate/can ventilate, or can intubate/can't ventilate situations. This is of particular relevance to anesthesia training, in that tools are provided to build scenarios that address many of the pathways in the difficult airway algorithm according to the American Society of Anesthesiologists (ASA).[16]

Cost Versus Fidelity

A basic assumption in simulation is that simulation effectiveness improves as the precision in replicating real-world environments improves. Model fidelity in terms of simulator output is often a trade-off between perceived educational benefit and the cost of engineering resources required to create the output.[8] Recent work in simulation has not supported this assumption. In some instances, higher fidelity has not led to improved training outcomes, and lower fidelity simulations, by contrast, have been found to be effective.[17] As technology in simulation advances, it is apparent that features of realism necessary to create valid scenarios for high-stakes assessments are not well defined, and these should be closely scrutinized when considerable effort is required to achieve higher degrees of fidelity.[18,19]

For example, a cardiovascular simulator that uses a hydromechanical system to generate brachial and radial arterial pulses for blood pressure measurements re-creates with a high degree of realism how clinicians interact with a patient when measuring blood pressure.[8] Participants would be able to cannulate the radial artery or use a conventional blood pressure cuff, as they would in real clinical practice. The engineering required to develop this, although available, along with the associated cost to maintain it, is not likely of significant educational benefit for training in anesthesia. A more simplified system that provides simulated cuff or arterial line pressures is often sufficient in developing scenarios of educational value.

COMPONENTS OF A SIMULATION CENTER

A simulation center is a facility designed to mimic real clinical environments. For anesthesia, simulation centers are typically designed as an operating room (OR), postanesthesia care unit (PACU), surgical intensive care unit, or any out-of-OR location where anesthesia is provided, such as an interventional radiology suite. A schematic floor plan of a simulation center is presented in Figure 25-2. It contains a set of rooms that are ideally located adjacent to one another to facilitate execution of simulation activities. Essential rooms for a simulation center include a control room, a simulation suite, and a

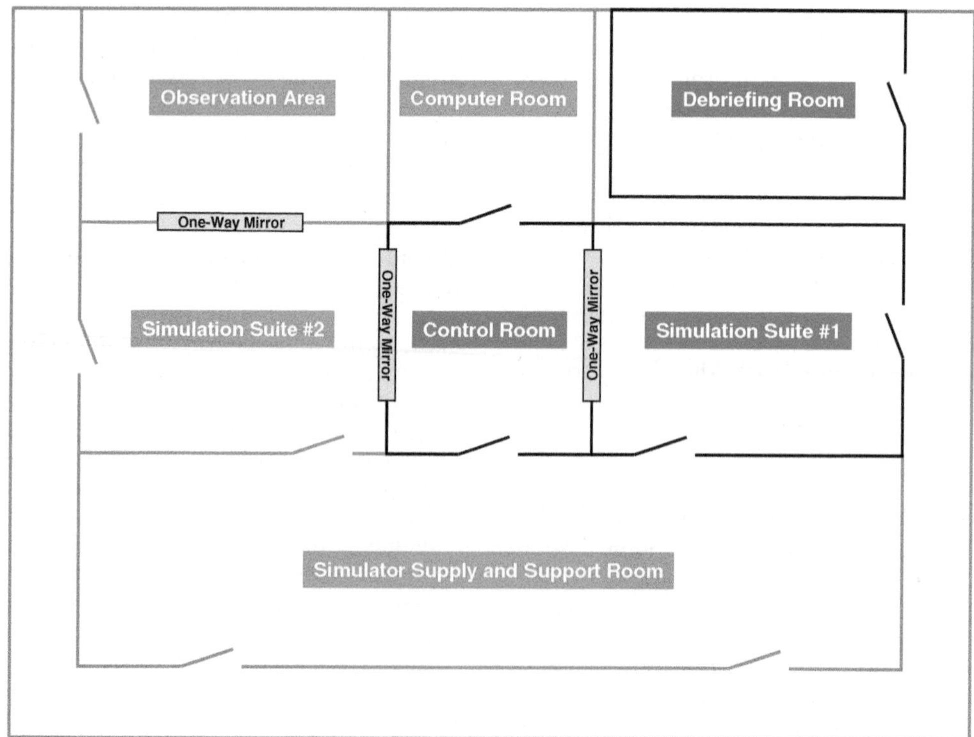

FIGURE 25-2 ■ Floor plan illustrating basic features of a simulation center. Blue and gold represent essential and useful rooms, respectively. Ideal room configuration places the control room adjacent to the simulation suite and in proximity to the debriefing room.

debriefing room. Other useful rooms include a computer room, an observation room, and a storage room. Each room has a unique function, with specific design considerations and a variety of available technologies to enhance functionality.

Facilities

Control Room

The control room represents the nerve center of a simulation center. It is equipped to monitor participant activities, control simulation equipment, and communicate with actors and other personnel in the simulation suite.

To monitor activities, participants can be instrumented with wireless microphones, or the simulation suites can be equipped with three to four strategically placed microphones. Input from these microphones is fed through an audio amplifier and is made available to simulation operators via either earphones or a speaker system in the control room. This component of the simulation control room is especially important when monitoring participants' communication with other participants and actors and their verbal expressions of diagnostic and therapeutic interventions, which may require a response in the progression of a simulated event. Additional monitoring is achieved with video cameras, and a simulation suite can be instrumented with one to three video cameras that are linked to the control room. Video displays within the control room are used to present real-time video collected from these cameras. Fixed cameras capture video from specific areas (e.g., the mannequin head and neck) within the simulation suite. More-expensive cameras provide pan, tilt, and zoom features, and they steer and focus the camera remotely from within the control room.

Physiologic data presented to participants in the simulation suite can be presented to control room personnel via a secondary display. Using a digital audiovisual mixer, video clips from the physiologic display can be overlaid onto video clips of the simulation suite in real time. Combined video from the simulation suite and physiologic monitor are recorded and used for debriefing, investigational studies, or presentation in real time to other participants in a remote location outside the simulation suite.

To control simulation equipment, the primary interface is through computer software that controls all possible responses in a mannequin and/or physiologic display. Additional diagnostic information can be introduced into the simulation suite through the use of secondary displays, such as chest radiograph, transesophageal echocardiography (TEE) video clips, data from an electronic medical record or a digital anesthesia record, and so on. The simulator operator also provides audio input as appropriate through a speaker system contained within the mannequin. This includes prerecorded responses and statements or scripted or impromptu responses offered by the operator. It is our experience that auditory feedback from the mannequin as scenarios develop improves simulation realism. Communication equipment is also used by the simulator operator to guide actors in the execution of key events to meet teaching or evaluation goals. This equipment consists of a wireless radio, earpiece, and microphone. To maintain realism, communication from the actor to control room personnel is minimized.

Simulation Suite

The suite is equipped with a mannequin, audio and video recording devices, and medical-grade gases (oxygen, air), and depending on the type of simulator, nitrogen and carbon dioxide pressurized gas tanks. The suite is often configured to mimic a clinical care station consistent with a given scenario. For example, to imitate an OR, the simulation suite is configured with conventional OR equipment, such as an operating table, anesthesia cart, anesthesia machine, physiologic monitors, IV poles, infusion pumps, surgical case cart and instrument table, suction canisters, defibrillator, OR lights, radio/digital music player, and so on. A schematic of equipment and information flow is presented in Figure 25-3.

Debriefing Room

The debriefing room provides accommodations for participants and simulation instructors to review a simulation scenario. A debriefing room is equipped with a large monitor and video player to play a recorded simulation. The video player allows operators to take advantage of event markers and quickly move to key portions of recorded video clips. The debriefing room should provide an environment that promotes reflection, an important component of experiential learning.

When teaching large groups, it is useful to have an observation room adjacent to a simulation suite with a one-way mirror. This maintains an element of realism such that observers are not inside the simulation suite along with the participants. The observation room is equipped with a display of the physiologic monitor and a speaker system so that observers can see physiologic data presented to participants and hear conversations, alarms, and other auditory data presented during a scenario.

Additional rooms that may be useful include a computer room to house computer systems at the appropriate temperature to protect them and to ensure optimal functionality. For large simulation centers, a storage room is also useful to accommodate props, back-up mannequins, costumes, part-task trainers, and as a location for simulation personnel to prepare items to be introduced into a scenario.

Several simulation management systems are available to facilitate capturing, assessing, and debriefing simulation activities. Both Laerdal and CAE Healthcare (METI products) have companion products for their respective simulation systems. B-Line Medical (Washington, DC) also offers a similar product designed to be used with a variety of simulation systems. Selected features of these systems are presented in Box 25-2.

Importance of People

A simulation program's success is a function of the people staffing a simulation center. S. Barry Issenberg wrote an

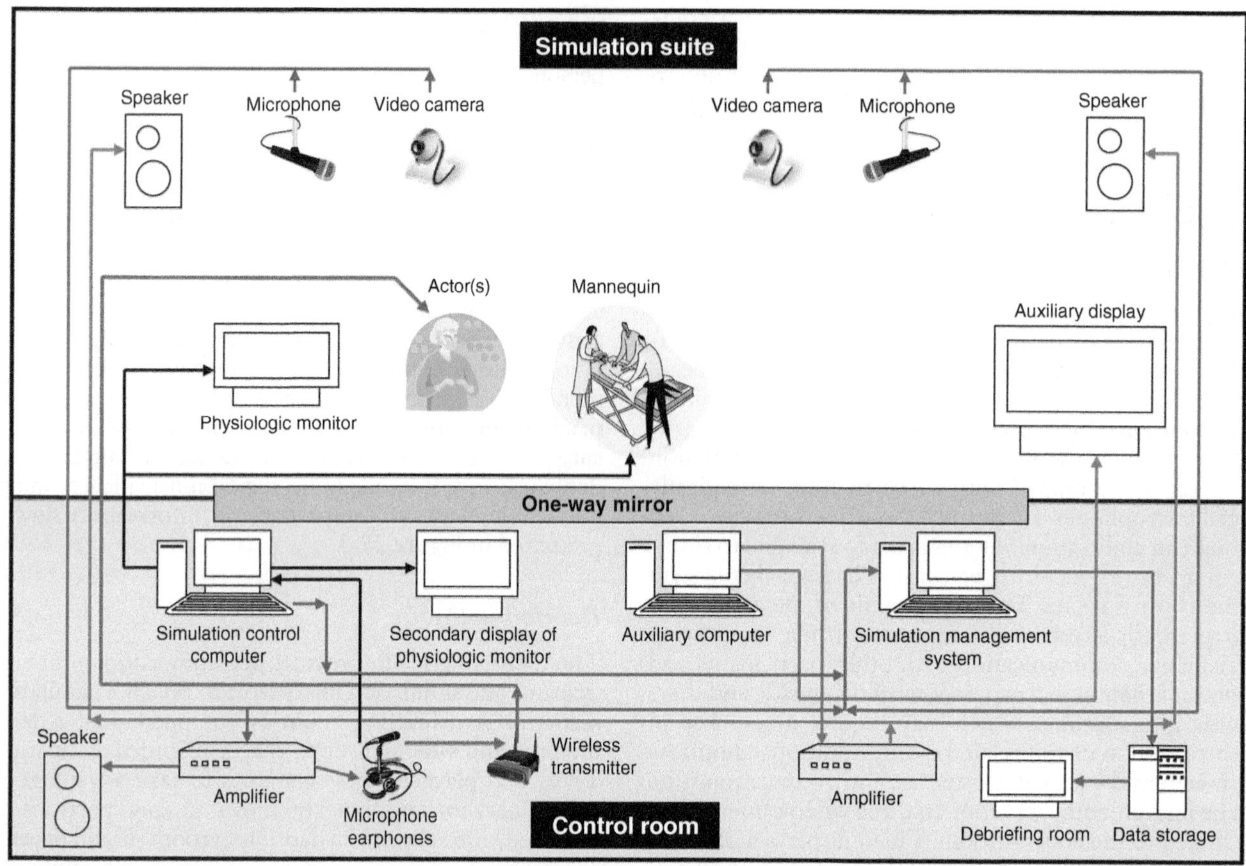

FIGURE 25-3 Schematic representation of equipment configuration in a high-resolution full-body simulation center. The *black lines* represent the flow of information from the simulation control computer to control the behavior of the mannequin, physiologic displays, and audio (voice) output from the mannequin. The *blue lines* represent the flow of audiovisual information captured from within the simulation suite by the simulation management system. Audio from the microphones is also broadcast over the control room speaker system or to earphones worn by the simulation operator. This system also captures events data (transitions from one simulated state to another, drug administration, vital signs, etc.) from the simulation control computer. Integrated simulation data are then archived in a storage device and made available as needed for playback and review in the debriefing room. The *red lines* represent the flow of data from an auxiliary computer capable of presenting additional audio (music) or visual information (transesophageal echocardiography clips) during a given scenario to an auxiliary screen or speakers within the simulation suite. The *green lines* represent the flow of audio data from the microphone in the control room to actors (confederates) in the simulation suite to guide the progress of the simulation or to provide real-time voice data to the mannequin. This figure represents only one of many useful configurations.

BOX 25-2 Components of Simulation Management Systems

- Capture audio and video feeds from multiple cameras and microphones within one simulation suite
- Audio and video capture from multiple simulation sites
- Simultaneous display of multiple camera views and physiologic data
- Integration of data from simulation systems with audio and video data; data from simulation systems can include waveform and discrete values from physiologic monitors, event markers, physiologic models used to simulate patient conditions, pharmacologic models used to simulate drug effect, and scenario programming
- Software to record, manage, play back, and archive simulations
- Tools to mark either programmed or observed events for review during debriefing
- Internet-based software to allow users to review recorded simulations at any location with Internet access
- Provides tools for scenario development and checklists for evaluation purposes

editorial entitled "The Scope of Simulation-Based Healthcare Education" and described three core components to ensure effective use of simulation-based education: 1) training resources, 2) trained educators, and 3) curricular institutionalization.[20] Training resources include simulation equipment and facilities as previously described in this chapter to meet a program's needs.

Trained educators, in this case anesthesiologists, have training in simulation-based education and in management and administration. When considering the minimum requirements for staffing a simulation program, staffing should include support of a director, simulation technician, and an educational specialist. Support consists of training opportunities, adequate "supported time" allotment to simulation activities, and clearly defined expectations of what a program will provide to an institution or department. Although simulation has been a part of anesthesia training for over two decades, relatively few centers offer instructor training, and no formal certification process exists to become a simulation-based educator in anesthesia. As simulation becomes more integrated into

BOX 25-3 Guidelines for Instructor Credentialing

- The director should be board certified in anesthesiology.
- Simulation educators should provide quality learning opportunities to American Society of Anesthesiologists members.
- Instructors should have experience in simulation-based teaching of anesthesia residents, faculty, and medical students.
- Instructors should be able to provide simulation experiences that involve team management and/or cognitive knowledge and procedural skills.
- Students should have experience with "debriefing" simulation exercises.
- The program should provide documentation of participant evaluations from students and fellow instructors who observed or who participated in simulation and debriefing exercises with specific questions directed at the effectiveness of the debriefing.
- Scholarly activities in simulation should be demonstrated to include presentation at national meetings, participation in workshops, development of peer-reviewed courses, or publication of topics in simulation.
- Qualifications of participants should be recognized (practicing anesthesiologists and Diplomates of the American Board of Anesthesiology).
- When possible, provide evidence of participant learning that validates the instructor's teaching ability.

institutional certification[3] and recertification processes, the demand for instructor training will likely increase.

Curricular institutionalization refers to a sponsoring institution's adoption of goals directed at patient safety and improving patient care. This includes institutional efforts to prevent medical errors and improve competencies. Among those competencies in anesthesia easily addressed through simulation are crisis resource management, acute management of adverse cardiopulmonary events, and skills in managing difficult airways.

Recent efforts by the American Board of Anesthesiology (ABA) to enhance the maintenance of certification in anesthesia programs now include a requirement for a simulation experience, and the ASA's Committee on Simulation has been asked to develop a mechanism by which simulation programs are endorsed so that they can offer the simulation training required by the ABA. In July 2006, the committee issued a white paper outlining their recommended approval process.[20a] In that white paper, the committee established guidelines for instructor credentialing. Key elements are presented in Box 25-3.

The simulation operator controls the mannequin and other equipment from within the control room. A skillful simulation operator has intimate knowledge of simulation equipment and its ability to create pathophysiologic states. The operator must also have a solid understanding of principles of cardiopulmonary physiology and clinical pharmacology to properly interact via the mannequin with participants in real time. The simulator operator must integrate events observed with programmed simulation event timelines. In some event-driven simulations, the operator must formulate responses based on previously established event-driven look-up tables to create a believable (high-fidelity) simulation. Figure 25-4 presents the often complex milieu of information that must be integrated in real time to seamlessly simulate clinical events. Figure 25-4 also illustrates the numerous sources of information available to anesthesia care providers and the importance of re-creating these sources in a clinically meaningful manner to enhance the immersive feel of the simulation.

Cost of Simulation-Based Education

Simulation centers range in size from a one-room facility usually mocked up as an OR to a complete virtual hospital and are expensive to build and operate. Costs depend on the size and scope of simulation activities the center will provide. Infrastructure development costs include floor space configured as a clinical venue, simulation management equipment, full-body simulation mannequins, task trainers, and props such as anesthesia machines, ventilators, beds, OR tables, anesthesia equipment, and infusion pumps . High-fidelity human patient simulators range in cost from $30,000 to $210,000 depending on the desired capability. Task trainers and virtual reality trainers are less expensive and range in cost from $1000 to $80,000. Maintenance and operation costs include faculty salaries, consumables, instructor training, and maintenance contracts. A maintenance contract for a high-fidelity human patient simulator, depending on the coverage, ranges between $10,000 and $18,000 for 3 years of coverage. A maintenance contract is advisable; in our experience, high utilization leads to frequent repairs and preventive maintenance requirements. Available simulation instructor courses range in cost from 1-day events for $1000 to week-long courses for more than $5000.

Data summarizing simulation center costs versus capacity and workload are not available in a central repository. Many simulation centers either have a sponsoring agency that offsets many of the costs or have had a large endowment from an entity interested in promoting simulation-based education in medicine. Many academic anesthesia departments share simulation facility resources with other departments within a medical school or with other schools (e.g., nursing schools) on a medical education campus. Some anesthesia programs operate their own simulation centers. Sources of revenue to simulation centers include course tuition, industry- or government-sponsored research, contributions from medical malpractice insurance companies,[2] medical institution support, and industry grants.

SIMULATION IMPLEMENTATION

Scenario Development

When formulating a scenario for a simulation, several components of the scenario merit consideration to optimize their educational value. The rationale for documenting a scenario in a rigorous and consistent format includes ensuring that the scenario content is reproducible and making sure it is easily shared among simulation programs. The simulation program at Duke University has developed its own template, which is free and available

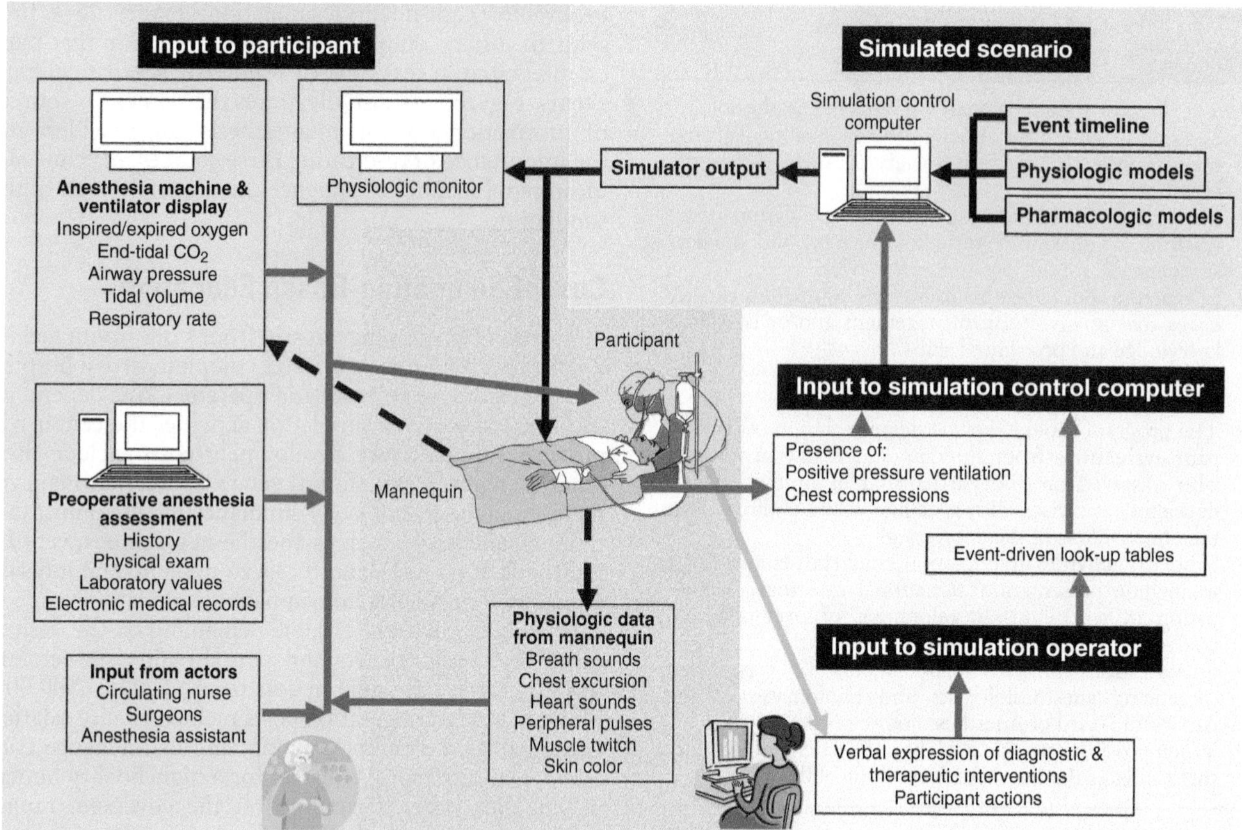

FIGURE 25-4 ■ Schematic of information flow within a simulation. The simulation control computer uses information from multiple sources (*solid black lines*) to control the mannequin and, with selected manufacturers, the physiologic monitor. The *dashed black lines* illustrate how data are transmitted from the mannequin to the participant and anesthesia machine. Participants may examine the simulated patient to auscultate the heart, and if the mannequin has an instrumented airway and is on mechanical ventilation, simulated data characterizing pulmonary mechanics are sent via the mannequin to the anesthesia machine ventilator. The *blue lines* represent information flow from devices, medical records, and actors within the simulation suite to the participant. The *green line* represents information the simulator operator observes and uses to provide input to the simulation control computer during a simulation. The *pink lines* represent data sent to the simulation control computer. Sources of information include the simulator operator, the mannequin, and the event look-up tables. Data from the mannequin are sent back to the simulation control computer as feedback to drive physiologic responses; that is, if the simulated patient is under neuromuscular blockade and is not mechanically ventilated, the patient develops hypoxia.

online at http://simcenter.duke.edu/support.html. An abbreviated version of the Duke template is presented in Box 25-4 that uses a comprehensive approach to documenting a scenario in a reproducible format and contains sections that address simulated patient demographics, curricular information, preparation requirements, and briefing information. Some examples of the scenarios include a venous air embolism during a sitting-position craniotomy,[21] trauma and awareness,[22] intraoperative apnea as a result of a medication error,[23] and defective anesthetic gas delivery.[24]

Importance of Debriefing

Debriefing is an effective form of learning following a simulation,[25] and it helps participants develop and integrate insights from their simulated experience into clinical practice.[26] It is an opportunity for reflection of what participants thought, felt, and did during simulation in order to improve future performance. Central to an effective debriefing are concise, respectful critiques that clarify participant perspectives. Rudolph and colleagues[26] suggest that a debriefing meet two criteria: that it create a context for learning and that it provide effective learning objectives.

Creating a context for learning is an approach in which simulation instructors establish rules of participation and clarify expectations. This generally consists of instructor feedback and trainee reflection on performance. This requires building an environment of psychological safety that is predictable and secure enough to describe and scrutinize thoughts, motivations, and goals. This environment allows participants to take interpersonal risks and permits exploration of difficult topics. Lastly, instructors should treat participants as capable professionals by taking a respectful and curious approach to participants' successes and failures and work on the premise that participants are intelligent, doing their best, and interested in learning.[26]

Effective objectives define a desired performance level against which actual performance can be compared. Concise feedback is used to describe the gap between actual and desired performance. Objectives should be specific, observable during simulation, and easy to assess. They should also lend themselves to the development of

BOX 25-4 Duke Template for Scenario Development

SECTION 1: DEMOGRAPHICS

Case Title:
Patient Name:
Scenario Name:
Simulation Developer(s):
Date(s) of Development:
Appropriate for the Following Learning Groups: identify specialty, training-level physician (faculty, residents, medical students), nurse anesthetics, or nursing

SECTION 2: CURRICULAR INFORMATION

Educational Rationale:
Learning Objectives: Categorized according to ACGME core competencies (medical knowledge, patient care, practice-based learning and improvement, interpersonal and communication skills, professionalism, and systems-based practice)
Guided Study Questions:
References Used (include PubMed identifier when possible):
Didactics (includes teaching adjuncts to include electronic presentations and Web sites):
Assessment Instruments:

SECTION 3: PREPARATION

Monitors Required: Noninvasive blood pressure cuff, arterial line, central venous catheter, five-lead ECG, temperature probe, capnograph, processed electroencephalogram monitor, other
Other Equipment Required: May include anesthesia machine, infusion pumps, bronchoscope, defibrillator, intravenous fluid warmer, nerve stimulator, transesophageal or transthoracic echocardiography machine, endotracheal tubes, laryngeal mask airways, and laryngoscopes
Supporting Files: May include chest radiographs, ECGs, echo clips, and assessment handouts
Time Duration: Setup, preparation, simulation, and debrief

SECTION 4: CASE STEM AND BACKGROUND AND BRIEFING INFORMATION

Consists of one to two paragraphs on pertinent patient and scenario information (for the learner); should include location, physician/help availability, family present, and such. The background and briefing information is for the facilitator/coordinator's eyes only.

SECTION 5: PATIENT DATA BACKGROUND AND BASELINE STATE

Patient History (follow standard history/physical examination format):
Review of Systems: Central nervous system, cardiovascular, pulmonary, renal/hepatic, endocrine, hematology/coagulation
Current Medications and Allergies:
Physical Examination: General, weight, height, vital signs, airway, lungs, and heart
Laboratory, Radiology, and Other Relevant Studies: hematocrit, chest radiograph, ECG
Baseline Simulator State: What underlying alterations in physiology would this patient have compared with the "perfect" 70-kg man or woman? Include target numbers along with vital signs, neurologic examination, respiratory function, cardiovascular function, gastrointestinal status, genitourinary status, metabolic state, and environmental conditions.
Table of Scenario States and Teaching Points: The table contains the simulator state (baseline; state 1, 2, 3; and so on), patient status (e.g., normal, myocardial ischemia, resolution), and student learning outcomes or actions desired and the trigger to move to the next state; these include notes to the simulation operator and teaching points for the instructor.

ACGME, Accreditation Council for Graduate Medical Education.
From Duke University, Durham, NC. Available at simcenter.duke.edu/support.html.

2- to 5-minute didactic lectures that address current evidence and best practices.[26]

Current concepts in debriefing suggest that a session consist of three phases: a *reactions* phase, an *analysis* phase, and a *summary* phase. During the reactions phase, participants respond to the scenario, the instructor clarifies the facts of the scenario, and participants are encouraged to analyze and discuss the scenario. This process may provide important clues about what is most concerning to the participant.[26]

During the analysis phase, educational specialists recommend four steps to analyze performance: 1) observe the gap between objectives and performance, 2) provide feedback on the performance gap, 3) investigate frames of reference underlying the gap, and 4) close the gap with didactics and discussion.[26] Providing feedback on and investigating performance gaps should have as the underlying assumption that mistakes are puzzles to be learned from, and the instructor is seeking to clarify the underlying frame of reference with honest inquiry ("I noticed X, and I was concerned about that because of Y, and I wonder how you saw it").[27]

Frame of reference, also called *cognitive frame* or *mental model,* refers to the underlying assumptions people use to filter, create, and apply meaning to the environment. Clinical frames shape actions. For example, if participants believe that the patient has gastroesophageal reflux disease, their actions will be very different than if they believe that the patient is having an acute myocardial infarction. Rudolph suggests that instructors "learn what frames drive trainee behaviors so that both their failures and successes can be understood as an ingenious, inevitable, and logical solution to the problem as perceived within their frames."[27]

Video recording of simulation sessions has become a widely accepted technique in debriefing. Although popular, the value of this technology is not clear. Savoldelli and colleagues[28] explored the utility of video-assisted feedback during debriefing compared with oral debriefing from the instructor or no debriefing at all. They found that although participants who received debriefing improved more than participants without debriefing, improvement tended to be lower in the video-assisted debriefing group than the oral debriefing group. They concluded that an instructor-based approach to debriefing is acceptable and may be preferable.

In summary, debriefing is a key element of simulation training and is as important, if not more important, than equipment used to create the simulated perioperative environment. Recent work has demonstrated that a well-conducted debriefing can influence participants' performance up to 9 months after the simulator session.[25,28]

Crisis Resource Management

Crisis resource management in anesthesiology evolved from the field of aviation and provides a framework for effective teamwork training. Core principles in crisis resource management include role clarity, communication, personnel support, and situational awareness.[29]

Role clarity means that people responding to an adverse event understand their role and perform specific functions. Role clarity, particularly of an appropriate team leader, should be established early in the management of a critical event. The team leader directs the action, rather than participating in procedures (unless absolutely necessary), and preserves a "bird's-eye view" to consider the entire situation. A leader should flatten the hierarchy so that information can easily flow from leader to support personnel and vice versa. Role clarity includes the need for good "followership" also; nonleaders should share observations and ideas regarding diagnoses and interventions, and they must avoid competing with the leader in role assignments.[30]

Effective communication in crisis resource management implements closed-loop dialogue. In this form of communication, leaders address support personnel, preferably by name and with eye contact if possible, and issue their request. The support person repeats the order back (e.g., "Start an IV line") and then confirms completion (e.g., "IV line started"). Poor communication was implicated in a series of 35 pediatric mock codes; in each was at least one order, given by the leader and assumed to be completed, that was discovered to be incomplete during debriefing. Assertive communication is encouraged, as opposed to "hint and hope," and it should be recognized that people can show deference to expertise and experience but still speak up in a respectful and nonthreatening manner.[30]

Management of personnel and resources includes calling for help early, requesting help from other team members, mutual performance monitoring to manage any performance decreases, and actively assisting other team members.[29,30] Cognitive aids and the patient's medical record are useful resources that are often overlooked.

Skills in situational awareness include repeated *situation assessments* and avoidance of *fixation errors:* situation assessments should be shared with other members of the team, so that all team members share the same mental model of the patient's condition; fixation errors are prevalent, and their defining characteristic is that clinicians focus on one element of an adverse event that persists over time—for example, the oxygen saturation. Fixation errors may include the "this and only this" error; that is, an unwillingness to consider alternative diagnoses. They may include the "everything but this" error, in which a diagnosis is avoided in favor of collecting further data. Lastly, "everything's okay" is the fixation error that avoids the recognition of any serious problem.[30,31]

Crisis resource management assumes that problems inevitably occur despite efforts to prevent them. This is particularly relevant to the specialty of anesthesia. Anesthesiologists may have more demands on their attention than can be addressed, and patients may require multiple simultaneous interventions. The OR is a dynamic, complex environment that can be influenced by many factors, some of which are not readily apparent. Some of these factors include latent errors, predisposing factors, and psychologic precursors. *Latent errors* refer to characteristics of an operating system that go undetected for a time and are identified once they combine with other factors to create a critical incident. Examples of latent errors include OR staff scheduling policies, look-alike drug labels on syringes, and equipment that is awkward to control in less than ideal circumstances. Examples of predisposing factors include preexisting recognized and unrecognized patient conditions or the elements of the planned surgical intervention, such as duration of the procedure, extent of blood loss, tissue injury, and organ dysfunction. Psychological precursors include fatigue, illness, injury, boredom, medications, abuse of drugs and alcohol, and environmental noise.[32]

Implementing crisis resource management training in anesthesia requires a carefully planned simulation scenario, a full complement of personnel to participate, and a well-trained instructor to conduct the simulation and debriefing sessions. The scenario should create a need for communication, leadership, division of labor, and time pressure. Ideally, the scenario should include all the clinical personnel typically found in the simulated clinical venue. For example, in the OR, this would include a surgeon, scrub nurse, circulating nurse, anesthesiologist, and anesthesia technician and other personnel as needed. Typically the role of the anesthesiologist is that of the participant in the "hot seat." Other roles are played by confederates (simulator center personnel) and/or other participants. The simulator operator orchestrates the development of a crisis and responds to input as needed from participants; confederates may have a script to follow to enhance the scenario. The instructor attends the simulation and provides guidance to the simulator operator and confederates to ensure that key elements of the scenario are enacted and that the scenario is clinically realistic. Following the scenario, the instructor conducts the debriefing session, focusing on elements of crisis resource management.

Interdisciplinary Teamwork

An emerging form of simulation in anesthesia combines simulation-based education with other specialties and clinicians in the perioperative environment. Rarely do anesthesiologists respond to an adverse event as the sole responder (Fig. 25-5). During most adverse events, surgeons, nurses, and other support personnel are present. Full-scale simulations of low-frequency but high-risk events, such as chemical gas exposure, or complex procedures known to be error prone, such as unanticipated aortic dissection during cannulation for coronary artery bypass, that focus on teamwork among clinicians will likely save lives. Although a few centers conduct

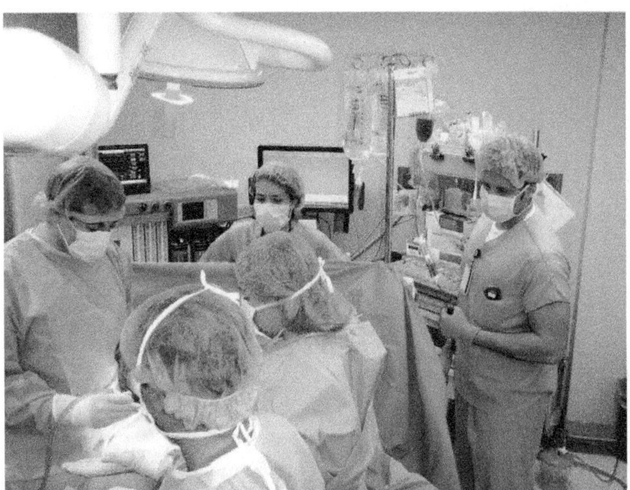

FIGURE 25-5 ■ Multidisciplinary high-fidelity human patient simulation in the operating room. Simulation training with an emphasis on teamwork seeks participation from surgeons, anesthesia care providers, circulating and scrub nurses, and support staff at the Center for Patient Simulation, University of Utah, Salt Lake City.

teamwork-based simulations, unfortunately, teamwork in health care is underdesigned and not well emphasized in clinical training.[18] For example, recent work has demonstrated that simulation evaluations with an emphasis on teamwork have revealed inadequacies in intensive care unit (ICU) team skills in managing sepsis and septic shock.[33] Future work is warranted in developing infrastructure, opportunities, and acceptance among health care teams to participate in teamwork-based simulations.

Limitations of Simulation

Any simulator system imposes multiple trade-offs by virtue of the system constructs, learning objectives, and cost and the availability of technology, physical space, and support staff. Participants in a simulation scenario must be familiar with any variables that may affect their care of the "patient," such as the presence of breath sounds in particular locations and their nonpathologic absence in others. Mathematical models of physiologic variables and responses to medications or procedures are estimates based on past experience and thus imperfectly represent reactions of every possible patient. Validity and reliability of participant assessments are increasingly difficult to achieve with increasing task complexity, because the closer control of variables in a scenario provides a more robust test of participant ability, whereas less instructor control provides greater fidelity.[32,34]

Participants often find themselves being hypervigilant, because they know that the simulator is an opportunity to test them, whereas others may be cavalier, thinking that it does not really matter much, because a simulator is not a real patient. The Heisenberg uncertainty principle, whereby observation changes the observed behavior, is extremely likely in simulation; but given the tremendous resources required to observe anesthesiologists routinely in the OR in hopes of assessing behavior, it is a limitation we must accept.[32]

OTHER TYPES OF SIMULATORS

Task Trainers

Practicing procedures such as spinal anesthesia, arterial or central line placement, and cricothyrotomy on a patient simulator can greatly increase the participant's comfort level with the procedure when faced with a real patient for the first time. Although no patient simulator is realistic enough to provide a completely accurate experience for the participant, students may increase efficiency and improve clinical skills.[35,36] Furthermore, the struggle to perform a procedure on a mannequin provides the instructor with an opening to discuss difficulties commonly encountered in clinical practice and their remediation.

Airway Trainers

A complete airway trainer will include an articulated neck and anatomically correct nasopharynx, oropharynx, and laryngopharynx. Such a device will allow endotracheal and esophageal intubations and the use of common airway adjuncts, such as laryngeal mask airways (LMAs) or lightwands, with appropriate chest rising or filling of the abdomen (Fig. 25-6). Some models, such as the Laerdal difficult airway trainer, will allow transtracheal jet ventilation and cricothyrotomy. Laerdal's airway trainer also allows the instructor to enlarge the tongue to increase difficulty with intubation. The RespiTrainer Advance (IngMar Medical, Pittsburgh, PA) includes the inflatable tongue and breakout teeth and also provides real-time ventilation parameters (volume, flow, and pressure) in both training and test modes. More differentiated partial task trainers, such as the Nasco Life/form (Fort Atkinson, WI) cricothyrotomy simulator, also exist.

Central Venous Vascular Access Trainers

Vascular access trainers include torsos for internal jugular and subclavian vein cannulation as well as femoral vein models. Blue Phantom (Advanced Medical Technologies, Redmond, WA) produces a torso amenable to ultrasound visualization of the internal jugular vein and carotid artery with options for a nonpulsatile artery, hand-pump arterial pulsations, and automated arterial pulsations (Fig. 25-7). The model can tolerate full placement of a central venous catheter given its self-healing skin and vessels. Self-healing skin has its limitations, however; after multiple cannulations, visible leakage from former sites makes identification of vessels easier. Use of the manufacturer's lubricant may lessen the amount of needle damage and extend the life of the simulated tissue, but manufacturers recommend replacing the self-healing skin after several hundred needle insertions. These issues may be more troublesome in the adult and child intraosseous part task trainers. Landmarks for cannulation of the subclavian vein can become misplaced and require some internal adjustment with padding. Within the neck and torso, the vein vessel length is truncated, and a guidewire can be advanced only a few centimeters past the access needle tip.

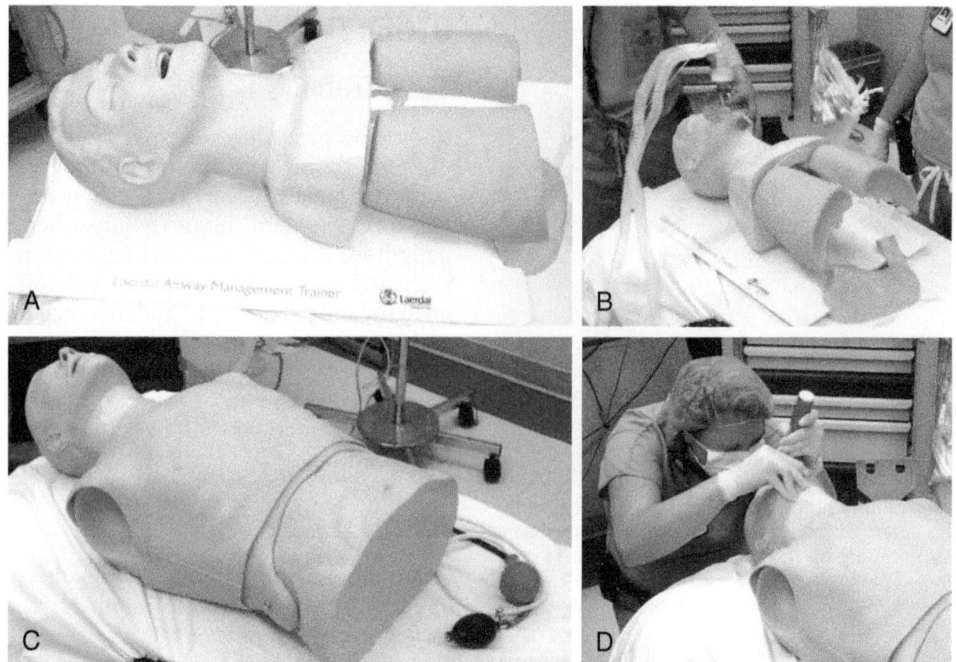

FIGURE 25-6 ■ The Airway Management Trainer and the Deluxe Difficult Airway Trainer (Laerdal Medical, Stavanger, Norway). **A,** Airway trainer with an exposed thoracic cavity allows visualization of the lungs, esophagus, and stomach. **B,** With bag/mask ventilation or mechanical ventilation, the lungs expand during positive pressure ventilation. **C,** Airway trainers consist of an anatomic airway, bronchial tree, inflatable lungs, esophagus, stomach, articulating cervical spine, and articulating mandible; a more advanced airway trainer is presented here. **D,** In addition to conventional laryngoscopy and tracheal intubation, a trainer can simulate an obstructed airway or tongue edema and can accommodate a surgical airway using the manual inflation bulbs (**C**).

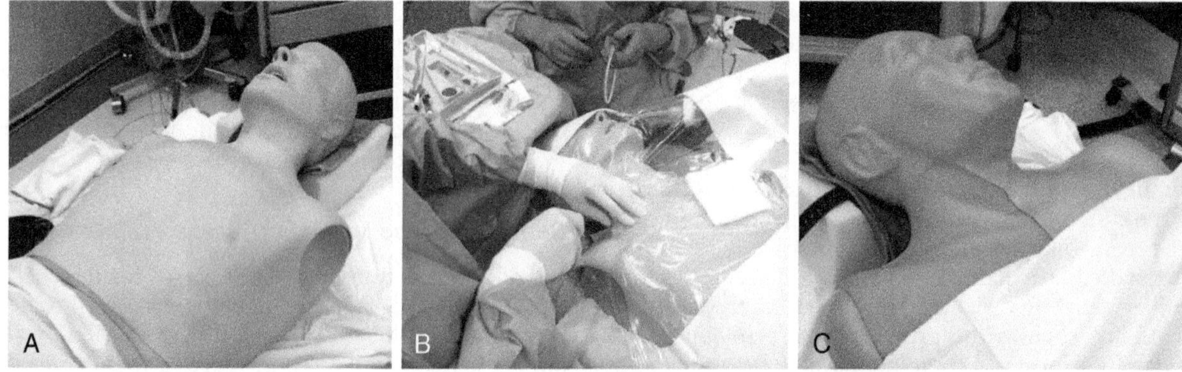

FIGURE 25-7 ■ Central line vascular access trainers consisting of a head, neck, and torso. The model presented in **A** simulates right subclavian central line access (Vascular Access Trainer; Laerdal Medical, Stavanger, Norway). A subclavian vein and lung and rib cage are simulated underneath the skin. Users can puncture the subclavian vein (**B**) but cannot thread a guidewire; the tubing that makes up the vein is not long enough. If the needle is misplaced, users can puncture the lung. Ultrasound imaging is not available on this model. The model presented in **C** simulates right internal jugular vein access (central venous access and regional anesthesia model, Blue Phantom; Advanced Medical Technologies, Redmond, WA). It accommodates ultrasound visualization of the carotid artery and internal jugular vein for ultrasound-guided insertion of a central line. The chest and neck on the right side have been modified for ultrasound imaging. This model also does not accommodate guidewire placement.

Ultrasound-Guided Peripheral Nerve Block Trainers

The neck and torso model produced by Blue Phantom also accommodates ultrasound visualization of components of the brachial plexus (Fig. 25-8). Both infraclavicular and interscalene views of the brachial plexus are available. This technology provides a platform for participants to learn basic skills in developing images of nerves in relation to vascular structures, understand differences between in- and out-of-plane needle insertion (i.e., the orientation of the needle insertion to the ultrasound beam), and short- and long-axis imaging of neurovascular structures. It also allows users to inject fluid through the needle to verify needle tip placement and simulate infusion of local anesthetic. The images developed using these "phantoms" do not include muscles. For example, when imaging the brachial plexus in the interscalene groove, landmarks such as the sternocleidomastoid muscle, anterior and middle scalene muscles, and the deep cervical fascia are not visualized.

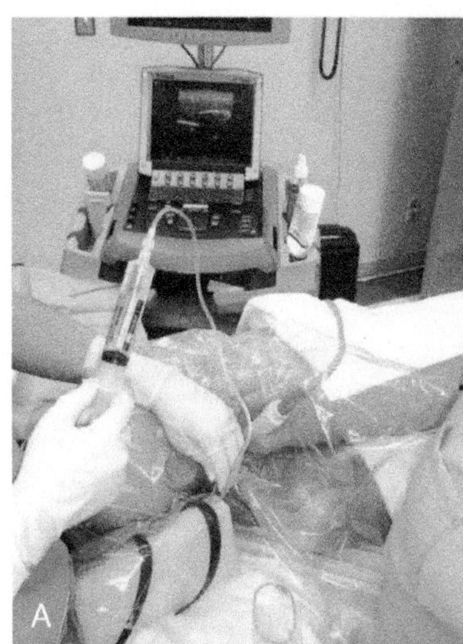

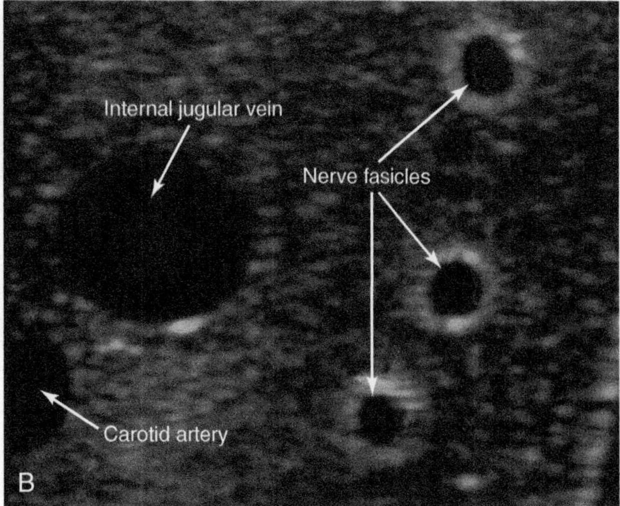

FIGURE 25-8 ■ The Blue Phantom ultrasound-guided regional anesthesia trainer, consisting of a head, neck, and torso, accommodates ultrasound imaging on the right neck (**A**) and has segments of the brachial plexus (central venous access and regional anesthesia model). **B,** Visualization of nerve fascicles in proximity to the right internal jugular vein and carotid artery when imaging from the interscalene groove. (Courtesy Blue Phantom, Redmond, WA.)

Radial Arterial Line Trainers

Arm and hand task trainers for radial arterial cannulation and IV placement consist of an isolated extremity with fluid-filled tubes embedded within the extremity to mimic vessels (Fig. 25-9). In our experience, a reasonable flash of simulated blood occurs with arterial and venous cannulation, and catheters can be threaded in a realistic manner with the Laerdal arm for arterial lines and the Nasco Life/form hand for IV cannulation. The arterial line trainer provides a palpable radial pulse, and a hand pump is used to create pulsations such that the pulse intensity and rate can be varied by the instructor. These simulators suffer from the same skin problems as with the central line access simulators; after multiple needle sticks, the puncture site becomes obvious and may develop leaks.

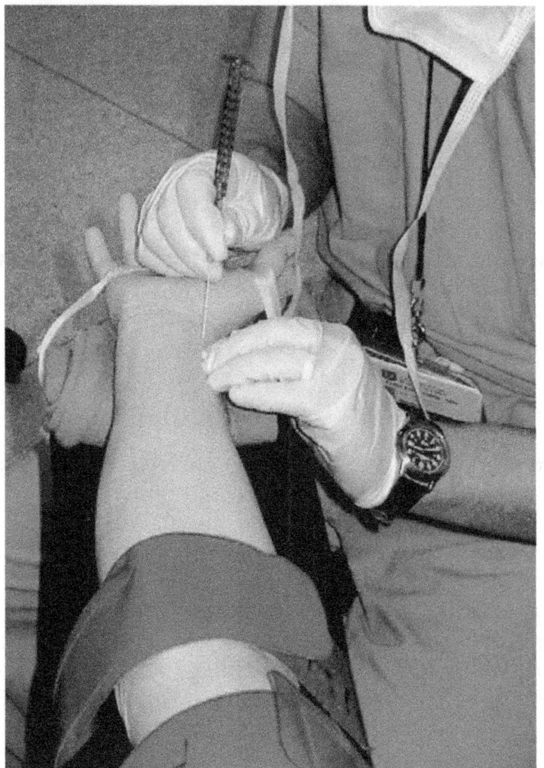

FIGURE 25-9 ■ A right arm radial arterial line trainer (Arterial Stick Arm Trainer; Laerdal Medical, Stavanger, Norway). A radial artery is simulated beneath the skin with manual squeezing of a pressure bulb. The task trainer accommodates a guidewire and allows cannulation of the vessel.

Neuroaxial Access Trainers

The Nasco Life/form Spinal Injection Simulator is a neuroaxial access trainer that provides a lower-torso segment that contains the tissue layers, vertebral bodies, iliac spines, and spinal column found in the lumbar spine (Fig. 25-10). The spinal column contains clear fluid, to mimic cerebral spinal fluid, and is connected to a bag of fluid placed above the simulator to generate pressure within the cerebral spinal column. The simulator accommodates spinal needle access of the spinal column and drainage of cerebral spinal fluid. A clear window over the lumbar spine allows visualization of the vertebral bodies underneath the skin and subcutaneous tissue. Self-healing skin over the L4-L5 interspaces can be quickly replaced when needed.

Trauma Task Trainers

Simulation trainers available for trauma evaluations include equipment that mimics an injured head (Mr. Hurt Head Trauma Trainer; Laerdal Medical) and a torso and abdomen (TraumaMan; Simulab, Seattle, WA). The head trauma trainer includes skull, facial, and cervical spine fractures, unequal pupils, hemotympanum, and a deviated trachea. It is used primarily for developing diagnostic skills during a trauma evaluation and does not provide options to practice therapeutic interventions. It can be transferred to an adult mannequin for full-body simulations. TraumaMan allows

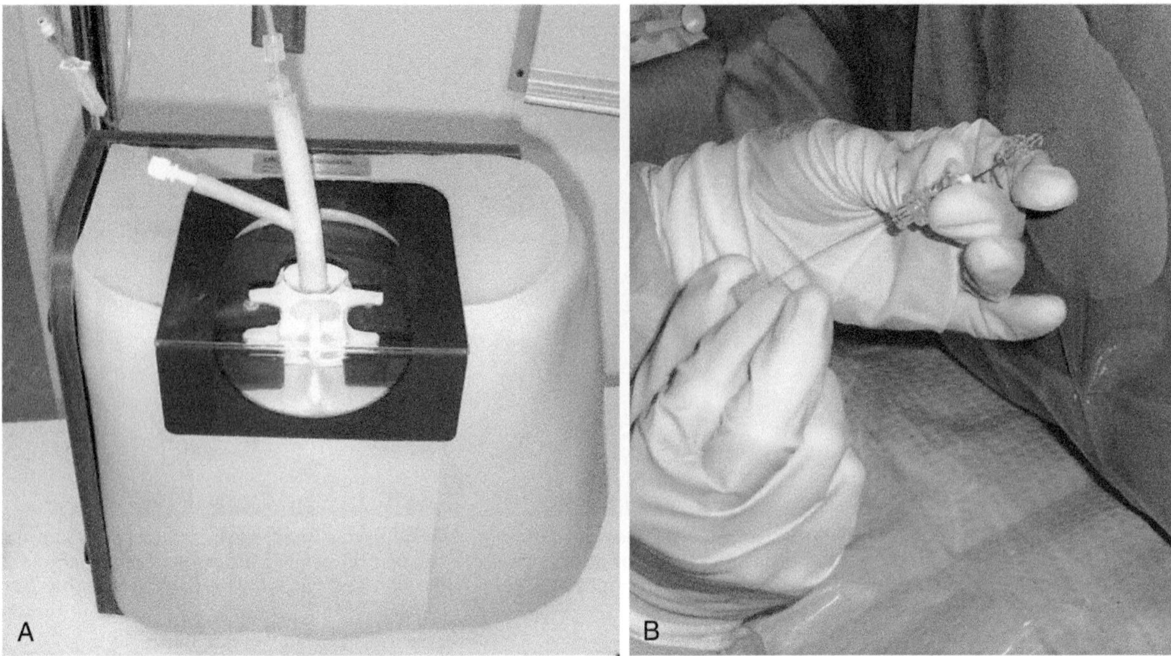

FIGURE 25-10 ■ Spinal injection trainer (Spinal Injection Simulator; Nasco Life/form, Fort Atkinson, WI). **A,** This trainer consists of a lumbar spine with vertebral bodies, spinal cord with dura, ligament tissue, subcutaneous tissue, and skin. **B,** It can accommodate needle puncture of the dura for aspiration of cerebral spinal fluid.

participants to perform numerous procedures in the neck, chest, and abdomen. It consists of simulated human tissue to include skin, subcutaneous tissue, muscle, and peritoneal and thoracic cavity organ mockups. It accommodates diagnostic peritoneal lavage, chest tube insertion, pericardiocentesis, IV cutdown, needle decompression of a tension pneumothorax, percutaneous tracheostomy, and cricothyrotomy.

Computer Screen–Based Simulators

Computer-based, Internet-based, or screen-based simulations have the advantage of being highly portable and, in the case of Internet-based simulations, accessible almost anywhere. Inherent in this flexibility is the ability of the participant to self-educate at a convenient time and place. Simulators in general, and particularly screen-based simulators, can address the needs of multiple participants at once on demand, rather than relying on the relatively scarce resource of a human patient with certain pathology. A screen-based simulator must provide a trade-off between scope and detail; the full spectrum of visual and auditory input from an OR cannot be represented on a computer screen with adequate detail, so various screen models may be used to circumvent this limitation. One example is a panoramic, dynamic background that allows the user to click and drag a portion of the background into view, like the simulated anesthesia application developed around neuromuscular blockade monitoring.[37]

A drawback of some computer-based simulators is that they disallow incorrect choices and provide a list of possible actions or medications rather than requiring participants to develop a plan de novo. However, as a teaching tool, computer-based simulators are reported by participants to have value and may be as effective as conventional didactic lectures, maybe even more effective.[38]

Case-Based Simulators

The Anesoft Corporation (www.anesoft.com) offers downloads and compact discs of various screen-based simulators, including cases in anesthesiology, critical care, advanced cardiac lifesaving, obstetrics, and pediatrics. Each simulator includes multiple case scenarios that address various clinical situations. The anesthesia simulator comprises 32 cases, ranging from a routine induction, to familiarize the user with the simulator interface, to elevated intracranial pressure, diabetic ketoacidosis, eclampsia, and malignant hyperthermia, among other conditions. The simulator includes a library of available drugs, which is extensive but not exhaustive, and photographs of relevant actions such as the mask being placed over the patient's face, the view on laryngoscopy, and the movement of the bellows on the anesthesia machine. The majority of the display is made up of the vital signs, similar to a display seen in the OR (Fig. 25-11). Anesoft's simulations may be completed for continuing medical education credits, and the company invites users to create and submit new cases, with technical and programming support from Anesoft.

Virtual Anesthesia Machine

The Center for Simulation, Safety, and Advanced Learning Technology at the University of Florida has created multiple screen-based simulations. The best known of these is the Virtual Anesthesia Machine, which includes animated schematics and photographs of the anesthesia machine. Simulations allow user input to vary fresh gas flows, vaporizer input, ventilator settings, and position of

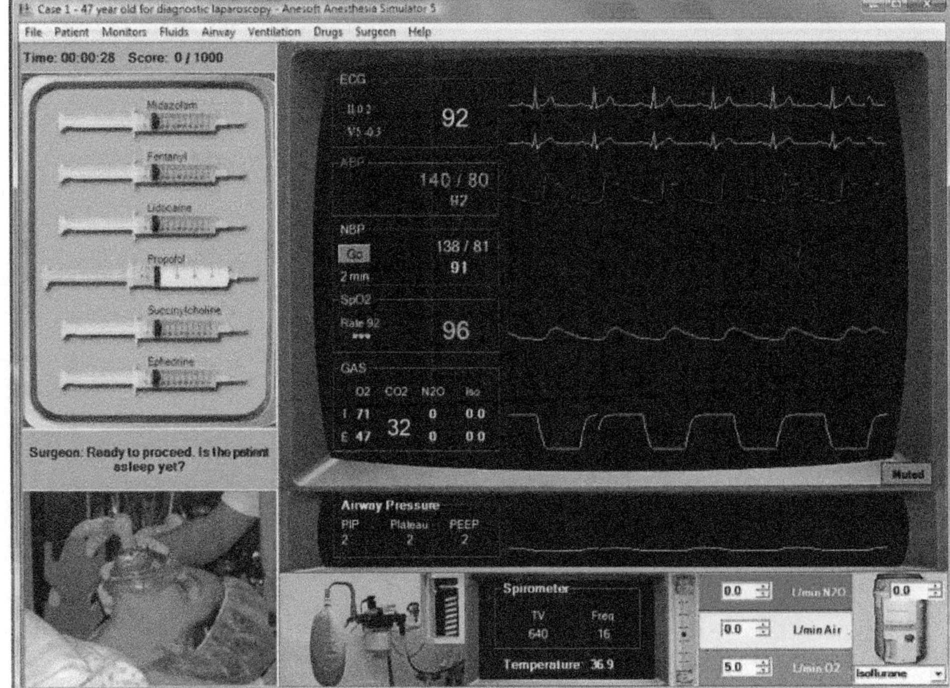

FIGURE 25-11 ■ Anesoft computer screen–based anesthesia simulator. This simulator offers multiple real-time, screen-based simulators that cover emergency situations in anesthesiology that include anaphylaxis, bronchospasm, and intracranial hypertension. This screen displays windows that simulate physiologic data, ventilator data, fresh gas flows, the potent inhaled agent vaporizer, and IV medications. It also provides a window that presents an image of the patient and operating room commentary. (Courtesy Anesoft, Issaquah, WA.)

the adjustable pressure-limiting valve. Moving circles indicate gas flow through valves, the carbon dioxide absorber, the reservoir bag, and into the patient. Users may experiment with changes to anesthesia machine controls and ventilator settings, and they can utilize various scenarios, such as a power failure. In addition to the Virtual Anesthesia Machine, simulations that illustrate various physiologic and pharmacokinetic principles are available, and continuing medical education credit is offered for some simulations.[37]

Bronchscopy Simulators

A screen-based bronchoscopy simulator is available on the Internet (www.thoracic-anesthesia.com) and includes a schematic map of the bronchial tree with simultaneous bronchoscopic video (Fig. 25-12). Users can control the direction of the bronchoscope using mouse clicks, and they can turn labels on the schematic and the video on or off. Selecting a labeled structure in the video portion replaces the bronchial tree schematic with the name of the labeled structure and a description of the anatomy. A quiz tests knowledge before and after using the simulator.

Clinical Pharmacology Simulators

Several software applications have been developed that illustrate in graphic form the time course of anesthetic drug concentration and, in more sophisticated systems, drug effect. Examples of these applications are presented in Table 25-4, and they have been developed and extensively used both for educational and research purposes. These applications provide users with a visual image of predicted plasma and effect-site concentrations for commonly used inhaled and IV anesthetics (Fig. 25-13). These tools allow users to "see" the time course of a bolus or continuous-infusion dosing regimen. They use population pharmacokinetic models to estimate drug concentrations, and for selected drugs, they can account for patient age, weight, and gender.

Gas Man is a computer-based program that was developed and distributed by a nonprofit organization, Med Man Simulations (www.gasmanweb.com/index.html). It is intended to teach uptake, distribution, and pharmacokinetics of inhaled anesthetics, accompanied by a written tutorial explaining the concepts and the computer simulations.[39,40] Gas Man graphically illustrates these principles over time and allows the user to experiment with various settings that include fresh-gas flow, inhaled agent, delivered anesthetic, minute ventilation, cardiac output, oxygen flush, and circuit characteristics (Fig. 25-14).

More sophisticated systems include tools that illustrate the effects of combined anesthetic techniques (desflurane and fentanyl) on patient responses such as level of responsiveness and analgesia and muscle relaxation.[41-44] With these tools, clinicians are able to visualize the onset and duration of effect, either in real time during patient care or off-line during educational activities designed to explore the behavior of various dosing regimens (Fig. 25-15). For example, users can explore the onset and duration of effect for 1) a fentanyl bolus alone, 2) a bolus in the presence of 1 minimum alveolar concentration (MAC) isoflurane, or 3) a 50 μg/kg/min propofol drip. This is an especially interesting area of development, given that both Dräger Medical (Telford, PA) and GE Healthcare (Waukesha, WI) have recently marketed drug display systems.[45] Limiting these simulation systems is their inability to account for changes in pharmacokinetics and pharmacodynamics as a result of chronic exposure to opioids, benzodiazepines, and disease states known to significantly alter cardiopulmonary physiology.

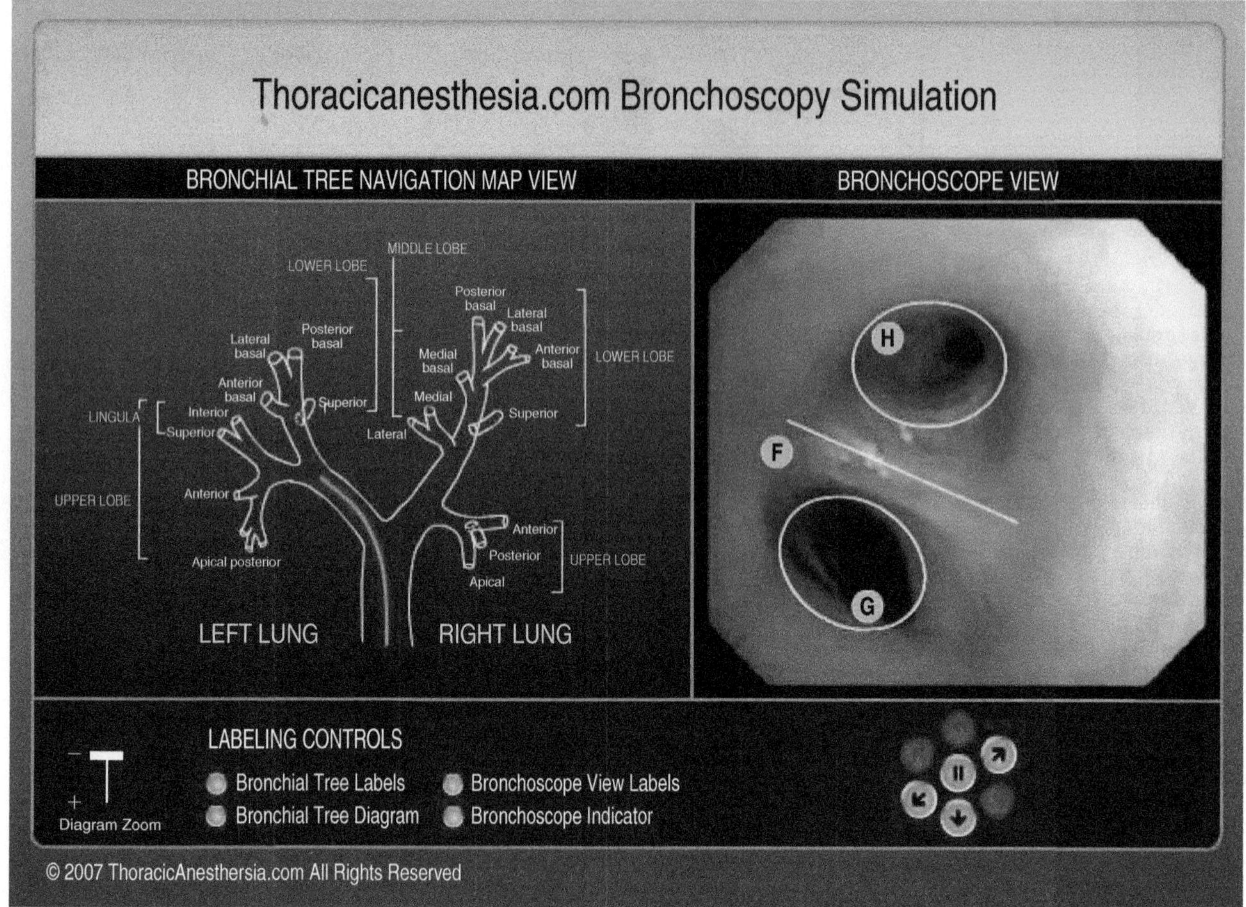

FIGURE 25-12 ■ Computer screen–based bronchoscopy simulator from www.thoracic-anesthesia.com. Dr. Peter Slinger at the University of Toronto developed this Internet-based bronchoscopy simulator to review bronchial anatomy. The user can direct the bronchoscope using the arrow buttons, while the schematic to the left tracks the bronchoscope position. The bronchoscopic view can be enhanced with labeled structures and text descriptions. (Courtesy Thoracic-anesthesia.com, Toronto, Canada.)

TABLE 25-4 **Examples of Computer-Based Anesthetic Drug Simulators**

Product Name	Manufacturer/Author
Gas Man (www.gasmanweb.com/software.html)	Med Man Simulations
Navigator (www.gehealthcare.com/euen/anesthesia/docs/Navigator_bro_M1 159810_eng.pdf)	GE Healthcare, Waukesha, WI
PK/PD Display (www.medvis.com/solutions.php)	Applied Medical Visualization, Salt Lake City, UT
PK/PD Tools (www.pkpdtools.com/doku.php)	Thomas Schnider, MD, Charles Minto, MD
Tivatrainer (eurosiva.org/tivatrainer/instructions_for_downloading.htm)	European Society for Intravenous Anesthesia
Two-compartment pharmacokinetic model with bolus: simulation (vam.anest.ufl.edu/simulations/simulationportfolio.php)	Center for Safety, Simulation and Advanced Learning Technologies, University of Florida
Smart Pilot Trainer (www.draeger.com/media/10/03/01/10030149/draeger_re view_97_1_anaesthesia_18-19.pdf)	Dräger Medical, Telford, PA
Target controlled infusion technology (STANPUMP; www.opentci.org/doku.p hp?id=code:code)	Steven L. Shafer, MD

PK/PD, pharmacokinetics/pharmacodynamics.

Virtual Reality

Virtual reality simulators are currently used in industries such as aviation, manufacturing, and retail store design. At its best, virtual reality provides an immersive experience in which an electronically displayed environment responds to participant movements with limited physical equipment, such as a head-mounted display and data gloves or a wand.

Virtual reality is being successfully used in industry to test and refine designs and train end users. A major difference between virtual reality in manufacturing and industry and virtual reality in medicine is that a plane or car designer has a thorough understanding of the physical

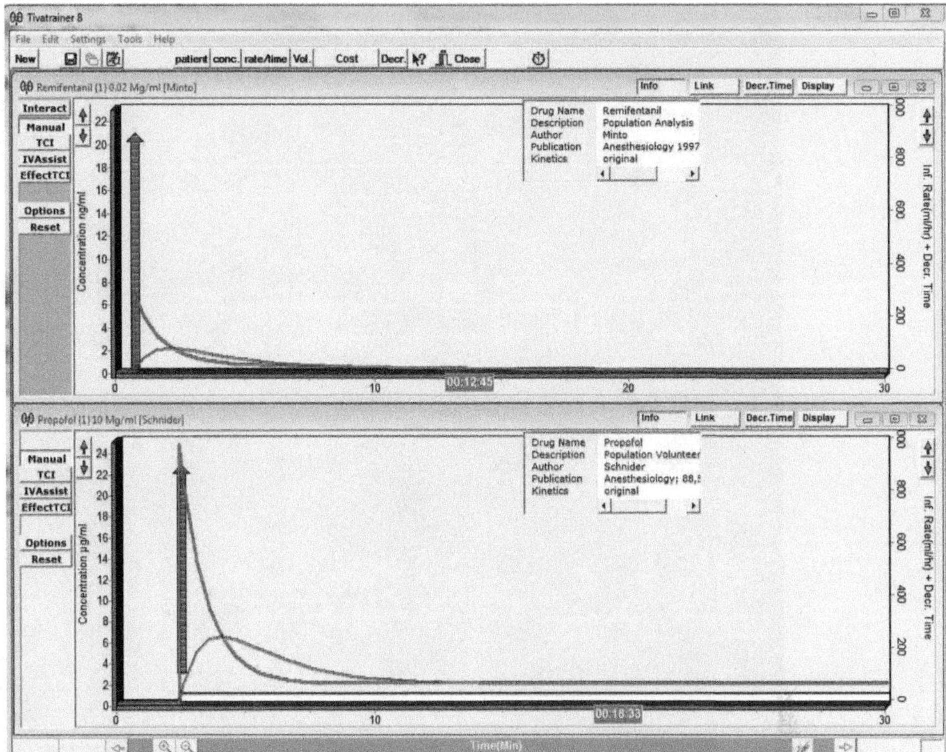

FIGURE 25-13 ■ Intravenous drug simulator. This TIVAtrainer from AstraZeneca (London, UK) presents users with estimates of plasma (*green line*) and effect site (*red line*) concentrations over time, following a bolus or continuous infusion of IV anesthetics. Concentration estimates are made using published population pharmacokinetic models.

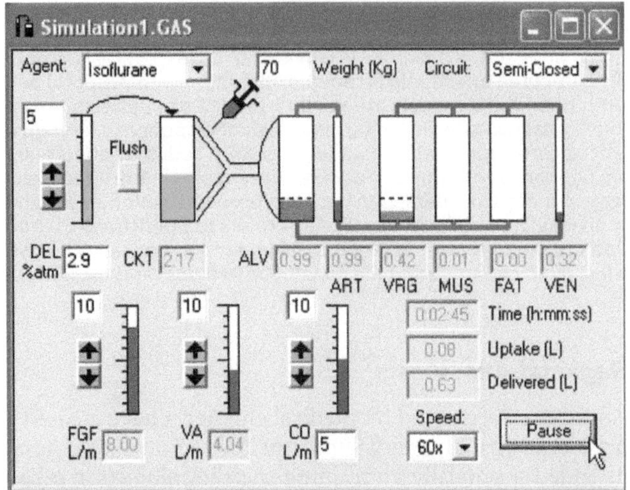

FIGURE 25-14 ■ Inhaled agent drug simulator. The GasMan simulator (www.gasmanweb.com/index.html) predicts inhalation agent concentrations over time in the alveolus (*ALV*); arterial blood (*ART*); vessel-rich organs, labeled *vessel-rich group* (*VRG*); muscle (*MUS*); fat (*FAT*); and venous blood (*VEN*). It allows users to adjust gas flow, vaporizer setting, and ventilatory settings for commonly used inhalation agents. (Courtesy Med Man Simulations, Boston, MA.)

components and mechanical stresses making up the prototype, a degree of knowledge that we approximate less fully with regard to a human patient. Even with that full understanding, however, an airplane will still undergo wind tunnel tests to further replicate real-life conditions. In medicine, virtual reality simulator use is increasing, particularly for surgical training, and virtual reality part task trainers are being developed for anesthesiology. Some examples of virtual reality simulation systems in anesthesia include fiberoptic bronchoscopy, TEE, and regional anesthesia simulators.

Fiberoptic Bronchoscopy

Manufacturers have developed simulation systems that provide an interface with a fiberoptic bronchoscope and a visual presentation of the bronchial tree as the scope is manipulated. The AccuTouch Flexible Bronchoscopy Simulator (Immersion Corporation, San Jose, CA) is a high-fidelity, computerized, virtual reality simulator with a model head, haptic feedback, and computer-generated bronchoscopy images that correlate with the movements and expected anatomic position of the bronchoscope. The simulator displays physiologic responses, such as bleeding of the mucosa from the patient being bumped with the bronchoscope and coughing if local anesthetic has not been administered. The simulator is limited by an inability to pass an endotracheal tube.[46] Simbionix (Cleveland, OH) has introduced the GI-Bronch Mentor (Fig. 25-16), a virtual reality simulator that includes an anatomic compass, three-dimensional bronchial maps, anatomy labels, and an anatomy atlas.

Virtual bronchoscopy has been studied several times to try to determine its utility. In 2002, Rowe and Cohen[47] stated that this simulator was effective at teaching the psychomotor skills necessary for fiberoptic intubation of children. Residents were evaluated on fiberoptic intubation skills before training on the simulator and after an average of 39 minutes of simulator practice. The control group was evaluated during two

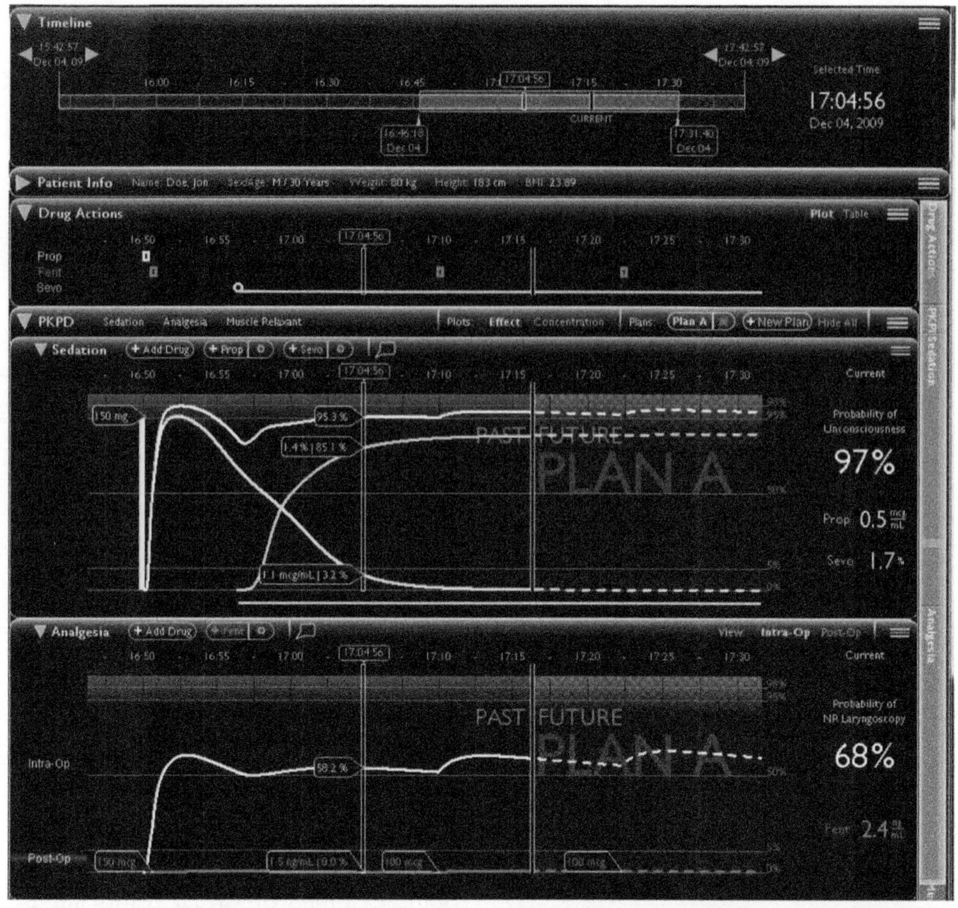

FIGURE 25-15 ■ Drug interaction display. This pharmacokinetic/pharmacodynamic (PK/PD) display (Medvis, Salt Lake City, UT) demonstrates drug effect over time—past, present, and future—as a result of a combined anesthetic technique, induction with propofol and fentanyl, followed by maintenance with sevoflurane and fentanyl. Combined PK/PD models are used to predict drug effects. Anesthetic effects are divided into probability of unconsciousness (*middle plot*), analgesia framed in terms of loss of response to laryngoscopy (*bottom plot*), and muscle relaxation (not shown). Fentanyl effects are represented by the *blue line*; sedative effects are represented by the *bright yellow line* for propofol and the *dark yellow line* for sevoflurane; and *white lines* represent drug interactions. For example, the white line on the analgesia plot illustrates the large synergistic interaction between propofol, sevoflurane, and fentanyl on analgesia and, to a lesser extent, the synergistic interaction on loss of consciousness. *PLAN A* refers to predictions of drug effect, if the dosing scheme presented in the "future" window is carried out (sevoflurane 1.8% with 100-μg fentanyl bolus). The two *vertical lines* represent a scrollable pointer to identify predicted drug effect at any point during the anesthetic (*left line*) and the current predictions (*right line*). (Courtesy Medvis, Salt Lake City, UT.)

sequential fiberoptic intubations with no additional training. The group who trained with the simulator had decreased time to successful intubation, spent less time viewing the mucosa, and touched the mucosa with the bronchoscope less often.[47]

A 2006 study by Goldmann and Steinfeldt[46] also examined the AccuTouch system and determined that novices trained on the simulator achieved similar times to reach the carina with a bronchoscope in a cadaver as experts (defined as anesthesia attendings having performed more than 50 fiberoptic intubations).

Interestingly, Chandra and colleagues[48] studied the use of the AccuTouch system compared with the use of a low-fidelity simulator, in which training was done with a fiberoptic bronchoscope on nonanatomic models, intended to improve fiberoptic bronchoscope manipulation. Evaluation of participants using a global rating scale, checklist assessment, and success of intubation were no different for the high-fidelity simulator in comparison with the low-fidelity simulator.

Regional Anesthesia

Anesthesiologists and biomedical engineers have created a prototype virtual reality simulator for regional anesthesia intended specifically for training anesthesiologists in celiac plexus blocks, a relatively rare procedure in which the needle is in proximity to several vital structures.[49] Using the National Library of Medicine's Visible Human Project male computed topography dataset,[50] they generated the visualized simulator dataset, which was then combined with the haptic data. Empiric haptic data were obtained on forces encountered in various tissue types with actual needle insertions on unfixed cadavers within 72 hours of death. This simulator consists of a head-mounted display coupled with the haptic feedback device to create a virtual patient on which to practice celiac plexus blocks. The visualized portion can have skin rendered opaque or transparent, with the patient positioned prone, supine, or upright.

A similar approach to virtual reality for regional anesthesia was reported by Grottke and colleagues.[51] Magnetic resonance imaging (MRI) and magnetic resonance angiogram

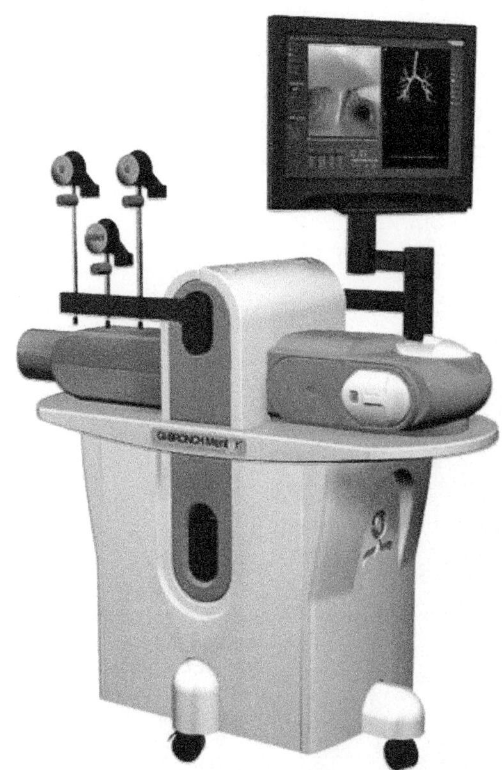

FIGURE 25-16 Virtual reality bronchoscopy simulator (GI-Bronch Mentor) includes a head and torso supine on a tabletop and a display. The head accommodates placement of a simulated bronchoscope. Images on the display are coordinated with the user's manipulation of the bronchoscope, and users are able to navigate through the bronchial airway trees of both the right and left lungs. (Courtesy Simbionix, Cleveland, OH.)

(MRA) scans from five subjects were acquired to create three-dimensional anatomic datasets and nerve models. This simulator is described as a high-fidelity simulation that can accommodate a range of input devices that include a tracking ball, a six-degrees-of-freedom mouse, a two-dimensional mouse, and customized haptic input devices.

Echocardiography Simulators

A simulation system from Blue Phantom offers a life-size mannequin head and torso that contains a nonbeating heart, ribs, lungs, liver, pericardial fluid, and major vessel structures. Using conventional ultrasound equipment, transesophageal and transthoracic images can be obtained. The heart phantom contains right and left atria and ventricles, all heart valves, and a left atrial appendage, and the mannequin accommodates drainage of pericardial fluid. When conducting a TEE, as users manipulate the probe within the esophagus (up, down, right/left rotation) and adjust the orientation of the transducer array, they are able to visualize heart structures.

Advances in computer graphics have led to the creation of a three-dimensional computer-generated virtual beating heart capable of generating TEE images (HeartWorks; Inventive Medical, London, UK). Simulation development was based on extensive characterization of cardiac structures from cadaveric hearts combined with graphic design animation to accurately reconstruct cardiac movements. The simulator consists of a head and torso mannequin, a simulated TEE probe, a display of the simulated ultrasound image, and a computer-generated model of the heart sliced open along the ultrasound beam (Fig. 25-17). As users manipulate the probe up and down or rotate it within the esophagus and manipulate the angle of the transducer array, they are able to develop images of a beating heart in a realistic manner. It was designed to be a training tool for practitioners learning how to do echocardiography, and it provides anatomically accurate ultrasound images. It also allows the user to capture all of the views recommended by the American College of Echocardiography to complete a basic exam.[52] Resolution of the virtual heart includes coronary vessel anatomy, valvular apparatus, muscle contractions, and large vessel anatomy. At present, TEE simulation technology provides models of normal cardiac function but no Doppler functionality (continuous wave, pulse wave, and color Doppler). It does not yet have a library of ultrasound images to represent pathologic states.

Dorfling and colleagues[53] have explored the integration of conventional TEE clips into high-resolution full-body simulation as part of resident training. In their technical report, they establish the feasibility of using previously recorded TEE clips that cover a range of cardiovascular states in the management of a pulmonary embolism, and they sequence the clips to match simulated hemodynamic states. The authors used a PowerPoint presentation to show the clips on an auxiliary display mounted on a cart in the simulation suite. They suggest that integrated echocardiography images during simulations of severe hemodynamic disturbances may improve resident understanding of cardiac pathophysiology that leads to unexplained perioperative hypotension.

Full-Scale Simulation

Little work has been done with complete virtual reality systems in anesthesia, although some work has been done in developing virtual reality environments for advanced cardiac lifesaving. Semeraro and colleagues[54] developed a prototype device that included the Laerdal advanced lifesaving mannequin, data gloves, and head-mounted display to increase realism of emergency cardiac scenarios. In their preliminary analysis of this technology, 39 participants managed a simulated patient who collapsed and required cardiac resuscitation in a virtual environment. They surveyed the participants regarding simulation realism, user friendliness, and educational value. A majority of participants (84%) found that the virtual reality experience achieved a high degree of realism and would be useful for health care training. They concluded that this combination was well liked by resuscitation experts and that realism was high. No studies have compared the educational value of this technology to conventional methods of teaching advanced cardiac lifesaving.

EMERGING ROLE OF SIMULATION IN ANESTHESIA

With growing interest across multiple disciplines, clinicians, educators, and researchers from all over the world

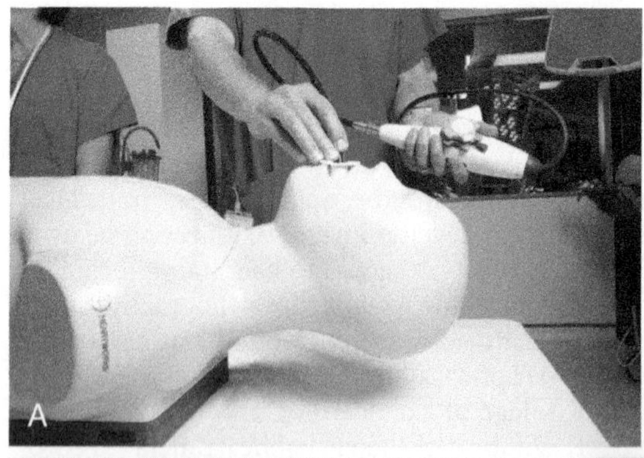

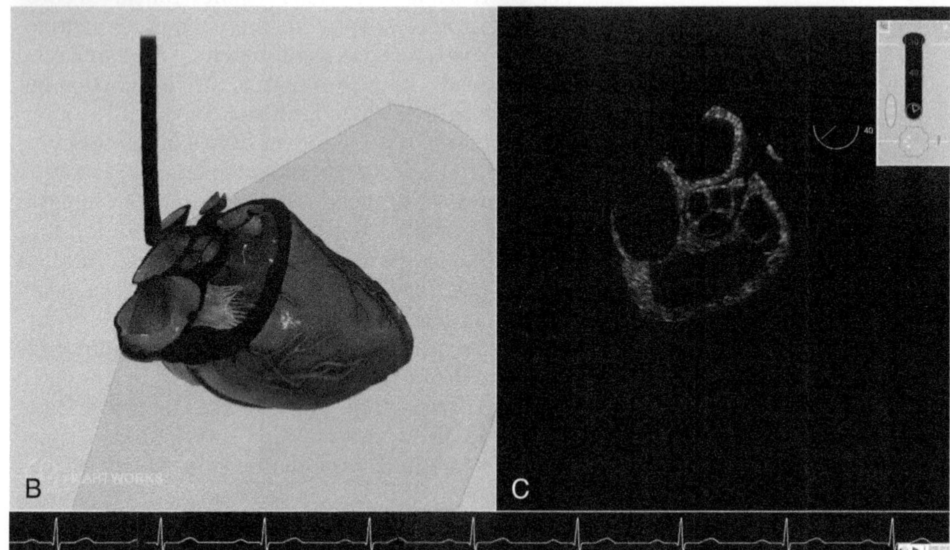

FIGURE 25-17 ■ **A,** The HeartWorks virtual reality simulator includes a head and torso and a simulated transesophageal echocardiography (TEE) probe. **B,** Users can visualize a beating heart from different views with a simulated TEE probe and display. The display provides a computer-rendered slice through the heart that shows the orientation of the ultrasound beam and animated cardiac tissues and an animated, simulated ultrasound image (**C**). (B, Courtesy HeartWorks by Inventive Medical Limited, London, UK.)

have come together to advance simulation use for training in health care. In 2003, two organizations focused on the advancement of medical simulation were formed. One was the Advanced Initiative for Medical Simulation (AIMS) and the other was the Society for Medical Simulation (SMS), which in 2006 changed its name to the Society for Simulation in Healthcare (SSH).[55]

AIMS holds an annual symposium in Washington, DC, to create a forum for federal legislators and policymakers to interact with leaders in the simulation community and to advocate for legislation to fund simulation programs.[56] SSH launched a multidisciplinary journal entitled the *Journal of Healthcare Simulation* in 2006, which recently gained citation by the National Library of Medicine. Since its inception, anesthesiologists have consistently contributed original work describing how simulation can be used to train, educate, and test anesthesia practitioners. The SSH also sponsors an annual meeting that in recent years has grown to encompass postgraduate training, workshops, training tracks, and scientific sessions with healthy contribution of abstracts from the scientific community.[56] Over the past decade, simulation in anesthesia has enjoyed increasing support from several prominent foundations that include the Anesthesia Patient Safety Foundation (APSF) and the Foundation for Anesthesia, Education, and Research. These foundations have sponsored numerous projects to explore new techniques in, and the benefits of, simulation training.

Perhaps a reflection of the increasing relevance of simulation in anesthesiology is the growing interest from agencies that certify anesthesia care providers in simulation as a means of demonstrating core skill sets. For example, the Australian and New Zealand College of Anaesthetists requires a simulation-based course entitled "Effective Management of Anaesthetic Crises" for trainees to be eligible for certification. The American Board of Anesthesiology is implementing a simulation component to their program for maintenance of certification in anesthesia, in which diplomates must complete a course in simulation training to recertify every 10 years.

As with other high-stakes professions, the use of simulation in anesthesia has followed the example of the aviation industry. With strong parallels in training individuals to acquire and process information in a time-sensitive manner, effectively communicate with others, and quickly provide solutions to avoid injury or death, simulation training in aviation has in many ways provided a road map for how simulation might be used in anesthesia. By comparison to commercial aviation, however, simulation has not enjoyed widespread acceptance among practicing anesthesia care providers.[57] Commercial pilots must submit to simulation-based evaluations on an annual basis with an interim 6-month in-flight evaluation. This level of recurring scrutiny has led to widespread consistency in the evaluation of pilot skill sets. Simulation technology in aviation has developed equipment for specific aircraft and geographic locations and unique flying conditions. Pilots are able to train on a specific aircraft simulator and then certify before piloting an actual flight. The corollaries in anesthesia are self-evident: different OR environments—interventional radiology procedure suites, cardiac catheterization laboratories, preoperative clinics—along with various anesthetic techniques that include moderate sedation, general anesthesia, and total IV anesthesia, plus a broad spectrum of patient comorbidities and surgical procedures. The reasons for poor acceptance are numerous, but some may be related to perceived or actual deficiencies in the technologies used in anesthesia-based simulations.

It has been demonstrated that fully trained anesthesiologists with years of clinical experience fail at managing critical events. In 1992, Schwid and O'Donnell[58] evaluated 10 anesthesiology residents, 10 academic anesthesiologists, and 10 private practice anesthesiologists and found that fewer than half adequately treated simulated episodes of anaphylaxis, myocardial ischemia, and cardiac arrest. Similarly, Henrichs and colleagues[59] in a recent study explored how 35 anesthesiologists and 26 certified registered nurse anesthetists responded when asked to manage eight simulated acute emergencies. Results in both groups were quite variable with only modestly higher scores in the anesthesiologist group. Practitioners in both groups failed to diagnose and treat several simulated intraoperative emergencies. The authors concluded that if their observations were reflective of clinical practice, performance in both groups was worrisome. In an accompanying editorial, Catherine McIntosh suggested that anesthesia care providers may suffer from the "Lake Wobegon effect." This comes from Garrison Keillor's radio variety show, *The Prairie Home Companion*, in which "the women are strong, the men are good looking, and the children are above average." This reflects a human tendency to overestimate achievements and capabilities relative to similar accomplishments of others. McIntosh[34] concluded that anesthesia skills in acute care "should be taught systematically, reinforced throughout clinicians' careers, and perhaps tested as a component of ongoing programs of maintenance of competency." In our opinion, this should occur more frequently than once every 10 years.

REFERENCES

1. Gaba DM: The future vision of simulation in health care, *Qual Saf Health Care* 13(Suppl 1):i2–i10, 2004.
2. McCarthy J, Cooper JB: Malpractice insurance carrier provides premium incentive for simulation-based training and believes it has made a difference, *APSF Newslett*, Spring 2007.
3. Weller J, Morris R, Watterson L, Garden A, et al: Effective management of anaesthetic crises: development and evaluation of a college-accredited simulation-based course for anaesthesia education in Australia and New Zealand, *Simul Healthc* 1:209–214, 2006.
4. *Certification and maintenance of certification*, Raleigh, 2009, American Board of Anesthesiology.
5. American College of Surgeons Committe on Trauma: *Advanced trauma life support for doctors*, ed 8, 2009, American College of Surgeons.
6. Campher D, Liu D, Brewer L, Jenkins S: *Comparison of respiratory mechanics on the METI Emergency Care Simulator and Human Patient Simulator using physiologically modeled lung volume* [abstract], Proceedings of the SimTec Health Care Simulation Conference, Melbourne, Australia, September 2009.
7. Reference deleted in proofs.
8. van Meurs WL, Good ML, Lampotang S: Functional anatomy of full-scale patient simulators, *J Clin Monit* 13:317–324, 1997.
9. Reference deleted in proofs.
10. Reference deleted in proofs.
11. Reference deleted in proofs.
12. Tooley MA, Lauder GR, Lovell AT: Abnormal drug responses with adrenaline on an educational paediatric simulator: the measurement of the responses and correction of the pharmacological model parameters, *Physiol Meas* 28:1237–1250, 2007.
13. Reference deleted in proofs.
14. Maran NJ, Glavin RJ: Low- to high-fidelity simulation: a continuum of medical education? *Med Educ* 37((Suppl 1):22–28, 2003.
15. Schwid HA: Anesthesia simulators: technology and applications, *Isr Med Assoc J* 2:949–953, 2000.
16. Practice guidelines for management of the difficult airway: an updated report by the American Society of Anesthesiologists Task Force on Management of the Difficult Airway, *Anesthesiology* 98:1269–1277, 2003.
17. Dieckmann P, Gaba D, Rall M: Deepening the theoretical foundations of patient simulation as social practice, *Simul Healthc* 2:183–193, 2007.
18. Devita MA: Society for simulation in healthcare presidential address, January 2009, *Simul Healthc* 4:43–48, 2009.
19. Rudolph JW, Simon R, Raemer DB: Which reality matters? Questions on the path to high engagement in healthcare simulation, *Simul Healthc* 2:161–163, 2007.
20. Issenberg SB: The scope of simulation-based healthcare education, *Simul Healthc* 1:203–208, 2006.

20a. American Society of Anesthesiologists: *White paper on simulation: ASA proposes approval of anesthesiology simulation programs*, 2006. Available at www.asahq.org/for-members/education-and-events/simulation-education/workgroup-correspondence-and-publications-to-asa-membership/white-paper-on-simulation-asa-proposes-approval-of-anesthesiology-simulation-programs.aspx.

21. Kimitian S, Aguilar D, Rudy S, Henry J, Sinz EH: Venous air embolism during sitting craniotomy, *Simul Healthc* 1:246–250, 2006.
22. Singh S, Sinz EH, Henry J, Murray B: Trauma and awareness, *Simul Healthc* 1:240–245, 2006.
23. Taekman JM, Hobbs E, Wright MC: Intraoperative apnea: medication error with disclosure (simulation case scenario), *Simul Healthc* 2:39–42, 2007.
24. Sposito JA, Hobbs E, Taekman J: Keep it flowing: a simulation involving defective anesthetic gas delivery equipment, *Simul Healthc* 2:241–245, 2007.
25. Morgan PJ, Tarshis J, LeBlanc V, et al: Efficacy of high-fidelity simulation debriefing on the performance of practicing anaesthetists in simulated scenarios, *Br J Anaesth* 103:531–537, 2009.
26. Rudolph JW, Simon R, Raemer DB, Eppich WJ: Debriefing as formative assessment: closing performance gaps in medical education, *Acad Emerg Med* 15:1010–1016, 2008.
27. Rudolph JW, Simon R, Rivard P, Dufresne RL, Raemer DB: Debriefing with good judgment: combining rigorous feedback with genuine inquiry, *Anesthesiol Clin* 25:361–376, 2007.
28. Savoldelli GL, Naik VN, Park J, et al: Value of debriefing during simulated crisis management: oral versus video-assisted oral feedback, *Anesthesiology* 105:279–285, 2006.
29. Blum RH, Raemer DB, Carroll JS, et al: Crisis resource management training for an anaesthesia faculty: a new approach to continuing education, *Med Educ* 38:45–55, 2004.
30. Hunt EA, Shilkofski NA, Stavroudis TA, Nelson KL: Simulation: translation to improved team performance, *Anesthesiol Clin* 25: 301–319, 2007.
31. Gaba DM, Fish KJ, Howard SK: *Crisis management in anesthesiology*, New York, 1994, Churchill Livingstone.
32. Gaba DM: Improving anesthesiologists' performance by simulating reality, *Anesthesiology* 76:491–494, 1992.
33. Mah JW, Bingham K, Dobkin ED, et al: Mannequin simulation identifies common surgical intensive care unit teamwork errors long after introduction of sepsis guidelines, *Simul Healthc* 4:193–199, 2009.
34. McIntosh CA: Lake Wobegon for anesthesia. Where everyone is above average except those who aren't: variability in the management of simulated intraoperative critical incidents, *Anesth Analg* 108:6–9, 2009.

35. Domuracki KJ, Moule CJ, Owen H, Kostandoff G, Plummer JL: Learning on a simulator does transfer to clinical practice, *Resuscitation* 80:346–349, 2009.
36. Batchelder AJ, Steel A, Mackenzie R, et al: Simulation as a tool to improve the safety of pre-hospital anaesthesia: a pilot study, *Anaesthesia* 64:978–983, 2009.
37. Lampotang S: Computer and web-enabled simulations for anesthesiology training and credentialing, *J Crit Care* 23:173–178, 2008.
38. Tan GM, Ti LK, Tan K, Lee T: A comparison of screen-based simulation and conventional lectures for undergraduate teaching of crisis management, *Anaesth Intensive Care* 36:565–569, 2008.
39. Garfield JM, Paskin S, Philip JH: An evaluation of the effectiveness of a computer simulation of anaesthetic uptake and distribution as a teaching tool, *Med Educ* 23:457–462, 1989.
40. Philip JH: Gas Man: an example of goal oriented computer-assisted teaching which results in learning, *Int J Clin Monit Comput* 3:165–173, 1986.
41. Bouillon TW, Bruhn J, Radulescu L, et al: Pharmacodynamic interaction between propofol and remifentanil regarding hypnosis, tolerance of laryngoscopy, bispectral index, and electroencephalographic approximate entropy, *Anesthesiology* 100:1353–1372, 2004.
42. Johnson KB, Syroid ND, Gupta DK, et al: An evaluation of remifentanil propofol response surfaces for loss of responsiveness, loss of response to surrogates of painful stimuli and laryngoscopy in patients undergoing elective surgery, *Anesth Analg* 106:471–479, 2008, table of contents.
43. Manyam SC, Gupta DK, Johnson KB, et al: Opioid-volatile anesthetic synergy: a response surface model with remifentanil and sevoflurane as prototypes, *Anesthesiology* 105:267–278, 2006.
44. Schumacher PM, Dossche J, Mortier EP, et al: Response surface modeling of the interaction between propofol and sevoflurane, *Anesthesiology* 111(4):790–804, 2009.
45. Johnson KB: Bringing advanced clinical pharmacology to the operating room: innovations in real-time visualization of the effects of anesthetic drugs, *Anesthesiology News* 26–27, July 2009.
46. Goldmann K, Steinfeldt T: Acquisition of basic fiberoptic intubation skills with a virtual reality airway simulator, *J Clin Anesth* 18:173–178, 2006.
47. Rowe R, Cohen RA: An evaluation of a virtual reality airway simulator, *Anesth Analg* 95:62–66, 2002.
48. Chandra DB, Savoldelli GL, Joo HS, Weiss ID, Naik VN: Fiberoptic oral intubation: the effect of model fidelity on training for transfer to patient care, *Anesthesiology* 109:1007–1013, 2008.
49. Martin DP, Blezek DJ, Robb RA: Simulating lower extremity nerve blocks with virtual reality, *Tech Reg Anesth Pain Manag* 3:58–61,1999.
50. Ackerman MJ: The Visible Human Project: a resource for anatomical visualization, *Stud Health Technol Inform* 52 Pt(2):1030–1032, 1998.
51. Grottke O, Ntouba A, Ullrich S, et al: Virtual reality-based simulator for training in regional anaesthesia, *Br J Anaesth* 103:594–600, 2009.
52. Shanewise JS, Cheung AT, Aronson S, et al: ASE/SCA guidelines for performing a comprehensive intraoperative multiplane transesophageal echocardiography examination: recommendations of the American Society of Echocardiography Council for Intraoperative Echocardiography and the Society of Cardiovascular Anesthesiologists Task Force for Certification in Perioperative Transesophageal Echocardiography, *Anesth Analg* 89:870–884, 1999.
53. Dorfling J, Hatton KW, Hassan ZU: Integrating echocardiography into human patient simulator training of anesthesiology residents using a severe pulmonary embolism scenario, *Simul Healthc* 1:79–83, 2006.
54. Semeraro F, Frisoli A, Bergamasco M, Cerchiari EL: Virtual reality enhanced mannequin (VREM) that is well received by resuscitation experts, *Resuscitation* 80:489–492, 2009.
55. Dawson S, Alverson D, Bowyer M, Eder-Van Hook J, Waters RJ: The complementary roles of the advanced initiative in medical simulation and the society for simulation in healthcare, *Simul Healthc* 2:30–32, 2007.
56. Gaba DM, Raemer D: The tide is turning: organizational structures to embed simulation in the fabric of healthcare, *Simul Healthc* 2:1–3, 2007.
57. Gaba DM: Out of this nettle, danger, we pluck this flower, safety: healthcare vs. aviation and other high-hazard industries, *Simul Healthc* 2:213–217, 2007.
58. Schwid HA, O'Donnell D: Anesthesiologists' management of simulated critical incidents, *Anesthesiology* 76:495–501, 1992.
59. Henrichs BM, Avidan MS, Murray DJ, et al: Performance of certified registered nurse anesthetists and anesthesiologists in a simulation-based skills assessment, *Anesth Analg* 108:255–262, 2009.
60. Blum RH, Raemer DB, Carroll JS, Dufresne RL, Cooper JB: A method for measuring the effectiveness of simulation-based team training for improving communication skills, *Anesth Analg* 100:1375–1380, 2005.
61. Boulet JR, Murray D, Kras J, et al: Reliability and validity of a simulation-based acute care skills assessment for medical students and residents, *Anesthesiology* 99:1270–1280, 2003.

PART VI

SPECIAL CONDITIONS

CHAPTER 26

CLOSED-CIRCUIT ANESTHESIA

James H. Philip

CHAPTER OUTLINE

PRINCIPLES

Introduction

The basic principle of closed-circuit anesthesia is maintenance of a constant anesthetic state by adding gases and vapors to the breathing circuit at the same rate that the patient's body removes those same substances. Often, the desired anesthetic state is first established using a high fresh gas flow (FGF) composed of gases, such as oxygen and nitrous oxide or air, and vapors (e.g., isoflurane, sevoflurane, desflurane). Once a steady state is attained, inspired and end-expired gas concentrations or tensions are noted, and FGF is reduced. Throughout this chapter, the words *tension* and *partial pressure* are used interchangeably. For gases, they have the same value as concentration. This is discussed under the section Partial Pressure. The circuit and patient gas tensions are maintained constant by adding oxygen, nitrous oxide, and agent vapor to the breathing circuit. In one common approach to closed-circuit maintenance, the amount of gas and vapor administered is determined empirically by titration. Several different titration endpoints can be used. Choices include maintenance of inspired tension, expired tension, and/or estimated anesthetic depth. When titrating against a defined endpoint, drugs can be added in a measured or quantified manner, or they can be added empirically without regard to the total amount administered. In closed-circuit anesthesia techniques, carbon dioxide is removed from exhaled gas, and the remaining exhaled gases and vapors are added to the FGF to produce inhaled gas. One advantage of this technique is that all gases exhaled are already warmed and humidified by the patient and are therefore well suited for rebreathing.[1] Another advantage is that oxygen consumption is monitored by titration. A final advantage is that cost is reduced dramatically.

In closed-circuit and low-flow anesthesia, inhaled gas is formed from two sources, and exhaled gas forms most of what the patient will breathe. In addition to exhaled gas, fresh gas is added in the correct quantity and composition to achieve the inspired gas tensions desired. The same inspired and expired gas tensions are established with a closed circuit as with a semiclosed or open (nonrebreathing) circuit. In this chapter the terms *open circuit* and *nonrebreathing circuit* are used interchangeably.

Closed-Circuit Anesthesia

Closed-circuit anesthesia can be viewed in several different ways. From one perspective, it is an anesthetic technique unlike all others. The classical closed-circuit literature describes theory and practice different from other techniques. In the classic closed-circuit approach, once a stable level of anesthesia is established with high-flow oxygen, nitrous oxide, and volatile agent, FGF is reduced to the patient's predicted oxygen consumption (243 mL/min for a 70-kg adult), predicted nitrous oxide uptake rate (approximately 100 mL/min after the first 30 min), and predicted inhaled agent uptake. Nitrous oxide and agent uptake rates are calculated according to a mathematical formula based on body weight.[2]

The traditional closed-circuit anesthesia literature uses anesthetic liquid injection or infusion rather than a vaporizer. Liquid agent is administered to the breathing circuit according to a prescribed time regimen.[3-5] Specifically, the drug administration rate is inversely proportional to the square root of time (t):

$$\text{Administration rate} = \text{Uptake} \propto Kt^{-0.5}$$

This empiric relationship was first noted by Severinghaus[6] for nitrous oxide in 1954 and was popularized by Lowe[5] beginning in 1972. Severinghaus's original data demonstrated that nitrous oxide uptake followed this power/function relationship fairly closely in the subjects he studied. Connor and Philip recently revalidated this mathematical relationship numerically[7] and analytically.[8]

A scientific explanation exists for this curious and unexpected relationship. It has long been known that body tissues perfused with blood of a constant drug concentration or vapor tension have an uptake rate that decreases with time. Specifically, theory and research[9] have demonstrated that uptake into each tissue takes the form of an exponential:

$$\text{Uptake} = K \times e^{-t/\tau}$$

where t is time and τ is the *time constant*, or the time required to achieve 63% of the final value in response to a step input; e is the base of natural logarithms (2.7183 and so on), and K is a predictable constant. It can easily be derived that

$$\tau = 0.69 \times t_{1/2}$$

and

$$t_{1/2} = 1.44\,\tau$$

where $t_{1/2}$ equals the time required to achieve half the final value in response to a step input.

Total body uptake is the sum of the individual uptakes by each tissue. In this case, uptake is the sum of a group of exponentials of different amplitudes (K_{tissue}) and time constants (τ_{tissue}). The sum of these exponentials is approximately equal to the power function, $K \times t^{-0.5}$. It must be emphasized that the exponential relationship for a single tissue is derived theoretically and can be demonstrated empirically. But the power/function relationship is an empiric one that approximates the multiple exponential functions that describe the uptake into diverse tissues.[7,8]

Partial Pressure, Tension, and Concentration

Throughout this chapter, the words *tension* and *partial pressure* are used interchangeably. This physical variable represents the effective pressure exerted by a gas, whether it is in the gas phase alone, in combination with another gas, or dissolved in blood or tissue.

Partial pressure is expressed in percent of 1 atmosphere (1 atm = 760 mm Hg). Expressing partial pressure this way serves several purposes. When partial pressure is expressed as percent of 1 atm, partial pressure and concentration have the same numeric value for gases. For example, 1 vol% isoflurane has an isoflurane tension of 1% of 1 atm, an expression often shortened to 1%. For blood and tissues, partial pressure is also expressed as a percent. By this definition, a tissue anesthetic measure of 1% does not represent 1% concentration; rather, it represents a partial pressure of 1% of 1 atm or 1% times 760 mm Hg, or 7.6 mm Hg in terms of absolute pressure.

Next, when partial pressure is expressed as a percent of one *standard* atmosphere (i.e., 760 mm Hg), the numbers and concepts work equally well at any atmospheric pressure. This is because the physiologic effects of inhaled anesthetics are the result of partial pressure and not concentration.[7,8] Thus, anesthetic tensions in the apparatus and patient are the variables that best explain kinetics in an understandable way.

When anesthetics are present in liquid or tissue, their concentrations are equal to their partial pressure × tissue/gas solubility × atmospheric pressure, according to Henry's law. According to Dalton's law, for multiple gases, this applies to each as if it were alone.

It is believed that the blood leaving each tissue compartment is in equilibrium with the tissues in that compartment, therefore the partial pressure in venous blood is equal to that in the tissues, as Graham's law states. The blood entering each compartment has the same partial pressure of all gases as the arterial blood has everywhere. In the absence of lung shunt, arterial partial pressure equals alveolar partial pressure. Clinicians measure end-tidal (ET) gas concentrations or partial pressures. End-tidal partial pressure equals alveolar partial pressure when there is no physiologic dead space. After an infinite amount of time, the partial pressure of anesthetic inspired gas, alveolar gas, arterial blood, all tissues, and all venous blood, including mixed venous blood, is equal. At this time, there is no blood uptake of anesthetic at all. Thus the inspired and expired partial pressures are equal as well. Thus, after an infinite amount of time, the partial pressure of anesthetic throughout the system, from vaporizer to all tissues, is the same.

The above paragraph is a simplification that serves well in most situations. Exploring this further, in the presence of lung shunt, arterial tension is closer to mixed venous tension than it would be otherwise. When physiologic dead space is present, some of the gas leaving the lungs is inspired gas, rather than alveolar gas. This makes end-tidal partial pressure closer to inspired partial pressure than it would otherwise be. These are temporary limitations. After an infinite amount of time, these effects disappear as well, and anesthetic tension is equal everywhere. Because the alive body continues to consume oxygen and produce carbon dioxide, this equalization does not occur with these gases.

Lowe Technique

In the classic Lowe[2] technique for closed-circuit anesthesia, a loading dose of anesthetic vapor is administered to the breathing circuit to bring circuit tension to that desired in the patient's alveoli. This level is somewhat higher than in the inspired gas. A unit dose for maintenance is then selected according to the patient's body weight and is proportional to body mass to the three-quarter power ($kg^{3/4}$), a relationship first shown by Kleiber[10] that has been further described by Brody.[11] Kleiber's law goes on to state that many parameters of metabolic and circulatory processes—oxygen consumption, carbon dioxide production, cardiac output, and daily liquid requirement—are proportional to body mass raised to the three-quarter power.

In Lowe's classic closed-circuit anesthesia, unit doses are administered at specific times with intervals between administrations increasing with time. These intervals, in minutes, are the sequence of odd integers {1, 3, 5, 7, 9, ...} This results in injections being made at 0, 1, 4, 9, 16, and 25 minutes. This is referred to as the *square root of time model*, in that these injection times are the series of numbers whose square roots are sequential integers. This strange number manipulation may seem farfetched; however, Connor and Philip[7,8] demonstrated that this relationship approximated the uptake of nitrous oxide shown by Severinghaus[6] with remarkable accuracy.

Even closed-circuit enthusiasts advise care and careful observation of the patient, as always. Lowe recommended that after 25 minutes, the square root of time method should be modified, and that the intervals between injections should not be lengthened as much (Lowe, personal communication, 1979). This is because after 25 minutes of anesthetic at constant depth, the rate of uptake becomes almost constant. By this time, fast (vessel-rich) tissues have equilibrated with arterial blood. Meanwhile, uptake into muscle and fat are diminishing slowly, more slowly than the square root of time, because of their long time constants.

It must be noted that the original 1972 theory and "cookbook" for closed-circuit anesthesia was written during the era of more primitive measurement and analysis (in 1972, the digital pocket calculator had not yet replaced the analog slide rule). Anesthetic agent analysis was uncommon, and the only clinically available device was the Dräger Narkotest (Dräger Medical, Telford, PA), which consisted of a slowly responding silicone rubber band in a box connected to a mechanical indicator.[12] The "rubber band in a box" stretched in proportion to the potency of the single or combined inhalation anesthetic tensions administered.

With each administration technique—open circuit, semiclosed circuit with high flow, semiclosed circuit with low flow, closed circuit with vaporizer, and closed circuit with liquid injection—each patient's inspired, end-expired, and alveolar anesthetic tensions are the same and are independent of administration technique. Thus from the patient's viewpoint, all inhalation anesthetic administration techniques are equivalent. The only difference is in the way the drugs are administered and the resulting waste or lack thereof.

Although the conventional closed-circuit literature used models created by fitting experimental data to particular mathematical formulations, this chapter does not rely on these. Rather it assumes that an anesthetic agent monitor is available and in use, measuring inspired and expired anesthetic concentrations. The dosage administration scheme is adjusted on the basis of a patient's measured and needed levels of inspired and expired vapor and nitrous oxide. Delivered oxygen flow is adjusted similarly. In the absence of a multigas monitor, closed-circuit anesthesia may still be employed, but greater vigilance and understanding of anesthetic depth and uptake of anesthetic and oxygen are required.

ANESTHESIA ADMINISTRATION AND MONITORING

Limitations and Solutions

Truly closed-circuit anesthesia cannot always be performed because of technical limitations of our gas delivery systems or gas monitors. In the 1980s, gas monitoring was often performed with a multiplexed mass spectrometer shared by 16 or 31 ORs, monitoring these rooms in succession. In that situation, sampled gas could not be returned to the patient from whom it was sampled. With the advent and commonality of stand-alone or integrated gas monitors with anesthesia delivery systems, there should be no such impediment. However, sampled gas return requires specific approval and is not available with anesthesia gas monitors by GE Healthcare (Waukesha, WI).

In 1963, Eger[13] introduced the concept of anesthesia at constant alveolar concentration and defined the term *minimum alveolar concentration* (MAC). As a foundation for his approach, he used the pharmacokinetic theory explained by Seymour Kety[14,15] in 1950. Eger showed that constant alveolar concentration or tension can be produced and maintained when inspired anesthetic concentration is adjusted properly. To compute the proper adjustment sequence, or continuum, he calculated anesthetic uptake into each organ group and adjusted inspired concentration to maintain alveolar concentration constant. Figure 26-1 shows the inspired concentration required to maintain 0.8% alveolar halothane, equal to 1 MAC.[13] Inspired halothane concentration is begun at 3.3% and is slowly and continuously reduced to 2% at 5 minutes, 1.5% at 20 minutes, and 1% at 3 hours.

A more realistic clinical endpoint is constant or desired anesthetic tension in the site of interest, the target organ, the brain, and the spinal cord. Producing a stepped or controlled change in brain anesthetic tension from its current level to any desired level is a useful clinical objective. This is equally true for high-flow, low-flow, and closed-circuit anesthesia.

Anesthesia Assessment and Adjustment

To the clinician who has used halothane, Eger's calculated time course of halothane administration is quite reasonable. It mimics what was administered to many patients. Of course, in today's clinical practice, the vaporizer is not adjusted according to the clock. Rather, the patient's depth of anesthesia is assessed by mental integration of many signs. The pupils are observed for dilation or constriction; and blood pressure, heart rate, and possibly processed electroencephalogram (EEG; e.g., bispectral

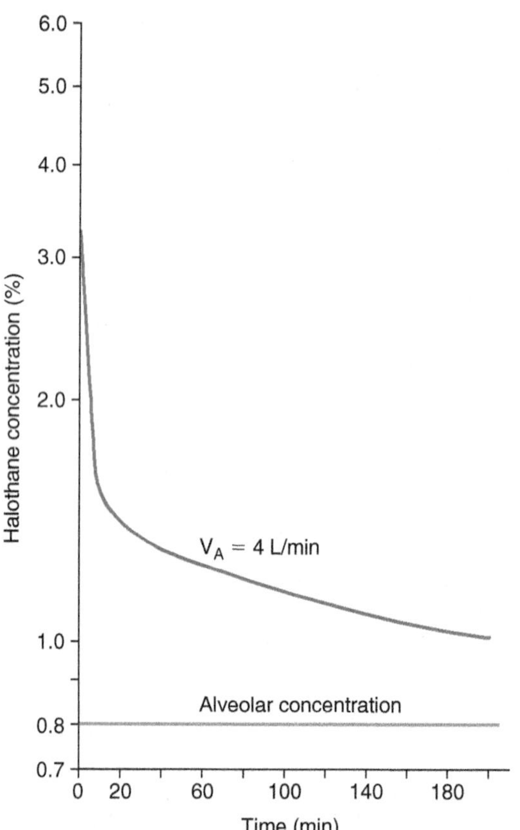

FIGURE 26-1 Inspired concentration required to maintain 0.8% alveolar halothane. Halothane inspired concentration begins at 3.3% and is slowly and continuously decreased to 2% at 5 minutes, 1.5% at 20 minutes, and 1% at 3 hours. V_A, alveolar ventilation. (From Eger EI II, Guadagni NP: Halothane uptake in man at constant alveolar concentration. *Anesthesiology* 1963; 24:299-304.)

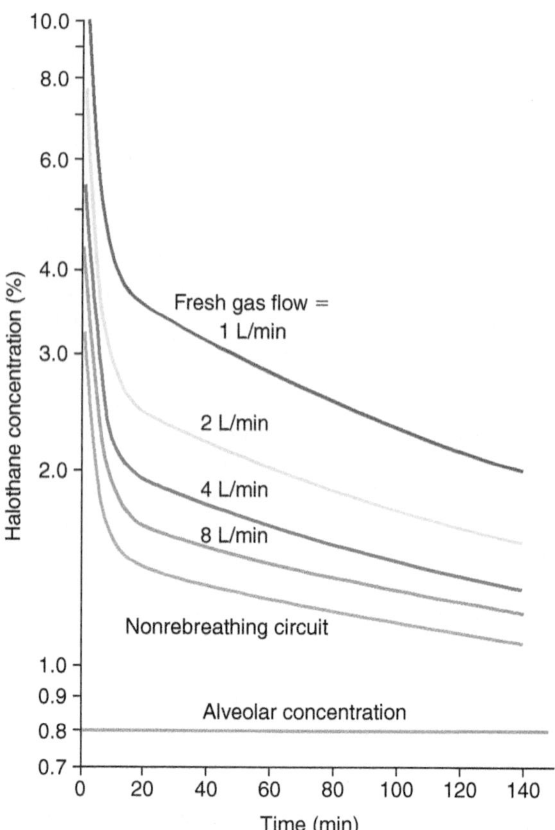

FIGURE 26-2 Semiclosed circuit vaporizer settings required for constant alveolar tension of 0.8% halothane at various fresh gas flows as calculated by Eger. (From Eger EI II, Guadagni NP: Halothane uptake in man at constant alveolar concentration. *Anesthesiology* 1963; 24:299-304.)

index, patient state index, entropy) and other variables are measured and evaluated. With the convenient availability of anesthetic agent monitors, most clinicians monitor expired anesthetic concentration (tension) as an important additional sign. This represents the anesthetic level in the end-expired gas as an approximation to that in the alveoli as an approximation to that in the blood. In the best of all situations, where end-tidal equals alveolar and arterial tension, the brain delay is still 3 to 5 minutes. This means that the measured end-tidal value predicts what the brain concentration will be in the near future. Likewise, view of the end-tidal value a few minutes previous is a real-time indicator of the brain and spinal cord values.

To achieve the "ideal" anesthetic, vaporizer setting and FGF are adjusted to maintain constant brain anesthetic tension. This is done by allowing a reasonable amount of alveolar overpressure during the period when anesthesia is being deepened (described later in this chapter). Finally, an estimate or measure of depth of anesthesia can be used.

High and Low Flows

Semiclosed Circuit Anesthesia

Eger's example (see Fig. 26-1) demonstrates anesthesia administration with a perfect nonrebreathing circuit (open circuit). In that system, inspired concentration is perfectly controlled. In contrast, a *semiclosed* breathing circuit with a carbon dioxide absorber is the one most commonly used around the world. With this circuit, inspired concentration or tension is dependent on FGF and vaporizer setting as well as by exhaled ventilatory flow and exhaled agent tension.

Figure 26-2 shows the semiclosed circuit vaporizer settings required for constant alveolar tension of 0.8% halothane at various FGFs as calculated by Eger.[13] As FGF into the semiclosed circuit is progressively decreased from 8 L/min to 1 L/min, vaporizer setting, and hence tension delivered to the breathing circuit, must be increased. This again is because inspired gas is a mixture of fresh gas from the anesthesia machine and gas exhaled from the patient. As FGF is decreased, a relatively higher fraction of exhaled gas is rebreathed. Because exhaled gas usually has a lower anesthetic tension than inspired gas, higher vaporizer settings are required to achieve the same inspired tension.

Note that at 1 L/min of FGF, the initial halothane vaporizer setting is more than 10%. This is difficult, if not impossible, to achieve with modern anesthesia delivery systems, because the vaporizer cannot deliver that high a concentration. It must be emphasized that the high concentration of anesthetic is delivered *to the breathing circuit,* where it mixes with the 0.8% in the patient's exhaled gas to produce an inspired concentration that

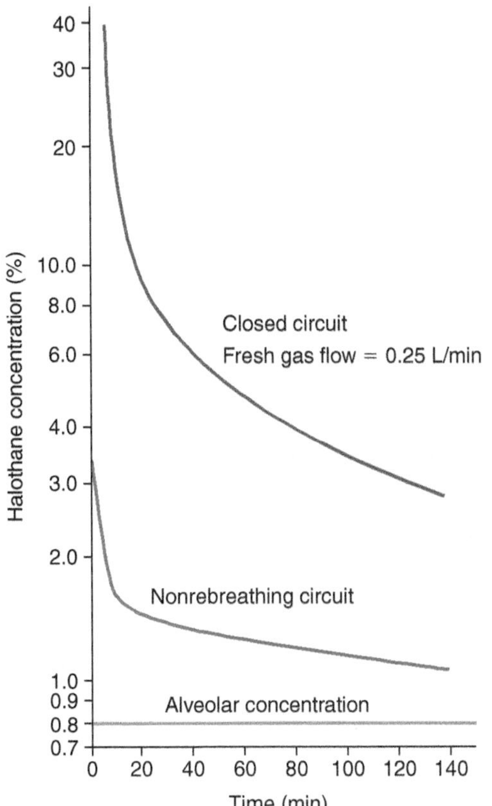

FIGURE 26-3 Vaporizer settings required to maintain constant alveolar tension of halothane for a nonrebreathing (open) circuit and a completely closed circuit with a fresh gas flow of 0.25 L/min.

must be the same 3.3% as was required in an open circuit. In the two cases, the time course of anesthesia induction is identical, because inspired anesthetic concentration is the same. The patient's body is not aware of how the anesthesiologist created the gas mixture breathed.

Nonrebreathing (Open-Circuit) and Closed-Circuit Anesthesia

Figure 26-3 shows vaporizer settings required to maintain constant alveolar tension for a nonrebreathing circuit (open circuit) and a completely closed circuit with an FGF of 0.25 L/min. With the closed circuit, the initial vaporizer setting is 40% halothane. In practice, this is impossible for several reasons. First, modern concentration-calibrated vaporizers can be set to administer no more than 5% halothane. Second, the vapor pressure of halothane at room temperature is only 0.33 atm (33%, or 243 mm Hg), thus 40% halothane cannot exist under these conditions. Nonetheless, 40% is the theoretical concentration required. This high concentration at the low FGF of 250 mL/min into a closed circuit produces the same 3.3% inspired concentration that will achieve the same 1 MAC (0.8% end-expired) anesthetic.

Liquid Injection Anesthesia

As discussed, 1 MAC anesthesia can be attained and maintained with a wide range of FGFs and required high-range of vaporizer settings. It also can be approximated with sequential injections of anesthetic liquid into the breathing circuit. In closed-circuit liquid injection anesthesia, the same inspired and expired tensions are desired. Because the liquid injection is in multiple boluses, the time course of inspired and expired tension is not as smooth. However, the brain's 3 minute time constant tends to provide constant anesthetic depth even with sequential liquid injections. The advantage of liquid injection is that the concentration limitation of the vaporizer can be overcome.

Some closed-circuit enthusiasts choose to inject liquid anesthetic into the breathing circuit with a syringe pump. For this technique to work, the same overall administration rate must be maintained as with closed-circuit liquid bolus injection. The earlier-described square-root-of-time model is still used, but the injection rate is adjusted to administer unit doses over successively longer time periods.

MODEL-ASSISTED UNDERSTANDING OF CLOSED-CIRCUIT ANESTHESIA

Gas Man (Med Man Simulations, Chestnut Hill, MA) is an educational computer program (www.gasmanweb.com/index.html)[16] designed to teach the pharmacokinetics of inhalation anesthetics. It has been shown to be an effective educational tool[17] and has been used to demonstrate various aspects of inhaled agent kinetics[18] and has been shown to be accurate.[19] Various models have been previously described to explain uptake and distribution,[20-23] and other programs are also available.[24]

The Gas Man picture represents the inhalation kinetics uptake and distribution models in schematic form and provides a static snapshot of the anesthetic tensions in body tissues (compartments). The Gas Man graph shows the time course of anesthetic tension in each compartment.

Figure 26-4 shows an annotated Gas Man picture (*top*) and Gas Man graph (*bottom*), which represent the time course and current state of the patient and breathing circuit after 15 minutes; here, it is at the end of 5% isoflurane anesthesia. The picture shows anesthetic tension in various locations of interest as well as flows that conduct drugs from compartment to compartment. Compartments are filled to heights that represent their respective partial pressures. In the equilibrium state, all compartments would become filled to the same height, because their partial pressures are equal.

In the graph of Figure 26-4 (*bottom*) it is apparent that tissues in the vessel-rich group rapidly equilibrate with and almost equal arterial anesthetic tension. Muscle and fat equilibrate more slowly. The anesthetic tension in mixed venous blood returning to the heart is dominated by blood coming from the vessel-rich group, which receives and returns 75% of the cardiac output. Muscle receives 20% and fat receives 5% of cardiac output, respectively. Anesthetic returning to the patient's alveoli is then either exhaled to the breathing circuit or recirculated to arterial blood according to the relationship between alveolar ventilation and cardiac output. Although this simple description of the Gas Man oversimplifies the situation, it is sufficient to explain both

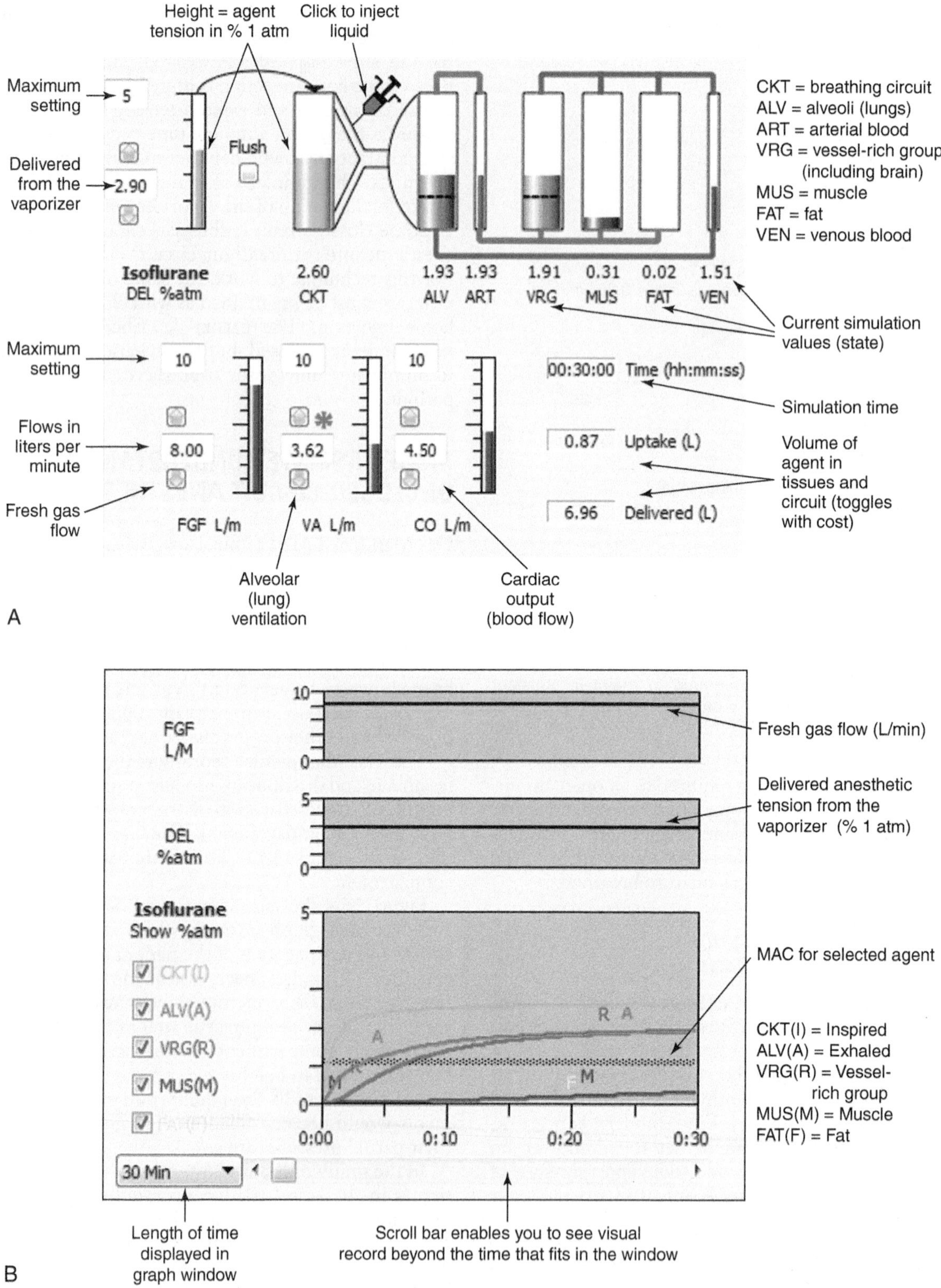

FIGURE 26-4 ■ Annotated Gas Man picture and graph (Med Man Simulations, Chestnut Hill, MA). **A,** The picture shows the current state; compartments are filled to heights that represent their respective partial pressures. **B,** Annotated graph shows the 30-minute time course of anesthesia. *MAC*, minimum alveolar concentration.

qualitative and quantitative aspects of inhalation anesthesia.

In addition to displaying the flow between compartments, Figure 26-4, *B*, provides additional information about simulation time, patient uptake of anesthetic, and quantity of anesthetic delivered to the breathing circuit. At the end of 15 simulated minutes, anesthetic uptake is 0.9 L isoflurane vapor, and volume delivered to the breathing circuit is 6.0 L. The difference between these two values, 5.1 L, is the volume discarded from the breathing circuit through the exhaust valve during the 15 minutes of anesthetic administration plus that which remains in the circuit. *Efficiency* is defined as the ratio of uptake to delivered quantities, expressed as a percent. Here, efficiency equals 0.9 L uptake divided by 6.0 L delivered, which equals 0.15, or 15%. It should be noted that 5.1 L (85%) of the nitrous oxide–oxygen–isoflurane mixture is discarded. This gas is collected by the waste anesthetic gas system in the OR, conducted to the hospital chimney, and released to the atmosphere.

The above example shows how the Gas Man screens can be interpreted. Furthermore, it shows the breathing circuit response to a constant vaporizer setting and a high FGF. This administration technique mimics what is clinically achieved when an attempt is made to provide constant inspired tension using a semiclosed circle system at high FGFs. Anesthesia, however, is not normally administered with a constant vaporizer setting or constant inspired tension. Rather, the trained clinician attempts to maintain anesthesia depth appropriate for surgical conditions by adjusting the vaporizer settings. This is done by observing the response of the patient's clinical signs and by interpreting whatever quantitative measurements are available. Although blood pressure and EEG measures and the like may be useful, there is at present no reliable quantified measure of anesthesia depth.

In an attempt to maintain constant anesthesia depth, constant anesthetic tension in the alveoli is a reasonable objective, and end-expired anesthetic tension or concentration is a good measure of alveolar tension.[13,25] The specific measurable objective in administering anesthesia with constant depth then is to maintain a constant end-expired anesthetic tension; this is now a quantifiable and achievable objective, accomplished by adjusting the vaporizer in whatever manner is required while observing the anesthetic agent monitor that displays inspired and end-expired anesthetic tensions.

CONTINUUM FROM HIGH-FLOW TO LOW-FLOW ANESTHESIA

The continuum from high-flow to low-flow anesthesia can also be well explained by the Gas Man model and simulation. Figure 26-5 shows the picture and graph representing constant alveolar tension for halothane administered with an open (nonrebreathing) circuit for 15 minutes. The inspired (equal to delivered for the open circuit) halothane tension is initially set to 3.3% and then gradually reduced to produce a flat alveolar tension curve. When this is done carefully, the time course of vaporizer setting and expired anesthetic tension or concentration is indistinguishable from that seen in Eger's example (Fig. 26-1).

Notice that in the Gas Man picture, after 15 minutes of anesthesia, the cumulative patient uptake of anesthetic is 0.6 L of halothane vapor. The volume of halothane delivered to the breathing circuit is 2.7 L, computed as if the FGF were 10 L/min. Also, the upper half of the Gas Man graph shows alveolar ventilation and cardiac output; delivered tension and FGF are not relevant to an open circuit. Delivered tension and FGF are displayed in this location when a semiclosed or closed system technique is simulated.

Figure 26-6 shows the picture and graph of isoflurane administered at constant alveolar isoflurane tension (1 MAC = 1.1%) achieved and maintained by appropriate vaporizer adjustment in a nonrebreathing (open) circuit. Initial inspired isoflurane tension is 2.9%, tapered to 1.5% after 15 minutes.

It was noted earlier that alveolar overpressure—that is, alveolar tension transiently above 1.0 MAC—is sometimes used to produce a more rapid increase in anesthetic tension in the vessel-rich tissue group (VRG), which includes the brain, spinal cord, and other fast organs (kidneys, liver, spleen). The VRG includes the target organ,

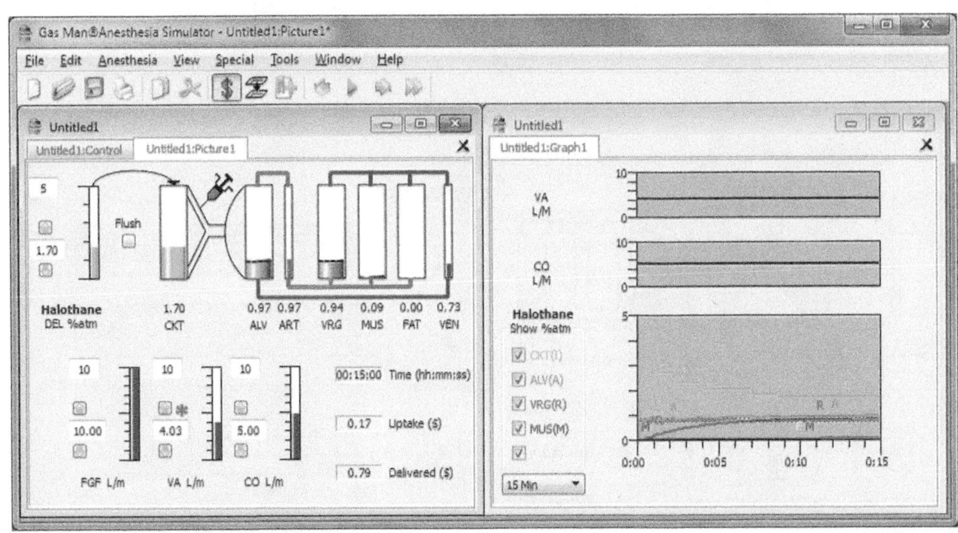

FIGURE 26-5 ■ Open-circuit constant alveolar halothane anesthetic. The Gas Man picture and graph (Med Man Simulations, Chestnut Hill, MA) show constant alveolar tension achieved and maintained with an open (nonrebreathing) circuit and careful adjustment of the vaporizer setting.

the patient's brain and spinal cord; this anesthetic tension is termed *VRG*. Only a brief period of overpressure is required, because VRG rapidly equalizes with arterial tension, which should by this time have fallen to the desired level. A common target for anesthesia in the brain is 1 MAC; another is 1.3 MAC.

Figure 26-7 shows the picture and graph of isoflurane administered at constant VRG isoflurane tension (1 MAC = 1.1%) achieved and maintained by appropriate vaporizer adjustment in a nonrebreathing (open) circuit. Initial inspired isoflurane tension is 5.0%, tapered to 1.5% after 15 minutes. Alveolar tension rises to about 2 MAC for about 2 minutes.

Figure 26-8 shows the picture and graph depicting constant brain isoflurane tension (1 MAC = 1.1%) achieved in a semiclosed circuit with an FGF of 10 L/min.

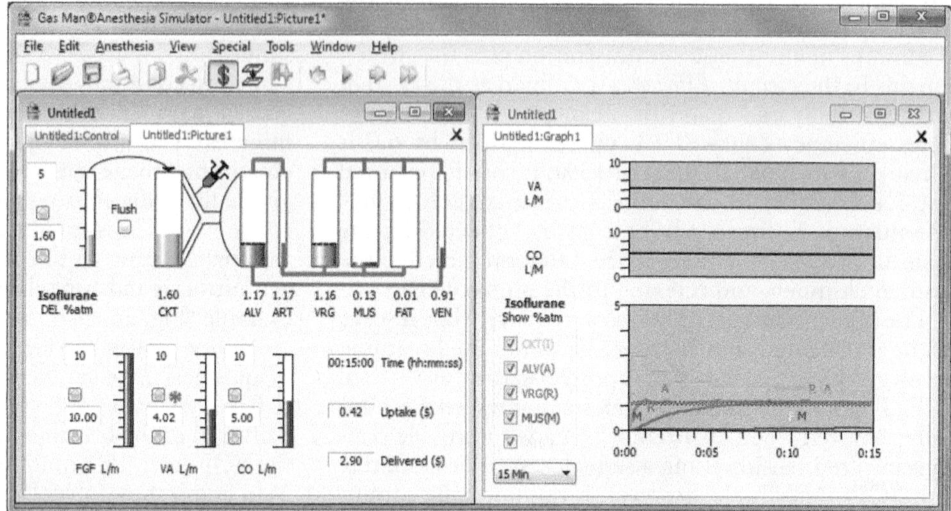

FIGURE 26-6 ■ Isoflurane open-circuit constant alveolar anesthetic tension. The Gas Man picture and graph (Med Man Simulations, Chestnut Hill, MA) show constant alveolar isoflurane tension achieved and maintained with an open (nonrebreathing) circuit and careful vaporizer adjustment. Note the relative similarity to the halothane open-circuit curve in Figure 26-5.

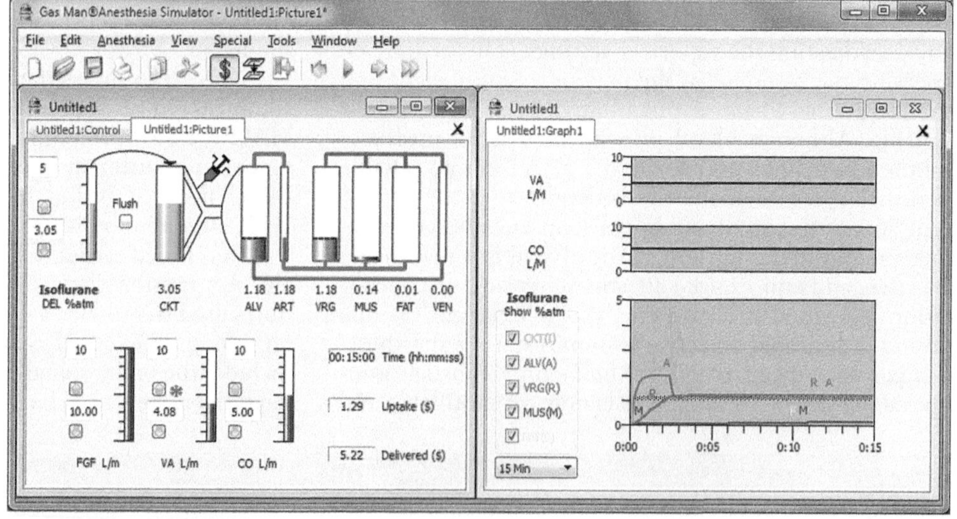

FIGURE 26-7 ■ Constant brain anesthetic tension achieved with an open circuit administering isoflurane. The Gas Man picture and graph (Med Man Simulations, Chestnut Hill, MA) show constant brain tension achieved and maintained with an open (nonrebreathing) circuit and careful vaporizer adjustment.

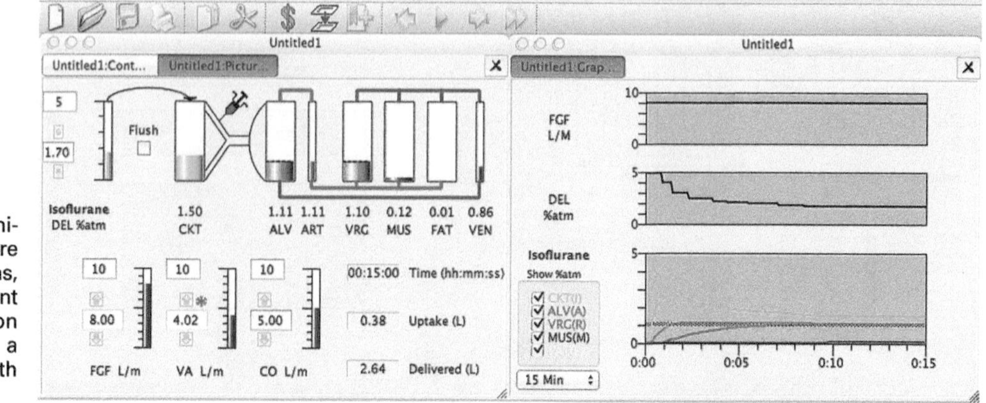

FIGURE 26-8 ■ High-flow semiclosed circuit. Gas Man picture and graph (Med Man Simulations, Chestnut Hill, MA) of constant alveolar isoflurane tension achieved and maintained with a high-flow semiclosed circuit with a fresh gas flow of 8 L/min.

The anesthetic tension delivered to the breathing circuit (DEL) begins at 5% isoflurane and is reduced to achieve and maintain a constant VRG tension of 1.1%. Just as with the open circuit, it is observed that inspired tension (I) begins at 2.9% and is reduced to approximately 1.5% at the end of 15 minutes. Alveolar tension rises to about 1.6% for about 3 minutes. Constant VRG tension is achieved with 3.3 L of vapor delivered to the breathing circuit, and the patient's tissue uptake is 0.4 L of vapor. The efficiency is thus about 12% (efficiency = 0.4 L uptake/3.3 L delivered, or 12.1%) Hence, in the common high-flow clinical situation, more than 80% of the anesthetic agent delivered to the breathing circuit is wasted.

Figure 26-9 shows a trend graph of airway anesthetic tension obtained during a high-flow induction with isoflurane, measured with an infrared agent analyzer. Inspired and end-tidal isoflurane tensions are represented by the upper and lower edges of the graph. The isoflurane vaporizer is set to 3%, 2.5%, and 2.2% at 0, 1, and 2 minutes, respectively. Note that constant alveolar anesthetic tension is achieved and maintained after the 3-minute "wash-in" of the patient's lungs.

Low-Flow Anesthesia

Use of the breathing circuit can be carried one step further. Instead of decreasing the vaporizer setting, FGF can be reduced to achieve the same decreasing inspired tension; Figure 26-10 shows this. FGF begins at 8 L/min while the vaporizer is set to 5% isoflurane (DEL). At the end of 2 minutes, rather than decreasing the vaporizer setting, FGF is decreased to 2 L/min. Then, several minutes later, the vaporizer setting (DEL) is decreased as needed. All adjustments are made while the alveolar anesthetic tension (A, dark green) is observed, and the FGF vaporizer setting is adjusted to achieve 1.1% (1 MAC) expired isoflurane. At the end of 15 minutes with this low-flow anesthetic technique, 1.2 L has been delivered to the breathing circuit, and uptake by the patient's tissues is 0.6 L. This anesthetic administration is then 33% efficient in terms of use of isoflurane vapor (i.e., 0.4/1.2 = 0.333). In other words, with the low-flow technique, the concentration inspired by the patient is identical to that inspired with the high-flow technique; patient response—end-expired anesthetic tension, alveolar tension, and anesthesia depth—are also unaffected. The only difference between the two techniques is the manner in which the appropriate gas mixture is created.

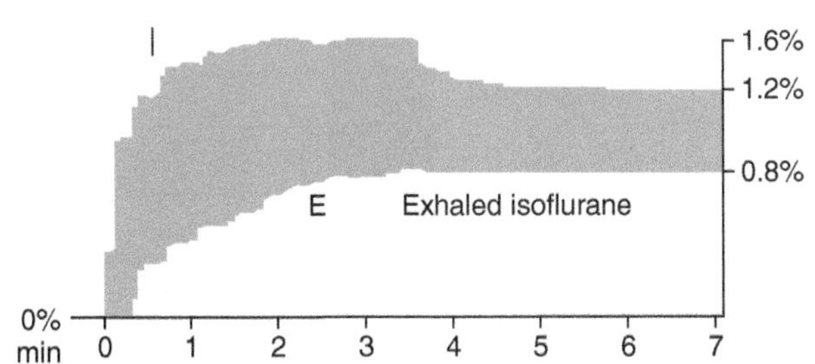

FIGURE 26-9 ■ Constant expired anesthetic tension shown on trend from multigas monitor. The graph shows the time course of airway anesthetic tension with the upper and lower edges representing inspired (*I*) and end-expired (*E*) isoflurane tensions.

CLOSED-CIRCUIT ANESTHESIA

FGF can be reduced to its minimum, thus achieving a completely closed circuit. Figure 26-11 illustrates this in schematic form. In the closed-circuit anesthesia technique, FGF is set equal to the patient's uptake of each and every gas used, including oxygen. When this is achieved, total volume is constant, and the concentration and tension of each substance is constant.

Oxygen uptake, usually referred to as *oxygen consumption*, is a particularly interesting result obtained using a closed circuit. The patient's oxygen consumption is equal to the flow of oxygen to the closed circuit. This equality is maintained by careful adjustment of oxygen flow.

Liquid Injection

To achieve closed-circuit anesthesia beginning with induction, or to accomplish rapid deepening during anesthesia, a modern concentration-calibrated, direct-reading vaporizer will not suffice. This is because the volume of its output at low FGF is insufficient to produce large or rapid changes in inspired tension. For this reason, *liquid* anesthetic agent is injected directly into the breathing circuit by many practitioners of the closed-circuit technique. The Gas Man model allows liquid injection to be simulated, while the student observes the resulting

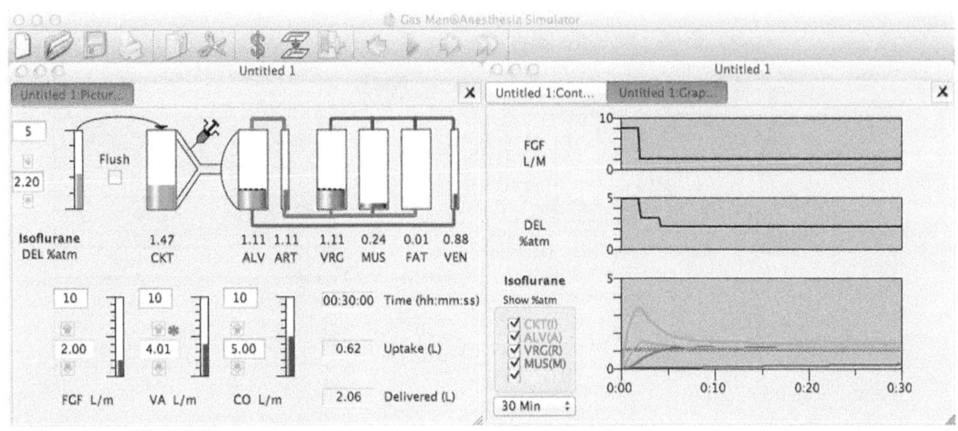

FIGURE 26-10 ■ Low-flow semi-closed circuit. Constant (1 MAC) alveolar isoflurane tension is achieved and maintained with a semiclosed circuit. First, high fresh gas flow ([FGF] 8 L/min) is used for 2 minutes. FGF is then reduced to 2 L/min (moderately low flow), and the vaporizer setting is reduced as needed to maintain a constant end-expired tension.

anesthetic tensions in the circuit and in the patient. Other practitioners increase FGF whenever they desire to change depth.

Figure 26-12 shows a Gas Man representation of closed-circuit anesthesia administered with 0.5 mL liquid isoflurane injections timed to achieve and maintain 1.1% exhaled anesthetic partial pressure. Each 0.5 mL of liquid isoflurane generates approximately 100 mL of vapor at room temperature. Liquid isoflurane is injected at empiric times with the objective of maintaining 1.1% alveolar partial pressure. Note that although inspired tension changes dramatically, and expired tension varies somewhat, brain tension (VRG on the picture, brown [R] on the graph) is quite stable over time. Alveolar tension can be smoothed by decreasing the liquid bolus volume and increasing the frequency of injection by converting to a continuous infusion of liquid anesthetic into the breathing circuit.

At the end of 30 minutes of empiric intermittent liquid injection, the graph in Figure 26-12 shows that patient uptake is again 0.6 L of isoflurane vapor. To achieve this, 0.9 L of vapor was delivered to the breathing circuit as nine individual 0.5 mL liquid injections. The discrepancy between the 0.9 L delivered and the 0.6 L uptake is anesthetic vapor that remains in the breathing circuit (CKT, 5 L) and the patient's lungs (ALV, 2 L). This same 0.3 L volume of anesthetic vapor was neglected in the previous descriptions for the sake of clarity. Other than storage in the circuit and lungs (alveoli), the efficiency of agent use is 100% when a closed-circuit technique is used as described.

Figure 26-13 shows a Gas Man representation of closed-circuit anesthesia administered with injections of liquid isoflurane according to Lowe's square-root-of-time model. Observe the 1.1% VRG (R) isoflurane tension that results. The first injection (0.5 mL) is made at time zero (first DEL spike). Subsequent (0.7 mL) injections are made at 1, 4, and 9 minutes. Note that bouncy but generally constant alveolar anesthetic tension (A, dark green) is achieved.

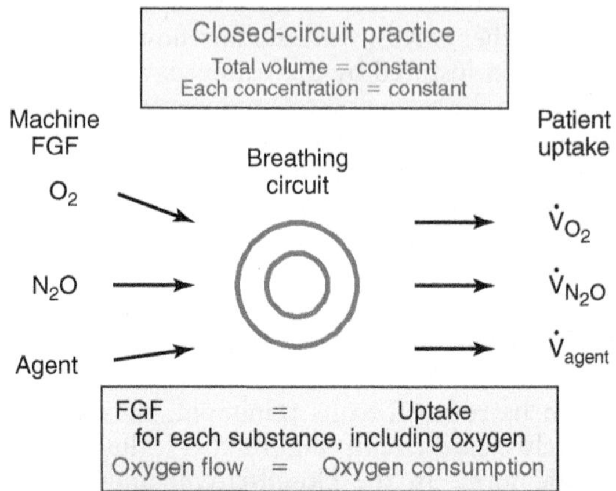

FIGURE 26-11 ■ The fundamental principle of closed-circuit anesthesia. Fresh-gas flow (*FGF*) to the breathing circuit is equal to the patient's uptake for each and every gas and vapor. As a result, the total volume is constant, and the concentration and tension (partial pressure) of each gas are constant. The patient's oxygen consumption can be estimated from the oxygen flow to the closed circuit.

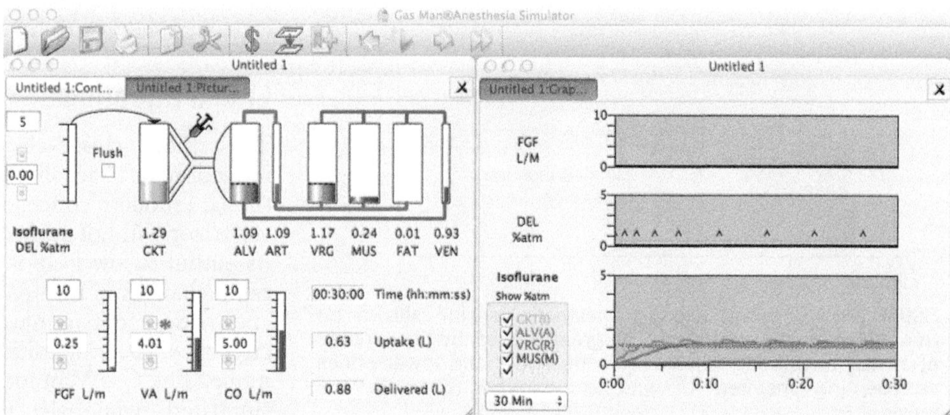

FIGURE 26-12 ■ Closed circuit with 0.5 mL injections of liquid isoflurane timed empirically from Gas Man (Med Man Simulations, Boston, MA). Each time alveolar tension fell to 1.0 %, a 0.5 mL injection of isoflurane was made in the Gas Man model.

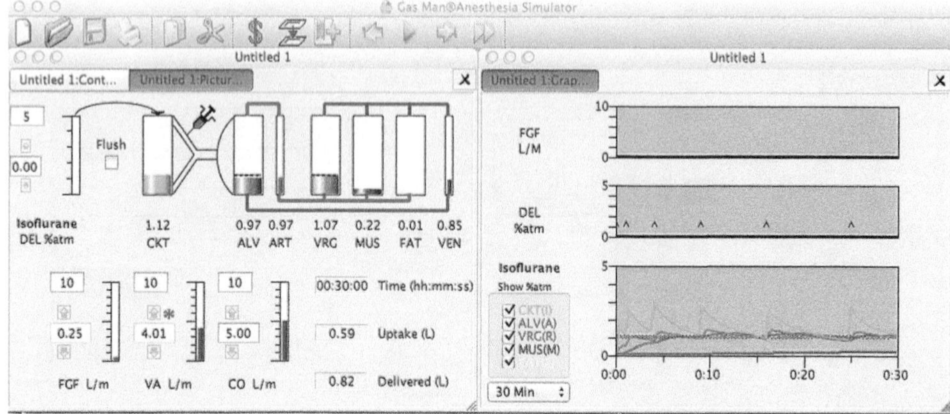

FIGURE 26-13 ■ Gas Man (Med Man Simulations, Boston, MA) simulation of the classic square root of time closed-circuit liquid injection technique. Liquid boluses at a 0.5 mL loading dose at time (t) = 0 followed by 0.7 mL maintenance dose injected at 1, 4, and 9 minutes. Note that the alveolar isoflurane tension remains near 1 MAC (1.1%) with injections made "by the clock."

At the end of 30 minutes of empiric intermittent liquid injection, patient uptake is again 0.6 L of isoflurane vapor (see Fig. 26-13). To achieve this, 0.8 L of vapor was delivered to the breathing circuit as five individual 0.7 mL liquid injections following a loading dose of 0.6 mL. The discrepancy between the 0.8 L delivered and the 0.4 L uptake is anesthetic vapor that remains in the breathing circuit (CKT, 6 L) and the patient's lungs (ALV, 2 L). This same 0.1 L anesthetic volume was neglected in the previous descriptions for the sake of clarity. Other than this, the efficiency of agent use is 100%. The slight differences in uptake in Figures 26-11, 26-12, and 26-13 are due to the slight differences in anesthetic tension maintained in VRG.

The initial (average) inspired concentration necessary to achieve 1.1% alveolar tension was approximately 2.9%, as in the previous examples. Average inspired tension was allowed to fall to 1.3% at the end of 30 minutes, as before, this time by lengthening the time between liquid injections. Inspired tension varied considerably between injections, but on the average, inspired tension was similar to that for higher flow systems.

The same principles apply to desflurane closed-circuit anesthesia. Figure 26-14 shows a Gas Man simulation of closed-circuit desflurane anesthesia with a 2.0 mL initial injection followed by 1.5 mL liquid desflurane injections at 1, 4, and 9 minutes. Figure 26-15 shows a Gas Man simulation of closed-circuit desflurane anesthesia with a 2.0 mL initial injection followed by 1.5 mL liquid desflurane injections at 1, 4, and 9 minutes. At 12 minutes, 1.0 MAC levels are achieved in alveolar gas and in the vessel-rich tissue group; the vaporizer is set to 16% desflurane, and no further liquid injections are required. The vaporizer setting needs to be reduced beginning at 30 minutes.

Choice of Anesthetic Agent

The choice of anesthetic agent should take into consideration the patient, surgery, and closed-circuit technique. Whenever a rebreathing circuit with carbon dioxide absorption is used, there is some expired admixture to FGF. As FGF is reduced toward that of a closed circuit, expired concentration plays a greater role and fresh-gas concentration plays a lesser role in determining inspired concentration. Inspired concentration is the flow-weighted average of fresh gas and expired gas concentrations. Low-solubility agents provide expired concentrations close to those of inspired concentrations. Thus they require relatively lower delivered (vaporizer) concentrations than agents of higher solubility. If the concentration required exceeds the maximum vaporizer setting, alternative administration techniques are required. Higher FGF can be used, and the closed-circuit technique abandoned, in favor of low, also called *minimal*, flow—at least until the vaporizer alone will suffice. Alternatively, a closed circuit can be achieved by injecting liquid anesthetic into the breathing circuit.

Only desflurane can consistently be used without the liquid injections required in a closed circuit. Desflurane's low blood/gas solubility (0.42) and vanishingly low metabolism make it well suited for low-flow and

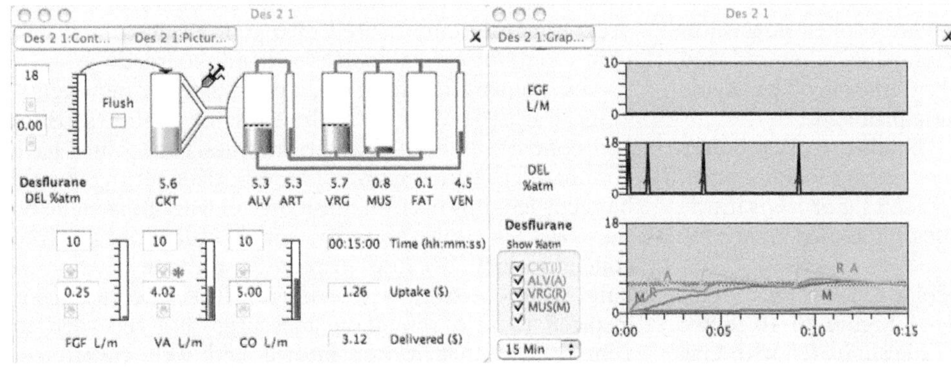

FIGURE 26-14 ▪ Gas Man simulation (Med Man Simulations, Boston, MA) of closed-circuit desflurane anesthesia with 2.0 mL initial injection followed by 1.5 mL liquid desflurane injections at 1, 4, and 9 minutes.

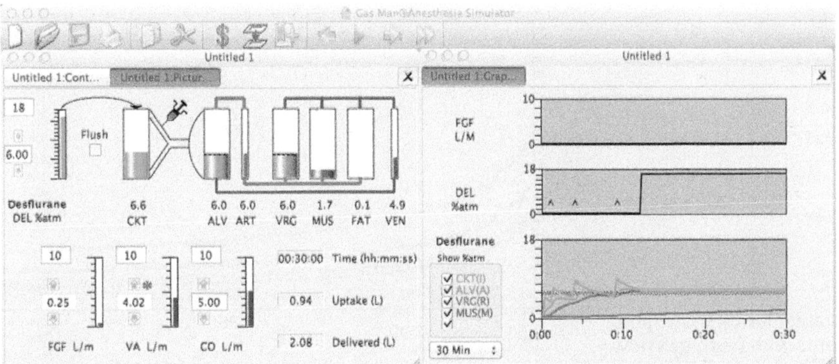

FIGURE 26-15 ▪ Gas Man (Med Man Simulations, Boston, MA) simulation of closed-circuit desflurane anesthesia with a 2.0 mL initial injection followed by 1.5 mL liquid desflurane injections at 1, 4, and 9 minutes. At 12 minutes, 1.0 MAC levels are achieved in the alveoli and vessel-rich group, the vaporizer is set to 16% desflurane, and no further liquid injections are required. The vaporizer setting needs to be reduced beginning at 30 minutes.

closed-circuit anesthesia. When used this way, it becomes quite economical. The maximum vaporizer setting of 18% exceeds that necessary to maintain anesthesia depth.

Sevoflurane has relatively low blood/gas solubility (0.67) and is used for closed-circuit anesthesia in countries where there is no regulation barring it.[26] In the United States, the Food and Drug Administration (FDA) package insert requires an FGF of 2 L/min for cases of a duration greater than 2 MAC × the number of hours (e.g., 1 MAC for 2 hours, 2 MAC for 1 hour). For less than this time × duration product, at least 1 L/min is required.

This FDA restriction is based on the increased heat produced by carbon dioxide absorption and the accompanying temperature rise in the carbon dioxide absorbent. Baralyme was removed from the U.S. market because of its substantial heat production.[27] In many countries, a variety of "cool" CO_2 absorbents are available that use lower or absent NaOH and KOH in combination with $CaCO_3$ or other absorbents.[27]

The resulting increased temperature increases the degradation of sevoflurane to compound A, which is toxic in swine.[27] Sevoflurane's use in low-flow and closed-circuit situations has not shown any clinical problems.[26] The maximum vaporizer setting of 8% is just sufficient to maintain anesthesia after adequate depth is attained.

Isoflurane's higher blood/gas solubility (1.3) requires high vaporizer settings during maintenance. Indeed, the maximum isoflurane vaporizer setting of 5% is insufficient to maintain 1 MAC anesthesia in a closed circuit for the first hour.

Both isoflurane and desflurane are broken down into compounds, including carbon monoxide, when exposed to high temperatures.[27] With the removal of Baralyme from the market, this is no longer a problem.[28]

Halothane's high blood/gas solubility (2.4) requires particularly high vaporizer settings during maintenance. The maximum halothane vaporizer setting of 5% is insufficient to maintain 1 MAC anesthesia in closed circuit for the first hour.

The ratio of delivered to alveolar tension for several agents was first explored by Zuntz.[9] Figure 26-16 shows the delivered/alveolar ratio over time simulated with Gas Man. Note that the higher the blood/gas solubility, the higher the delivered/alveolar tension ratio.

Practical Aspects of Administration

The practical aspects of administration of closed-circuit anesthesia must be known and understood for this technique to be used effectively. Many contemporary anesthesia machines available in the United States are not designed to facilitate or allow closed-circuit techniques and thus need modification before or during use; all GE Healthcare anesthesia machines fall into this category. In the United States, the Dräger Apollo and Fabius can provide fully closed-circuit anesthesia because there is no lower limit to FGF, and return of sampled gas is facilitated by a built-in sampled gas-return port.

In some countries, GE Healthcare and Dräger both provide low-flow anesthesia machines with end-tidal control of agent and end-tidal (GE Aisys) or inspired (Dräger Zeus) control of oxygen. Neither of these provides fully closed-circuit anesthesia.

Likewise, the anesthetic record must be adapted for the closed-circuit technique. It is important for the anesthetic record to capture FGFs and vaporizer settings as well as measured inspired and end-expired concentrations. When low-flow or closed-circuit anesthesia is administered, certain additional variables need to be recorded on the anesthetic record. First, the flows of nitrous oxide, air, and oxygen must be recorded to explain what is really administered to the breathing circuit separate and distinct from the resulting inspired concentrations of oxygen, nitrous oxide, and balance gas, which is predominantly unmeasured nitrogen. Expired tidal volume should be carefully observed and recorded.

With older anesthesia delivery systems, patient ventilation was dependent on both ventilator volume settings and concurrent FGF. Newer anesthesia machines have eliminated this interaction. The vaporizer setting should be recorded, however, because the adjustment is made by the anesthesia care provider, and it influences inspired concentration. Because inspired anesthetic tension is quite different from that delivered from the vaporizer, inspired tension should be measured and recorded to demonstrate that it was known and well controlled.

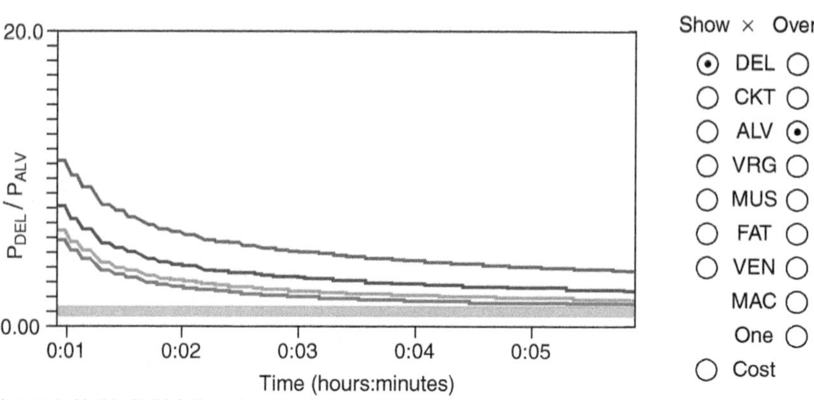

FIGURE 26-16 Delivered/alveolar tension ratio. The ratio for several agents with fresh gas flow of 6 L/min are simulated using the Gas Man (Med Man Simulations, Chestnut Hill, MA) overlay. The higher the blood/gas solubility, the higher the delivered/alveolar tension ratio. Time interval shown is 1 minute to 6 minutes.

Finally, expired anesthetic tension should be controlled and recorded to assist in patient management. The need to monitor and record expired-agent tension applies irrespective of FGF; it is equally applicable to high-flow techniques. When all three of these variables—vaporizer setting, inspired tension, and expired tension—are recorded, the anesthetic record documents the patient's receipt of a safe and effective anesthetic. All closed-circuit concentrations and flows should be recorded without reservation. Closed-circuit anesthesia has been shown to be as safe as a high-flow technique.[29]

Practical administration of closed-circuit anesthesia follows the basic principle of the technique: deliver gases and vapors at a rate equal to tissue uptake while maintaining alveolar tension at the desired level (Figure 26-11). For most adult patients, the following regimens work as a first approximation. As with any clinical technique, changes are made to adapt delivery to each patient, surgery, and anesthetic agent.

Isoflurane

Inhalation anesthesia with isoflurane is induced with high flows and is maintained for approximately 20 minutes. During this time, alveolar anesthetic tension is established at the desired level; mechanical ventilation is usually used. Before flows are reduced, exhaled tidal volume, inspired and expired agent tensions, and inspired oxygen concentration are carefully measured and recorded on the anesthetic record. Breathing circuit gas is then transferred from the ventilator to the reservoir bag by switching between the two reservoirs during mechanical or manual ventilation. This is described below. In this way, if a switch between these two is necessary later in the anesthetic, the same concentrations are breathed from either ventilation source. Flows are then reduced as described below.

Inhalation anesthesia with isoflurane can be induced with a closed-circuit technique from the outset, but a liquid circuit injection is required. I prefer avoiding nitrous oxide and making sequential 0.5 mL isoflurane injections into the inspired limb of the breathing circuit while observing inspired and expired tension on a breath-by-breath basis. Liquid anesthetic is injected whenever inspired or expired tension falls below the desired level. The location of the liquid injection is described below.

Desflurane

Desflurane can be conveniently used with closed-circuit anesthesia. Inhalation induction is avoided for clinical reasons, and desflurane is introduced after the airway is secured with a tracheal tube or supraglottic airway.

Desflurane anesthesia is easily begun with an FGF of about 1 L/min. I prefer oxygen-enriched air and the avoidance of nitrous oxide. When air is predominantly used, an FGF of 1 L/min air is supplemented to oxygen flow slightly in excess of estimated oxygen consumption. This oxygen flow is 200 mL/min in adults. Thus FGF is 1.25 L/min. With this flow rate, a vaporizer setting of 18% desflurane causes inspired and expired desflurane concentrations to rise slowly and smoothly. After about 8 minutes, the inspired concentration reaches 8%, and the expired concentration reaches 6%. At this time the vaporizer setting or FGF can be reduced. At 1.2 L/min FGF, the vaporizer setting can be reduced to 9% to 10%.

With oxygen administration during initiation of desflurane anesthesia, it is convenient to reduce the vaporizer setting to maintain inspired and expired concentrations as desired. With this technique, oxygen concentration falls to about 85% with inspired gas containing residual nitrogen, which emerges from tissues during anesthesia.

With oxygen-enriched air administration during initiation of desflurane anesthesia, inspired and expired desflurane concentrations are established before inspired oxygen is controlled to fall to the desired level, typically below 30%. I prefer to reduce inspired oxygen to the FiO_2, where arterial oxygen saturation falls to 98%, rather than 100%, to be sensitive to lung shunt and be ready to reduce it. To make this safe, the pulse oximeter oxygen saturation (SpO_2) audible alarm is set to 95%. SpO_2 becomes a sensitive indicator of lung shunt of any source. This transforms SpO_2 from a statistical safety monitor into a clinical monitor that is useful to detect many problems at an early stage. Inspired oxygen concentration is typically between 21% and 35%, depending on lung shunt and other physiology. Past authors have suggested higher inspired oxygen concentrations. The danger of administering 1 L/min air without supplemental oxygen is described under "Avoiding Hypoxia" below.

Flow Control

When a high-flow technique is used first, FGF is reduced to provide a completely closed circuit. The adjustable pressure-limiting (APL), or pop-off, valve is closed to keep gas from leaving the circuit, should the reservoir bag be used later. On older anesthesia machines, in which tidal volume and FGF were related, set tidal volume was increased to provide an undiminished exhaled tidal volume. With newer anesthesia machines that directly control inspired tidal volume, this adjustment is no longer necessary.

With agent plus nitrous oxide plus oxygen anesthesia in adults, oxygen flow is reduced to 200 mL/min, and nitrous oxide is reduced to 100 mL/min. This approximates patient uptake for these gases. With isoflurane, the vaporizer is set to 3% to provide the approximately 9 mL/min isoflurane vapor required for 0.5 MAC contribution of isoflurane. With desflurane, the vaporizer setting is 5% to provide the approximately 16 mL/min desflurane vapor required for the 0.5 MAC contribution of desflurane.

With agent plus air plus oxygen anesthesia, oxygen flow is reduced to 200 mL/min to approximate oxygen uptake, and air is turned off because there is no nitrogen uptake or elimination when circuit gas concentrations are near that of air. With isoflurane, the vaporizer is set to 5%, which does not quite supply the 18 mL/min required to maintain 1 MAC anesthesia. Either FGF must be increased periodically or liquid isoflurane must be injected occasionally. With desflurane, the vaporizer is set to approximately 14% to supply the 32 mL/min desflurane vapor required to maintain 1 MAC anesthesia.

The ventilator is adjusted so that no gas leaves the breathing circuit at the end of exhalation; the exact technique depends on the ventilator used and is described below. Typically, the ascending (standing) bellows is adjusted to prevent it from rising to the mechanical stop that initiates discharge of excess gas. A mark can be placed on the bellows housing to signify the correct end-expired bellows position. This represents a volume mark. Deviation of the bellows from this volume mark signifies inequality between total volume delivered to the circuit and volume taken up by the patient. This deviation suggests that total FGF should be modified in some way.

Changes in concentrations of gases and vapors disclose what should be changed, the direction of change, and the magnitude of change. A change in measured F_IO_2 suggests that a change should be made in the flow ratio of oxygen to the other gas (nitrous oxide or air). A change in inspired agent tension suggests that a change should be made in the administration of anesthetic agent. This agent administration may have been in the form or vapor or liquid. If administration is in the form of vapor from a vaporizer, the vaporizer setting should be changed. If administration is in the form of periodic liquid injection, this suggests a change in interval of the same unit dose, adjustment of the unit dose using the same interval, or some combination of change of dose and interval. If administration is in the form of a continuous liquid injection into the breathing circuit, the rate of injection is altered.

The quantification of these adjustments is not immediately obvious. When the volume of the ventilator bellows changes, flows of nitrous oxide and oxygen are adjusted in proportion to their concentrations in the breathing circuit, *not* according to their proportion in fresh gas. For example, if the respiratory gas monitor indicates an inspired concentration of 66% nitrous oxide and 33% oxygen, it is in this ratio that additional gas must be added to maintain the same inspired oxygen concentration. Therefore the adjustments in oxygen flow are accompanied by adjustments in nitrous oxide that in this case happen to be twice as large. That is, when oxygen flow is increased by 100 mL/min, nitrous oxide flow is increased by 200 mL/min.

When a decrease in FiO_2 is noted in the absence of a change in circuit volume, oxygen flow is increased, and nitrous oxide flow is decreased, this time by equal amounts to keep circuit volume constant. Simultaneous changes in FiO_2 and circuit volume require mixed compensation, which is a combination of the two techniques described.

Finally, when inspired or expired agent tension requires an increase, the vaporizer setting is increased, or additional liquid is injected into the breathing circuit. To lighten anesthesia, the vaporizer is turned off, or a liquid injection dose is withheld or delayed. An activated charcoal filter may be used to adsorb volatile agent.[30-35] Charcoal functions best when a pair of filters are placed in the inspiratory and expiratory limbs of the circuit.[35] Anesthesia may also be lightened by flushing the breathing circuit briefly with oxygen. When a nitrous oxide plus oxygen plus agent anesthetic is used, the agent dilution should be done with a mixture of oxygen and nitrous oxide, with flows proportional to their circuit concentrations. When an agent plus air plus oxygen anesthetic is administered, air plus oxygen is the appropriate gas for agent dilution; the latter two cannot be done simply with today's anesthesia delivery systems. In each case the resulting change in inhaled tensions of all gases and vapors should be observed and controlled. Because lightening anesthesia happens most often near the end of anesthesia, increasing inspired oxygen concentration may be desired, and oxygen flush or increased flow can be used. This is especially true for agent plus air plus oxygen anesthesia; however, this might not be appropriate for agent plus nitrous oxide plus oxygen anesthesia.

During the administration of any anesthetic, switching between mechanical and manual ventilation (i.e., controlled and spontaneous, respectively) is often desired. This change influences closed-circuit anesthesia in several ways. First, if the content of the reservoir bag and bellows is different, switching modes will produce a change in gas composition. This usually is not desired. Such a change is averted by emptying whichever gas reservoir is not in use, bellows or reservoir bag, and transferring circuit gases back into the empty reservoir (bellows or bag) when convenient. This is done in a manner that will be described below.

When a change in the volume in the ventilator bellows or reservoir bag is desired, this can be accomplished by switching between bag and ventilator. To do this, the clinician maintains a partially filled reservoir bag throughout the case. Meanwhile, the patient is ventilated mechanically. Whenever it becomes necessary to compensate for accumulated circuit volume change, gas is transferred between bellows and bag. This is done by transferring gas via the patient's lungs during exhalation. Deft adjustment of the bag/bellows selector lever is required. The same technique is used to fill the out-of-use reservoir bag or ventilator bellows, as introduced above.

With the earlier Ohmeda (GE Healthcare) breathing circuit assembly (Modulus 2 Plus), when the selector valve was moved 5% of the way from "Vent" to "Bag," the ventilator and bag were connected to each other, and gas could be easily transferred without using the patient's lungs as a temporary reservoir. With newer anesthesia delivery systems, this is no longer possible. With the GE Aestiva, using the patient's lungs can successfully act as a transfer volume. This is because the switch to ventilator mode interposes a momentary expiratory pause, during which the patient's lungs can empty into the ventilator bellows. When transferring gas from the bellows to the reservoir bag, switching the mode from "Vent" to "Bag" at the beginning of exhalation fills the reservoir bag and leaves the ventilator bellows partly empty.

With the GE Advanced Breathing System (ABS) Aespire, Avance, and Aisys workstations, switching to mechanical ventilation mode begins instantly with the inspiratory phase of ventilation. Thus the patient's first tidal volume may be increased above the set tidal volume under some conditions.

With the Dräger FGF decoupling machines (e.g., Fabius, Apollo, and in some countries, Julian), the reservoir bag is in the expiratory limb of the breathing circuit during mechanical and manual/spontaneous ventilation. Therefore the bag contains gases and vapors of the correct concentration and sufficient volume to switch ventilation modes at any time. In these Dräger anesthesia delivery systems, the clinician must be aware that switching from vent to bag creates a moment in which the reservoir bag positive-pressure relief valve is open. Squeezing the reservoir bag during this period results in lost volume from the circuit to the scavenger interface. With high-flow anesthesia, this is not a problem; but with low-flow or closed-circuit anesthesia, this will leave the reservoir bag empty, and it will not refill. Thus the user must delay squeezing the reservoir bag until the valve closes (about 1 second).

RESPIRATORY GAS SAMPLING

Respiratory gas sampling for analysis complicates low-flow and closed-circuit administration unless pure sampled gas is returned to the breathing circuit. This can be done simply and conveniently by connecting the sampled gas return tube to the expiratory limb or to the carbon dioxide absorber itself using a reusable or disposable adapter. This connection exists as an FDA-approved feature in newer Dräger anesthesia delivery systems (e.g., Tiro, Fabius GS, and Apollo). This connection does not exist in GE anesthesia delivery systems. This connection is already made in the Dräger Apollo.

Although a truly closed circuit cannot be achieved without gas return, circuit loss to sampling can be compensated by the addition of fresh gas to offset the loss. An excessive gas sampling rate can produce negative pressure in the breathing circuit and can deplete the volume necessary for patient ventilation.[36,37] To compensate for gas sampling without sample gas return, the anesthesiologist increases nitrous oxide, oxygen, and agent flows by an amount equal to the respective rate of removal by the gas sampling system. This total sampling flow varies slightly among manufacturers and models, but it is usually between 200 and 300 mL/min total flow.

Correcting for sample gas loss requires certain considerations. Sample gas composition equals circuit composition, which is a mixture of inspired and expired gas, weighted according to the inspiratory and expiratory times. Throughout most of the duration of the anesthesia, inspired and expired values do not differ by an amount that affects this minor correction. Because all of the exhaled gas is rebreathed (with carbon dioxide removed), circuit composition is dominated by the composition of exhaled gas with slight alteration by fresh gas.

When breathing circuit composition is 66% nitrous oxide, 33% oxygen, and 0.5% isoflurane, gas sampled from the breathing circuit will approximate this composition. Thus if the sampling rate is 250 mL/min, an additional 165 mL/min (250×0.66) nitrous oxide, 82 mL/min oxygen, and 2 mL/min isoflurane must be added to compensate for the loss of sampled gas. The total resulting flows and concentrations are 265 mL/min nitrous oxide, 282 mL/min oxygen, and 18 mL/min isoflurane, or 3% of FGF. Rounding off for convenience, with nonreturn airway gas sampling, FGF is adjusted to 300 mL/min oxygen and 300 mL/min nitrous oxide, and the vaporizer is set to 3% (halothane or isoflurane) as a reasonable starting point.

When the breathing circuit composition is desflurane 6% in oxygen, oxygen flow is increased by 300 mL/min to a total of 500 mL/min. When the breathing circuit composition is desflurane 6% in 25% oxygen, to a first approximation, the sample gas is compensated with pure air. This is then corrected with a decrease of 50 mL/min air and an increase of 50 mL/min oxygen. Most anesthesia machines do not have the precision to do this well.

Whenever nitrous oxide is administered to a closed circuit, concentration or tension of oxygen in the breathing circuit must be monitored even more carefully than usual. This is because in a closed circuit, inspired oxygen concentration depends on both gas delivered from the anesthesia machine (FGF) and that exhaled by the patient. Inspired oxygen tension or concentration must be monitored to ensure the safety of gases inspired by the patient. When low flows are used, oxygen concentration alarms should be set tightly above and below the desired FiO_2. Expired as well as inspired oxygen concentration monitoring is advisable when possible, and arterial oxygen saturation should always be monitored, as for any other anesthetic; this is discussed further in the section "Avoiding Hypoxia." When air is added to a closed circuit, usually because of sample gas discard, FiO_2 must be monitored and alarmed very carefully.

In contrast to high-flow systems, in which FGF to the circuit replaces carbon dioxide–laden exhaled gas, closed-circuit anesthesia requires effective carbon dioxide absorption. Thus, carbon dioxide monitoring (capnography) is even more important with low flows than with high flows. A functioning carbon dioxide absorber must always be ensured, which is accomplished by monitoring inspired partial pressure of carbon dioxide ($PiCO_2$). A carbon dioxide level of more than 5 mm Hg is cause for concern. When this is seen, I advise an increase in FGF to twice the minute ventilation, ensuring that $PiCO_2$ falls to approximately zero. If it does, the carbon dioxide absorbent should be presumed to be used up and no longer effective. Carbon dioxide absorbent should be replaced at this time; if this is accomplished by an exchange of carbon dioxide absorber assembly, the original absorbent should be retained briefly. If the new carbon dioxide absorbent exhibits the same $PiCO_2$ greater than 5 mm Hg, the carbon dioxide absorbent is not the problem. Rather, the problem is usually an inappropriate estimation of inspired concentration by the gas monitor; in rare cases, it might represent a breathing circuit valve malfunction. If the carbon dioxide absorbent is changed, recognize that the volatile agent absorbed in the absorbent granules and stored in the absorbent empty spaces must be replaced by additional anesthetic agent. Careful addition of vapor or liquid should be performed while observing inspired agent tension and bringing it to what it was before the absorbent change. Do not rely on expired agent tension, because its change will be slow and will lead to not fully replacing the lost agent.

Liquid Agent Injection

Where to inject liquid agent is an interesting question. Early writings advocated injecting into the expiratory limb of the circuit to avoid unmonitored and unknown changes in inspired tension. Careful monitoring of airway anesthetic tension allows liquid injection closed-circuit

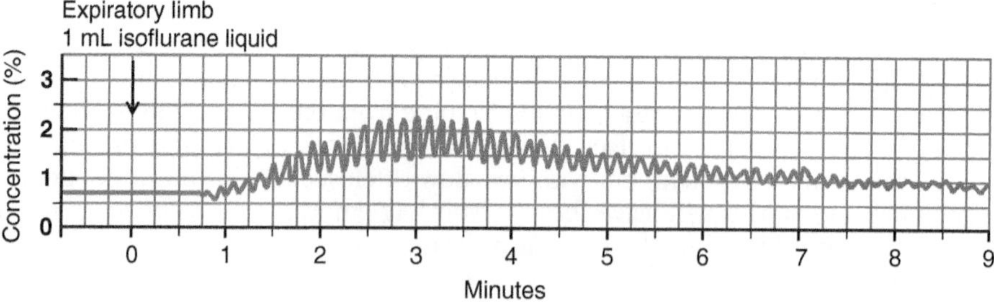

FIGURE 26-17 ■ Expiratory limb injection. Time course of airway anesthetic tension after injection of 1.0 mL liquid isoflurane into the expiratory limb of the breathing circuit. Peaks are inspired tension and troughs are expired tension. Inspired tension begins to rise 1 minute after injection. Inspired and expired tensions begin to rise 2.5 minutes after injection and reach peak values 3 minutes after injection.

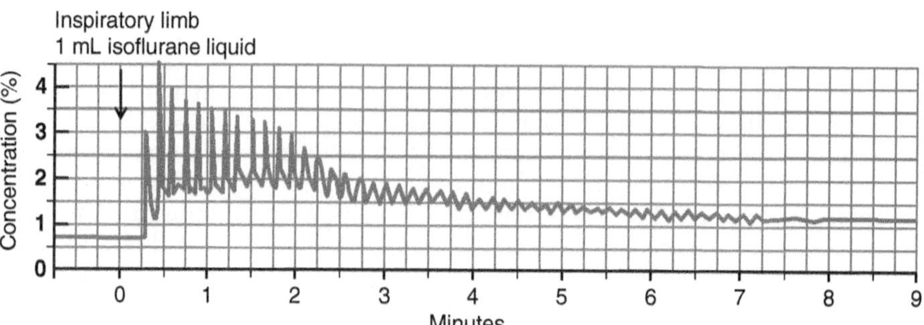

FIGURE 26-18 ■ Inspiratory limb injection. Time course of airway anesthetic tension after injection of 1.0 mL liquid isoflurane into the inspiratory limb of the breathing circuit. Peaks are inspired tension and troughs are expired tension. Inspired tension rises to 4.5% two breaths after injection. Expired tension peaks after two breaths at 1.7% after two breaths (1.2% above its value two breaths earlier) and remains at this level for several minutes.

anesthesia to be performed simply and safely. Figure 26-17 shows the time course of airway anesthetic tension in response to a 1.0 mL injection of liquid isoflurane into the expiratory limb of the breathing circuit connected to a 70-kg patient undergoing surgery. With this agent monitor, concentration rises with each inspiration and falls with each expiration. Thus the peaks and troughs represent inspired and end-tidal anesthetic tensions, respectively. Separate curves connecting all the peaks and all the troughs would follow the "I" and "E" curves of the isoflurane simulations in Figs. 26-12 and 26-13. Note that inspired tension does not rise for 1 minute, and an additional 1.5 minutes elapses before peak inspired tension is reached. At the peak, inspired tension rises by 1.5% from its baseline of 0.5%. Meanwhile, expired tension rises by 0.7% from 0.5% to 1.2%.

With the advent of breath-by-breath monitors of anesthetic agents, it became obvious that injection in the inspiratory limb is possible and advantageous. Figure 26-18 shows the result of a 1.0 mL liquid isoflurane injection into the inspiratory limb of the circuit in the same patient. Inspired tension peaks at 4.4% above baseline after two breaths (15 seconds). Expired tension rises by 1.2% within two breaths and remains constant for about 2 minutes, and 3 minutes after injection, the two tracings that depict injection in the two circuit locations become quite similar. A note of caution is in order here: when injected into either the inspired or the expired limb, *liquid anesthetic must never be allowed to reach the patient.* Conventional breathing circuits with a dependent section between the carbon dioxide absorber and the patient easily achieve this. Continuous, breath-by-breath gas monitoring helps the clinician ensure that inspired and expired tensions are as desired and expected. Figure 26-19 shows alternate injections of 0.5 mL of liquid isoflurane into the inspiratory and expiratory limbs of the circuit. In each case, injection into the inspiratory limb resulted in an inspired peak within two breaths, whereas injection into the expiratory limb resulted in an

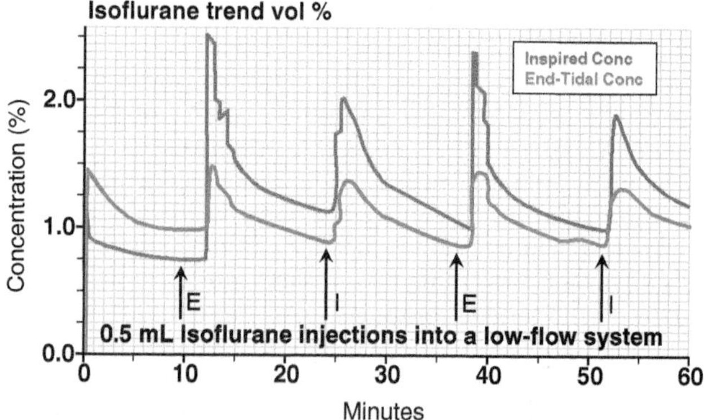

FIGURE 26-19 ■ Alternate injections into the inspiratory (I) and expiratory (E) circuit limbs. In each case, inspiratory limb injection resulted in an inspired peak within two breaths, and expiratory limb injection resulted in end-tidal peak approximately 90 seconds after injection. The red tracing represents inspiratory isoflurane tension, and the blue tracing represents tidal expiratory isoflurane tension.

inspired peak approximately 90 seconds after injection. Injection into the inspiratory limb provides superior control of inspired and expired anesthetic tension. An exhaled limb injection may be acceptable when constant depth is the goal. Figure 26-20 shows a 6 minute trend graph of inspired and expired desflurane concentration after 1 mL desflurane liquid injections were made into the inspired circuit limb adjacent to the carbon dioxide absorber. Note that inspired tension rises to 3% quickly. This small rise in inspired tension does not generally elicit a sympathetic response.

Many anesthesiologists use a concentration-calibrated vaporizer for closed-circuit anesthesia. Some adjust the vaporizer by intermittently selecting between full on and full off. With low flow through a concentration-calibrated vaporizer, the time constant (τ) for circuit tension change is long, because τ is equal to circuit volume divided by circuit flow in a fully mixed circuit. With a volume of 8 L (6 L circuit + 2 L lung volume or functional residual capacity

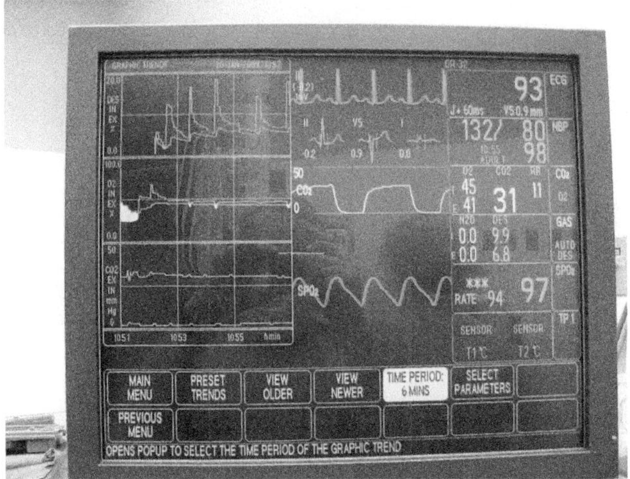

FIGURE 26-20 Solar 8000i physiologic monitor (GE Healthcare, Waukesha, WI). Display of a 6-minute graph of inspired and expired desflurane (*top left*), oxygen (*middle left*), and carbon dioxide (*bottom left*). Injections of 1 mL desflurane are made in the inspired limb of the breathing circuit.

[FRC]) and a flow of 0.25 to 0.5 L/min, τ is between 32 and 16 minutes. Because of this, even a drastic change in vaporizer setting produces a very slow change in the composition of inspired gas. If faster control is desired, either FGF must be increased or liquid must be injected.

Closed-circuit anesthesia can also be administered via measured-flow vaporizers (e.g., Copper Kettle and Vernitrol). However, because of the potential for error in the calculations required,[38] and the fact that these vaporizers are considered obsolete, their use is discouraged (see also Chapter 3).[38]

The initial administration of inhaled agents can be performed by liquid injection. With desflurane, a convenient liquid volume for adults is 1.0 mL. Figure 26-20 is a screen shot of the 6-minute graph of inspired and expired desflurane concentration. When the same administration sequence is viewed over a 15-minute window, the bumps in inspired and expired concentration are smoothed, and the inspired and expired curves appear just as they would with careful vaporizer use with high or low FGF.

LACK OF BUILDUP OF TOXIC SUBSTANCES

When high flows are used during anesthesia, gases in the breathing circuit are replaced frequently. Thus any gases that might accumulate in the breathing circuit are removed and replaced with fresh gas. In a closed circuit, all substances entering the breathing circuit remain there unless taken up by the patient, carbon dioxide absorbent, or circuit materials.

Circuit contaminants can arise from several sources.[39] Anesthetics by themselves or in reaction with soda lime can produce unintended substances. Specifically, halothane produces two metabolites, 2-chloro-1,1,1-trifluoroethane (CF_3CH_2Cl) and 2-chloro-1,1-difluoroethylene (CF_2CHCl), and they produce a metabolite decomposition product, 2-bromo-2-chloro-1,1-difluoroethylene (CF_2CBrCl). Concentrations in a closed circuit are no higher than in a semiclosed circuit, and the decomposition product is not present in an absorbent-free Bain circuit, although these substances are not believed to be a hazard.[40,41]

Enflurane,[42] isoflurane,[43] and desflurane[44] are stable enough to warrant no special concern during closed-circuit anesthesia. Sevoflurane[45] has been shown to produce three breakdown products in soda lime. The first is compound A, or fluoromethyl 2,2-difluoro-1-(trifluoromethyl)-vinyl ether, alternatively called 1,1,1,3,3-pentafluoroisopropenyl fluoromethyl ether, or PIFE ($F_2C{=}C[CF_3]OCH_2F$). The second is compound B, or fluoromethyl 2-methoxy-2,2 difluoro-1-(trifluoromethyl)-ethyl ether, alternatively called 1,1, 1,3,3-pentafluoro-3-methoxy-isopropyl fluoromethyl ether, or PMFE ($H_3COCF_2CH[CF_3]OCH_2F$). The third is hexafluoroisopropanol, or HFIP. In a closed circuit, PIFE and HFIP concentrations remain low; the safety of PMFE in a closed-circuit system is still under investigation.

Patients can produce substances that would be better removed from the breathing circuit than rebreathed. One such product is carbon monoxide.[46] In addition, tissue nitrogen continues to be released into the breathing circuit[47] at a rate of approximately 10 mL/min and accounts for a slow asymptotic rise in circuit nitrogen toward 10% without exceeding this value.[48] Acetone, methane, and other inert gases also build up.[49] However, values attained are less than those allowed for chronic occupational exposure.[50] It is possible that the breathing circuit should be flushed periodically with a high FGF, although the need for this has not been established.

During laparoscopy or other surgeries in which carbon dioxide is used to distend a body space (insufflation), carbon dioxide is absorbed. This absorption is not accompanied by increased oxygen consumption; therefore FGF does not need to be increased. When oxygen consumption changes for any reason, this will be detectable by changes in circuit volume and gas composition. Thus in situations such as shock or decreased oxygen consumption in shock, changes in oxygen consumption may be observed. The information obtained from closed-circuit anesthesia provides insight into changing physiology.

Substances can also enter the breathing circuit from other sources. For example, acrylic monomer is exhaled when joint prostheses are surgically cemented. During this period, the closed circuit should be interrupted, and high FGF should be used to prevent rebreathing of this chemical.

Some gas monitors sample room air or calibration gases intermittently. The Ohmeda Rascal and Rascal II (GE Healthcare) self-zero with argon and room air periodically. Argon buildup is insignificant, as is nitrogen accumulation.[48] The electronic paramagnetic oxygen monitors used in some multigas monitors entrain room air for continuous calibration. If the instrument combines calibration gas with sampled patient gas, gas returned from the instrument contains room air, and nitrogen accumulation in the closed circuit is noticeable and significant. This problem makes the GE Healthcare gas monitors problematic for closed-circuit anesthesia administration.[51]

Avoiding Hypoxia

During anesthesia, hypoxia must be avoided, so its likelihood must be reduced to as close to zero as possible. It is

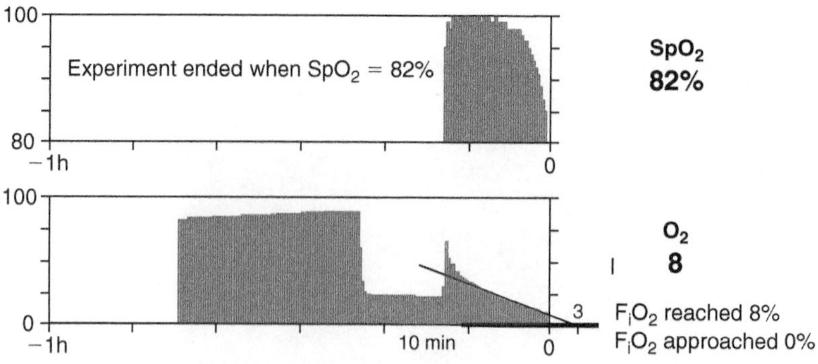

FIGURE 26-21 Graph of the fraction of inspired oxygen (FiO_2) and pulse oximeter value (SpO_2) over time. An 84-kg patient breathing fresh gas flow at 1 L/min air plus 0.050 L/min oxygen from a semiclosed breathing circuit (Ohmeda Modulus 2 Plus or Modulus CD anesthesia machine with GMS absorber assembly; GE Healthcare, Waukesha, WI). After 12 minutes, FiO_2 fell to 8%, SpO_2 fell to 82%, and the demonstration was terminated. The patient had no ill effects. The early exponential fall describes a first order, proportional uptake, process. The later linear fall implies zero order, constant uptake, process.

crucial to understand how inspired hypoxia can develop during closed-circuit and even low-flow anesthesia.

In a closed circuit, as long as oxygen administration exceeds oxygen uptake, inspired oxygen concentration rises. In steady state, oxygen administration exactly equals oxygen uptake, and FiO_2 remains constant. This is a fundamental principle of closed-circuit anesthesia.

In low-flow non–closed-circuit situations, oxygen delivery in excess of uptake is *not* sufficient to avoid falling FiO_2 and inspired hypoxia. This is because in all non–closed-circuit situations, gas leaves the breathing circuit, and this gas includes oxygen. Thus a 1 L/min FGF of air inevitably leads to inspired hypoxia in a 70-kg patient. This is because a 70-kg awake patient consumes about 250 mL/min oxygen, and this value falls to about 210 mL/min under anesthesia. With an FGF of 1 L/min of air, 790 mL/min nitrogen and 210 mL/min oxygen are delivered to the breathing circuit. Thus oxygen delivery exactly equals oxygen uptake. But each minute, uptake of oxygen is 210 mL, and uptake of nitrogen is zero. Thus the *net* flow to the breathing circuit is 790 mL/min nitrogen and 0 mL/min oxygen. Breathing circuit oxygen concentration therefore falls, and it falls linearly, because oxygen is taken up at a constant rate until life ceases or is diminished. Thus in a breathing circuit and patient lungs with a combined volume of 8 L, FiO_2 will fall 2.6%/min ([0.21 L/min]/8 L = 0.026/min). Figure 26-21 shows the graph of FiO_2 and SpO_2 over time in an 84 kg subject breathing FGF at 1 L/min air plus 0.050 L/min oxygen from a semiclosed breathing circuit (Ohmeda Modulus 2+ CD anesthesia machine with a GMS absorber assembly). After 12 minutes, FiO_2 fell to 8% and SpO_2 fell to 82% when the demonstration was terminated.

MACHINE REQUIREMENTS

For an anesthesia machine to facilitate administration of closed-circuit anesthesia, several specifications should be met (Box 26-1).

USING TODAY'S TECHNOLOGY: PRACTICALITIES

As of 2012, anesthesia machines generally did not meet all the requirements for closed-circuit anesthesia; some needs were met, but some were not. The two largest manufacturers that supply the U.S. market and the rest of the world have introduced anesthesia machines that provide control of end-tidal anesthetic agent concentration and control of inspired (Dräger) or end-expired (GE Healthcare) oxygen concentration. To maintain constant levels of these variables, such machines use low to very low FGFs but not a closed circuit. To change these variables, they use an FGF higher than what most anesthesiologists practicing closed-circuit anesthesia with an older machine would use.

GE Healthcare anesthesia delivery systems have a particular limitation. Their gas monitoring module draws a reference flow of room air to the oxygen sensor at a rate of 27 to 45 mL/min. This additional air exits with the sampled gas. In the United States, where end-tidal control is not available, sample gas return is not FDA approved; however, in others countries, it is. Clinicians performing manual closed-circuit anesthesia have always returned sampled gas to the breathing circuit to quantify the true closed-circuit flows. With GE Healthcare gas monitors, when sampled gas is returned to the circuit, its room-air content lowers circuit concentration of oxygen, agent, and nitrous oxide while increasing circuit volume and making the bellows rise. This breaks the simplicity and accuracy of closed-circuit anesthesia whenever monitors such as this are used, no matter what anesthesia delivery system is used.

BOX 26-1 Desired Attributes for a Closed-Circuit Anesthesia Delivery System

Leak-free gas delivery system
Leak-free breathing circuit
Leak-free ventilator
Low to no gas flow capability
Accurate and precise gas flow control and measurement
Accurate and precise agent delivery down to closed-circuit flow
Sample gas return not contaminated with other substances
Sample gas return approved by the U.S. Food and Drug Administration
Ability to transfer gases between manual and ventilator reservoirs
Quantitative volatile agent delivery
Tidal volume independent of fresh gas flow
Delivered agent concentration independent of fresh gas flow
Display of gas and vapor uptake and delivery

An additional limitation of the Aisys machine is that it does not allow FGF less than 200 mL/min and only allows FGF to be changed 50 mL/min at a time. When one of the goals of closed circuit-anesthesia is to quantify oxygen and agent delivery, this precision is not sufficient. The letter "X" in the module number designates that the gas monitoring module computes oxygen uptake and carbon dioxide exhalation. This is computed using the on-airway gas monitoring connection.

With Aisys it is difficult to provide manual breaths intermixed with ventilator breaths in that the reservoir bag contains an older concentration than does the ventilator bellows. Mechanical techniques of transferring gas between bag and bellows by giving a breath to the patient from one source and causing the patient to breathe to the other is difficult because of the immediate inspiratory ventilator phase when the "Bag/Mechanical" switch is set to mechanical ventilation.

Dräger Apollo, the highest technology Dräger machine available in the United States, allows closed-circuit anesthesia to be performed. That is, flows can be reduced to near zero, there is no electronic limitation of resolution; the vaporizer functions properly over the whole range of flows; and there is no room air contamination of the sampled gas, which is returned to the circuit whether low FGF is used or not. Also, the reservoir bag is in the circuit during both mechanical and manual ventilation; thus ventilation can be switched from bag to ventilator at any time and not change breathing circuit concentration of any gas. A fresh gas wizard encourages FGF as low as 0.5 L/min but gives a warning with lower FGF, even when it is within reasonable closed-circuit ranges, well above the patient's metabolic and distributive needs.

Dräger Fabius and Tiro series machines have all the Apollo features except the low-flow wizard. They do not come with an integral gas monitor, so the closed-circuit practitioner should choose one that does not entrain room air into the sample gas return. Dräger Zeus is approved and available in many countries, including Canada. It uses very different technology than other anesthesia machines and uses low but not closed-circuit flows.

Most other anesthesia machines on the world market will allow conventional closed-circuit anesthesia. With some, the user must implement sample gas return with an appropriate connector. New standards for small connectors are in the process of change.

To provide liquid injection, adapters are typically purchased specially or are fabricated by the user. Many configurations are used,[52] but none is ideal. Figure 26-22 shows an example of a system I use for inspiratory liquid injection and expiratory sample gas return. Here it is implemented on a Dräger Fabius GS anesthesia machine. The plastics shown are all compatible with both sevoflurane and desflurane. The Cardinal Health (Miamisburg, OH) bronchodilator inhaler product has a Silastic cover over a tiny hole, which allows liquid anesthetic injection through the silastic cover via a needle. In addition to plastic/anesthetic compatibility concerns, components for liquid injection must be selected to reduce the likelihood of unintentional overdose from unintended excess liquid agent being injected into the circuit. The plastic syringe shown provides the static friction that glass lacks. The 23-gauge standard needle (shown) or a 22-gauge spinal needle provides resistance to liquid flow, and the bend in the needle inverts the syringe to offset the effect of gravity on the plunger.

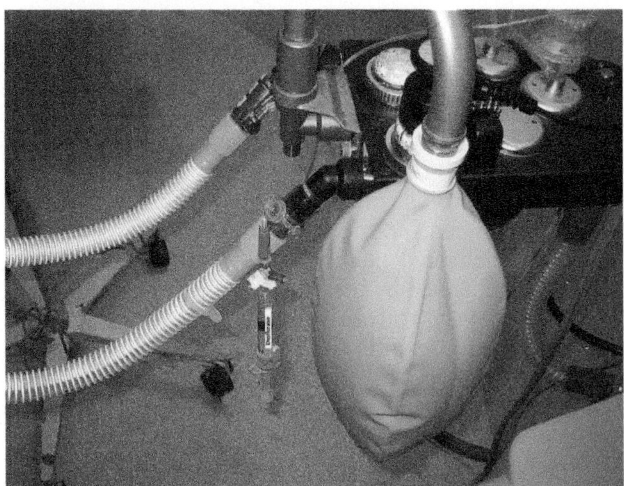

FIGURE 26-22 ■ Liquid anesthetic agent injection system that can be used in a closed-circuit system. Note that the syringe barrel is up. This averts the possibility that vaporized anesthetic forces liquid anesthetic into the breathing circuit, which presents a hazard with desflurane.

Whenever desflurane liquid is placed in a syringe, the syringe should never be directed downward. When the syringe is directed downward, any liquid formed from vaporization will push liquid desflurane out of the bottom of the syringe and into the breathing circuit. Desflurane has a vapor/liquid volume ratio of 209. Therefore, if 1 mL of vapor is formed at the top of the syringe, it will force 1 mL of liquid desflurane out of the bottom of the syringe; this liquid volume will form 209 mL of desflurane vapor. When the desflurane syringe is directed upward, when 1 mL of vapor is formed, only that 1 mL of vapor leaves the syringe and enters the breathing circuit. To attach the syringe to the breathing circuit, it is useful to bend the needle that links the syringe to the breathing circuit adapter. This holds it in place while pointing the syringe upward. The presence of a bent needle, a clear caution label, and the statement of the drug name combine to increase the safety of this technique. If a syringe pump is to be used for liquid infusion into the breathing circuit, a bent 22-gauge spinal needle allows reasonable freedom of motion for the pump. Some syringe pump infusion tubing sets are not compatible with any inhaled anesthetic liquid, so special caution must be exercised when using them. One example is the tubing for the Infuse-OR syringe pump (Baxter, Deerfield, IL), which is well suited for agent injection by bolus plus infusion.

IDIOSYNCRASIES OF CONTEMPORARY ANESTHESIA MACHINES

Some contemporary anesthesia machines make the administration of closed-circuit anesthesia difficult. The aging Dräger Narkomed series presents several unique impediments. FGF below 300 mL/min is difficult to produce, and nitrous oxide cannot be administered without sounding an alarm when oxygen flow is below 1 L/min. The bag/ventilator selector valve has a water-venting hole that must be occluded to prevent a slow loss of reservoir-bag gas to the room during mechanical ventilation. On this machine, end-expiratory bellows height determines delivered tidal volume. Specifically, inspiration is accomplished by bellows descent from its starting volume downward to zero volume. Thus as circuit volume changes, end-expiratory bellows height changes, and tidal volume changes follow.

The aging Ohmeda Modulus II (GE Healthcare) machine facilitates closed-circuit administration in several ways. An optional factory or field modification provides calibrated oxygen flow as low as 50 mL/min. Calibration resolution is no better than 50 mL/min, however. Up to 75% nitrous oxide can be delivered at any oxygen flow, and concentrations above this are prevented by a chain linking the oxygen and nitrous oxide flow-control needle valves (see Chapter 2). The 75% limitation still precludes closed-circuit nitrous oxide induction, which requires 2 L/min nitrous oxide for a brief period, while oxygen consumption is only 250 mL/min.

The Modulus II system has no intentional circuit leaks, and incorrect bellows position (within limits) does not affect tidal volume during mechanical ventilation. This is accomplished by a fixed volume of driving gas compressing the bellows, which delivers the actual inspired tidal volume. Inspired tidal volume diminishes only when volume in the bellows is insufficient. This causes an alarm to sound.

The separate control for ventilator setting and ventilator-in-circuit provides a unique but subtle advantage. In low-flow or closed-circuit circumstances, when the ventilation source is switched from bag to ventilator, it is important that there be sufficient gas in the ventilator bellows to provide the set tidal volume; insufficient bellows volume at the transition time is a significant problem in many anesthesia delivery systems. This transition is accomplished with the Modulus II by squeezing the reservoir bag to give a tidal volume to the patient and sliding the "Bag/Vent" lever to "Vent." The patient's exhaled tidal volume then fills the bellows. As soon as the bellows is sufficiently filled (~1 second) and the ventilator is turned on by the clinician, a proper tidal volume is delivered. The danger of independent controls for mechanical connection and ventilator operation made this independence dangerous, and it is not present on later machines. However, bellows filling from the patient's exhaled gas could be accomplished if there were a 1- to 2-second delay before inspiration began when the combined switch was set to "Vent."

Anesthesia Machines in the United States

Dräger Apollo, Fabius, and Tiro are all capable of FGF down to 100 mL/min. Apollo has sample gas returned to the breathing circuit via internal connections, so the user need not make any changes. Apollo guides the user to use flows less than 500 mL in excess of patient uptake. The Datex-Ohmeda (GE Healthcare) Aestiva allows FGF down to zero, but there is no connection for sample gas return. The Datex-Ohmeda Aespire and Avance allow FGF as low as 50 mL/min, but there is no connection for sample gas return. The Aisys has 200 mL/min minimum oxygen flow with 50 mL/min increments. Aisys air flow is zero, 100 mL/min, and higher with 50 mL/min increments. There is no connection for sample gas return, and if sample gas is returned from a GE monitor, room airflow of 10 to 40 mL/min accompanies it. This makes Aisys difficult to use for closed-circuit anesthesia. Box 26-1 shows closed-circuit attributes of anesthesia delivery systems available in the United States as of the time of this writing.

THE FUTURE

The future of closed-circuit anesthesia is uncertain. Although it has been practiced and advocated for many years, closed-circuit anesthesia is currently used only in a few centers and only by a small number of individuals in the United States. Obstacles to its practice fall into two categories: technological and philosophical.

The technological encumbrances to closed-circuit anesthesia were described earlier in this chapter. They make closed-circuit administration inconvenient. Philosophical encumbrances usually center on issues of safety. Even though this issue has been adequately addressed,[29,53,54] lack of an obvious relationship between control settings and inspired gas is disconcerting to many practitioners. Monitoring of inspired and expired gas tensions and exhaled volume becomes more critical. Finally, a greater understanding of drug kinetics is required for a full understanding of the technique.

In Europe, closed-circuit anesthesia has had equipment to support it.[55] The PhysioFlex[56,57] anesthesia machine (Dräger Medical) was introduced in the late 1980s. It provided automated closed-circuit anesthesia. The Dräger Zeus was introduced in 2003 in Europe, and it provides near–closed-circuit anesthesia when possible while controlling end-expired anesthetic concentration and inspired oxygen concentration. The Zeus was introduced in Canada in 2011.

SUMMARY

Closed-circuit anesthesia is a technique that maintains a constant anesthetic state by adding gases and vapors to the breathing circuit at the same rate that the patient's body redistributes (stores) or eliminates them. Some practitioners use liquid anesthetic injection at prescribed time intervals using the empiric square-root-of-time model; others monitor and maintain inspired or expired anesthetic tensions using a gas monitor that returns analyzed gas to the breathing circuit. A commercial almost–closed-circuit anesthesia machine is available in Europe.

REFERENCES

1. Bengston JP, Bengston A, Stenqvist O: The circle system as a humidifier, *Br J Anaesth* 63:453–457, 1989.
2. Lowe HJ: *Dose regulated Penthrane (methoxyflurane) anesthesia*, Chicago, 1972, Abbott Laboratories.
3. Lowe HJ, Mackrell TN, Mostert JW, et al: Quantitative closed circuit anesthesia, *Anesthesiol Rev* 12:16–19, 1974.
4. Aldrete JA, Lowe HJ, Virtue RW, editors: *Low flow and closed system anesthesia*, New York, 1979, Grune and Stratton.
5. Lowe HJ, Ernst EA: *The quantitative practice of anesthesia: use of closed circuit*, Baltimore, 1981, Williams & Wilkins.
6. Severinghaus JW: The rate of uptake of nitrous oxide in man, *J Clin Invest* 33:1183–1189, 1954.
7. Connor CW, Philip JH: The Severinghaus square root of time relationship for anesthetic uptake and its implications for the stability of compartmental pharmacokinetics, *Physiol Meas* 29:685–701, 2008. Available online at http://iopscience.iop.org/0967-3334/29.
8. Connor CW, Philip JH: Closed-form solutions for the optimum equivalence of first-order compartmental models and their implications for classical models of closed-circuit anesthesia, *Physiol Meas* 30:N11–N21, 2009.
9. Zuntz N: Zu Pathogenese und Therapie der durch rasche luft druck anderungen erzeliegten krankheiten, *Fortschr Med* 15:632, 1897.
10. Kleiber M: Body size and metabolism, *Hilgardia* 6:315–353, 1932.
11. Brody S: *Bioenergetics and growth*, New York, 1945, Reinhold.
12. Lowe HJ, Hagler K: Clinical and laboratory evaluation of an expired anesthetic gas monitor (Narko-test), *Anesthesiology* 34: 378–382, 1971.
13. Eger EI II, Guadagni NP: Halothane uptake in man at constant alveolar concentration, *Anesthesiology* 24:299–304, 1963.
14. Kety SS: The physiological and physical factors governing the uptake of anesthetic gases by the body, *Anesthesiology* 11:517–526, 1950.
15. Kety SS: The theory and application of the exchange of inert gas at the lungs and tissues, *Pharmacol Rev* 3:1–41, 1951.
16. Philip JH: Gas Man: an example of goal-oriented computer-assisted teaching which results in learning, *Int J Clin Mon* 3:165–173, 1986.
17. Garfield JM, Paskin S, Philip JH: An evaluation of the effectiveness of a computer simulation of anesthetic uptake and distribution as a teaching tool, *Med Educ* 23:457–462, 1989.
18. Eger EI, Shafer SL: Context-sensitive decrement times for inhaled anesthetics, *Anesth Analg* 101:688–696, 2005.
19. Bouillon T, Shafer S: (Editorial) Hot air or full steam ahead? An empirical pharmacokinetic model of potent inhaled agents, *Br J Anaesth* 84:429–431, 2000.
20. Eger EI II: *Anesthetic uptake and action*, Baltimore, 1974, Williams & Wilkins.
21. Mapleson WW: An electrical analogue for the uptake and exchange of inert gases and other agents, *J Appl Physiol* 18:197–204, 1963.
22. MacKrell TN: An electrical teaching model. In Papper EM, Kitz RJ, editors: *Uptake and distribution of anesthetic agents*, New York, 1963, McGraw-Hill, pp 215–223.
23 Leroux JG, Booij LH: Model-based administration of inhalation anaesthesia 1. Developing a system model, *Br J Anaesth* 86:12–28, 2001.
24. Gravenstein JS: Training devices and simulators, *Anesthesiology* 69:295–297, 1988.
25. Eger EI, Bahlman SH: Is the end-tidal anesthetic partial pressure an accurate measure of the arterial anesthetic partial pressure? *Anesthesiology* 35:301–303, 1971.
26. Bito H, Ikeda K: Closed-circuit anesthesia with sevoflurane in humans: effects on renal and hepatic function and concentrations of breakdown products with soda lime in the circuit, *Anesthesiology* 80:71–76, 1994.
27. Kharasch ED, Powers KM, Artru AA: Comparison of Amsorb, sodalime, and Baralyme degradation of volatile anesthetics and formation of carbon monoxide and compound A in swine in vivo, *Anesthesiology* 96:173–182, 2002.
28. ECRI Health Devices Alerts, October 8, 2004, Vol 28, No. 41.
29. Ernst EA, MacKrell TN, Pearson JD, et al: Patient safety: a comparison of open and closed anesthesia circuits [abstract], *Anesthesiology* 67(3A):A474, 1987.
30. Epstein HG: Removal of ether vapour during anaesthesia, *Lancet*114–116, 1944.
31. Hawes DW, Ross JAS, White WC, et al: Servo-control of closed circuit anaesthesia, *Br J Anaesth* 54:229–230, 1982.
32. Ernst EA: Use of charcoal to rapidly decrease depth of anesthesia while maintaining a closed circuit, *Anesthesiology* 57:343, 1982.
33. Baumgarten RK: Simple charcoal filter for closed circuit anesthesia, *Anesthesiology* 63:125, 1985. (letter).
34. Jantzen JP: More on black and white granules in the closed circuit, *Anesthesiology* 69:437–438, 1988. (letter).
35. Birgenheier N, Stoker R, Westenskow D, Orr J: Activated charcoal effectively removes inhaled anesthetics from modern anesthesia machines, *Anesth Analg* 112:1363–1370, 2011.
36. Huffman LM, Riddle RT: Mass spectrometer and/or capnograph use during low-flow, closed circuit anesthesia administration [letter], *Anesthesiology* 66:439–440, 1987.
37. Mushlin PS, Mark JB, Elliott WR, et al: Inadvertent development of subatmospheric airway pressure during cardiopulmonary bypass, *Anesthesiology* 71:459–462, 1989.
38. Keenan RL, Boynan CP: Cardiac arrest due to anesthesia: a study of arrest incidents and causes, *JAMA* 253:2373, 1985.
39. Morita S: Inspired gas contamination by non-anesthetic gases during closed-circuit anesthesia, *Journal of the Society for Closed Circuit Anesthesia* 2:24–25, 1985.
40. Sharp JH, Trudell JR, Cohen EN: Volatile metabolites and decomposition products in man, *Anesthesiology* 50:2, 1979.
41. Eger EI II: Dragons and other scientific hazards, *Anesthesiology* 50:1, 1979. (editorial).
42. Eger EI II: *Enflurane: a compendium and reference*, ed 3, Madison, WI, 1985, Anaquest.
43. Eger EI II: *Isoflurane: a compendium and reference*, ed 2, Madison, WI, 1985, Anaquest.
44. Eger EI II: Stability of I-653 in soda lime, *Anesth Analg* 66:983–985, 1987.
45. Hanaki C, Fujii K, Morio M, et al: Decomposition of sevoflurane by soda lime, *Hiroshima J Med Sci* 36:61–67, 1987.
46. Speiss W: To what degree should we be concerned about carbon monoxide accumulation in closed circuit anesthesia? *Journal of the Society for Closed Circuit Anesthesia* 1:8, 1984.
47. Barton FL, Nunn JF: Use of refractometry to determine nitrogen accumulation in closed circuits, *Br J Anaesth* 47:346–349, 1975.
48. Philip JH: Nitrogen buildup in a closed circuit [abstract], *Anesthesiology* 73:A465, 1990.
49. Bengston JP, Sonander H, Stenqvist O: Denitrogenation and low flow anesthesia, *Journal of the Society for Closed Circuit Anesthesia* 5:8–9, 1988.
50. Morita S, Latta W, Hambro K, et al: Accumulation of methane, acetone and nitrogen in the inspired gas during closed-circuit anesthesia, *Anesth Analg* 64:343–347, 1985.
51. Hendrickx JF, van Zundert AA, de Wolf AM: Influence of the reference gas of paramagnetic oxygen analyzers on nitrogen concentrations during closed-circuit anesthesia, *J Clin Monit Comput* 14(6):381–384, 1998.
52. Aldrete JA: Vaporizing adaptors as injection ports for closed anesthesia system, *Journal of the Society for Closed Circuit Anesthesia* 2:26–28, 1985.
53. Petrella WK: Enhanced discovery of anesthesia related events: an analysis of 400 consecutive low-flow and closed-circuit cases, *Journal of the Society for Closed Circuit Anesthesia* 6:14–15, 1989.
54. Hylani MA: Closed circuit anesthesia, *Middle East J Anesthesiol* 8:505–510, 1986.
55. Droh R, Spintge R: *Closed-circuit system and other innovations in anaesthesia*, Berlin, 1986, Springer-Verlag.
56. Rolly G, Versichelen L, Verkaaik, et al: Mass spectrometry analysis of a new closed circuit anesthesia apparatus (PhysioFlex), *Journal of the Society for Closed Circuit Anesthesia* 6:5–6, 1989.
57. Verkaail AP, Erdmann W: Respiratory diagnostic possibilities during closed circuit anaesthesia, *Acta Anaesthesiol Belg* 41:177–188, 1990.

CHAPTER 27

ANESTHESIA DELIVERY IN THE MRI ENVIRONMENT*

Keira P. Mason • Robert S. Holzman

CHAPTER OUTLINE

OVERVIEW

Familiarity with anesthesia equipment, the environment, and basic monitoring principles are vital to the safe and successful administration of anesthesia in the magnetic resonance imaging (MRI) environment. Equipment design and knowledge of the principles of monitoring in the MRI environment requires a thorough understanding of the effects of the magnetic field and the underlying principles behind the challenges, limitations, and even the location of MR imaging equipment.

In 1986, the American Society of Anesthesiologists (ASA) first established standards for monitoring during anesthesia and subsequently delineated specific standards for the delivery of anesthesia and sedation in sites distant to the operating room (OR).[1] Recognizing that not all care in areas outside the OR require anesthesia, the ASA and other nonanesthesia specialty societies followed with guidelines for sedation and analgesia. In the 1990s, the American Academy of Pediatrics (AAP),[2] American College of Emergency Physicians (ACEP),[3] and American Academy of Pediatric Dentists (AAPD)[4] published sedation guidelines. In 1996, the ASA introduced their guidelines for the administration of sedation and analgesia by nonanesthesiologists; these guidelines were updated in 2010.[5,6]

The Joint Commission has published guidelines to encourage uniformity and documentation of monitoring at locations throughout the hospital.[5] The delivery of anesthesia and sedation in the MRI environment would fall under the guidelines and regulations not only of the ASA but also of The Joint Commission, other specialty organizations, and the Center for Medicaid and Medicare Services (CMS). In 2009 the CMS published its *Revised Hospital Anesthesia Services Interpretive Guidelines—State Operations Manual* (SOM); these were subsequently updated in 2010 and 2011.[7,8] This document defined deep sedation as falling under anesthesia services. The term *deep sedation* was clearly defined: "a drug-induced depression of consciousness during which patients cannot be easily aroused but respond purposefully following repeated or painful stimulation. The ability to independently maintain ventilatory function may be impaired. Patients may require assistance in maintaining a patent airway, and spontaneous ventilation may be inadequate. Cardiovascular function is usually maintained."

Accordingly, the CMS guidelines indicate that the administration of deep sedation should be limited to a 1) qualified anesthesiologist; 2) doctor of medicine or osteopathy (other than an anesthesiologist); 3) dentist, oral surgeon, or podiatrist qualified to administer anesthesia under state law; 4) certified registered nurse anesthetist (CRNA), or 5) anesthesiologist's assistant under the supervision of an anesthesiologist who is immediately available if needed.[7] These guidelines triggered the restructuring of those sedation programs that had been delivering sedation by providers no longer approved by the CMS. One such example is Boston Children's Hospital, which in November 2010 replaced registered nurses with nurse anesthetists, pediatricians, and anesthesiologists as the providers of deep sedation. Coincident with this restructuring, anesthesiologists have now become more prevalent providers in the MRI environment with a coincident sensitivity to the importance of establishing guidelines for safe practices in the MRI environment.

Many of the challenges encountered with anesthesia delivery and physiologic monitoring in the MRI environment have now been addressed. Technologic advances over the past decade have yielded monitoring, equipment, and devices that are more consistent, reliable, and valuable in the magnetic environment. As anesthesiologists

*Portions of this chapter are from Mason KP, Holzman RS: Anesthesia and sedation for procedures outside the operating room. In Davis PJ, Cladis F, Motoyama EK, editors: *Smith's Anesthesia for Infants and Children*, ed 8, Philadelphia, 2011, Elsevier, pp 1041-1057.

become more prevalent in the MRI environment, they have coincidentally taken a more active role in the design, layout, space allotment, and equipment acquisition of new MRI units.

This chapter outlines some of the basic principles of magnetic fields as well as the challenges and limitations to delivering anesthesia, deep sedation, or monitored anesthesia in the MRI environment. It includes a detailed review of the latest monitors, equipment, and devices.

MRI PHYSICS AND CLINICAL APPLICATIONS

Imaging by magnetic resonance was first described by Rabi in 1939, the first human images were produced in 1977, and the first commercial scanner was introduced in 1990.[9-11] The physics behind MR imaging relies on the integrity of the magnetic field. Atoms with an odd number of protons and/or neutrons are capable of acting as magnets. When they are aligned in a static magnetic field, they can be subjected to radiofrequency (RF) energy that alters their original orientation. With removal of the RF pulse, the nuclei rotate back to their original alignment (relaxation), and the energy released can be detected and transformed into an image. Hydrogen is the atom most often used for imaging, as it is present in most tissues as water and long-chain triglycerides.

The application of MRI studies is far reaching, and MRI is used for the evaluation of neoplasms, trauma, skeletal abnormalities, and vascular anatomy.[12] Brain MRIs are frequently performed to evaluate developmental delay, behavioral disorders, seizures, failure to thrive, apnea/cyanosis, hypotonia, and mitochondrial and metabolic disorders. MR angiography (MRA) and MR venography (MRV) are especially helpful in evaluating vascular flow and can sometimes replace invasive catheterization studies for follow-up or initial evaluations of vascular malformations, interventional treatment, or radiotherapy.[13] Functional MRI (fMRI) is an evolving technology that measures the hemodynamic or even metabolic response related to neural activity in the brain or spinal cord, and fMRI is often able to localize sites of brain activation. As a result, it is now dominating brain mapping techniques because of its low invasiveness and lack of radiation exposure.[14-17]

Some fMRI studies require cognitive facility that demands a conscious and responsive patient. It is unclear how fMRI studies of children unable to respond appropriately, either because of age or cognitive compromise, will evolve in pediatric anesthesiology practice. Recently, dynamic MRI airway studies have used three-dimensional (3D) reconstruction of the images to visualize areas of airway collapse, tracheomalacia, or compromise.[18,19]

Historically, anesthetic management of children in the MRI suite has been highly dependent on and somewhat limited by the availability of monitors and anesthesia gas machines suitable for use in an MR suite.[20-22] The American College of Radiology (ACR) established guidelines to minimize the risk of MRI-related mishaps but did not address the needs of the anesthesiologist.[23] These guidelines were written in response to fatalities that occurred when loose, ferromagnetic oxygen cylinders became projectiles when inadvertently brought into the MRI suite with a patient in the bore of the magnet.[24] In 2008 the ASA assembled a task force composed of anesthesiologists and a radiologist with MRI expertise. This Task Force on Anesthetic Care for Magnetic Resonance Imaging created a practice advisory on anesthetic care for magnetic resonance imaging,[25] in which the MRI environment was acknowledged as a hazardous environment that challenges both the delivery of anesthesia and the ability of the anesthesiologist to monitor the patient. This document establishes important recommendations for safe practice and consistency of anesthesia care in the MRI environment. Most important, this practice advisory includes all sedation, monitored anesthesia care, general anesthesia, critical care, and ventilatory support. Conditions of *high-risk imaging* were defined as imaging in patients with risks related to health, equipment, procedure, or surgery. MRI-guided interventions, cardiac imaging, and airway imaging were all identified as high-risk procedures. The advisory was designed to promote patient and health care provider safety, prevent MRI mishaps, recognize limitations in physiologic monitoring, optimize patient management, and identify potential equipment and health risks.[25]

Anesthetic management depends on the availability of support personnel, equipment, and monitors; the personal style and comfort level of the anesthesiologist; and, of course, the patient's medical history. Requiring a general anesthetic solely to ensure motionless conditions for a radiologic imaging study is often a frightening concept for parents to embrace. They frequently equate pain and surgical interventions to the need for anesthesia and are reluctant to expose their child to a general anesthetic for an MRI study. Children younger than 5 years most commonly require moderate to deep sedation or an anesthetic to ensure motionless conditions. Pentobarbital, chloral hydrate, propofol, and dexmedetomidine have all been described as successful alternatives to inhalation anesthesia.[26-31]

In the presence of a magnetic field, anesthesiologists must be aware of many personal items, usually taken for granted, that can be a hazard: clipboards, pens, watches, scissors, clamps, credit cards, eyeglasses, paper clips, and so on.[20-22] As early as 1985, up to 24% of all MRI centers cited a projectile-related accident.[32] However, projectiles are not the only concern. Conventional electrocardiographic (ECG) monitoring is not possible during MRI because as the lead wires traverse the magnetic field, image degradation occurs; most importantly, however, the ECG leads may inductively heat and cause patient burns. Fiberoptic ECG monitoring is necessary to minimize the risk of patient burns; but even with fiberoptic cables, it is important to recognize that the connections between the ECG pads and the telemetry box are still hard wired, and careful attention must be paid to prevent frays, overlap, exposed wires, and knots in the cables.[33]

To prevent patient injury, care must be used to avoid creating a conductive loop between the patient and a conductor (ECG monitoring/gating leads, plethysmographic gating wire, and fingertip attachment). During the scan, no exposed wires or conductors can touch the patient's skin, and no imaging coil can be left unconnected to the magnet. Pulse oximeters are also not conventional, rather they are fiberoptic. Failure to remove the conventional pulse oximeter probes and adhesives has resulted in second- and third-degree burns.[33,34]

Average noise levels of 95 dB have been measured in a 1.5 Tesla (T) MRI machine, comparable to noise levels of very heavy traffic (92 dB) or light road work (90 to 110 dB). Exposure to this level of noise has not been considered hazardous if limited to less than 2 hours per day,[35] although both temporary[36] and permanent[37] hearing loss after an MRI scan have been reported. The 3-T magnet offers the advantage of less image degradation and improved neuroskeletal and musculoskeletal imaging. As the field strength increases, so does the noise.[38] In fact, the peak sound-pressure level of a 3-T magnet exceeds 99 dB, the level approved by the International Electrotechnical Commission. Noise reduction did not differ between earplugs and headphones, although the combination of both was more effective at reducing sound.[38] Earplugs or MRI-compatible headphones should be offered to all pediatric patients and are required for all patients imaged in the 3-T magnet.

Additional challenges in the 3-T environment occur with fMRI: the noise of the magnet can interfere with the acoustic stimulation generated for purposes of obtaining the fMRI.[39,40] Video goggles compatible with the 1.5-T and 3-T environments (Resonance Technology, Los Angeles) may be worn by the patient during MR imaging to provide a 3D virtual reality system complete with audio integration (see MRI Video Goggles section below). The introduction of this integrated audio-video headset has revolutionized the ability to offer distraction to patients, so that many more patients are now able to tolerate imaging without adjuvant sedation or anesthesia.

Although studies in mice[41] and dogs[42] suggest that exposure to magnetic fields may increase body temperature, it is unlikely that static magnetic fields up to 1.5 T have any effect on core body temperature in adult humans,[43] although this may be of greater concern in infants and small children, such as in cardiac MRI studies that require a long scan time. The specific absorption rate (SAR) is measured in watts per kilogram and is used to follow the effects of RF heating. The Food and Drug Administration (FDA) allows an SAR of 0.4 W/kg averaged over the whole body.[44] Ex vivo exposure of large metal prostheses to fields over six times that experienced in MRI have not revealed any appreciable heating.[45] To date, no conclusive evidence has shown that RF is a significant clinical issue in magnets up to 3 T.

The biologic effects of MRI should be considered when offering parents of pediatric patients the opportunity to be present in the MRI suite during the induction of anesthesia or throughout a deep sedation. Although there are no reports implicating MRI in chromosomal aberrations, pregnant women, particularly during the critical periods of organogenesis, are generally not permitted in the MRI environment except in cases of a need for an emergent study or for fetal imaging. MRI scans during pregnancy are discouraged by the ACR during the first and second trimester, unless fetal imaging is required or the MRI is necessary for emergent medical care.[46] Studies in amphibians demonstrate that exposure to magnetic fields as high as 4 T do not cause any defects in embryologic development,[47] and most hospital MRI machines are 1.5 to 3 T.

Important MRI safety issues include implanted objects (i.e., cardiac pacemakers), ferromagnetic attraction creating "missiles," noise, biologic effects of the magnetic field, thermal effects, equipment issues, and claustrophobia. Some stainless steel may contain ferritic, austenitic, and martensitic components.[48-50] Martensitic alloys contain fractions of a crystal phase known as *martensite*, which has a body-centered cubic structure, is prone to stress corrosion failure, and is ferromagnetic. Austenite is formed in the hardening process of low-carbon and alloyed steels and has ferromagnetic properties. Iron, nickel, and cobalt are also ferromagnetic. For this reason, the components of *any* implanted device should be carefully researched prior to entering the magnet.

In addition, an external magnetic field may exert translational (attractive) and rotational (torque) forces on stainless steel or surgical stainless objects. Intracranial aneurysm clips, cochlear and stapedial implants, shrapnel, orthodontic devices (braces), intraorbital metallic bodies, and prosthetic limbs may move and potentially dislodge. Special precautions should be taken with cochlear implants in the 3-T environment, because those nonremovable magnets may suffer demagnetization in the scanner. Patients implanted with such devices should only undergo 3-T imaging after special precautions are taken.[51]

It is important to note that some eye makeup and tattoos may contain metallic dyes and may therefore cause ocular, periorbital, and skin irritation.[47,52] In addition, some tissue expanders used in reconstructive surgery have a magnetic port to help identify the location for intermittent injections of saline.[53] Bivona tracheostomy tubes usually contain ferrous material, although this is not specified in the package insert; these should be replaced with a Shiley tube prior to entering the MRI environment.

In the presence of an external magnetic field, ferromagnetic objects can develop their own magnetic field and become projectiles. The attractive forces created between the intrinsic and extrinsic magnetic fields can propel the ferromagnetic object toward the MRI scanner. Special note should be made of the magnet strength. Over the past few years, 1.5-T magnets have been supplanted by 3-T magnets. The field strength and magnetic force generated by a 3-T scanner is unforgiving to the careless or inadvertent introduction of a ferrous object into the environment. Placing a magnet outside the MRI scanner can be a crude, helpful, and sometimes inaccurate way to test an object. If the object is not attracted to the magnet, this is *not* an absolute indication that no ferrous material is present. More sophisticated and sensitive detectors of ferrous material have been introduced that include hand-held detectors and walk-through detectors, similar to those at airports. None of these methods of detection should supplant or eliminate the careful, methodical, face-to-face screening that should be performed on everyone and everything prior to entry into the MRI suite. Some unusual objects that have found their way into the MRI suite to become projectiles include a metal fan, pulse oximeter, shrapnel, wheelchair, cigarette lighter, stethoscope, pager, hearing aid, vacuum cleaner, calculator, hair pin, oxygen tank, prosthetic limb, pencil, insulin infusion pump, keys, watches, and steel-tipped and steel-heeled shoes.[54]

Small objects can usually be easily removed from the magnet, but large objects may be subject to so much attractive force from the magnet that it is impossible to remove them by manual force. In these circumstances, the only way to release an object attached to the scanner is by quenching the magnet, which will eliminate the magnetic field over a matter of minutes. This process is not without substantial risk: as helium gas is vented, condensation and considerable noise fills the suite. All personnel are required to vacate the suite during a quench because of a risk of hypoxic conditions, should the helium inadvertently enter the room. The specific indications for quenching a magnet were detailed in 1997 in the ACR's guidance document for safe MR practices: "Quenching the magnet (for superconducting systems only) is not routinely advised for cardiac or respiratory arrest or other medical emergency, since quenching the magnet and having the magnetic field dissipate could easily take more than a minute. Because of the risks to personnel, equipment, and physical facilities, manual magnet quenches are to be initiated only after careful consideration and preparation."[23]

Cardiac pacemakers present a special hazard in and around the MRI scanner, especially in patients who are pacemaker dependent. Most pacemakers have a reed relay switch that can be activated when exposed to a magnet of sufficient strength,[55] which could convert the pacemaker to the asynchronous mode. This is an extremely dangerous situation: At least two cases are known of patients with pacemakers who died from cardiac arrest in an MRI scanner. The autopsy of one patient determined that the death was the result of an interruption of the pacemaker in the magnetic environment.[56]

In addition to the risk of pacemaker malfunction, the risk exists for torque on the pacer or pacing leads to create a disconnect or microshock.[57] Recent studies demonstrate that with careful preparation, select patients with permanent pacemakers and implantable cardioverter-defibrillators may safely undergo imaging in the 1.5-T environment without any inhibition or activation of their device.[58] In February 2011, the first and only MRI conditional pacemaker was approved by the FDA. The Revo MRI SureScan Pacing System (Medtronic, Minneapolis, MN) is available for between $5000 and $10,000 and requires specific training of the cardiologist and radiologist prior to use.

The ACR formed a Blue Ribbon Panel on MRI Safety in 2001 to review existing safety practices and issue new guidelines. ACR guidance documents were published in 2002 and updated in 2004 and again in 2007.[23] Pediatric safety concerns were specifically addressed in the 2007 document, with specific emphasis on patient screening, sedation, and monitoring issues. Implanted cardiac pacemakers or implantable cardioverter-defibrillators (ICDs) were considered a relative contraindication to MRI, and patients with such devices should only be scanned in locations staffed with radiologists and cardiologists of appropriate expertise. The recommendation was for radiology and cardiology personnel, along with a fully stocked emergency cart, to be readily available with a programmer to adjust the device if necessary. Following the MRI, a cardiologist should confirm function of the device and recheck it within 1 to 6 weeks. In general, heart valves are not ferromagnetic and are not a contraindication to MRI. It is critical that everyone entering the vicinity of the MRI scanner fill out a screening form that specifically lists every possible implantable device, alerting the MRI staff to any potential hazards.

It is important to note that the magnetic field may affect the ECG. Changes in the T wave are not due to biologic effects of the magnetic field but rather to superimposed induced voltages. This effect of the magnetic field on the T wave is not related to cardiac depolarization because no changes to the P, Q, R, or S waves have ever been observed in patients exposed to fields up to 2 T, and no reports have been made of MRI affecting heart rate,[59] ECG recording,[60] cardiac contractility,[61] or blood pressure.[62] One study, however, found that humans exposed to a 2-T magnet for 10 minutes developed a 17% increase in the cardiac cycle length (CCL), which represented the duration of the R-R interval. The CCL reverted to preexposure length within 10 minutes of removing the patient from the magnetic field.[63] The implications of this finding are unclear, and this change in CCL in patients with normal hearts may be of no consequence; however, the implications of this finding for patients with fragile dysrhythmias or sick sinus syndrome have yet to be determined.

In 2008, The Joint Commission recognized the potential and existent hazards of the MRI environment when they published a Sentinel Event Alert that identified five MRI-related incidents and four MRI-related deaths, one from a projectile and three from cardiac events.[64] The alert specifically identified eight types of possible injury and was designed to prevent accidents and injuries in the MRI suite (Box 27-1).

It is important to recognize the ACR designation of the different zones as they pertain to the proximity of the MRI scanner. In 2002, four zones were defined relative to the magnet that were important in identifying and demarcating the safety precautions that should be taken for each zone (Table 27-1).[65]

In 1997, the FDA Center for Devices and Radiological Health (CDRH) proposed the terms *MR safe* and *MR compatible* to identify devices and equipment that could be safely brought into the MR environment. These terms were presented in the document entitled "A Primer on Medical Device Interactions with Magnetic Resonance Imaging Systems."[66]

MR safe indicates a device that did not pose a patient safety risk in the MR environment, but it does not indicate whether the MR quality will be affected; *MR compatible* devices were defined as not posing a patient safety risk *or* affecting the quality of the MR image. Furthermore, the FDA stressed that the MR environment in which the device was tested—including the static, gradient (time varying), and RF electromagnetic fields—must be specified when describing the safety and compatibility of a device. The terminology was redefined and clarified by the FDA in 2008 by eliminating the term *MR compatible* and replacing it with *MR conditional*.[67] The terminology

BOX 27-1 Accidents and Injuries in the MRI Suite

- "Missile effect" or "projectile" injury in which ferromagnetic objects (those having magnetic properties) such as ink pens, wheelchairs, and oxygen canisters are pulled into the MRI scanner at rapid velocity.
- Injury related to dislodged ferromagnetic implants such as aneurysm clips, pins in joints, and drug infusion devices.
- Burns from objects that may heat during the MRI process, such as wires (including lead wires for both implants and external devices) and surgical staples, or from the patient's body touching the inside walls (the bore) of the MRI scanner during the scan.
- Injury or complication related to equipment or device malfunction or failure caused by the magnetic field. For example, battery-powered devices (laryngoscopes, microinfusion pumps, monitors, etc.) can suddenly fail to operate; some programmable infusion pumps may perform erratically; and pacemakers and implantable defibrillators may not behave as programmed.
- Injury or complication from failure to attend to patient support systems during the MRI. This is especially true for patient sedation or anesthesia in MRI arenas. For example, oxygen canisters or infusion pumps run out, and staff must either leave the MRI area to retrieve a replacement or move the patient to an area where a replacement can be found.
- Acoustic injury from the loud knocking noise that the MRI scanner makes.
- Adverse events related to the administration of MRI contrast agents.
- Adverse events related to cryogen handling, storage, or accidental release in superconducting MRI system sites.

From The Joint Commission: *Preventing accidents and injuries in the MRI suite*, 2008. Available at http://www.jointcommission.org/assets/1/18/SEA_38.pdf.

TABLE 27-1 Zone Definitions

Zone I	All areas that are freely accessible to the general public. This area is typically outside the MR environment itself and is the area through which patients, health care personnel, and other employees of the MR site access the MR environment.
Zone II	The interface between the publicly accessible uncontrolled zone I and the strictly controlled zone III. Typically, the patients are greeted in zone II and are not free to move throughout zone II at will but rather are under the supervision of MR personnel. It is in zone II that patient histories, answers to medical insurance questions, and answers to MR imaging screening questions are typically obtained.
Zone III	The region in which free access by unscreened non-MR personnel or ferromagnetic objects or equipment can result in serious injury or death as a result of interactions between individuals or equipment and the MR scanner's particular environment. These interactions include but are not limited to those with the MR scanner's static and time-varying magnetic fields. All access to zone III is to be strictly restricted, with access to regions within it, including zone IV (see below), controlled by and entirely under the supervision of MR personnel.
Zone IV	The MR scanner magnet room. By definition, zone IV will always be located within zone III, because it is the MR magnet and its associated magnetic field, which generates the existence of zone III.

MR, magnetic resonance.

From Practice advisory on anesthetic care for magnetic resonance imaging: a report by the Society of Anesthesiologists Task Force on Anesthetic Care for Magnetic Resonance Imaging. Anesthesiology *2009; 110:459-479.*

was associated with color-coded and identifiable icons that could be used to identify all equipment and materials as *MR safe*, *MR conditional*, or *MR unsafe*. These icons were consistent with international standards for colors and shapes of safety signs (Table 27-2).[68] The terms are clear: *MR safe* items pose no known hazards in all MRI environments, regardless of field strength; *MR conditional* items pose no known hazards, but this depends on the specified MR environment; and *MR unsafe* items represent a hazard in any MR environment and should be kept out. All equipment monitors and materials should be clearly labeled with one of these identifying icons to ensure the safety of the patient, health care worker, and equipment.

MRI ANESTHESIA EQUIPMENT AND PHYSIOLOGIC MONITORS

A variety of choices of anesthesia equipment, supplementary devices, and physiologic monitors are currently available. Although most are designated as MRI conditional or MRI safe, differences between the options may have important implications on the delivery of anesthesia. The more substantive and commonly utilized choices available are reviewed below. It is important to recognize that despite the technologic advances in monitors and equipment, some limitations remain; for example, a continued limitation in the MRI environment is the ability to monitor a pulmonary artery catheter. To date, the FDA has not approved any pulmonary artery catheter for the MR environment, and no monitor or device with MR conditional labeling is yet equipped with electronic record keeping, which still needs an interface to download data.

Physiologic Monitors

Invivo

Invivo (Gainesville, FL) is a branch of Philips Electronics that produces the Expression, an MR conditional physiologic monitor approved by the FDA in 2009 (Fig. 27-1). The Expression is approved for function at the 5000 gauss (G) line and is MRI conditional with 1.5- and 3-T magnets to 5000 G. In general, for an actively shielded 1.5-T scanner, this monitor could be adjacent to the bore of the magnet and approximately 1 foot from the bore of a 3-T scanner.

The main monitor weighs 16 lb inclusive of the battery and has up to 8 hours of battery life. In addition to the main monitor is a remote monitor that communicates and interacts with the main monitor. This monitor is usually placed in zone 3, which enables the health care provider to monitor the patient during MRI without being exposed to the noise and magnetic field of zone 4.

TABLE 27-2 Requirements for Colored Magnetic Resonance Icons

Icon Geometric Shape and Appearance	Meaning
A square MR or MR	MR Safe
An equilateral triangle with rounded outer corners MR	MR Conditional
A circle with a diagonal bar MR	MR Unsafe

From ASTM F2503-08, Standard Practice for Marking Medical Devices and Other Items for Safety in the Magnetic Resonance Environment. Copyright ASTM International, 100 Barr Harbor Drive, West Conshohocken, PA, 19428.

At this time, the Expression is the only monitor on the market that offers core temperature monitoring. A disposable probe is fiberoptic and may be used for axillary, rectal, or esophageal temperature monitoring in the 1.5-T and 3-T MRI scanners. Invivo monitors are unique in that they offer wireless ECG and pulse oximetry monitoring. These wireless modules are operated by batteries that hold a charge for up to 8 hours. The batteries of the monitor display remaining power in time and not percentages, facilitating the planning of battery replacement and charge. Two ECG leads may be monitored simultaneously, and the company claims to have developed algorithms to minimize artifact that can occur during advanced imaging sequences. A pneumatic respiration monitor encircles the chest circumferentially and is able to detect respiratory rate, and the pulse oximeter offers a variety of different size probes: two alligator-style clips for older children and adults and four adhesive disposable probes for neonates and infants. The disposable probes offer an advantage particularly in those children who are immunocompromised or infectious. The monitor offers both disposable and reusable noninvasive blood pressure cuffs for the limbs and thigh as well as invasive blood pressure capability that can display two locations simultaneously, such as arterial and intracranial blood pressure.

The monitor displays adaptive trend arrows to indicate the direction of change in blood pressure, temperature, and heart rate. The main monitor is equipped with a large blinking red light visible up to 360 degrees to facilitate visualization of any triggered alarms, which include physiologic thresholds and low battery.

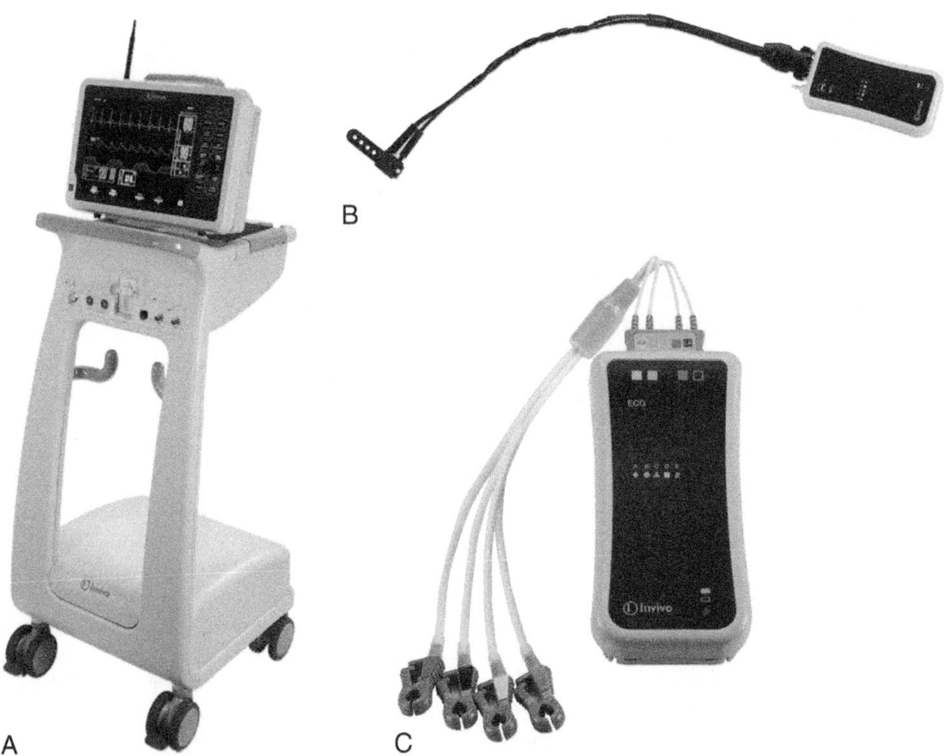

FIGURE 27-1 ■ **A,** Invivo Expression (Philips Electronics, Gainesville, FL) system, including wireless pulse oximeter (**B**) and wireless electrocardiograph (**C**).

Medrad

The Veris monitor by Medrad (Warrendale, PA) is a physiologic monitor approved by the FDA in 2004 (Fig. 27-2). It has an MRI conditional label and is restricted to a minimum of 2000 to 500 G, depending on monitor configuration. This is a six-channel monitor, able to display up to six waveforms at one time. The ECG consists of fiberoptic carbon fiber leads, virtually eliminating the risk of heat-related injury. Unlike the Expression, the Veris monitor uses an ECG module that is not wireless; it uses nonremovable batteries that can hold a charge for up to 40 hours, and charging of the battery requires charging of the ECG module. The respiratory rate is extracted from the capnograph, which is presented as a filled-in solid waveform, in contrast to the linear tracing of the Expression. The Veris can monitor up to two invasive arterial pressures, and a fiberoptic probe enables two separate, simultaneous measurements of cutaneous temperature. Two inhalation agents may be monitored and displayed simultaneously, which is particularly useful following the administration of a long general anesthetic with agents of different pharmacokinetic profiles. In addition, a variety of noninvasive blood pressure cuffs are available for both adults and children, both disposable and reusable.

In contrast to the fiberoptic technology of the Invivo pulse oximeter, the Veris is not wireless. The pulse oximeter probes that operate similar to a clothespin come in multiple sizes for both adults and children and clip on the finger or encircle the entire finger as a band. A fully charged monitor has a battery life of up to 10 hours, and the remote monitor is equipped with both audible and visible alarm indicators, is not detachable, and is mounted on a rolling stand. It requires AC power and is not battery operated.

Intravenous Infusion Delivery Systems

Two noteworthy intravenous (IV) infusion delivery systems are available for use in the MRI environment. Both use linear peristaltic technology. The Continuum (Medrad) has FDA conditional approval and may be used in the 1.5- and 3-T environment with a 3000-G limitation (see Fig. 27-2). It can be programmed in any of three modes: continuous infusion and two dose modes, either weight based or non–weight based. Alarms, both audible and visual, identify when the pump is within the 2000-G line, when there are errors in delivery or function, or when the battery is low. These alarms also may be used to identify the impending completion of a programmed dose. The entire unit must be charged because there is no removable battery, and the unit will not operate from mains with a depleted battery. A fully charged unit can deliver up to 24 hours of continuous usage at rates below 15 mL/h. It can detect air bubbles of between 0.4 and 1.0 mL but has no inlet occlusion/pressure sensing. The Continuum is FDA approved to deliver within an accuracy of 10% at ranges of 1 to 1200 mL/h and has a remote monitor that uses fiberoptic technology and a Certo Wireless network to direct the communication between the monitor and the remote (see Fig. 27-2, *D*). The remote can be used to control all but the initial program, which must be controlled at the main pump. One remote may operate up to 27 infusion pumps by changing wireless channels. The display of the remote is in color, and it can follow no more than three pumps per channel selection. These infusion pumps must be mounted securely to a wheel-locked Medrad IV pole, which can hold up to three pumps.

The MRidium 3860 infusion system (IRadimed, Winter Park, FL) uses ultrasonic motor technology and has FDA MR conditional approval for 1.5- and 3-T MRI systems up to 10,000 G. It can be programmed in multiple modes, both continuous infusion and dose modes (weight and non–weight based or over time). The system has bubble/air detection as well as inlet and outlet occlusion and pressure sensing with full alarm reporting and history. MRidium also offers an integrated pulse oximeter as an option that uses Masimo technology, which can monitor and display oxygen saturation both inside and outside the MRI environment (Fig. 27-3). A reusable fiberoptic pulse oximeter with three probe sizes and a 7.5-foot cable extends from the back of the pump to the patient. The MRidium also has a wireless remote control that allows programming and viewing of the pump, and it can accommodate one attached "side car," allowing for delivery of a second IV infusion. The MRidium delivers at rates from 0.1 to 1400 mL/h, and the battery is removable for charging and has a life of up to 12 hours. Both the Continuum and MRidium can accommodate customized medication programs. The MRidium can also come with preset options for dexmedetomidine, dobutamine, adenosine, and propofol delivery in their respective appropriate units at generally accepted dosing.

Anesthesia Machines

The Dräger Fabius MRI (Dräger Medical, Telford, PA) anesthesia workstation was FDA approved in 2008 as MRI conditional for the 1.5-T and 3-T environment up to a field strength of 400 G (Fig. 27-4). The Fabius is equipped with a Teslameter that emits an acoustic signal when the machine reaches the 400 G perimeter. The Fabius is equipped with two vaporizers and uses an electronically controlled ventilator able to deliver multiple modes of ventilation in the MRI suite. These include spontaneous, volume- and pressure-controlled, pressure-support mode, synchronized intermittent mechanical ventilation (SIMV), and SIMV with pressure support. The ventilator may be mounted on either the right or left side to accommodate the logistics of a particular MRI environment. The alarms, large and visible, are equally flexible with respect to ease of use and visibility: they are redundant on both the right and left side. The Fabius is on wheels to facilitate easy mobility in the MRI suite. It has castors around each wheel, however, to reduce unwanted movement. Two vaporizers may be mounted on the Fabius simultaneously. The machine can be equipped with either an interlock or an autoexclusion system to ensure that only one vaporizer is turned on at a time. The Fabius is plugged into the wall and accommodates pin indexed E cylinders and gas from a central source. Even without a power supply, the Fabius can still

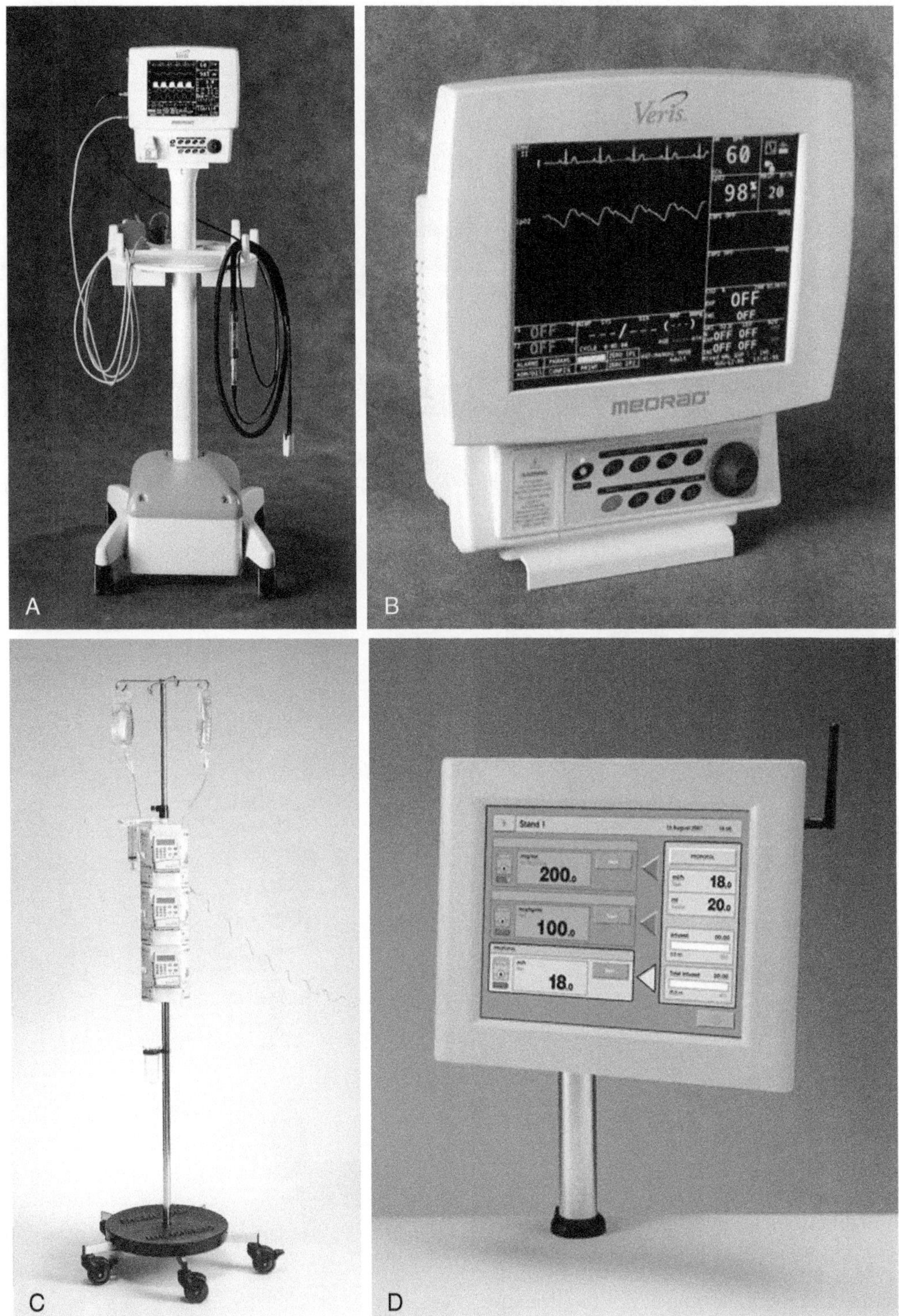

FIGURE 27-2 ■ Veris (**A**) (Medrad, Warrendale, PA) magnetic resonance monitor (**B**) and remote display **C,** Medrad Continuum, a three-unit modular intravenous fluid administration system, and wireless remote display (**D**).

deliver gas and permit the use of vaporizers. The internal battery can function for a minimum of 45 minutes in the event of a power failure. The ventilator is piston driven, so even in the event of a compressed gas supply failure, the ventilator will still function to ventilate the patient by entraining room air. This is a significant advancement in the safe delivery of anesthesia in the MRI environment. Gas-driven bellows ventilators require a supply of compressed gas to function; in the event of a gas supply failure, they would be unable to function. Manual ventilation using the reservoir bag would also not be possible.

Ohmeda

The Datex-Ohmeda Aestiva 5 (GE Healthcare, Waukesha, WI) is an MRI compatible anesthesia workstation

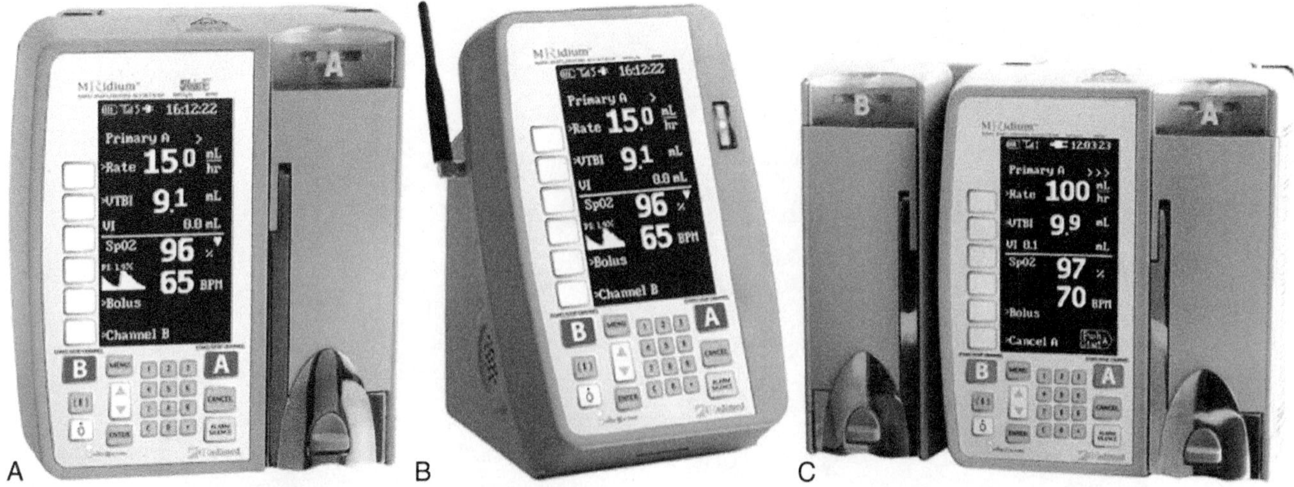

FIGURE 27-3 ■ MRidium pump (IRadimed, Winter Park, FL). **A,** Pump 3860, 3860+ with pulse oximetry. **B,** MRidium remote 3865 wireless. **C,** The Side Car pump module can be attached to Model 3860 MRidium MRI infusion pump to provide a second channel for infusion delivery.

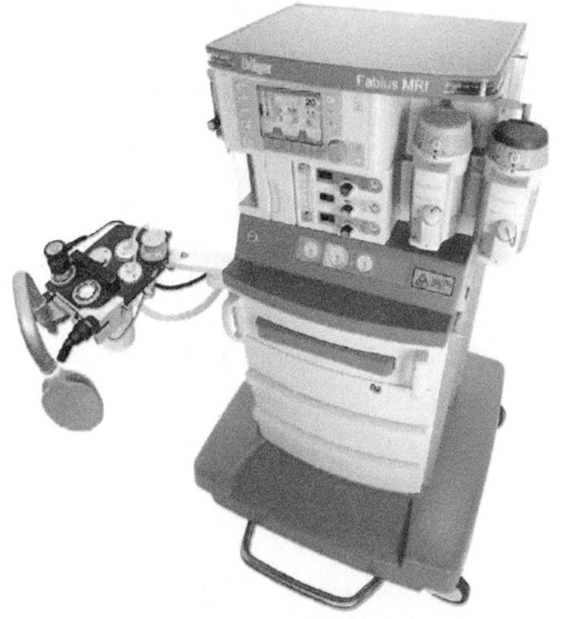

FIGURE 27-4 ■ Dräger Fabius (Dräger Medical, Telford, PA).

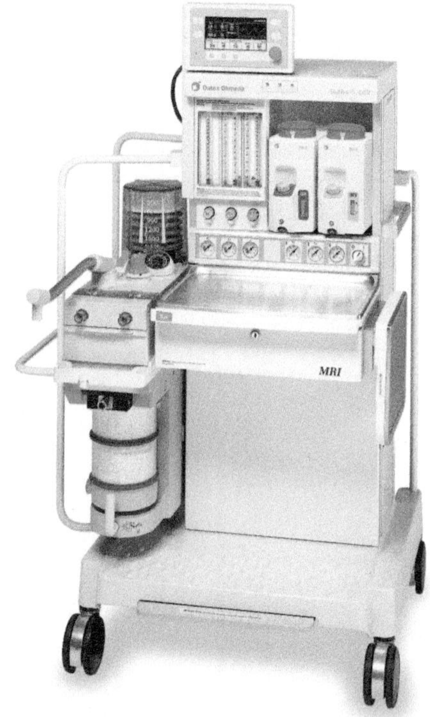

FIGURE 27-5 ■ Datex-Ohmeda Aestiva/5 (GE Healthcare, Waukesha, WI).

that was FDA approved in 2000 for use within both a 1.5-T and 3-T magnetic field environment up to a field strength of 300 G (Fig. 27-5). In 2005, GE Healthcare was the first to provide spontaneous support modes of ventilation in the MRI environment, adding PSVPro (Pressure Support Ventilation) and SIMV with pressure-support ventilation. In addition, the Aestiva offers volume-controlled ventilation, pressure-controlled ventilation, and electronic positive end-expiratory pressure (PEEP)—all are a part of the Aestiva SmartVent, which uses a digitally controlled flow valve similar to some intensive care unit (ICU) ventilators on the market (GE Healthcare Engstrom Carestation, Dräger Evita, Maquet Servo I, Puritan Bennett 840) to optimize the delivery of targeted pressures.

The Aestiva MRI model has a gauss alarm that warns when the system is too close to the magnet. The breathing system is fully integrated to minimize the risk of misconnects or disconnects. All gases, nitrous oxide included, automatically shut off when the system is powered down. The vaporizer back bar accommodates two Tec 5 or Tec 7 vaporizers, and the interlock system ensures that only one is in use at a time.

Important limitations, restrictions, and precautions exist when using a ventilator in the MRI suite. Desflurane cannot be delivered in the MRI environment, regardless of the anesthesia delivery system, because the use of desflurane requires an additional power supply, whose unshielded cables can create artifact on MR images.

There is still no flexible arm for the reservoir bag; thus anesthesia providers are still limited and inflexible in their ability to position themselves to facilitate hand ventilation. There are currently no FDA-approved anesthesia machines for use in an open MR system. It is not inherently obvious that an MRI conditional anesthesia machine approved for 1.5- and 3-T environments cannot be used in the 0.35-, 0.7-, or 1-T field strength of the open magnet. However, because of the fringe fields in these environments, an unapproved anesthesia machine would be unsafe even in the lower strength magnets. General MRI safety requires that all service of the anesthesia machines be done *outside* the MRI environment. Changing of vaporizers, repairs, annual service checks, and exchanges of gas cylinders (even if MRI safe) should be done with the anesthesia machine removed from the MRI suite.

MRI VIDEO GOGGLES

The availability in 2000 of FDA-approved MRI safe audio and video systems (CinemaVision, Resonance Technology, Los Angeles) for the 1.5- and 3-T environment revolutionized the ability to advance patient care and MR imaging capability (Fig. 27-6). This system is composed of goggles worn over the eyes and an audio system worn over the ears that enable the user to observe and listen to videos with accompanying sound. The goggles are plastic, and information is transferred with fiberoptic technology. There are two transducers: one in the MRI suite to receive the fiberoptics from the connected headset and a second in the MRI control room to transmit and receive information. The transducer outside of the MRI scanner is equipped with a digital screen, radio tuner, and DVD player. The display is based on liquid crystal diode (LCD) technology. The video goggles are designed to create a virtual environment for the patient during the MRI procedure, providing goggles for visualization as well as headphones to provide acoustics. A microphone is attached to the headset, providing the patient with the ability to communicate with those in the MRI control room during the MRI study. The microphone, similar in design to those used by pilots, is sensitive enough to detect respirations. The headphones attenuate but do not eliminate all MRI-associated noise. For example, in the 3-T magnet, a 110-dB sound can be attenuated to 70 dB with the application of headphones. These headphones have provided some patients who are claustrophobic, anxious, or generally too young to remain motionless with an alternative to sedation, anxiolytics, or anesthesia. With the addition of headphones for audio, patients can attach an mp3 music player or video device and have the option of undergoing an MRI with the distraction of the video goggles.

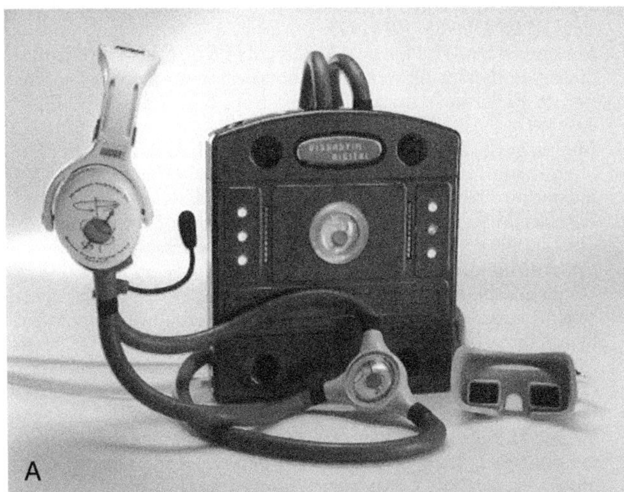

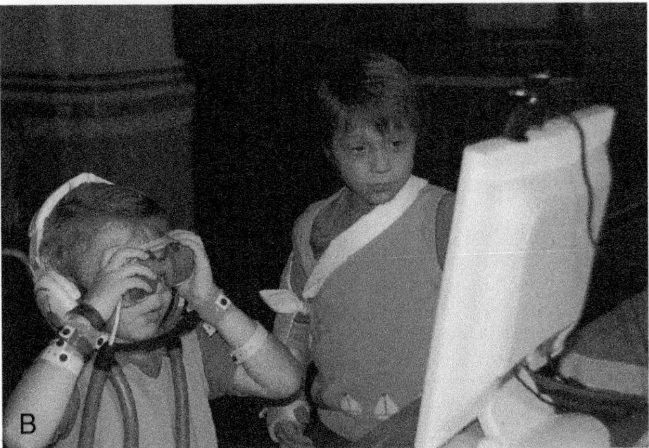

FIGURE 27-6 ■ CinemaVision (Resonance Technology, Los Angeles, CA). **A,** Earphone, headset, and video apparatus. **B,** Children becoming familiar with the system.

These goggles have also revolutionized the ability to perform sophisticated MRI studies that have been described as "functional imaging." For example, the goggles can come with built-in cameras that can track eye movements. Thus in response to specified audio or visual stimulation, the camera can track the eye response and relay the information to a computer, and it can take up to 60 photos per second. By tracking the center of the pupil, precise eye movements can be followed and compared with specific images of the brain. A newer set of goggles can come with visual stimulation capabilities, which have improved optics compared with the video goggles. These optics enable text of various fonts to be sent to the patients, either to one eye or to both. Each eye can be exposed (simultaneously or sequentially) to different stimuli, and 3D images may also be relayed. The visual display can be extremely clear, with more than 1 million pixels in a half-inch area. The camera in these goggles can take up to 1000 photos per second. These goggles are also used for fMRI, superimposing the functional data with the anatomic data from the MRI study to compare brain activity responses to stimulation. This technology has been used for preoperative assessment to determine or predict which areas and functions of the brain will be spared or sacrificed.

The demand for anesthesia and sedation services in the MR environment is increasing, particularly as ORs are being constructed that accommodate intraoperative MR imaging.[69-71] The challenges of providing anesthesia in an MRI-equipped OR are largely based on the suite's location. Most of these MR ORs are separate and physically distant from the main surgical ORs. This distance facilitates the ability to appropriately screen all personnel entering this OR as well as to implement MRI safety standards and guidelines. These surgical suites are commonly reserved only for those procedures that require intraoperative MRI. There are some institutions, such as Boston Children's Hospital, that have the MR OR integrated into the main surgical OR environment. Adjacent to the main surgical ORs, this area is at a greater risk of having personnel unfamiliar with the MR environment obtain access. Steps to limit this include a separate keycard or password access to the MR OR and requisite MR safety training of any personnel who enter the environment, environmental service personnel included. Other challenges include the desire to use this MR-equipped OR as a normal surgical OR when it is not in use for an MR-guided procedure. Accommodating these requests requires that the OR be equipped to either perform non–MR-guided surgery with nonferrous equipment or to have the MRI unit withdrawn into a "garage" housing. When housed in this garage, there may or may not be a magnetic field in the OR. This is dependent on how the room is constructed. Obviously the OR personnel must be aware of whether the magnetic field is always on. Regardless, this OR must be vigilantly policed before the start of any MR-guided procedures for any ferrous objects that may have been brought into the OR during prior procedures.

A complete knowledge of the MRI environment, appropriate equipment, ASA guidelines for providing anesthesia services in the MRI environment, and the subtleties of the imaging studies required are all necessary for patient care. The incidence of adverse events in the MRI environment relative to other sites distant to the OR is unknown. It is interesting to note, however, that differences between office-based facilities and surgical centers exist.

Comparative outcomes analysis in Florida cites a higher incidence of adverse events in the office-based setting when compared with outpatient surgical centers.[72] Although these outcomes cannot be directly compared with the MRI environment, they may be reflective of an increased risk when MRI units are at off-site locations. Sedation, monitored anesthesia care, and general anesthesia are all choices that carry risks. Historically, an avoidance of a general anesthesia has been thought to minimize the risk of adverse outcomes. However, closed-claims analysis has shown that monitored anesthesia care poses a risk equal to that of general anesthesia with respect to severity of injury, death, and permanent brain damage. Furthermore, 24% of all monitored anesthesia care claims involve oversedation and respiratory depression.[73] In summary, anesthesia care providers must recognize that as the demand for off-site services increases, so also should their ability to understand the environment and do careful risk analysis when selecting patients and formulating a plan of care.

REFERENCES

1. Standards for basic anesthetic monitoring. In *American Society of Anesthesiologists 1998 Directory of Members*, 63rd ed, Park Ridge, IL, 1996, ASA, p 438.
2. American Academy of Pediatrics Committee on Drugs: Guidelines for monitoring and management of pediatric patients during and after sedation for diagnostic and therapeutic procedures, *Pediatrics* 89:1110–1115, 1992.
3. Sacchetti A, Schafermeyer R, Geradi M, et al: Pediatric analgesia and sedation, *Ann Emerg Med* 23:237–250, 1994.
4. Guidelines for the elective use of pharmacologic conscious sedation and deep sedation in pediatric dental patients, *Pediatr Dent* 15:297–301, 1993.
5. Practice guidelines for sedation and analgesia by non-anesthesiologists: A report by the American Society of Anesthesiologists Task Force on Sedation and Analgesia by Non-Anesthesiologists, *Anesthesiology* 84:459–471, 1996.
6. *Granting Privileges for Deep Sedation to Non-Anesthesiologist Sedation Practitioners*. Approved by the ASA House of Delegates on October 20, 2010. Available at http://www.asahq.org/publicationsAndServices/sgstoc.htm.
7. Department of Health & Human Services [DHHS], Centers for Medicare & Medicaid Services [CMS] Manual System: Pub. 100–07, State Operations Provider Certification. Transmittal 59: Clarification of the Interpretive Guidelines for the Anesthesia Services Condition of Participation. May 21, 2010. Available at https://www.cms.gov/transmittals/downloads/R59SOMA.pdf.
8. DHHS, CMS Manual System: Pub 100–07, State Operations Provider Certification. Appendix A, 42 CFR, Section 482.52. Revised hospital anesthesia services interpretive guidelines. Available at http://www.cms.gov/SurveyCertificationgeninfo/downloads/SCLetter11_10.pdf.
9. Bloch F, Hansen WW, Packard ME: Nuclear induction, *Phys Rev* 69:127, 1946.
10. Purcell EM, Torry HC, Pound CV: Resonance absorption by nuclear magnetic moments in a solid, *Phys Rev* 69, 1946.
11. Edelman R, Kleefield J, Wentz K, Atkinson D: Basic principles of magnetic resonance imaging. In Edelman R, Hesselink J, editors: *Clinical magnetic resonance imaging*, Philadelphia, 1990, WB Saunders.
12. Barnes P: Imaging of the central nervous system in pediatrics and adolescence, *Pediatr Clin North Am* 39:743, 1992.
13. Edelman RR, Warach S: Magnetic resonance imaging (Part II), *N Engl J Med* 328:785–791, 1993.
14. Macdonald PA, Macdonald AA, Seergobin KN, et al: The effect of dopamine therapy on ventral and dorsal striatum-mediated cognition in Parkinson's disease: support from functional MRI, *Brain* 134:1447–1463, 2011.
15. Miettinen PS, Pihlajamaki M, Jauhiainen AM, et al: Effect of cholinergic stimulation in early Alzheimer's disease: functional imaging during a recognition memory task, *Curr Alzheimer Res*, 2011.
16. Pavuluri MN, Passarotti AM, Lu LH, Carbray JA, Sweeney JA: Double-blind randomized trial of risperidone versus divalproex in pediatric bipolar disorder: fMRI outcomes, *Psychiatry Res*, 2011.
17. Wilde EA, Newsome MR, Bigler ED, et al: Brain imaging correlates of verbal working memory in children following traumatic brain injury, *Int J Psychophysiol*, 2011.
18. Mahmoud M, Gunter J, Sadhasivam S: Cine MRI airway studies in children with sleep apnea: optimal images and anesthetic challenges, *Pediatr Radiol* 39:1034–1037, 2009.
19. Saigusa H, Suzuki M, Higurashi N, Kodera K: Three-dimensional morphological analyses of positional dependence in patients with obstructive sleep apnea syndrome, *Anesthesiology* 110:885–890, 2009.
20. Karlik SJ, Heatherley T, Pavan F, et al: Patient anesthesia and monitoring at a 1.5 T MRI installation, *Magn Reson Med* 7:210–221, 1988.
21. Menon DK, Peden CJ, Hall AS, Sargentoni J, Whitwam JG: Magnetic resonance for the anaesthetist. Part I: Physical principles, applications, safety aspects, *Anaesthesia* 47:240–255, 1992.
22. Tobin JR, Spurrier EA, Wetzel RC: Anaesthesia for critically ill children during magnetic resonance imaging, *Br J Anaesth* 69:482–486, 1992.
23. Kanal E, Barkovich A, Bell C, et al: ACR guidance document for Safe MR Practices: 2007, *AJR Am J Roentgenol* 188:1–27, 2007.
24. Chaljub G, Kramer L, Johnson RR, et al: Projectile cylinder accidents resulting from the presence of ferromagnetic nitrous oxide or oxygen tanks in the MR suite, *AJR Am J Roentgenol* 177:27–30, 2001.
25. American Society of Anesthesiologists Task Force on Anesthetic Care for Magnetic Resonance Imaging, Ehrenwerth J, Singleton MA, Bell C, et al: Practice advisory on anesthetic care for magnetic resonance imaging: a report by the American Society of Anesthesiologists Task Force on Anesthetic Care for Magnetic Resonance Imaging, *Anesthesiology* 110:459–479, 2009.

26. Mason KP, Zurakowski D, Zgleszewski SE, et al: High-dose dexmedetomidine as the sole sedative for pediatric MRI, *Paediatr Anaesth* 18:403–411, 2008.
27. Mason KP, Zgleszewski SE, Prescilla R, Fontaine PJ, Zurakowski D: Hemodynamic effects of dexmedetomidine sedation for CT imaging studies, *Paediatr Anaesth* 18:393–402, 2008.
28. Mason KP, Zurakowski D, Karian VE, et al: Sedatives used in pediatric imaging: comparison of IV pentobarbital with IV pentobarbital with midazolam added, *AJR Am J Roentgenol* 177:427–430, 2001.
29. Mason KP, Zurakowski D, Connor L, et al: Infant sedation for MR imaging and CT: oral versus intravenous pentobarbital, *Radiology* 233:723–728, 2004.
30. Yamamoto LG: Initiating a hospital-wide pediatric sedation service provided by emergency physicians, *Clin Pediatr (Phila)* 47:37–48, 2008.
31. Guenther E, Pribble CG, Junkins EP Jr, et al: Propofol sedation by emergency physicians for elective pediatric outpatient procedures, *Ann Emerg Med* 42:783–791, 2003.
32. Pavlicek W: Safeguarding against MRI hazards, *Diag Imaging* 2:166, 1985.
33. Shellock FG: Biological effects and safety aspects of magnetic resonance imaging, *Magn Reson Q* 5:243–261, 1989.
34. Brow TR, Goldstein B, Little J: Severe burns resulting from magnetic resonance imaging with cardiopulmonary monitoring: risks and relevant safety precautions, *Am J Phys Med Rehabil* 72:166–167, 1993.
35. Gangarosa RE, Minnis JE, Nobbe J, Praschan D, Genberg RW: Operational safety issues in MRI, *Magn Reson Imaging* 5:287–292, 1987.
36. Brummett R, Talbot J, Charuhas P: Potential hearing loss resulting from MR imaging, *Radiology* 169:539–540, 1988.
37. Kanal E, Shellock F, Talagala L: Safety considerations in MR imaging, *Radiology* 176:593–606, 1990.
38. Hattori Y, Fukatsu H, Ishigaki T: Measurement and evaluation of the acoustic noise of a 3 Tesla MR scanner, *Nagoya J Med Sci* 69:23–28, 2007.
39. Ravicz ME, Melcher JR, Kiang NY: Acoustic noise during functional magnetic resonance imaging, *J Acoust Soc Am* 108:1683–1696, 2000.
40. Menendez-Colino LM, Falcon C, Traserra J, et al: Activation patterns of the primary auditory cortex in normal hearing subjects: a functional magnetic resonance imaging study, *Acta Otolaryngol* 127:1283–1291, 2007.
41. Sperber D, Oldenbourg R, Dransfeld K: Magnetic field induced temperature change in mice, *Naturwissenschaften* 71:100–101, 1984.
42. Shuman W, Haynor D, Guy A, et al: Superficial- and deep-tissue temperature increases in anesthetized dogs during exposure to high specific absorption rates in a 1.5-T MR imager, *Radiology* 167:551–554, 1988.
43. Shellock FG, Schaefer DJ, Gordon CJ: Effect of a 1.5 T static magnetic field on body temperature of man, *Magn Reson Med* 3:644–647, 1986.
44. Food and Drug Administration: *Guidelines for evaluating electromagnetic exposure risk for trials of clinical NMR systems*, Washington, DC, 1982, Food and Drug Administration.
45. Davis P, Crooks L, Arakawa M, et al: Potential hazards in NMR imaging: heating effects of changing magnetic fields and RF fields on small metallic implants, *Am J Roentgenol* 137:857–860, 1981.
46. Woodard PK, Bluemke DA, Cascade PN, et al: American College of Radiology: ACR practice guideline for the performance and interpretation of cardiac magnetic resonance imaging (MRI), *J Am Coll Radiol* 3:665–676, 2006.
47. Prasad N, Wright D, Ford J, Thornby J: Safety of 4-T MR imaging: study of effects on developing frog embryos, *Radiology* 174:251–253, 1990.
48. Persson B, Stahlberg F: Safety aspects of magnetic resonance examinations, *Int J Technol Assess Health Care* 1:647–665, 1985.
49. Dujovny M, Kossovsky N, Kossowsky R, et al: Aneurysm clip motion during magnetic resonance imaging: in vivo experimental study with metallurgical factor analysis, *Neurosurgery* 17:543–548, 1985.
50. American Society for Metals Committee for Wrought Stainless Steels: *Wrought stainless steels*, ed 8, Metals Park, OH, 1961, American Society for Metals.
51. Majdani O, Leinung M, Rau T, et al: Demagnetization of cochlear implants and temperature changes in 3.0T MRI environment, *Otolaryngol Head Neck Surg* 139:833–839, 2008.
52. Scherzinger A, Hendee W: Basic principles of magnetic resonance imaging—an update, *West J Med* 143:782–792, 1985.
53. Liang M, Narayanan K, Kanal E: Magnetic ports in tissue expanders—a caution for MRI, *Magn Reson Imaging* 7:541–542, 1989.
54. Kanal E: An overview of electromagnetic safety considerations associated with magnetic resonance imaging, *Ann NY Acad Sci* 649:204–224, 1992.
55. Pavlicek W, Geisinger M, Castle L, et al: The effects of nuclear magnetic resonance on patients with cardiac pacemakers, *Radiology* 147:149–153, 1983.
56. Center for Devices and Radiological Health: *MR product reporting program and medical device report program*, Washington, DC, 1989, U.S. Food and Drug Administration.
57. Erlebacher J, Cahill P, Pannizzo F, Knowles R: Effect of magnetic resonance imaging on DDD pacemakers, *Am J Cardiol* 57:437–440, 1986.
58. Nazarian S, Roguin A, Zviman MM, et al: Clinical utility and safety of a protocol for noncardiac and cardiac magnetic resonance imaging of patients with permanent pacemakers and implantable-cardioverter defibrillators at 1.5 Tesla, *Circulation* 114:1277–1284, 2006.
59. Beischer: Vectorcardiogram and aortic blood flow of squirrel monkeys in a strong superconductive electromagnet. In Barnothy M, editor: *Biological effects of magnetic fields*, New York, 1969, Plenum, p 241.
60. McRobbie D, Foster M: Cardiac response to pulsed magnetic fields with regard to safety in NMR imaging, *Phys Med Biol* 30:695–702, 1985.
61. Gulch R, Lutz O: Influence of strong static magnetic fields on heart muscle contraction, *Phys Med Biol* 31:763–769, 1986.
62. Tenforde T, Gaffey C, Moyer B, Budinger T: Cardiovascular alterations in Macaca monkeys exposed to stationary magnetic fields: experimental observations and theoretical analysis, *Bioelectromagnetics* 4:1–9, 1983.
63. Jehenson P, Duboc D, Lavergne T, et al: Change in human cardiac rhythm induced by a 2 T static magnetic field, *Radiology* 166:227–230, 1988.
64. The Joint Commission: *Preventing accidents and injuries in the MRI suite*, 2008. Available at http://www.jointcommission.org/assts/1/18/SEA38.pdf..
65. Kanal E, Borgstede J, Barkovich A, et al: American College of Radiology white paper on MR safety, *AJR Am J Roentgenol* 178:1335–1347, 2002.
66. United States Food and Drug Administration, Center for Devices and Radiological Health: A primer on medical device interactions with magnetic resonance imaging systems. Available at http://www.fda.gov/MedicalDevices/DeviceRegulationandGuidance/GuidanceDocuments/ucm107721.htm.
67. Guidance for Industry and FDA Staff: Establishing safety and compatibility of passive implants in the magnetic resonance (MR) environment, Document issued August 21, 2008. Available at http://www.fda.gov/downloads/MedicalDevices/DeviceRegulationandGuidance/GuidanceDocuments/ucm107708.pdf.
68. American Society for Testing and Materials International: *Designation: F2503-08, Standard Practice for Marking Medical Devices and Other Items for Safety in the Magnetic Resonance Environment*, West Conshohocken, PA, 2005, American Society for Testing and Materials International.
69. Senft C, Schoenes B, Gasser T, et al: Feasibility of intraoperative MRI guidance for craniotomy and tumor resection in the semisitting position, *J Neurosurg Anesthesiol*, 2011.
70. Corn SB: Spinal anaesthesia for a paediatric patient undergoing an image guided invasive procedure in the open configuration magnetic resonance imaging unit, *Paediatr Anaesth* 7:155–157, 1997.
71. Cox RG, Levy R, Hamilton MG, et al: Anesthesia can be safely provided for children in a high-field intraoperative magnetic resonance imaging environment, *Paediatr Anaesth* 21:454–458, 2011.
72. Vila H Jr, Soto R, Cantor AB, Mackey D: Comparative outcomes analysis of procedures performed in physician offices and ambulatory surgery centers, *Arch Surg* 138:991–995, 2003.
73. Bhananker SM, Posner KL, Cheney FW, et al: Injury and liability associated with monitored anesthesia care: a closed claims analysis, *Anesthesiology* 104:228–234, 2006.

CHAPTER 28

Anesthesia at High Altitude

Gerardo Bosco • Enrico Camporesi

CHAPTER OUTLINE

OVERVIEW

In the course of common anesthetic practice, it is unusual to worry about alterations in total environmental pressure, because the majority of anesthetic procedures are conducted normally, within a limited pressure range. In fact, most organized hospital settings have developed in a narrow span of altitudes not far from sea level, although a significant portion of the world's population continues to live at high altitude. In recent years, traditional surgical and anesthetic techniques have been expanded to countries in development, such as Nepal in Asia, the Andean Highlands of South America, and elevated African regions such as Zimbabwe. Utilization of gas-based anesthesia has increased at altitudes where total barometric pressure is reduced.

It is interesting to explore low barometric pressure at high altitudes with attention to the physiologic changes commonly associated with anesthesia, and the results provide principles and insights applicable to daily practice at "normal" environmental pressure. The first part of the chapter provides a description of the principal physiologic challenges introduced by low pressure; the second part summarizes anesthetic considerations at low barometric pressures.

GASES AROUND THE BODY

The pressure exerted by gas molecules on all surfaces of the body constitutes the *environmental pressure*. This pressure is the result of both the atmospheric gases prevailing at any one site and the composition of the gases in the column of air above the location. Total environmental pressure at sea level amounts to 760 mm Hg (14.7 lb/in^2 atmospheric [psia]). This value undergoes frequent, often daily changes; at most, it ranges up and down by 10 to 15 mm Hg as a consequence of weather fluctuations. The composition of atmospheric air, on the other hand, is singularly constant in its original constituents and is summarized in Table 28-1.

Only water vapor content varies significantly as a function of total humidity, and the partial pressure of the water molecules may contribute various amounts to the total pressure. Water vapor pressure (P_{H_2O}) depends on available water molecules in the atmosphere at a certain temperature. At 0° C, air that is fully saturated has a water vapor pressure of approximately 5 mm Hg, whereas at body temperature (37° C), the water vapor pressure is increased to 47 mm Hg. Whatever humidity and temperature prevail in the gas outside the body, as soon as air is inspired and equilibrated with moist tracheal gas, it is rapidly fully saturated and is heated or cooled to body temperature. Water vapor is added to gases in the airways by the moist linings of the respiratory tract.

The addition of water vapor to atmospheric gases and the usual heating of the inspired gas to body temperature both induce substantial changes in the partial pressure of all gases and, in particular, to the partial pressure of oxygen (PaO_2) (Table 28-2). Nitrogen and oxygen are the only gases present in substantial concentration in dry air. Moist, warm tracheal air contains significant amounts of water vapor.

TABLE 28-1 Composition of Atmospheric Gas (Dry, Sea Level)

Gas	mm Hg	% of Total
Nitrogen	594	78.09
Oxygen	159	20.95
Carbon dioxide	0.2	0.03
Other inert gases	7	0.93
Water vapor	0	0.00
Total	760.2	100.00

TABLE 28-2 Approximate Composition of Inspired Gases at Atmospheric Pressure at Sea Level

Gas	Dry Air (mm Hg)	Moist Tracheal Air (mm Hg)	Alveolar Gas (mm Hg)
Nitrogen	601	564	568
Oxygen	159	149	105
Carbon dioxide	0.2	0.2	40
Water vapor	0	47	47
Total	760	760	760

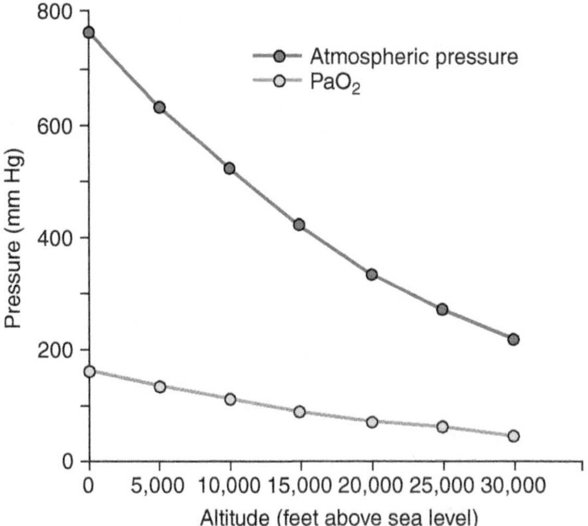

FIGURE 28-1 Effects of altitude on total barometric pressure and partial pressure of oxygen (PaO_2). Note that PaO_2 is a fixed proportion (20.95%) of total barometric pressure. At sea level, PaO_2 is 159 mm Hg; this value is approximately halved at 18,000 feet.

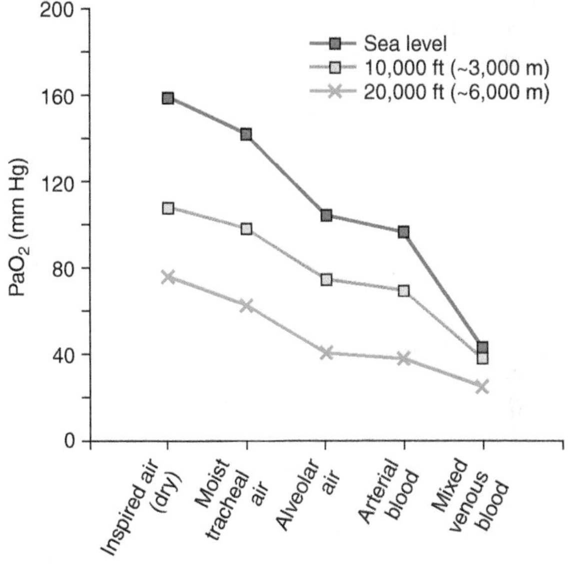

FIGURE 28-2 Effect of altitude on partial pressure of oxygen (PaO_2) in the respiratory and blood compartments. Average values are shown at sea level, 10,000 feet, and 20,000 feet. Although changes in the gas phase and in arterial blood are reduced in physical proportion, mixed venous PaO_2 changes that occur with altitude are reduced by adaptive responses, mainly an increase in cardiac output. Thus mixed venous blood and tissue values reflect much smaller changes in PaO_2 than does arterial blood.

Because the total barometric pressure is unchanged in the trachea, water vapor displaces each of the other gases, thereby decreasing their partial pressures. Alveolar gas contains approximately 100 to 105 mm Hg of oxygen. Commonly, oxygen is taken up by the blood in the lungs, and carbon dioxide is released into the alveoli. During respiratory processes, the gases are primarily moved by convection from the atmosphere to the alveolar space and back to the exhaled gas outside the body. In the alveolar compartment, diffusion is the primary mechanism for oxygen and carbon dioxide exchange. Therefore changes in oxygen partial pressure in the inspired gas lead to proportional changes in the alveolar PaO_2.

High-altitude environments are characterized by a decreased barometric pressure and a reduced partial pressure of inspired oxygen compared with sea level values. While breathing air, there is a large range of total atmospheric pressure changes still compatible with adequate gas exchange, from pressures on the highest mountains (about 300 mm Hg total pressure) to those at several hundred feet underwater (about 6 to 7 times 760 mm Hg). The limits can be extended, especially at altitude, by slow adaptive phenomena that require several days to weeks to unfold fully; these phenomena are in part under hereditary control.

REDUCED ENVIRONMENTAL PRESSURE

Acute awareness of the adverse effects of the low barometric pressure of high altitude is recorded in literature regarding the Spanish invasion of South America; these effects were commonly attributed to the "thinness of the air." Acute mountain sickness at an elevation of about 10,000 feet was first described in 1671 by the physiologist Borelli.

Acute exposure to altitude can be achieved in a decompression chamber, by rapid ascent in an airplane, or by a brisk climb on a mountain. The decrease in total barometric pressure with altitude and the attendant reduction in inspired PaO_2 are shown in Figure 28-1; Figure 28-2 illustrates the approximate values for PaO_2 in inspired air, moist tracheal air, alveolar gas, and arterial and mixed venous blood. High altitude (HA) significantly affects the human body because of a decrease in the PaO_2 in an environment of low ambient barometric pressure. A whole spectrum of disturbances and diseases was described for sojourners into HA. On one hand, the lack of oxygen generally triggers physiologic mechanisms and may result in a well-compensated state called *acclimatization*. The extent to which a person adapts to this depends on the rate and extent of the ascent and the baseline physiologic status of the individual. On the other hand, *high-altitude illness* (HAI) refers to the set of symptoms that range from mild to severe, sometimes even life-threatening consequences, such as cerebral and pulmonary edema.

Acclimatization

Acclimatization is a physiologic state that tends to improve oxygen transport and utilization at HA. An essential adaptation to acute HA hypoxia is hyperventilation. In the range of altitude from 10,000 to 15,000 feet, the increase in altitude causes an increase in ventilation proportional to the decrease in density of the air. Thus the increase in ventilation approximates the amount required to produce equivalent delivery of oxygen to the alveolar spaces. This is achieved by an increase in respiratory rate and tidal volume.[1] The arterial hypoxia results in stimulation of peripheral chemoreceptors, which causes an increase in alveolar ventilation. Carbon dioxide is washed out of the alveoli at an increased rate, and the arterial partial pressure of carbon dioxide ($PaCO_2$) is decreased. The reduction of $PaCO_2$ leads to a respiratory alkalosis with an associated increase of arterial pH, and these changes stimulate the excretion of bicarbonate from the blood and the kidneys. This increase in ventilation is generally sustained for several days, and it may not reach a plateau until several days at altitude. As a consequence, during the following days, the blood bicarbonate is reduced, and a new level appropriate for the level of hyperventilation is established, with a near normal pH. Thus the respiratory alkalosis is compensated.

The respiratory adaptations and the bicarbonate excretion affect the electrolyte status of spinal fluid and alter subsequent ventilatory responses. As the bicarbonate is excreted from the blood, bicarbonate is also lost from cerebrospinal fluid (CSF). In view of this decreased buffer capacity, changes in carbon dioxide in the CSF result in faster changes in hydrogen ion concentration and lead to an increased sensitivity to carbon dioxide. At this point in adaptation, ventilatory sensitivity to carbon dioxide is enhanced. Gradually, the respiratory system adapts (respiratory acclimatization) to hypoxia, resulting in an increase in the hypoxic ventilatory response. A resetting of the arterial $PaCO_2$ set point also occurs. These processes result in restoration of normoxia with persistent hyperventilation and hypocapnia.[2] Overall, the hypocapnia is beneficial for oxygen transport, because it shifts the dissociation curve to the left with increased affinity of hemoglobin (Hb) for oxygen; this enhances the oxygenation of blood at the lung. Extreme altitude results in an arterial PaO_2 in the range of 20 mm Hg, a profound depression of the central nervous system (CNS) is unmasked, and ventilatory drive is depressed.

Other Effects

Additional effects on lung function have been demonstrated with exposure to altitude, including an increase in pulmonary diffusing capacity, an increase in pulmonary blood flow to the apical lung regions, larger lung volumes with increased vital and total lung capacity, hypoxic pulmonary vasoconstriction, and an increase in pulmonary vascular pressures. *Hypoxic pulmonary vasoconstriction* is a vasomotor response of small, muscular pulmonary arteries that tends to increase resistance to flow in areas of alveolar hypoxia, thereby improving ventilation/perfusion (V/Q) match and reducing the shunt fraction. As a result, prolonged arterial hypoxia increases right-ventricular pressure for extended periods of time and induces right ventricular hypertrophy, with predictable electrocardiographic (ECG) changes of right-axis deviation and right ventricular strain.

Hemoglobin concentration increases rapidly at altitude, within hours; this is because of rapidly rising hemoconcentration. Eventually, however, a real increase in erythropoiesis and a true increase in red cell mass ensues that may not be fully realized for several weeks. As the red cell mass and hemoglobin concentration rise, the erythropoietin level decreases. Because of the sigmoid shape of the oxygen dissociation curve, up to 3000 m (9843 feet) of elevation, oxygen saturation is maintained; beyond 3000 m (9843 feet), the arterial PaO_2 falls steeply, resulting in lower oxygen saturation. Soon after the development of the hypoxic state, production of 2,3 diphosphoglycerate (2,3-DPG) increases, which shifts the hemoglobin dissociation curve to the right and allows for more effective extraction in the capillaries.

Cardiac output is characteristically increased as a result of an increase in the heart rate in response to hypoxia. This response adapts during continuing exposure as cardiac output decreases as a result of diuresis and a lower plasma volume. Tissue blood flow tends to increase as a result of increased nitric oxide (NO) concentration in the plasma, which causes vasodilation.[3] A corresponding increase in organ blood flow occurs that includes pulmonary, cardiac, and cerebral blood flow. Increased pulmonary blood flow leads to failure of red blood corpuscles to fully equilibrate with the alveolar gas, which augments any existing hypoxia. HA may induce a hypercoagulable state as a result of polycythemia and platelet activation, which increases the risk of thromboembolic events.[4]

In acclimatization, a state of improved oxygen transport and utilization combats the HA hypoxia; molecular responses involved include activation of gene coding for proteins involved in oxygen transport (hypoxia inducible factor 1 [HIF-1])[5] and growth of blood vessels (vascular endothelial growth factor [VEGFA])[6] in the heart.

Despite these adaptive responses to altitude, no significant change occurs in either resting oxygen consumption or in the ability to perform high levels of exercise at moderate altitude. At altitudes in excess of 10,000 feet, exercise tolerance is limited with acute exposure, and other symptoms of acute hypoxia manifest themselves by interference with several organ systems.

TABLE 28-3 **High-Altitude Illness and Various Clinical Syndromes**

Syndrome	Special Features	Prevention	Clinical Features	Management
Mild acute mountain sickness (AMS); includes high-altitude headache	Most recover	Slow ascent or staging*; acetazolamide†	Headache, reduced appetite, nausea, vomiting, edema, insomnia, dizziness, fatigue	Stop ascent, rest, and acclimatize for at least a day; if symptoms do not improve, descend ≥500 m Acetazolamide, 125-250 mg bid Symptomatic treatment as necessary with analgesics (aspirin, ibuprofen) and antiemetics
Moderate to severe AMS	Similar to AMS but increased in severity	Slow ascent or staging*; acetazolamide†	Headache, reduced appetite, nausea, vomiting, edema, insomnia, dizziness, fatigue	As for AMS, *plus*: Oxygen supplementation (if available) Dexamethasone 4 mg PO, IM, or IV q6h Hyperbaric therapy
High-altitude cerebral edema	A medical emergency (vasogenic cerebral edema)	Slow ascent or staging*; acetazolamide†	Ataxia, altered consciousness, papilledema, focal deficits	As for AMS, *plus*: Immediate descent or evacuation Minimize exertion and keep warm Consider tracheal intubation to protect airway or if respiration is inadequate
High-altitude pulmonary edema	Occurs within first few days; increased pulmonary capillary pressure and exudate in alveoli because of inhomogeneous HPV	Slow ascent; for susceptible persons, nifedipine, tadalafil, or dexamethasone are prophylactic	Fatigue, dyspnea, cough, cyanosis	As for AMS, *plus*: Nifedipine, 10 mg PO q4h by titration to response, or 10 mg PO once, followed by 30-mg ER q12-24h Nitric oxide therapy *and/or*: Tadalafil 10 mg bid or sildenafil 50 mg q8h; various other modalities to lower pulmonary arterial pressure
Chronic mountain sickness	Known as *Monge syndrome;* the result of excessive erythrocytosis, pulmonary hypertension leading to cor pulmonale leading to CHF	A public health problem in the Andean plateau; abatement includes modifying risk factors (e.g., smoking, obesity, pollution, lung disease)	Headache, dizziness, dyspnea, palpitations, localized cyanosis, burning sensation in the palms and soles, venous dilation, joint and muscle pain, lack of mental concentration, memory changes	Phlebotomy for transient relief Descent to lower altitude ACEIs, domperidone, acetazolamide, and respiratory stimulants (medroxyprogesterone and almitrine) Nifedipine and sildenafil to reduce pulmonary artery pressure

*Several days are spent at an intermediate altitude of 200 m.

†Produces a state of bicarbonate diuresis and thereby augments the ventilatory response to hypoxia; may also produce tissue respiratory acidosis and diuresis and inhibits carotid body response to carbon dioxide.

ACEI, angiotensin-converting enzyme inhibitor; bid, twice per day; CHF, congestive heart failure; ER, extended-release; HPV, hypoxic pulmonary vasoconstriction; IM, intramuscular; IV, intravenous; PO, by mouth.

Modified from Leissner KB, Mahmood FU: Physiology and pathophysiology at high altitude: considerations for the anesthesiologist, *J Anesth* 23:543-553, 2009; and Moon RE, Camporesi EM: Clinical care in extreme environments: at high and low pressure and in space. In Miller R, Eriksson L, Fleisher LA, Wiener-Kronish J, editors: *Miller's anesthesia*, ed 7, Philadelphia, 2010, Elsevier.

High-Altitude Illness

HAI is composed of a group of syndromes that develop as a result of continuous exposure to hypoxia, and it is generally divided into four categories: 1) acute mountain sickness, 2) high-altitude cerebral edema, 3) high-altitude pulmonary edema, and 4) chronic mountain sickness. The risk of HAI is directly proportional to the rate of ascent and the altitude reached; therefore a gradual ascent to promote acclimatization may be the best strategy to prevent HAI. Guidelines suggest that above an altitude of 2500 m (8200 feet), the altitude at which a person sleeps should not be increased by more than 600 meters (1970 feet) per day[7] (Table 28-3).[4,8]

Gamow Bag

The Gamow bag is a rescue product for high-altitude climbers and trekkers that can be used for the treatment of moderate to extreme altitude sickness.[9] A Gamow bag is an inflatable pressure bag large enough to fit a person inside. By inflating the bag with a foot pump, the effective altitude can be decreased by as much as 7000 feet, thus relieving the symptoms of *acute mountain sickness* (AMS). The

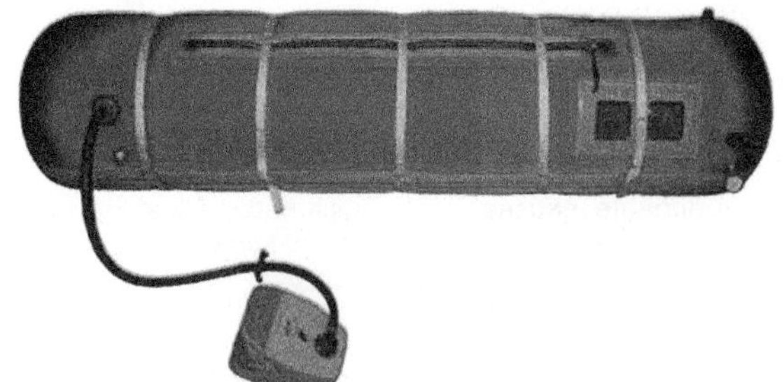

FIGURE 28-3 ■ The Gamow bag.

Gamow bag is also used for treatment of life-threatening *high-altitude pulmonary edema* (HAPE) and *high-altitude cerebral edema* (HACE). Gamow bags are constructed of durable nylon and are reinforced with circular nylon straps. A lengthwise zipper allows patients access into the bag, and the four clear windows allow visual contact during treatment. The bag is pressurized with ambient air to 2 psi by use of a foot pump powered by healthy partners standing outside the bag (Fig. 28-3).

Gamow bag treatments for altitude sicknesses are used to provide temporary relief in the hope that it will give the patient enough time and strength to descend to a lower altitude, alleviating the need for a full-blown lifesaving rescue effort by everyone on the mountain. Descent to a lower altitude is generally recommended in most cases.

Pregnancy and Altitude

Because the fetus in utero does not derive oxygen directly from the low barometric pressure at HA, it seems to be little affected by acute exposure to altitudes up to 2500 to 3000 m and suffers no adverse effects. Adaptation to chronic exposure to HA includes a decrease in villous membrane thickness and an increase in placental capillary volume. Infants born at HA are suddenly exposed to the hypoxic environment, whereas the transition to adult circulation occurs more gradually,[10] with a higher incidence of patent foramen ovale (PFO) and patent ductus arteriosus. Increased incidence of acute respiratory distress syndrome (ARDS) and pulmonary arterial hypertension that requires oxygen and/or mechanical ventilation is also seen.

ANESTHETIC PROBLEMS AND ALTITUDE

Two main problems can be identified in the administration of anesthetics at altitude: the relative hypoxic background of air at lower ambient pressure, especially before and after anesthetic administration, and the prevailing technical problems associated with delivery of anesthetic vapors from vaporizers when the total ambient pressure is reduced. Significant alterations in the effectiveness of intravenous (IV) agents and of regional anesthetic techniques have not been reported, and these agents and techniques may still be used with the some precautions as at sea level.

Pressure Considerations

The effective anesthetic power of nitrous oxide is also reduced as total barometric pressure decreases. It has been shown that analgesia induced by 50% N_2O is reduced by nearly 50% at 5000 feet, and it becomes insignificant at 10,000 feet.[11,12] Therefore nitrous oxide is not a useful anesthetic gas at altitude. In fact, Safar and Tenicela[13] and James and White[14] condemned the use of nitrous oxide for anesthesia at altitude.

Although total IV anesthesia (TIVA) seems to be safer than inhalational anesthetics, at HA all anesthetics and opiates still potentially depress the respiratory drive. In addition, the regular dose of these drugs may show increased respiratory depression in unacclimatized individuals. Thus the anesthetic technique least likely to suppress ventilation should be applied, especially in the field, where monitoring facilities and supplemental O_2 may not be readily available.

Regional anesthesia seems to be a safe option when applicable, but regional anesthesia can compromise respiratory function when it affects the phrenic nerve. Because of this, caution must be exercised during the performance of brachial plexus and stellate ganglion block. Increased incidence of postdural puncture headache with subarachnoid block has been reported, possibly owing to hypovolemia, along with increased and altered sensitivity to CSF pressure; otherwise, effects are similar to those seen when such procedures are performed at sea level.

At an altitude approximating 5000 feet, the partial pressure of oxygen in air is reduced from the sea-level value of approximately 160 mm Hg to about 125 mm Hg. While room air is breathed at altitude, arterial PaO_2 is consequently lowered to approximately 80 mm Hg in normal individuals. Powell and Gingrich[11] recommended administering a gas mixture that contains no less than 40% oxygen during anesthesia at an altitude of 1 mile (approximately 5000 feet) to compensate for the reduced arterial PaO_2 commonly observed during anesthesia. When this altitude is doubled to about 10,000 feet, the inspired PaO_2 is reduced to 110 mm Hg, and PaO_2 is reduced to 65 mm Hg in air. At this hypoxic level, alveolar ventilation increases, and $PaCO_2$ is steadily reduced (34 mm Hg at rest).

It is important to remember that long-term adapted residents are more tolerant to hypoxemia and have increased hematocrit, pulmonary hypertension, and low $PaCO_2$ and biocarbonate (HCO_3) concentrations. These values are the baseline and should be maintained throughout the procedure.

Machine Considerations

Vapors and Vaporizers at Altitude

The saturated vapor pressure (SVP) of a volatile anesthetic agent depends only on temperature[15] and is practically independent of total environmental pressure. Consequently, for a given vaporizer temperature, the concentration of a given mass of vapor increases as the barometric pressure is reduced, because the same mass of volatile agent is vaporized in a less and less dense carrier gas. However, the partial pressure of the agent (expressed in millimeters of mercury) remains unchanged, and so does its biologic effect on the neural tissue where the anesthetic effect is produced (see also Chapter 3).

With modern vaporizers, the partial pressure of the vapor should remain unaltered by barometric pressure changes. In fact, McDowall[16] showed that the output of the FluoTec Mark 2 (Cyprane, Keighley, United Kingdom) vaporizer differed by only a small amount from the theoretical prediction, and those changes could be attributed to the slight change in the density of the carrier gas. However, Safar and Tenicela[13] studied the Foregger vaporizer (Foregger Company, Roslyn Heights, NY) at 10,000 feet and showed, contrary to the theory, that a higher partial pressure of gas was produced at increased altitude. Twenty years later, James and White[14] studied this with a more precise analytical technique, using the Engström EMMA vapor analyzer, whose principle of operation is a vibrating lipophilic-coated piezoelectric crystal. They studied the accuracies of a FluoTec Mark 2 vaporizer and a Dräger Vapor halothane vaporizer (Dräger Medical, Telford, PA) inside a pressure chamber simulating altitude but were unable to show differences in halothane partial pressure with decreased environmental pressure. These authors concluded that, because the reading of the vapor analyzer remained constant, the last two types of vaporizers produced a relatively constant partial pressure of halothane even at reduced environmental pressure (see also Chapter 3).

Concentration-calibrated variable bypass vaporizers—such as the Datex-Ohmeda Tec series (Tec 4, 5, and 7; GE Healthcare, Waukesha, WI) and the Dräger Vapor 19.n and 2000 series—set to deliver a given concentration in volumes percent at 1 atm pressure at an altitude where ambient pressure is less than 1 atm (<760 mm Hg) will deliver a higher concentration in volumes percent than that set on the dial. However, when that concentration (vol%) is converted to agent partial pressure, which determines effect or potency, the increase is proportionately smaller than the increase in volumes percent. For example, when gas flows from the anesthesia machine's flowmeters into a variable-bypass vaporizer set to deliver 1% isoflurane at 20° C and 760 mm Hg ambient pressure, that gas flow is split in the ratio of 46:1 for bypass–to–vaporizing chamber flow (see Chapter 3 for derivation of split ratios). It will be assumed that the split ratio remains unchanged with changes in altitude. The SVP of isoflurane at 20° C is 240 mm Hg, and atmospheric pressure is 760 mm Hg; therefore the concentration of isoflurane that emerges from the vaporizing chamber is 32% (240/760). When atmospheric pressure is 500 mm Hg (~⅔ atm), the concentration of isoflurane that emerges from the vaporizing chamber would be 48% (240/500). Because the bypass flow remains constant (same split ratio), the concentration of isoflurane that emerges from the vaporizer would be approximately 2% by volume, *almost double* the dial setting. However, consider the partial pressures of isoflurane, because it is this value in the CNS that determines anesthetic depth or potency. At 1 atm, 1% partial pressure of isoflurane is 1% × 760, or 7.6 mm Hg. At ⅔ atm, the partial pressure of isoflurane would be 2% of 500, or 10 mm Hg—*1.3 times* that at 1 atm. This effect on agent concentration occurs because isoflurane vapor is added after the vaporizer's incoming gas flow has been split.

The Tec 6 and Dräger D-Vapor vaporizers are different from the traditional variable-bypass vaporizers described above in that these vaporizers always deliver the dialed-in concentration in volumes percent regardless of ambient pressure. At altitude, therefore, the percent desflurane (Pdes) delivered will be less. Thus 10% desflurane at 1 atm represents a Pdes of 10% × 760, or 76 mm Hg. At ⅔ atm, 10% desflurane has a Pdes of 10% of 500, or 50 mm Hg. Thus to obtain the same Pdes (potency) as at 1 atm, the vaporizer dial setting must be increased to 15% because 15% × 500 is 75 mm Hg.

Gas Analyzers

Most of the gas analyzers used by anesthesiologists are based on one of the various physical properties of the agent being measured. Most analyzers respond to the number and activity of molecules of the agent present, independently of the presence of additional gas molecules. Such instruments, therefore, measure partial pressure, not concentration of agents. Most often, however, such devices are traditionally calibrated in percentages. This calibration scale might introduce important errors that must be prevented when specialized equipment will be used at increasing altitudes (see Chapter 8).

Oxygen Analyzers

All oxygen analyzers in current use—paramagnetic, fuel cell, and oxygen electrode devices—respond to partial pressure of oxygen alone and produce alterations of the total measurement output as barometric pressure changes. An oxygen analyzer calibrated at sea level to measure 21% oxygen in air gives a reading of 17.4% oxygen when reading air at 5000 feet. Of course, the analyzer must be recalibrated at altitude to read 21% when air is injected. If the oxygen activity were to be presented as partial pressure (e.g., mm Hg of oxygen), the device would indeed reflect oxygen availability to the patient's lungs and blood at any pressure. As noted above, the key issue is that air at an altitude above 5000 feet is relatively hypoxic, and it approaches a clinically significant hypoxic level at 10,000 feet. The same principle applies in hyperbaric conditions: compressed air at 5 atm contains 21% oxygen, but total oxygen exerts a partial pressure of approximately 800 mm Hg (21% × 5 × 760, or 798 mm Hg).

Carbon Dioxide Analyzers

Carbon dioxide analyzers most frequently operate on the principle of infrared absorption. As indicated above, most analyzers have scales that read in percentages, although the sensitive element is responding to the increasing partial pressure of carbon dioxide. By the use of precise gas mixtures, it is possible to calibrate these analyzers to read exact percentages at a fixed altitude. If, however, the analyzer is calibrated at sea level, and the same gas containing a fixed percentage of carbon dioxide is injected into the analyzer at a different altitude, the reading of the analyzer decreases in the percentage scale in proportion to the total barometric pressure.

Gas Density and Flow. Alteration of total barometric pressure induces a proportional change in gas density. In fact, density reflects closely the number of molecules per unit volume. Gas flowmeters and variable-flow resistors used to produce oxygen-enriched mixtures represent critical devices that use indicators that depend on gas density. Some ventilators deliver tidal volumes that are lower than set volumes during volume-control ventilation because of decreased gas density and viscosity at HA.

Flowmeters

The action of most flowmeters is due to the decrease in pressure that occurs when a gas passes through a fixed resistance, an indication of total gas flow. If this fixed resistance is represented by an orifice, resistance depends primarily on gas density. However, if the fixed resistance is of a laminar nature, viscosity becomes the prime determinant of the magnitude of the pressure reduction provided by the flow. Most flowmeters currently in use utilize a floating bobbin supported by a stream of gas inside a tube with a tapered diameter.

The density of a gas changes in proportion to the change in total barometric pressure, but viscosity changes relatively little, or not at all, because viscosity depends mostly on temperature. In a tapered tube at low levels of flow, the movement of the bobbin primarily depends on laminar flow. As the float moves up the tube, the resistance makes it behave progressively more like an orifice. In practice, only minor errors, usually 1% per every 1000 feet of altitude, have been reported for most gas flowmeters, such that minor corrections to the total flow can be easily applied.[17] However, if total environmental pressure changes by more than 1 atm, Halsey and White[18] recommended a complete recalibration, because a single correction factor will be significantly in error. The following equation can be used to derive an approximate correction factor, both at altitude and at increased pressure:

$$F_1 = F_0 \times \sqrt{(d_0 d_1)}$$

In this expression, F_1 is flow at the present ambient pressure, F_0 indicates flow on the scale calibrated at sea level, d_0 is density of gas at sea level, and d_1 is density of gas at the present pressure. The correction factor may be significant at increased pressure but seldom exceeds 10% at altitudes up to 5000 feet.

James and White[14] tested oxygen and nitrous oxide flow indicators (despite the warning not to use N_2O at altitude) and measured the percentage error at flowmeter settings that ranged from 1 to 8 L/min. They demonstrated that errors were larger at higher flow settings and ranged from 3% to 8% at 5000 feet but from 5% to 20% at 10,000 feet. This is an issue when oxygen and nitrous oxide are used together at high flows, because flowmeters tend to under-read the actual flow rate. The result is a hypoxic mixture that results from the mix of a flow of oxygen with a higher flow of nitrous oxide.[14] An oxygen analyzer calibrated at HA can be used to monitor the final output.

High-Flow Oxygen Enrichment and Other Devices

Fixed-orifice Venturi devices are commonly used to provide an enriched gas mixture with elevated oxygen content. Fixed settings—usually 28%, 35%, or 40%—are produced by variable orifices, which produce different amounts of entrainment of air into an oxygen stream. Most of these devices "run rich" at altitude, because the total gas density decreases.[14] Therefore the Venturi-type mask might be used safely at altitude, provided the flowmeter used to quantitate total oxygen flow is properly calibrated for the altitude at which it is being used.

During the rewarming phase of cardiopulmonary bypass, the low barometric pressure becomes a critical factor for adequate oxygenation. The reduction in the ambient PaO_2 has a significant deleterious effect on the performance of the oxygenator used, although this can be overcome by having a low priming volume, low pressure drop, and sufficient gas transfer to provide safe oxygenation at HA in the oxygenator.

According to Boyle's law, pressure is inversely proportional to volume, and as a result of a decrease in pressure at HA, up to a 30% increase in volume of air is seen in the tracheal tube cuff and within a laryngeal mask airway (LMA). During rapid ascent to altitudes commonly experienced during aeromedical transport, this may cause ischemic injury to the tracheal or pharyngeal mucosa. Removal of air from the cuff or filling the cuff with water may be indicated.

RECOMMENDATIONS FOR ANESTHESIA AT ALTITUDE

It is important to use anesthetics, analgesics, and tranquilizers judiciously, because they have the potential to decrease the ventilatory drive. They should be carefully titrated to effect. Ketamine seems to be a good anesthetic option, because it produces a dissociative state of anesthesia with minimal respiratory depression and does not interfere with the pharyngeal or laryngeal reflexes. Although oxygen desaturation and central apnea have been reported, supplemental oxgyen and respiratory monitoring can be implemented. There is a theoretical risk of worsening pulmonary vascular resistance; however, propofol, the most popular induction agent, seems to be safe, although there is a need for a higher dose than usual.[19]

The major risk of anesthesia at HA is that anesthetized patients can become hypoxic despite the fact that adequate oxygen concentrations are being administered. The effectiveness of nitrous oxide is so reduced by the decrease in partial pressure at altitude that no significant contribution by nitrous oxide to the anesthetic mixture is of clinical use. In addition, it is important to maintain a higher concentration of oxygen both during and after administration of the anesthetic to support adequate oxygenation. It is suggested that 30% oxygen be the minimum at 5000 feet, and that 40% oxygen be the minimum at 10,000 feet, for both intraoperative anesthetic management and postoperative recovery.

The problem may be compounded by inaccuracies in flow measurement, because the only way to obtain accurate flow rates at fixed altitude is to use flowmeters appropriately calibrated at altitude. Sea level–calibrated equipment may produce small errors at 5000 feet, but it certainly will deviate significantly, up to 20% at 10,000 feet. Finally, it is important to think of oxygenation and anesthetic vapor activity in terms of partial pressures of oxygen and partial pressures of anesthetic agent, rather than as volumetric percentages.

Gastric emptying is significantly delayed at HA and increases the risk for aspiration. Rapid-sequence induction and full-stomach precautions should be considered. Temperature homeostasis should be maintained at HA, because hypothermia-related causes of coagulopathy and hypothermia-induced vasoconstriction can mask hypovolemia. In addition, hypovolemia may be present because of insufficient water intake, a dry environment, increased surgical blood loss as a result of capillary ooze attributed to higher venous pressure, vasodilation and dense capillaries, increased set point of the plasma osmolality/plasma vasopressin relationship, and decreased aldosterone secretion mediated through the release of atrial natriuretic factor (ANF).

IV lines should be completely cleared of air bubbles, because right-to-left shunts develop frequently through a PFO in the setting of pulmonary vasoconstriction. Antithrombotic prophylaxis should be strongly considered for postsurgical patients because of the risks of hypercoagulability produced as a result of acclimatization to HA. Substrate metabolism at HA favors carbohydrate oxidation, thus the body depends more on blood glucose levels, because carbohydrate oxidation generates more adenosine triphosphate (ATP) per molecule of oxygen than fat utilization.[4] Glucose levels should be checked, because HA may increase glucose consumption.

The ambient temperature of the operating room must be raised, and it should be warm upon arrival of the patient. IV fluids should be warmed, warm-water baths should be prepared for areas of frostbite, and warming blankets should be applied. Humidification of inspired gases reduces evaporative heat loss and helps to warm the patient. Furthermore, heated peritoneal, bladder, or colonic lavage and extracorporeal circulatory rewarming may be used. Patients need to be monitored carefully during rewarming because of potential cardiac arrhythmia as a result of cold blood returning to the heart and peripheral vasodilation leading to hypotension and shock.

COMMON MEDICAL PROBLEMS AND COMMERCIAL FLIGHTS

The number of people traveling by air has increased to reach close to 2 billion annually in recent years[20] with a corresponding increase in the frequency of in-flight emergencies. The exact figures are not known, but the reported incidences of in-flight emergencies vary from 1 to 75 reported events per 1 million passengers[21] to 1 per 39,600 passengers.[22] Common in-flight emergencies include syncope, trauma as a result of turbulence and objects falling from the overhead bin, nausea, vomiting, hyperventilation, and dizziness.

Most events are minor, but a few—myocardial infarction, respiratory failure secondary to exacerbation of reactive airway disease, and pulmonary embolism—can be life threatening. From 0.01 to 0.8 deaths per million passengers have been reported,[8] but the actual figure may be even more staggering, because there is no mandatory reporting of all the emergencies and their outcomes. Contributory factors may be that older and sicker people are traveling in increased numbers. Many sick passengers are certified by physicians for air travel per the comprehensive medical guidelines set by the Aerospace Medical Association.[23] The right of a person to fly cannot be denied unless that person is deemed a hazard to the safety of other passengers, and it is more common than before to see people who have obstructive and restrictive lung diseases with supplemental oxygen and passengers with obstructive sleep apnea on noninvasive ventilator support on board an aircraft.[24] For passengers at risk of hypoxemia who intend to use pulse oximetry during the flight, recommendations are that they have a prior medical evaluation and a plan of management.[25]

In-Flight Environment and Its Clinical Implications

The scope of an anesthesiologist has expanded from the operating room to various other locations, and anesthesiologists have established themselves as perioperative physicians and trauma specialists. With the knowledge of physiology combined with the skill of airway management and routine handling of emergencies, an anesthesiologist is in a unique position to handle an emergency in the vicinity, and one such vicinity is inside an aircraft. Therefore the anesthesiologist must be aware of the challenges that can arise here, in case there is an emergency.

Most flights ascend to an altitude between 7300 and 13,000 meters, and the internal environment is regulated to keep the barometric pressure consistent with an altitude of 2400 m (8000 feet) and the temperature equivalent to that of sea level, which is well tolerated by most individuals. At 2400 m, the barometric pressure is 565 mm Hg, and there is some amount of hypoxia—partial pressure of alveolar oxygen (P_AO_2) is 118 mm Hg, PaO_2 is 60 mm Hg, and the arterial oxygen saturation (SaO_2) is 89%.

Patients with baseline hypoxemia as a result of lung or heart diseases may experience significant hypoxemia. The arterial PaO_2 falls onto the steep portion of the hemoglobin dissociation curve, toward the left, and such patients should be considered for in-flight O_2 administration.

The air in the cabin of an aircraft has decreased relative humidity (<10%). This dry air can exacerbate reactive airway diseases such as asthma and can also augment dehydration secondary to insensible water loss. As cabin pressure decreases, gas contained within closed spaces expands during flight. Because of this air expansion in the middle ear and sinus spaces, symptoms such as transient decrease in hearing acuity or minor ear and sinus pain are experienced by a few people. Spontaneous rupture of bronchogenic cysts, pulmonary bullae,[26] and wound dehiscence have been reported. Medical devices that contain air spaces, such as tracheal tube cuffs and feeding tubes, will expand as cabin pressure decreases.

Spreading of communicable diseases, especially upper respiratory tract infections, is common during commercial flight. This is mainly due to the number of people in close proximity within a confined environment, because the air inside the cabin is relatively free of contaminants.[27] During long-distance flights, deep venous thrombosis (DVT) is a potential risk because of venous stasis secondary to immobility and hyperviscosity secondary to dehydration. But its relation to air travel is doubtful, because its incidence is not greater in air travelers than in the general population.[28] Yet it seems prudent to advise susceptible passengers to walk around during long flights, exercise the calf muscles while seated, prevent dehydration, and consider the use of compressive stockings. Early signs of a dislodged thrombus into the pulmonary circulation may be breathlessness, and a person must have a high index of suspicion for this, especially if is associated with acute pleuritic chest pain in a susceptible individual. It is interesting to note that the incidence of children becoming ill is much less when compared with adults.[29]

In-Flight Emergency Management

Flight crews are well trained in handling in-flight emergencies. Indeed, the safety of all passengers on board the flight is the responsibility of the flight crew. The routine management of an ill passenger during flight consists of obtaining the patient's history, assessing his or her status, and making provisions for the patient's comfort. Meanwhile, immediate availability to the patient of oxygen and medical equipment on board should be ensured, and flight personnel should delegate responsibility, request medical assistance when appropriate, and suggest diversion of the flight if it will be of benefit to the patient.

Aircraft are required to carry emergency medical kits, basic first aid kits, automated external defibrillators (AEDs), and supplemental oxygen as per the Federal Aviation Administration (FAA) minimum standards. To provide a PaO_2 equivalent to sea level at an altitude of 2400 meters (8000 feet), the FiO_2 should be 28%, which is achieved by a flow rate of 2 L/min. It must be remembered that the emergency equipment on board is limited in scope and variable in nature to manage the emergencies encountered.

If a physician must volunteer during an in-flight emergency, proof of identity must be provided, and treatment must be administered in concordance with ground medical personnel in liaison with the cabin crew members. The goal of in-flight medical assistance is to stabilize the patient and advise the flight crew as to a diagnosis and necessary treatment. In addition, when appropriate, the volunteer should seek consultation from ground-based medical support personnel and suggest diversion of the aircraft.[24] It is very important that the volunteer physician clearly document the event and patient history for the continuum of care. The crew must cater to the needs of other passengers in addition to caring for the sick; they must also comply with the regulations governing aviation and with the laws of the aircraft's country of registration, and they must act in accordance with physicians on the ground. The law does protect a physician acting as a Good Samaritan when there is no monetary benefit involved, but the quality of care should not have been compromised.[29]

Most airlines function on the basis of contacting their ground base first, which is a medical consulting service that consists of physicians trained in aerospace and emergency medicine; they must also request assistance from volunteering physicians on board if advised to do so by their ground-based medical personnel. If a flight must be diverted to a nearby airport in an emergency, the crew will contact the ground-based medical personnel, and ultimately the captain of the aircraft makes the decision for the flight diversion based on the airline policy and FAA regulations. The legislation governing these aspects and the responsibility of the medical consultants on the ground is complex and unclear.

Flying During Pregnancy

Flying is not contraindicated in an uncomplicated pregnancy, but there are some precautions that a pregnant traveler should consider. Excessive flying should be avoided, and a pregnant traveler should rest as much as possible while in the air; in addition, it is important to make comfortable arrangements: get a seat with more leg room, wear support hose and shoes with adjustable straps in case the feet swell, plan to walk in the aisles, take frequent bathroom breaks, and drink adequate water. Travelers should be wary of dehydration on airplanes, which can be worse during pregnancy. Certain conditions in pregnancy—such as severe anemia, sickle cell disease, clotting disorders, and placental insufficiency—can increase the risk of problems.

According to the American College of Obstetricians and Gynecologists, air travel is safest for pregnant women during the second trimester. It is best not to travel before 12 weeks' gestation because of morning sickness and possible increased risk of miscarriage, although many pregnant women have no trouble flying in the first trimester. After 28 weeks, when the risk of going into labor increases, most airlines require a letter from a doctor stating the patient's fitness for air travel while pregnant and confirming the estimated due date. If more than 36 weeks' pregnant, many airlines will not let pregnant patients fly because of the increased risk of delivering on board.

SPACEFLIGHT

Spaceflight involves the launch of a space vehicle, after which it accelerates to orbital speed and for a period of time stays in space in an environment known as *microgravity*, where there is an absence of gravitational forces. The International Space Station is a research lab set up in space, and experiments have been continuously conducted in the microgravity environment there since November 2000 by crewmembers who are replaced at regular intervals. Here, we will cover the physiologic changes that occur during spaceflight and its anesthetic implications, should a crewmember require medical treatment that involves anesthesiologists; these implications may be applicable to the astronauts for a long time after their return to earth.

The space station and space shuttle often operate in microgravity, and pressure is maintained close to the

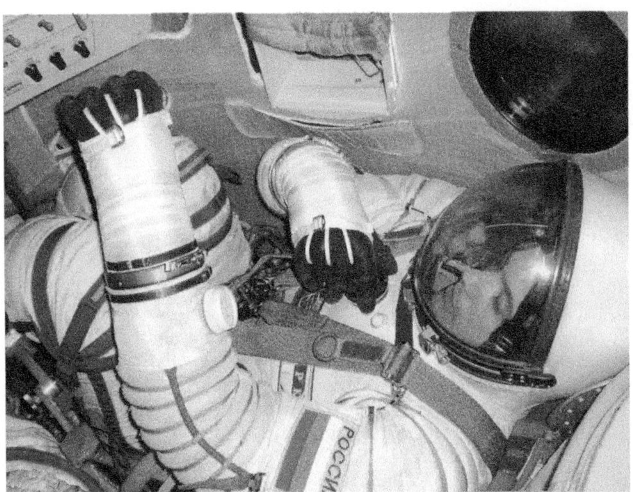

FIGURE 28-4 Astronaut in spacesuit preparing for extravehicular activity. (Courtesy Dr. Landolfi.)

atmospheric pressure at sea level, which is about 760 mm Hg. The pressure in a space suit, however, is 222 mm Hg, which places the wearer at potential risk of decompression sickness as a result of the pressure change. Astronauts use space suits during extravehicular activity, and they breathe 100% oxygen to combat hypoxia (Fig. 28-4).

In the microgravity environment, central redistribution of blood occurs with reduced venous pressure and an increase in left-ventricular end-diastolic volume. In addition, facial edema occurs along with a diuresis that depletes up to 20% or more of plasma volume.[30] Most astronauts experience transient nausea, vomiting, dizziness, and drowsiness shortly after reaching space. Skeletal muscle atrophy can occur after short missions, and cardiac muscle atrophy[31] occurs after several days in space. Both renal stones from hypercalciuria and osteoporosis as a result of a loss of significant amounts of calcium from bones may occur during long spaceflights as an effect of lack of weight bearing.

Sudden exposure to zero atmospheric pressure, which could occur as a result of a tear in the space suit, causes ebullism and generalized bubble formation.[8] If an unprotected human were to slip into the cold and airless void of space, using our knowledge of outer space, data from experiments, and extrapolations from accidents over the years, scientists were able to make some reasonable conclusions about what would happen.

A number of injuries would begin to occur immediately; although relatively minor at first, they would accumulate rapidly into a life-threatening combination. Expansion of gases within the lungs and digestive tract would be the first effect. Because water is converted into vapor immediately in the absence of atmospheric pressure, moisture in the mouth and eyes would quickly boil away. Water in the muscle and soft tissue would evaporate also, causing some parts of the body to swell to twice their usual size after a few moments. Within seconds the reduced pressure would cause the nitrogen dissolved in the blood to form gaseous bubbles, a painful condition known to divers as "the bends." The first few seconds may not be life threatening, and "useful consciousness" would gradually fade as the effects of brain hypoxia set in. The gas exchange that normally takes place in the lungs would work in reverse, evolving oxygen out of the blood and into the alveoli as a result of the low atmospheric pressure. After about 10 seconds, loss of vision and impaired judgment occur, and the cooling effect of evaporation will lower the temperature of the mouth and nose to near freezing. Unconsciousness and convulsions would follow a few seconds later, followed by cyanosis, stupor, and unresponsiveness. Without intervention, the blood pressure would fall, the blood itself would begin to boil, and the heart would stop beating. There are no reports of successful resuscitation beyond that threshold.

Emergency care in space involves numerous challenges. First off, it is difficult to confine fluids; as a result, conventional vaporizers would have to be redesigned for use under conditions of microgravity. In addition, the risk of aspiration is increased, because acid reflux is more common in microgravity under general anesthesia. Also, the air-fluid interface generates bubbles, and IV fluids must have the air bubbles removed during administration, or fluids must be degassed before the flight. Hypotension may not be adequately treatable because of limited supplies, preexisting hypovolemia, and increased G-forces on reentry. Securing an airway may be difficult or unsuccessful because of facial edema and the insecure position of both the patient and the intubator. Scavenging the anesthetic gases and oxygen in space is another issue.

After landing, nausea and vomiting recur, and some degree of orthostatic intolerance is experienced by most astronauts.[32] Such orthostasis may be due to hypovolemia, enhanced endothelial nitric oxide synthase expression, and downregulation of α-adrenergic receptors. In addition, some loss of pressor response to phenylephrine has been observed.[33] Cardiovascular deconditioning, ventricular atrophy, and changes in arterial stiffness may also play a role. Although the physiologic response of anesthesia in space is not exactly known, the immediate postflight hemodynamic response to general or neuraxial anesthesia may include variable degrees of resistant hypotension.

The atrophy that occurs because of the effect of loss of gravity, immobilization, and disuse of the skeletal muscles result in proliferation of extrajunctional acetylcholine receptors. As a result astronauts may be sensitive to succinylcholine with an exaggerated hyperkalemia response and a risk of cardiac arrest. They may also be resistant to nondepolarizing neuromuscular blocking drugs. The most common electrolyte abnormalities reported after spaceflight are hypokalemia and hypomagnesemia.[34]

Thus the environment of space, limited in terms of area and resources available, makes any kind of medical treatment a logistical challenge. The anesthesiologist at present seems to be just an emergency care provider, should a need arise. Any further role in routine anesthetic management in space has a long way to go, along with developments in the active fields of robotics, surgery, and on-board diagnostics. It is important to realize the fact that even during a short spaceflight, astronauts have altered physiology that continues beyond their return to earth. Therefore it is best to avoid administration of elective anesthesia to astronauts after their return and to provide time for the altered physiology to normalize.

REFERENCES

1. Basu CK, Selvamurthy W, Bhaumick G, Gautam RK, Sawhney RC: Respiratory changes during initial days of acclimatization to increasing altitudes, *Aviat Space Environ Med* 67:40–45, 1996.
2. Hupperets MD, Hopkins SR, Pronk MG, et al: Increased hypoxic ventilatory response during 8 weeks at 3800 m altitude, *Respir Physiol Neurobiol* 142:145–152, 2004.
3. Erzurum SC, Ghosh S, Janocha AJ, et al: Higher blood flow and circulating NO products offset high altitude hypoxia among Tibetans, *Proc Natl Acad Sci U S A* 104(17):593–598, 2007.
4. Leissner KB, Mahmood FU: Physiology and pathophysiology at high altitude: considerations for the anesthesiologist, *J Anesth* 23:543–553, 2009.
5. Fukuda R, Zhang H, Kim JW, et al: HIF-1 regulates cytochrome oxidase subunits to optimize efficiency of respiration in hypoxic cells, *Cell* 129:111–122, 2007.
6. Forsythe JS, Hang BH, Iyer NV, et al: Activation of vascular endothelial growth factor gene transcription by hypoxia-inducible factor 1, *Mol Cell Biol* 16:4604–4613, 1999.
7. Hackett PH, Roach RC: High-altitude illness, *N Engl J Med* 345:107–114, 2001.
8. Moon RE, Camporesi EM: Clinical care in extreme environments: at high and low pressure and in space. In Miller R, Eriksson L, Fleisher LA, Wiener-Kronish J, editors: *Miller's anesthesia*, ed 7, Philadelphia, 2010, Churchill Livingstone.
9. Cymerman A, Rock PB: Medical problems in high mountain environments: a handbook for medical officers. USARIEM-TN94-2. U.S. Army Research Institute, Department of Environmental Medicine, Thermal and Mountain Medicine Division Technical Report. Available at archive.rubicon-foundation.org/7976.
10. Niermeyer S: Cardiopulmonary transition in the high altitude infant, *High Alt Med Biol* 4(2):225–239, 2003.
11. Powell JN, Gingrich TF: Some aspects of nitrous oxide anesthesia at an altitude of one mile, *Anesth Analg* 48:680–685, 1969.
12. James MFM, Manson EDM, Dennett JE: Nitrous oxide analgesia and altitude, *Anaesthesia* 37:285–288, 1982.
13. Safar P, Tenicela R: High altitude physiology in relation to anesthesia and inhalation therapy, *Anesthesiology* 25:515–531, 1964.
14. James MFM, White JF: Anesthetic considerations at moderate altitude, *Anesth Analg* 63:1097–1105, 1984.
15. Hill DW: *Physics applied to anesthesia* ed 4, Boston, 1980, Butterworths. pp 336–337.
16. McDowall DG: Anaesthesia in a pressure chamber, *Anaesthesia* 19:321–336, 1964.
17. Friedman MD, Lightstone PJ: The effect of high altitude on flowmeter performance [abstract], *Anesthesiology* 55:A117, 1981.
18. Halsey MJ, White DC: Gas and vapour supply. In Gray TC, Nunn JF, Utting JE, editors: *General anaesthesia*, ed 4, London, 1980, Butterworths, pp 953–961.
19. Puri GD, Jayant A, Dorje M, Tashi M: Propofol-fentanyl anaesthesia at high altitude: anaesthetic requirements and haemodynamic variations when compared with anaesthesia at low altitude, *Acta Anaesthesiol Scand* 52:427–431, 2008.
20. IATA Annual Report. Available at http://www.iata.org/pressroom/documents/annual-report-2011.pdf.
21. Delaune EF 3rd, Lucas RH, Illig P: In-flight medical events and aircraft diversions: one airline's experience, *Aviat Space Environ Med* 74:62–68, 2003.
22. Cummins RO, Schubach JA: Frequency and types of medical emergencies among commercial air travelers, *JAMA* 261:1295–1299, 1989.
23. Aerospace Medical Association: *Air Transport Medicine Committee: Medical guidelines for airline travel*, ed 2, Alexandria, VA, 2003, Aerospace Medical Association.
24. Ruskin KJ, Hernandez AK, Barash PG: Management of in-flight medical emergencies, *Anesthesiology* 108:749–755, 2008.
25. Dillard TA, Bansal AK: Commentary: pulse oximetry during airline travel, *Aviat Space Environ Med* 78:143–144, 2007.
26. Closon M, Vivier E, Breynaert C, et al: Air embolism during an aircraft flight in a passenger with a pulmonary cyst: a favorable outcome with hyperbaric therapy, *Anesthesiology* 101:539–542, 2004.
27. Zitter JN, Mazonson PD, Miller DP, Hulley SB, Balmes JR: Aircraft cabin air recirculation and symptoms of the common cold, *JAMA* 288:483–486, 2002.
28. Adi Y, Bayliss S, Rouse A, Taylor RS: The association between air travel and deep vein thrombosis: systematic review and meta-analysis, *BMC Cardiovasc Disord* 4:7, 2004.
29. 105th Congress, public law 170, Avaiation Medical Assistance Act of 1998. Available at http://www.gpo.gov/fdsys/pkg/PLAW-105publ170/html/PLAW-105publ170.htm.
30. Leach CS, Alfrey CP, Suki WN, et al: Regulation of body fluid compartments during short-term space flight, *J Appl Physiol* 81:105–116, 1996.
31. Tuday EC, Berkowitz DE: Microgravity and cardiac atrophy; no sex discrimination, *J Appl Physiol* 103:1–2, 2007.
32. Buckey JC Jr, Lane LD, Levine BD, et al: Orthostatic intolerance after spaceflight, *J Appl Physiol* 81:7–18, 1996.
33. Meck JV, Waters WW, Zeigler MG, et al: Mechanisms of post-spaceflight orthostatic hypotension: low alpha1-adrenergic receptor responses before flight and central autonomic dysregualtion post flight, *Am J Physiol Heart Circ Physiol* 286:H1486–H1495, 2004.
34. Leach CS, Alexander WC, Johnson PC: Endocrine, electrolyte, and fluid volume changes associated with Apollo missions. In Johnston RS, Dietlein LF, Berry CA, editors: *Biomedical results of Apollo*, Washington, DC, 1975, Biotechnology, pp 163–184.

CHAPTER 29

Anesthesia in Difficult Locations and in Developing Countries

Roger Eltringham • Collin Sprenker • Enrico Camporesi

CHAPTER OUTLINE

INHALATIONAL ANESTHESIA IN DIFFICULT LOCATIONS

Modern anesthesia workstations are complex and sophisticated pieces of medical equipment. They have evolved over many years to improve performance and reduce the risk of accidents and mishaps. The most recent workstations offer the ability to administer a wide range of volatile agents using a variety of breathing circuits. In addition, physiologic functions can be monitored and displayed, trends can be observed, and both audible and visual alarms can be set to predetermined limits to reduce risks to an absolute minimum.

Although these developments have led to improved standards of safety in wealthy countries, these advantages have not been mirrored in poorer countries. These sophisticated machines are unaffordable in many countries such that even when donated, major problems obstruct their successful deployment. These machines are designed to work in ideal conditions, and additional problems encountered in the most impoverished areas of the world often cannot be overcome. An anesthetic machines' success in such an environment relies on its ability to function in the absence of oxygen, electricity, and regular servicing by skilled technicians.

It is important to adapt to adverse situations, and extensive technical support may not be available. There have been no overwhelming military or natural catastrophes in the United States in recent years; in addition, emergency medical crews are able to extricate victims from practically any accident without limb amputation, and patients in remote areas who require surgery can usually be transported to facilities equipped with standard anesthesia equipment.

This chapter reviews some of the equipment that can be used for anesthesia under mobile disaster circumstances and in isolated and economically deprived conditions, although techniques for providing anesthesia are not described in detail. Anesthesia equipment must be compact, portable, and robust. Surgery can be performed in a hazardous location but must be rapid and essential. In an emergency, evacuation of even mass casualties should be prompt. Cost is not a limiting factor, and anesthesia is normally administered by an expert anesthesia specialist using intravenous (IV) inductions followed by volatile inhaled agents if indicated. Regional anesthesia for surgery in conscious patients may not be as useful under these conditions as when it is used as an analgesic supplement or in more controlled conditions.

DRAW-OVER BREATHING SYSTEM

The oldest method of providing inhalational anesthesia involves breathing air, perhaps enriched with oxygen, drawn over a volatile anesthetic agent. This principle was first used when a handkerchief containing anesthetic was held to the face, with various Schimmelbusch types of masks, with the Flagg can, and with numerous hand-held or table-top inhalers. Few vaporizers were calibrated to deliver a known concentration of anesthetic agent. This knowledge was not considered essential for anesthesia, because more reliance was placed on clinical signs than on achieving a specified minimum alveolar concentration (MAC) in the end-tidal gas.

For a volatile agent to be vaporized, a carrier gas must pass through a vaporizing chamber. It can be driven through the chamber by positive pressure from a cylinder or central supply, as in continuous-flow anesthesia, or through the chamber by negative pressure generated by the patient`s inspiratory effort.

For use in isolated hospitals, oxygen cylinders must be transported over long distances on roads that may be impassable for prolonged periods, and supplies may run out altogether. In the absence of oxygen, the administration of inhalational anesthesia by continuous flow is impossible. Draw-over anesthesia offers an alternative that is used especially in military and disaster situations when no local facilities exist.[1]

A draw-over system has the following basic components: 1) a reservoir tube, 2) a vaporizer, 3) a self-inflating bag, 4) a nonrebreathing valve, and 5) an optional reservoir tube (Fig. 29-1).The reservoir generally consists of a section of corrugated tubing about 1 m in length, one end of which is attached to the vaporizer; the other end is open to the atmosphere. There is a side arm for the addition of supplementary oxygen, if it is available; while the patient is breathing out, the oxygen flows into the reservoir to be incorporated into the next breath. Plenum vaporizers are unsuitable for draw-over anesthesia, because the resistance to spontaneous breathing is too high. Vaporizers designed for draw-over anesthesia must have a sufficiently low resistance to enable spontaneous respiration to occur. The Epstein-Macintosh-Oxford (EMO) vaporizer is an example of an early draw-over vaporizer designed for use with ether (Fig. 29-2). Later models include the Oxford miniature vaporizer (Penlon Inc., Minnetonka, MN; Fig. 29-3) and the DiaMedica (Minneapolis, MN) vaporizer, both of which can be used with halothane, isoflurane, and other volatile agents. The self-inflating bag for controlled or assisted ventilation is separated from the vaporizer by a one-way valve. When the bag is compressed, the valve ensures that the contents are directed toward the patient and that they cannot reenter the vaporizer. A nonrebreathing valve is situated as close to the patient as possible to minimize the dead space. The function of the valve is to ensure that only the anesthetic mixture is inhaled during inspiraction and that it is not diluted with atmospheric air. During exhalation, the valve directs the exhaled mixture into the atmosphere and prevents it from reentering the breathing system.

Several types of nonrebreathing valves are on the market, including Laerdal Medical (Stavanger, Norway), Ambu (Ballerup, Denmark), and Ruben (Intersurgical Ltd., Workingham, UK) valves. A scavenging system can be connected to the expiratory port of the nonrebreathing valve. When using a face mask in draw-over anesthesia, an airtight seal is essential during inspiration to create the required negative pressure. In some circumstances,

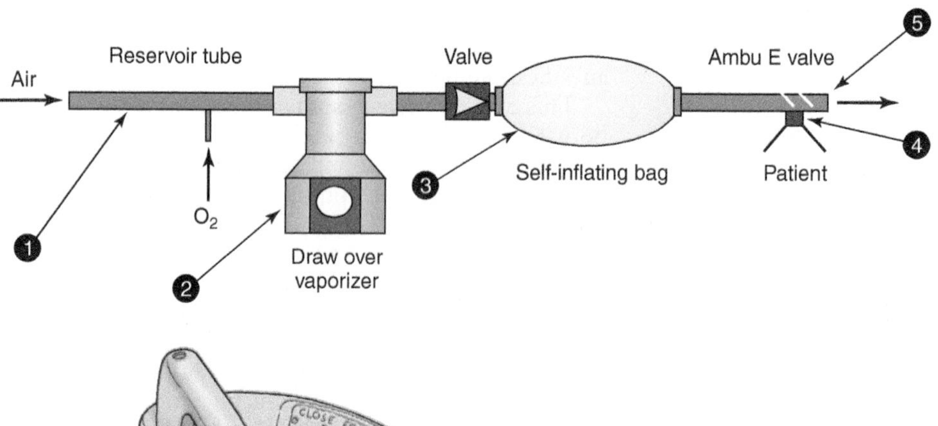

FIGURE 29-1 Components of a draw-over system.

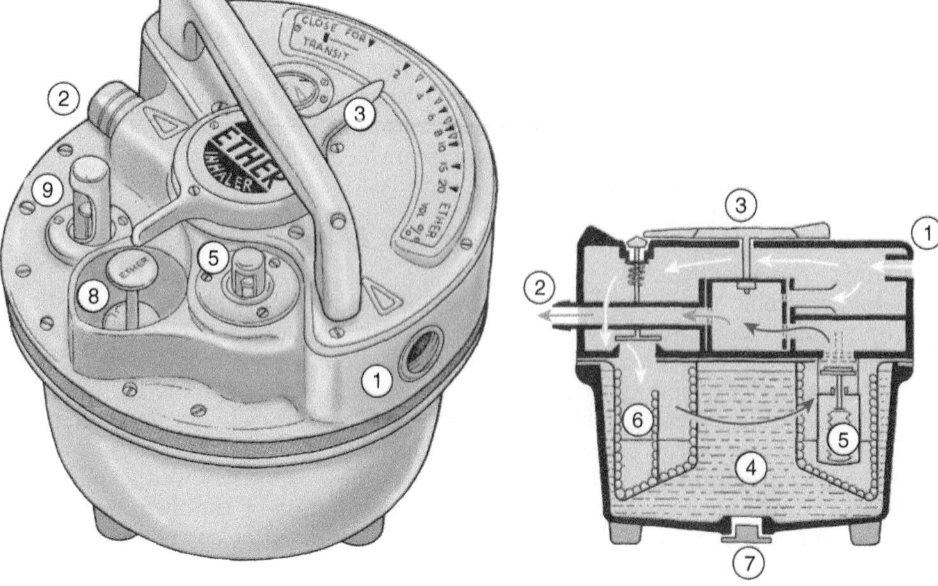

FIGURE 29-2 Schematic of the Epstein-Macintosh-Oxford vaporizer. *1,* Inlet port; *2,* outlet port; *3,* concentration control; *4,* water jacket; *5,* thermocompensator valve; *6,* vaporizing chamber; *7,* filling port for water; *8,* filling port for anesthetic; *9,* anesthetic level indicator. (From Dobson MB: *Anaesthesia at the district hospital.* Geneva, 1988, World Health Organization. Reproduced by permission.)

such as an inhalation induction of anesthesia in uncooperative children or in the presence of facial trauma, an airtight seal may be impossible to achieve. In these circumstances, the draw-over system can be converted to a continuous-flow system by occluding the open end of the reservoir.[2] The same maneuver is required in small children (<10 kg) for whom the resistance to breathing through the vaporizer is excessive. In these patients the draw-over breathing circuit can be replaced by an Ayres T-piece system attached directly to the vaporizer.

OXYGEN CONCENTRATOR

Cylinders of oxygen are expensive, hazardous to transport, and contain a limited volume. On the other hand, air costs nothing, does not require transport, and the supply does not run out. Therefore it is logical to use atmospheric air as the source of oxygen whenever possible, which can be done effectively by the use of an oxygen concentrator similar to the type used for domestic oxygen therapy (Fig. 29-4).

Function

The function of an oxygen concentrator depends on the ability of zeolite granules to absorb nitrogen from compressed air. Atmospheric air is first drawn into the concentrator through a filter and is compressed to a pressure of 20 psi. It then passes through a column containing granules of zeolite, where the nitrogen is absorbed, and the residual oxygen is directed to the patient. Two columns of zeolite are used in parallel so that the supply of compressed air can be directed to each of the columns alternately: one

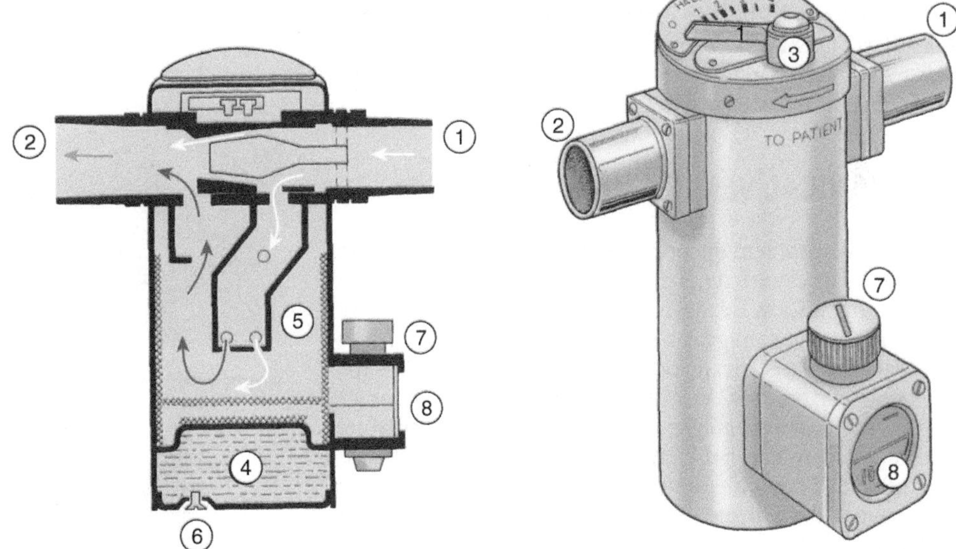

FIGURE 29-3 ■ Schematic of the Oxford miniature vaporizer (Penlon Inc., Minnetonka, MN). *1,* Inlet port; *2,* outlet port; *3,* concentration control; *4,* heat sink; *5,* vaporizing chamber; *6,* filling port for water; *7,* filling port for anesthetic; *8,* anesthetic level indicator. (From Dobson MB: *Anaesthesia at the district hospital.* Geneva, 1988, World Health Organization. Reproduced by permission.)

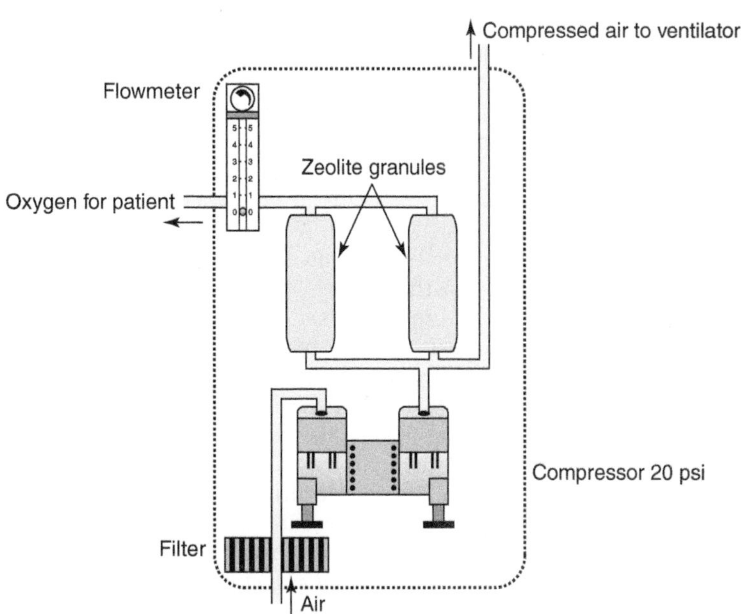

FIGURE 29-4 ■ Oxygen concentrator.

column contains air at 20 psi, and the zeolite is absorbing nitrogen and allowing oxygen to pass to the patient. At the same time, the pressure in the other column is reduced to atmospheric pressure, and the nitrogen is automatically released into the surroundings. In this way a continuous supply of oxygen at a concentration of up to 95% can be produced indefinitely. Unlike soda lime, zeolite granules do not become exhausted or require changing but can be used for many years. Early oxygen concentrators were able to produce a supply of oxygen at 5 L/min, but modern concentrators can supply 10 L/min or more.

One of the advantages of using an oxygen concentrator in place of cylinders is economy. At a rate of 5 L/min, oxygen from a concentrator costs about $0.01/hr, whereas cylinder oxygen costs approx $2.00/hr. When utilization is notoriously high, such as in intensive care and neonatal units, huge savings are possible if a concentrator can be used as source of oxygen.[3]

The basic design of the early oxygen concentrator for domestic oxygen therapy can be modified as required for anesthetic use. For example, there can be additional outlets for air or oxygen for the patient or for oxygen under sufficient pressure to drive a ventilator.

MECHANICAL VENTILATORS

A persistent problem encountered in poor countries is that the supply of electricity is prone to interruption, often for prolonged periods. Even when the supply is not completely interrupted, the voltage can vary by as much as 30%. Most ventilators are electrically powered and depend on the supply being continuous. As an alternative to electrically powered ventilators, several gas-driven ventilators are available. Although these are satisfactory when oxygen supplies are guaranteed, in poor countries, one disadvantage is their extravagant oxygen consumption. Many ventilators, such as the Penlon Nuffield 400 series, require a supply of oxygen equal to the patient's entire minute volume; thus it is not ideal in situations of limited supply.[4]

In 1995, Dr. Roger Manley developed the Manley Multivent (Penlon), a ventilator specifically for use in poor countries with limited facilities.[5] It was a simple gas-driven ventilator in which the volume of driving gas required was reduced to a minimum. It consisted of a set of bellows under a metal beam (Fig. 29-5).

Function

In the simple gas-driven ventilator, one end of the beam was attached to the top of the bellows, while the other rotated around a fulcrum. A piston was situated below the beam close to the fulcrum, and the piston was driven upward from below by compressed gas, causing the bellows to expand and fill with the anesthetic mixture. An adjustable weight above the beam then compressed the bellows, delivering the anesthetic to the patient.

The driving gas for the Manley Multivent could be either compressed air or oxygen. Because the distance between the piston and the fulcrum was much less than the distance between the bellows and the fulcrum, the ventilator required only one seventh of the minute volume delivered to the patient for driving gas. This was particularly valuable when supplies were limited.

When oxygen is the driving gas, still further economy is possible; once it has driven the piston upward, the gas can be recycled and added to the inspiratory mixture. In other words, the oxygen is used twice: first to drive the ventilator and subsequently to supplement the inspired gas mixture. This method of driving a ventilator is extremely economical and has been incorporated into other gas-driven ventilators.[6] Using the Glostavent (DiaMedica), it has been shown that a single E-sized oxygen cylinder containing 680 L of oxygen can ventilate the lungs of an adult and can supplement the inspired mixture with 35% oxygen for approximately 12 hours.[7] These three components—the oxygen concentrator, draw-over system, and gas-driven ventilator—can be combined in a single anesthetic machine as, for example, in the Glostavent (Fig. 29-6).

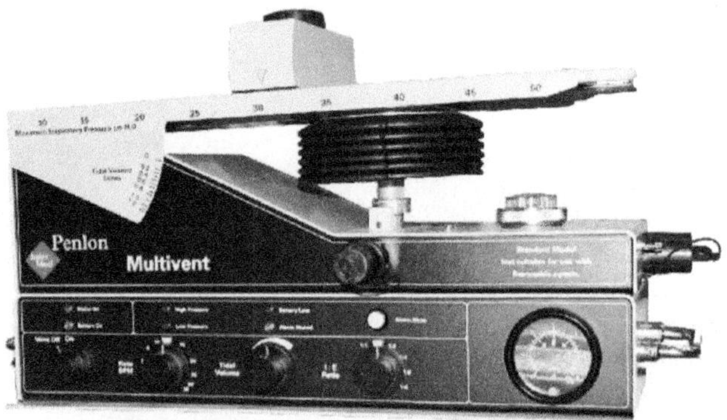

FIGURE 29-5 Manley Multivent (Penlon Inc., Minnetonka, MN).

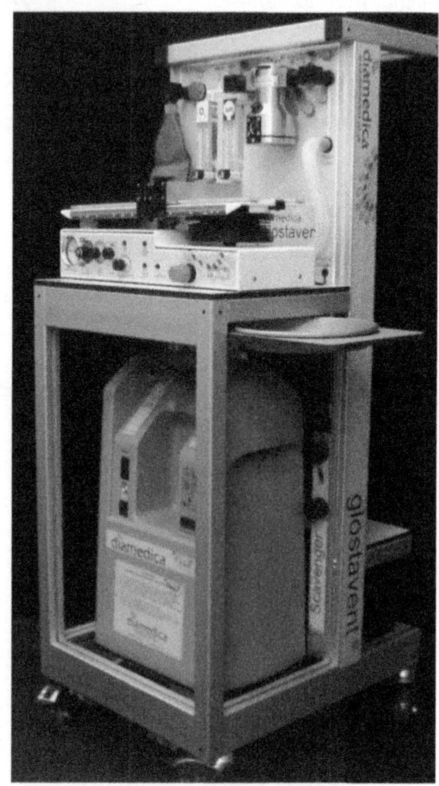

FIGURE 29-6 Glostavent anesthesia machine (DiaMedica, Minneapolis, MN).

Two additional features further increase the versatility of anesthesia machines in difficult situations: 1) an uninterruptable power supply (UPS) that will neutralize severe fluctuations in voltage and maintain supply for up to 20 minutes in the event of a complete interruption of electricity and 2) a cylinder of oxygen kept in reserve for use only if prolonged electrical failure incapacitates the oxygen concentrator.

When this combination of features is used in a single machine, it can be used both for the administration of anesthesia in an operating room and for long-term ventilation in an intensive care unit (ICU) or postoperative recovery room. This combination is also ideal for use in isolated hospitals with limited facilities, because it can continue to function without interruption for prolonged periods in the absence of oxygen or electricity.

Under normal circumstances, when electricity is available, it is much cheaper to use the concentrator both as the source of oxygen for the patient and for pressure to drive the ventilator. Only if the electrical supply is interrupted, causing the oxygen concentrator to stop, is the reserve cylinder used as the source of oxygen for the breathing circuit and for pressure to drive the ventilator. The changeover of supply from concentrator to cylinder occurs automatically and requires no action on the part of the anesthesiologist.

RECENT DEVELOPMENTS

As awareness of the problems of providing anesthesia in the developing world has become more widespread, the interest in improving the performance of anesthesia machines been renewed. As a result of an extensive research program, various components of the Glostavent have been improved.[8]

The draw-over system has been the focus of most attention. Although the tri-service apparatus (TSA) has been used successfully for many years and in many fields of conflict, significant improvements have been made to the various components. The efficiency of the reservoir has been increased by three additions (Fig. 29-7): a valve at the open end prevents spillage of oxygen; a reservoir bag increases the volume of the reservoir; and a pressure relief valve set at 5 cm H_2O prevents distention of the reservoir bag. These modifications contribute to the conservation of oxygen by totally eliminating waste. If the flow rate of added oxygen exceeds the patient's minute volume, the reservoir bag becomes distended, and the valve at the open end of the reservoir closes.

These additions have also enabled the system to function in either a draw-over or continuous-flow mode without the need for a change in the breathing system. The mode in use at any time is determined by the ratio of the fresh-gas flow to the patient's respiratory minute volume. If the flow of fresh gas entering the reservoir is less than the patient's respiratory minute volume leaving the reservoir, then the pressure in the reservoir becomes subatmospheric, air is drawn in, and the system operates in draw-over mode. To transfer to continuous flow mode, it is only necessary to increase the fresh-gas flow until it exceeds the patient's respiratory minute volume. The pressure in the reservoir then rises, and the flow becomes continuous.

VAPORIZERS

One of the first vaporizers used for draw-over anesthesia was the EMO, which was used with ether (see Fig. 29-2). The EMO vaporizer was produced in 1956 by Epstein and Macintosh as an improved version of the Oxford ether vaporizer, which was itself inspired by the Flagg can.[9] It incorporates many ingenious features, requires routine maintenance only every 5 years, and is ubiquitous in developing countries. It is still in production and in common use but is not discussed here in detail because it can be used only with ether or methoxyflurane (1/10 calibration scale), neither of which is commonly used to provide clinical anesthesia in the United States. As ether was gradually phased out, the EMO was replaced by the Oxford miniature vaporizer (OMV; see Fig. 29-3), which is calibrated for use with halothane, isoflurane, and trichloroethylene.

Although the OMV has been used successfully in the British army for many years, it is gradually being replaced by the DiaMedica Draw-Over Vaporizer (DDV), which has many advantages.[10] These include a greater consistency of output, higher concentrations of volatile agents, and a larger reservoir. In addition, an alternative version of the vaporizer is now available that can deliver a concentration of up to 8% sevoflurane, which greatly facilitates gaseous induction in field conditions.

Valves

The traditional nonrebreathing valves all have the disadvantages that come with adding bulk in the vicinity of the patient's airway. A tendency to cause kinking of the endotracheal tube and obstruction of the airway requires

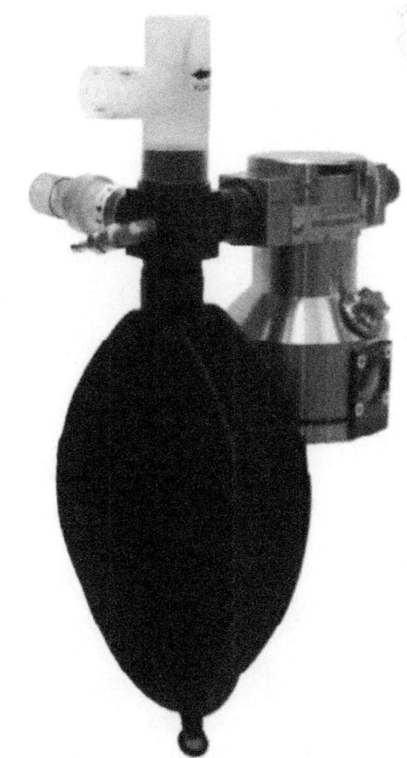

FIGURE 29-7 ■ Reservoir unit for draw-over system.

frequent intervention by the anesthesiologist. The situation is exacerbated when more bulk is added with an additional scavenging tube, although this problem has been eliminated with the introduction of the DiaMedica Draw-Over Valve.[11] The valve is located at the anesthesia machine, well away from the patient's airway, thus eliminating the need for inconvenient bulk in this area. Further improvement in the delivery system can be achieved by replacing the separate inspiratory and expiratory breathing tubes with a single, lightweight, double-lumen tube (Vital Signs Limb-O, GE Healthcare, Waukesha, WI) that connects directly with the endotracheal tube, laryngeal mask airway (LMA), or face mask.

PORTABLE ANESTHESIA MACHINES

Although the new draw-over machines, such as the Glostavent, are able to deliver safe anesthesia in hospitals whose facilities are severely limited and unreliable, demand also exists for the administration of anesthesia under field conditions—that is, where there are no facilities at all—and where everything required by the anesthesiologists must be carried into position.

To be suitable for use in such situations, an anesthetic machine must be specifically designed to be able to overcome additional hazards and limitations. It must be lightweight, easy to assemble and operate, able to use a variety of inhalational agents, and economical in its utilization of oxygen; in addition, it must contain a minimal number of parts that could malfunction.

The TSA is an example of such a machine, and it has given reliable service in many fields of conflict over the past 40 years. However, recent innovations in draw-over anesthesia have led to the introduction of a new lightweight anesthetic machine, known as the *portable Glostavent*, or DPA01 (Fig. 29-8),[12] which has a reservoir unit that consists of a small, hollow block of acetyl with five openings, one of which is connected to the entry port of the vaporizer; the other is connected to a 2-L oxygen reservoir bag. Attached to the other openings are a pressure relief valve, a nonreturn valve at the air inlet port to prevent spillage of oxygen into the atmosphere, and a connecting piece for the oxygen supply. There is also a DiaMedica vaporizer, self-inflating bag, and nonrebreathing valve, as in the standard version of the Glostavent.

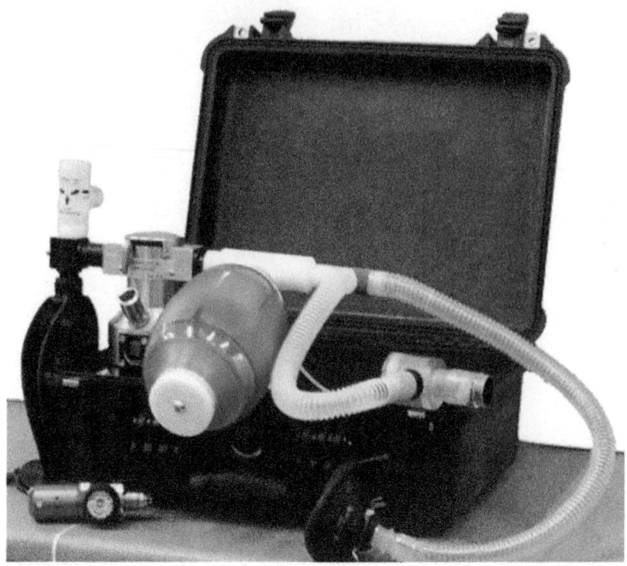

FIGURE 29-8 ■ DPA 02 portable anesthetic machine (DiaMedica, Minneapolis, MN).

The DPA01 weighs less than 10 kg and fits in a polymer container the size of a small suitcase (44 × 50 × 20 cm). The hermetically sealed container is manufactured to a military standard (defstan 81/41) and is waterproof as well as dust, shock, and corrosion proof. It incorporates all the components required for draw-over anesthesia, including many of the recent improvements introduced into the Glostavent.

A portable anesthetic machine should be suitable for use with any size patient, whether the patient requires controlled or spontaneous respiration, and it should be able to deliver sufficient concentrations of volatile agent to facilitate inhalational induction when required. The portable Glostavent fulfils all of these requirements, and it is inexpensive, lightweight, and versatile; the DPA01 has been recommended as a worthy successor to the TSA for use in adverse conditions.

TOTAL INTRAVENOUS ANESTHESIA

Another alternative method to anesthesia in austere environments is the exclusive use of IV agents. The equipment required for total IV anesthesia (TIVA) is lightweight, familiar, and portable: sterile syringes, needles, an infusion apparatus, and drugs. TIVA is the most common method of producing anesthesia in the field for short surgical procedures, such as the amputation of a trapped, unsalvageable limb. Ketamine is usually the primary IV anesthetic, and it is also effective when given intramuscularly; more recently, satisfactory experience has been described with propofol infusions. Administered by competent personnel, TIVA has proven very satisfactory over a large number of cases, both in emergencies and for elective surgery.[13]

TIVA can be provided with many combinations of drugs to achieve hypnosis, analgesia, and muscle relaxation without undue cardiovascular depression. The ablation of the autonomic reflex to surgery, which is necessary when the viscera are stimulated, can be achieved with a sympatholytic drug such as labetalol. The next major development in this field will be the introduction of a drug capable of producing surgical depths of anesthesia without significant respiratory depression or unwanted psychogenic effects. Ketamine was originally marketed as such, as were thiopental and propofol. Stereospecific isomers of ketamine show some promise, as do receptor-specific opioids.

TIVA has a major advantage over inhalational anesthesia when contamination of the ambient atmosphere is a problem. In addition, if high inspired oxygen concentrations are needed, (i.e., in the presence of major thoracic trauma or smoke inhalation), and oxygen supplies are limited, a closed-circle system utilizing minimal quantities of fresh oxygen can most easily be used in conjunction with

IV anesthesia. One E cylinder of oxygen (containing 660 L when filled to a pressure of 1900 psig) will last for approximately 40 hours at a flow rate of 250 mL/min, roughly one average week of anesthesia. With the advent of fast-acting IV drugs; portable, robust, and dependable infusion pumps; and drugs that reverse residual anesthesia, it is surprising that TIVA is not more popular, both for elective and field surgery. Despite its attractive simplicity, the technique requires practice and familiarity to achieve sufficient expertise. The requisite of multiple essential drugs, all of which need to be kept sterile, is also a disadvantage in field use. Especially in primitive surroundings, in which patients must recover without expert supervision, inhalational and perhaps regional anesthesia are still more popular than TIVA for mass casualties.

REGIONAL AND LOCAL ANESTHESIA

As with TIVA, equipment to provide regional and local anesthesia is compact and portable and must be kept sterile. Disposable syringes, needles, and microcatheters of practically every configuration are readily available, as are a wide variety of local anesthetic preparations. However, major regional anesthesia requires careful planning and constant practice, which will often preclude its use in field situations for anything other than the provision of analgesia for musculoskeletal injuries. Nevertheless, in more static situations, regional anesthesia may be preferred, especially for mass casualties, when facilities and personnel for general anesthesia are scarce. In one field hospital dispatched to Armenia immediately after the earthquake of December 7, 1988, regional anesthesia was used for 14 of 26 surgical procedures carried out under difficult circumstances. These 14 anesthetics consisted of four epidurals and six intravenous regional and four local infiltrations.[14]

Apparatus for regional anesthesia in the field does not differ from hospital equipment. If improvisation is necessary to avoid repeating the disasters of adhesive arachnoiditis caused by detergent residues of a generation ago, the skill of honing dull needles must be relearned, along with the knowledge how to clean and resterilize needles. Many articles describe techniques for regional anesthesia in difficult situations.[15,16]

MONITORING

One of the major disadvantages of administering general or regional anesthesia in the absence of a reliable electricity supply is that sophisticated electronic monitors cease to function when the electricity supply fails. Even when electricity is available, the accuracy of the monitors cannot be guaranteed in the absence of regular calibration and servicing by highly trained engineers.

Fortunately, the draw-over system has several built-in safety features that contribute to safety if monitors are unreliable or nonexistent. First, it is impossible to administer a hypoxic mixture accidentally because the room air being inhaled already contains 21% oxygen, to which further oxygen is then added; so the resulting inspired concentration will increase rather than decrease. Second, the concentration of volatile agent inhaled by the patient is identical to that leaving the vaporizer. It is not diluted by an unknown concentration in the expired mixture as occurs when low flows of fresh gas are used in a circle system, and where monitoring of the inspired concentration is essential. Third, the levels of carbon dioxide are not influenced by such factors as the condition of soda lime or the adequacy of fresh gas flow rates, as is the case in other breathing systems. When using a draw-over system, carbon dioxide levels are proportional to the respiratory activity, which can be observed clinically. These built-in safety features enable the administration of draw-over anesthesia with more confidence while using conscientious clinical monitoring than by relying on sophisticated monitors that are not calibrated and are dependent on an irregular supply of electricity.

The semiclosed circle system is often advocated for economic reasons because low flows of fresh gas can be used. It is true that lower oxygen flow rates can be used with correspondingly lower rates of evaporation of volatile agent. However, this must be weighed against the cost of the soda lime and purchase of monitors, and it has been shown that savings are in fact minimal.[17]

REFERENCES

1. Jowitt MD: Anaesthesia in the Falklands, *Ann Royal Coll Surg* 66:197–200, 1984.
2. Dobson M, editor: *Anaesthesia in the district hospital*, ed 2, Geneva, 2000, World Health Organization.
3. Binh HS, Thang C: Experience with the Glostavent in Viet Nam, *WFSA Newslett* 8(2):27, 2005.
4. Davey AJ, Moyle JTB, Ward CS, editors: *Ward's anaesthesia equipment*, ed 3, Philadelphia, 1992, W.B. Saunders, p 235.
5. Manley R: A new ventilator for developing countries and difficult locations, *World Anaesth Newslett* 5:10–11, 1991.
6. Eltringham RJ, Varvinski A: An anaesthetic machine designed to be used in developing countries and difficult situations, *Anaesthesia* 52:668–672, 1997.
7. Bailey TM, Webster S, Tully R, Eltringham R, Bordeaux C: An assessment of the efficiency of the Glostavent ventilator, *Anaesthesia* 64:899–902, 2009.
8. Beringer RM, Eltringham RJ: The Glostavent; evolution of an anaesthetic machine for developing countries, *Anaesth Intensive Care* 36:442–448, 2008.
9. Macintosh RR: Saved by the Flagg 2.1. In Atkinson RS, Boulton TB, editors: *The history of anaesthesia*, Park Ridge, NJ, 1989, Parthenon Publishing Group.
10. English WA, Tully R, Muller GD, Eltringham RJ: The Diamedica Draw-Over Vaporizer; a comparison of a new vaporizer with the Oxford Miniature Vaporizer, *Anaesthesia* 64:84–92, 2009.
11. Payne S, Tully R, Eltringham R: A new valve for draw-over anaesthesia, *Anaesthesia* 65:1080–1084, 2010.
12. Tully R, Eltringham R, Walker IA, Bartlett AJ: The portable Glostavent: a new anaesthetic machine for use in difficult situations, *Anaesth Intensive Care* 12(1):27–28, 2010.
13. Restall J, Tully AM, Ward PJ, et al: Total intravenous anaesthesia for military surgery: a technique using ketamine, midazolam and vecuronium, *Anaesthesia* 43:46–49, 1988.
14. Donchin Y, Wiener M, Grande CM, et al: Military medicine: trauma anesthesia and critical care on the battlefield, *Crit Care Clinics* 6:185–202, 1990.
15. Breckenmeier CC, Lee EH, Shields CH, et al: Regional anesthesia in austere environments, *Regional Anesth Pain Med* 28(4):321–327, 2003.
16. Boulton TB: Local anaesthesia in difficult environments. In Lofstrom JB, Sjostrand U, editors: *Local anaesthesia and regional blockade*, Amsterdam, 1988, Elsevier.
17. Drake M: A comparison of the cost of inhalational anaesthesia using various breathing systems, *Anaesthesia Points West* 42(1):51–54, 2009.

PART VII

SAFETY, STANDARDS, AND QUALITY

CHAPTER 30

HAZARDS OF THE ANESTHESIA DELIVERY SYSTEM

James B. Eisenkraft

CHAPTER OUTLINE

PERSPECTIVE

Failure of the anesthesia delivery system alone is a rare cause of anesthesia-related injury or death of a patient. More commonly, the delivery system is misused, the operator errs, or the delivery system fails in combination with the anesthesiologist being unaware that failure has taken place. In most cases of anesthesia machine failure, a temporal window of opportunity exists during which the anesthesiologist can detect the problem and correct it before the patient is harmed. Therefore a sound understanding of the anesthesia delivery system and the ways in which it can fail or be misused provides the basis for safe anesthesia practice.

Critical Incidents

The critical incident (CI) technique was first described by Flanagan in 1954[1] and was developed to reduce loss of military pilots and aircraft during training. It was modified and introduced into anesthesia by Cooper and colleagues,[2] who interviewed staff and resident anesthesiologists in a large metropolitan teaching hospital. They collected and analyzed 1089 descriptions of CIs during anesthesia.[3] A mishap was labeled a CI when it was clearly an occurrence that could have led, if not discovered or corrected in time, or did lead to an undesirable outcome, ranging from increased length of hospital stay to death or permanent disability. Other CI study inclusion criteria were that each incident involved an error by a member of the anesthesia team or failure of the anesthetist's equipment to function properly; it occurred during patient care; it could be clearly described; and the incident was clearly preventable. Of the 1089 CIs, 70 represented errors or failures that had contributed in some way to a "substantive negative outcome" (SNO) defined as mortality, cardiac arrest, canceled operative procedure, or extended stay in the postanesthesia care unit (PACU), intensive care unit (ICU), or in the hospital. Although 30% of all CIs were related to equipment failures that included breathing circuit disconnections and misconnections, ventilator malfunctions, and gas flow-control errors, only three SNOs (4.3%) involved equipment failure, suggesting that human error was the predominant problem. Although equipment failures rarely cause death, CIs related to equipment are common and have prompted improvements in equipment design and construction and in system and patient monitoring.[4]

Many studies have demonstrated that anesthesia caregivers perform poorly when it comes to identifying problems with their anesthesia delivery systems. Buffington and colleagues[5] intentionally created five faults in a standard anesthesia machine and then invited 190 attendees at a Postgraduate Assembly of the New York State Society of Anesthesiologists to identify them within 10 minutes. The average number of discovered faults was 2.2; 7.3% of participants found no faults, and only 3.4% found all five. The authors concluded that greater emphasis was needed in educational programs on the fundamentals of anesthesia machine design and detection of hazards.

In an effort to improve patient safety and ensure proper use of the anesthesia machine, the American Society of Anesthesiologists (ASA), the Anesthesia Patient Safety Foundation (APSF), and others support the use of checklists to enable the anesthesia practitioner to ensure that the anesthesia delivery system is functioning normally prior to the start of an anesthetic. In 1986, the U.S. Food and Drug Administration (FDA)—in cooperation with the ASA, machine experts, and manufacturers—published a generic apparatus checklist to enable the practitioner to check out anesthesia equipment thoroughly prior to use (see Chapter 32).[6] March and Crowley[7] evaluated the FDA recommended checklist and individual practitioner checklists in order to determine whether the existence of the FDA checklist would improve detection of anesthesia machine faults. Participants in this study were given machines with four faults that were detectable if the FDA checklist was used properly. The results of the study revealed that 25.8% of faults were found with the practitioner's checklist, and 29.9% were found with the FDA checklist. In either case the results were poor and indicated that the mere introduction of the FDA checklist in 1986 did not improve the ability of these anesthesiologists to detect machine faults. However, it should be noted that in this study, no attempt was made to ensure that the FDA checklist was used properly during the checkout procedure.

Kumar and colleagues[8] conducted a random inspection of 169 anesthesia machines and ancillary monitors in 45 hospitals in Iowa. The machines ranged in age between 1 and 28 years, the oldest being 1958 vintage. Five machines had no back-up source of oxygen, 60 had no functioning oxygen analyzer, 15 had gas leaks of greater than 500 mL/min (two proximal to the common gas outlet, 13 in the patient circuit). In addition, 14 of the 383 vaporizers tested did not meet the manufacturer's calibration standards, and 20 had been added downstream of the machine common gas outlet. Of the 123 machines with ventilators, 16 had no alarm for low airway pressure, and only 31 had a high-pressure alarm. Of the ventilators surveyed, 59% were of the hanging bellows design; 41% had a standing bellows. Of these 123 machines, 95.5% had a scavenging system, but in 24.3% the scavenging circuit connectors were indistinguishable from the breathing circuit connectors, a potentially hazardous situation.[7] The use of these old machines increases the risk for development of problems related to the delivery system; in addition, equipment users may not be as educated as they should be in their ability to detect such problems.

In 1993, the Australian Anaesthesia Patient Safety Foundation published results of the Australian Incident Monitoring Study (AIMS) that had collected information on 2000 CIs.[9] Of these, 177 incidents (9%) were due to equipment failure in general, and 107 (60%) involved the anesthesia delivery system.[10] Failures included problems with unidirectional valves, ventilator malfunctions, gas or electrical supplies, circuit integrity, vaporizers, absorbers, and pressure regulators. Concerning the problems with ventilation, it was recommended that critical areas be doubly or triply monitored and that monitoring equipment be self-activating.[11]

Adverse Outcomes

In the absence of mandatory reporting systems and concerns for litigation, it is difficult to accurately estimate the frequency of adverse outcomes associated with use of anesthesia delivery systems. Case vignettes have provided some insight into how adverse outcomes have arisen and led to development of standards for monitoring.[12] The role of equipment failures leading to malpractice litigation in the United States has been studied by the ASA Closed Claims Project (CCP), a structured evaluation of adverse anesthetic outcomes obtained from the closed claims files of 35 U.S. professional liability insurance companies. A 1997 analysis of 3791 claims,[13] of which 76% occurred during the period 1980 through 1990, found that gas delivery equipment problems accounted for 72 (2%) of 3791 claims. Of these 72, 39% were related to the breathing circuit, 17% to ventilators, 21% to vaporizers, 11% to gas tanks or lines, and 7% to the anesthesia machine. Death or brain damage occurred in 76% of the 72 cases. Initiating events were circuit misconnects, disconnects, and gas delivery system errors. The primary mechanism of injury was inadequate oxygenation in 50% of the claims, excessive airway pressure in 18%, and anesthetic overdose in 13%. Misuse was judged to have occurred in 75%, and equipment failure occurred in only 24%. Anesthesia caregivers were considered responsible in 70% of use error cases, and ancillary staff (e.g., technicians) were found to have contributed in 30%. Predominant mechanisms of injury were hypoxemia, excessive airway pressure, and anesthetic agent overdose. Overall, the reviewers deemed 78% of claims to have been preventable by better use of monitoring. Payment or settlements were made in 76% of the claims (median payment was $306,000; range, $542 to $6,337,000), and claims were notable for their high severity of injury, high cost, and prominent role of equipment misuse.

As of May 2012, the CCP database included 9536 claims, of which 115 were related to anesthesia gas delivery equipment.[14] The most recent gas delivery system claim was for an event in 2003. Thus far, however, it appears that gas delivery equipment problems are decreasing as a proportion of total claims. Anesthesia gas delivery claims represented 4% of all claims from the 1970s, 3% from the

1980s, 1% from the 1990s, and 1% from 2000 through 2010. Only 39 anesthesia gas delivery system claims were reported from 1990 through 2010. These include 4 supplemental oxygen line events, 7 anesthesia machine problems, 13 vaporizer problems, 5 ventilator problems, and 10 breathing circuit problems. The outcomes in anesthesia gas delivery equipment claims from 1990 through 2008 seem to be less severe than earlier claims. During that time, 38% of anesthesia gas delivery system claims resulted in severe injury or death, compared with 80% from 1970 through 1989 ($P < .001$). Among the 39 claims from 1990 through 2010 were 10 deaths, 5 cases of permanent brain damage, 6 cases of pneumothorax, and 9 awareness claims. Payments reflect the lower severity of injury, with a median payment (in 2011 dollars) of $199,000 in the 1990 through 2010 claims period compared with $802,750 (adjusted to 2011 dollars) for earlier gas delivery equipment claims. Thirty-two (82%) of the 39 post-1990 claims resulted in payment.

With patient safety as the primary concern, over the past several years, the basic gas machine has evolved into the present, more sophisticated anesthesia delivery system/workstation. The most current voluntary consensus standard describing the features of a modern machine is that published in 2000, and republished in 2005, by the American Society for Testing and Materials, ASTM F1850-00, which describes the requirements for anesthesia workstations and their components.[15] This standard supersedes ASTM F1161-88, first published in 1988 and reapproved in 1994.[16] It is anticipated that patient safety will be enhanced with the use of a state-of-the-art anesthesia gas delivery system together with adoption of the Standards for Basic Anesthetic Monitoring, first published by the ASA in 1986 and periodically updated.[17] As in the case of monitoring standards, however, absolute confirmation may be difficult.

COMPLICATIONS

Complications caused by the anesthesia delivery system may be operator induced (misuse) or attributable to failure of a component. Issues with oxygen delivery and carbon dioxide elimination, circuit pressure and volume, inhaled anesthetic agent doses, humidification of inhaled gases, and electrical failure are discussed in detail here.

Hypoxemia

For the purposes of this chapter, *hypoxemia* is defined as an arterial partial pressure of oxygen (PaO_2) less than 60 mm Hg, and it may be caused by problems with the anesthesia delivery system or by problems with the patient. If the patient is adequately ventilated, and the alveolar oxygen concentration is as expected, the problem is with the patient. Pulmonary conditions that cause shunting, venous admixture, ventilation/perfusion (V/Q) mismatch, or, less likely, diffusion defects can cause hypoxemia. Examples of these conditions are pneumonia, atelectasis, pulmonary edema, pneumothorax, hemothorax, pyothorax, pulmonary embolism, alveolar proteinosis, and bronchospasm. In addition, conditions that decrease mixed venous oxygen, such as anemia and shock, may also cause or contribute to hypoxemia (Box 30-1).

The anesthesia delivery system may cause hypoxemia by failing to deliver sufficient oxygen to the lungs, thereby reducing the alveolar oxygen concentration (Box 30-2). Inadequate ventilation, caused by either apnea or low minute ventilation, is a well-described cause of alveolar hypoxia. Problems can arise from failure to initiate manual or mechanical ventilation or from failure to recognize a major leak or disconnection in the breathing circuit, even though ventilation is attempted. The anesthesia delivery system may also cause hypoxemia by delivering insufficient oxygen from the machine to the breathing circuit.[18]

Insufficient or low inspired oxygen concentrations can be definitively detected via the use of an oxygen analyzer. The oxygen analyzer is a critical monitor, because although it may appear that pure oxygen is being delivered from the oxygen flowmeter, if the gas in the flowmeter is not oxygen, the patient will receive a hypoxic gas mixture.[19] Without the oxygen analyzer, this condition would not be recognized. Although certainly a valuable patient monitor, the pulse oximeter does not replace the

BOX 30-1 Causes of Inadequate Arterial Oxygenation

Failure to deliver adequate oxygen to the alveoli
Inadequate alveolar ventilation
Low FiO_2
Intrapulmonary pathology
Shunt
Ventilation/perfusion mismatch
Diffusion defects

BOX 30-2 Causes of Failure to Deliver Oxygen to the Alveoli

UPSTREAM OF THE MACHINE

- Liquid oxygen reservoir empty or filled with hypoxic gas (e.g., nitrogen)
- Crossed hospital pipelines
- Crossed hoses or adapters in the operating room
- Closed pipeline valves
- Disconnected oxygen hose
- Failure of backup hospital oxygen reserve

WITHIN THE MACHINE OR CIRCUIT

- Cylinder filled with hypoxic gas
- Empty oxygen cylinder
- Incorrect cylinder on oxygen yoke
- Crossed pipes within the machine
- Closed oxygen cylinder valve
- Oxygen flowmeter off
- Failure of proportioning system
- Oxygen leak within the machine or flowmeter
- Incompetent or absent circuit unidirectional valves
- Breathing circuit leak
- Closed-system anesthesia with inadequate fresh oxygen supply
- Inadequate ventilation

oxygen analyzer. A low oxygen saturation (SpO_2) reading on a properly functioning pulse oximeter merely indicates that the patient's hemoglobin is poorly saturated with oxygen. However, only the oxygen analyzer in the breathing circuit would be able to determine that the cause was inadequate delivery of oxygen to the patient. Therefore, these two monitors are complementary, and both must be used to ensure patient safety.

The oxygen analyzer is not without limitations. For it to act as a valuable safety device, it must have an adequate power source and be properly calibrated. In addition, it must be positioned such that it is sampling the gases that the patient will breathe. An analyzer placed by the inspiratory unidirectional valve may indicate a normal oxygen concentration, but if there is a disconnection between that point and the patient, the patient will not receive that gas. For this reason it is critical that the anesthesiologist understand the equipment design and the limitations of this device. The analyzer must function normally, the circuit valves must be present, the circuit must be intact, and the patient must be ventilated if the reading on the oxygen analyzer is to reflect the oxygen being delivered to the alveoli. Vigilant observation of patient ventilation, the integrity of the breathing system, and the oxygen analyzer ensure proper delivery of oxygen to the patient.

The gas entering the anesthesia machine from the hospital pipeline gas supply system or the oxygen cylinders may contain a gas other than oxygen. The central liquid oxygen reservoir may be filled with a gas other than oxygen (e.g., liquid nitrogen),[20] or the pipelines throughout the hospital may be crossed, so that nitrous oxide or some other gas may be flowing through the oxygen pipeline.

Placement of a nitrous oxide wall adapter on one end of an oxygen hose would allow that hose to be connected to the wall's nitrous oxide source and the anesthesia machine's oxygen inlet, in which case nitrous oxide would flow through the oxygen flowmeter on the machine.[21,22] During use of an anesthesia workstation, if it is suspected that a gas other than pure oxygen is being delivered via the pipeline, the pipeline hose must be disconnected, and the back-up oxygen tank must be opened. If the tank is opened but the pipeline remains connected, oxygen will not flow from the tank because of the difference in pressures between the pipeline (usually 55 psig) and the tank's first-stage regulator (45 psig).

Most contemporary anesthesia workstations are equipped with an auxiliary oxygen flowmeter and oxygen outlet, for example, for connecting a nasal cannula. It must be recognized that no analysis of the gas flowing from this outlet exists, and it is *presumed* to be oxygen. In the event of a pipeline crossover, the hypoxic gas would also be delivered from the auxiliary oxygen flowmeter. Mudumbai and colleagues[23] used medical simulation to investigate the response of 20 third-year anesthesia residents to an anesthesia machine pipeline crossover scenario. A significant number used the auxiliary oxygen flowmeter as a presumed external source of oxygen in their response to this crisis, which contributed to delays in definitive treatment.

In one case report, a modification of the gas-specific oxygen quick-connect on a wall outlet oxygen flowmeter allowed it to be connected to a nitrous oxide wall outlet. When a self-inflating resuscitation bag was connected to the wall outlet (presumed to be) oxygen flowmeter, in the course of resuscitating two patients, the anesthesia caregivers unknowingly delivered nitrous oxide with catastrophic outcomes.[24] In the event that a gas presumed to be oxygen is being delivered in the absence of an oxygen analyzer, if the patient does not appear to be responding appropriately, the possibility of a wrong gas must always be considered, and the clinician should ventilate instead with room air.

Because of potential problems with the wall oxygen source, it has been suggested that only oxygen cylinders be used. However, this approach overlooks the possibility that an oxygen cylinder may be empty, the valve may be faulty, a tank key may not be available, or the tank may contain a gas other than oxygen.[25,26] A nitrous oxide or other gas cylinder may be attached to the oxygen hanger yoke if the pin index system is defeated, either by removal of a pin or by placement of more than one washer between the yoke and the cylinder. Lorraway and colleagues[27] studied a total of 20 second- and fourth-year anesthesia residents in a simulation of an oxygen pipeline supply failure. They found that the majority of participants either did not know how to change the oxygen cylinder or did not attempt it, even after prompting; this demonstrates an apparent basic deficiency in their training. Finally, crossed pipes within the anesthesia machine would allow a gas other than oxygen into the oxygen flowmeter.[28] Delivery of a hypoxic gas via the oxygen pipeline or from a cylinder has been the basis for some now classic movies (e.g., "Green for Danger," 1946; "Coma," 1978).

Turning on the oxygen flow control valve may result in no oxygen gas flow.[29] The hospital's central oxygen system may be empty, shut down, or otherwise unavailable to deliver oxygen.[30,31] In one report, separation of a brazed joint between the stainless steel liquid oxygen storage vessel and the brass pipe fitting connection to the hospital oxygen pipeline resulted in spillage of 8000 gallons of liquid oxygen into the atmosphere.[32] Fortunately in this case, a bulk liquid oxygen storage tank in another location maintained the oxygen supply to the facility.

The oxygen hose to the anesthesia machine may become disconnected from the wall, and the back-up cylinders may be empty, absent, or turned off.[33] The oxygen flow control valve or oxygen piping in the machine may be obstructed, thereby preventing the flow of oxygen to the flowmeter.[34,35] In addition, the flowmeter bobbin or rotameter may become stuck, and it may appear that gas is flowing from that flowmeter even when it is not. Leaks in the oxygen flowmeter tube or in the low-pressure portion of the anesthesia machine can permit loss of oxygen before it reaches the common gas outlet of the machine.[36-39]

Contemporary anesthesia workstations are equipped with proportioning systems that prevent the delivery of a less than 25% oxygen mixture when nitrous oxide is being administered. Older anesthesia machines may not have these safety design features and should be considered obsolete. Because the oxygen fail-safe system is sensitive to the *pressure*, rather than the *flow*, of oxygen, it is possible on older anesthesia machines for the nitrous oxide flowmeter to be turned on without the oxygen flowmeter also being turned on (Fig. 30-1). This could lead to the

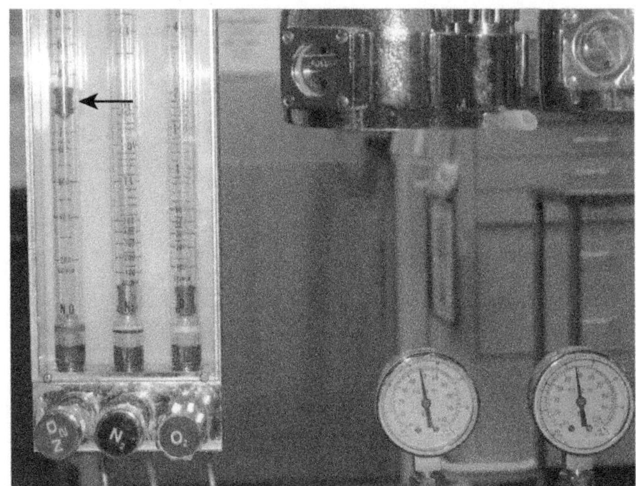

FIGURE 30-1 ■ The fail-safe system (pressure sensor shutoff valve/oxygen failure protection device). The fail-safe system is pressure sensitive but not flow sensitive. Because the supply *pressure* of oxygen is adequate (2000 psig from the tank and therefore 45 psig in the machine), nitrous oxide may flow to its flowmeter and beyond at 4 L/min (arrow), even though the oxygen flow control valve is turned off and there is no flow of oxygen.

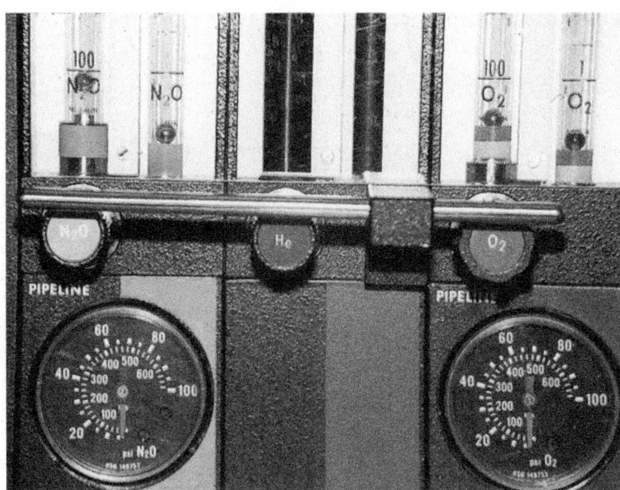

FIGURE 30-2 ■ Three-gas anesthesia machine with flowmeter for helium. The proportioning system functions only between N_2O and O_2 flows. In addition, if a helium-oxygen mixture (75% He, 25% O_2) were being administered and the helium tank were to become depleted, a hyperoxic mixture would be delivered to the patient circuit.

delivery of a hypoxic gas mixture in the breathing circuit; the oxygen analyzer would detect this problem, and the anesthesiologist would have to recognize it and respond by adding oxygen to the mixture. Such a machine would, however, be considered unsafe per the ASA guidelines for determining anesthesia machine obsolescence.[40]

Although nitrous oxide–oxygen proportioning systems help to prevent the delivery of hypoxic mixtures, they are not foolproof and cannot be relied on entirely as the only method to prevent a hypoxic mixture. The Ohmeda Link-25 proportion limiting system (GE Healthcare, Waukesha, WI) causes the oxygen flow control valve to open further and increase flow if a hypoxic mixture would otherwise result when only oxygen and nitrous oxide are being used. This system can fail if the needle valve is broken in the closed position or if the linkage between the flowmeter controls fails.[41,42] A limitation of all oxygen–nitrous oxide proportioning systems is that they do not analyze the gas flowing through the oxygen flowmeter, nor do they prevent administration of a hypoxic gas mixture if the machine has flowmeters for a third or fourth gas that is hypoxic (e.g., helium, carbon dioxide; Fig. 30-2).

Abnormalities in the anesthesia breathing circuit can lead to a hypoxic mixture. Absent or incompetent unidirectional valves in the circle system will permit rebreathing of exhaled gas, which would present the patient with a hypoxic mixture if these gases were insufficiently mixed with fresh gas. In the Mapleson circuits (see Chapter 4), loss of the fresh gas supply from the machine leads to severe rebreathing of a hypoxic mixture as the patient uses up the oxygen and replaces it with carbon dioxide. Failure of the fresh gas supply in the circle system results in a breathing mixture that becomes progressively hypoxic, as the oxygen is consumed and only nitrous oxide remains.[43-45]

Leaks in the breathing circuit lead to loss of gases, especially during positive-pressure ventilation. If a hanging (descending) bellows ventilator is used, the lost gas may be replaced with entrained room air as the bellows descends by gravity during exhalation (Fig. 30-3). A standing bellows collapses if a significant leak develops in the breathing circuit. In addition, system leaks can lead to severe hypoventilation. The sources of leaks may be valve housings, circuit hoses, pressure monitoring and gas sampling lines, connection sites, pressure relief valves, and carbon dioxide absorbers. Leaks can also be caused by subatmospheric pressure being applied to the system from a scavenger suction or by a catheter that has unintentionally been passed into the trachea alongside the tracheal tube. A leak in the ventilator bellows might allow the drive gas in the ventilator bellows housing to enter the patient circuit. Depending on the gas used, this could affect the composition of the breathing mixture.[46]

Closed-system or low-flow anesthesia can lead to the delivery of a hypoxic mixture. The total flow of gas is adjusted to compensate for the uptake of nitrous oxide and oxygen. However, if the oxygen content of the circuit gases is not carefully monitored, the uptake of nitrous oxide may be low, and that of oxygen may be high. The resultant mixture could become hypoxic.

Hyperoxia

Administration of a mixture that contains more oxygen than desired results in hyperoxia, which may be caused by insufficient nitrous oxide or air administered from the flowmeters; in addition, flowmeter leaks and inaccurate flowmeters may cause gases to be lost, with resultant high oxygen concentrations. A leak in a ventilator bellows that allows injection of pressurizing or drive-gas oxygen into the bellows (e.g., Datex-Ohmeda 7000, 7800, and 7900 series ventilators; GE Healthcare) may cause the inspired oxygen concentration to increase.[47,48] Administration of helium and oxygen via separate flowmeters during laser surgery of the airway could be hazardous if the helium supply becomes depleted, or if the oxygen flush were operated, in which case a hyperoxic gas mixture would result that could lead to a fire (see Fig. 30-2).[49]

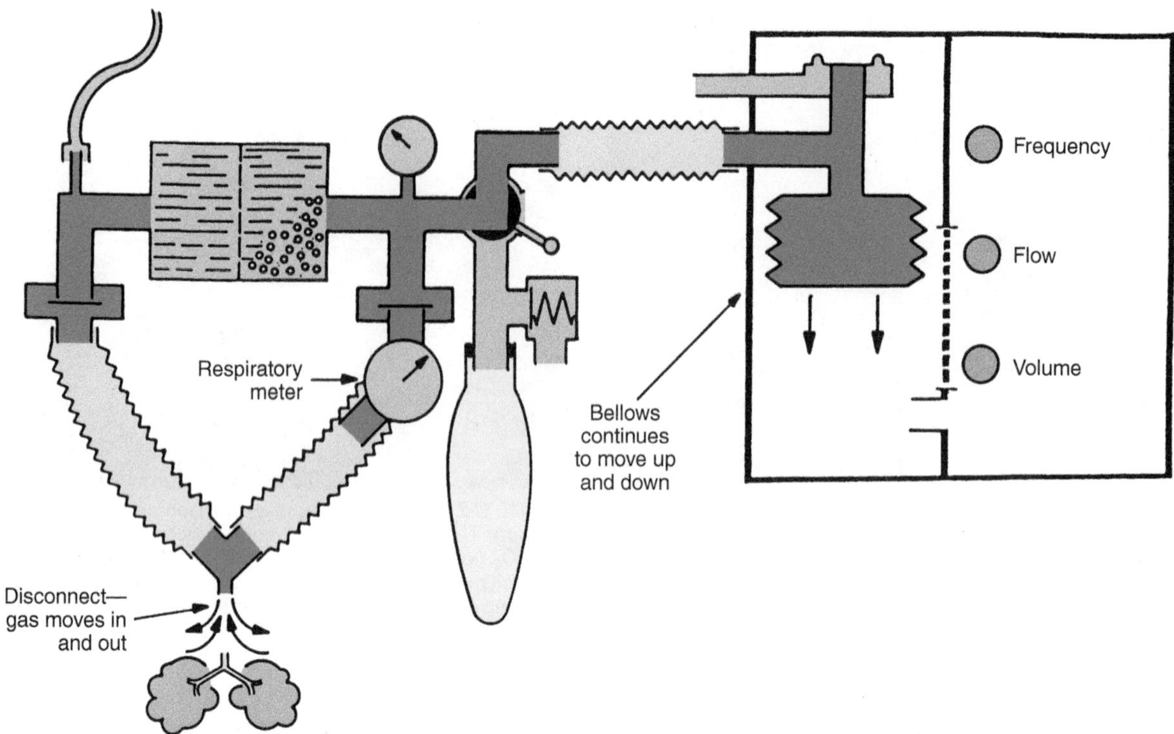

FIGURE 30-3 ■ Hanging (descending) bellows ventilator. In the event of a disconnection, room air will be drawn into the circuit as the bellows fills during exhalation.

Hyperoxia may be undesirable or even dangerous in certain situations. It has been suggested that bleomycin induces sensitivity to oxygen toxicity and that the minimum fraction of inspired oxygen (FiO_2) that can maintain an SpO_2 of 90% or greater should be used in these patients.[50] Similarly, when a fire risk is present, such as in airway or head and neck procedures, the FiO_2 should be kept to the minimum compatible with an acceptable SpO_2.[51,52] In such situations, use of an oxygen analyzer with an appropriately set high oxygen concentration alarm is essential.

Hypercarbia

When carbon dioxide production exceeds elimination, the arterial carbon dioxide tension increases until an equilibrium is achieved. During anesthesia, patient factors or delivery system conditions may cause hypercarbia.

Patients breathing spontaneously are prone to hypercarbia because of the depressant effects of anesthetics on the central respiratory center, weakness from muscle relaxants, and motor blockade during spinal or epidural anesthesia. Complete or partial airway obstruction can cause hypercarbia. Pulmonary conditions that cause a large shunt and increased metabolic production of carbon dioxide without a concomitant increase in ventilation also cause hypercarbia.

The anesthesia delivery system can be a source of hypercarbia. Apnea caused by failure to ventilate either manually or mechanically raises the carbon dioxide concentration. Ventilating with an inadequate tidal volume or respiratory rate reduces alveolar ventilation and leads to hypercarbia. Leaks in the machine, circuit, and ventilator and failure to fill the bellows may also lead to hypoventilation (Box 30-3).

BOX 30-3 Patient Factors Causing Hypercarbia During Spontaneous Breathing

- Central respiratory depression
- Muscle relaxants
- Motor blockade (regional anesthesia)
- Airway obstruction
- Severe pulmonary shunting
- Delivery system problems
- Apnea (failure to initiate or continue controlled ventilation)
- Inadequate minute ventilation (low tidal volume or respiratory rate)
- Increased apparatus dead space
- Missing or incompetent unidirectional valves
- Incorrectly assembled circle system
- Exhausted carbon dioxide absorbent or channeling
- Carbon dioxide absorber bypass open (certain older systems)
- Unintended administration of carbon dioxide
- Inadequate fresh gas flow in a system without carbon dioxide absorption

The anesthesia breathing circuit may contain insufficient gas if the pipeline gas source fails. However, this problem can be overcome by use of the reserve gas cylinders on the anesthesia machine. Inside the machine, leaks may develop either at the oxygen yoke or from a faulty check valve that permits gas to escape into the room. It is also possible for gas to leak from the pipes, flowmeters, vaporizers, vaporizer selector switches, and vaporizer mounts on the machine.

The interface hose from the anesthesia machine (common gas outlet) to the breathing circuit and the breathing circuit itself may be sources of a leak, and disconnections and leaks of sufficient magnitude lead to hypercarbia. Flow of gas from the machine to the circuit may be obstructed either in the machine or in the interface hose.[53-56] Leaks in valve housings, tracheal tubes, ventilator hoses, reservoir bags, ventilator bellows, and system relief valves can reduce the volume in the breathing system and cause hypercarbia.[57-60]

Subatmospheric pressure applied to the breathing system can reduce the system volume and cause hypercarbia. Sources of subatmospheric pressure include vacuum hoses on scavenger interfaces, nasogastric tubes that have been placed in the trachea and suctioned, and sampling catheters from sidestream gas analysis systems (see Chapter 8).[61]

The anesthesia ventilator can cause hypercarbia if the settings are such that inadequate alveolar ventilation is provided. Either the rate may be too low or the tidal volume may be too small. On ventilators that allow the clinician to set the tidal volume, ventilatory rate, inspiratory-to-expiratory ratio, and flow of compressing gas independently of each other, smaller tidal volumes than desired may be delivered. The reason for this is that the ventilator may cycle to exhalation before the bellows is emptied completely; therefore it fails to deliver the preset volume to the patient. Factors that can cause this problem are high respiratory rate, low inspiratory/expiratory (I:E) ratio, low rate of inflow of the ventilator driving gas, and decreased pulmonary compliance. This problem can be discovered by careful observation of the ventilator bellows and monitoring of the exhaled tidal volume.

Poor pulmonary compliance also causes volume to be lost, because some of the tidal volume expands the compliant breathing circuit tubing. This "compression" volume is included in the tidal volume measured by a breathing system expiratory limb spirometer during exhalation, but it does not contribute to the alveolar ventilation. Pressure-preset ventilators may cycle to exhalation before an adequate tidal volume has been delivered. This also causes hypercarbia if it is unrecognized; therefore it is important to monitor the tidal volume and minute ventilation and not to assume that the volume set on the ventilator will in fact be delivered to the patient.

Fresh gas flows continuously from the anesthesia machine into the breathing system, but gas can leave the circuit only during exhalation. With older ventilator models used for anesthesia (e.g., Dräger AV-E [Dräger Medical, Telford, PA], Ohmeda 7000), the fresh gas entering the circuit during the inspiratory phase of ventilation is added to the tidal volume delivered by the ventilator, so that the patient receives a larger tidal volume than was set on the ventilator. These are described as *tidal volume and I:E ratio change-uncompensated* ventilators, in contrast to the more recent ventilator designs that use fresh gas decoupling or computerized compensation to ensure that changes in fresh gas flow (FGF), respiratory rate, or I:E ratio do not change the tidal volume that the patient receives. During use of an uncompensated ventilator, if the patient is normocarbic and the FGF is decreased, or if the I:E ratio is changed such that exhalation is prolonged, the result is a decreased tidal volume (less augmentation by the fresh gas inflow) and an increase in partial pressure of carbon dioxide ($PaCO_2$; Fig. 30-4).[62,63]

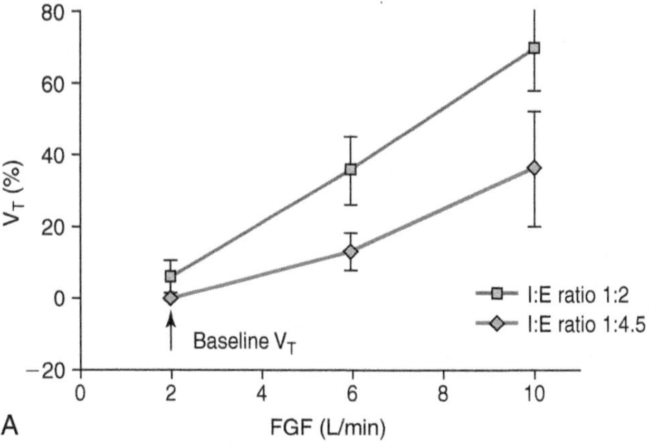

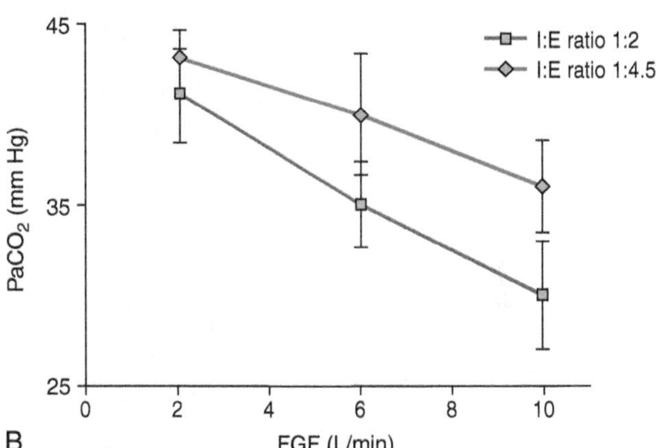

FIGURE 30-4 **A,** Effect of fresh gas flow (FGF) and inspiratory/expiratory (I:E) ratio on partial pressure of carbon dioxide ($PaCO_2$) in patients during mechanical ventilation using an anesthesia ventilator with fixed-rate and bellows tidal volume. Note that as FGF increases, or the I:E ratio increases from 1:4.5 to 1:2, $PaCO_2$ decreases. This is due to an increase in alveolar ventilation caused by an increase in tidal volume. Conversely, a decrease in FGF or I:E ratio results in an increase in $PaCO_2$. The volume of gas added to the circuit during each inspiration is that exiting the ventilator bellows plus the FGF entering the circuit during inspiration (when the ventilator relief valve is closed). The latter volume is $I/(I + E) \times FGF/f$, where *f* is the respiratory rate. Patient tidal volume, which determines alveolar ventilation and therefore $PaCO_2$, is determined by the above formula, less gas compressed in the circuit during inspiration. This volume is calculated as circuit compliance times peak inspiratory pressure. **B,** Effect of FGF and I:E ratio on measured tidal volume (V_T) during mechanical ventilation using an anesthesia ventilator at fixed rate and bellows tidal volume. As FGF or I:E ratio increases, the measured V_T increases because during inspiration the fresh gas inflow is added to the delivered bellows tidal volume. All data are mean ± standard deviation. (From Scheller MS, Jones BR, Benumof JL: The influence of fresh gas flow and I:E ratio on tidal volume and $PaCO_2$ in ventilated patients. *J Cardiothoracic Anesth* 1989;3:564.)

The carbon dioxide absorber may cause hypercarbia by providing a source of leaks from the circuit or by failing to absorb the carbon dioxide produced by the patient. The absorber may not be closed and sealed properly; improperly applied gaskets and absorbent granules on the gaskets can prevent the absorber canister from being sealed, and failure to close the handle on the absorber canister can also cause a huge leak.[64] Exhausted granules and channeling of gas through the absorber prevent the absorption of carbon dioxide, which causes rebreathing of exhaled CO_2 and hypercarbia. Machines equipped with absorber bypass switches can allow the exhaled carbon dioxide to be deliberately rebreathed. If this is not monitored carefully, the patient may become hypercarbic. Some contemporary workstations use detachable and disposable cartridges of CO_2 absorbent. Removal of such a cartridge to facilitate buildup of CO_2 at the end of a case is effectively the same as activating the absorber bypass switch on older machines (Fig. 30-5). The clinician must remember to replace the absorber cartridge in the circuit once the CO_2 is as desired and before starting the next case.

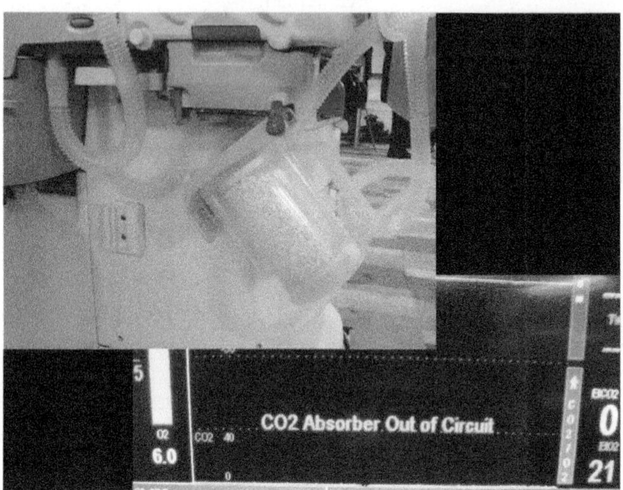

FIGURE 30-5 ■ Removal of absorber cartridge, allowing carbon dioxide to build up in the breathing system. In this workstation a warning appears on the screen.

The color of the dye (e.g., ethyl violet) in the carbon dioxide absorbent indicates whether the absorbent has been exhausted. However, it has been noted that the ethyl violet indicator can be photodeactivated by fluorescent lights and can thereby give the false impression that the absorbent is fresh when it is in fact exhausted.[65] Some anesthesia workstations are capable of controlled delivery of carbon dioxide (Fig. 30-6). Unintentional or improper use of the carbon dioxide flowmeter may cause hypercarbia.[66-68]

Hypercarbia has also been reported when an anesthesia machine nitrous oxide hose with an N_2O quick-connect fitting was connected to a CO_2 wall outlet in the operating room (OR). In this case the manufacturer-specific (Ohmeda) quick-connects for CO_2 and N_2O happened to be mirror images of one another, so that rotating the N_2O hose connection through 180 degrees allowed it to be inserted into the CO_2 wall outlet (Fig. 30-7).[69]

By increasing apparatus dead space, the anesthesia breathing circuit can increase dead space ventilation and act as a cause of hypercarbia. Specifically, the unidirectional inspiratory and expiratory valves may be absent or broken, or they may malfunction in the open position (Fig. 30-8). Large-volume tubes (e.g., "goosenecks") placed between the Y-piece of the breathing circle and the airway increase apparatus (mechanical) dead space and may cause hypercarbia if compensatory ventilatory maneuvers (i.e., larger tidal volumes) are not used (Fig. 30-9).

The components of the circle breathing circuit must be arranged in such a way as to prevent rebreathing. Three

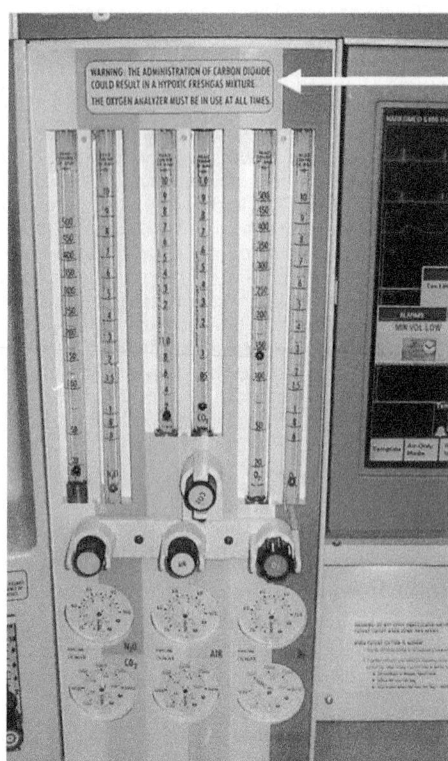

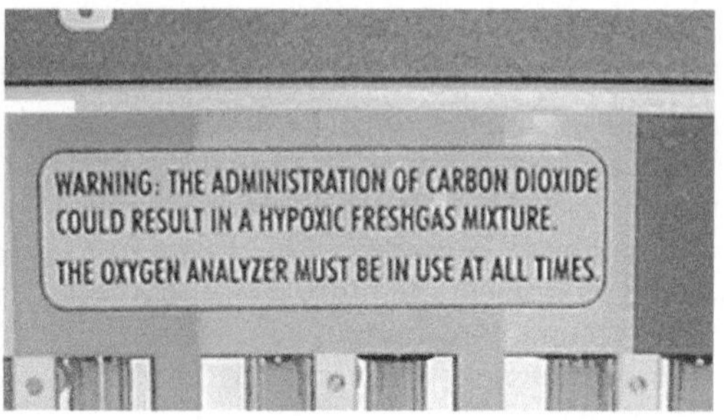

FIGURE 30-6 ■ Anesthesia workstation with CO_2 flowmeter. Note the warning label above the rotameter bank.

arrangements of the circle system must be avoided: 1) the fresh gas inlet must not be placed between the patient and the expiratory unidirectional valve; 2) the adjustable pressure-limiting (APL, or "pop-off") valve must not be placed between the patient and the inspiratory unidirectional valve; and 3) the reservoir bag must not be between the patient and the inspiratory or expiratory unidirectional valves.[70]

The Mapleson systems will permit the rebreathing of carbon dioxide, and hypercarbia will develop if appropriate precautions are not taken. For example, the Mapleson A circuit (the Magill attachment) should be used only with spontaneously breathing patients, and the FGF must be at least 0.7 times the minute ventilation. In addition, the hose between the patient and the reservoir bag must be long enough so that exhaled carbon dioxide does not reach the bag (Fig. 30-10).[71]

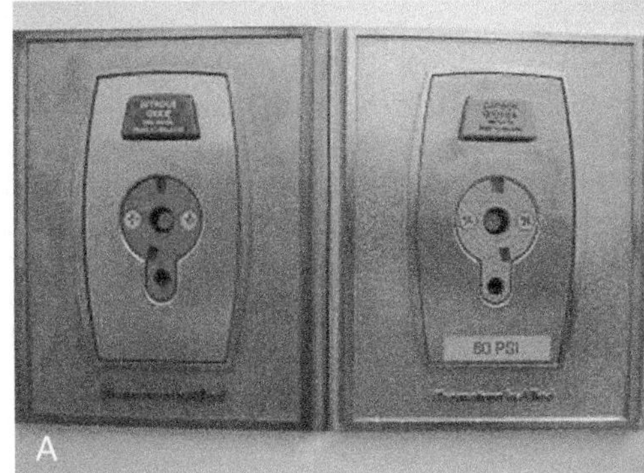

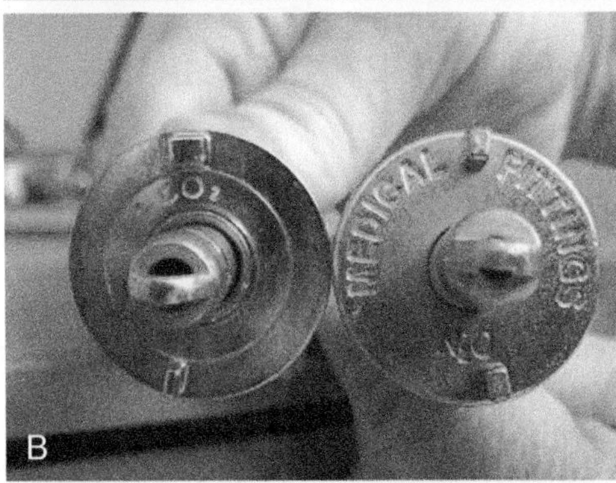

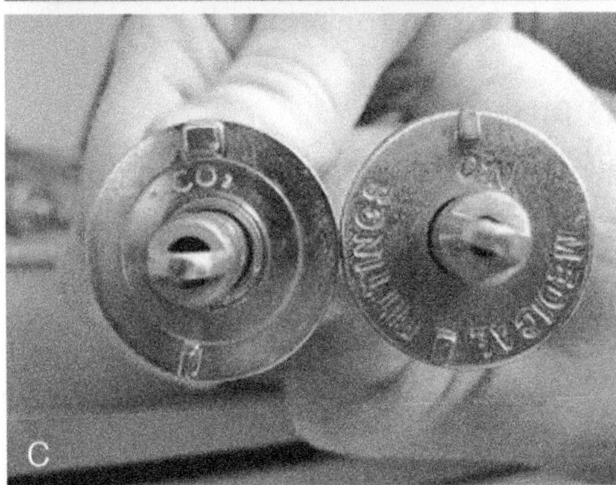

FIGURE 30-7 Ohmeda (GE Healthcare, Waukesha, WI) quick connectors for N_2O and CO_2 are mirror images of each other. **A,** Wall outlets. **B,** Hose connectors. **C,** Rotation of N_2O connector through 180 degrees permitted connection to CO_2 wall outlet. (From Ellett AE, Shields JC, Ifune C, Roa N, Vannucci A: A near miss: a nitrous oxide–carbon dioxide mix-up despite current safety standards. *Anesthesiology* 2009;110:1429.)

The Mapleson B and C systems always permit the rebreathing of exhaled carbon dioxide because exhaled gas is directed into a blind pouch. To prevent hypercarbia with these systems, FGFs of 1.5 to 2.5 times normal minute ventilation must be used, and the patient must be hyperventilated (see Fig. 30-10). If the patient is breathing spontaneously, the metabolic work performed increases. However, controlled ventilation with these circuits does not create this problem, because the work of breathing is not being performed by the patient.

The T-piece systems—Mapleson D, E, and F—function similarly (Fig. 30-11). FGFs of 2.5 to 3 times minute ventilation prevent rebreathing at calculated normal minute ventilation. Alternatively, reduced FGFs can be used, but hypercarbia is prevented by hyperventilation. If the fresh gas connection is disrupted, hypercarbia will occur. This may be an especially difficult problem with the Bain circuit (coaxial Mapleson D), because the disconnected or kinked inner hose may go unnoticed (Fig. 30-12; see also Chapters 4 and 17).[41,72-74]

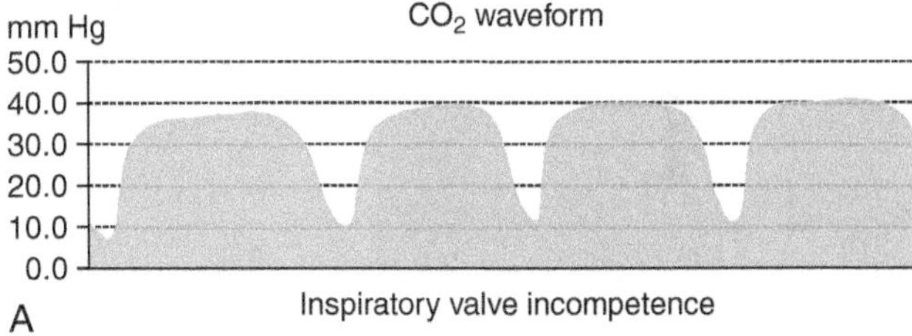

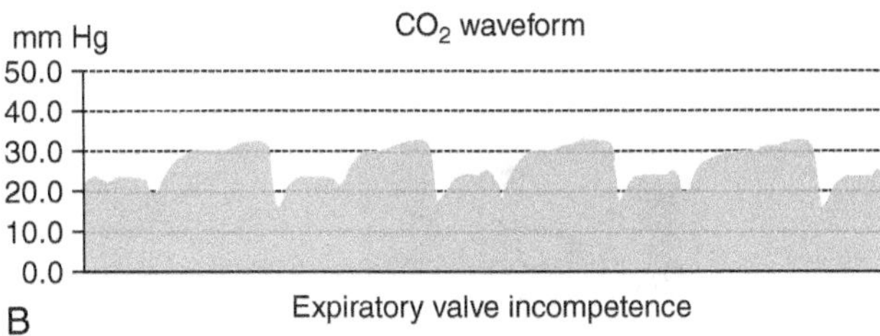

FIGURE 30-8 Incompetent unidirectional valves in a circle system. Capnograms from subject breathing from circle system. **A,** When inspiratory valve is incompetent. **B,** When expiratory valve is incompetent.

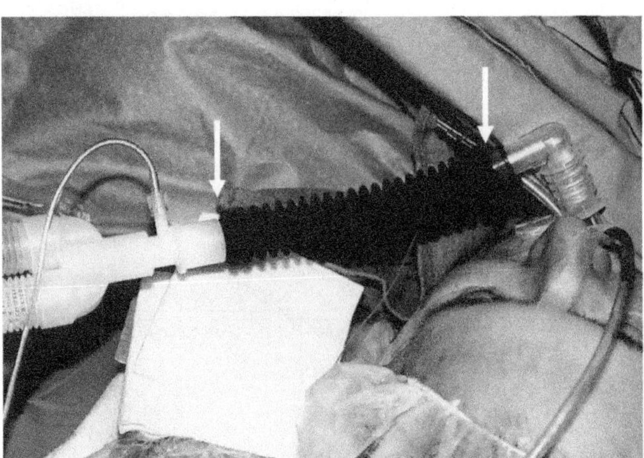

FIGURE 30-9 Insertion of "goose neck" connection between the Y-piece and a patient's airway increases apparatus (mechanical) dead space.

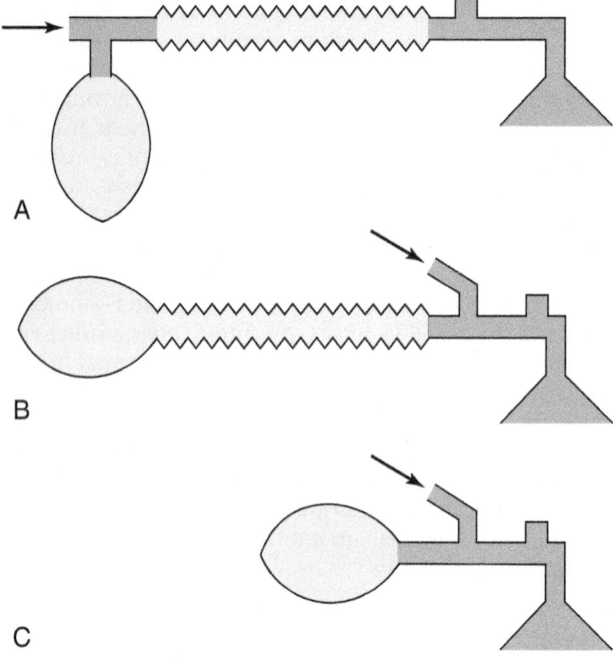

FIGURE 30-10 ■ Mapleson A, B, and C rebreathing systems.

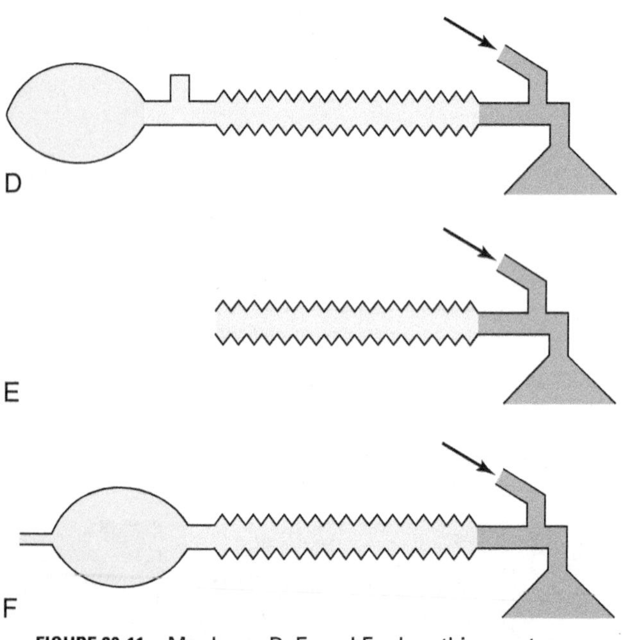

FIGURE 30-11 ■ Mapleson D, E, and F rebreathing systems.

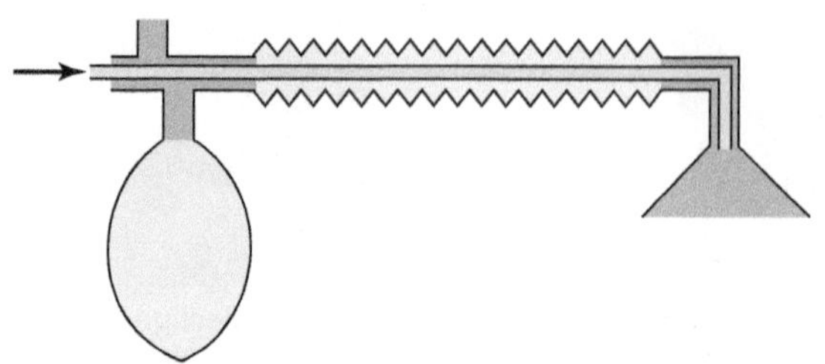

FIGURE 30-12 ■ Bain circuit (coaxial version of Mapleson D).

Hypocarbia

When carbon dioxide elimination exceeds production, $PaCO_2$ decreases. When equilibrium between the two processes is achieved, a new steady state develops, and $PaCO_2$ stabilizes. General anesthesia, neuromuscular blocking agents, and hypothermia reduce the metabolic rate. If minute ventilation is not decreased, the patient becomes hypocarbic. In addition, hyperventilation in general causes hypocarbia.

Hyperventilation and the resultant hypocarbia can be caused by simply having either the tidal volume, ventilatory rate, or both set too high. The FGF, which contributes to the minute ventilation in uncompensated ventilators (see above), will cause the patient to become hypocarbic if its contribution is not taken into account when the ventilator settings are chosen. In patients with very compliant lungs, the contribution of the FGF may be significant. The driving gas from the ventilator may increase ventilation if there is a hole in the bellows. This is more significant with the Dräger AV-E ventilator, because drive gas—a mixture of oxygen and entrained room air—flows into the bellows housing throughout the inspiratory time, whereas with the Datex-Ohmeda ventilators, the drive gas is oxygen, and drive-gas volume is determined by the set tidal volume. With the Dräger AV-E ventilator, drive gas that enters the breathing circuit via a hole in the bellows increases the volume of gas delivered to the patient and also affects the composition of the circuit gases. The result is hyperventilation of the patient's lungs with an unintended gas mixture.

CIRCUIT PRESSURE AND VOLUME PROBLEMS

Essential to anesthesia delivery, oxygenation, and ventilation of the patient is adequate movement of gases between the delivery system and the patient's lungs. Four basic causes of failure of this function have been described by Schreiber[18] and include 1) occlusion in the ventilatory pathway, inspiratory or expiratory; 2) insufficient gas in the breathing system; 3) failure to initiate artificial ventilation when required; and 4) disconnection in the breathing system during mechanical ventilation.

Occlusions

The anesthesia circle breathing system is composed of a number of tubes that may become occluded.[75] In general, the cause of such occlusions can be found outside the tube, within the wall, or within the lumen of the tube. Tubing misconnections have become less common since the introduction of standard diameters; however, if adapters are used, misconnections are still possible. By standard, breathing circuit tubing connections are 22 mm in diameter, waste gas scavenging tubing is 19 or 30 mm in diameter, and the common gas outlet and tracheal tube connectors are 15 mm in diameter. Accessories added to the circuit may cause an obstruction to the gas pathway. Filters placed in the circuit, incorrectly connected humidifiers, manufacturing defects in tubing, and failure to completely remove plastic wrapping from breathing system components before connecting them into the circuit have all been reported as causes of total occlusion of the breathing circuit (Fig. 30-13).[76-80]

A freestanding positive end-expiratory pressure (PEEP) valve may cause obstruction if it is placed in the inspiratory limb of a circle system. The PEEP valves that use a weighted ball, such as those made by the Boehringer Company (Wynnewood, PA), are designed to be mounted vertically on the expiratory side of a circle system. In one case, the weighted-ball PEEP valve was erroneously placed horizontally and was reversed in the expiratory limb between the circuit and the exhalation unidirectional valve. When the oxygen flush was operated, the metal ball was driven downstream, totally obstructing the PEEP valve and circuit, preventing exhalation, and causing increased intrathoracic pressure. In another case, the PEEP valve was placed on the inspiratory side in reversed fashion; this caused total obstruction on the inspiratory side of the circuit and prevented inspiration (Fig. 30-14).[81] Because of such potentially fatal errors, freestanding PEEP valves must be used with great caution, if they must be used at all. Freestanding bidirectional PEEP valves are safer, because incorrect placement will not cause total breathing circuit obstruction.[82]

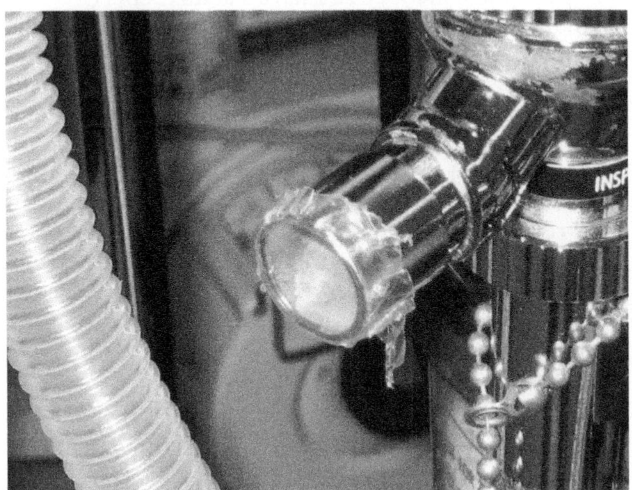

FIGURE 30-13 ■ Disposable circuit with plastic packaging intact. Plastic that is not removed before connecting the circuit to the inspiratory port on the absorber canister would cause complete obstruction to inspiration.

Although total occlusion of the breathing circuit should activate a pressure or volume alarm in most cases, depending on the system used, these alarms may be fooled when the tracheal tube is totally occluded. Consider a breathing circuit with a pressure-monitoring system that incorporates a fixed setting of +65 cm H_2O for the high-pressure alarm limit threshold, such as that used on some older anesthesia machines. When the tracheal tube becomes totally obstructed because of a kink or total intraluminal obstruction, the pressure rises in the circuit, which satisfies the low-pressure alarm. However, unless the pressure reaches +65 cm H_2O, the high-pressure alarm is not activated. The peak pressure achieved in the circuit during inspiration depends on the inspiratory flow control setting, which determines the driving pressure available to compress the bellows, the preset tidal volume, the inspiratory time, and the fresh gas inflow rate

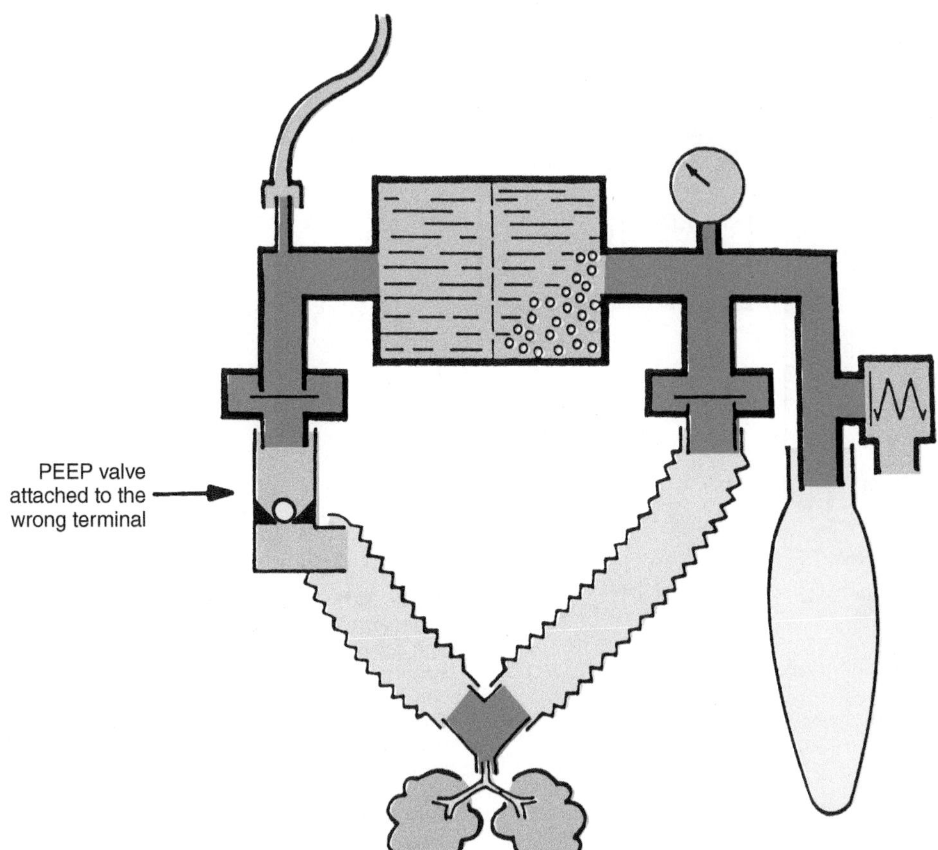

FIGURE 30-14 ■ Erroneous insertion of positive end-expiratory pressure (*PEEP*) valve on inspiratory port causes complete obstruction to inspiration.

from the anesthesia machine. At low ventilator inspiratory flow settings, the driving pressure of the ventilator may be 50 cm H_2O or less; when combined with normal rates of fresh gas inflow from the machine, this may result in failure of the peak inspiratory pressure to reach the high-pressure alarm threshold of +65 cm H_2O. During exhalation, excess gas is released normally from the patient circuit. The volume alarm may also be fooled in this situation, depending on its low-limit threshold setting. In the system described, the low-volume alarm threshold was fixed at 80 mL. The situation described above involved total failure to ventilate the patient and resulted in an adverse outcome.[12] In contemporary practice this should be immediately detectable by continuous capnometry by pressure and volume alarms whose thresholds can be set close to the normal values for that particular patient. An appropriately set high-pressure limit on the ventilator should prevent an adverse outcome in such a situation.

Misconnections and obstructions should be preventable and may be detected by testing of the breathing circuit before use; this should be done with all accessories in place and in spontaneous, assisted, and controlled ventilation modes. These procedures are described in the recommended preuse checkout. Occasionally, however, an obstruction can develop because of failure of a component during the case, so there is no substitute for monitoring and vigilance.[83]

Insufficient Gas in the Breathing System

An insufficient volume of gas in the breathing system may be caused by inadequate delivery or excessive loss. Inadequate delivery may be due to failure of gas delivery to the machine or from the common gas outlet.[84] A decrease in oxygen supply pressure to the machine may cause a decrease in gas flows set at the flowmeters, and flow setting errors may also occur. A disconnection, misconnection, or obstruction between the machine's common gas outlet and the patient circuit have a similar effect.

An inadequate volume of gas in the circuit may also be caused by excessive removal. An active waste-gas scavenging system uses wall suction to remove waste gases from the scavenging interface. Excess negative pressure may be applied to the circuit if the negative-pressure relief ("pop-in") valve or valves on the interface should become occluded.[85] A similar situation can arise with an open-reservoir scavenging system if the relief ports become occluded while suction is applied to the interface. A high subatmospheric pressure in the scavenging system may open the circuit APL valve, transmitting the subatmospheric pressure to the patient circuit. If a ventilator were being used, unrelieved excess negative pressure in the scavenging system would in most cases tend to hold the ventilator pressure relief valve to its seat, preventing its opening on exhalation and causing high pressure to develop in the circuit (Fig. 30-15).

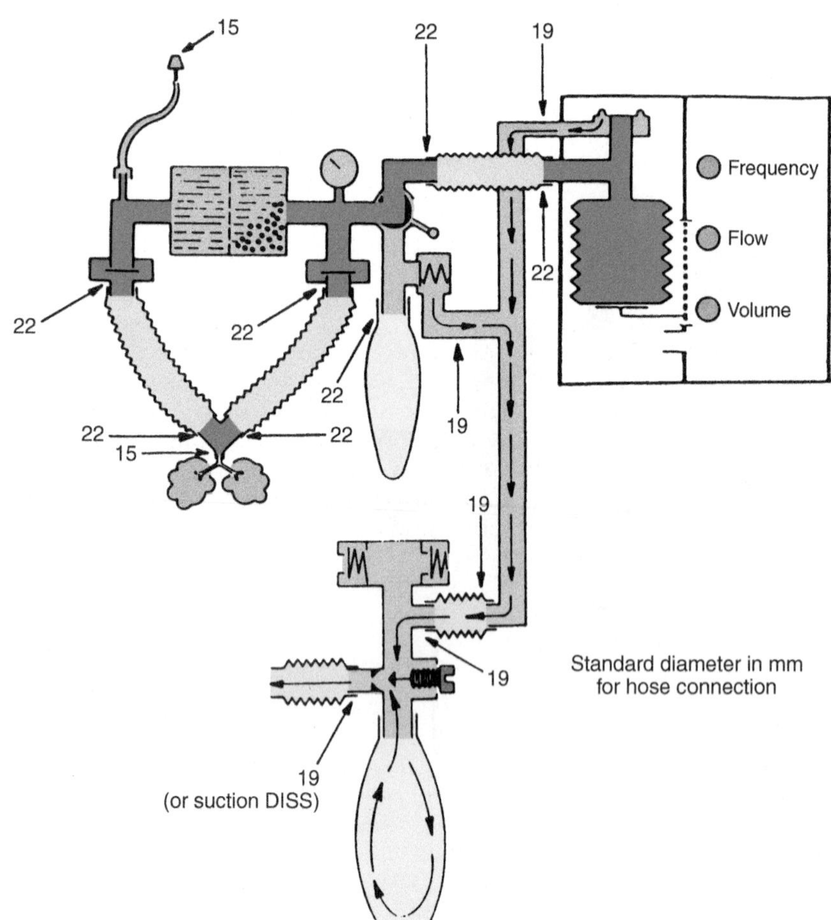

FIGURE 30-15 Diameters (in millimeters) for hose terminals in the anesthesia breathing and scavenger systems. Unrelieved subatmospheric pressure from the scavenger system can be applied directly to the patient circuit through the adjustable pressure-limiting valve. This creates subatmospheric pressure in the breathing circuit and, consequently, in the lungs. DISS, diameter index safety system (connector). (From Schreiber P: *Safety guidelines for anesthesia systems,* Telford, PA, 1985, Dräger Medical.)

A sidestream-sampling (diverting) gas analyzer connected to the patient circuit has been reported as the cause of excessive negative pressure in a breathing circuit, where the FGF of 50 mL/min during cardiopulmonary bypass was less than the analyzer's gas sampling rate of 250 mL/min.[61] The gas sampling rates of commonly used sidestream-sampling gas analyzers vary between about 50 mL/min and 300 mL/min. Although the potential for creating negative pressure in the circuit exists if low FGF rates are being used, contemporary analyzers are designed to sound an alarm and limit the negative pressure that can be generated.

Excess gas removal by a sampling device during spontaneous ventilation creates a subatmospheric pressure in the circuit that in turn causes the APL valve to close. This prevents the scavenging system negative-pressure relief valve or valves from relieving the negative pressure in the circuit. In one study, albeit from 1987, the maximum circuit subatmospheric pressure achieved by sidestream-sampling devices during testing ranged from -1 to -148 mm Hg.[61] If transmitted to the patient's airway, such low pressures have the potential to cause negative-pressure barotrauma and cardiovascular dysfunction.

Excessive volume loss resulting in negative pressures in the breathing system may arise if hospital suction is applied through the working channel of a fiberoptic bronchoscope that has been inserted into the circuit through an airway diaphragm adapter; this can also occur with a suction catheter that has been accidentally advanced alongside the tracheal tube into the trachea.

Inadequate circuit volume and negative pressure may occur during spontaneous ventilation in the presence of a low FGF rate and inadequate size of reservoir bag, such as a pediatric size used with an adult patient. During inspiration, the reservoir bag will collapse, and a negative pressure will be created in the circuit. Circuit APL valves usually have a minimum opening pressure that is slightly greater than that needed to distend the reservoir bag. If the bag were the correct size but noncompliant, or if the APL valve were to have a low opening pressure, most of the gas would exit through the APL valve during exhalation rather than fill the bag. The net result would be an inadequate reservoir volume for the next inspiration. Modern circuit pressure monitors incorporate a subatmospheric pressure alarm such that when pressure is less than -10 cm H_2O at any time, audible and visual alarms are triggered.

Failure to Initiate Artificial Ventilation

Failure to initiate artificial ventilation is usually attributable to an operator error. The error may be a failure to turn on the ventilator, for example, after tracheal intubation or separation from cardiopulmonary bypass; unintentionally setting a respiratory rate of zero breaths/min; failure to select the "automatic" (ventilator) setting on the manual/automatic selector switch in the circuit; or failure to connect the ventilator circuit hose, either at the patient circuit connector by the selector switch or at the bag mount. Because some older circuit volume and pressure alarms must be deliberately enabled or are enabled only when the ventilator is on, these monitors will fail to detect that the ventilator has not been turned on. In this respect, continuous capnography provides the most sensitive monitor of ventilation. If the delivery system incorporates a standing-bellows ventilator, failure to connect the ventilator tubing to the circuit will cause the bellows to collapse.

With either a standing or hanging bellows design, when a ventilator is turned on but the "manual" (bag) mode is selected at the selector switch, the bellows will attempt to empty during inspiration against a total obstruction—the closed selector switch—and its failure to empty will be readily observed. Failure to ventilate in this situation is sounded by both low pressure and volume alarms in the breathing system. Some older designs of circle system lack a manual/automatic selector switch, and the APL valve must be closed to effect intermittent positive-pressure ventilation (IPPV) when the ventilator hose is connected to the bag mount. In such a case, failure to close the APL valve is yet another cause of failure to initiate IPPV.

Even if the breathing system incorporates a selector switch, there are occasions when the primary anesthesia ventilator fails, and a freestanding ventilator may be brought in to provide IPPV. The foregoing considerations apply if the new ventilator is connected to the circuit via the bag-mount connection; that is, the "manual" mode is selected, and the APL valve is closed.

Leaks and Disconnections in the Breathing System

Breathing circuit disconnections and leaks are among the most common causes of anesthesia mishaps.[3,13] Anesthesia breathing systems contain numerous basic connections, and as more monitors, humidifiers, filters, and gas flow and gas sampling adapters are added, additional connections are needed. Each connection is a potential disconnection. Disconnections cannot be totally prevented; in the past, some have considered the 15-mm connector between the tracheal tube and the circuit to be a "safety fuse" to prevent unintentional extubation, although most now prefer a secure system that does not disconnect. Circuit disconnections and their detection have been the subject of several reviews.[86] Cooper and colleagues[2] found that disconnections of the patient from the machine were responsible for 7.5% of critical incidents involving human error or equipment failure. Of these disconnections, about 70% occured at the Y-piece.[2,87]

The risks of disconnection are reduced by secure locking of connecting components; use of disconnect alarms (pressure, volume, and capnography); and, most importantly, user education. Making secure friction connections, such as those between the tracheal tube and elbow adapter or between the adapter and the Y-piece, requires that the clinician use a pushing and twisting motion rather than merely pushing the two units together. When a disconnection occurs, the anesthesiologist must systematically trace the flow of gases through the breathing system, looking for the disconnection in the same way as would be done in the event of an obstruction situation or no gas flow.

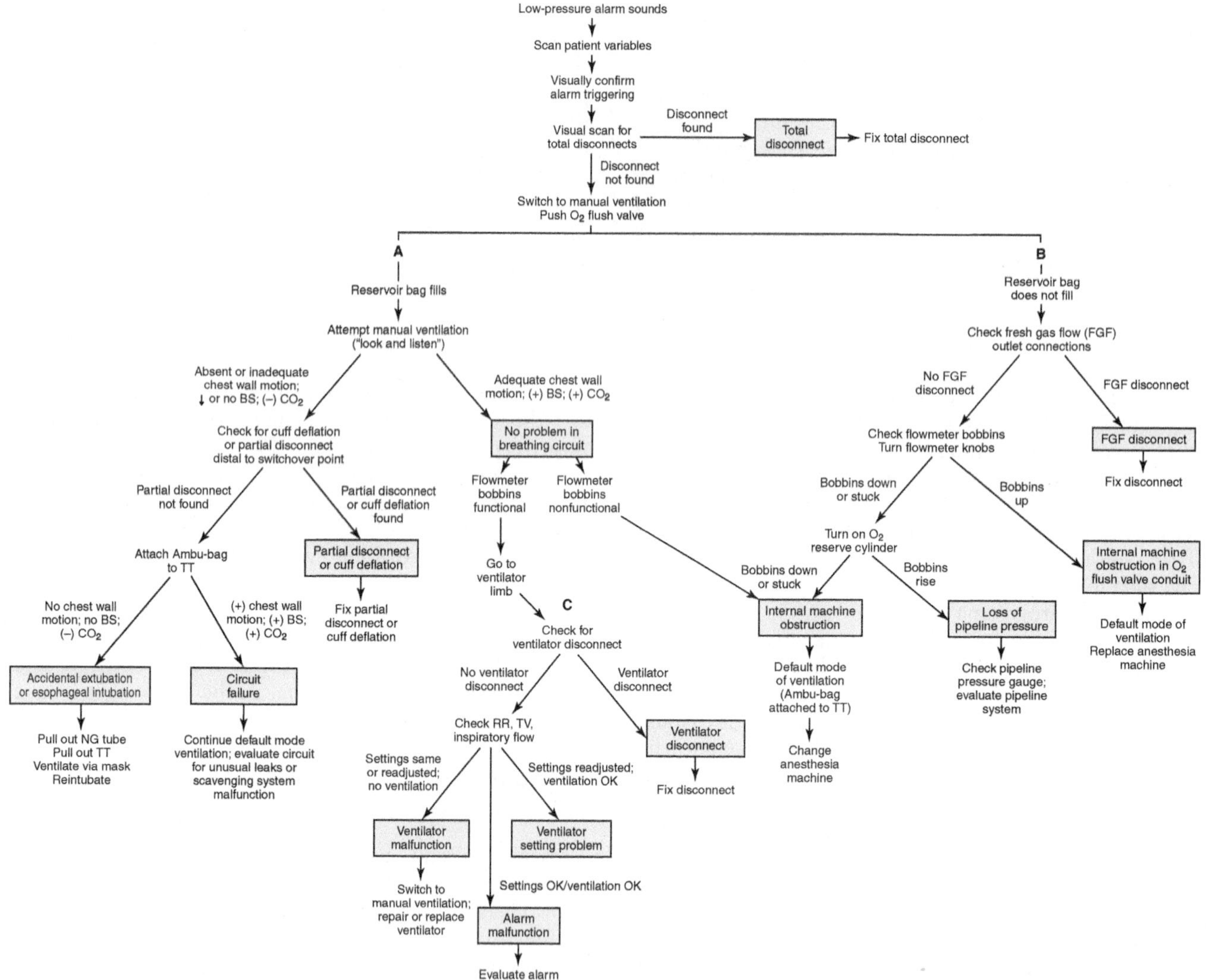

FIGURE 30-16 ■ Response algorithm for a low-pressure alarm condition. The three limbs of the algorithm are the breathing circuit limb (*A*), the fresh gas flow (*FGF*) limb (*B*), and the ventilator limb (*C*). BS, breath sounds; NG, nasograstric; *RR*, respiratory rate; TT, tracheal tube; *TV*, tidal volume. (From Raphael DT, Weller RS, Doran DJ: A response algorithm for the low-pressure alarm condition. *Anesth Analg* 1988;67:876-883. Reproduced by permission of the International Anesthesia Research Society.)

Most disconnections are detectable by the basic breathing system monitors of pressure, volume, and flow. Pressure monitors sound an alarm if the peak inspiratory pressure in the circuit fails to reach the threshold low setting. The alarm setting on the monitor should be user adjustable, and the user should be able to set it to a level just below the usual peak inspiratory pressure. Most monitors now provide a continuous graphic display of the circuit pressure and alarm threshold or thresholds. A response algorithm for the low-pressure alarm condition has been proposed (Fig. 30-16).[88]

The breathing circuit low-pressure alarm can be "fooled" if it is not set at the correct sensitivity. Thus a circuit disconnection at the Y-piece combined with sufficient resistance at the patient-connector end may not trigger the low-pressure alarm if inspiratory gas flow from the ventilator bellows is high enough for the pressure to cross the low-pressure alarm threshold. Examples include unintended extubation of a patient who has a small-diameter tracheal tube, in which case the tube connector offers a high resistance to gas flow, and occlusion of the open patient connector by the surgical drapes. A circuit low-pressure alarm sensing pressure in the absorber may be fooled in the presence of high resistance between the inspiratory tubing connector and the Y-piece, such as may be attributable to a cascade humidifier in the inspiratory limb of the circle.[89] Humidifiers may also represent the source of a detectable leak in the anesthesia circuit.

A breathing circuit low-pressure alarm is less likely to be fooled when a standing bellows ventilator is being used, because failure of the bellows to fill adequately during exhalation will lead to lower peak pressures on the next inspiration (Fig. 30-17). With the hanging bellows design, the peak inspiratory pressure with a disconnect tends to be higher than with a standing bellows ventilator disconnect, the hanging bellows having filled completely during exhalation. A pressure alarm set to an inappropriately low threshold is therefore more likely to be fooled by a hanging bellows ventilator.

The common gas outlet of the anesthesia machine was a site of disconnections before the standard use of retaining devices. The diameter of the tubing connecting the

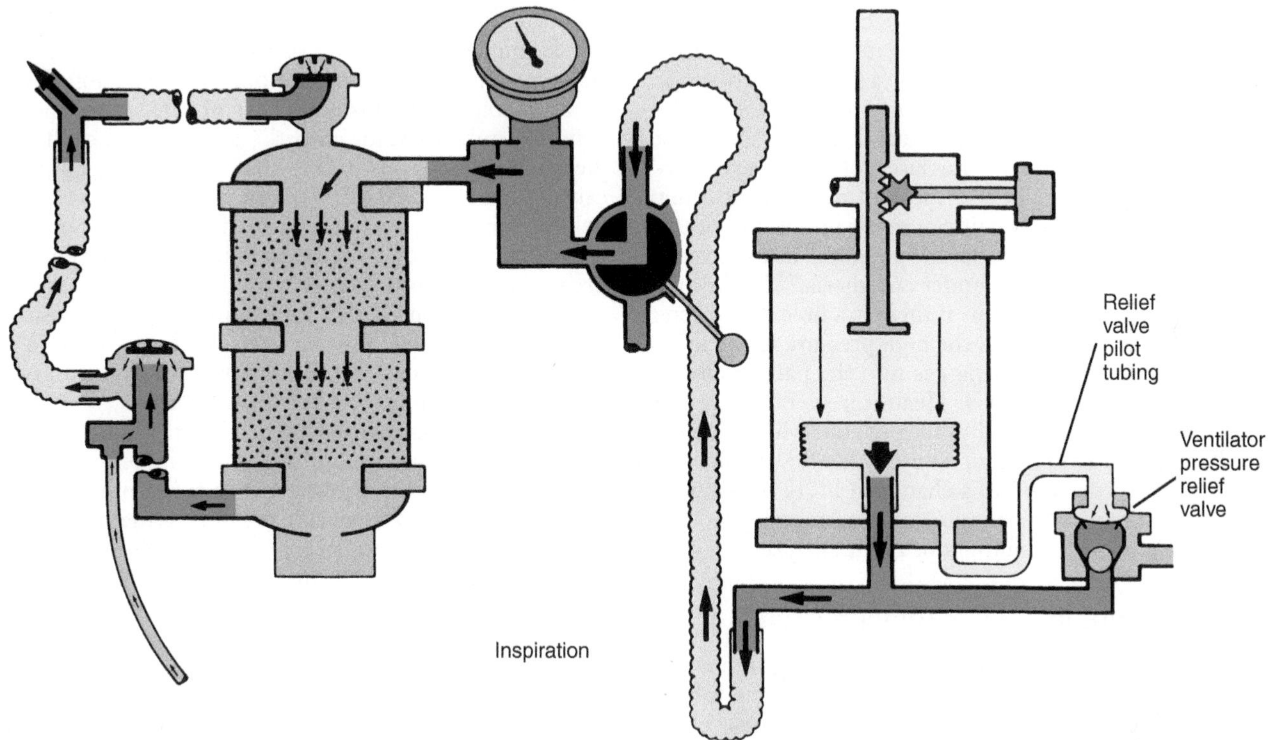

FIGURE 30-17 ■ AV-E standing bellows ventilator in inspiratory cycle. When a disconnect in the breathing circuit occurs with the standing bellows ventilator, the bellows falls and does not reexpand until the circuit is made gas tight again. (Courtesy Dräger Medical, Telford, PA.)

common gas outlet with the circuit is relatively narrow and offers relatively high resistance to gas flow compared with the 22 mm diameter circuit tubing. If a hanging-bellows ventilator were being used with a large tidal volume setting, the machine-to-circuit connector tubing resistance may be such that during inspiration, the low-pressure alarm limit would be exceeded despite the leak.[90] During exhalation, room air would be entrained via the fresh gas inflow tubing to refill the bellows (see Fig. 30-3). A disconnection of this tubing may also lead to a hypoxic gas mixture in the circuit, as air is entrained and oxygen is consumed. Detection of this type of disconnection, which is associated with air entrainment, is aided by an oxygen analyzer with an appropriately set low concentration alarm threshold located in the patient circuit.

If the circuit low-pressure alarm has been set as recommended, to just below the peak inspiratory pressure, it should be recognized that more false-positive alarms will be generated. Thus, when a tidal volume–uncompensated ventilator is used with a set tidal volume, a decrease in FGF, I:E ratio, or inspiratory flow rate or an increase in respiratory rate will decrease the peak inspiratory pressure and thereby trigger the alarm. However, a false-positive alarm with an appropriate response is preferable to failing to detect a potentially hazardous situation, provided that the user does not permanently silence the alarm.

Leaks from the breathing circuit, other than those attributable to component disconnection, may also result in inadequate exchange of gas between the system and patient. Leaks may arise in any component because of cracking, incorrect assembly, or malfunction of a system component, particularly the ventilator pressure relief valve.[91] Sometimes the design of a component may make a leak more likely. In the Fabius and Apollo workstations (Dräger Medical), lifting the APL valve allows gas to leave the circuit. Several incidents of tubing becoming trapped under the APL valve that resulted in a leak and failure to ventilate have been reported.[92-95] As a result the APL valve has been redesigned, and for those machines with the older design, an upgrade is available.

During inspiration, the ventilator pressure relief valve is normally held closed by the pressure of the driving gas from the bellows housing. If this valve is not held closed during inspiration, gas in the patient circuit may be vented to the scavenging system rather than going to the patient. Incompetence of the ventilator pressure relief valve has been reported in connection with pilot-line disconnection or occlusion and valve damage.[96] In such a situation, the loss of volume from the circuit would be detected by appropriately set pressure and volume alarms, but the source of the leak might be less obvious. If a closed-reservoir scavenging system is in use, the diagnosis is made by observation of the scavenging system reservoir bag. The bag normally fills during exhalation, as gas is released from the patient circuit, and it empties during inspiration, when the ventilator pressure relief valve is closed. If the ventilator pressure relief valve is incompetent, the scavenging system reservoir bag will be seen to fill during the inspiration, as the ventilator bellows empties its contained gas into the scavenging system.

Leaks and malfunctions in the patient circuit are sometimes first detected by an airway gas monitor, when the composition of the gas mixture in the breathing system deviates significantly from that expected. Application of negative pressure to the circuit by a malfunctioning scavenging system, or intermittently by a hanging bellows or piston ventilator during exhalation, may cause entrainment of air into the breathing system through a small leak otherwise unrecognized by pressure, volume, or even carbon dioxide monitoring.[97,98] A leak of room air or other gases into the patient circuit can result in dilution of the anesthesia gas mixture and has the potential, in an extreme case, to induce awareness under anesthesia.[99] Leaks into the patient circuit may occur if there is a hole in the ventilator bellows. In this case, the high pressure in the driving-gas circuit forces driving gas into the patient circuit during inspiration. With GE Healthcare ventilators, the diluting gas is normally 100% oxygen; but with a Dräger AV-E, it is a mixture of air and oxygen.[100,101] Such an event might be detected by a change in FiO_2, peak inspiratory pressure, tidal or minute volume, or end-tidal carbon dioxide or with a multigas or agent analyzer.

High Pressure in the Breathing System

The anesthesia machine provides a continuous flow of gas to the patient circuit. Whenever circuit gas inflow rate exceeds outflow rate, excessive pressures can develop. If these pressures are transmitted to the patient's lungs, severe cardiovascular compromise, barotrauma, and even pneumothorax may arise.[102,103]

During spontaneous ventilation, high pressure may be caused by 1) inadequate opening, or even complete closure, of the APL valve; 2) kinking or occlusion of the tubing between the APL valve and the scavenging interface; or 3) malfunction of the interface positive-pressure relief valve. During spontaneous ventilation, the bag will distend to accommodate the excess gas. Reservoir bags are highly distensible and limit the maximum circuit pressure to approximately 45 cm H_2O. Nevertheless, such an airway pressure could produce hypotension by inhibiting venous return. Increases in circuit pressure will be more rapid when the fresh gas inflow rate is high; for example, during prolonged use of the oxygen flush.[104]

Excessive pressure in the circuit may occur during use of an anesthesia ventilator. During inspiration, the ventilator pressure relief valve is normally held closed (see Fig. 30-17). Thus a high inspiratory gas-flow rate will be associated with increased peak pressures in the circuit. To protect the patient's lungs from excessive pressure, all contemporary ventilators incorporate a high-pressure alarm and high-pressure limit.

There are many reports of ventilator malfunctions causing excessive circuit pressures. Failure of the ventilator to cycle from inspiration to expiration results in driving gas continuing to enter the bellows housing (Dräger Medical), or it causes gas to enter but not leave (Datex-Ohmeda). This causes the ventilator pressure relief valve to remain closed, and excess pressure build ups within the circuit. The pressure increase is limited by the driving-gas pressure prevailing in the bellows housing.[105] In Dräger AV-E ventilators, this pressure depends on the setting of the inspiratory flow-control knob. Other reported causes of the ventilator pressure relief valve failing to open normally include mechanical obstruction of the driving-gas exhaust system (e.g., blocked Dräger AV-E muffler),[106] kinking of a Dräger AV-E ventilator pressure relief valve pilot line during inspiration, failure of a solenoid valve causing persistent inhalation, and diffusion of nitrous oxide into the space between the two pieces of rubber constituting the relief valve diaphragm, causing insidious PEEP.[107] Even with normal ventilator bellows function, high pressures in the circuit may be caused by occlusion of the tubing between the ventilator pressure relief valve outlet and the scavenging system or by obstruction of the scavenging interface positive-pressure relief valve. In such cases, as the pressure in the patient circuit rises, the ventilator bellows empties less completely and may even become distorted.

High pressures arising in the circuit are detected by the circuit pressure monitor, which incorporates two types of alarms: a continuing-pressure alarm is annunciated usually when the circuit pressure remains in excess of +15 cm H_2O for more than 10 seconds, and a high-pressure alarm is annunciated when the circuit pressure exceeds the high-pressure threshold limit, which in contemporary monitors is set by the user but often has a default setting of +40 cm H_2O, depending on the unit. When either of these alarms is annunciated during mechanical ventilation, a problem should be suspected with the ventilator circuit. In the absence of a high-pressure limit feature, circuit pressure can be immediately relieved by disconnection of the patient from the circuit at the Y-piece, inspiratory hose, or expiratory hoses or by selecting the manual (bag) mode and relieving pressure by opening the APL valve. The incorporation of safety relief valves into the circuit as a protection against high pressures is now the norm, and the opening threshold is set usually to about 5 cm H_2O above peak inspiratory pressure. The pressure limit must be set according to the patient, because too low a setting may preclude the ability to ventilate a patient with poor total thoracic compliance.

Pressure-limiting devices differ among some of the older model ventilators. The Datex-Ohmeda 7800 series ventilators incorporate an inspiratory high-pressure limit such that when the selected threshold is exceeded (the pressure measured in the patient circuit downstream of the inspiratory unidirectional valve), the ventilator cycles to expiration, driving-gas circuit pressure falls to zero, and excess patient-circuit gas is discharged to the scavenging system via the ventilator pressure relief valve. The basic model Dräger AV-E ventilators were not pressure limited, but a pressure-limit control is available and may be retrofitted to certain standing bellows–design AV-E units.[108] The Dräger AV-E pressure-limit control device senses the pressure in the patient circuit at the bellows, and whenever the threshold high-pressure limit is exceeded, a valve opens in the driving-gas circuit (bellows housing) to release excess driving gas to the atmosphere, thereby limiting driving-gas pressure such that patient circuit pressure does not exceed the set limit for the remainder of the inspiration. The time cycling (I:E ratio and set ventilatory rate) of the Dräger AV-E is therefore maintained, in contrast to the Datex-Ohmeda 7000/7800 series ventilators.[109] Both the Dräger AV-E and Datex-Ohmeda approaches to limiting pressure in the patient circuit require a normally functioning ventilator pressure relief valve, because it is through this valve, the opening pressure of which is controlled by the pressure in the driving-gas circuit, that excess gas and pressure is relieved from the patient circuit. If the pressure relief valve or its outflow path should become obstructed, neither the Dräger AV-E nor the Datex-Ohmeda pressure-limiting mechanisms would be effective in relieving pressure in the patient circuit.

ANESTHETIC AGENT DOSAGE AND ADMINISTRATION PROBLEMS

Adverse outcomes may arise as a result of an anesthetic agent overdosage or underdosage or administration of an incorrect agent. Hazards of vaporizer malfunction causing anesthetic overdosage or underdosage are caused by incorrect handling, incorrect agent use, human error, and, rarely, internal breakdown of the vaporizer itself.

Liquid Agent in the Fresh Gas Piping

Lethal anesthetic agent overdosage may occur when excessive amounts of saturated vapor or even liquid agent enter 1) the bypass portion of the vaporizer, 2) the machine piping between the vaporizer and the common gas outlet, 3) the interface hose, or 4) the breathing circuit.[110] The overdosage situation was more likely when measured-flow vaporizers (Copper Kettle [Puritan-Bennett; Covidien, Mansfield, MA], Verni-Trol [Ohio Medical Products, Gurnee, IL]) were used because calculation or flow-setting errors could easily arise. In addition, some older designs of vaporizers could be overfilled, so that excess liquid could enter the fresh gas piping. Fortunately, measured-flow systems are no longer in use and are considered obsolete. Modern vaporizers are concentration calibrated and are designed to prevent overfilling (see also Chapter 3).

Tilting or tipping of a vaporizer may cause liquid agent to enter the bypass of the vaporizer or the machine piping. One milliliter of liquid potent volatile agent produces approximately 200 mL of vapor at 20° C (see Chapter 3). For example, if 1 mL of liquid isoflurane were to enter the common gas piping, it would require approximately 20 L of fresh gas to dilute the resulting vapor to a concentration of 1%, or a minimum alveolar concentration (MAC) of approximately 0.8. It is easy to appreciate how a relatively small volume of liquid agent in the wrong place could have a profound effect on a patient.

If a vaporizer has been tilted or tipped, and there is concern that liquid agent may have leaked into the piping of the machine, then with no patient connected to the system, the vaporizer should be drained and then flushed with a high flow rate of oxygen from the anesthesia machine flowmeter (*not* the oxygen flush, which bypasses the vaporizer); the vaporizer dial should be set to a *high* concentration during this procedure.[111,112] If any doubt still exists as to the safe function of the vaporizer, it must be withdrawn from clinical service until certified safe for use by an authorized service representative. Additional caution is needed with a halothane vaporizer that has been tipped. Liquid halothane contains thymol, a sticky preservative that does not evaporate. Thymol entering the flow control and temperature-compensating parts of a variable-bypass vaporizer could cause vaporizer malfunction even after the halothane has been flushed out of these parts.

Modern vaporizers are mounted on the back bar of the anesthesia machine. Contemporary anesthesia vaporizers, such as the Dräger Vapor 2000 series and Datex Tec 7 series (GE Healthcare) have antispill designs. In the case of the Dräger Vapor 2000 vaporizers, the dial must be set to the T (transport) position to remove the vaporizer from the anesthesia workstation. In this position, the vaporizer sump is isolated from the other parts. GE's Aladin cartridges also have antispill mechanisms and can be safely tilted when removed from the workstation, but they must be withdrawn from the slot in the workstation during filling to prevent overflow of liquid agent into the workstation, which can occur despite the workstation's overflow protection mechanism. In the event liquid agent overwhelms the overflow mechanisms and enters the workstation parts of the vaporizer, the vaporizer shuts down, and no agent is delivered.

Overfilling of a vaporizer, which led to a halothane overdose and neurologic impairment in a 3-year-old boy, has been reported in connection with incorrect use of an agent-specific key-fill device.[113,114] When used correctly, the keyed bottle adaptor must be screwed tightly onto the bottle to ensure a gas-tight joint. The other end of the adapter is inserted into the vaporizer fill port and tightened; then with the concentration dial turned to OFF, the filler control is opened, the bottle is raised, and liquid agent flows into the vaporizer, displacing air from the vaporizer to flow back into the bottle via the air return tube. Overfilling is prevented, because the intake of air into the bottle stops when filling has reached the maximum safe level in the vaporizer sump; and because the vaporizer dial is in the OFF position, the air space at the top of the vaporizer sump is sealed. Slow filling of the vaporizer by the correct method described has resulted in individuals speeding up the process by loosening the seal between the agent bottle and key-fill adapter and turning the vaporizer on; this dangerous practice has led to the overfilling of vaporizers with adverse outcomes.

Design of the Concentration Dial

Anesthetic agent overdosage may also occur if a vaporizer delivers unexpectedly high concentrations. With all contemporary concentration-calibrated variable-bypass vaporizers, as well as the electronic Tec 6 and D-Vapor, output concentration *increases* when the dial is turned *counterclockwise*.[16] In some older designs of vaporizers, turning the dial *clockwise* increases the concentration; and some machines may still be in use that are equipped with the older design or, worse, a combination of the two designs, which might therefore present a hazard if the dial is turned inappropriately (Fig. 30-18).

Confusion can also occur with certain models of GE Healthcare workstations equipped with the electronically controlled Aladin vaporizing system. In the Datex ADU workstation, agent concentration is increased by turning the concentration wheel *counterclockwise*, as is the convention for mechanical vaporizers. The Aisys Carestation also uses the Aladin vaporizing system, but in this workstation, the "com wheel" is turned *clockwise* to increase the agent concentration (Fig. 30-19, *B*). This can lead to setting errors, especially in institutions that have both Aisys and ADU workstations. It is therefore important that the anesthesiologist deliberately observe the dial and concentration mark settings when adjusting agent concentration.

Incorrect Filling of Vaporizers

Anesthetic agent overdosage or underdosage can occur if an agent-specific vaporizer is filled wholly or partially with an incorrect agent. If an empty concentration-calibrated vaporizer designed for one agent is filled with an agent for which it was not designed, the vaporizer concentration output may be erroneous.[115,116] If a vaporizer designed for an agent with relatively low saturated vapor pressure (SVP) at room temperature (20° C; e.g., sevoflurane, 160 mm Hg; enflurane, 175 mm Hg) is filled with an agent that has a relatively high SVP (e.g., isoflurane, 239 mm Hg; halothane, 241 mm Hg), the output concentration will be greater than that set on the dial. The opposite occurs if a vaporizer designed for isoflurane or halothane is filled with sevoflurane or enflurane.

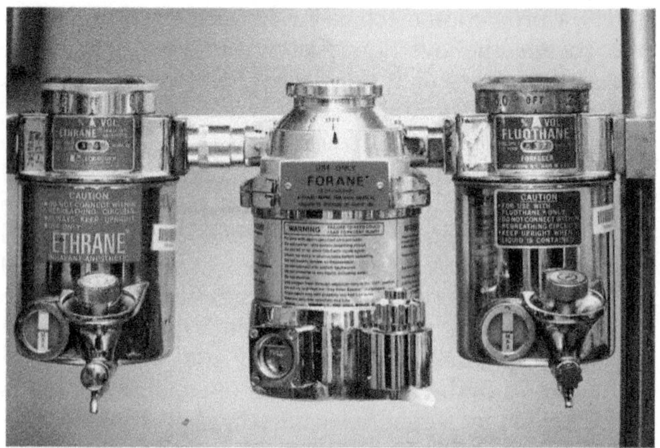

FIGURE 30-18 Three concentration-calibrated vaporizers mounted in series on the backbar of a now-obsolete anesthesia machine. In the absence of an interlock device, all three can be turned on simultaneously so that vapor from an upstream vaporizer can enter the vaporizing chambers of those downstream. On the two outer vaporizers, concentration is increased by turning the dial *clockwise,* whereas in the center vaporizer, the modern convention is followed in that concentration is increased by turning the dial *counterclockwise.*

Theoretically, an extremely dangerous condition would arise if a vaporizer designed for methoxyflurane, an agent with an SVP of only 20.3 mm Hg at 20° C and an MAC of 0.16, were filled with halothane. A methoxyflurane vaporizer filled with halothane and set to deliver 1% methoxyflurane (6 MAC of methoxyflurane) would deliver 14.8% (approximately 20 MAC) halothane! Fortunately, methoxyflurane and its vaporizers are no longer available.

The outputs of erroneously filled vaporizers are shown in Chapter 3, Table 3-4. Erroneous filling affects the output concentration and consequently the MAC or potency output of the vaporizer.[117] Thus a sevoflurane vaporizer set to 2% (1 MAC) but filled with isoflurane will deliver almost 3% (2.5 MAC) of isoflurane—that is, 2.5 times the anticipated anesthetic potency output (see Chapter 3, Table 3-4).

Erroneous filling of vaporizers may be prevented by careful attention to the specific agent and the vaporizer when filling is performed. Patented agent-specific fill devices, analogous to the quick-connect systems for medical gases, are available for all potent volatile anesthetic agents. Liquid anesthetic agents other than desflurane are packaged in bottles that have agent-specific collars. An agent-specific filling device has one end that fits the collar on the agent bottle and another end that fits only the vaporizer designed for that agent. Despite agent-specific fill devices, problems with erroneous fitting of a collar to the wrong bottle have been reported.[117]

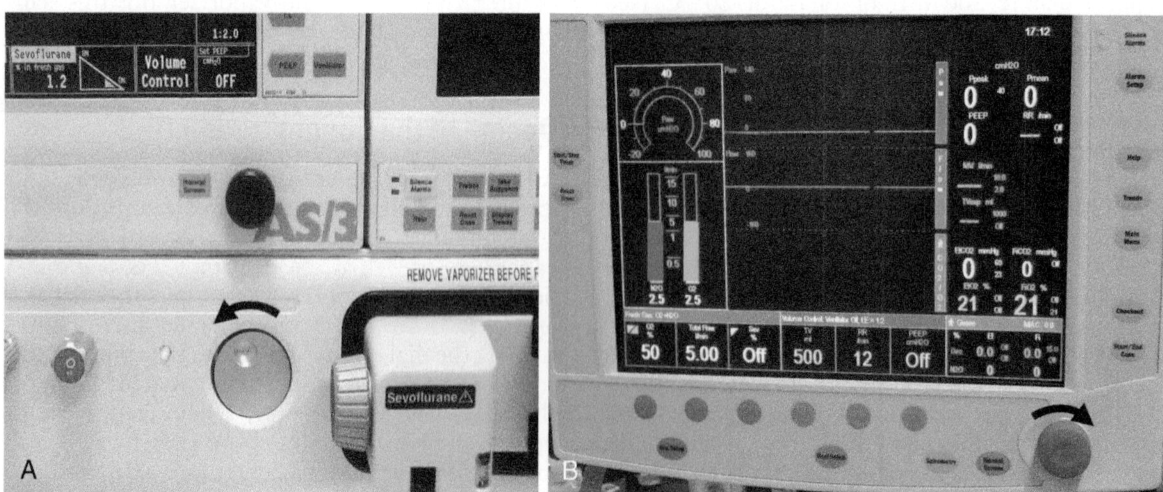

FIGURE 30-19 **A,** Aladin vaporizer concentration dial on Datex ADU workstation (GE Healthcare, Waukesha, WI) is turned *counterclockwise* to increase agent concentration. **B,** Aladin vaporizer concentration dial on GE Aisys Carestation is turned *clockwise* to increase agent concentration.

Desflurane has a very high SVP at room temperature (669 mm Hg) and boils at 22.8° C. Erroneously filling a modern flow-splitting variable-bypass vaporizer, such as a Tec 7 or Vapor 2000, with desflurane could lead to very high concentration outputs of this agent. The theoretical consequences of erroneously filling a vaporizer with desflurane have been reported by Andrews and colleagues.[118] They calculated that the most hazardous filling error would occur if an enflurane vaporizer were misfilled with desflurane. The calculated desflurane output of a misfilled enflurane vaporizer at a dial setting of 1% and a temperature of 22° C is 57.8%, or 9.6 MAC. For a misfilled isoflurane vaporizer at a dial setting equivalent to 1 MAC at 22° C, the calculated desflurane output is 10.2 MAC. A small increase in temperature would lead to a drastically increased output concentration, and the situation could become uncontrolled and potentially lethal if the temperature exceeded 22.8° C and desflurane were to boil.

Perhaps a more likely scenario is when an agent-specific vaporizer partially filled with a correct agent is topped off with an incorrect agent.[117] This situation is more complex and less easily predicted in terms of vaporizer output, and significant errors can arise in delivered vapor administration. Halothane, enflurane, and isoflurane do not react chemically when mixed, but they do influence each other's ease of vaporization. Halothane facilitates the vaporization of both enflurane and isoflurane and in the process is itself more likely to vaporize. The clinical consequences depend on the potencies of each of the mixed agents and on the delivered vapor concentrations. If a halothane vaporizer 25% full is refilled to 100% with isoflurane and set to deliver 1%, the halothane output is 0.41% (0.51 MAC), and the isoflurane output is 0.9% (0.78 MAC; see Chapter 3, Table 3-5).[119] In this case, the output potency of 1.29 MAC is not far from the 1.25 MAC (1% halothane) expected.

On the other hand, an enflurane vaporizer 25% full and set to deliver 2% (1.19 MAC) enflurane topped off to 100% with halothane has an output of 2.43% (3.03 MAC) halothane and 0.96% (0.57 MAC) enflurane.[117] This represents a total MAC of 3.6, or three times that intended. This illustrates why it is so important to avoid erroneous filling of vaporizers. If erroneous filling is suspected, the vaporizer should be emptied and, if necessary, serviced, flushed, and refilled with the correct agent.

Simultaneous Use of More Than One Vaporizer

Contemporary anesthesia vaporizers and their mounting systems incorporate an interlock system to prevent simultaneous use of more than one vaporizer and agent. Older anesthesia machine designs had up to three variable-bypass vaporizers arranged in series, such that fresh gas passed through each vaporizer, albeit through the bypass flow, to reach the common gas outlet of the anesthesia machine. Without an interlock device, which would have permitted only one vaporizer to be in use at any time, it was possible to have all three vaporizers on simultaneously (see Fig. 30-18). Apart from potentially delivering an anesthetic overdose to the patient, the agent from the upstream vaporizer could contaminate the agent or agents in the downstream vaporizers.[120,121] During subsequent use, the output of the downstream vaporizer would be contaminated, and the concentration of the emerging gas and vapor mixture would be indeterminate—and it might even be lethal. With such in-series arrangements, care must be taken to ensure that only one vaporizer is on at any time; and to minimize risk in case cross-contamination should occur, the sequence of vaporizers from upstream to downstream should be such that the agent that has the lowest SVP is upstream; that is, it is farthest from the patient. The correct series sequence would therefore be 1) sevoflurane, 2) enflurane, 3) isoflurane, and 4) halothane, with halothane being closest to the common gas outlet of the anesthesia machine. The standard use of safety-interlock devices prevents the in-series arrangement and its potential consequences. Vaporizers are neither in series nor parallel because only one can be connected to the machine's low-pressure system at any one time. The above discussion should therefore be of historical interest only (see Box 30-4, item D).

Although vaporizer interlock/exclusion systems are standard safety features on modern machines, failures of these systems have been reported. Failure may result in more than one vaporizer being on at the same time.[122] Exclusion of the selected vaporizer has been described with a Select-a-tec system (GE Healthcare).[122] It is therefore important that the anesthesiologist check the interlock system periodically for correct function.

The safety features of the vaporizer interlock system can also be defeated if a freestanding vaporizer is used in series with the FGF but downstream of the common gas outlet. Such arrangements, configured by the user, are potentially dangerous and should never be used.[123]

Pumping Effect

The now obsolete measured-flow vaporizers and some other, older designs of concentration-calibrated vaporizers were subject to the so-called pumping effect, which could result in increased output concentrations during mechanical ventilation when low FGF rates were in use. The explanation for this effect is that during positive-pressure ventilation, increased pressure in the vaporizer caused bypass gas to enter the vaporizing chamber, thereby increasing output. Contemporary vaporizing systems are designed to be compensated for or protected against the pumping effect. In certain models of Datex-Ohmeda anesthesia machines (GE Healthcare), vaporizer protection is afforded by an outlet check valve located just upstream of the common gas outlet; this configuration prevents increases in pressure in the patient circuit from being transmitted back into the machine and thence to the vaporizer.

Malignant Hyperthermia: Preparation for Susceptible Patients

If an anesthesia machine is to be used for a patient who is susceptible to malignant hyperthermia (MH), it has been recommended that the vaporizers be removed and

BOX 30-4 Recommendations for Preparing an Anesthesia Workstation for a Malignant Hyperthermia–Susceptible Patient

Remove vaporizer(s)
Replace breathing circuit and all hoses
Replace CO_2 absorbent
Replace ventilator components (bellows, connecting tubes)
Purge workstation with oxygen 10 mL/min, ventilating model lung with tidal volume 500 mL at a rate of 10 breaths/min
Purge time is workstation model specific (see Table 30-1)
Use activated charcoal filters on inspiratory and expiratory sides of circle breathing system
Use fresh gas flow of 10 L/min throughout the procedure
A decrease in fresh gas flow can result in a rebound in concentration of anesthetic

TABLE 30-1 Reported Purge Times Using an Oxygen Flow of 10 mL/min to Reach a 5 ppm Concentration of Anesthetic

Workstation	Time (min)	Reference
Ohmeda Excel 210	7	126
Datex ADU AS/3	30	127
Dräger Apollo	70	128
Dräger Narkomed GS	18	129
Dräger Fabius GS	50	130
GE Aestiva (sevoflurane)	51	131
GE Aestiva (desflurane)	71	131
GE Aisys (sevoflurane)	55	131
GE Aisys (desflurane)	69	131

that the machine be purged with oxygen before use. The Malignant Hyperthermia Association (MHA) has provided specific instructions on purging anesthesia machines of volatile agents to reduce the risk of exposure. However, these recommendations were developed from studies of older-generation machines. A major barrier to validating any guidelines for purging anesthesia machines is that a maximum "safe" concentration of potent inhaled volatile agent to which an MH-susceptible patient can be exposed is not known and likely never will be. In pigs an anesthetic concentration of 5 ppm is known not to trigger MH; therefore recent studies of purging anesthesia workstations have used this concentration as their endpoint. Modern anesthesia workstations are more complex and contain more gas-absorbing materials. A recent review of the literature concluded that current MHA guidelines[124] for the United States were inadequate to prepare newer-generation workstations, which require more time for purging of anesthetic gases, autoclaving or replacement of parts, and modifications to the gas delivery system. A review of study recommendations for preparing an anesthesia machine for the MH-susceptible patient has been published.[125] The authors proposed that new protocols be developed for each model of new workstation to prepare for an MH-susceptible patient.[125] Current recommendations are summarized in Box 30-4 and Table 30-1.[126-131]

Use of Activated Charcoal Filters

As an alternative to purging the anesthesia workstation, Birgenheier and colleagues[132] studied the efficacy of placing activated charcoal filters (Vapor-Clean; Dynasthetics, Salt Lake City) on both the inspiratory and expiratory sides of the circle system of several contaminated anesthesia machines and measured the time needed to flush the machine so that the delivered concentrations of isoflurane, sevoflurane, and desflurane would be less than 5 ppm. They also simulated a case in which MH is diagnosed 90 minutes after induction of anesthesia, and they measured how well activated charcoal filters limit further exposure. They found that the filters decreased the concentration of volatile anesthetic delivered by a contaminated machine to an acceptable level in less than 2 minutes, and the concentrations remained well below 5 ppm for at least 60 minutes. These authors concluded that activated charcoal filters provide an alternative approach to the 10 to 104 minutes of flushing time normally required to prepare a machine used previously to deliver a volatile anesthetic. Whether these filters should become standard of care is discussed in an editorial in the same journal issue.[133]

POSSIBLE MALFUNCTIONS

Anesthetic Agent Dosing Problems

Anesthetic agent underdosage may occur that results in light anesthesia, patient movement, or even awareness. Common causes include forgetting to turn the vaporizer on, especially after it has been turned off for refilling; an empty vaporizer; an incorrect concentration setting; or an incorrect agent in the vaporizer.

The unintentional delivery of high concentrations of anesthetic vapor may be caused by any kind of internal malfunction of the vaporizer. Therefore regular checking of function and output calibration are essential, and such checking should ideally be performed in the normal use environment of the vaporizer.

Although numerous design features have helped to make modern vaporizing systems safer for the patient, ideally, an agent-specific gas analyzer with user-adjustable high- and low-concentration alarm limits should be used in the patient circuit to monitor inhaled concentrations. A variety of such units using various technologies are available (see Chapter 8).

Incompatibility problems have been reported between Penlon Sigma Delta vaporizers and sevoflurane.[134] One is a variable degree of corrosion of the plastic key-fill stoppers with resultant leakage of anaesthetic gas on both low- and high-pressure leak testing. Another problem relates to a yellow discoloration of the sevoflurane in the gauge chamber and partial disintegration of the indicator ball. It was found that different manufacturers of sevoflurane use formulations with different amounts of water content, varying between 357 ppm water in Ultane and 19 ppm in Minrad sevoflurane. Degradation and hydrogen fluoride production associated with the low-water sevoflurane formulations were accompanied by physical corrosion of the vaporizers, specifically etching of the sight glass and degradation of the metal filler port shoe, leading to possible leakage of sevoflurane.[135] In September 2006 in the United Kingdom, Penlon recalled and replaced the affected vaporizers. Penlon altered the manufacturing process to use a polytetrafluoroethylene (PTFE) plastic–coated internal surface, but some older Penlon vaporizers may remain in circulation and may be subject to Lewis acid degradation.[136-138]

Desflurane Vaporizer Problems

The Tec 6 heated and pressurized desflurane vaporizer was introduced in 1993. Associated with the novel design, some new problems have been reported as the device has evolved. In particular there have been occasional reports of anesthetic agent overdosage because of a faulty control valve, which led to a recall of some Tec 6 vaporizers in 1994.[139] A gas leak problem after the Tec 6 was turned off, associated with an inability to subsequently turn on the Tec 6 or other vaporizers mounted on the same machine, led to another change in design.[140] There have been further sporadic reports of desflurane overdosage because of Tec 6 malfunctions, including one that led to cardiac arrest.[141,142]

Unusual yellow discoloration has been reported in the sight-glass display level of some D-Vapor desflurane vaporizers when filled for the first time with desflurane.[143] An investigation by the manufacturer of desflurane (Suprane, Baxter Healthcare, Deerfield, IL) found that the discoloration resulted from oxidation of butylated hydroxytoluene (BHT), an antioxidant present in many polymers, including those in the closure mechanism of Suprane bottles (Saf-T-Fill), and that the vaporizer itself was not the cause.

The Aladin vaporizing system used on Datex-Ohmeda (GE Healthcare) workstations can also deliver desflurane. There is one report of this system, set to 5% with a 5 L/min gas flow, delivering 14% desflurane for about 2 minutes following decrease of the FGF to 0.70 L/min.[144] The cause of the problem was thought to be that the one-way valve that prevents backflow of saturated vapor from the cassette via the inspiratory channel toward the bypass channel may have failed to close after lowering the FGF (see Chapter 3, Fig. 3-36). This problem may be more significant when desflurane is used, because the pressure in the desflurane Aladin cassette may exceed 1 atm due to its high vapor pressure when the temperature is greater than 22.8° C (boiling point of desflurane at 1 atm pressure).

Humidification Problems

Humidification of the inspired gases is desirable because it 1) prevents heat loss caused by evaporation of water from the tracheobronchial tree, 2) maintains moisture in the conducting airways and thereby facilitates ciliary function, and 3) prevents insensible water loss from the patient by evaporation. Humidity can be provided by heat and moisture exchange (HME) devices connected to the tracheal tube and by moistening of the inside of the breathing tubes and reservoir bag with water before use.[145,146] In addition, unheated water vaporizers can be used to provide moisture to the patient. However, the disadvantage of any system that does not use heat is that it will cool as evaporation takes place, and the amount of humidity generated will therefore be reduced.

Heated humidifiers (vaporizers) are devices through which the inspired gases are passed in order to saturate the gases with water at the temperature of the humidifier. The dry gases either bubble through the humidifier or pass over the surface of the water. The heat is usually provided by electricity.

The advantage of this type of system is that the inspired gases become saturated with water at an increased temperature. However, as the gas cools upon leaving the humidifier, condensation occurs in the tubing, and the amount of humidity delivered to the patient decreases. The condensation problem can be managed by heating the gases in the inspiratory hose either externally or internally with a heating wire. Keeping the distance from the humidifier to the patient as short as possible also decreases the amount of condensation (see also Chapter 7).

Another technique is to heat the humidifier to a temperature above body temperature, so that as the inspired gases cool in the inspiratory tubing, they enter the tracheal tube at the desired temperature. This technique must be used carefully to avoid burning the patient's tracheobronchial tree. It is therefore mandatory to monitor the temperature of the inspired gases at the tracheal tube to ensure that the gases are not too hot. Because gases delivered to the patient have at most 100% relative humidity, there is little chance that the patient will experience fluid overload when a heated humidifier is used. Another problem with this technique is that water will condense ("rain out") into the tubing as the gases cool. A significant amount of water can collect in the tubing, which can cause increased resistance to breathing or be accidentally delivered to the patient.

Hazards associated with the HME, or "artificial nose," include misconnection, obstruction, and disconnection.[147,148] A heated humidifier may cause bulk water delivery to the patient, thermal trauma to the airway, or obstruction of the breathing circuit, or it may become an electrical or fire hazard. These devices are electrically powered, and thermostat failure may lead to superheating of the gases in the humidifier, causing the plastic inspiratory tubing to soften.[149] A soft inspiratory hose may become completely occluded or may develop a hole, resulting in a large leak and thereby preventing ventilation of the patient. This problem can be avoided by making sure that the gas flow through the humidifier is initiated before the humidifier is turned on.[150]

Although fire in the OR is an uncommon event, a 2010 report of two fires in one brand of heated humidified circuit drew further attention to this potential danger. The authors considered that the inherent dangers of such a circuit did not warrant their continued use.[151]

Humidity can also be provided with a nebulizer technique. Nebulizers create droplets of water either by a jet of gas over the surface of the water or ultrasonically. Unlike the heated vaporizer, the nebulizer creates three hazards: 1) it can act as a nidus for bacterial transmission, 2) respiratory resistance may increase, and 3) the patient can become overhydrated. Therefore extreme care should be taken in cleaning the nebulizer; sterile water must be used, and the amount of water delivered must be carefully monitored. In addition, because of the risk of increased respiratory resistance, nebulizers should probably not be used with patients who are breathing spontaneously.

When using heated humidifiers or nebulizers, the anesthesiologist should guard against 1) fluid overload, 2) thermal injury, 3) additional sites for disconnection within the breathing circuit, 4) obstruction of gas flow, 5) burning of the equipment because of electrical malfunction, 6) shock hazards, and 7) the risk of infection transmission via the nebulizer.

Electrical Failure

Contemporary anesthesia workstations rely on electrical and mechanical devices to function. The power cord of the machine uses 90 to 130 V at 50 to 60 Hz alternating current (AC). On the workstation itself are usually at least four convenience receptacles that can provide electrical power for such additional equipment as monitors, anesthesia information management systems (AIMS), and infusion pumps that do not draw large amounts of current. There is also a rechargeable battery that acts as a back-up power source in case the external power fails.

The preoperative check of a workstation includes a status review of the AC power and the reserve battery (Fig. 30-20). A discharged battery may require up to 16 hours to recharge, so cases should not be started if either of these is not functioning. The ON/OFF switch on a traditional machine mechanically activates the flow of gases through the flowmeters and turns on the electrical power. In the event of an electrical power failure, having the switch turned on allows gases to flow to the flowmeters. The battery provides power to the electrical devices built into the machine; these include the ventilator, the alarm system, and the integral monitors. External electrical appliances plugged into the convenience receptacles are not powered by the battery.

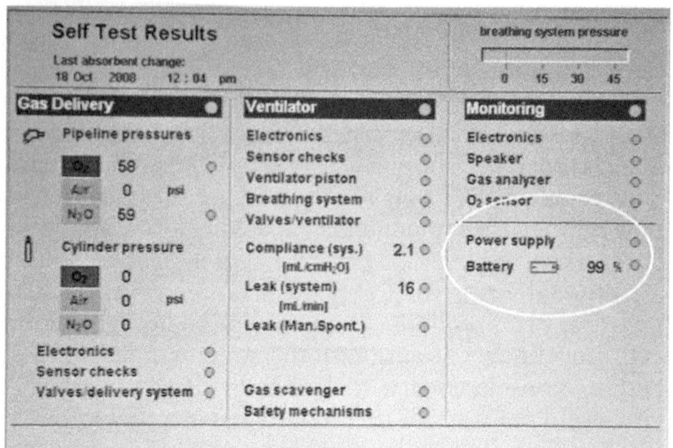

FIGURE 30-20 ■ Battery charge indicator during preuse checkout.

Usually the back-up battery provides power for approximately 40 minutes. When its voltage drops to below about 10 V, all power to the machine ceases in order to prevent a deep discharge of the battery. Failure of the battery would cause the monitors, alarm system, and ventilator on the machine to stop functioning. Manual ventilation would then be required.

In some institutions the anesthesia workstation and AIMS are connected to an uninterruptible power supply (UPS; Fig. 30-21), which extends the amount of time the workstation can function in the event direct current (DC) power is lost. The workstation and/or UPS should be connected to a wall outlet that would be energized by the institution's emergency generator power supply in the event power is lost from the electric utility company.

Leaving the machine power on with the electrical cord disconnected from the wall is a common cause of battery discharge. This should be discovered on the preuse check of the equipment, and ideally the machine should not be used until the battery has been recharged. Another source of trouble is accidentally plugging the power cord from the machine into one of the machine convenience receptacles; in essence, the machine is plugged into itself and has no external power supply. The anesthesiologist is alerted to this problem if the AC power failure indicator is activated and the "battery in use" warning light is on.

The electrical portion of the machine has several circuit breakers, which generally protect circuits for the AC power supply, the battery, and the convenience receptacles. When any of the electrical systems of the machine malfunction, the circuit breakers should be checked to determine whether they have been tripped. The anesthesiologist is sometimes responsible for anesthesia machine

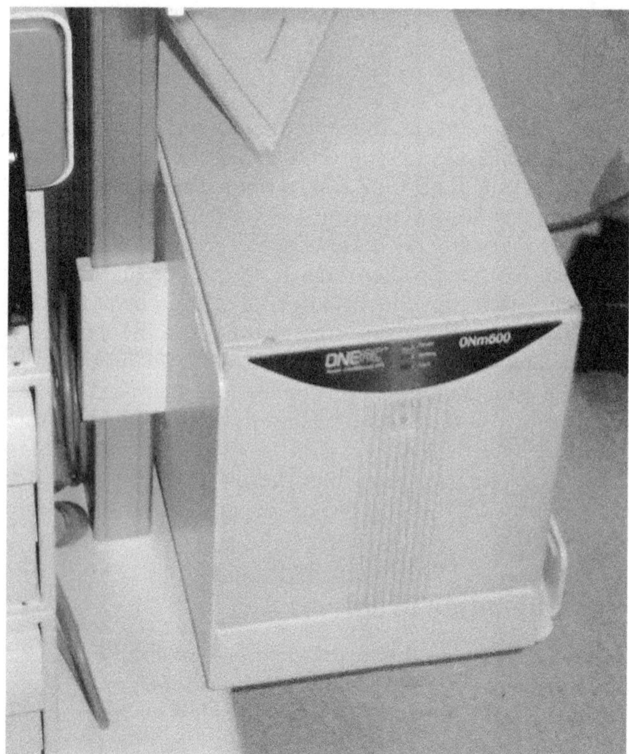

FIGURE 30-21 ■ Uninterruptible power supply unit.

electrical failure. In one reported case, the anesthesiologist had intended to turn off the ventilator but instead turned off the main power switch to the machine. The effect was to turn off the gas flow, the alarm system, and the ventilator. In this situation, because the alarm system no longer functioned, it was up to the anesthesiologist, through vigilance, to recognize that the machine had been turned off and to intervene appropriately.[152]

With contemporary anesthesia workstations being dependent on electrical power, it is important to plan for such failures to ensure patient safety. Recent reports and an editorial have highlighted this topic and have proposed a preparedness checklist.[153-155] Total electrical failure in the OR affects all equipment that does not have a battery back-up system. This includes all monitors, the anesthesia machine, the cardiopulmonary bypass machine, and the electric lights. All institutions should have an emergency plan for this type of utility failure. A sentinel alert from The Joint Commission requires that each health care facility must assess the risk of electrical power failure, at various degrees of magnitude and impact severity, and make plans to deal with such an emergency.[156] For more information, see Chapter 31.

Electromagnetic interference (EMI) is another potential cause of delivery system failure and has been reported to cause ventilator failure.[157] The design of contemporary electronic equipment makes EMI less likely, and all equipment is tested for EMI. Modern cellular telephones do not appear to interfere with OR equipment.

Hazards from Interactions with Carbon Dioxide Absorbent

Since 1990, there have been several reports of patients who developed increased levels of carboxyhemoglobin in response to accumulation of carbon monoxide in the circle system, generated when desflurane, enflurane, and to a lesser extent isoflurane interact with dry (desiccated) carbon dioxide absorbent, particularly Baralyme (no longer being manufactured).[158] Although no case of patient harm has been reported to date, carbon monixide represents a potential hazard of which the anesthesia caregiver should be aware.[159] Measures to decrease this potential hazard include using absorbent that has the standard complement of water or addition of liquid water to the top of the absorbent. Fresh gas should be turned off at the end of each case to prevent desiccation of the absorbent, and consideration should be given to replacing the absorbent more frequently, especially if the machine has been left unused for some time, such as over a weekend.

Another approach is to use a carbon dioxide absorbent that does not contain strong bases, such as barium hydroxide ($BaOH_2$) and potassium hydroxide (KOH).[160,161] For example, Amsorb (Armstrong Medical, Coleraine, Northern Ireland) is a carbon dioxide absorbent that does not contain a strong base and does not form carbon moxide or compound A in vitro. It also turns purple when desiccated, which is an additional advantage.

Desiccated Baralyme acting on sevoflurane can produce absorber temperatures that exceed 300° C, and it can lead to both fires and explosions.[162-165] Animal studies and a bench model demonstrate fires and explosions with sevoflurane, and there are now several reports of fires and explosions in clinical practice with sevoflurane, but none with desflurane or isoflurane. In one case, a patient was injured. In late 2004, the manufacturer of Baralyme discontinued its distribution, which should minimize or even eliminate the problems of fire and explosion. The risk of fire and explosion is considered to be much less with soda lime, although it has been suggested that the absorber temperature be routinely monitored using a skin probe.[166]

PREVENTION OF COMPLICATIONS

Complications from the anesthesia delivery system are uncommon, but when they do occur, they are usually due to user error rather than actual equipment failure.[167] Contemporary anesthesia workstations incorporate many safety design features, and older systems that are obsolete should no longer be used. Criteria for determining obsolescence of an anesthesia machine have been published by the ASA (Box 30-5). User

BOX 30-5 American Society of Anesthesiologists Guidelines for Determining Anesthesia Machine Obsolescence (June 2004)

The following guidelines have been developed to assist anesthesia providers and other health care personnel, administrators, and regulatory bodies in determining when an anesthesia machine is obsolete. Anesthesia equipment can become obsolete if essential components wear out and cannot be replaced. It may also become obsolete as a result of changes in medical practices, changes in the training and experience of anesthesia providers, or development of new safety features.

An anesthesia machine should not be considered obsolete solely because it has reached an arbitrary age. Furthermore, a machine should not be expected to meet all of the performance and safety requirements specified in U.S. or international equipment standards published after the machine was manufactured. It is the responsibility of the anesthesia provider to determine whether a machine's failure to meet newer standards represents a sufficient threat to patient safety to render the machine obsolete.

The ASA Standards for Basic Anesthetic Monitoring[17] apply to all anesthesia care. The equipment necessary to accomplish this monitoring may be integral to the anesthesia machine or separate from it. The criteria for defining obsolescence described in this document relate only to the gas and vapor delivery portion of the machine. Integral monitors (e.g., electrocardiograph, oxygen monitor, blood pressure monitor, pulse oximeter, carbon dioxide monitor) should be considered separately and are not addressed in these guidelines.

These guidelines apply only to existing machines and are not intended to unduly restrict the design of machines in the future. It is recognized that future machines may incorporate different safety mechanisms than those in use today to accomplish the same goals.

Continued

BOX 30-5 American Society of Anesthesiologists Guidelines for Determining Anesthesia Machine Obsolescence (June 2004)—cont'd

Absolute Criteria

An anesthesia machine shall be considered to be obsolete if any of the following criteria apply.

I. Lack of Essential Safety Features

A. Minimum oxygen ratio device (O_2/N_2O proportioning system) on a machine that can deliver nitrous oxide
Rationale: Hypoxia has been a major cause of patient death or severe brain injury during anesthesia. An anesthesia machine that cannot deliver oxygen must automatically be rendered incapable of delivering nitrous oxide as well.

B. Oxygen failure safety ("fail-safe") device
Rationale: One of the most serious mishaps that occurred with anesthesia machines in the past was depletion of the oxygen supply, usually from an exhausted cylinder, without the user being aware. The result was delivery of a hypoxic mixture, and this mishap can occur even with piped gas supplies. An oxygen fail-safe device prevents this hazard by stopping the flow of nitrous oxide when there is a loss of oxygen supply pressure.

C. Oxygen supply pressure failure alarm
Rationale: Although the supply of oxygen from a pipeline system or cylinders is usually very reliable, interruptions in that supply can occur. Given the critical nature of oxygen delivery, the operator of an anesthesia machine should be made aware immediately of the failure of the central oxygen supply so that appropriate remedial measures (e.g., opening a cylinder, reducing the use of oxygen, obtaining additional cylinders) can be taken.

D. Vaporizer interlock device
Note 1: This does not apply to an anesthesia machine that allows only one vaporizer to be mounted at a time.
Note 2: It may be possible to add a vaporizer interlock device to a machine.
Rationale: Turning on two vaporizers at the same time can result in dangerously high anesthetic vapor concentrations being delivered and contamination of the downstream vaporizer.

E. Pin-index safety system
Rationale: This system is needed to prevent mounting a cylinder on an incorrect yoke.

F. Noninterchangeable, gas-specific (e.g., diameter-index safety system) connectors on the gas pipeline inlets
Rationale: These connectors are needed to prevent attachment of an incorrect gas delivery hose to the machine.

II. Presence of Unacceptable Features

A. Measured flow (flowmeter-controlled) vaporizers (e.g., Copper Kettle, Verni-trol)
Rationale: These vaporizers have not been manufactured for some time, and servicing for them is no longer available. Many anesthesia providers are not sufficiently familiar with them to use them correctly, which may result in delivery of inadequately low or dangerously high anesthetic vapor concentrations. Some of these vaporizers lack the side-fill feature needed to prevent accidental overfilling and spilling of liquid anesthetic into the breathing system.

B. More than one flow control knob for a single gas delivered to the common gas outlet of the machine
Note: This does not include the flow control knob for an auxiliary oxygen flowmeter.
Rationale: Having more than one flow control knob for a gas may result in an unintended high or low flow of gas being delivered. Parallel flowmeters may cause ambiguity, because on all recently manufactured machines, flowmeters are in series, with one flow control knob for each gas delivered to the machine's common gas outlet.

C. Vaporizer with rotary concentration dial such that the anesthetic vapor concentration increases when the dial is turned clockwise
Note: It may be possible to replace an unacceptable vaporizer without replacing the entire machine.
Rationale: All vaporizers manufactured in recent years are designed to deliver increased vapor concentration when the dial is turned counterclockwise. Uniformity in vaporizer controls will prevent errors and increase safety.

D. Connection(s) in scavenging systems of the same diameter (i.e., 15 mm or 22 mm) as a breathing system connection
Note: It may be possible to replace an unacceptable scavenging connection without replacing the entire machine.
Rationale: Having 15 or 22 mm diameter connections in the scavenging system can result in incorrect connections between the breathing system and the scavenging system, potentially resulting in negative or high pressure in the breathing system. Current standards mandate 30 (preferred) or 19 mm connections in the scavenging system.

III. Adequate Maintenance no Longer Possible

A. The manufacturer or certified service personnel will not or cannot service the machine with acceptable replacement parts so that it performs within the tolerances to which it was originally designed.
Note 1: Although a manufacturer may declare that its own subsidiaries will no longer service, support, or certify a particular machine, the essential core components of the machine may still be serviceable.
Note 2: Obtaining acceptable replacement parts can be a problem. In some cases, it may be possible to obtain the parts from the party who supplied them to the machine manufacturer. Alternatively, such parts may be obtained from machines that have already been taken out of service.
Note 3: When a manufacturer declares that it will no longer provide support for a machine, responsibility is typically transferred to the user (health care facility) and/or the third party who services the machine.
Rationale: A machine that cannot be serviced or for which replacement parts are not available cannot be maintained according to the standards and specifications to which it was originally designed and is dangerous.

Relative Criteria

A. Consideration should be given to replacing an anesthesia machine if any of the following safety features are lacking:
1. Means to isolate the adjustable pressure-limiting (APL) valve during mechanical ventilation
Note: Isolation of the APL valve can be done in a number of ways (e.g., mechanically, electronically).
Rationale: The APL valve is designed for use with manual, not mechanical, ventilation. If an APL valve is left open and is not isolated from the breathing system

BOX 30-5 American Society of Anesthesiologists Guidelines for Determining Anesthesia Machine Obsolescence (June 2004)—cont'd

during mechanical ventilation, a portion of the inspired tidal volume may be lost.

2. Oxygen flow control knob that is fluted and larger than the other flow control knobs

Rationale: Current standards mandate that the oxygen flow control knob be larger than other flow control knobs and that it be fluted. Alterations to gas flows may be performed during low-light conditions or when the anesthesia provider is not looking directly at the machine. Tactile identification of the oxygen flow control knob should reduce errors.

3. Oxygen flush control protected from accidental activation

Note: Protection can be either by placement or design of the control.

Rationale: Accidental activation of the oxygen flush can result in barotrauma.

4. Main ON/OFF switch for electrical power to integral monitors and alarms

Rationale: Current standards mandate that the main power switch, when turned on, enables integral monitors and alarms. Operators unfamiliar with older anesthesia machines may not appreciate that monitors and alarms are not automatically enabled and may neglect to turn on one or several of them if they are not activated by a single switch.

5. Antidisconnection device at the fresh gas outlet

Rationale: Disconnection of the fresh gas inflow to the breathing system may lead to undesirable anesthetic or oxygen concentrations delivered to the patient, or it may create a significant leak in the breathing system with rapid loss of gas. Depending on the mode of ventilation (spontaneous or controlled), disconnection of the fresh gas hose may not be immediately apparent.

6. Airway pressure alarm for detecting sustained positive pressure, negative pressure, and high peak pressure

Note: An alarm for detecting disconnections (low-pressure alarm) is a criterion of the ASA Standards for Basic Anesthetic Monitoring.

Rationale: These pressure conditions represent an immediate threat to patient safety and need to be brought to the immediate attention of the anesthesia provider.

I. Problems with Maintenance

A. The maintenance history indicates that problems with the machine (e.g., increasing frequency of service calls, machine frequently not available for use) are impacting clinical service in a manner that is unacceptable to the institution or that threatens patient safety.

Note: Maintenance records or logs should be kept for all anesthesia machines in clinical use, and problems should be documented. These records should be reviewed regularly to determine what types of problems are occurring with each machine, how often they occur, and their effect on the anesthesia practice.

II. Potential for Human Error

A. Differences between older and newer machines can be a source of confusion and error if certain features, such as automatic activation of monitors and alarms by a main ON/OFF switch, are present on some machines but not on others or are in different locations on the machines.

Rationale: Having certain machine features in different locations on different machines can create confusion and increase the likelihood of operator error. Anesthesia providers more familiar with anesthesia machines manufactured recently may mistakenly expect that certain features are present on older machines, and it may not be readily apparent that they are different. Standardization of anesthesia machines throughout an institution should be considered.

III. Inability to Meet Practice Needs

A. The machine cannot accept vaporizers for newer potent inhaled volatile agents.

Note: A vaporizer should never be placed downstream of the common gas outlet. This is a dangerous practice.

B. The machine cannot deliver fresh gas flows that are low enough for current anesthetic techniques.

C. The integral anesthesia ventilator is incapable of safely and effectively ventilating the lungs of the target patient population.

Rationale: New agents, techniques, and/or ventilators may not be compatible with older anesthesia machines. If their use is considered to be necessary for optimal patient management, a new anesthesia machine should be obtained.

When it has been determined that a machine is obsolete, it should not be placed somewhere in the facility where it might be used clinically (for example, as an oxygen delivery device). A machine that has been determined to be obsolete should either be destroyed or donated to a worthy party (e.g., a developing country, zoo, or laboratory). If the latter course is followed, it would be prudent to obtain legal advice about potential liability relating to the donation. It is also prudent to ensure that the recipient possesses the infrastructure (e.g., electrical power, medical gases), access to drugs and supplies (e.g., volatile anesthetics, circuits, replacement parts), technical expertise, and training to safely use the machine.

Rationale: Placing an obsolete machine where it might be used would involve many hazards. Many of the hazards noted above are related to the possible misuse of an older anesthesia machine by personnel unfamiliar with its idiosyncrasies and deviations from more modern machines. Placement of an obsolete anesthesia machine in a location where it would be used only infrequently during high-acuity situations, possibly by personnel without anesthesia training, can only magnify these risks. User expectations that it is a "modern" machine with "modern" safety features will still be present. The presence of an anesthesia machine in an atypical location may tempt personnel unfamiliar with the machine to modify it. Nonanesthesia personnel may avoid using it because they are not familiar with it.

The need to provide positive-pressure ventilation with oxygen in remote locations can be met by using an oxygen cylinder or flowmeter connected to a pipeline outlet and a nonrebreathing bag. This is inexpensive, easy to use, and can easily be made available in remote locations.

Based on Standards for Basic Anesthetic Monitoring.[17] Available from the American Society of Anesthesiologists, Park Ridge IL, and online at http://www.ASAhq.org. Variances from the recommendations contained in this document may be acceptable based on the judgment of the responsible anesthesiologist. The recommendations are designed to encourage quality patient care and safety in the workplace but cannot guarantee a specific outcome. They are subject to revision from time to time as warranted by the evolution of technology and practice.

education/in-servicing is essential if sophisticated equipment, such as a computerized anesthesia workstation, is to be used appropriately.[168] Education of medical as well as ancillary (nursing/technical) staff is also important, because they may unwittingly contribute to the occurrence of a complication.[169,170]

Excellent written and interactive electronic materials are available from some manufacturers of anesthesia workstations and serve to supplement the personal in-servicing of users and operators of new equipment.[171,172]

Preuse Checkout of the Delivery System

The purpose of the preanesthetic checkout is to determine that all the necessary equipment is present and functioning as expected before the induction of anesthesia. The importance of this is self-evident; moreover, its usefulness is supported in the anesthesia literature, which describes anesthesia machine malfunctions that could have been discovered before the case began had a thorough check of the equipment been performed.[173]

When the delivery system is checked before the start of anesthesia, it should be set up in the way it will be used during the case. Moving the machine after the case has begun, modifying the breathing circuit with a humidifier, or adding other components can affect the performance of the anesthesia delivery system. Inspecting the machine in the condition in which it will be used during the operation minimizes this type of problem. However, the preoperative equipment check does not guard against the problem of intraoperative equipment failure, so the anesthesiologist must be vigilant in the monitoring of equipment performance and must be ready to intervene in any hazardous situation.

Studies have shown that anesthesia providers often fail to properly perform the preuse checkout of their anesthesia delivery system[174] and that instructional review improves residents' performance of the checkout.[175] This may be due to the complexity of previously published checkouts.[176] The preuse checking of anesthesia equipment has been associated with a decreased risk of severe postoperative morbidity and mortality.[177]

As the anesthesia workstation evolved since publication of the FDA 1993 checkout recommendations, it became clear that a single checkout recommendation could not apply to all delivery systems. In 2004, a subcommittee of the ASA Committee on Equipment and Facilities was formed to develop a guideline that described what items should be checked rather than describing the methodology of checking. Seven requirements were identified as the underlying rationale for the guideline:

1. Reliable delivery of oxygen at any appropriate concentration up to 100%
2. Reliable means of positive-pressure ventilation
3. Back-up ventilation equipment available and functioning
4. Controlled release of positive pressure in the breathing circuit
5. Anesthesia vapor delivery (if intended as part of the anesthetic plan)
6. Adequate suction
7. Means to conform to standards for patient monitoring

The new checkout guidelines were approved by the ASA in 2007 and were published in 2008 (see Chapter 32, Table 32-2).[178] (For a more detailed description of the checkout guidelines, see Chapter 32.[179]) Suggested preuse checkouts for a number of contemporary workstations are also available at the ASA web site (www.asahq.org).

The ASA guidelines indicate which items could be checked by a technician alone and which must be checked in conjunction with the anesthesia provider. Notwithstanding the role of the technician, the guidelines emphasize, however, that the ultimate responsibility for ensuring that equipment functions properly lies with the anesthesia provider.

The new electronic workstations have preuse checkouts in which many of the checks are automated, but some must be completed by the user. It is essential that the user understand how to perform the required tasks. For example, the user must correctly assemble and connect the breathing system to the workstation. The automated checkout is then able to pressurize the system to measure compliance and check for leaks but not necessarily to check for correct gas flow through the components. It may be possible for a breathing system to be incorrectly assembled, be gas tight, yet not permit any gas to flow to the patient.

Some anesthesia workstations (Dräger Narkomed 6400, Apollo, and Fabius GS; Datascope [now Mindray Medical, Mahwah, NJ] Anestar) use fresh gas decoupling (FGD) to ensure that changes in FGF do not affect the desired (dialed-in) tidal volume delivered to the patient's airway. During the inspiratory phase of IPPV, only gas from the piston chamber (Dräger) or bellows (Anestar) is delivered to the inspiratory limb of the circle system, because the decoupling valve closes to divert FGF into the reservoir bag. FGD circuits differ from the traditional circle system in design and therefore may be associated with different problems, including detection of an air leak into the breathing system during the exhalation phase of positive-pressure ventilation[180] and failure of the FGD valve, resulting in failure to ventilate in the ventilator (but not in manual/bag mode; see Fig. 30-22).[181] All indicated and required monitors must be available and used correctly with alarm limits and alarm volumes set appropriately for the individual patient's situation. Anesthesia equipment should be regularly serviced by authorized personnel, and the equipment should be updated as necessary to conform to any existing requirements. A 2004 statement concerning guidelines to determine anesthesia machine obsolescence has been published by the ASA.[182]

A preuse checkout of the delivery system should be developed by each institution to suit local needs. Item 1 on any preuse checkout should be that a back-up means of ventilation should be made immediately available, and its function should be verified. Testing the function of the self-inflating resuscitation bag during the preuse checkout is essential. Occasionally, a bag is found to be faulty; either it does not generate positive pressure when it is squeezed, or it does not release positive pressure when it is longer being squeezed. Thus in the event of a delivery system failure, the patient's lungs can be ventilated with room air (or oxygen if a tank is available) using a self-inflating resuscitation bag.[183]

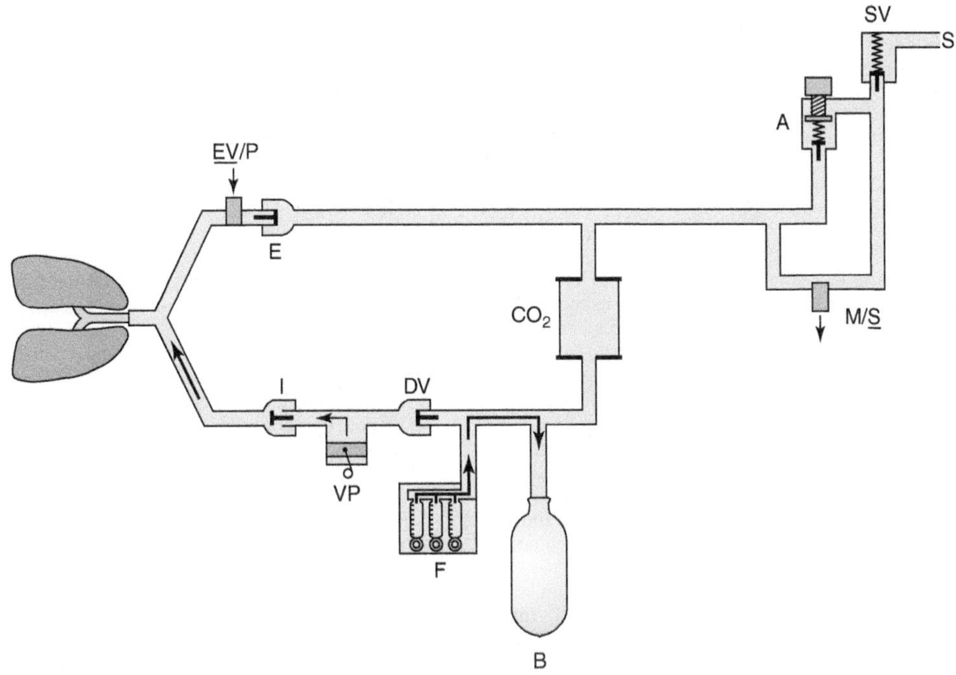

FIGURE 30-22 ■ Fresh gas decoupling breathing system as used in a Fabius GS workstation (Dräger Medical, Telford, PA). The fresh gas decoupling valve (*DV*) is located between the ventilator piston (*VP*) and the fresh gas inflow (*F*). During positive-pressure inspiration, anesthesia gas in the ventilator chamber is driven into the breathing circuit by the ventilator piston. The positive pressure causes the DV to close, directing fresh gas inflow into the reservoir bag (*B*). If the decoupling valve fails to close, gas inflow from the ventilator takes the path of least resistance into the reservoir bag, rather than past the inspiratory unidirectional valve (*I*), to ventilate the patient's lungs. Ventilation of the lungs is possible in bag mode. *EV/P*, expiratory valve/positive end-expiratory pressure valve; *A*, adjustable pressure limit (APL) valve; *M/S*, APL bypass valve; *SV*, scavenging valve; *S*, scavenging system. (Courtesy Michael A. Olympio, MD.)

Recent studies suggest that awareness is increasing regarding the importance of the preuse checkout and management of machine-related critical incidents.[184-187] Simulation of anesthesia equipment failure has been used to assess residents' performance in the management of these scenarios.[188] At least one national anesthesiology board has even incorporated aspects of the preuse checkout into the objective structured clinical evaluation component of its board examination in anesthesiology.[189]

The anesthesia delivery system may cause complications to the patient because of misuse or component failure. Anesthesia equipment failure and misuse represent a small proportion of anesthesia-related malpractice claims, but when they occur, the severity of injury is great. Use error is more common than pure equipment failure. The delivery system continues to evolve as more is learned about patient safety and as design and monitoring features are added. Clearly, a basic understanding of the structure and function of the delivery system will enhance patient safety by avoiding misuse and facilitating troubleshooting or alternative techniques if a component fails.

REFERENCES

1. Flanagan JC: The critical incident technique, *Psychol Bull* 51:327–358, 1954.
2. Cooper JB, et al: Preventable anesthesia mishaps, *Anesthesiology* 49:399–406, 1978.
3. Cooper JB, et al: An analysis of major errors and equipment failures in anesthesia management, *Anesthesiology* 60:34–42, 1984.
4. Sykes MK: Incidence of mortality and morbidity due to anaesthetic equipment failure, *Eur J Anaesthesiol* 4:198–199, 1987.
5. Buffington CW, Ramanathan S, Turndorf H: Detection of anesthesia machine faults, *Anesth Analg* 63:79–82, 1984.
6. *Anesthesia apparatus checkout recommendations*, Rockville, MD, 1986, U.S. Food and Drug Administration.
7. March MG, Crowley JJ: An evaluation of anesthesiologists' present checkout methods and the validity of the FDA checklist, *Anesthesiology* 75:724–729, 1991.
8. Kumar V, Hintze MS, Jacob AM: A random survey of anesthesia machines and ancillary monitors in 45 hospitals, *Anesth Analg* 67:644–649, 1988.
9. Webb RK, Currie M, Morgan CA, et al: The Australian Incident Monitoring Study: an analysis of 2000 incident reports, *Anaesth Intensive Care* 21:520–528, 1993.
10. Webb RK, Russell WJ, Klepper I, Runciman WB: The Australian Incident Monitoring Study. Equipment failure: an analysis of 2000 incident reports, *Anaesth Intensive Care* 21:673–677, 1993.
11. Russell WJ, Webb RK, Van de Walt JH, Runciman WB: The Australian Incident Monitoring Study. Problems with ventilation: an analysis of 2000 incident reports, *Anaesth Intensive Care* 1:617–620, 1993.
12. Eichhorn JH: Prevention of intraoperative anesthesia accidents and related severe injury through safety monitoring, *Anesthesiology* 70:572–527, 1989.
13. Caplan RA, Vistica MF, Posner KL, Cheney FW: Adverse anesthetic outcomes arising from gas delivery equipment: a closed claims analysis, *Anesthesiology* 87:741–748, 1997.
14. Posner Karen L: ASA Closed Claims Project, Personal communication, May 2012.
15. American Society for Testing and Materials (ASTM): Standard specification for particular requirements for anesthesia workstations and their components (ASTM F1850-00). West Conshohocken, PA, 2005, ASTM.
16. ASTM: *Specification for minimum performance and safety requirements for components and systems of anesthesia gas machines (ASTM F1161-88)*, Philadelphia, 1989, ASTM.
17. American Society of Anesthesiologists (ASA): Standards for basic anesthetic monitoring. Approved by the ASA House of Delegates on October 21, 1986; last amended on October 20, 2010, with an effective date of July 1, 2011. Park Ridge, IL, ASA.

18. Schreiber P: *Safety guidelines for anesthesia systems*, Telford, PA, 1985, North American Dräger.
19. Abraham ZA, Basagoitia J: A potentially lethal anesthesia machine failure, *Anesthesiology* 66:589–590, 1987 (letter).
20. Feeley TW, Hedley-Whyte J: Bulk oxygen and nitrous oxide delivery systems: design and dangers, *Anesthesiology* 44:301–305, 1976.
21. O'Connor CJ, Hobin KF: Bypassing the diameter-indexed safety system, *Anesthesiology* 71:318–319, 1989.
22. Anderson B, Chamley D: Wall outlet oxygen failure, *Anaesth Intensive Care* 15:468–469, 1987. (letter).
23. Mudumbai SC, Fanning R, Howard SK, Davies MF, Gaba DM: Use of medical simulation to explore equipment failures and human-machine interactions in anesthesia machine pipeline supply crossover, *Anesth Analg* 110:1292–1296, 2010.
24. "Surgery mix-up causes 2 deaths." *New Haven Register*, January 20, 2002.
25. Jawan B, Lee JH: Cardiac arrest caused by an incorrectly filled oxygen cylinder: a case report, *Br J Anaesth* 64:749–751, 1990.
26. Holland R: Wrong gas disaster in Hong Kong, *APSF Newslett* 4:26, 1989.
27. Lorraway PG, Savoldelli GL, Joo HS, et al: Management of simulated oxygen supply failure: is there a gap in the curriculum? *Anesth Analg* 102:865–867, 2006.
28. Bonsu AK, Stead AL: Accidental cross-connexion of oxygen and nitrous oxide in an anaesthetic machine, *Anaesthesia* 38:767–769, 1983.
29. Lacoumenta S, Hall GM: A burst oxygen pipeline, *Anaesthesia* 38:596–597, 1983. (letter).
30. Carley RH, Houghton IT, Park GR: A near disaster from piped gases, *Anaesthesia* 39:891–893, 1984.
31. Bancroft ML, du Moulin GC, Hedley-White J: Hazards of hospital bulk oxygen delivery systems, *Anesthesiology* 52:504–510, 1980.
32. Schumacher SD, Brockwell RC, Andrews JJ, Ogles D: Bulk liquid oxygen supply failure, *Anesthesiology* 100:186–189, 2004.
33. Feeley TW, Hedley-Whyte J: Bulk oxygen and nitrous oxide delivery systems: design and dangers, *Anesthesiology* 44:301–305, 1976.
34. Beudoin MG: Oxygen needle valve obstruction, *Anaesth Intensive Care* 16:130–131, 1988. (letter).
35. Khalil SN, Neuman J: Failure of an oxygen flow control valve, *Anesthesiology* 73:355–356, 1990.
36. Williams AR, Hilton PJ: Selective oxygen leak: a potential cause of patient hypoxia, *Anaesthesia* 41:1133–1134, 1986.
37. Hanning CD, Kruchek D, Chunara A: Preferential oxygen leak: an unusual case, *Anaesthesia* 42:1329–1330, 1987 (letter).
38. Moore JK, Railton R: Hypoxia caused by a leaking rotameter: the value of an oxygen analyser, *Anaesthesia* 39:380–381, 1984 (letter).
39. Cole AG, Thompson JB, Fodor IM, et al: Anaesthetic machine hazard from the Selectatec block, *Anaesthesia* 38:175–177, 1983. (letter).
40. ASA: *Guidelines for determining anesthesia machine obsolescence*, Park Ridge, IL, June 2004, ASA Committee on Equipment and Facilities.
41. Richards C: Failure of a nitrous oxide–oxygen proportioning system, *Anesthesiology* 71:997–999, 1989.
42. Goodyear CM: Failure of nitrous oxide-oxygen proportioning device, *Anesthesiology* 72:397–398, 1990.
43. Ghanooni S, Wilks DH, Finestone SC: A case report of an unusual disconnection, *Anesth Analg* 62:696–697, 1983.
44. Henshaw J: Circle system disconnection, *Anaesth Intensive Care* 16:240, 1988 (letter).
45. Horan BF: Unusual disconnection, *Anaesth Intensive Care* 15:466–467, 1987 (letter).
46. Ripp CH, Chapin JW: A bellows leak in an Ohio anesthesia ventilator, *Anesth Analg* 64:942, 1985 (letter).
47. Ripp CH, Chapin JW: A bellows leak in an Ohio anesthesia ventilator, *Anesth Analg* 64:942, 1985 (letter).
48. Spoor J: Ventilator malfunction, *Anaesth Intensive Care* 14:329, 1986 (letter).
49. Pashayan AG, Gravenstein JS, Cassisi NJ, McLaughlin G: The helium protocol for laryngotracheal operations with CO_2 laser: a retrospective review of 523 cases, *Anesthesiology* 68:801–804, 1988.
50. Mathes DD: Bleomycin and hyperoxia exposure in the operating room, *Anesth Analg* 81:624–629, 1995.
51. ASA Task Force on Operating Room Fires: Practice advisory for the prevention and management of operating room fires, *Anesthesiology* 108:786–801, 2008.
52. ECRI Institute: New clinical guide to surgical fire prevention, *Health Devices* 38(10), 2009.
53. Wan YL, Swan M: Exotic obstruction, *Anaesth Intensive Care* 18:274, 1990 (letter).
54. Boscoe MJ, Baxter RC: Failure of anaesthetic gas supply, *Anaesthesia* 38:997–998, 1983 (letter).
55. Hogan TS: Selectatec switch malfunction, *Anaesthesia* 40:66–69, 1985.
56. Milliken RA, Bizzarri DV: An unusual cause of failure of anesthetic gas delivery to a patient circuit [letter], *Anesth Analg* 63:1047–1048, 1984.
57. Eisenkraft JB, Sommer RM: Flapper valve malfunction, *Anesth Analg* 67:1132, 1988 (letter).
58. Sommer RM, Bhalla GS, Jackson JM, et al: Hypoventilation caused by ventilator valve rupture, *Anesth Analg* 67:999–1001, 1988.
59. Lamarche Y: Anaesthetic breathing circuit leak from cracked oxygen analyzer sensor connector [letter], *Can Anaesth Soc J* 32:682–683, 1985.
60. Gravenstein D, Wilkhu H, Liem EB, Tilman S, Lampotang S: Aestiva ventilation mode selector switch failures, *Anesth Analg* 104:860–862, 2007.
61. Mushlin PS, Mark JB, Elliott WR, et al: Inadvertent development of subatmospheric airway pressure during cardiopulmonary bypass, *Anesthesiology* 71:459–462, 1989.
62. Ghani GA: Fresh gas flow affects minute volume during mechanical ventilation, *Anesth Analg* 63:619, 1984.
63. Scheller MS, Jones BR, Benumof JL: The influence of fresh gas flow and I:E ratio on tidal volume and $PaCO_2$ in ventilated patients, *J Cardiothoracic Anesth* 3:564–567, 1989.
64. Birch AA, Fisher NA: Leak of soda lime seal after anesthesia machine check [letter], *J Clin Anesth* 1:474–476, 1989.
65. Andrews JJ, Johnston RV, Bee DE, et al: Photodeactivation of ethyl violet: a potential hazard of sodasorb, *Anesthesiology* 72:59–64, 1990.
66. Nunn JF: Carbon dioxide cylinders on anaesthetic apparatus, *Br J Anaesth* 65:155–156, 1990.
67. Razis PA: Carbon dioxide: a survey of its use in anaesthesia in the U.K, *Anaesthesia* 44:348–351, 1989.
68. Todd DB: Dangers of CO2 cylinders on anesthetic machines, *Anaesthesia* 50:911–912, 1995.
69. Ellett AE, Shields JC, Ifune C, Roa N, Vannucci A: A near miss: a N_2O-CO_2 mix-up despite current safety standards, *Anesthesiology* 110:1429, 2009.
70. Eger EI 2nd: Anesthetic systems: construction and function. In Eger EI, editor: *Anesthetic uptake and action*, Baltimore, 1974, Williams & Wilkins, pp 206–227.
71. Conway CM: Anaesthesia breathing systems. In Scurr CF, Feldman S, editors: *Scientific foundations of anaesthesia*, London, 1982, Heinemann, pp 557–566.
72. Forrest PR: Defective anaesthetic breathing circuit, *Can J Anaesth* 34:541–542, 1987 (letter).
73. Jackson FJ: Tests for co-axial systems [letter], *Anaesthesia* 43:1060–1061, 1988.
74. Hewitt AJ, Campbell W: Unusual damage to a Bain system [letter], *Anaesthesia* 41:882–883, 1986 (letter).
75. Goldman JM, Phelps RW: No flow anesthesia [letter], *Anesth Analg* 66:1339, 1987.
76. Koga Y, Iwatsuki N, Takahashi M, et al: A hazardous defect in a humidifier, *Anesth Analg* 71:712, 1990.
77. Schroff PK, Skerman JH: Humidifier malfunction: a cause of anesthesia circuit occlusion, *Anesth Analg* 67:710–711, 1988.
78. Spurring PW, Small LF: Breathing system disconnexions and misconnexions: a review of some common causes and some suggestions for improved safety, *Anaesthesia* 38:683–688, 1983.
79. Olympio MA, Stoner J: Tight mask fit could have prevented "airway" obstruction, *Anesthesiology* 77:822–825, 1992.
80. Peady CJ: Another report of obstruction of a heat and moisture exchange filter, *Can J Anesth* 49:1001, 2002.
81. Arellano R, Ross D, Lee K: Inappropriate attachment of PEEP valve causing total obstruction of ventilation bag, *Anesth Analg* 67:1050–1051, 1987.

82. ECRI Institute: PEEP valves in anesthesia circuits, *Health Devices* 13:24, 1983.
83. Anagnostou JM, Hults S, Moorthy SS: PEEP valve barotrauma, *Anesth Analg* 70:674–675, 1990.
84. Goldman JM, Phelps RW: No flow anesthesia [letter], *Anesth Analg* 66:1339, 1987.
85. Sharrock NE, Leith DE: Potential pulmonary barotrauma when venting anesthetic gases to suction, *Anesthesiology* 46:152–154, 1977.
86. Adams AP: Breathing system disconnections, *Br J Anaesth* 73:46–54, 1994.
87. Sara CA, Wark HJ: Disconnection: an appraisal, *Anaesth Intensive Care* 14:448–452, 1986.
88. Raphael DT, Weller RS, Doran DJ: A response algorithm for the low-pressure alarm condition, *Anesth Analg* 67:876–883, 1988.
89. Slee TA, Pavlin EG: Failure of a low-pressure alarm associated with use of a humidifier, *Anesthesiology* 69:791–793, 1988.
90. Ghanooni S, Wilks DH, Finestone SC: A case report of an unusual disconnection, *Anesth Analg* 62:696–697, 1983.
91. Eisenkraft JB: Potential for barotrauma or hypoventilation with the Dräger AV-E ventilator, *J Clin Anesth* 1:452–456, 1989.
92. Kibelbek MJ: Cable trapped under Dräger Fabius automatic pressure limiting valve causes inability to ventilate, *Anesthesiology* 106:639–640, 2007.
93. Hennefent S, Suslowicz B: Circuit leak from capnograph sampling line lodged under APL valve, *Anesth Analg* 111:578, 2010.
94. Robards C, Corda D: A potential hazard involving the gas sampling line and the adjustable pressure limiting valve on the Dräger Apollo anesthesia workstation, *Anesth Analg* 111:579, 2010.
95. Vijayakumar A, Saxena DK, Pillay AS, Darsow R: Massive leak during manual ventilation: adjustable pressure limiting valve malfunction not detected by pre-anesthetic checkout, *Anesth Analg* 111:579–580, 2010.
96. Choi JJ, Guida J, Wu WH: Hypoventilatory hazard of an anesthetic scavenging device, *Anesthesiology* 65:126–127, 1986.
97. Lanier WL: Intraoperative air entrainment with Ohio Modulus anesthesia machine, *Anesthesiology* 64:266–268, 1986.
98. Sandberg WS, Kaiser S: Novel breathing system architecture: new consequences of old problems, *Anesthesiology* 100:755–756, 2004.
99. Baraka A, Muallem M: Awareness during anaesthesia due to a ventilator malfunction, *Anaesthesia* 34:678–679, 1979.
100. Waterman PM, Pautler S, Smith RB: Accidental ventilator-induced hyperventilation, *Anesthesiology* 48:141, 1978.
101. Longmuir J, Craig DB: Inadvertent increase in inspired oxygen concentration due to defect in ventilator bellows, *Can Anaesth Soc J* 23:327–329, 1976.
102. Dean HN, Parsons DE, Raphaely RC: Bilateral tension pneumothorax from mechanical failure of anesthesia machine due to misplaced expiratory valve, *Anesth Analg* 50:195–198, 1971.
103. Sears BE, Bocar ND: Pneumothorax resulting from a closed anesthesia ventilator port, *Anesthesiology* 47:311–313, 1977.
104. Sprung J, Samaan F, Hensler T, et al: Excessive airway pressure due to ventilator control valve malfunction during anesthesia for open heart surgery, *Anesthesiology* 73:1035–1038, 1990.
105. Sprung J, Samaan F, Hensler T, Atlee JL 3rd, Kampine JP: Excessive airway pressure due to ventilator control valve malfunction during anesthesia for open heart surgery, *Anesthesiology* 73:1035–1038, 1990.
106. Roth S, Tweedie E, Sommer RM: Excessive airway pressure due to a malfunctioning anesthesia ventilator, *Anesthesiology* 65:532–534, 1986.
107. Henzig D: Insidious PEEP from a defective ventilator gas evacuation outlet valve, *Anesthesiology* 57:251–252, 1982.
108. *Pressure limit control, operator's instruction manual*, Telford, PA, 1988, North American Dräger.
109. *Ohmeda 7000 electronic anesthesia ventilator, service manual*, Madison, WI, 1985, Ohmeda, The BOC Group.
110. Kopriva CJ, Lowenstein E: An anesthetic accident: cardiovascular collapse from liquid halothane delivery, *Anesthesiology* 30:246, 1969.
111. *Dräger Vapor 19.n operating instructions*. Lübeck, Germany, 1998, Drägerwerk AG.
112. *Ohmeda Tec 5 continuous flow vaporizer: operation and maintenance manual*, Madison, WI, 1989, Ohmeda.
113. Sinclair A, van Bergen J: Vaporizer overfilling, *Can J Anesth* 40:77–78, 1993.
114. Hardy JF: Vaporizer overfilling, *Can J Anesth* 40:1–3, 1993.
115. Bruce DL, Linde HW: Vaporization of mixed anesthetic liquids, *Anesthesiology* 60:342–346, 1984.
116. Chilcoat RT: Hazards of mis-filled vaporizers: summary tables, *Anesthesiology* 63:726–727, 1985.
117. Riegle EV, Desertspring D: Failure of the agent-specific filling device, *Anesthesiology* 73:353–354, 1990.
118. Andrews JJ, Johnston RV Jr, Kramer GC: Consequences of misfiling contemporary vaporizers with desflurane, *Can J Anaesth* 40:71–76, 1993.
119. Korman B, Ritchie IM: Chemistry of halothane-enflurane mixtures applied to anesthesia, *Anesthesiology* 63:152–156, 1985.
120. Dorsch SE, Dorsch JA: Chemical cross-contamination between vaporizers in series, *Anesth Analg* 52:176–180, 1973.
121. Silvasi DL, Haynes A, Brown ACD: Potentially lethal failure of the vapor exclusion system, *Anesthesiology* 71:289–291, 1990.
122. Cudmore J, Keogh J: Another Selectatec switch malfunction, *Anaesthesia* 45:754–756, 1990.
123. Marks WE, Bullard JR: Another hazard of freestanding vaporizers: increased anesthetic concentration with reversed flow of vaporizing gas, *Anesthesiology* 45:445, 1976.
124. Beebe JJ, Sessler DI: Preparation of anesthesia machines for patients susceptible to malignant hyperthermia, *Anesthesiology* 69:395–400, 1988.
125. Kim TW, Nemergut ME: Preparation of modern anesthesia workstations for malignant hyperthermia-susceptible patients: a review of past and present practice, *Anesthesiology* 114:205–212, 2011.
126. Prinzhausen H, Crawford MW, O'Rourke J, Petroz GC: Preparation of the Drager Primus anesthetic machine for malignant hyperthermia-susceptible patients, *Can J Anaesth* 53:885–890, 2006.
127. Schonell LH, Sims C, Bulsara M: Preparing a new generation anaesthetic machine for patients susceptible to malignant hyperthermia, *Anaesth Intensive Care* 31:58–62, 2003.
128. Crawford MW, Prinzhausen H, Petroz GC: Accelerating the washout of inhalational anesthetics from the Drager Primus anesthetic workstation: Effect of exchangeable internal components, *Anesthesiology* 106:289–294, 2007.
129. Gunter JB, Ball J, Than-Win S: Preparation of the Drager Fabius anesthesia machine for the malignant hyperthermia susceptible patient, *Anesth Analg* 107:1936–1945, 2008.
130. Whitty RJ, Wong GK, Petroz GC, et al: Preparation of the Drager Fabius GS workstation for malignant hyperthermia-susceptible patients, *Can J Anaesth* 56:497–501, 2009.
131. Jones C, Bennett K, Kim TW, et al: Preparation of Datex-Ohmeda Aestiva and Aisys anaesthetic machines for use in malignant hyperthermia-susceptible patients, *Anaesth Intensive Care* 40:490–497, 2012.
132. Birgenheier N, Stoker R, Westenskow D, Orr J: Activated charcoal effectively removes inhaled anesthetics from modern anesthesia machines, *Anesth Analg* 112:1363–1370, 2011.
133. Block FE Jr: Malignant hyperthermia and charcoal absorbent: too hot to handle, *Anesth Analg* 112:1270–1271, 2011.
134. O'Neill B, Hafiz MA, De Beer DA: Corrosion of Penlon sevoflurane vaporizers, *Anaesthesia* 62:421, 2007.
135. Saltarelli M: Abbott addresses sevoflurane formulation, *APSF Newslett* 22(4), 2008.
136. Kharasch ED, Subbarao GN, Cromack KR, Stephens DA, Saltarelli MD: Sevoflurane formulation water content influences degradation by Lewis acids in vaporizers, *Anesth Analg* 108:1796–1802, 2009.
137. Kharasch E, Subbarao GN, Cromack KR, et al: "Dry" sevoflurane and the falling sky (or lack thereof), *Anesth Analg* 110:254–255, 2010.
138. Baker MT: Sevoflurane-Lewis acid stability, *Anesth Analg* 108:1725–1726, 2009.
139. Riddle R: Tec 6 recall, *Anesthesiology* 81:791–792, 1994.
140. Salahadin A, Acquadro MA: Technical failure of desflurane vaporizer Tec 6, *Anesthesiology* 81:226–227, 1995.
141. Kayser D, Khodja M, Marguerite G: Delivery of desflurane by a Tec 6 vaporizer at a concentration superior to that posted on the regulating valve, *Ann Fr Anesth Reanim* 18:691–693, 1999.

142. Geffroy JC, Gentili ME, Le Pollès R, Triclot P: Massive inhalation of desflurane due to vaporizer dysfunction, *Anesthesiology* 103:1096–1098, 2005.
143. Schulte TE, Ellis SJ: Discolored desflurane in the vaporizer, *Anesth Analg* 110:644–645, 2010.
144. Hendrickx JFA, Carette RM, Deloof T, De Wolf AM: Severe ADU desflurane vaporizing unit malfunction, *Anesthesiology* 99:1459–1460, 1993.
145. Bickler PE, Sessler DI: Efficiency of airway heat and moisture exchangers in anesthetized humans, *Anesth Analg* 71:415–418, 1990.
146. Turner DA, Wright EM: Efficiency of heat and moisture exchangers, *Anaesthesia* 42:1117–1119, 1987 (letter).
147. Bengtsson M, Johnson A: Failure of a heat and moisture exchanger as a cause of disconnection during anaesthesia, *Acta Anaesthesiol Scand* 33:522–523, 1989.
148. Prasad KK, Chen L: Complications related to the use of a heat and moisture exchanger, *Anesthesiology* 72:958, 1990.
149. Ward CF, Reisner LS, Zlott LS: Murphy's law and humidification, *Anesth Analg* 62:460–461, 1983.
150. Shroff PK, Skerman JH: Humidifier malfunction: a cause of anesthesia circuit occlusion, *Anesth Analg* 67:710–711, 1988 (letter).
151. Laudanski K, Schwab WK, Bakuzonis CW, Paulus DA: Thermal damage of the humidified ventilator circuit in the operating room: analysis of plausible causes, *Anesth Analg* 111:1433–1436, 2010.
152. Maurer WG: A disadvantage of similar machine controls, *Anesthesiology* 75:167–168, 1991.
153. Carpenter T, Robinson ST: Response to partial power failure in the operating room, *Anesth Analg* 110:1644–1646, 2010.
154. Yasny J, Soffer R: A case of power failure in the operating room, *Anesth Prog* 52:65–69, 2005.
155. Eichhorn JH, Hessel EA: Electrical power failure in the operating room: a neglected topic in anesthesia safety, *Anesth Analg* 110:1519–1521, 2010.
156. The Joint Commission: Sentinel event alert. Preventing adverse events caused by emergency electrical power system failures, Sept 6, 2006, Issue 37. Available at http://www.accreditationcenter.com/details_print.cfm?content_id=65355.
157. *Urgent medical device safety alert*, Madison, WI, 1991, Ohmeda, a BOC Health Care Company.
158. Fang ZX, Ei Eger 2nd, Laster MJ, et al: Carbon monoxide production from degradation of desflurane enflurane, isoflurane, halothane and sevoflurane by soda lime and Baralyme, *Anesth Analg* 80:1187–1193, 1995.
159. Berry PD, Sessler DI, Larson MD: Severe carbon monoxide poisoning during desflurane anesthesia, *Anesthesiology* 90:613–616, 1999.
160. Kharasch ED, Powers KM, Artru AA: Comparison of Amsorb, sodalime, and Baralyme degradation of volatile anesthetics and formation of carbon monoxide and compound A in swine in vivo, *Anesthesiology* 96:173–182, 2002.
161. Olympio MA: Carbon dioxide absorbent desiccation conference convened by APSF, *APSF Newsletter* 20(2):4, 2005.
162. Laster M, Roth P, Eger EI 2nd: Fires from the interaction of anesthetics with desiccated absorbent, *Anesth Analg* 99:769–774, 2004.
163. Wu J, Previte JP, Adler E, et al: Spontaneous ignition, explosion, and fire with sevoflurane and barium hydroxide lime, *Anesthesiology* 101:534–537, 2004.
164. Castro BA, Freedman LA, Craig WL, Lynch C 3rd: Explosion within an anesthesia machine: Baralyme, high fresh gas flows and sevoflurane concentration, *Anesthesiology* 101:537–539, 2004.
165. Fatheree RS, Leighton BL: Acute respiratory distress syndrome after an exothermic Baralyme-sevoflurane reaction, *Anesthesiology* 101:531–533, 2004.
166. Woehlck HJ: Sleeping with uncertainty: anesthetics and desiccated absorbent [editorial], *Anesthesiology* 101:276–278, 2004.
167. Eisenkraft JB: A commentary on anesthesia gas delivery equipment and adverse outcomes. Editorial, *Anesthesiology* 87:731–733, 1997.
168. Olympio MA: Formal training and assessment before using advanced medical devices in the OR, *APSF Newslett* 22:63, 2008.
169. Singh S, Loeb RG: Fatal connection: death caused by direct connection of oxygen tubing into tracheal tube connector, *Anesth Analg* 99:1164–1155, 2004.
170. Wax DB, Bhagwan S, Beilin Y: Tension pneumothorax and cardiac arrest from an improvised oxygen delivery system, *J Clin Anesth* 19:546–548, 2007.
171. *Explore! The anesthesia system.* Aisys. Datex-Ohmeda, a Division of GE Healthcare, Waukesha, WI, 2005.
172. The Dräger Academy. Basics of Respiration and Ventilation. Accessed online at http://www.draeger.com/local/products/draeger_academy_intl/index.html.
173. Eng TS, Durieux ME: Case report: automated machine checkout leaves an internal gas leak undetected: the need for complete checkout procedures, *Anesth Analg* 114:144–146, 2012.
174. Larson ER, Nuttall GA, Ogren BD, et al: A prospective study on anesthesia machine fault identification, *Anesth Analg* 104:154–156, 2007.
175. Olympio MA, Goldstein MM, Mathes DD: Instructional review improves performance of anesthesia apparatus checkout procedures, *Anesth Analg* 83:618–622, 1996.
176. FDA: *Anesthesia Apparatus Checkout Recommendations*, Available at http://www.vam/anest.ufl.edu/fdacheckout.html.
177. Arbous MS, Meursing AE, van Kleef JW, et al: Impact of anesthesia management characteristics on severe morbidity and mortality, *Anesthesiology* 102:257–268, 2005.
178. Feldman JM, Olympio MA, Martin D, Striker A: New guidelines available for pre-anesthesia checkout, *APSF Newslett* 23(1):1, Spring 2008.
179. American Society of Anesthesiologists (ASA): *Pre-anesthesia checkout design guideline*, Park Ridge, IL, 2008, ASA.
180. Sandberg WS, Kaiser S: Novel breathing system architecture: new consequences of old problems, *Anesthesiology* 100:755–756, 2004.
181. Ortega RA, Zambricki ER: Fresh gas decoupling valve failure precludes ventilation in a Draeger Fabius GS anesthesia machine, *Anesth Analg* 104:1000, 2007.
182. American Society of Anesthesiologists (ASA): *Guidelines for determining anesthesia machine obsolescence*, Park Ridge, IL, 2004, ASA.
183. Stefan A, Ianchulev SA, Comunale ME: To do or not to do a preinduction check-up of the anesthesia machine, *Anesth Analg* 101:774–776, 2005.
184. Mudumbai SC, Fanning R, Howard SK, et al: Use of medical simulation to explore equipment failures and human–machine interactions in anesthesia machine pipeline supply crossover, *Anesth Analg* 110:1292–1296, 2010.
185. Lorraway PG, Savoldelli GL, Joo HS, et al: Management of simulated oxygen supply failure: is there a gap in the curriculum? *Anesth Analg* 102:865–867, 2006.
186. Weller J, Merry A, Warman G, et al: Anaesthetists' management of oxygen pipeline failure: a room for improvement, *Anaesthesia* 62:122–126, 2007.
187. DeMaria S Jr, Blasius K, Neustein SM: Missed steps in the preanesthetic set-up, *Anesth Analg* 113:84–88, 2011. Epub 2011 Apr 5.
188. Waldrop WB, Murray DJ, Boulet JR, Kras JF: Management of anesthesia equipment failure: a simulation-based resident skill assessment, *Anesth Analg* 109:462–433, 2009.
189. BenMenachem E, Ezri T, Ziv A, et al: Identifying and managing technical faults in the anesthesia machine: lessons learned from the Israeli Board of Anesthesiologists, *Anesth Analg* 112:864–866, 2011.

CHAPTER 31

ELECTRICAL AND FIRE SAFETY*

Jan Ehrenwerth • Harry A. Seifert

CHAPTER OUTLINE

The myriad electrical and electronic devices in the modern operating room (OR) greatly improve patient care and safety. However, these devices also subject both the patient and OR personnel to increased risks. To reduce the risk of electrical shock, most ORs have electrical systems that incorporate special safety features. It is incumbent upon the anesthesiologist to have a thorough understanding of the basic principles of electricity and an appreciation of the concepts of electrical safety applicable to the OR environment.

PRINCIPLES OF ELECTRICITY

One basic principle of electricity is known as *Ohm's law*, which is represented by the following equation, where E is electromotive force (in volts [V]), I is current (in amperes [A]), and R is resistance (in ohms [Ω]):

$$E = I \times R$$

Ohm's law forms the basis for the following physiologic equation:

$$BP = CO \times SVR$$

Here, the blood pressure (*BP*) of the vascular system is analogous to voltage, the cardiac output (*CO*) is analogous to current, and the systemic vascular resistance (*SVR*) is analogous to the forces opposing the flow of electrons. Electrical power (P) is measured in watts. Power is the product of the voltage (*E*) and the current (*I*), as defined by the formula:

$$P = E \times I$$

The amount of electrical work done is measured in watts multiplied by a unit of time. The watt-second (a joule [J]) is a common designation for electrical energy expended in doing work. The energy produced by a defibrillator is measured in watt-seconds (joules). The kilowatt-hour is used by electrical utility companies to measure larger quantities of electrical energy.

Wattage can be thought of as a measure not only of work done but also of heat produced in any electrical circuit. Substituting Ohm's law in the formula:

$$P = E \times I$$

$$P = (I \times R) \times I$$

$$P = I^2 \times R$$

Thus, power (in watts) is equal to the square of the current I (amperage) multiplied by the resistance, R. With these formulas, it is possible to calculate the number of amperes and the resistance of a given device if the wattage and the voltage are known. For example, a 60 W

*This chapter and the images contained herein were developed in whole for *Clinical Anesthesia* (ed. 7, Wolters Kluwer Health/Lippincott Williams & Wilkins; Barash PG, Cullen BF, Stoelting RK, et al., editors) and *Anesthesia Equipment: Principles and Applications* (ed. 2, Elsevier; Ehrenwerth J, Eisenkraft JB, Berry JM, editors) with permission of the editors and publishers.

lightbulb operating on a household 120 V circuit would require 0.5 A of current for operation. Rearranging the formula so that I equals P/E:

$$I = 60W/120\ V$$

$$I = 0.5\ A$$

Using this in Ohm's law (R = E/I), the resistance can be calculated to be 240 Ω:

$$R = 120\ V/0.5\ A$$

$$R = 240\ \Omega$$

It is obvious from the previous discussion that 1 V of electromotive force (EMF) flowing through a 1 Ω resistance will generate 1 A of current. Similarly, 1 A of current induced by 1 V of electromotive force will generate 1 W of power.

Direct and Alternating Currents

Any substance that permits the flow of electrons is called a *conductor*. Current is characterized by electrons flowing through a conductor. If the electron flow is always in the same direction, it is referred to as *direct current* (DC). However, if the electron flow reverses direction at a regular interval, it is termed *alternating current* (AC). Either of these types of current can be pulsed or continuous in nature.

The previous discussion of Ohm's law is accurate when applied to DC circuits. However, when dealing with AC circuits, the situation is more complex because the flow of the current is opposed by a more complicated form of resistance, known as *impedance*.

Impedance

Impedance, designated by the letter Z, is defined as the sum of the forces that oppose electron movement in an AC circuit. Impedance consists of resistance (ohms [Ω]) but also takes capacitance and inductance into account. In actuality, when referring to AC circuits, Ohm's law states that voltage equals current multiplied by impedance:

$$E = I \times Z$$

An *insulator* is a substance that opposes the flow of electrons. Therefore an insulator has a high impedance to electron flow, whereas a conductor has a low impedance to electron flow.

In AC circuits the capacitance and inductance can be important factors in determining the total impedance. Both capacitance and inductance are influenced by the frequency (cycles per second, or hertz [Hz]) at which the AC current reverses direction. The impedance is directly proportional to the frequency (f) times the inductance (*IND*):

$$Z \propto (f \times IND)$$

In addition, the impedance is inversely proportional to the product of the frequency (f) and the capacitance (*CAP*):

$$Z \propto 1/(f \times CAP)$$

As the AC current increases in frequency, the net effect of both capacitance and inductance increases. However, because impedance and capacitance are inversely related, total impedance decreases as the product of the frequency and the capacitance increases. Thus as frequency increases, impedance falls and more current is allowed to pass.

Capacitance

A *capacitor* consists of any two parallel conductors separated by an insulator (Fig. 31-1). A capacitor has the ability to store charge. *Capacitance* is the measure of a substance's ability to store charge. In a DC circuit the capacitor plates are charged by a voltage source (i.e., a battery), and there is only a momentary current flow. The circuit is not completed, and no further current can flow unless a resistance is connected between the two plates and the capacitor is discharged.

In contrast to DC circuits, a capacitor in an AC circuit permits current flow even when the circuit is not completed by a resistance. This is because of the nature of AC circuits, in which the current flow is constantly being reversed. Because current flow results from the movement of electrons, the capacitor plates are alternately charged—first positive and then negative, with every reversal of the AC current direction—resulting in an effective current flow as far as the remainder of the circuit is concerned, even though the circuit is not completed.

Because the effect of capacitance on impedance varies directly with the AC frequency in hertz, the greater the AC frequency, the lower the impedance. Therefore, high-frequency currents (0.5 to 2 million Hz), such as those used by electrosurgical units (ESUs), will cause a marked decrease in impedance.

Electrical devices use capacitors for various beneficial purposes. However, a phenomenon known as *stray capacitance* is capacitance that was not designed into the system but is incidental to the construction of the equipment. All AC-operated equipment produces stray capacitance. An ordinary power cord, for example, that consists of two insulated wires running next to each other will generate significant capacitance simply by being plugged into a 120 V circuit, even though the piece of equipment is not turned on. Another example of stray capacitance is found in electric motors. The circuit wiring in electric motors generates stray capacitance to the metal housing of the motor. The clinical importance of capacitance will be emphasized later in the chapter.

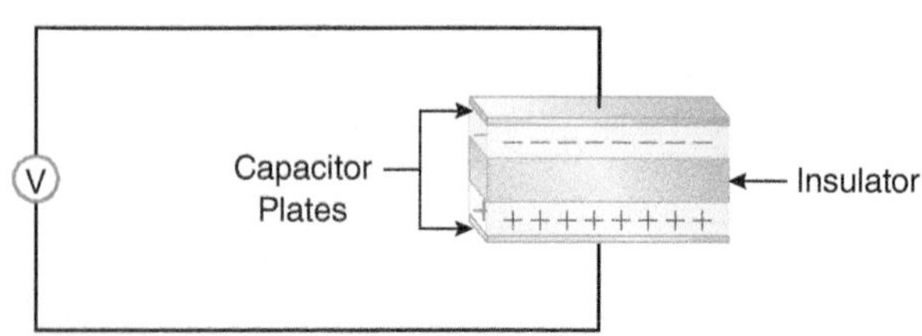

FIGURE 31-1 ■ A capacitor consists of two parallel conductors separated by an insulator. The capacitor is capable of storing charge supplied by a voltage source (*V*).

Inductance

Whenever electrons flow in a wire, a magnetic field is induced around the wire. If the wire is coiled repeatedly around an iron core, as in a transformer, the magnetic field can be very strong. *Inductance* is a property of AC circuits in which an opposing EMF can be electromagnetically generated in the circuit. The net effect of inductance is to increase impedance. Because the effect of inductance on impedance also depends on AC frequency, increases in frequency will increase the total impedance. Therefore the total impedance of a coil will be much greater than its simple resistance.

ELECTRICAL SHOCK HAZARDS

Alternating and Direct Currents

Whenever an individual contacts an external source of electricity, an electric shock is possible. An electric current can stimulate skeletal muscle cells to contract and thus can be used therapeutically in devices such as pacemakers or defibrillators. However, casual contact with an electrical current, whether AC or DC, can lead to injury or death. Although it takes approximately three times as much DC as AC to cause ventricular fibrillation, this by no means renders DC harmless. Devices such as an automobile battery or a DC defibrillator can be sources of direct current shocks.

In the United States, utility companies supply energy in the form of alternating currents of 120 V at a frequency of 60 Hz. The 120 V of EMF and 1 A of current are the effective voltage and amperage in an AC circuit. This is also referred to as *root-mean-square* (RMS). It takes 1.414 A of peak amperage in the sinusoidal curve to give an effective amperage of 1 A. Similarly, it takes 170 V (120 × 1.414) at the peak of the AC curve to get an effective voltage of 120 V. The 60 Hz refers to the number of times in 1 second that the current reverses its direction of flow. Both the voltage and current waveforms form a sinusoidal pattern (Fig. 31-2).

To have the completed circuit necessary for current flow, a closed loop must exist, and a voltage source must drive the current through the impedance. If current is to flow in the electrical circuit, there has to be a *voltage differential*, or a drop in the driving pressure across the impedance. According to Ohm's law, if the resistance is held constant, the greater the current flow, the larger the voltage drop must be.

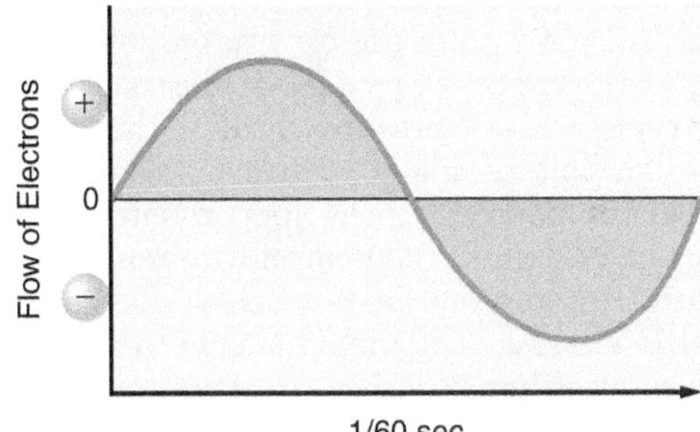

FIGURE 31-2 ■ Sine wave flow of electrons in a 60 Hz alternating current.

The power company attempts to maintain the line voltage constant at 120 V. Therefore by Ohm's law, the current flow is inversely proportional to the impedance. A typical power cord consists of two conductors: one, designated as *hot*, carries the current to the impedance; the other is *neutral*, and it returns the current to the source. The potential difference between the two is effectively 120 V (Fig. 31-3). The amount of current flowing through a given device is frequently referred to as the *load*. The load of the circuit depends on the impedance. A very high impedance circuit allows only a small current to flow and thus has a small load. A very low impedance circuit will draw a large current and is said to carry a large load. A *short circuit* occurs when there is a zero impedance load with a very high current flow.[1]

Source of Shocks

Electrical accidents or shocks occur when a person becomes part of, or completes, an electrical circuit. To receive a shock, a person must contact the electrical circuit at two points, and there must be a voltage source that causes the current to flow through the individual (Fig. 31-4).

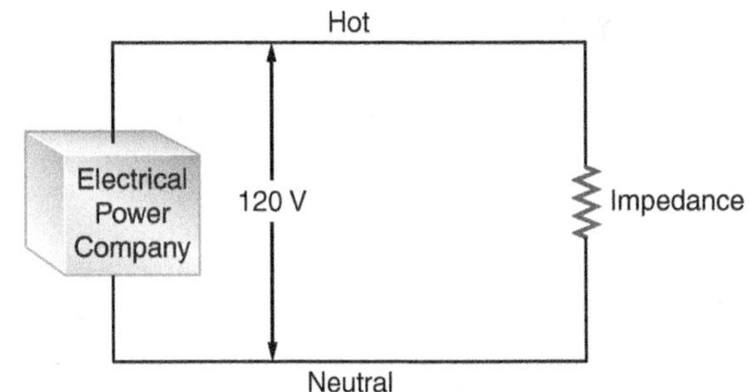

FIGURE 31-3 ■ A typical alternating current (AC) circuit. A potential difference of 120 V exists between the hot and neutral sides of the circuit. The current flows through a *resistance,* which in AC circuits is more accurately referred to as *impedance,* and then returns to the electrical power company.

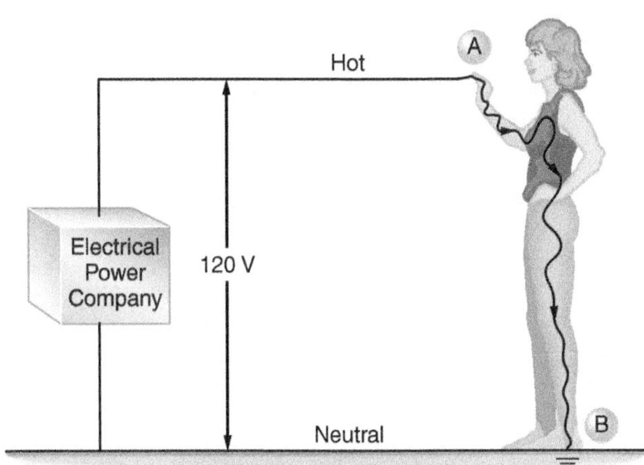

FIGURE 31-4 ■ An individual can complete an electrical circuit and receive a shock. If the person is standing on the ground (point B), by coming in contact with the hot side of the circuit (point A), the contact point and the ground provide the two contact points necessary for a completed circuit. The severity of the shock received depends on the individual's skin resistance.

When an individual comes in contact with a source of electricity, injury occurs in one of two ways. First, the electrical current can disrupt the normal electrical function of cells. Depending on its magnitude, the current can contract muscles, alter brain function, paralyze respiration, or disrupt normal heart function, leading to ventricular fibrillation. The second mechanism involves the dissipation of electrical energy throughout the body's tissues. An electrical current passing through any resistant substance raises the temperature of that substance. If enough thermal energy is released, the temperature will rise sufficiently to produce a burn. Accidents involving household currents usually do not result in severe burns. However, in accidents involving very high voltages (i.e., power transmission lines), severe burns are common.

The severity of an electrical shock is determined by the amount of current (amperes) and the duration of the current flow. For the purposes of this discussion, electrical shocks are divided into two categories: *macroshock* refers to large amounts of current flowing through a person, which can cause harm or death; *microshock* refers to very small amounts of current. Concern for injury with microshock applies only to the electrically susceptible patient, an individual who has an external conduit that is in direct contact with the heart; this can be a pacing wire or a saline-filled catheter, such as a central venous or pulmonary artery catheter. In the case of the electrically susceptible patient, even minute amounts of current (microshocks) can cause ventricular fibrillation.

Table 31-1 shows the effects typically produced by various currents following a 1-second contact with a 60 Hz current. When an individual contacts a 120-V household current, the severity of the shock will depend on his or her skin resistance, the duration of the contact, and the current density. Skin resistance can vary from a few thousand to 1 million Ω. If a person with a skin resistance of 1000 Ω contacts a 120 V circuit, he or she would receive 120 mA of current, which would probably be lethal. However, if that same person's skin resistance is 100,000 Ω, the current flow would be 1.2 mA, which would barely be perceptible.

$$I = E/R = 120\ V/1000\ \Omega = 120\ mA$$

$$I = E/R = 120\ V/100{,}000\ \Omega = 1.2\ mA$$

The longer an individual is in contact with the electrical source, the more dire the consequences because more energy will be released, and more tissue will be damaged. Also, there will be a greater chance of ventricular fibrillation from excitation of the heart during the vulnerable period of the electrocardiogram (ECG) cycle.

Current density is a way of expressing the amount of current applied per unit area of tissue. The diffusion of current in the body tends to be in all directions. The greater the current or the smaller the area to which it is applied, the higher the current density. In relation to the heart, a current of 100 mA (100,000 μA) is generally required to produce ventricular fibrillation when applied to the surface of the body. However, only 100 μA (0.1 mA) is required to produce ventricular fibrillation when that minute current is applied directly to the myocardium through an instrument with a very small contact area, such as a pacing wire electrode. In this case, the current density is a thousandfold greater when applied directly to the heart; therefore only 1/1000 of the energy is required to cause ventricular fibrillation. An electrically susceptible patient can be electrocuted with currents well below 1 mA, which is the threshold of perception for humans.

The frequency at which the current reverses is also an important factor in determining the amount of current an individual can safely contact. Utility companies in the United States produce electricity at a frequency of 60 Hz, because higher frequencies cause greater power loss through transmission lines, and lower frequencies cause a detectable flicker from light sources.[2] The "let go" current is defined as that current above which sustained muscular contraction occurs and at which an individual would be unable to let go of an energized wire. The let-go current for 60 Hz AC power is 10 to 20 mA,[1,3,4] whereas at a frequency of 1 million Hz, up to 3 A (3000 mA) is generally considered safe. It should be noted that very high frequency currents do not excite contractile tissue; consequently, they do not cause cardiac dysrhythmias.

It can be seen that Ohm's law governs the flow of electricity. For a completed circuit to exist, a closed loop must exist with a driving pressure to force a current through a resistance, just as in the cardiovascular system, in which BP must drive the cardiac output through the peripheral resistance. Figure 31-5 illustrates that a hot wire carrying a 120 V pressure through the resistance of a 60 W lightbulb produces a current flow of 0.5 A. The voltage in the neutral wire is approximately zero volts, whereas the current in the neutral wire remains at 0.5 A. This correlates with our cardiovascular analogy, in which a mean BP decrease of 80 mm Hg between the aortic root and the right atrium forces a cardiac output of 6 L/min through a systemic vascular resistance of 13.3 resistance units. However, the flow—in this case, the cardiac output, or in the case of the electrical model, the current—is

TABLE 31-1 Effects of 1 Second Contact of 60 Hz Current on an Average Human

Current	Effect
Macroshock	
1 mA (0.001 A)	Threshold of perception
5 mA (0.005 A)	Accepted as maximum harmless current intensity
10 to 20 mA (0.01-0.02 A)	"Let go" current before sustained muscle contraction
50 mA (0.05 A)	Pain, possible fainting, mechanical injury; heart and respiratory functions continue
100 to 300 mA (0.1-0.3 A)	Ventricular fibrillation will start, but respiratory center remains intact
6,000 mA (6 A)	Sustained myocardial contraction followed by normal heart rhythm; temporary respiratory paralysis; burns if current density is high
Microshock	
100 μA (0.1 mA)	Ventricular fibrillation
10 μA (0.01 mA)	Recommended maximum 60 Hz leakage current

still the same everywhere in the circuit. That is, the cardiac output on the arterial side is the same as the cardiac output on the venous side.

Grounding

To fully understand electrical shock hazards and their prevention, the clinician must have a thorough knowledge of the concepts of grounding. These concepts of grounding probably constitute the most confusing aspects of electrical safety, because the same term is used to describe several different principles. In electrical terminology, the term *grounding* is applied to two separate concepts. The first is the grounding of electrical *power*, and the second is the grounding of electrical *equipment*. Thus the concepts that power can be grounded or ungrounded and that power can supply electrical devices that are themselves grounded or ungrounded are not mutually exclusive. It is vital to understand this point as the basis of electrical safety. Whereas electrical *power* is grounded in the home, it is usually ungrounded in the OR (Table 31-2). In the home, electrical *equipment* may be grounded or ungrounded, but it should always be grounded in the OR.

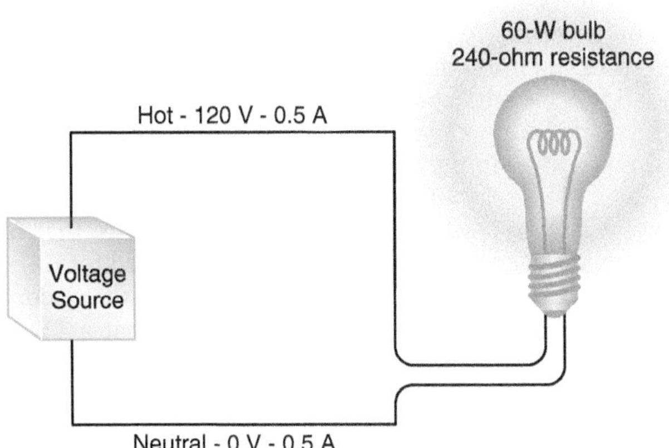

FIGURE 31-5 ■ A 60 W lightbulb has an internal resistance of 240 Ω and draws a 0.5 A current. The voltage drop in the circuit is from 120 V in the hot wire to zero in the neutral wire, but the current is 0.5 A in both the hot and neutral wires.

ELECTRICAL POWER: GROUNDED

Electrical utilities universally provide power that is grounded (by convention, the earth-ground potential is zero, and all voltages represent a difference between potentials); that is, one of the wires supplying the power to a home is intentionally connected to the earth. The utility companies do this as a safety measure to prevent electrical charges from building up in their wiring during electrical storms. This also prevents the very high voltages used in transmitting power by the utility from entering the home in the event of an equipment failure in their high-voltage system.

The power enters the typical home via two wires attached to the main fuse box or circuit breaker box at the service entrance. The "hot" (electrified) wire supplies power to the hot distribution strip. The neutral wire is connected to the neutral distribution strip and to a service entrance ground (i.e., a pipe buried in the earth; Fig. 31-6). From the fuse box, three wires leave to supply the electrical outlets in the house. In the United States, the hot wire is color-coded black and carries a 120 V above-ground potential. The second wire is the neutral wire color-coded white; the third wire is the ground wire, which is either color-coded green or is uninsulated (bare wire). The ground and the neutral wires are attached at the same point in the circuit breaker box and are also connected to a cold-water pipe (Figs. 31-7 and 31-8). Thus, this grounded power system is also referred to as a *neutral grounded power system*. The black wire is not connected to the ground, because this

TABLE 31-2 Differences Between Power and Equipment Grounding in the Home and the Operating Room

	Power	Equipment
Home	Grounded	May or may not be grounded
Operating room	Ungrounded	Grounded

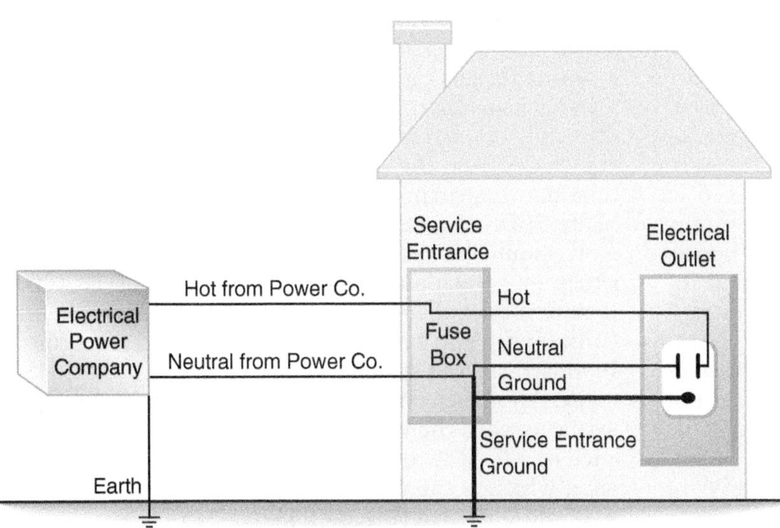

FIGURE 31-6 ■ In a neutral grounded power system, the electric company supplies two lines to the typical home. The neutral wire is connected to ground by the power company and is also connected to a service entrance ground when it enters the fuse box or breaker panel. Both the neutral and ground wires are connected together in the supply box at the neutral bus bar, which is also attached to the service entrance ground.

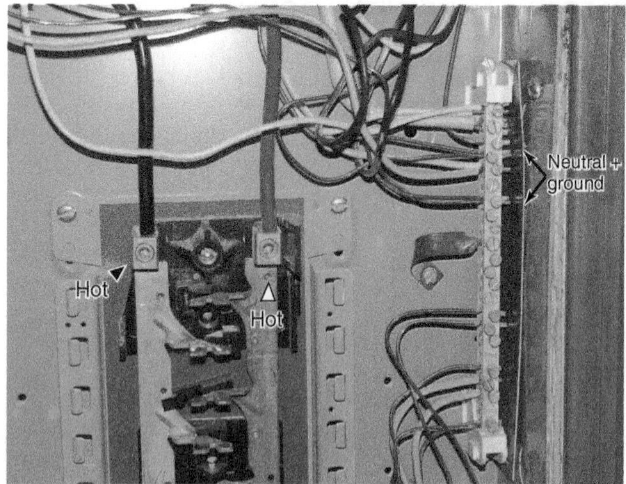

FIGURE 31-7 ■ Inside a breaker panel with the circuit breakers removed. The *arrowheads* indicate the hot wires energizing the strips where the circuit breakers are located. The *arrows* point to the neutral bus bar, where the neutral and ground wires are connected.

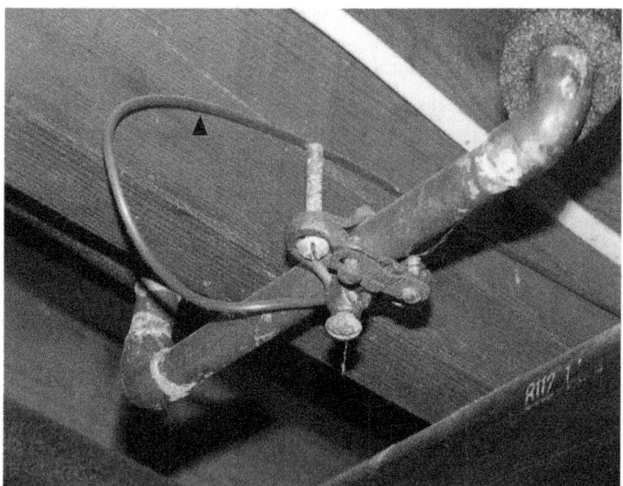

FIGURE 31-8 ■ A ground wire from the circuit breaker (*arrowhead*) attached to a cold-water pipe.

would create a short circuit. The black wire is attached to the hot distribution strip (i.e., 120 V above ground) on which the circuit breakers or fuses are located. From here, numerous branch circuits supply electrical power to the outlets in the house. Each branch circuit is protected by a circuit breaker or fuse that limits current to a specific maximum amperage. Most electrical circuits in the house are 15 or 20 A circuits. These typically supply power to the electrical outlets and lights in the house. Several higher amperage circuits are also provided for certain devices, such as electric stoves or clothes dryers. These devices are powered by 240 V circuits, which can draw from 30 to 50 A of current. The circuit breaker or fuse will interrupt the flow of current on the hot side of the line in the event of a short circuit, or if the demand placed on that circuit is too high. For example, a 15 A branch circuit is capable of supporting 1800 W of power.

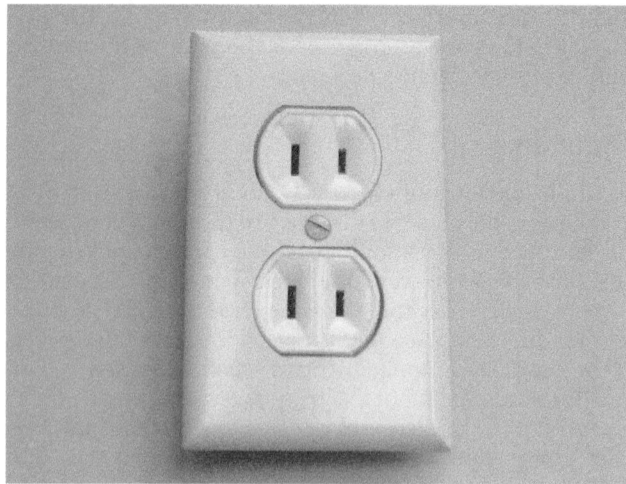

FIGURE 31-9 ■ An older style electrical outlet. Only two wires are present, a hot and a neutral. There is no ground wire.

$$P = E \times I$$

$$P = 120\ V \times 15\ A$$

$$P = 1800\ W$$

Therefore if two 1500 W hair dryers were simultaneously plugged into one outlet, the load would be too great for a 15 A circuit, and the circuit breaker would open (trip), or the fuse would melt. This is designed to prevent the supply wires in the circuit from melting and starting a fire. The amperage of the circuit breaker on the branch circuit is determined by the thickness of the wire that it supplies. If a 20 A breaker is used with wire rated for only 15 A, the wire could melt and start a fire before the circuit breaker would trip. It is important to note that a 15 A circuit breaker does not protect an individual from lethal shocks; the 15 A of current that would trip the circuit breaker far exceeds the 100 to 200 mA that will produce ventricular fibrillation.

The wires that leave the circuit breaker supply the electrical outlets and lighting for the rest of the house. In older homes the electrical cable consists of two wires, a hot and a neutral, which supply power to the electrical outlets (Fig. 31-9). In newer homes, a third wire has been added to the electrical cable (Fig. 31-10). This third wire is either green or uninsulated (bare) and serves as a ground wire for the power receptacle (Fig. 31-11). On one end, the ground wire is attached to the receptacle (Fig. 31-12); on the other, it is connected to the neutral distribution strip in the circuit breaker box along with the neutral (white) wires (Fig. 31-13).

It should be realized that in both the old and new situations, the power is grounded. That is, a 120 V potential exists between the hot (black) and the neutral (white) wire and between the hot wire and the ground. In this case, the ground is the earth (Fig. 31-14). In modern home construction, a 120 V potential difference exists between the hot and the neutral wire, and a difference of 120 V is found between the equipment ground wire, which is the third wire, and also between the hot wire and the earth (Fig. 31-15).

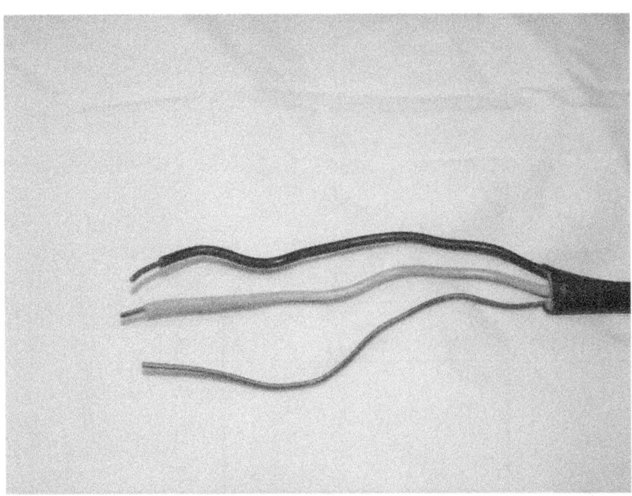

FIGURE 31-10 ■ Modern electrical cable in which a third wire, or ground, has been added. Wires from top to bottom are *hot, neutral,* and *ground.*

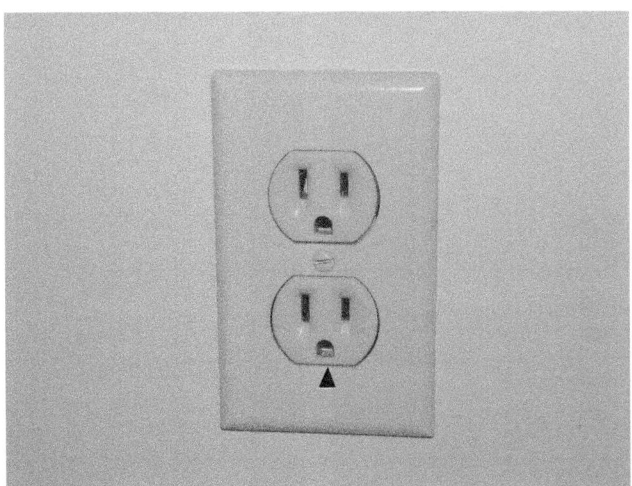

FIGURE 31-11 ■ Modern electrical outlet in which the ground wire is present. The *arrowhead* points to the part of the receptacle where the ground wire connects.

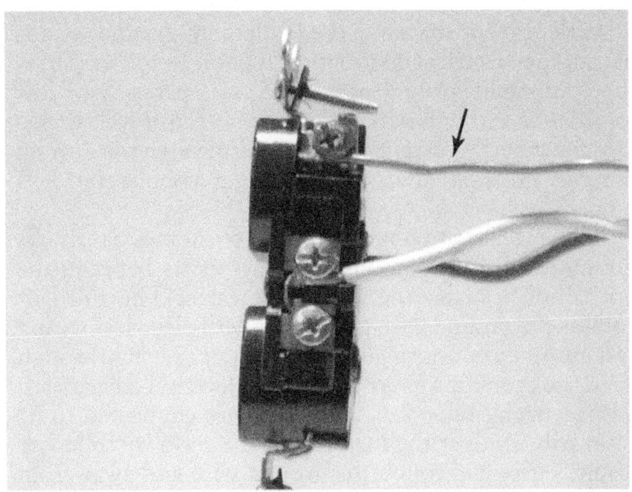

FIGURE 31-12 ■ Detail of modern electrical power receptacle. The *arrow* points to the ground wire (bare wire), which is attached to the green grounding screw on the power receptacle.

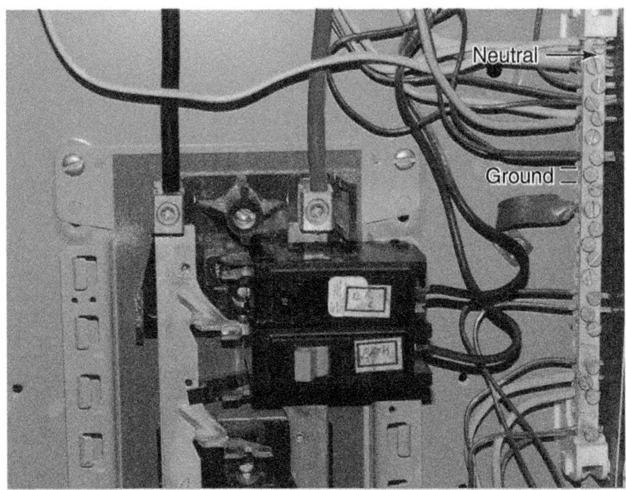

FIGURE 31-13 ■ The ground wires (bare wires) from the power outlet are run to the neutral bus bar, where they are connected with the neutral wires (white wires; *arrow*).

A 60 W lightbulb can be used as an example to further illustrate this point. Normally, the hot and neutral wires are connected to the two wires of the lightbulb socket, and throwing the switch will illuminate the bulb (Fig. 31-16). Similarly, if the hot wire is connected to one side of the bulb socket, and the other wire from the lightbulb is connected to the equipment ground wire, the bulb will still illuminate. If there is no equipment ground wire, the bulb will still light if the second wire is connected to any grounded metallic object, such as a water pipe or a faucet. This illustrates the fact that the 120 V potential difference exists not only between the hot and the neutral wires but also between the hot wire and any grounded object. Thus in a grounded power system, the current will flow between the hot wire and any conductor with an earth ground.

As previously stated, current flow requires a closed loop with a source of voltage. For an individual to receive an electric shock, he or she must contact the loop at two points. Because we may be standing either on the ground or in contact with an object that is referenced to the ground, only one additional contact point is necessary to complete the circuit and thereby receive an electrical shock. This is an unfortunate and inherently dangerous consequence of grounded power systems. Modern wiring systems have added the third wire, the equipment ground wire, as a safety measure to reduce the severity of a potential electrical shock. This is accomplished by providing an alternate, low-resistance pathway through which the current can flow to the ground.

Over time the insulation covering the wires may deteriorate. It is then possible for a bare, hot wire to contact the metal case or frame of an electrical device. The case would then become energized and would create a shock hazard to anyone coming in contact with it. Figure 31-17 illustrates a typical short circuit, in which the individual has come in contact with the hot (electrified) case of an instrument. This illustrates the type of wiring found in older homes: there is no ground wire in the electrical outlet, nor is the electrical apparatus equipped with a ground

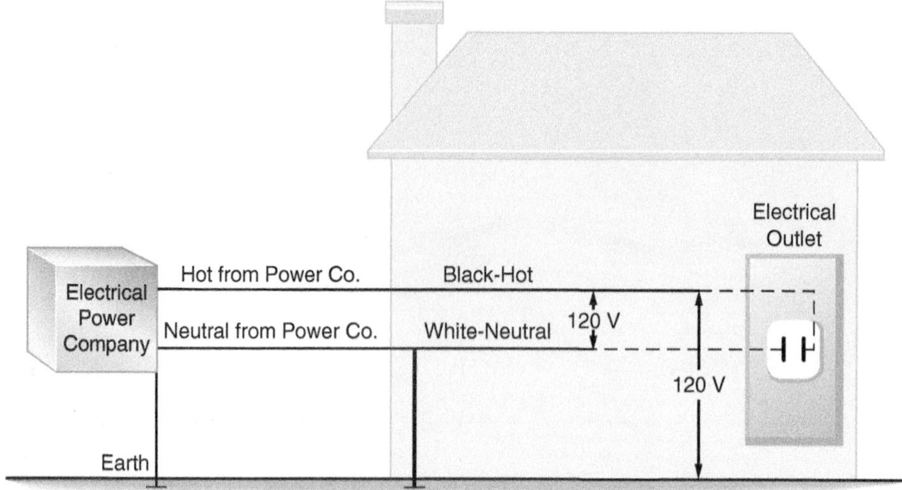

FIGURE 31-14 ■ Diagram of a house with older style wiring that does not contain a ground wire. A 120 V potential difference exists between the hot and the neutral wires and between the hot wire and the earth.

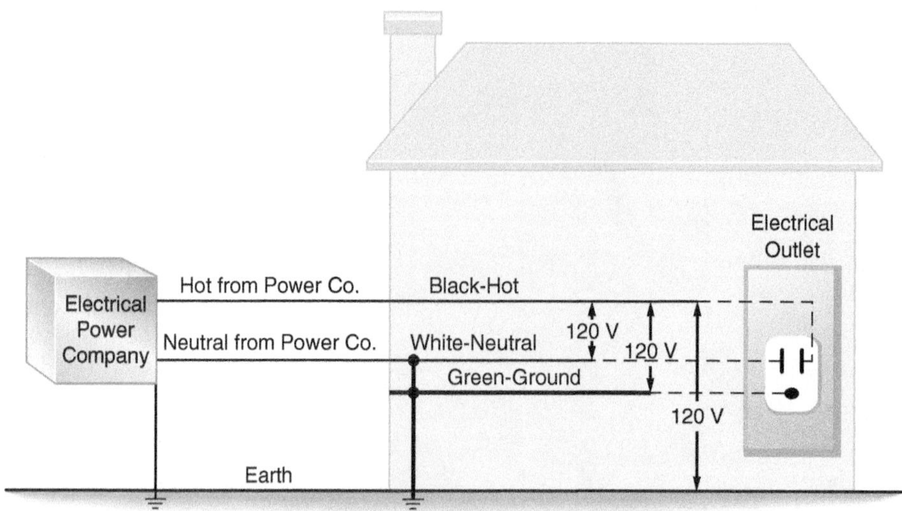

FIGURE 31-15 ■ Diagram of a house with modern wiring in which a third wire, or ground, has been added. The 120 V potential difference exists between the hot and neutral wires, the hot and the ground wires, and the hot wire and the earth.

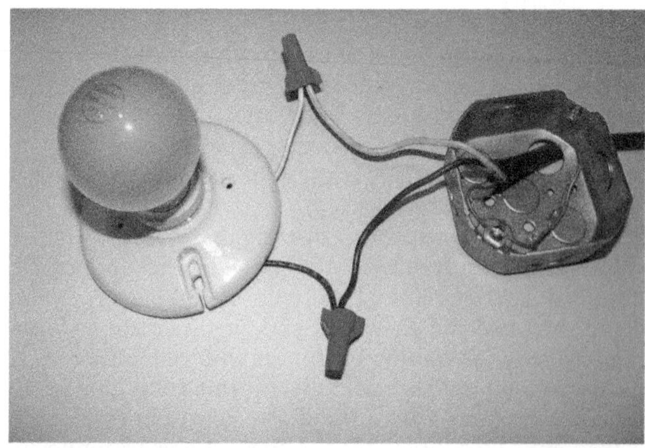

FIGURE 31-16 ■ A simple lightbulb circuit. The hot (*black*) and neutral (*white*) wires are connected with the corresponding wires from the lightbulb fixture.

wire. Here, the individual completes the circuit and receives a severe shock. Figure 31-18 illustrates a similar example, except that now the equipment ground wire is part of the electrical distribution system. In this example, the equipment ground wire provides a pathway of low impedance through which the current can travel; therefore most of the current would travel through the ground wire. In this case, the person may get a shock, but it is unlikely to be fatal.

The electrical power supplied to homes is always grounded. A 120 V potential always exists between the hot conductor and the ground or earth. The third or equipment ground wire used in modern electrical wiring systems does not normally have current flowing through it. In the event of a short circuit, an electrical device with a three-prong plug (i.e., a ground wire connected to its case) will conduct the majority of the short-circuited or "fault" current through the ground wire and away from the individual. This provides a significant safety benefit to someone accidentally contacting the defective device. If a large enough fault current exists, the ground wire

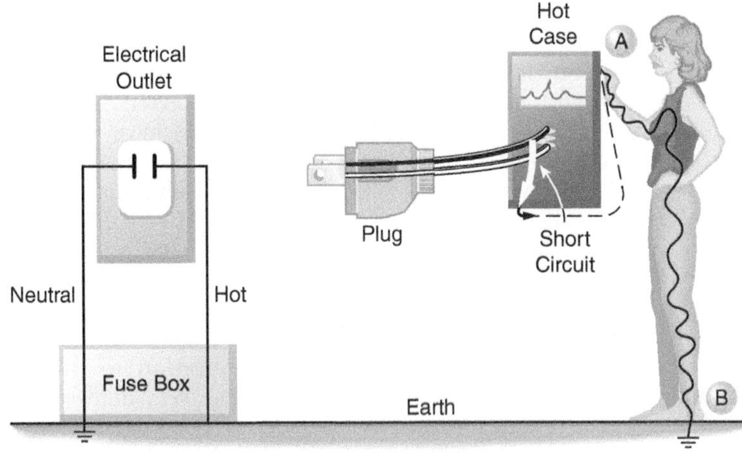

FIGURE 31-17 ■ When a faulty piece of equipment without an equipment ground wire is plugged into an electrical outlet that also does not contain a ground wire, the case of the instrument will become hot. An individual touching the hot case (point A) will receive a shock because he or she is standing on the earth (point B), completing the circuit. The current (*dashed line*) will flow from the instrument through the individual touching the hot case.

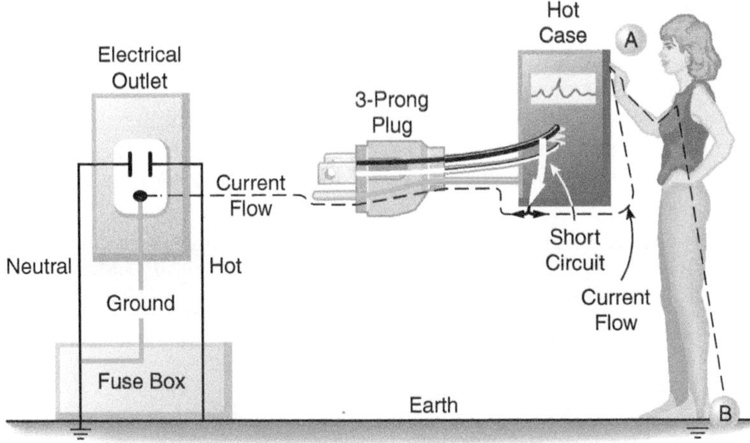

FIGURE 31-18 ■ When a faulty piece of equipment with an equipment ground wire is properly connected to an electrical outlet with a grounding connection, the current (*dashed line*) will preferentially flow down the low-resistance ground wire. An individual touching the case (point A) while standing on the ground (point B) will still complete the circuit; however, only a small part of the current will go through the individual.

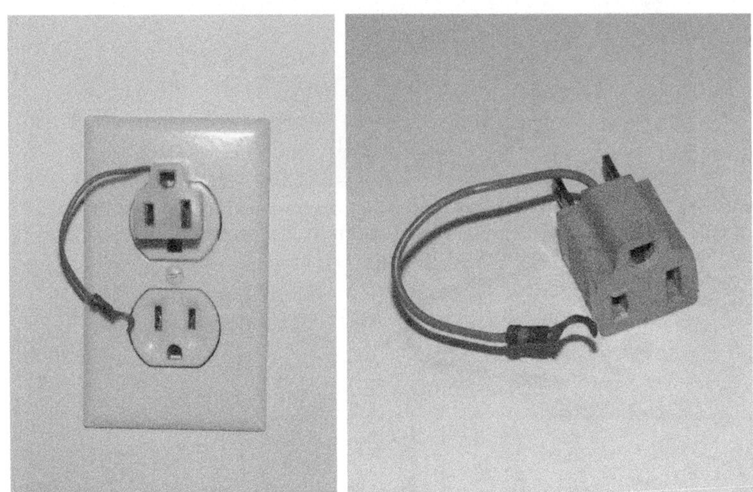

FIGURE 31-19 ■ *Right,* A "cheater plug" that converts a three-prong power cord to a two-prong cord. *Left,* The wire attached to the cheater plug is rarely connected to the screw in the middle of the outlet. This defeats the purpose of the equipment ground wire.

also will provide a means to complete the short circuit back to the circuit breaker or fuse, and this will either melt the fuse or trip the circuit breaker. Thus, in a grounded power system, it is possible to have either grounded or ungrounded equipment, depending on when the wiring was installed and whether the electrical device is equipped with a three-prong plug that contains a ground wire. Obviously, attempts to bypass the safety system of the equipment ground should be avoided. Devices such as a "cheater plug" (Fig. 31-19) should never be used because they defeat the safety feature of the equipment ground wire.

ELECTRICAL POWER: UNGROUNDED

Numerous electronic devices, together with power cords and puddles of saline solution on the floor, make the OR an electrically hazardous environment for both patients and personnel. Bruner and colleagues[5] found that 40% of electrical accidents in hospitals occurred in the OR. The complexity of electrical equipment in the modern OR demands that electrical safety be a factor of paramount importance. To provide an extra measure of safety from macroshock, the power supplied to most ORs is ungrounded. In this ungrounded power system, the current is isolated from ground potential. The 120 V potential difference exists only between the two wires of the isolated power system (IPS), but no circuit exists between the ground and either of the isolated power lines.

Supplying ungrounded power to the OR requires the use of an *isolation transformer* (Fig. 31-20). This device uses electromagnetic induction to induce a current in the ungrounded or secondary winding of the transformer from energy supplied to the primary winding. No direct electrical connection exists between the power supplied by the utility company on the primary side and the power induced by the transformer on the ungrounded, or secondary, side. Thus, the power supplied to the OR is isolated from ground (Fig. 31-21). Because the 120 V potential exists only between the two wires of the isolated circuit, neither wire is hot or neutral with reference to ground; in this case, they are simply referred to as *line 1* and *line 2* (Fig. 31-22). Using the example of the lightbulb, if the two wires of the bulb socket are connected to the two wires of the IPS, the bulb will illuminate. However, if one of the wires is connected to one side of the isolated power, and the other wire is connected to the ground, the light will not illuminate. If the wires of the IPS are connected, the short circuit will trip the circuit breaker. In comparing the two systems, standard grounded power has a direct connection to ground, whereas the isolated system imposes a very high impedance to any current flow to ground. The added safety of this system can be seen in Figure 31-23. In this case, a person has come in contact with one side of the IPS (point A). Because standing on the ground (point B) does not constitute a part of the isolated circuit, the individual does not complete the loop and will not receive a shock. This is because the ground is part of the primary circuit, and the person is contacting only one side of the isolated secondary circuit. The person does not complete either circuit; that is, the person does not have two contact points; therefore this situation does not pose an electric shock

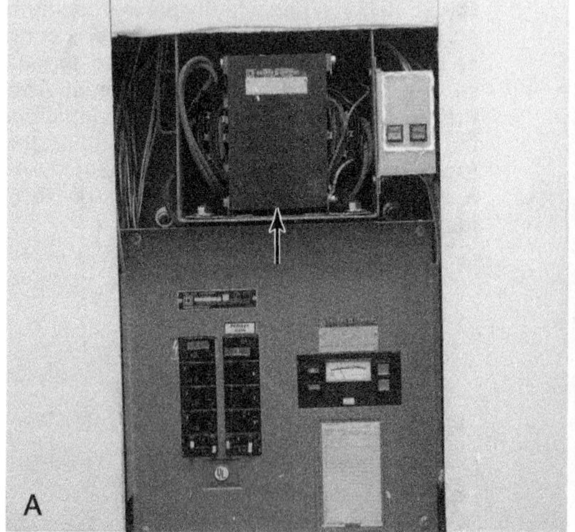

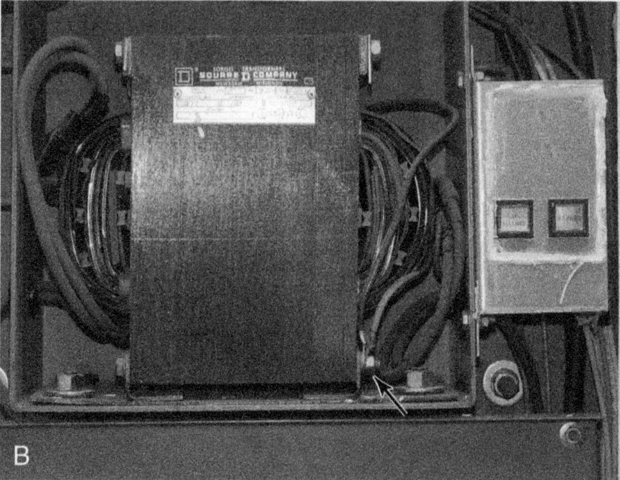

FIGURE 31-20 ■ **A,** Isolated power panel showing circuit breakers, line isolation monitor, and isolation transformer (*arrow*). **B,** Detail of an isolation transformer with the attached warning lights. The *arrow* points to ground wire connection on the primary side of the transformer. Note that no similar connection exists on the secondary side of the transformer.

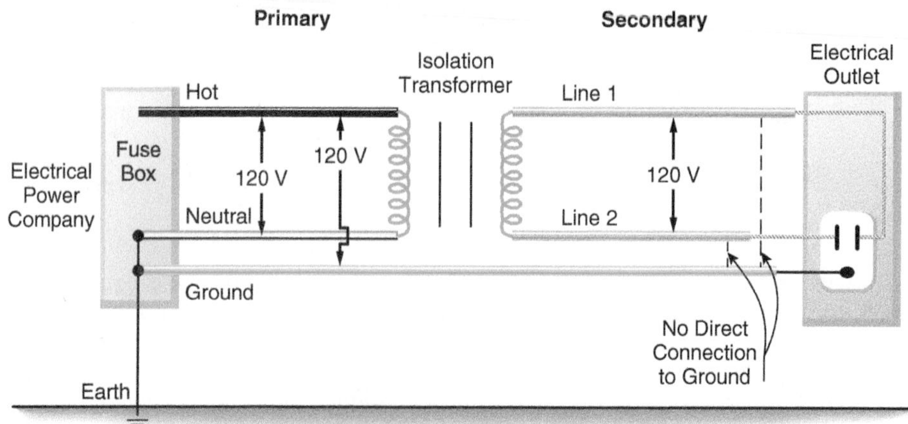

FIGURE 31-21 ■ In the operating room, the isolation transformer converts the grounded power on the primary side to an ungrounded power system on the secondary side of the transformer. A 120 V potential difference exists between line 1 and line 2. There is no direct connection from the power on the secondary side to ground. The equipment ground wire, however, is still present.

hazard. Of course, if the person contacts both lines of the IPS, an unlikely event, he or she would receive a shock.

If a faulty electrical appliance with an intact equipment ground wire is plugged into a standard household outlet, and the home wiring has a properly connected ground wire, the amount of electrical current that will flow through a person is considerably less than what will flow through the low-resistance ground wire. Here, an individual would be fairly well protected from a serious shock. However, if that ground wire were broken, the person might receive a lethal shock. No shock would occur if the same faulty piece of equipment were plugged into the IPS, even if the equipment ground wire were broken. Thus the IPS provides a significant amount of protection from macroshock. Another feature of the IPS is that the faulty piece of equipment, even though it may be partially short-circuited, will not usually trip the circuit breaker. This is an important feature, because the faulty piece of equipment may be part of a life-support system for a patient. It is important to note that even though the power is isolated from ground, the case or frame of all electrical equipment is still connected to an equipment ground. The third wire, the equipment ground wire, is a necessary component of any electrical safety program.

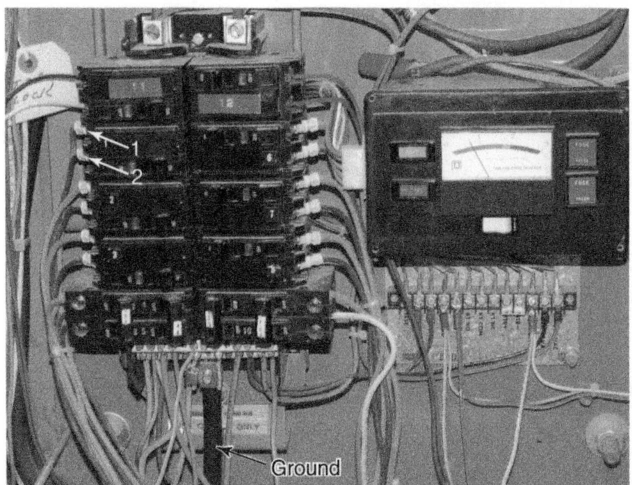

FIGURE 31-22 Detail of the inside of a circuit breaker box in an isolated power system. The bottom arrow points to ground (*green*) wires meeting at the common ground terminal. Arrows 1 and 2 indicate lines 1 and 2 (*orange and brown*) from the isolated power circuit breaker. Neither line 1 nor line 2 is connected to the same terminals as the ground wires. This is in marked contrast to Figure 31-13, where the neutral and ground wires are attached at the same point.

Figure 31-24 illustrates a scenario involving a faulty piece of equipment connected to the IPS. This does not represent a hazard; it merely converts the isolated power back to a grounded power system as exists outside the OR. In fact, a *second* fault is necessary to create a hazard.

The previous discussion assumes that the IPS is perfectly isolated from ground. Actually, perfect isolation is impossible to achieve; all AC-operated power systems and electrical devices manifest some degree of capacitance. As previously discussed, electrical power cords, wires, and electrical motors exhibit capacitive coupling to the ground wire and metal conduits, and they leak small amounts of current to ground (Fig. 31-25). This so-called *leakage current* partially ungrounds the IPS; this does not usually amount to more than a few milliamperes in an OR, so a person coming in contact with one side of the IPS would receive only a very small shock (1 to 2 mA). Although this amount of current would be perceptible, it would not be dangerous.

LINE ISOLATION MONITOR

The *line isolation monitor* (LIM) is a device that continuously monitors the integrity of an IPS. If a faulty piece of equipment is connected to the IPS, this will, in effect, change the system back to a conventional grounded system. Also, the faulty piece of equipment will continue to function normally. Therefore it is essential that a warning system be in place to alert personnel that the power is no longer ungrounded. The LIM continuously monitors the isolated power to ensure that it is indeed isolated from ground, and the device has a meter that displays a continuous indication of the integrity of the system (Fig. 31-26). The LIM is actually measuring the impedance to ground of each side of the IPS. As previously discussed, with perfect isolation, impedance would be infinitely high, and no current would flow in the event of a first-fault situation ($Z = E/I$; if $I = 0$, then $Z = \infty$). Because all AC wiring and all AC-operated electrical devices have some capacitance,

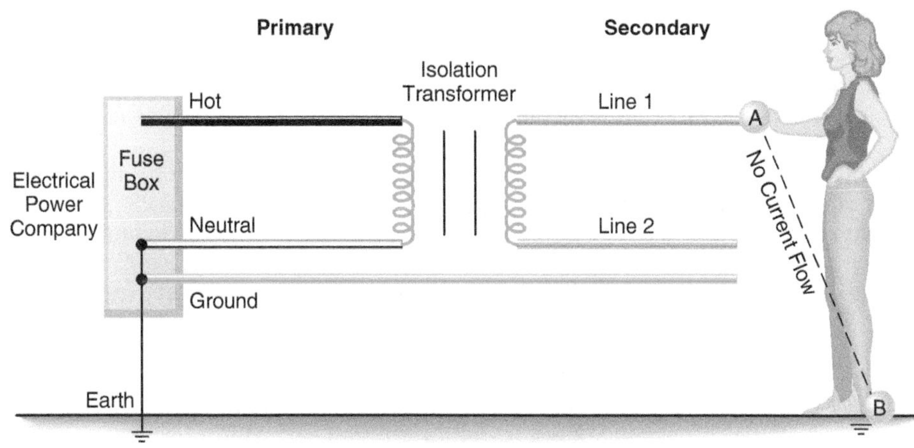

FIGURE 31-23 A safety feature of the isolated power system (IPS). An individual in contact with one side of the IPS (point A) and standing on the ground (point B) will not receive a shock. In this instance, the individual is not contacting the circuit at two points and thus is not completing the circuit. Point A is part of the IPS, and point B is part of the primary or grounded side of the circuit.

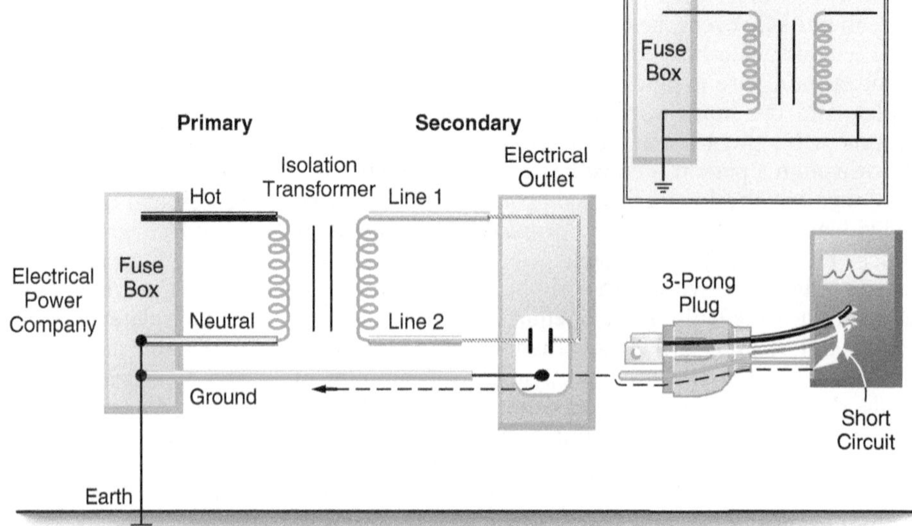

FIGURE 31-24 ■ A faulty piece of equipment plugged into the isolated power system (IPS) does not present a shock hazard. It merely converts the IPS into a grounded power system. The *inset* illustrates that the IPS is now identical to the grounded power system. The *dashed line* indicates current flow in the ground wire.

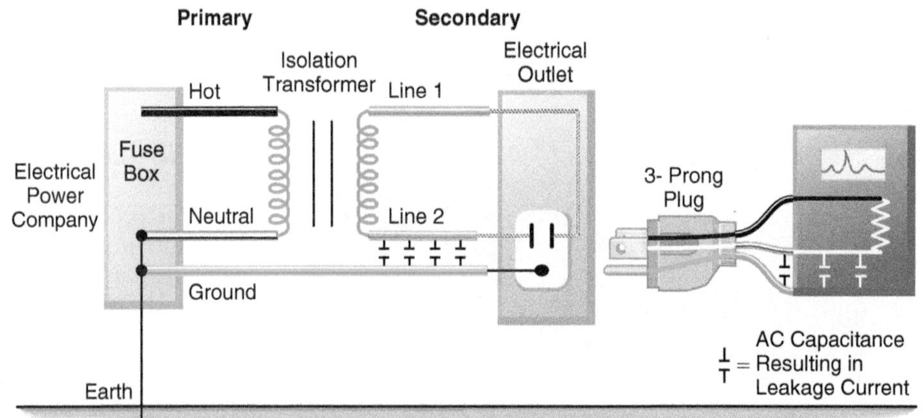

FIGURE 31-25 ■ The capacitance that exists in alternating current (AC) power lines and AC-operated equipment results in small "leakage currents" that partially degrade the isolated power system.

small leakage currents are present that partially degrade the isolation of the system. The meter of the LIM will indicate (in milliamperes) the total amount of leakage in the system resulting from capacitance, electrical wiring, and any devices plugged into the IPS.

The reading on the LIM does not mean that current is actually flowing; rather it indicates how much current would flow in the event of a first fault. The LIM is set to alarm at 2 or 5 mA, depending on the age and brand of the system. Once this preset limit is exceeded, visual and audible alarms are triggered to indicate that the isolation from ground has been degraded beyond a predetermined limit (Fig. 31-27). This does not necessarily mean that a hazardous situation exists; rather it shows that the system is no longer totally isolated from ground; a second fault is required to create a dangerous situation. For example, if the LIM were set to alarm at 2 mA, using Ohm's law, the impedance for either side of the IPS would be 60,000 Ω:

$$Z = E/I$$

$$Z = 120\ V/0.002\ A$$

$$Z = 60{,}000\ \Omega$$

Therefore if either side of the IPS had less than 60,000 Ω impedance to ground, the LIM would trigger an alarm. This might occur in two situations. In the first, a faulty piece of equipment is plugged into the IPS. In this case, a true fault to ground exists from one line to the ground. Now the system would be converted to the equivalent of a grounded power system. This faulty piece of equipment should be removed and serviced as soon as possible, although it could still be used safely if it were essential for the care of the patient. It should be remembered, however, that continuing to use this faulty piece of equipment would create the potential for a serious electrical shock. This would occur if a second faulty piece of equipment were simultaneously connected to the IPS.

The second situation involves connecting many perfectly normal pieces of equipment to the IPS. Although each piece of equipment has only a small amount of leakage current, if the total leakage exceeds 2 mA, the LIM will trigger an alarm. Assume that 30 electrical devices are present in the OR, and each has 100 μA of leakage current; the total (30 × 100 μA) would be 3 mA. The impedance to ground would still be 40,000 Ω (120/0.003), and the LIM alarm would sound in this instance, because the 2 mA set point was violated. However, the system is

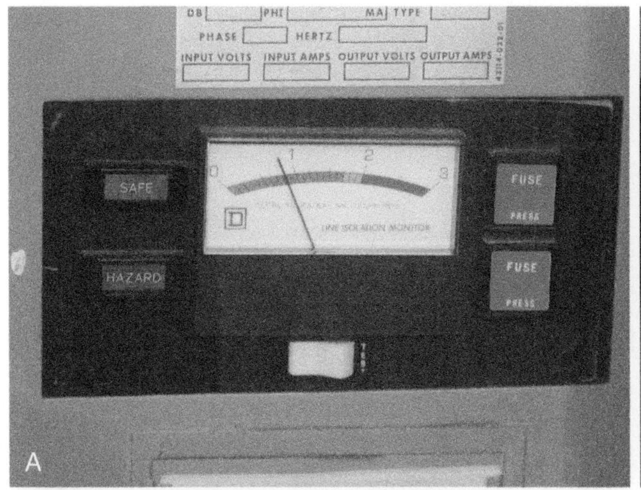

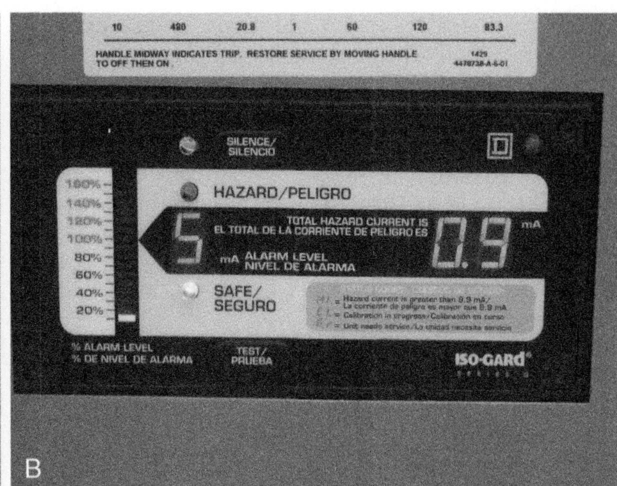

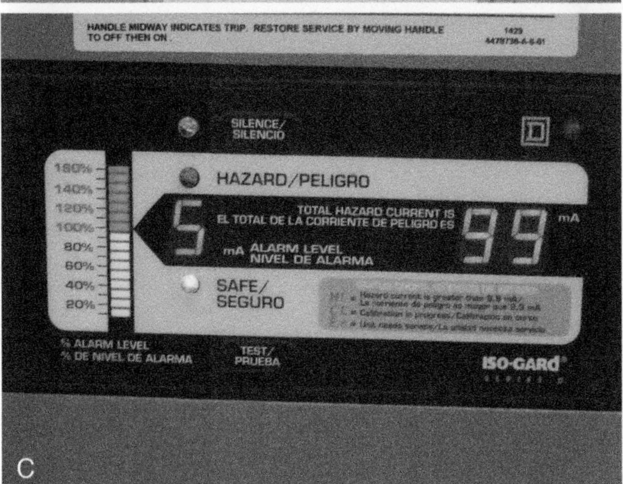

FIGURE 31-26 ▪ The meter of the line isolation monitor (LIM) is calibrated in milliamperes. If the isolation of the power system is degraded such that more than 2 mA of current (5 mA in newer systems) could flow, the hazard light will illuminate, and a warning buzzer will sound. Note the button for testing the hazard warning system. **A,** Older LIM that will trigger an alarm at 2 mA. **B,** Newer LIM that will trigger an alarm at 5 mA. **C,** The LIM alarm is triggered, and the red hazard stripe is illuminated; the number on the right shows 9.9 mA of potential current flow.

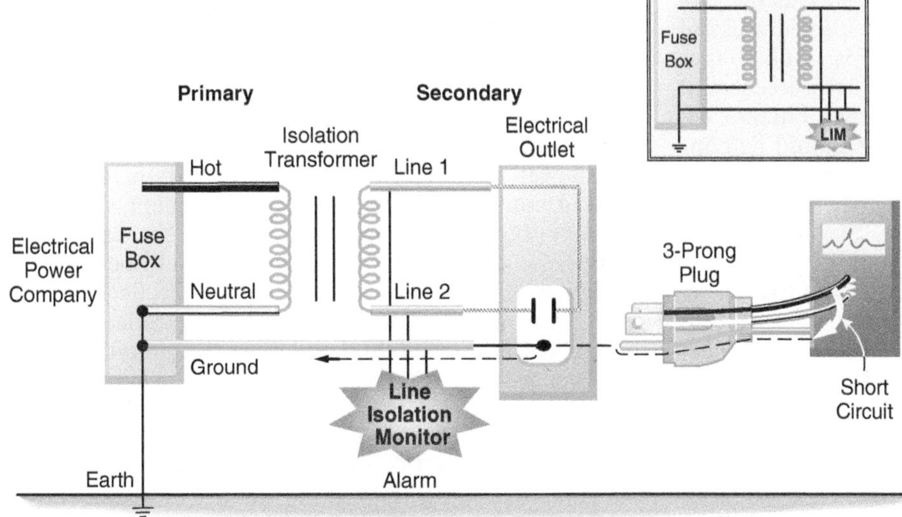

FIGURE 31-27 ▪ When a faulty piece of equipment is plugged into the isolated power system, it will markedly decrease the impedance from line 1 or line 2 to ground. This will be detected by the line isolation monitor, which will sound an alarm.

still safe and represents a state significantly different from that in the first situation. For this reason, the newer LIMs are set to alarm at 5 mA instead of 2 mA.

The newest LIMs are referred to as *third-generation monitors*. The *first-generation monitor*, or *static LIM*, was unable to detect balanced faults (i.e., a situation in which there are equal faults to ground from both lines 1 and 2). The *second-generation monitor*, or *dynamic LIM*, did not have this problem but could interfere with physiologic monitoring. Both of these monitors would trigger an alarm at 2 mA, which led to annoying "false" alarms. The third-generation LIM corrects the problems of its predecessors and has the alarm threshold set at 5 mA.[6] Proper functioning of the LIM depends on having both equipment ground wires intact and its own connection to ground. First- and second-generation LIMs could not detect the loss of the LIM ground connection. The third-generation LIM can detect this loss of ground to the monitor. In this case, the LIM alarm would sound, and the red hazard light would illuminate, but the LIM meter would read zero; this condition will alert the staff that the LIM needs to be repaired. In any event, the LIM still cannot detect broken equipment ground wires. An example of the third-generation LIM is the Iso-Gard, made by Square D (Monroe, NC).

The equipment ground wire is again an important part of the safety system. If this wire is broken, a faulty piece of equipment plugged into an outlet would operate normally, but the LIM would not alarm. A second fault could therefore cause a shock without any alarm from the LIM. Also, in the event of a second fault, the equipment ground wire provides a low-resistance path to ground for most of the fault current (see Fig. 31-24). The LIM will only be able to register leakage currents from pieces of equipment that are connected to the IPS and that have intact ground wires.

If the LIM alarm is triggered, the first thing to do is to check the gauge to determine whether it is a true fault; the other possibility is that too many pieces of electrical equipment have been plugged in, and the 2 mA limit has been exceeded. If the gauge is between 2 and 5 mA, it is probable that too much electrical equipment has been plugged in. If the gauge reads over 5 mA, most likely a faulty piece of equipment is present. The next step is to identify the faulty equipment, which is done by unplugging each piece of equipment until the alarm ceases. If the faulty piece of equipment is not of a critical nature, it should be removed from the OR. If it is a vital piece of life-support equipment, it can be safely used. (Note: if a critical piece of life-support equipment, such as the cardiopulmonary bypass machine, is the suspected cause of the alarm, do not disconnect it until it is no longer needed.) It must be remembered that the protection of the IPS and the LIM is no longer operative. Therefore if possible, no other electrical equipment should be connected during the remainder of the case, or at least until the faulty piece of equipment can be safely removed.

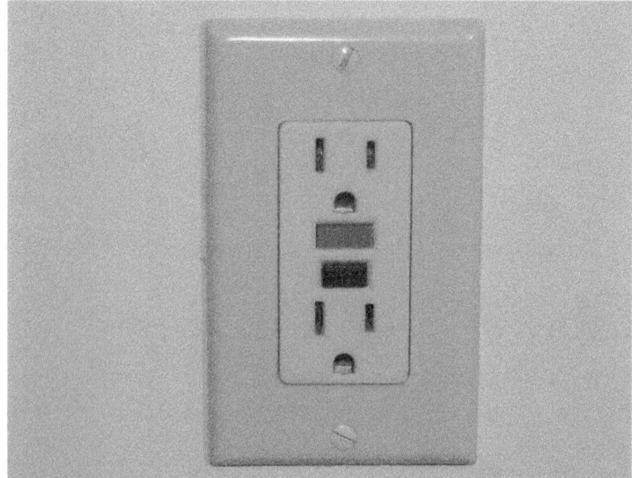

FIGURE 31-28 ■ A ground fault circuit interrupter electrical outlet with integrated test (black) and reset (red) buttons.

FIGURE 31-29 ■ Special ground fault circuit interrupter circuit breaker. Note the distinguishing red test button.

GROUND FAULT CIRCUIT INTERRUPTER

The ground fault circuit interrupter (GFCI, or occasionally GFI) is another popular device used to prevent individuals from receiving an electrical shock in a grounded power system. Electrical codes for most new construction require that a GFCI circuit be present in potentially hazardous (e.g., wet) areas such as bathrooms, kitchens, or outdoors. The GFCI may be installed as an individual power outlet (Fig. 31-28), or a special circuit breaker may be installed to which all the individual protected outlets are connected at a single point. The special GFCI circuit breaker is located in the main breaker box and can be distinguished by its red test button (Fig. 31-29). As Figure 31-5 demonstrates, the current flowing in both the hot and neutral wires is usually equal. The GFCI monitors both sides of the circuit for the equality of current flow; if a difference is detected, the power is immediately interrupted. If an individual should contact a faulty piece of equipment such that current flowed through the person, an imbalance between the two sides of the circuit would be created, which would be detected by the GFCI. Because the GFCI can detect very small current differences (in the range of 5 mA), the GFCI will open the circuit within a few milliseconds, thereby interrupting the current flow before a significant shock occurs. Thus the GFCI provides a high level of protection at a very modest cost. If the OR has a GFCI that tripped, an attempt should first be made to reset it by pushing the reset button; this is because a surge may have caused the GFCI to trip. If it cannot be reset, the equipment must be removed from service and checked by the biomedical engineering staff. It is essential that when GFCIs are used in an OR, only one outlet should be protected by each GFCI. They should never be "daisy-chained" such that one GFCI protects multiple outlets.

The disadvantage of using a GFCI in the OR is that it interrupts the power without warning. A defective piece

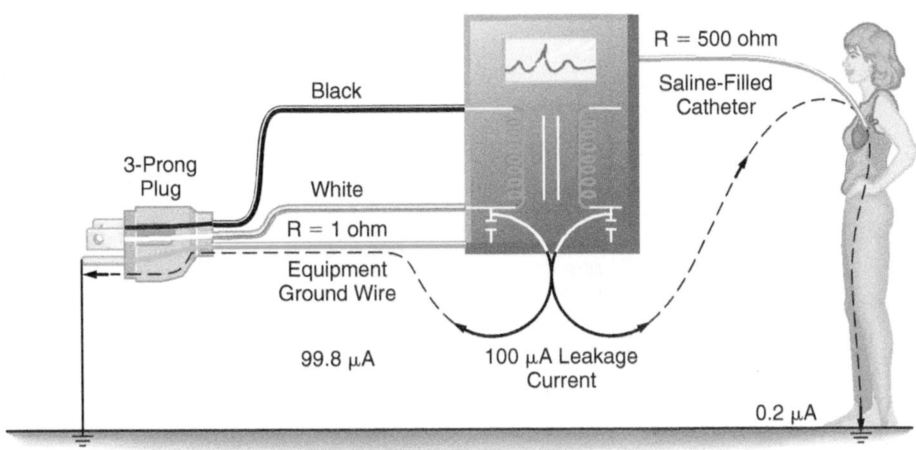

FIGURE 31-30 The electrically susceptible patient is protected from microshock by the presence of an intact equipment ground wire. The equipment ground wire provides a low-impedance path in which the majority of the leakage current (*dashed lines*) can flow. R, resistance.

of equipment could no longer be used, which could be a problem if it were essential for life support; whereas if the same faulty piece of equipment were plugged into an IPS, the LIM would alarm, but the equipment could still be used.

DOUBLE INSULATION

One instance in which it is acceptable for a piece of equipment to have only a two-prong and not a three-prong plug is when the instrument has what is termed *double insulation*. These instruments have two layers of insulation and usually have a plastic exterior. Double insulation is found in many home power tools and is seen in hospital equipment such as infusion pumps. Double-insulated equipment is permissible in the OR with IPSs; however, if water or saline should get inside the unit, it could present a hazard because the double insulation is bypassed. This is even more serious if the OR has no isolated power or GFCIs.[7]

MICROSHOCK

As previously discussed, macroshock involves relatively large amounts of current applied to the surface of the body. The current is conducted through all the tissues in proportion to their conductivity and area in a plane perpendicular to the current. Consequently, the "density" of the current (amperes per meter squared) that reaches the heart is considerably less than what is applied to the body surface. However, an electrically susceptible patient—one who has a direct external connection to the heart, such as through a central venous pressure catheter or transvenous cardiac pacing wires—may be at risk from very small currents; this is called *microshock*.[8] The catheter orifice or electrical wire with a very small surface area in contact with the heart produces a relatively large current density at the heart.[9] Stated another way, even very small amounts of current applied directly to the myocardium will cause ventricular fibrillation. Microshock is a particularly difficult problem because of the insidious nature of the hazard.

In the electrically susceptible patient, ventricular fibrillation can be produced by a current that is below the threshold of human perception. The exact amount of current necessary to cause ventricular fibrillation in this type of patient is unknown. Whalen and colleagues[10] were able to produce fibrillation with 20 μA of current applied directly to the myocardium of dogs. Raftery and colleagues[11] produced fibrillation with 80 μA of current in some patients. Hull[12] used data obtained by Watson and collagues[13] to show that 50% of patients would fibrillate at currents of 200 μA. Because 1000 μA (1 mA) is generally regarded as the threshold of human perception with 60 Hz AC, the electrically susceptible patient can be electrocuted with one tenth of the normally perceptible currents. This is not only of academic interest but also of practical concern, because many cases of ventricular fibrillation from microshock have been reported.[14-18]

The stray capacitance that is part of any AC-powered electrical instrument may result in significant amounts of charge buildup on the case of the instrument. If an individual simultaneously touches the case of an instrument where this has occurred in the electrically susceptible patient, he or she may unknowingly cause a discharge to the patient that results in ventricular fibrillation. Once again, the equipment ground wire constitutes the major source of protection against microshock for the electrically susceptible patient. In this case, the equipment ground wire provides a low-resistance path by which most of the leakage current is dissipated instead of stored as a charge.

Figure 31-30 illustrates a situation involving a patient with a saline-filled catheter in the heart with a resistance of about 500 Ω. The ground wire with a resistance of 1 Ω is connected to the instrument case, and a leakage current of 100 μA will divide according to the relative resistances of the two paths: in this case, 99.8 μA will flow through the equipment ground wire, and only 0.2 μA will flow through the fluid-filled catheter. This extremely small current does not endanger the patient. However, if the equipment ground wire were broken, the electrically susceptible patient would be at great risk, because all 100 μA of leakage current could flow through the catheter and cause ventricular fibrillation (Fig. 31-31). Currently, electronic equipment is permitted 100 μA of leakage current.

Modern patient monitors incorporate another mechanism to reduce the risk of microshock for electrically

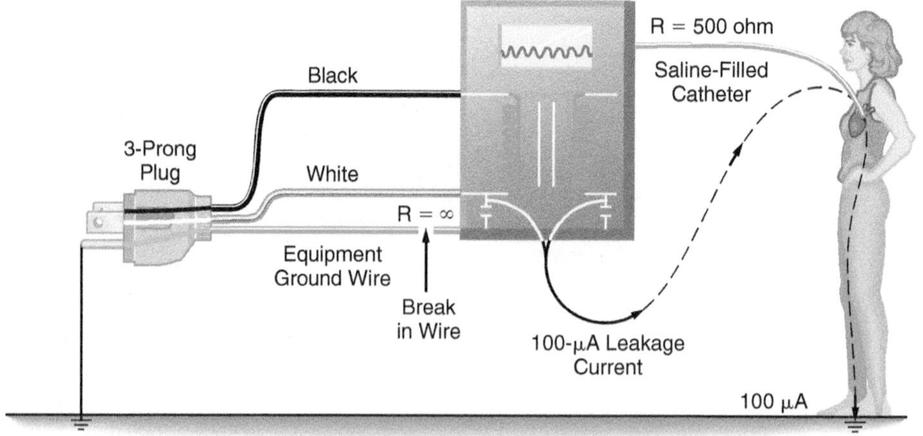

FIGURE 31-31 ■ A broken equipment ground wire results in a significant hazard to the electrically susceptible patient. In this case, the entire leakage current can be conducted to the heart and may result in ventricular fibrillation. R, resistance.

susceptible patients.[19] This mechanism involves electrically isolating all direct patient connections from the power supply of the monitor by placing a very high impedance between the patient and any device. This limits the amount of internal leakage through the patient connection to a very small value; the standard currently is less than 10 μA. For instance, the output of an ECG monitor's power supply is electrically isolated from the patient by placing a very high impedance between the monitor and the patient's ECG leads.[20] Isolation techniques are designed to inhibit hazardous electrical pathways between the patient and the monitor while allowing the passage of the physiologic signal.

An intact equipment ground wire is probably the most important factor in preventing microshock. There are, however, other things that the anesthesiologist can do to reduce the incidence of microshock, such as to never simultaneously touch an electrical device and a saline-filled central catheter or external pacing wires. When handling a central catheter or pacing wires, it is best to insulate oneself by wearing rubber gloves. Also, never let any external current source, such as a nerve stimulator, come into contact with the catheter or wires. Finally, be alert to potential sources of energy that can be transmitted to the patient; even stray radiofrequency current from the ESU (cautery) can, under the right conditions, be a source of microshock.[21] It must be remembered that the LIM is not designed to provide protection from microshock. The microampere currents involved in microshock are far below the LIM threshold of protection. In addition, the LIM does not register the leakage of individual monitors but rather indicates the status of the total system. The LIM reading indicates the total amount of leakage current resulting from the entire capacitance of the system. This is the amount of current that would flow to ground in the event of a first-fault situation.

The essence of electrical safety is a thorough understanding of all the principles of grounding; the objective of preventing injury is to make it difficult for electrical current to pass through people. For this reason, both the patient and the anesthesiologist should be isolated from ground as much as possible. That is, their resistance to current flow should be as high as is technologically feasible.

In the inherently unsafe electrical environment of an OR, several measures can be taken to help protect against contacting hazardous current flows. First, the grounded power provided by the utility company can be converted to ungrounded power by means of an isolation transformer. The LIM will continuously monitor the status of this isolation from ground and will issue a warning when the isolation of the power (from ground) has been lost, in the event that a defective piece of equipment is plugged into one of the isolated circuit outlets. In addition, the shock that an individual could receive from a faulty piece of equipment is determined by the capacitance of the system and is limited to a few milliamperes. Because all equipment plugged into the IPS has an equipment ground wire attached to the case of the instrument, this equipment ground wire will provide an alternative low-resistance pathway to enable potentially dangerous currents to flow to ground. Thus the patient and the anesthesiologist should be as insulated from ground as much as possible, and all electrical equipment should be grounded.

The equipment ground wire serves three functions. First, it provides a low-resistance path for fault currents to reduce the risk of macroshock. Second, it dissipates leakage currents that are potentially harmful to the electrically susceptible patient. Third, it provides information to the LIM on the status of the ungrounded power system. If the equipment ground wire is broken, a significant factor in the prevention of electrical shock is lost. Additionally, the IPS will appear safer than it actually is, because the LIM is unable to detect broken equipment ground wires.

Because power cords, plugs, and receptacles are subjected to greater abuse in the hospital than in the home, the Underwriters Laboratories (Melville, NY) has issued a strict specification for special "hospital grade" plugs and receptacles (Fig. 31-32). The plugs and receptacles that conform to this specification are marked by a green dot.[22] The hospital-grade plug is one that can be visually inspected or easily disassembled to ensure the integrity of the ground wire connection; molded opaque plugs are not acceptable. Edwards[23] reported that of 3000 non–hospital-grade receptacles installed in a new hospital building, 1800 (60%) were found to be defective after 3 years. When 2000 of the non–hospital-grade

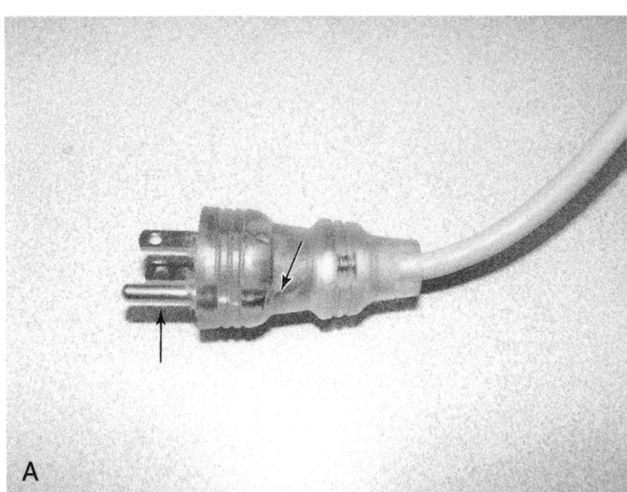

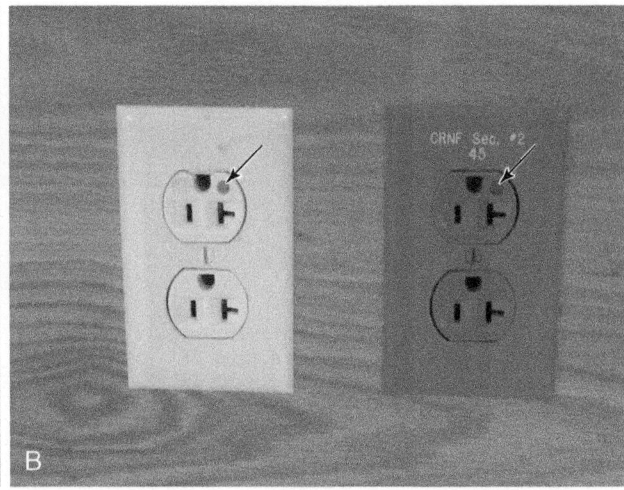

FIGURE 31-32 ■ **A,** A hospital-grade plug that can be visually inspected. The *arrow* points to the equipment ground wire, whose integrity can be readily verified. Note that the prong for the ground wire (*arrow*) is longer than the hot or neutral prong, so that it is the first to enter the receptacle. **B,** The arrows point to the green dot, denoting a hospital-grade power outlet. The red outlet on the right is connected to the emergency power (generator) system.

receptacles were replaced with hospital-grade receptacles, no failures occurred after 18 months of use.

ELECTROSURGERY

On that fateful October day in 1926, when Dr. Harvey W. Cushing first used an electrosurgical (ESU) machine invented by Professor William T. Bovie to resect a brain tumor, the course of modern surgery and anesthesia was forever altered.[24] The ubiquitous use of electrosurgery attests to the success of Professor Bovie's invention. However, this technology was not adopted without a cost. The widespread use of electrocautery has, at the very least, hastened the elimination of explosive anesthetic agents from the OR. In addition, as every anesthesiologist is aware, few things in the OR are immune to interference from the "Bovie." The high-frequency electrical energy generated by the ESU interferes with everything from the ECG signal to cardiac output computers, pulse oximeters, and even implanted cardiac pacemakers.[25]

The ESU operates by generating currents of a very high frequency—in the radiofrequency range, anywhere from 500,000 to 1 million Hz. Heat is generated whenever a current passes through a resistance, and the amount of heat produced (H) is proportional to the square of the current and inversely proportional to the area through which the current passes ($H = I^2/A$).[26] By concentrating the energy at the tip of the "Bovie pencil," the surgeon can produce either a cut or a coagulation at any given spot. This very-high-frequency current behaves differently from the standard 60 Hz AC current and can pass directly across the precordium without causing ventricular fibrillation.[26] This is because high-frequency currents have a low tissue penetration and do not excite contractile cells.

Although the ESU is used safely hundreds of thousands of times each year, there is evidence that under certain circumstances it has been the cause of ventricular fibrillation.[27-30] The mechanism is thought to be low frequency (50 to 60 Hz) "stray current" generated when the ESU is activated. Current in the 50 to 60 Hz range can cause ventricular fibrillation. These cases have been associated with use of the coagulation mode, when the surgeon is using the device near the heart, and when the patient has a conductor in the heart such as a central venous pressure or pulmonary artery catheter. However, the exact mechanism has not been proven.

The large amount of energy generated by the ESU can pose other problems to the operator and the patient. Cushing became aware of one such problem. He wrote, "Once the operator received a shock which passed through a metal retractor to his arm and out by a wire from his headlight, which was unpleasant to say the least."[31] The ESU cannot be safely operated unless the energy is properly routed from the ESU through the patient and back to the unit. Ideally, the current generated by the active electrode is concentrated at the ESU tip, constituting a very small surface area. This energy has a high current density and is able to generate enough heat to produce a therapeutic cut or coagulation. The energy then passes through the patient to a dispersive electrode of large surface area that returns the energy safely to the ESU (Fig. 31-33).

One unfortunate quirk in terminology concerns the return (dispersive) plate of the ESU. This plate, often incorrectly referred to as a *ground plate*, is actually a dispersive electrode of large surface area that safely returns the generated energy to the ESU via a low current density pathway. When inquiring whether the dispersive electrode has been attached to the patient, OR personnel frequently ask, "Is the patient grounded?" Because the aim of electrical safety is to isolate the patient from ground, this expression is worse than erroneous; it can lead to confusion. Because the area of the return plate is large, the current density is low; therefore, no harmful heat is generated, and no tissue destruction occurs. In a properly functioning system, the only tissue effect is at the site of the active electrode held by the surgeon.

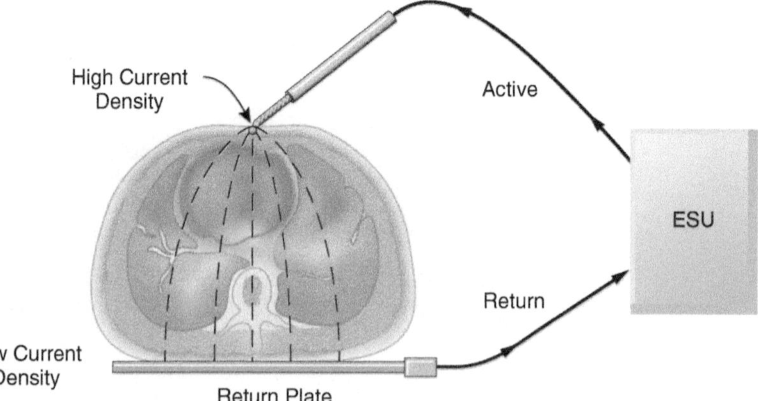

FIGURE 31-33 ■ A properly applied electrosurgical unit (ESU) return plate. The current density at the return plate is low, resulting in no danger to the patient.

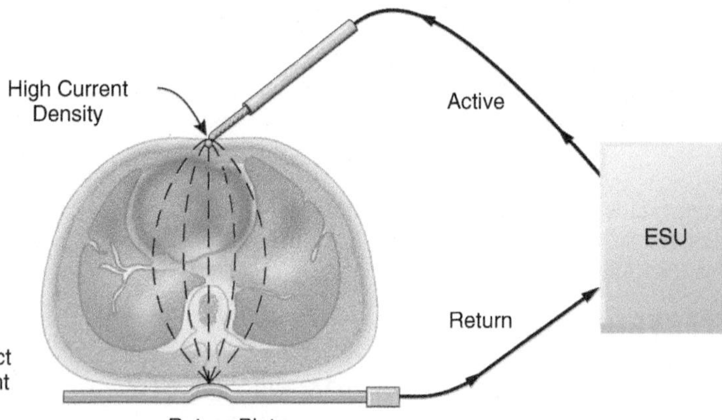

FIGURE 31-34 ■ An improperly applied electrosurgical unit (ESU) return plate. Poor contact with the return plate results in a high current density and a possible burn to the patient.

Problems can arise if the electrosurgical return plate is improperly applied to the patient or if the cord connecting the return plate to the ESU is damaged or broken. In these instances, the high-frequency current generated by the ESU will seek an alternate return pathway. Anything attached to the patient, such as ECG leads or a temperature probe, can provide this alternate return pathway. The current density at the ECG pad will be considerably higher than normal, because its surface area is much less than that of the ESU return plate; this may result in a serious burn at this alternate return site. Similarly, a burn may occur at the site of the ESU return plate if it is not properly applied to the patient, or if it becomes partially dislodged during the operation (Fig. 31-34). This is not merely a theoretical possibility but is evidenced by the numerous case reports involving patients who have received ESU burns.[32-37]

The original ESUs were manufactured with the power supply connected directly to ground by the equipment ground wire. These devices made it extremely easy for ESU current to return by alternate pathways. The ESU would continue to operate normally even without the return plate connected to the patient. In most modern ESUs, the power supply is isolated from ground to protect the patient from burns.[38] It was hoped that by isolating the return pathway from ground, the only route for current flow would be via the return electrode. Theoretically, this would eliminate alternate return pathways and greatly reduce the incidence of burns. However, Mitchell[39] found two situations in which the current could return via alternate pathways, even with the isolated ESU circuit. If the return plate were left either on top of an uninsulated ESU cabinet or in contact with the bottom of the OR table, the ESU could operate fairly normally, and the current would return via alternate pathways. It should be recalled that the impedance is inversely proportional to the capacitance times the current frequency. The ESU operates at 500,000 to more than 1 million Hz, which greatly enhances the effect of capacitive coupling and causes a marked reduction in impedance. Therefore even with isolated ESUs, the decrease in impedance allows the current to return to the ESU by alternate pathways. In addition, the isolated ESU does not protect the patient from burns if the return electrode does not make proper contact with the patient. Although the isolated ESU does provide additional patient safety, it is by no means foolproof protection against the patient receiving a burn.

Preventing patient burns from the ESU is the responsibility of all professional staff in the OR. Not only the circulating nurse but also the surgeon and the anesthesiologist must be aware of proper techniques and be vigilant to potential problems. The most important factor is the proper application of the return plate; it is essential that the return plate has the appropriate amount of electrolyte gel and an intact return wire. Reusable return plates must be properly cleaned after each use, and disposable plates must be checked to ensure that the electrolyte has not dried out during storage. In addition, it is prudent to place the return plate as close as possible to the site of the operation; ECG pads should be placed as far from the site of the operation as is feasible. In addition, OR personnel must be alert to the potential for pools of flammable "prep" solutions, such as alcohol and acetone, to ignite when the ESU is used. If the ESU must be used on a patient with a demand pacemaker, the return electrode should be located below the thorax; in addition, preparations for treating potential dysrhythmias should be available, including a defibrillator, an external pacemaker, and a magnet to convert the pacemaker to a fixed rate. It is best to keep the pacemaker out of the path between the surgical site and the dispersal plate.

The ESU has also caused other problems in patients with pacemakers, including reprogramming and microshock.[40,41] If the surgeon requests higher than normal power settings on the ESU, this should alert both the circulating nurse and the anesthesiologist to a potential problem. The return plate and cable must be immediately inspected to ensure that it is functioning and properly positioned. If this does not correct the problem, the return plate should be replaced.[42,43] If the problem remains, the entire ESU should be taken out of service. Finally, an ESU that is dropped or damaged must be removed immediately from the OR and thoroughly tested by a qualified biomedical engineer. Following these simple safety steps will prevent most patient burns from the ESU.

The previous discussion concerned only *unipolar* ESUs; a second type of ESU, in which the current passes only between the two blades of a pair of forceps, is also used. This type of device is referred to as a *bipolar* ESU. Because the active and return electrodes are the two blades of the forceps, it is not necessary to attach another dispersive electrode to the patient, unless a unipolar ESU is also being used. The bipolar ESU generates considerably less power than the unipolar device and is mainly used for ophthalmic and neurologic surgery.

In 1980 Mirowski and colleagues[44] reported the first human implantation of a device to treat intractable ventricular tachydysrhythmias. This device, known as the *automatic implantable cardioverter-defibrillator* (AICD), is capable of sensing ventricular tachycardia and ventricular fibrillation and automatically defibrillating the patient. Since 1980, thousands of patients have received AICD implants.[45,46] Because some of these patients may come in for noncardiac surgery, it is important that the anesthesiologist be aware of potential problems.[47] The use of a unipolar ESU may cause electrical interference that could be interpreted by the AICD as a ventricular tachydysrhythmia. This would trigger a defibrillation pulse to be delivered to the patient and would likely cause an actual episode of ventricular tachycardia or ventricular fibrillation. The patient with an AICD is also at risk for ventricular fibrillation during electroconvulsive therapy.[47] In both cases, the AICD should be disabled by placing a magnet over the device or by use of a specific protocol to shut it off; the device can be reactivated by reversing the process. In any event, it is best to consult with someone experienced with the device before starting surgery. Also, an external defibrillator and a noninvasive pacemaker should be in the OR whenever a patient with an AICD is anesthetized.

Electrical safety in the OR is a matter of combining common sense with some basic principles of electricity. Once OR personnel understand the importance of safe electrical practices, they are able to develop a heightened awareness to potential problems. All electrical equipment must undergo routine maintenance, service, and inspection to ensure that it conforms to designated electrical safety standards. Records of these test results must be kept for future inspection, because human error can easily compound electrical hazards. Starmer and colleagues[48] cited one case concerning a newly constructed laboratory, where the ground wire was not attached to a receptacle. In another study Albisser and colleagues[49] found a 14% (198 of 1424) incidence of improperly or incorrectly wired outlets.

Potentially hazardous situations should be recognized and corrected before they become a problem. For instance, electrical power cords are frequently placed on the floor where they can be crushed by various carts or the anesthesia machine. These cords could be located overhead or placed in an area of low traffic flow. Multiple-plug extension boxes should not be left on the floor where they can come in contact with electrolyte solutions. These could easily be mounted on a cart or on the anesthesia machine. Pieces of equipment that have been damaged or have obvious defects in the power cord must not be used until they have been properly repaired. If everyone is aware of what constitutes a potential hazard, dangerous situations can be prevented with minimal effort.

Sparks generated by the ESU may provide the ignition source for a fire with resulting burns to the patient and OR personnel. This is a particular risk when the ESU is used in an oxygen-enriched environment as may be present in the patient's airway or in close proximity to the patient's face. The administration of high-flow nasal oxygen to a sedated patient during procedures on the face and eye is particularly hazardous. Most plastics that would not burn in room air, such as tracheal tubes and components of the anesthetic breathing system, will ignite in the presence of oxygen or nitrous oxide. Tenting of the drapes to allow dispersion of any accumulated oxygen or its dilution by room air or use of a circle anesthesia breathing system with minimal to no leak of gases around the anesthesia mask will decrease the risk of ignition from a spark generated by a nearby ESU.

Conductive Flooring

In the past, conductive flooring was mandated for ORs where flammable anesthetic agents were being administered to minimize the buildup of static charges that could cause a flammable anesthetic agent to ignite. The standards have now been changed to eliminate the necessity for conductive flooring in anesthetizing areas where flammable agents are no longer used.

ENVIRONMENTAL HAZARDS

A number of potential electrical hazards in the OR are of concern to the anesthesiologist. The potential for electrical shock is present not only for the patient but also for OR personnel. In addition, cables and power cords to electrical equipment and monitoring devices can become hazardous through wear and misuse. Finally, all OR personnel should have a plan that outlines what to do in the event of a power failure.

Today's OR is populated with literally dozens of pieces of electrical equipment. It is not uncommon to have numerous power cords lying on the floor, where they are vulnerable to damage. If the insulation on the power cable becomes damaged, it is fairly easy for the hot wire to come in contact with a piece of metal equipment. If the OR does not have isolated power, that piece of equipment can become energized and pose a potential electrical shock hazard.[50] Having isolated power minimizes the risk to the patient and OR personnel. Clearly, getting electrical power cords off the floor is desirable. This can be accomplished by having electrical outlets in the ceiling or by having ceiling-mounted articulated arms that contain electrical outlets. Also, the use of multiple-outlet extension boxes that sit on the floor can be hazardous and should be avoided. In addition, these can become contaminated with fluids, which could easily trip the circuit breaker. In one case, it apparently tripped the main circuit breaker for the entire OR and resulted in a loss of all electrical power except for the overhead lights.[51]

Modern monitoring devices have many safety features incorporated into them. Virtually all of them have isolated the patient input from the power supply of the device. This is frequently done with optocoupler isolation circuits, an important feature that was lacking in the original ECG monitors. In the early days, patients could actually become part of the electrical circuit of the monitor. Relatively few problems have been experienced with patients and monitoring devices since the advent of isolated inputs. However, between 1985 and 1994, the Food and Drug Administration (FDA) received approximately 24 reports in which infants and children had received an electrical shock, including five children who died by electrocution.[52,53] These electrical accidents occurred because the electrode lead wires from either an ECG monitor or an apnea monitor were plugged directly into a 120 V electrical outlet instead of the appropriate patient cable. In 1997, the FDA issued a new performance standard for electrode lead wires and patient cables that requires exposed male connector pins from the electrode lead wires to be eliminated. Therefore, the lead wires must have female connections, and the connector pins must be housed in a protected patient cable (Fig. 31-35). This effectively eliminates the possibility of the patient being connected directly to an AC source, because no connector pins on the lead wires are exposed.

All health care facilities are required to have a source of emergency power. This generally consists of one or more electrical generators configured to start up automatically and provide power to the facility within 10 seconds after detecting a loss of power from the utility company. The facility is required to test these generators on a regular basis. However, in the past, not all health care facilities tested them under actual load. There are numerous anecdotal reports of generators not functioning properly during an actual power failure. If the generators are not tested under actual load, it is possible that

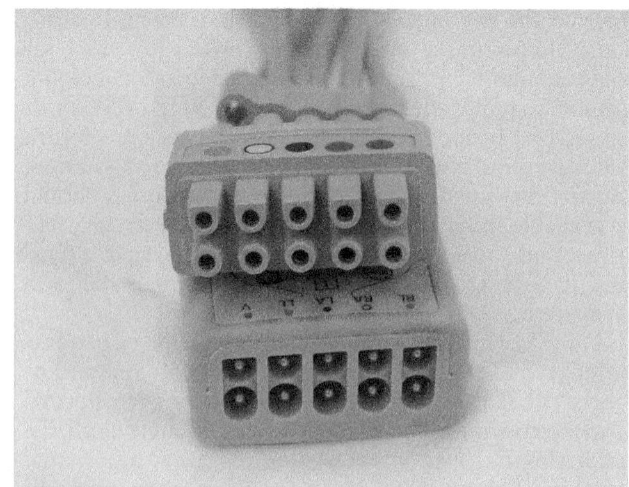

FIGURE 31-35 ■ The current standard for patient lead wires (*top*) requires a female connector. The patient cable (*bottom*) has shielded connector pins that the lead wires plug into.

many years will pass before a real power outage puts a severe demand on the generator. If the facility has several generators and one of them fails, the increased demand on the others may be enough to cause them all to fail in rapid succession. Under the current National Fire Protection Association (NFPA) 99 standards, hospitals must test their emergency power supply systems (generators) under connected load once a month for at least 30 minutes. If the generator is oversized for the application and cannot be loaded to at least 30% of its rating, it must be load-banked and run for a total of 2 hours every year. A fairly recent requirement is for emergency power supply systems to be tested once every 3 years for 4 continuous hours, with a recommendation that this be performed during peak usage of the system.[54,55]

Although all hospitals are required to have emergency generators to power essential equipment in the event of a power failure, they do not function in every circumstance. If there is a loss of power from the electrical utility, this is detected by a relay switch, which causes a series of events to activate the transfer of the power generation to the backup system. This usually happens seamlessly. However, if the transfer switch or the generator fails, there will be no back-up electricity.

Another cause of partial or total power failure has to do with construction mishaps. As hospitals frequently remodel, add new wings, or upgrade existing facilities, there is always a chance that the power will be accidentally interrupted, such as from a worker tripping a GFCI or a relay failure that causes a power transfer to a nonworking generator.[56,57] Because the electrical utility is still supplying power, the generators may not be activated.

It is vitally important that each OR have a contingency plan for a power failure. There should be a supply of battery-operated light sources available in each OR. A laryngoscope can serve as a readily available source of light until flashlights and such can be located. The overhead lights in the OR should also be connected to some sort of battery-operated lighting system. Most anesthesia machines have a back-up battery that will last

30 to 60 minutes. If the power failure lasts longer than that, the anesthesiologist must plan how to continue the anesthetic. The newer electronic machines may be more problematic than older traditional machines, because they may have electronic gas or vaporization systems. The department should have a supply of battery-powered monitors, but it is unlikely there will be enough for every OR. Syringe pumps typically have a battery, and BP can be taken with a manual sphygmomanometer. Because many ORs use automated drug-dispensing systems, these devices will not work without power and a communication link to the hospital information system. In reality, the back-up generators will usually supply power in the event of an emergency. However, there are many circumstances in which a hospital could experience partial or total power loss. And although the cost of preparing for these contingencies is relatively small, the benefits can be invaluable in an emergency.

ELECTROMAGNETIC INTERFERENCE

Rapid advances in technology have led to an explosion in the number of wireless communication devices in the marketplace. These devices include cellular telephones, cordless telephones, walkie-talkies, and wireless Internet access devices. All of these devices have something in common: they emit electromagnetic interference (EMI). The problem with this most commonly manifests when traveling on airplanes: most airlines require that these devices be turned off when the plane is taking off or landing, and in some cases during the entire flight, because of a concern that the EMI emitted by these devices may interfere with the plane's navigation and communication equipment.

In recent years, the number of people who own these devices has increased exponentially. Indeed, in some hospitals, such devices form a vital link in both the regular and emergency communication systems. It is not uncommon for physicians, nurses, paramedics, and other personnel to have their own cellular telephones. In addition, patients and visitors may also have cellular telephones and other types of communication devices. Hospital maintenance and security personnel frequently have walkie-talkie–type radios, and some hospitals have even instituted an in-house cellular telephone network that augments or replaces the paging system. However, concern has been raised that the EMI emitted by these devices may interfere with implanted pacemakers and various types of monitoring devices and ventilators in critical care areas.[58] One patient death was reported when a ventilator malfunctioned secondary to EMI.[59]

Several studies have been done to find out whether cellular telephones cause problems with cardiac pacemakers. One report by Hayes and colleagues[60] studied 980 patients with five different types of cellular telephones. They conducted more than 5000 tests and found that in more than 20% of the cases, they could detect some interference from the cellular telephone. Patients were symptomatic in 7.2% of the cases, and clinically significant interference occurred in 6.6% of the cases. When the telephone was held in the normal position over the ear, clinically significant interference was not detected. In fact, the interference that caused clinical symptoms occurred only if the telephone was directly over the pacemaker. Other studies have demonstrated changes such as erroneous sensing and pacer inhibition.[61,62] Again, these occurred only when the telephone was close to the pacemaker. The changes were temporary, and the pacemaker reverted to normal when the cellular telephone was moved to a safe distance. Currently, the FDA guidelines are that the cellular telephones be kept at least 6 inches from the pacemaker. Therefore, a patient with a pacemaker should not carry a cellular telephone in a shirt pocket adjacent to the pacemaker. There appears to be little risk if hospital personnel carry a cellular telephone if they ensure that it is kept at a reasonable distance from patients with a pacemaker.

AICDs comprise another group of devices of concern to biomedical engineers. Fetter and colleagues[63] conducted a study of 41 patients who had AICDs. They concluded that cellular telephones did not interfere with AICDs, although they did recommend keeping the cellular telephone at least 6 inches from the device.

EMI extends well beyond that of cellular telephones. Walkie-talkies, which are frequently used by hospital maintenance and security personnel; paging systems; police radios; and even televisions all emit EMI that could potentially interfere with medical devices. Although anecdotal reports abound, the amount of available scientific information on this problem is scant. Reports of interference include ventilator and infusion pumps that have been shut down or reprogrammed, interference with ECG monitors, and even an electronic wheelchair that was accidentally started because of EMI. It is a difficult problem to study because of the many different types of devices that emit EMI and the vast array of medical equipment with the potential to interact with these devices. Even though a device may seem safe in the medical environment, if two or three cellular telephones or walkie-talkies are brought together in the same area at the same time, unanticipated problems or interference may result.

Any time a cellular telephone is turned on, it is actually communicating with the cellular network even though a call is not in progress; therefore the potential to interfere with devices exists. The Emergency Care Research Institute (ECRI) reported in October 1999 that walkie-talkies were far more likely to cause problems with medical devices than cellular telephones.[64] This is because they operate on a lower frequency than cellular telephones and have a higher power output. The ECRI recommends that cellular telephones be maintained at a distance of 1 m from medical devices, while walkie-talkies be kept at a distance of 6 to 8 m.

Some hospitals have made restrictive policies on the use of cellular telephones, particularly in critical care areas.[65] These policies are supported by scant scientific documentation and are nearly impossible to enforce; indeed, the ubiquitous presence of cellular telephones carried by hospital personnel and visitors makes enforcing a ban virtually impossible. Even when people try to comply with the ban, failure is nearly inevitable because the general public is usually unaware that a cellular telephone in the standby mode is still communicating with the tower and generating EMI.

The real solution is to "harden" devices against EMI. This is difficult to do because of the many different frequencies over which these devices operate, and education of medical personnel is essential; when working in an OR or critical care area, all personnel must be alert to the fact that electronic devices and pacemakers can be interfered with by EMI. Creating a restrictive policy would certainly irritate personnel and visitors, and, in some cases, may actually compromise emergency communications.[66]

CONSTRUCTION OF NEW OPERATING ROOMS

Frequently, an anesthesiologist is asked to consult with hospital administrators and architects in designing new ORs or remodeling older facilities. In the past a strict electrical code was enforced because of the use of flammable anesthetic agents. This code included a requirement for IPSs and LIMs. The NFPA revised its standard for health care facilities in 1984 (NFPA 99-1984), and the new standards did not require IPSs or LIMs in areas designated for use of nonflammable anesthetic agents only.[67,68] Although not mandatory, NFPA standards are usually adopted by local authorities when revising their electrical codes.

This change in the standard created a dilemma. The NFPA 99-2012 Health Care Facilities Code mandates that "wet procedure locations shall be provided with special protection against electrical shock." Section 6.3.2.2.8.2 further states that "this special protection shall be provided as follows: (1) Power distribution system that inherently limits the possible ground-fault current due to a first fault to a low value, without interrupting the power supply. (2) Power distribution system in which the power supply is interrupted if the ground-fault current does, in fact, exceed the trip value of a Class A GFCI."[69]

The decision of whether to install isolated power hinges on two factors. The first is whether the OR is considered a wet location, and, if so, whether an interruptible power supply is tolerable. When power interruption is tolerable, a GFCI is permitted as the protective means. However, the standard also states that "the use of an isolated power system (IPS) shall be permitted as a protective means capable of limiting ground fault current without power interruption."

Most people who have worked in an OR would attest to its being a wet procedure location. The presence of blood, body fluids, and saline solutions spilled on the floor all contribute to making this a wet environment. The cystoscopy suite serves as a good example.

Once the premise that the OR is a wet location is accepted, it must be determined whether a GFCI can provide the means of protection. The argument against using GFCIs in the OR is illustrated by the following example. Assume that during an open heart procedure, the cardiopulmonary bypass pump and the patient monitors are plugged into outlets on the same branch circuit. Also assume that during bypass, the circulating nurse now plugs in a faulty headlight. If there is a GFCI protecting the circuit, the fault will be detected, and the GFCI will interrupt all power to the pump and the monitors. This undoubtedly would cause a great deal of confusion and consternation among the OR personnel and may place the patient at risk for injury. The pump would have to be manually operated while the problem was being resolved. In addition, the GFCI could not be reset, nor could power be restored, until the headlight was identified as the cause of the fault and unplugged from the outlet. However, if the OR were protected with an IPS and LIM, the same scenario would cause the LIM to alarm, but the pump and patient monitors would continue to operate normally. There would be no interruption of power, and the problem could be resolved without risk to the patient.

It should be realized that a GFCI is an active system. That is, a potentially hazardous current is already flowing and must be actively interrupted, whereas the IPS (with LIM) is designed to be safe during a first-fault situation. Thus, it is a passive system, because no mechanical action is required to activate the protection.[70]

Many hospital administrators and engineers wanted to eliminate IPSs in new OR construction by advocating that they were unnecessary and costly. They also grossly inflated the maintenance costs of the IPS. In fact the maintenance costs of modern systems are minimal, and the instillation costs are approximately 1% to 2% of the cost of constructing a new OR. The American Society of Anesthesiologists (ASA) and others, however, had advocated for the retention of IPSs.[70-73] In 2006, through its representatives to NFPA-99 and its technical committee on electrical systems, the ASA launched a major campaign to have ORs default to being a wet procedure location. This was vigorously opposed by the American Hospital Association and the American Society of Healthcare Engineers. The final version of the NFPA-99 2012 edition contains the following language: "Section 6.3.2.2.8.4 ORs shall be considered to be a wet procedure location, unless a risk assessment conducted by the health care governing body determines otherwise." In addition section 6.3.2.2.8.7 states: "Operating rooms defined as wet procedure locations shall be protected by either isolated power or ground fault circuit interrupters." Although this code applies only to new or remodeled ORs, it is nonetheless a major victory for the ASA, our patients, and OR personnel. In the event that the health care facility wants to classify an ORs as a "dry" location, they will have to do a risk assessment, and the NFPA-99 annex (A.6.3.2.2.8.4) states that among others, this should include clinicians.[69]

Although not perfect,[74] the IPS and LIM do provide both the patient and OR personnel with a significant amount of protection in an electrically hazardous environment. IPSs provide clean stable voltages, which are important for sensitive diagnostic equipment.[75] Also, modern microprocessor-based LIMs require only yearly, instead of monthly, testing.

The value of the IPS is illustrated in a report by Day[76] in 1994 of four instances of electrical shock to OR personnel in a 1-year period. The operating suite had been renovated and the IPS removed, and it was not until the OR personnel received a shock that a problem was discovered. Also, in 2010, Wills and colleagues[77] reported an incident in which an OR nurse received a severe electrical shock while plugging in a piece of equipment. This case further illustrates the consequences of having a wet floor in an OR with no IPS or GFCIs.

Anesthesiologists need to be aware of these new regulations and must strongly encourage others that new ORs be constructed with IPSs. The relatively small cost savings that the alternative would represent do not justify the elimination of such a useful safety system. The use of GFCIs in the OR environment can be acceptable if carefully planned and engineered. To avoid the loss of power to multiple instruments and monitors at one time, each outlet must be an individual GFCI. If that is the case, a fault will result in only one piece of equipment losing power. Using GFCIs also precludes the use of multiple plug strips in the OR.

Finally, in 2011, August[78] reported on the opening of 24 new ORs in his facility. To their dismay, they found that the electrical service panels outside each OR were locked, and that the ORs had been reclassified as "dry" locations without the knowledge of the anesthesia department. Barker[79] also reported an incident in which a postanesthesia critical care unit (PACU) monitor overheated and was billowing smoke. An attempt to shut off the power was met with a locked circuit breaker box. As a result, Barker also commented on the need to have ORs designated as wet procedure locations.

It is hoped that with the new NFPA-99 code, far fewer new ORs will be designated as "dry" locations, especially without the knowledge of the anesthesia department. It should be remembered that electrical safety is the concern of everyone in the OR. Accidents can be prevented only if appropriate safety equipment in the OR has been properly installaed and maintained and if OR personnel understand the concepts of electrical safety and are vigilant in their efforts to detect new hazards.[80]

FIRE SAFETY

Fires in the OR are just as much a danger today as they were 100 years ago, when patients were anesthetized with flammable anesthetic agents.[81,82] Because the potential consequences of a fire or explosion with ether or cyclopropane were well known and potentially devastating, OR fire safety practices were routinely followed.[83,84]

Today, the risk of an OR fire is probably as great or greater than in the days of ether and cyclopropane, in part because of the routine use of potential sources of ignition, including electrosurgical cauteries, in an environment rich in fuel sources (i.e., flammable materials) and oxidizers such as oxygen and nitrous oxide. Although the number of OR fires that occur annually in the United States is unknown, some estimates suggest that there are 550 to 650 fires each year, with as many as 5% to 10% associated with serious injury or death.[85] In contrast to the era of flammable anesthetics, there currently appears to be a lack of awareness of the potential for an OR fire. In response to the risks presented by this situation, in 2008 the ASA released a practice advisory on the prevention and management of operating room fires (Box 31-1).[86]

BOX 31-1 Recommendations for the Prevention and Management of Operating Room Fires

PREPARATION

Train personnel in operating room fire management.
Practice responses to fires (fire drills).
Ensure that fire management equipment is readily available.
Determine if a high-risk situation exists.
The team decides how to prevent/manage a fire.
Each person is assigned a task (e.g., remove endotracheal tube, disconnect circuit).

PREVENTION

Allow flammable skin preparations to dry before draping.
Configure surgical drapes to avoid buildup of oxidizer.
The anesthesiologist collaborates with the team throughout the procedure to minimize oxidizer-enriched environment near ignition source.
Keep oxygen (O_2) concentration as low as clinically possible.
Avoid nitrous oxide (N_2O).
Notify surgeon if oxidizer and ignition source are in proximity to each other.
Moisten gauze and sponges near any ignition source.

MANAGEMENT

Look for early warning signs of a fire, such as a pop, flash, or smoke.
Stop the procedure and have each team member immediately carry out an assigned task.

AIRWAY FIRE

Simultaneously remove the endotracheal tube and stop gases/disconnect circuit.
Pour saline into airway.
Remove burning materials.
Mask ventilate the patient, assess injury, consider bronchoscopy, and reintubate.

FIRE ON THE PATIENT

Turn off gases.
Remove drapes and burning materials.
Extinguish flames with water, saline, or fire extinguisher.
Assess patient's status, devise care plan, assess for smoke inhalation.

FAILURE TO EXTINGUISH

Use carbon dioxide fire extinguisher.
Activate the fire alarm.
Consider evacuation of the room: once outside, close the doors and do not reopen them.
Turn off the medical gas supply to room.

RISK MANAGEMENT

Preserve the scene.
Notify hospital risk manager.
Follow local regulatory reporting requirements.
Treat the fire as an adverse event.
Conduct fire drills regularly.

Modified from American Society of Anesthesiologists: Practice advisory for the prevention and management of operating room fires, approved by the ASA House of Delegates in October 2007. Park Ridge, IL, American Society of Anesthesiologists. Published in *Anesthesiology* May 2008.

For a fire to start, three components are necessary: the limbs of the "fire triad" are heat or an ignition source, fuel, and an oxidizer (Fig. 31-36).[87] A fire occurs when a fuel reacts chemically with an oxidizer, rapidly combining to release energy in the form of heat and light. Many heat and ignition sources are present in the OR, such as the ESU, lasers, and the ends of fiberoptic light cords. The main oxidizers in the OR are air, oxygen, and nitrous oxide. Oxygen and nitrous oxide function equally well as oxidizers, so a combination of 50% oxygen and 50% nitrous oxide would support combustion, as would 100% oxygen. Fuel for a fire can be found everywhere in the OR: paper drapes, which have largely replaced cloth drapes, are much easier to ignite and can burn with greater intensity.[88,89] Other sources of fuel include gauze dressings, endotracheal tubes, gel mattress pads, and even facial or body hair (Box 31-2).[90]

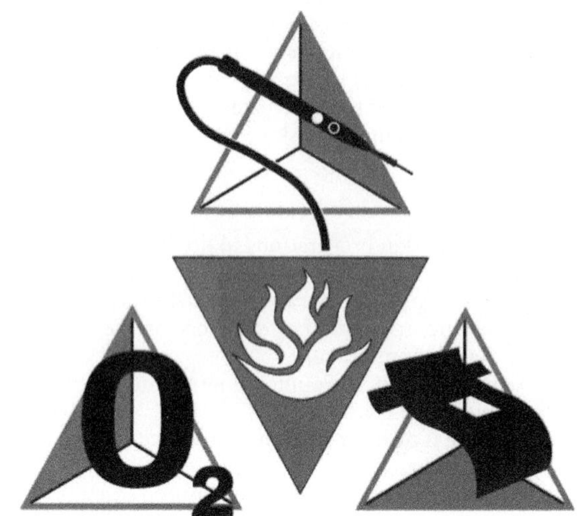

FIGURE 31-36 ■ The fire triad. (Copyright ECRI Institute. Used with permission.)

Fire prevention is accomplished by not allowing all three of the elements of the fire triad to come together at the same time.[91] The challenge in the OR is that frequently each of the limbs of the fire triad is controlled by a different individual. For instance, the surgeon is frequently in charge of the ignition source, the anesthesiologist is usually administering the oxidizer, and the OR nurse frequently controls the fuel sources. It is not always evident to any one individual that all of these elements may be coming together at the same time. This is especially true where the possibility exists for oxygen or an oxygen–nitrous oxide mixture to be delivered around the surgical site. In these circumstances, the risk of an OR

BOX 31-2 Fuel Sources Commonly Found in the Operating Room

"Prep" Agents
- Alcohol
- Degreasers (acetone, ether)
- Adhesives (tincture of benzoin, Aeroplast)
- Chlorhexidine digluconate (Hibitane)
- Iodophor (Dura-Prep)

Drapes, Covers, and Special Clothing
- Patient drapes (paper, plastic, cloth)
- Equipment drapes (paper, plastic, cloth)
- Blankets and sheets
- Pillows, mattresses, and padding
- Gowns
- Masks
- Shoe covers
- Gloves (latex, nonlatex)
- Clothing
- Compression (antiembolism) stockings

Patient
- Hair
- Alimentary tract gases (methane, hydrogen)
- Desiccated tissue

Dressings
- Gauze and sponges
- Petrolatum-impregnated dressings
- Xeroform
- Adhesive tape (cloth, plastic, paper)
- Elastic bandages
- Stockingettes
  - Sutures
  - Steri-Strips
  - Collodion

Ointments
- Petrolatum
- Antibiotics (bacitracin, neomycin, polymyxin B)
- Nitropaste (Nitro-Bid)
- EMLA
- Lip balms

Anesthesia Equipment
- Breathing circuit hoses
- Masks
- Endotracheal tubes
- Oral and nasal airways
- Laryngeal mask airways
- Nasogastric tubes
- Suction catheters and tubing
- Scavenger hoses
- Volatile anesthetics
- Carbon dioxide absorbers
- Intravenous tubing
- Pressure monitor tubing and plastic transducers

Other Equipment
- Charts and records
- Cardboard, wooden, and particle board boxes and cabinets
- Packing materials (cardboard, styrofoam)
- Fiberoptic cable covers
- Wire covers and insulation
- Fiberoptic endoscope coverings
- Sphygmomanometer cuffs and tubing
- Pneumatic tourniquet cuffs and tubing
- Stethoscope tubing
- Vascular shunts (Gore-Tex, Dacron)
- Dialysis and extracorporeal circulation circuits
- Wound drains and collection systems
- Mops and brooms

fire is markedly increased, and the need for communication among the surgeon, anesthesiologist, and OR nurses throughout the procedure is essential.

Several dangers may result from an OR fire. The most obvious is that the patient and OR personnel can sustain severe burns. However, a less obvious but potentially more deadly risk can be posed by the products of combustion, called *toxicants*. When materials such as plastics burn, a variety of injurious compounds can be produced. These include carbon monoxide, ammonia, hydrogen chloride, and even cyanide. Toxicants can produce injury by damaging airways and lung tissue, and they can cause asphyxia. OR fires can often produce significant amounts of smoke and toxicants, but they may not cause enough heat to activate overhead sprinkler systems. If enough smoke is produced, OR personnel may have to evacuate the area. Thus it is essential to have a carefully planned and considered evacuation plan prepared ahead of time for both the OR personnel and the patient.

OR fires can be divided into two different types. The more common type of fire occurs *in* or *on* the patient, especially during high-risk procedures in which an ignition source is used in an oxidizer-rich environment. These would include airway fires—including endotracheal tube fires; fires in the oropharynx, which may occur during a tonsillectomy; fires in the breathing circuit—and fires that occur during laparoscopy. In 2005, Katz and Campbell[92] reported on a fire during a thoracotomy. A dry gauze lap pad was set on fire because 100% oxygen was present in the thoracic cavity while the surgeon was using the electrocautery. Cases that involve stripping of the pleura or resection of pulmonary blebs can easily result in high concentrations of oxygen in the thoracic cavity when the lung is reinflated because of gas leakage. Solutions to this problem include making sure that the lap pads are always wet, and if the surgeon needs the lung inflated, then doing continuous positive airway pressure (CPAP) with air instead of oxygen will greatly reduce the risk of a fire.

Fires that occur on patients mainly involve head and neck surgery done under regional anesthesia or monitored anesthesia care when the patient is receiving high flows of supplemental oxygen. Because these fires occur in an oxygen-enriched environment, items such as surgical towels, drapes, or even the body hair can be readily ignited and produce a severe burn. Oxygen-enriched atmospheres lower the ignition temperature for any fuel source.[85] In addition, such fires will burn more vigorously and spread faster. The other type of OR fire is one that is remote from the patient. This would include an electrical fire in a piece of equipment or a carbon dioxide (CO_2) absorber fire.

There no such thing as an inflammable material in the presence of an oxygen-enriched environment. Wolf and colleagues[93] tested a number of surgical drape materials in 21%, 50%, and 95% oxygen. They found that the higher the concentration of oxygen, the more readily the material could be set on fire. In 50% and 95% oxygen, all the materials burned. In the case of a cotton huck towel, the time to ignition in 21% oxygen was a mean of 12 seconds. The same material ignited in 0.1 seconds in 95% oxygen.

The two major ignition sources for OR fires are the ESU and the laser. However, the ends of some fiberoptic light cords can also become hot enough to start a fire if they are placed on paper drapes. Although the ESU is responsible for igniting the majority of the fires,[94] it is the laser that has generated the most attention and research. *Laser* is an acronym for *light amplification by stimulated emission of radiation*. A laser consists of an energy source and material that the energy excites to emit light.[95-97] The material that the energy excites is called the *lasing medium*, and it provides the name for the particular type of laser (e.g., argon, yttrium-aluminum-garnet [YAG]). The important property of laser light is that it is coherent radiation, meaning that is monochromatic (a single wavelength), coherent (photons are in phase with each other), and collimated (the beam does not disperse as the distance from the source increases). This coherent light can be focused into very small spots that have very high power density.

Many different types of medical lasers are available, and each has a specific application. The argon laser is used in eye and dermatologic procedures, because argon is absorbed by hemoglobin and has a modest tissue penetration of between 0.05 and 2.0 mm. The potassium-titanyl-phosphate (KTP) or frequency-doubled YAG lasers are also absorbed by hemoglobin and have tissue penetrations similar to that of the argon laser. The tunable dye laser has a wavelength that is easily changed, and it can be used in different applications, particularly in dermatologic procedures. The neodymium-doped YAG (Nd:YAG) laser is the most powerful of the medical lasers. Because the tissue penetration is between 2 and 6 mm, it can be used for tumor debulking, particularly in the trachea and mainstem bronchi or in the upper airway. The energy can be transmitted through a fiberoptic cable placed down the suction port of a fiberoptic bronchoscope. The laser can then be used in a contact mode to treat a tumor mass. The CO_2 laser has very little tissue penetration and can be used where great precision is needed. Carbon dioxide is also absorbed by water, so minimal heat is dispersed to surrounding tissues. The CO_2 laser is used primarily for procedures in the oropharynx and in and around the vocal cords. The helium–neon laser (He-Ne) produces an intense red light and thus can be used for aiming the CO_2 and the Nd:YAG lasers; because it has very low power, it presents no significant danger to OR personnel.

One of the most devastating types of OR fires occurs when an endotracheal tube is ignited *in* the patient.[98-103] If the patient is being ventilated with oxygen and/or nitrous oxide, the endotracheal tube will essentially emit a blowtorch-type of flame that can result in severe injury to the trachea, lungs, and surrounding tissues (Fig. 31-37). Red rubber, polyvinyl chloride (PVC), and silicone endotracheal tubes all have *oxygen-flammability indexes*, defined as the minimum oxygen fraction in nitrogen that will just support a candlelike flame for a given fuel source using a standard ignition source[104] of less than 26%.[105] Historically, anesthesiologists attempted to improve the safety of these tubes by wrapping red rubber or PVC tubes with some sort of reflective tape. However, tape-wrapped tubes often became kinked, gaps formed in the tape and expose areas of the tube to the laser, and non–laser-resistant tape was sometimes unintentionally used. To prevent these problems during high-risk

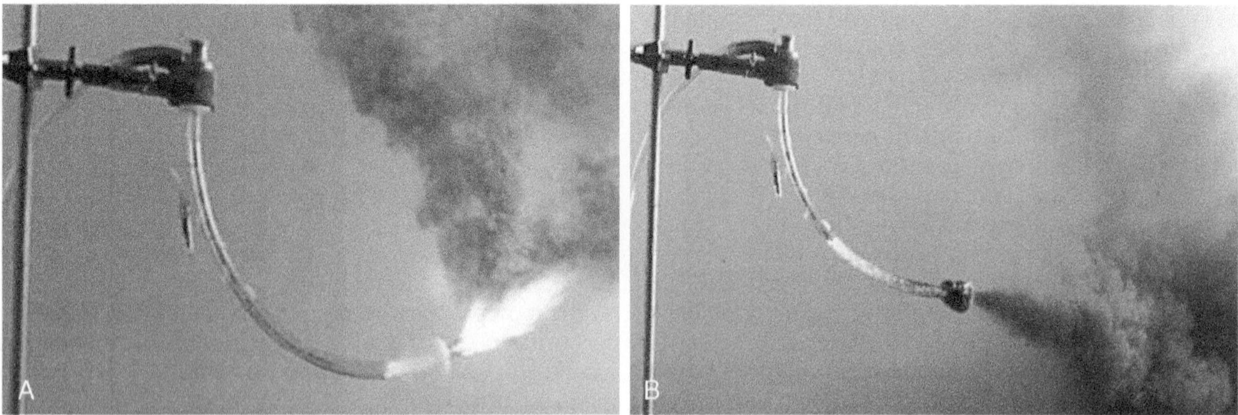

FIGURE 31-37 ■ A, Burning endotracheal (ET) tube with a high concentration of O_2 or O_2/N_2O will exhibit a "blowtorch" effect. B, A burning ET tube will produce a large amount of debris. (Copyright ECRI Institute. Used with permission.)

procedures, laser-resistant endotracheal tubes have been developed.[106-108] Anesthesiologists can now use an endotracheal tube designed to be resistant to ignition by the specific type of laser that will be used during surgery. For instance, when using the CO_2 laser, the LaserFlex (Mallinckrodt, St. Louis, MO; Fig 31-38) is an excellent choice. This is a flexible metal tube that has two cuffs that can be inflated with saline colored with methylene blue. The methylene blue enables the surgeon to easily recognize if one of the cuffs has been penetrated. The LaserFlex tube is highly resistant to being struck by the laser. If the Nd:YAG laser is being used, then the Lasertubus (Rüsch, Duluth, GA) can be used (Fig. 31-39). The Lasertubus has a soft rubber shaft covered by a corrugated silver foil that is in turn covered in a Merocel sponge jacket. In order to provide maximum protection, the Merocel (Medtronic; Mystic, CT) must be kept moist with saline. Of note, only the portion of the tube covered with the Merocel is laser resistant.

Another potential source of ignition for an OR fire is the ESU.[109,110] A typical example of how an ESU could cause ignition would be during a tonsillectomy in a child in whom the anesthesiologist was using an uncuffed, flammable endotracheal tube. In this case, the oxygen or oxygen–nitrous oxide mixture could leak around the endotracheal tube and pool at the operative site, providing an oxidizer-enriched environment. When the surgeon uses the ESU or laser to cauterize the tonsil bed, the combination of a high concentration of oxidizer (O_2 or an O_2/N_2O mixture), fuel (endotracheal tube), and ignition source (the ESU or laser) could easily start a fire.[111,112]

The best way to prevent this type of fire is to take steps to prevent the three legs of the fire triad from coming together. For example, mixing the oxygen with air will keep the inspired oxygen concentration as low as possible, thus reducing the available oxidizer. Another possibility would be to place wet pledgets around the endotracheal tube, which would prevent the escape of oxygen or oxygen–nitrous oxide mixture from the trachea into the operative field; this reduces the available oxidizer and would keep the endotracheal tube and tissues from becoming desiccated, thus reducing their suitability as fuel sources. However, the pledgets must be kept moist, lest they dry out and become an additional source of fuel for a fire.

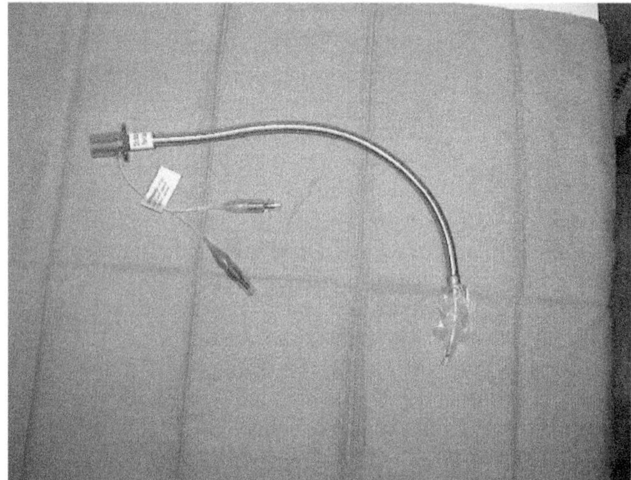

FIGURE 31-38 ■ LaserFlex laser-resistant endotracheal tube (Mallinckrodt Inc., St. Louis, MO).

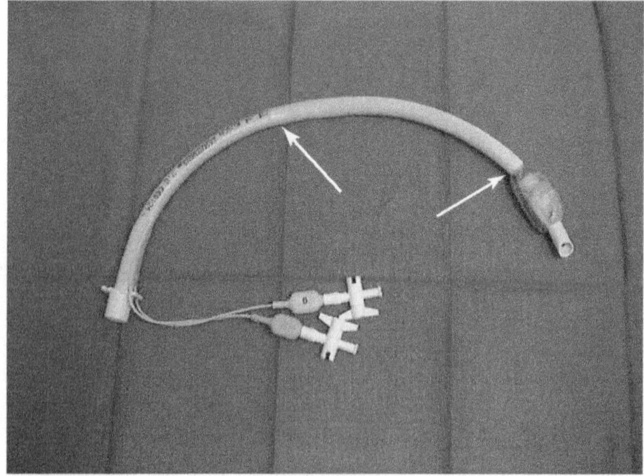

FIGURE 31-39 ■ Lasertubus laser-resistant endotracheal tube (Rüsch, Duluth, GA). *Arrows* denote laser-resistant covering.

A related situation that requires a different solution can arise when a critically ill patient requires a tracheostomy.[113,114] These patients may require very high concentrations of inspired oxygen to maintain tissue oxygenation so that any decrease in inspired oxygen concentration or interruption of ventilation would not be tolerated. In this circumstance, the best option for preventing a fire would be to avoid the use of electrocautery (ignition source) when the surgeon enters the trachea.

The Nd:YAG laser can be used to treat tumors of the lower trachea and mainstem bronchi. Most commonly, the surgeon will use a fiberoptic bronchoscope (FOB) and pass the laser fiber through the suction port of the bronchoscope. The FOB can be used in conjunction with a rigid metal bronchoscope or can be passed through an 8.5 or 9.0 mm PVC endotracheal tube. A special laser-resistant tube would not be used in this circumstance, because the FOB and laser fiber pass through the endotracheal tube and focus on tissue distal to the tube. Fire safety precautions available in this setting include titrating the concentration of inspired oxygen to as low a concentration as the patient can tolerate, while maintaining a saturation of between 90% and 95%, ideally keeping the inspired oxygen below 30%, keeping the tip of the endotracheal tube and FOB away from the site of surgery and out of the "line of fire" of the laser, and removing charred and desiccated tissue from the surgical field.

The use of a rigid metal bronchoscope instead of an endotracheal tube will eliminate the possibility of setting the tube on fire but does not eliminate the possibility of setting the FOB on fire. This would also necessitate the use of a jet Venturi system to ventilate the patient, which would in turn deliver an inspired oxygen concentration of between 40% and 60%.

A number of basic safety precautions should be taken whenever a laser is used in surgery. Because laser light can be reflected off any metal surface, it is important that all OR personnel wear protective goggles specific to the type of laser being used. The anesthesiologist must be aware that laser goggles may make it difficult to read certain monitor displays. In addition, it is important that the patient's eyes be covered with wet gauze or eye packs. In addition, OR personnel should wear high-filtration masks, because the laser "plume" may contain vaporized virus particles or chemical toxins. Finally, all doors to the OR should bear warning signs that a laser is in use, and all windows should be covered with black window shades.

Laparoscopic surgery in the abdomen is another potential risk for a surgical fire. Ordinarily, the abdomen is insufflated with carbon dioxide, which does not support combustion. It is important to verify that, indeed, only carbon dioxide is being used, as erroneous inclusion of oxygen can be disastrous.[115,116] Also, nitrous oxide administered to the patient as part of the anesthetic can, over 30 minutes, diffuse into the abdominal cavity and attain a concentration that could support combustion.[117] In fact, when sampling the abdominal gas contents after 30 minutes, the mean nitrous oxide concentration was 36%; however, in certain patients it reached a concentration of 47%. Both methane and hydrogen are flammable gases that are frequently present in bowel gas in significant concentrations. Methane concentration in bowel gas can be up to 56%, and hydrogen has been reported as high as 69%. With the maximum abdominal concentration of 47% nitrous oxide mixed with carbon dioxide, it would require the maximum of 56% of methane to be flammable. Therefore, this represents a relatively small hazard. In contrast, a concentration of 69% hydrogen is flammable if the nitrous oxide concentration is above 29%. Therefore a fire is possible if the surgeon enters the bowel while using the ESU, with a high concentration of hydrogen and an intraabdominal nitrous oxide content above 29%.

In recent years, fires *on* the patient seem to have become the most frequent type of OR fire. These cases occur most often during surgery in and around the head and neck, where the patient is receiving monitored anesthesia care, and supplemental oxygen is being administered by either a face mask or nasal cannula.[118-122] In these cases, the oxygen can collect under the drapes if it is not properly vented; and when the surgeon uses the ESU or the laser, a fire can easily start. There are many things that can act as fuel, such as the surgical towels, paper drapes, disinfecting preparation solutions, sponges, plastic tubing from the oxygen face mask, and even the body hair. These fires start very quickly and can turn into an intense blaze in only a few seconds. Even if the fire is quickly extinguished, the patient will usually sustain significant burns.

The majority of OR fires occur with monitored anesthesia care during head and neck surgery. Invariably, this involves an oxygen-enriched atmosphere, because 75% of surgical fires are oxygen enriched. Currently, the Anesthesia Patient Safety Foundation (APSF) and ECRI Institute recommend that there be no open delivery of oxygen during these cases.[85,123] If the patient needs increased levels of sedation during a time when the surgeon is using the ESU or laser, the airway should be secured with a laryngeal mask airway (LMA) or an endotracheal tube. Occasionally exceptional cases exist, in which the patient and the anesthesiologist need to communicate. An example of this might be a carotid endarterectomy or an awake craniotomy. In these cases it may be safe to use an FiO_2 up to 30%. Preferably, the patient should receive only room air during these cases.

The most important principle that the anesthesiologist has to keep in mind to minimize the risk of fire is to titrate the inspired oxygen to the lowest amount necessary to keep patient's oxygenation within safe levels. If the anesthesia machine has the ability to deliver air, the nasal cannula or face mask can be attached to the anesthesia circuit using a small (No. 3 or 4) 15-mm endotracheal tube adapter[124] attached to the right-angle elbow of the circuit. If the anesthesia machine is equipped with an auxiliary oxygen flowmeter that has a removable nipple adapter, a humidifier can be installed in place of the nipple adapter. The humidifier has a Venturi mechanism through which room air is entrained; thus the oxygen concentration delivered to the face mask can be varied from 28% to 100%. Finally, if this machine has a common gas outlet that is easily accessible, a nasal cannula or face mask can be attached at this point using the same small (3 or 4 mm) endotracheal tube adapter (Fig. 31-40). If it is necessary to deliver more than 30% oxygen to the patient, delivering 5 to 10 L/min of air under the drapes will dilute the oxygen, and the oxygen should always be discontinued at least 1 minute before the surgeon uses the ESU. Also, the bipolar ESU is preferable to the monopolar ESU, and it is important that the drapes be arranged in such a manner that no oxygen buildup can occur beneath them. Tenting the drapes and having the surgeon use an adhesive sticky drape that seals the operative site from the oxygen flow are steps that will help reduce the risk of a fire.

It is possible to discontinue the use of oxygen before the surgeon plans to use the electrocautery or laser. This would have to be done several minutes beforehand in order to allow any built-up oxygen to dissipate. If the surgeon is planning to use the electrocautery or laser during the entire case, this may not be practical. Also, the bipolar ESU is preferable to the monopolar ESU in this situation.

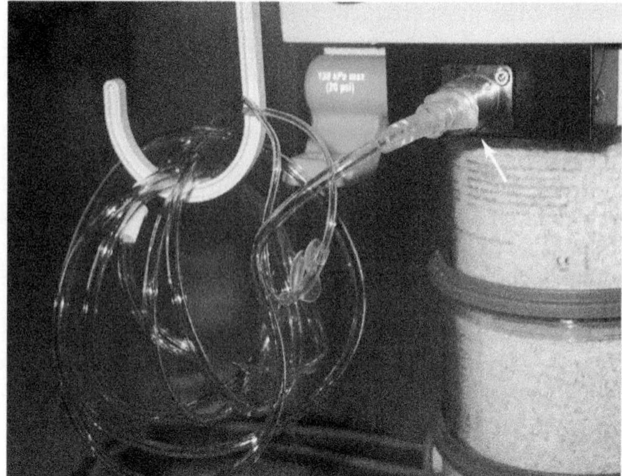

FIGURE 31-40 ■ A nasal cannula connected to the alternate fresh gas outlet *(arrow)* on a Datex-Ohmeda Aestiva (GE Healthcare, Waukesha, WI) anesthesia machine.

Some newer surgical preparation solutions can contribute to surgical fires.[125,126] These solutions typically come prepackaged in a "paint stick" applicator with a sponge on the end; the DuraPrep (St. Paul, MN) consists of iodophor mixed with 74% isopropyl alcohol, which is highly flammable and can easily provide fuel for an OR fire. In 2001, Barker and Polson[118] reported just such a case. In a laboratory re-creation, they found that if the DuraPrep had been allowed to dry completely (4 to 5 min), the fire would not have occured (Fig. 31-41). The other problem with these types of preparation solutions is that small pools of the solution can accumulate if the person doing the preparation is not careful. The alcohol in these small puddles will continue to evaporate for a period of time, and the alcohol vapors are also extremely flammable. Flammable skin preparation solutions should be allowed to dry and puddles should be wiped up before the site is draped (Fig. 31-42).

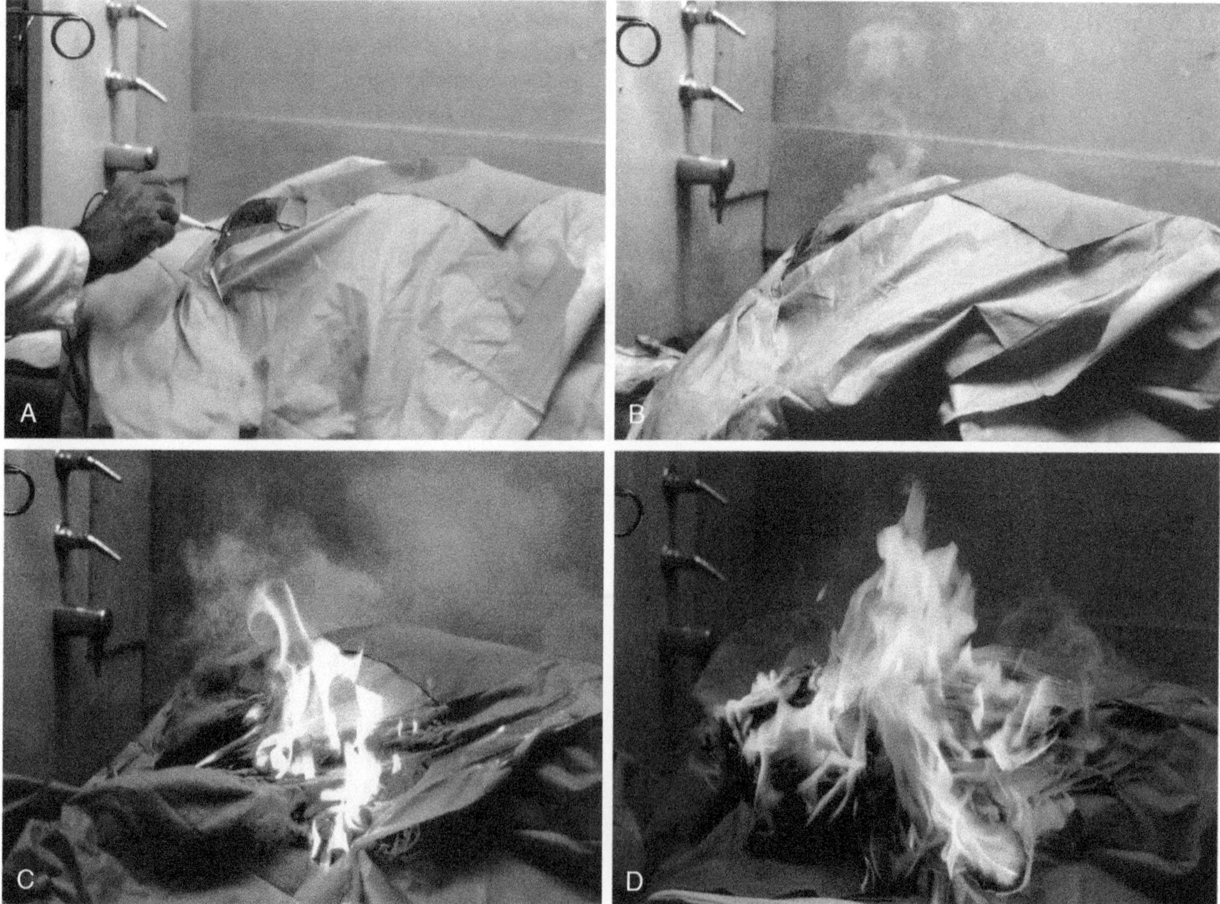

FIGURE 31-41 ■ Simulation of fire caused by electricosurgical unit (ESU) electrode during surgery. A, Mannequin prepared and draped for surgery. An ESU monopolar pencil electrode is applied to the operative site at the start of surgery. B, Six seconds after ESU application, smoke appears from under the drapes. C, Fourteen seconds after ESU application, flames burst through the drapes. D, Twenty-four seconds after ESU application, the patient's head and drapes in flames. (From Barker SJ, Polson JS: Fire in the operating room: a case report and laboratory study. *Anesth Analg* 2001; 93:960. Used with permission.)

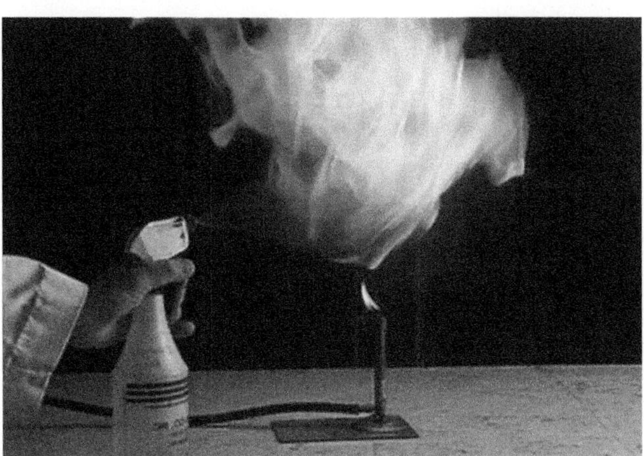

FIGURE 31-42 ■ A demonstration of the intense heat and flame present in an alcohol fire. (Photograph courtesy Marc Bruley, ECRI Institute. Reprinted with permission. Copyright 2009, ECRI Institute, www.ecri.org.)

It is important to bear in mind that halogenation of hydrocarbon anesthetics confers relative, but not absolute, resistance to combustion. Even the newer, "nonflammable" volatile anesthetics can, under certain circumstances, present fire hazards. For example, sevoflurane is nonflammable in air but can serve as a fuel at concentrations as low as 11% in oxygen and 10% in nitrous oxide.[127] In addition, sevoflurane and desiccated carbon dioxide absorbent, both soda lime and Baralyme, can undergo exothermic chemical reactions that have been implicated in several fires that involved the anesthesia breathing circuit.[128-131] In 2003, the manufacturer of sevoflurane published a "Dear Health Care Provider" letter and advisory alert.[132] To prevent futures fires, the manufacturer of sevoflurane has recommended that anesthesiologists use several measures to prevent fire that include avoiding the use of desiccated carbon dioxide absorbent and monitoring the temperature of the absorbers and the inspired concentration of sevoflurane. If elevated temperatures or an inspired sevoflurane concentration that differs unexpectedly from the vaporizer setting is detected, it is recommended that the patient be disconnected from the anesthesia circuit and monitored for signs of thermal or chemical injury and that the carbon dioxide absorbent be removed from the circuit and/or replaced.

Another way to prevent this type of fire is to use a carbon dioxide absorbent that does not contain a strong alkali, as do soda lime and Baralyme (no longer manufactured). Amsorb (Amstrong Medical Limited, Coleraine, UK) is a carbon dioxide absorbent that contains calcium hydroxide and calcium chloride but no strong alkali.[133] In experimental studies, Amsorb was found to be unreactive with currently used volatile anesthetics, and it did not produce carbon monoxide or compound A with desiccated absorbent; therefore it will not interact with sevoflurane and undergo an exothermic chemical reaction.

If a fire does occur, it is important to extinguish it as soon as possible. The first step is to interrupt the fire triad by removing one component. This is usually best accomplished by removing the oxidizer from the fire. Therefore if an endotracheal tube is on fire, disconnecting the circuit from the tube or disconnecting the inspiratory limb of the circuit will usually result in the fire immediately going out. Simultaneously the surgeon should remove the burning tracheal tube. Once the fire is extinguished, the airway is inspected via bronchoscopy, and the patient may be reintubated.

If the fire is *on* the patient, the most rapid and effective method to extinguish it is with a basin of saline. A sheet or towel may also be used. If the drapes are burning, particularly paper drapes, they must be removed and put on the floor. Paper drapes are impervious to water, thus throwing water or saline on them will do little to extinguish the fire. Once the burning drapes are removed from the patient, the fire can then be extinguished with a fire extinguisher. In most OR fires, the sprinkler system is not activated, because sprinklers are not located directly over the OR table, and OR fires seldom get hot enough to activate them.

All OR personnel should receive OR fire safety education, which should include training in institutional fire safety protocols and learning the location and operation of the fire extinguishers. Fire safety education, including fire drills, allows each member of the OR team to learn and practice what his or her responsibilities and actions should be if a fire were to occur. Fire drills are an important part of the plan and can help personnel become familiar with the exits, evacuation routes, locations of fire extinguishers, and how to shut off medical gas and electrical supplies. Although institutional fire safety protocols vary, the general principles of responding to an OR fire can be summarized by the mnemonic ERASE: ***e***xtinguish, ***r***escue, ***a***ctivate, ***s***hut, and ***e***valuate. Generally speaking, the team should first attempt to *extinguish* any fire on, in, or near the patient; depending on the situation, this may include the use of saline or a carbon dioxide fire extinguisher (this will be discussed later). If the initial attempts at extinguishing the fire are unsuccessful, the patient and all other persons at risk should be *rescued*, the OR should be evacuated if possible, and someone should *activate* the fire alarm. Once the OR is emptied of personnel, the doors should be *shut*, and the medical gas supply to the room should be *shut* off. The patient should then be *evaluated*, and any injuries should be appropriately managed.

Fire extinguishers are divided into three classes, termed *A*, *B*, and *C* based on the types of fires for which they are best suited. *Class A* extinguishers are used on paper, cloth, and plastic materials; *class B* extinguishers are used for fires when liquids or greases are involved; and *class C* extinguishers are used for energized electrical equipment. A single fire extinguisher may be useful for any one, two, or all three types of fires. Probably the best fire extinguisher for the OR is the carbon dioxide extinguisher, which can be used on class B and C fires and some class A fires. Other extinguishers provide a water mist or new environmentally friendly fluorocarbons, and these have replaced the Halon fire extinguisher. Finally, many ORs are equipped with a fire hose that supplies pressurized water at a rate of 50 gallons/min. Such equipment is best left to the fire department to use, except to *rescue* someone from a fire. In order to effectively use a fire extinguisher, the acronym *PASS* can be helpful: it stands for *pull* the pin to activate the fire extinguisher, *aim* at the base of the fire, *squeeze* the trigger, and *sweep* the extinguisher back and forth across the base of the fire. When responding to a fire, the acronym *RACE* is useful: it stands for *rescue*, *alarm*, *confine*, and *extinguish*. Clearly, having a plan that everyone is familiar with will greatly facilitate extinguishing any fire and will minimize harm to patients, personnel, and equipment. However, neither fire drills nor the presence and use of fire extinguishers should be relied on to provide a fire-safe operating environment. Only through heightened awareness, continuing education, and ongoing communication can the fire triad be avoided and the risk of an OR fire minimized.

REFERENCES

1. Harpell TR: Electrical shock hazards in the hospital environment: their causes and cures, *Can Hosp* 47:48, 1970.
2. Buczko GB, McKay WPS: Electrical safety in the operating room, *Can J Anaesth* 34:315, 1987.
3. Wald A: Electrical safety in medicine. In Skalak R, Chien S, editors: *Handbook of bioengineering*, New York, 1987, McGraw-Hill, p 34.
4. Dalziel CF, Massoglia FP: Let-go currents and voltages, *AIEE Trans* 75:49, 1956.
5. Bruner JMR, Aronow S, Cavicchi RV: Electrical incidents in a large hospital: a 42 month register, *JAAMI* 6:222, 1972.
6. Bernstein MS: Isolated power and line isolation monitors, *Biomed Instrum Technol* 24:221, 1990.
7. Gibby GL: Shock and electrocution. In Lobato EB, Gravenstein N, Kirby RR, editors: *Complications in anesthesiology*, Philadelphia, 2008, Wolters Kluwer/Lippincott Williams & Wilkins, p 780.
8. Weinberg DI, Artley JL, Whalen RE, et al: Electric shock hazards in cardiac catheterization, *Circ Res* 11:1004, 1962.
9. Starmer CF, Whalen RE: Current density and electrically induced ventricular fibrillation, *Med Instrum* 7:158, 1973.
10. Whalen RE, Starmer CF, McIntosh HD: Electrical hazards associated with cardiac pacemaking, *Ann N Y Acad Sci* 111:922, 1964.
11. Raftery EB, Green HL, Yacoub MH: Disturbances of heart rhythm produced by 50-Hz leakage currents in human subjects, *Cardiovasc Res* 9:263, 1975.
12. Hull CJ: Electrocution hazards in the operating theatre, *Br J Anaesth* 50:647, 1978.
13. Watson AB, Wright JS, Loughman J: Electrical thresholds for ventricular fibrillation in man, *Med J Aust* 1:1179, 1973.
14. Furman S, Schwedel JB, Robinson G, et al: Use of an intracardiac pacemaker in the control of heart block, *Surgery* 49:98, 1961.
15. Noordijk JA, Oey FJI, Tebra W: Myocardial electrodes and the danger of ventricular fibrillation, *Lancet* 1:975, 1961.
16. Pengelly LD, Klassen GA: Myocardial electrodes and the danger of ventricular fibrillation, *Lancet* 1:1234, 1961.
17. Rowe GG, Zarnstorff WC: Ventricular fibrillation during selective angiocardiography, *JAMA* 192:947, 1965.
18. Hopps JA, Roy OS: Electrical hazards in cardiac diagnosis and treatment, *Med Electr Biol Eng* 1:133, 1963.
19. Baas LS, Beery TA, Hickey CS: Care and safety of pacemaker electrodes in intensive care and telemetry nursing units, *Am J Crit Care* 6:301, 1997.
20. Leeming MN: Protection of the electrically susceptible patient: a discussion of systems and methods, *Anesthesiology* 38:370, 1973.
21. McNulty SE, Cooper M, Staudt S: Transmitted radiofrequency current through a flow directed pulmonary artery catheter, *Anesth Analg* 78:587, 1994.
22. Cromwell L, Weibell FJ, Pfeiffer EA: *Biomedical instrumentation and measurements*, ed 2, Englewood Cliffs, NJ, 1980, Prentice-Hall, p 430.
23. Edwards NK: Specialized electrical grounding needs, *Clin Perinatol* 3:367, 1976.
24. Goldwyn RM: Bovie: the man and the machine, *Ann Plast Surg* 2:135, 1979.
25. Lichter I, Borrie J, Miller WM: Radio-frequency hazards with cardiac pacemakers, *Br Med J* 1:1513, 1965.
26. Dornette WHL: An electrically safe surgical environment, *Arch Surg* 107:567, 1973.
27. Klop WM, Lohuis PJ, Strating RP, Mulder W: Ventricullar fibrillation caused by electrocoagulation during laparoscopic surgery, *Surg Endosc* 16:362, 2002.
28. Fu Q, Cao P, Mi WD, Zhang H: Ventricular fibrillation caused by electrocoagulation during thoracic surgery, *Acta Anaesthesiol Scand* 54:256, 2010.
29. Yan CY, Cai XJ, Wang YF, Yu H: Ventricular fibrillation caused by electrocoagulation in monopolar mode during laparoscopic subphrenic mass resection, *Surg Endosc* 25:309–311, 2011.
30. Dalibon N, Pelle-Lancien E, Puyo P, Leclerc JF, Fischler M: Recurrent asystotle during electrocauterization: an uncommon hazard in common situations, *Eur J Anaesthesiol* 22:476–478, 2005.
31. Cushing H: Electro-surgery as an aid to the removal of intracranial tumors: with a preliminary note on a new surgical-current generator by W.T. Bovie, *Surg Gynecol Obstet* 47:751, 1928.
32. Meathe EA: Electrical safety for patients and anesthetists. In Saidman LJ, Smith NT, editors: *Monitoring in anesthesia*, ed 2, Boston, 1984, Butterworth, p 497.
33. Rolly G: Two cases of burns caused by misuse of coagulation unit and monitoring, *Acta Anaesthesiol Belg* 29:313, 1978.
34. Parker EO: Electrosurgical burn at the site of an esophageal temperature probe, *Anesthesiology* 61:93, 1984.
35. Schneider AJL, Apple HP, Braun RT: Electrosurgical burns at skin temperature probes, *Anesthesiology* 47:72, 1977.
36. Bloch EC, Burton LW: Electrosurgical burn while using a battery-operated Doppler monitor, *Anesth Analg* 58:339, 1979.
37. Becker CM, Malhotra IV, Hedley-Whyte J: The distribution of radiofrequency current and burns, *Anesthesiology* 38:106, 1973.
38. Jones CM, Pierre KB, Nicoud IB, Stain SC, Melvin WV: *Electrosurgery. Curr Surg* 63:458–463, 2006.
39. Mitchell JP: The isolated circuit diathermy, *Ann R Coll Surg Engl* 61:287, 1979.
40. Titel JH, El Etr AA: Fibrillation resulting from pacemaker electrodes and electrocautery during surgery, *Anesthesiology* 29:845, 1968.
41. Domino KB, Smith TC: Electrocautery-induced reprogramming of a pacemaker using a precordial magnet, *Anesth Analg* 62:609, 1983.
42. Damaged reusable ESU return electrode cables, *Health Devices* 14:214, 1985.
43. Sparking from and ignition of damaged electrosurgical electrode cables, *Health Devices* 27:301, 1998.
44. Mirowski M, Reid PR, Mower MM, et al: Termination of malignant ventricular arrhythmias with an implanted automatic defibrillator in human beings, *N Engl J Med* 303:322, 1980.
45. Crozier IG, Ward DE: Automatic implantable defribrillators, *Br J Hosp Med* 40:136, 1988.
46. Elefteriades JA, Biblo LA, Batsford WP, et al: Evolving patterns in the surgical treatment of malignant ventricular tachyarrhythmias, *Ann Thorac Surg* 49:94, 1990.
47. Carr CME, Whiteley SM: The automatic implantable cardioverter-defibrillator, *Anaesthesia* 46:737, 1991.
48. Starmer CF, McIntosh HD, Whalen RE: Electrical hazards and cardiovascular function, *N Engl J Med* 284:181, 1971.
49. Albisser AM, Parson ID, Pask BA: A survey of the grounding systems in several large hospitals, *Med Instrum* 7:297, 1973.
50. McLaughlin AJ, Campkin NT: Electrical safety: a reminder (letter), *Anaesthesia* 53:608, 1998.
51. Nixon MC, Ghurye M: Electrical failure in theatre—a consequence of complacency? *Anaesthesia* 52:88, 1997.
52. Medical Devices; Establishment of a Performance Standard for Electrode Lead Wires and Patient Cables, *Federal Register* 62:25477, 1997.
53. Emergency Care Research Institute: FDA establishes performance standards for electrode lead wires, *Health Devices* 27:34, 1998.
54. National Fire Protection Association: NFPA 99, Health Care Facilities Code, 2012 Edition, Article 6.4.4.1.1.2 Maintenance and Testing of Alternate Power Source and Transfer Switches. Quincy, MA.
55. National Fire Protection Association: NFPA 110, Standard for Emergency and Standby Power Systems, Chapter 8, Quincy MA.
56. Carpenter T, Robinson ST: Response to a partial power failure in the operating room, *Anesth Analg* 110:1644–1646, 2010.

57. Eichhorn JH, Hessel EA: Electrical power failure in the operating room: a neglected topic in anesthesia safety, *Anesth Analg* 110:1519–1521, 2010.
58. Jones RP, Conway DH: The effect of electromagnetic interference from mobile communication on the performance of intensive care ventilators, *Eur J Anaesthesiol* 22:578, 2005.
59. Lawrentschuk N, Bolton DM: Mobile phone interference with medical equipment and its clinical relevance: a systematic review, *Med J Aust* 181:145, 2004.
60. Hayes DL, Wang PJ, Reynolds DW, et al: Interference with cardiac pacemakers by cellular telephones, *N Engl J Med* 336:1473, 1997.
61. Schlegel RE, Grant FH, Raman S, Reynolds D: Electromagnetic compatibility study of the *in vitro* interaction of wireless phones with cardiac pacemakers, *Biomed Instrum Technol* 32:645, 1998.
62. Chen WH, Lau CP, Leung SK, et al: Interference of cellular phones with implanted permanent pacemakers, *Clin Cardiol* 19:881, 1996.
63. Fetter JG, Ivans V, Benditt DG, Collins J: Digital cellular telephone interaction with implantable cardioverter-defibrillators, *J Am Coll Cardiol* 21:623, 1998.
64. Emergency Care Research Institute: Cell phones and walkie-talkies: Is it time to relax your restrictive policies? *Health Devices* 28:409, 1999.
65. Adler D, Margulies L, Mahler Y, Israeli A: Measurements of electromagnetic fields radiated from communication equipment and of environmental electromagnetic noise: impact on the use of communication equipment within the hospital, *Biomed Instrum Technol* 32:581, 1998.
66. Schwartz JJ, Ehrenwerth J: Electrical safety. In Lake CL, Hines RH, Blitt C, editors: *Clinical monitoring: practical applications for anesthesia and critical care*, Philadelphia, 2000, WB Saunders.
67. Kermit E, Staewen WS: Isolated power systems: historical perspective and update on regulations, *Biomed Tech Today* 1:86, 1986.
68. National Fire Protection Association: *National electric code (ANSI/NFPA 70-1984)*, Quincy, MA, 1984, NFPA.
69. *National Fire Protection Association, NFPA-99, Health Care Facilities Code*, Quincy, MA, 2012, NFPA, 2012 Edition.
70. Bruner JMR, Leonard PF: *Electricity, safety and the patient*, Chicago, 1989, Year Book Medical Publishers. p 300.
71. Matjasko MJ, Ashman MN: All you need to know about electrical safety in the operating room. In Barash PG, Deutsch S, Tinker J, editors: *ASA refresher courses in anesthesiology*, vol. 18, Philadelphia, 1990, JB Lippincott, p 251.
72. Lennon RL, Leonard PF: A hitherto unreported virtue of the isolated power system (letter), *Anesth Analg* 66:1056, 1987.
73. Barker SJ, Doyle DJ: Electrical safety in the operating room: dry versus wet, *Anesth Analg* 110:1517–1518, 2010.
74. Gilbert TB, Shaffer M, Matthews M: Electrical shock by dislodged spark gap in bipolar electrosurgical device, *Anesth Analg* 73:355, 1991.
75. Van Kerchhove K: Re-evaluating the isolated power equation, *Electrical Products and Solutions* 25–27, March 2008.
76. Day FJ: Electrical safety revisited: a new wrinkle, *Anesthesiology* 80:220, 1994.
77. Wills JH, Ehrenwerth J, Rogers D: Electrical injury to a nurse due to conductive fluid in an operating room designated as a dry location, *Anesth Analg* 110:1647–1649, 2010.
78. August DA: Locked out of a box and a process, *Anesth Analg* 112:1248–1249, 2011.
79. Barker SJ: In response to August DA, *Anesth Analg* 112:1249, 2011.
80. Litt L, Ehrenwerth J: Electrical safety in the operating room: important old wine, disguised in new bottles, *Anesth Analg* 78:417, 1994.
81. Seifert HA: Fire safety in the operating room. In Eisenkraft JB, editor: *Progress in anesthesiology*, Philadelphia, 1994, W.B. Saunders.
82. Neufeld GR: Fires and explosions. In Orkin K, Cooperman LH, editors: *Complications in anesthesiology*, Philadelphia, 1983, Lippincott, p 671.
83. Moxon MA: Fire in the operating room, *Anaesthesia* 41:543, 1986.
84. Vickers MD: Fire and explosion hazards in operating theatres, *Br J Anaesth* 50:659, 1978.
85. ECRI Institute: New clinical guide to surgical fire prevention, *Health Devices* 38(10):314–332, 2009.
86. Caplan RA, Barker SJ, Connis RT, et al: Practice advisory for the prevention and management of operating room fires, *Anesthesiology* 108:786–801, 2008.
87. de Richemond AL: The patient is on fire! *Health Devices* 21:19, 1992.
88. Cameron BG, Ingram GS: Flammability of drape materials in nitrous oxide and oxygen, *Anesthesiology* 26:218, 1971.
89. Johnson RM, Smith CV, Leggett K: Flammability of disposable surgical drapes, *Arch Ophthalmol* 94:1327, 1976.
90. Simpson JI, Wolf GL: Flammability of esophageal stethoscopes, nasogastric tubes, feeding tubes, and nasopharyngeal airways in oxygen- and nitrous oxide–enriched atmospheres, *Anesth Analg* 67:1093, 1988.
91. Ponath RE: Preventing surgical fires, *JAMA* 252:1762, 1984.
92. Katz J, Campbell L: Fire during thoracotomy: a need to control the inspired oxygen concentration, *Anesth Analg* 101:612, 2005.
93. Wolf G, Sidebotham GW, Lazard JLP: Laser ignition of surgical drape materials in air 50% oxygen, and 95% oxygen, *Anesthesiology* 100:1167–1171, 2004.
94. Food and Drug Administration: Surgical Fires Reported January 1995–June 1998. FDA Databases MDR/MAUDE, 1999.
95. Rampil IJ: Anesthetic considerations for laser surgery, *Anesth Analg* 74:424, 1992.
96. Pashayan AG, Ehrenwerth J: Lasers and electrical safety in the operating room. In Ehrenwerth J, Eisenkraft JB, editors: *Anesthesia equipment: principles and applications*, St. Louis, 1993, Mosby.
97. Emergency Care Research Institute: Lasers in medicine—an introduction, *Health Devices* 13:151, 1984.
98. Casey KR, Fairfax WR, Smith SJ, et al: Intratracheal fire ignited by the Nd:YAG laser during treatment of tracheal stenosis, *Chest* 84:295, 1983.
99. Burgess GE, LeJeune FE: Endotracheal tube ignition during laser surgery of the larynx, *Arch Otolaryngol* 105:561, 1979.
100. Cozine K, Rosenbaum LM, Askanazi J, et al: Laser induced endotracheal tube fire, *Anesthesiology* 55:583, 1981.
101 Geffin B, Shapshay SM, Bellack GS, et al: Flammability of endotracheal tubes during Nd:YAG laser application in the airway, *Anesthesiology* 65:511, 1986.
102 Hirshman CA, Smith J: Indirect ignition of the endotracheal tube during carbon dioxide laser surgery, *Arch Otolaryngol* 106:639, 1980.
103 Krawtz S, Mehta AC, Weidemann HP, et al: Nd:YAG laser-induced endobronchial burn, *Chest* 95:916, 1989.
104. Goldblum KB: Oxygen index: Key to precise flammability ratings, *Soc Plastics Engineers J* 25:50–52, 1969.
105. Wolf GL, Simpson JI: Flammability of endotracheal tubes in oxygen and nitrous oxide enriched atmosphere, *Anesthesiology* 67:236, 1987.
106. de Richemond AL: Laser resistant endotracheal tubes: protection against oxygen-enriched airway fires during surgery? In Stoltzfus JM, McIlroy K, editors: *Flammability and sensitivity of material in oxygen-enriched atmospheres*, vol 5, Philadelphia, 1991, American Society for Testing and Materials, p 157. ASTM STP 1111.
107. Emergency Care Research Institute (ECRI): Airway fires: reducing the risk during laser surgery, *Health Devices* 19:109, 1990.
108. Emergency Care Research Institute: Laser-resistant tracheal tubes (evaluation), *Health Devices* 21:4, 1992.
109. Aly A, McIlwain M, Ward M: Electrosurgery-induced endotracheal tube ignition during tracheotomy, *Ann Otol Rhinol Laryngol* 100:31, 1991.
110. Simpson JI, Wolf GL: Endotracheal tube fire ignited by pharyngeal electrocautery, *Anesthesiology* 65:76, 1986.
111. Gupte SR: Gauze fire in the oral cavity: a case report, *Anesth Analg* 51:645, 1972.
112. Snow JC, Norton ML, Saluja TS, et al: Fire hazard during CO_2 laser microsurgery on the larynx and trachea, *Anesth Analg* 55:146, 1975.
113. Lew EO, Mittleman RE, Murray D: Tube ignition by electrocautery during tracheostomy: Case report with autopsy findings, *J Forensic Sci* 36:1586, 1991.
114. Marsh B, Riley DH: Double-lumen tube fire during tracheostomy, *Anesthesiology* 76:480, 1992.
115. Neuman GG, Sidebotham G, Negoianu E, et al: Laparoscopy explosion hazards with nitrous oxide, *Anesthesiology* 78:875, 1993.
116. Di Pierro GB, Besmer I, Hefermehl LJ, et al: Intra-abdominal fire due to insufflating oxygen instead of carbon dioxide during

robot-assisted radical prostatectomy: case report and literature review, *Eur Urol* 58:626–628, 2010.

117. Greilich PE, Greilich NB, Froelich EG: Intraabdominal fire during laparoscopic cholecystectomy, *Anesthesiology* 83:871, 1995.
118. Barker SJ, Polson JS: Fire in the operating room: a case report and laboratory study, *Anesth Analg* 93:960, 2001.
119. Bruley ME, Lavanchy C: Oxygen-enriched fires during surgery of the head and neck. *Symposium on flammability and sensitivity of material in oxygen-enriched atmospheres (ASTM STP 1040)*, Philadelphia, 1989, American Society for Testing and Materials, p 392.
120. de Richemond AL, Bruley ME: Head and neck surgical fires. In Eisele DW, editor: *Complications in head and neck surgery*, St. Louis, 1993, Mosby.
121. ECRI: Fires during surgery of the head and neck area (hazard), *Health Devices* 9:50, 1979.
122. Ramanathan S, Capan L, Chalon J, et al: Mini-environmental control under the drapes during operations on eyes of conscious patients, *Anesthesiology* 48:286, 1978.
123. Anesthesia Patient Safety Foundation: Prevention and Management of Operating Room Fires (Video), Apsf.org, 2010.
124. Lampotang S, Gravenstein N, Paulus DA, Gravenstein D: Reducing the incidence of surgical fires: supplying nasal cannulae with sub-100% O_2 gas mixtures from anesthesia machines, *Anesth Analg* 101:1407–1412, 2005.
125. Patel R, Chavda KD, Hukkeri S: Surgical field fire and skin burns caused by alcohol-based skin preparation, *J Emerg Trauma Shock* 3(3):305, 2010.
126. Prasad R, Quezado Z, St. Andre A, O'Grady NP: Fires in the operating room and intensive care unit: awareness is the key to prevention, *Anesth Analg* 102:172–174, 2006.
127. Wallin RF, Regan BM, Napoli MD, Stern IJ: Sevoflurane: a new inhalational anesthetic agent, *Anesth Analg* 54:758, 1975.
128. Fatheree RS, Leighton BL: Acute respiratory syndrome after an exothermic baralyme-sevoflurane reaction, *Anesthesiology* 101:531, 2004.
129. Castro BA, Freedman LA, Craig WL, Lynch C: Explosion within an anesthesia machine: baralyme, high fresh gas flows and sevoflurane concentration, *Anesthesiology* 101:537, 2004.
130. Wu J, Previte JP, Adler E, et al: Spontaneous ignition, explosion and fire with sevoflurane and barium hydroxide lime, *Anesthesiology* 101:534, 2004.
131. Abbott A: *Dear healthcare provider (letter)*, Available at http://www.fda.gov/downloads/Safety/MedWatch/SafetyInformation/SafetyAlertsforHumanMedicalProducts/UCM169499.pdf.
132. Murray JM, Renfrew CW, Bedi A, et al: Amsorb: a new carbon dioxide absorbent for use in anesthetic breathing systems, *Anesthesiology* 91:1342, 1999.
133. Laster M, Roth P, Eger EI: Fires from the interaction of anesthetics with desiccated absorbent, *Anesth Analg* 99:769, 2004.

CHAPTER 32

Machine Checkout and Quality Assurance

Steven G. Venticinque • John H. Eichhorn

CHAPTER OUTLINE

OVERVIEW

Although the large majority of anesthesia critical incidents and catastrophes involve human error, some events involve overt equipment failure or failure of the anesthesia provider to discover an equipment problem. Most equipment problems in anesthesia practice are preventable, and this chapter is intended to help practitioners achieve that goal.

The analogy between administering general anesthesia and piloting a commercial jet may be somewhat overused, but it is singularly relevant in this context. The aviation industry has developed extraordinarily thorough plans involving "acute" and "chronic" interactions with its principal equipment, the commercial passenger jetliner. The acute component is the immediate preflight check to verify that a particular aircraft should fly safely that day on a given trip; the chronic component is the elaborate scheme of scheduled preventive maintenance, repair, exchange of old parts for new, and safety inspections of structural components. These are all oriented toward ensuring that the aircraft will fly safely for the designated interval of weeks or months covered by that particular action. In anesthesia practice, the analogy is obviously appropriate to an anesthesia equipment quality assurance (QA) program. The acute effort is the preanesthetic equipment check, and the chronic component is the vital and ongoing QA mechanism that involves preventive maintenance, testing for safe function, and the detection of expected wear prior to the failure of a piece of equipment.

Preflight checkout procedures in aviation have changed as technology has advanced. Aircraft systems have become more automated, and modern "glass cockpit" instrument displays have reduced the workload involved in operating multiple complex systems. This has allowed two crew members to do work that previously required three or more, with increased reliance on automated systems that function with minimal pilot input. Anesthesia equipment has also evolved rapidly, with increasing reliance on automated systems to function properly with minimal input by the anesthesia professional. Nevertheless, human vigilance will remain important as the ultimate watchdog and guarantor of machine safety.

BACKGROUND

Because the practice of anesthesia is heavily dependent on the correct functioning of a large number of diverse pieces of equipment, and because anesthesia professionals usually have technical and mechanical proclivities, reports of problems with anesthesia equipment have been prominent in the anesthesia literature virtually since its inception. A great many of the "classic" traditional problems that had been common since recognizable anesthesia machines came into use—such as fresh gas rotameter leaks, ventilator leaks, and disconnections of poorly designed hose or tubing connectors—have been largely eliminated by the adoption and implementation of rigorous so-called voluntary design and fabrication standards by anesthesia machine manufacturers.[1] By no means does this suggest that equipment problems do not arise today. On the contrary, some problems—such as absent, broken, or stuck unidirectional breathing system valves, or failure to remove the wrapper on prepackaged carbon dioxide absorbent inner canisters—are still a concern today. Also, because of the increasing complexity and integration of multiple parts and functions that had been separate (replaceable) components of anesthesia delivery systems, scrupulous attention to acute and chronic QA of anesthesia equipment is more important than ever. However, many of the details and the specific problems have changed, and advances have been made in the study of human interaction with the anesthesia system. Improving the "user friendliness" of anesthesia technology and study of the human factors in both routine and crisis anesthesia situations has been made possible in part by major growth and development of almost frighteningly realistic high-fidelity patient simulators—mannequins in particular, but also screen-based computer programs—that enable trials and modification of equipment and protocols without patient risk. Further, current simulators allow specific training of anesthesia professionals to deal with extremely rare catastrophic situations.[2] Although required to be familiar with and prepared to react to these challenges, everyone hopes to never encounter them in real life, such as crossed oxygen and nitrous oxide pipelines.[3]

Although historic perspectives are valuable with regard to anesthesia equipment, current concerns are more important than reproducing a litany of hundreds of problems that have been identified with anesthesia equipment over the years. Classic treatises on anesthesia equipment provide useful references for reviewing the spectrum of defects and problems that have been reported with anesthesia equipment.[4] Rendell-Baker[5] edited a classic monograph that described 48 specific safety-related problems with anesthesia machines. Among these, in order of frequency, were problems with 1) the vaporizer, 2) the breathing system, 3) the gas flowmeters, 4) the mechanical functions of the machine, and 5) human engineering. In another classic, Spooner and Kirby[6] outlined some of the data collected by the ECRI Institute regarding the role of equipment in anesthesia accidents. In the American Society of Anesthesiologists (ASA) Closed Claims Study, one report noted that only 2% of claims were apparently caused by the gas delivery equipment; however, 76% of those involved catastrophic adverse outcomes.[7] These data again suggest that a combination of the occasional overt device failure along with a large component of various types of human error lead to anesthesia mishaps.

Further, classic pioneering work by Cooper and associates[8] suggested that among anesthesia critical incidents, 82% involved human error, and only 14% resulted from overt equipment failure. Of course, many of the human errors involved unrecognized problems with the equipment, such as breathing system disconnection, that were not classic equipment failures—and that would not necessarily have been prevented or mitigated by the preanesthetic checkout (PAC) of the anesthesia equipment. Among the equipment failures, 20% involved the breathing circuit, 18% airway components, 12% laryngoscopes, and 12% the anesthesia machine. Failure to perform a normal checkout was cited 22 times on a list of 481 factors associated with 359 incidents. Follow-up studies of 1089 preventable critical incidents found that only 4% of incidents with substantive negative outcomes involved equipment failure.[9] Of all incidents reported in the various parts of the study, 11% to 19% involved equipment failure. However, 129 (22%) of 583 instances of human error involved anesthesia machine use, indicating that the interaction of the anesthesiologist with normally functioning equipment accounts for many problems. Minimizing this type of problem by eliminating defects in the delivery system prior to the start of any anesthetic is the goal of a thorough preuse anesthesia equipment checkout.

Many other studies have also implicated the failure to perform an adequate PAC of the equipment as a factor in critical incidents and accidents. For example, 1 of the 11 cases reported in the analysis of severe anesthesia injuries at the Harvard teaching hospitals was caused by a misconnection of a vaporizer that had just been returned from servicing, a condition that would have been detected by a thorough preuse checkout of the anesthesia equipment.[10]

PREANESTHESIA CHECKOUT

Historical Perspective

It is a well-accepted dictum that a thorough and stepwise anesthesia apparatus checkout should be performed prior to the delivery of anesthesia. Even in surveys that identify poor provider compliance with PAC procedures, most participants feel that such checks improve patient safety.[11] This perception is indeed correct, as it has been clearly demonstrated that a PAC performed with a checklist and protocol is associated with a decreased risk of perioperative morbidity and mortality.[12] It is important to note that a PAC is a *checklist*. The obvious industry parallel is aviation, in which a strict adherence to pre-event checklists (e.g., before start, at takeoff, on approach) is known to enhance compliance with important steps and procedures and to save lives. The unfortunate difference between anesthesiology and aviation is that pilots seem to use checklists much more regularly, possibly in part because the pilot of an airplane is always the first one to a crash scene. Through leadership and the personal effort of many, great progress has been made over the past decades in enhancing the knowledge of the anesthesia workstation and in introducing anesthesia equipment preuse checkout guidelines. What is striking, however, is that despite these efforts, our overall performance in "preflighting" the anesthesia workstation seems to be less than optimal. This is both troubling and perplexing given the pivotal role that the anesthesia machine plays in anesthesia practice and patient safety, and the fact that anesthesia professionals, by nature, are savvy about and comfortable with technology.

Data predating the first publication of the U.S. Food and Drug Administration (FDA) Anesthesia Apparatus Checkout Recommendations in 1986 demonstrated a low level of proficiency by anesthesiologists in detecting life-threatening machine problems. Using a machine with five intentionally created faults, researchers found that anesthesiologists detected on average only 2.2 serious problems (44%); and 7.3% found no faults at all despite knowing ahead of time that the machine was intentionally altered.[13] At that time, available preuse checkout procedures for anesthesia machines were provided and promoted by individual machine manufacturers. Given the design and engineering perspectives of the manufacturers and their liability concerns, the machine-specific checkout recommendations were not entirely "user friendly," nor were they well suited for clinical application. This also parallels current times, when manufacturer checkout recommendations still tend to be long and sometimes unwieldy, making them difficult to use routinely.

Prompted by a series of anesthesia machine–related accidents, in 1984 the FDA met with representatives from the ASA, anesthesia equipment experts, and anesthesia machine manufacturers to discuss methods of reducing patient risk during anesthesia.[14,15] During that meeting the FDA was asked to take the lead in the development of the first generic anesthesia apparatus checkout recommendations. This general guideline was intended to instruct users on how to perform a preuse checkout, to promote the concept of a preuse checkout, and to create a framework that providers could modify to meet their local needs.[14] This first preuse checkout was released in final form in August of 1986. These recommendations contained 25 primary items, with some having up to six subitems. The guideline intended that a comprehensive checkout be accomplished at the beginning of the day ("day check") followed by an abbreviated check prior to subsequent cases ("case check"). The 1986 PAC guideline was fairly detailed, proved to be very time consuming, and was found to be not extensively used.[16]

In an attempt to evaluate compliance with the 1986 checklist, the FDA surveyed anesthesiology providers at 125 hospitals in four states and found that only 70% of facilities acknowledged they had a documented anesthesia machine preuse checkout at their site.[17] Only 73% of the sites reported that a preuse checkout was routinely carried out at the beginning of each day or shift, and only 59% reported that a preuse checkout was accomplished between cases. Of those hospitals that acknowledged having a documented checkout, only 26% used the FDA's version. The issuance of the 1986 recommendations also did not appear to improve the ability of anesthesiologists to detect anesthesia machine faults. Testing this hypothesis, March and Crowley[15] showed that 188 anesthesiologists, using their own methods, could detect only one of four preset faults. When the same subjects used the FDA checklist to asses a different set of failures, detection performance improved only modestly. The authors concluded that the introduction of the FDA checklist did not improve the ability of anesthesiologists to detect anesthesia machine faults.

Recognizing that there was poor compliance with the 1986 guideline, the FDA revised the PAC in the early 1990s, working once again with anesthesiology professional organizations and industry. Other factors, including the development of monitoring standards by the ASA, the retirement of many older machines, and the introduction of newer-generation anesthesia machines following the new American Society for Testing and Materials (ASTM) specifications also provided impetus for the update of the guidelines.[16] The revised checklist was issued in 1993 and included only 14 major steps, many with several bulleted instructions (Fig. 32-1).[18] Although the checklist was fairly comprehensive and universal, a stated intent of the authors, similar to the 1986 version, was to encourage users to "modify [the guideline] to accommodate differences in equipment design and variations in local clinical practice" and to subject modifications to local peer review. It also encouraged users to "refer to the operator's manual for the manufacturer's specific procedures and precautions," particularly when addressing the machine's low-pressure system leak test.[18] Even without modification, the 1993 PAC was applicable to most machines of the day and was nicely formatted to fit onto a single page. It is interesting to note that like the 1986 guideline, the FDA did not mandate the use of the 1993 Anesthesia Apparatus Checkout Recommendations. It was made clear in the Federal Register in 1994 that the FDA recommendations only offered guidance and encouraged modification to accommodate differences in equipment design and variations in local clinical practice.[19] Even though the FDA authorized the matter, it did not undertake direct regulatory action.

Although the data are limited, evidence that the 1993 PAC recommendations led to improved user compliance and better detection of machine faults was not forthcoming. When anesthesiology providers of different backgrounds and experience levels were asked to use their own anesthesia preuse checkout procedures to check a fault-laden machine, and then went on to check another sabotaged machine using the 1993 FDA checkout procedure, researchers detected no difference in the rate of fault detection using either method.[20] In fact, despite having the FDA checklist in hand, 41% of the participants could not identify more than 50% of the faults. Using a prospective crossover design, Blike and Biddle[21] found that anesthesiology providers missed "easy" anesthesia machine faults 30% of the time and "difficult" anesthesia faults 62% of the time when provided with the FDA checklist. Larson and colleagues[22] observed 87 participants at a "nationally attended anesthesia meeting" when they were asked to perform a checkout on an anesthesia machine with preset faults. The average number of faults detected by all participants was 3.1 of 5 total faults. Interestingly, the authors showed a *negative* correlation between level of experience and the ability to detect faults. In other controlled settings, where anesthesiologists would be anticipated to be thorough and accurate

1993 FDA Anesthesia Apparatus Checkout Recommendations

This checkout, or a reasonable equivalent, should be conducted before administration of anesthesia. These recommendations are only valid for an anesthesia system that conforms to current and relevant standards and includes an ascending bellows ventilator and at least the following monitors: capnograph, pulse oximeter, oxygen analyzer, respiratory volume monitor (spirometer) and breathing system pressure monitor with high and low pressure alarms. This is a guideline which users are encouraged to modify to accommodate differences in equipment design and variations in local clinical practice. Such local modifications should have appropriate peer review. Users should refer to the operator's manual for the manufacturer's specific procedures and precautions, especially the manufacturer's low pressure leak test (step 5).

Emergency Ventilation Equipment

***1. Verify backup equipment is available and functioning.**

High Pressure System

***2. Check initial status of low Pressure System.**

a. Open O_2 cylinder and verify at least half full (about 1000 psi).
b. Close cylinder.

***3. Check central pipeline supplies.**

a. Check that hoses are connected and pipeline gauges read about 50 psi.

Low Pressure System

***4. Check initial status of low pressure system.**

a. Close flow control valves and turn vaporizers off.
b. Check fill level and tighten vaporizers' filler caps.

***5. Perform leak check of machine low pressure system.**

a. Verify that machine master switch and flow control valves are OFF.
b. Attach "suction bulb" to common (fresh) gas outlet.
c. Squeeze bulb repeatedly until fully collapsed.
d. Verify bulb stays fully collapsed for at least 10 seconds.
e. Open one vaporizer and repeat c and d as above.
f. Remove suction bulb and reconnect fresh gas hose.

***6. Turn on machine master switch and all other necessary electrical equipment.**

***7. Test flowmeters.**

a. Adjust flow of all gases through their full range, checking for smooth operation of floats and undamaged flow tubes.
b. Attempt to create a hypoxic O_2/N_2O mixture and verify correct changes in flow and/or alarm.

Scavenging System

***8. Adjust and check scavenging system.**

a. Ensure proper connections between the scavenging system and both APL (pop-off) valve and ventilator relief valve.
b. Adjust waste gas vacuum (if possible).
c. Fully open APL valve and occlude Y piece.
d. With minimum O_2 flow, allow scavenger reservoir bag to collapse completely and verify that absorber pressure gauge reads about zero.
e. With the O_2 flush activated allow the scavenger reservoir bag to distend fully, and then verify that the absorber pressure gauge reads < 10 cm H_2O.

Breathing System

***9. Calibrate O_2 monitor.**

a. Ensure monitor reads 21% in room air.
b. Verify low O_2 alarm is enabled and functioning.
c. Reinstall sensor in circuit and flush breathing system with O_2
d. Verify that monitor now reads greater than 90%.

10. Check initial status of breathing system.

a. Set selector switch to "bag" mode.
b. Check that breathing circuit is complete, undamaged and unobstructed.
c. Verify that CO_2 absorbent is adequate.
d. Install breathing circuit accessory equipment (e.g., humidifier, PEEP valve) to be used during the case.

11. Perform leak check of the breathing system.

a. Set all gas flows to zero (or minimum).
b. Close APL (pop-off) valve and occlude Y piece.
c. Pressurize breathing system to about 30 cm H_2O with O_2 flush.
d. Ensure that pressure remains fixed for at least 10 seconds.
e. Open APL (pop-off) valve and ensure that pressure decreases.

Manual and Automatic Ventilation System

12. Test ventilation system and unidirectional Valves.

a. Place a second breathing bag on Y piece.
b. Set appropriate ventilator parameters for next patient.
c. Switch to automatic ventilation (ventilator) mode.
d. Fill bellows and breathing bag with O_2 flush and then turn ventilator ON.
e. Set O_2 flow to minimum, other gas flows to zero.
f. Verify that during inspiration bellows delivers appropriate tidal volume and that during expiration bellows fills completely.
g. Set fresh gas flow to about 5 L/min.
h. Verify that the ventilator bellows and simulated lungs fill, and empty appropriately without sustained pressure at end expiration.
i. Check for proper action of unidirectional valves.
j. Exercise breathing circuit accessories to ensure proper function.
k. Turn ventilator OFF and switch to manual ventilation (Bag/APL) mode.
l. Ventilate manually and ensure inflation and deflation of artificial lungs and appropriate feel of system resistance and compliance.
m. Remove second breathing bag from Y piece.

Monitors

13. Check, calibrate and/or set alarm limits of all monitors.

-Capnometer
-Pulse oximeter
-Oxygen analyzer
-Respiratory volume monitor (spirometer) pressure monitor with high and low airway alarms

Final Position

14. Check final status of machine.

a. Vaporizers off
b. APL valve open
c. Selector switch to "Bag"
d. All flowmeters to zero
e. Patient suction level adequate
f. Breathing system ready to use

* If an anesthesia provider uses the same machine in successive cases, these steps need not be repeated or may be abbreviated after the initial checkout.

FIGURE 32-1 The Food and Drug Administration (FDA) 1993 anesthesia apparatus checkout recommendations. Users of the guideline were encouraged to modify the checklist to accommodate for differences in machine design and then subject the changes to peer review. The FDA also encouraged users to refer to the operator's manual to identify manufacturer-specific procedures and precautions to modify the checklist.

regarding the checkout procedure, the data also indicate poor performance. Olympio and colleagues[23] observed anesthesiology residents checking out the machine and noted a low performance rate (69%), which improved by only 12% after focused instructional review. It is important to note that the residents knew in advance that their performance would be evaluated. In another experimental setting, Armstrong and colleagues[24] observed anesthesiologists in a simulator who knew only that they were involved in a study to evaluate the simulator as a testing tool, and they were aware that simulated patient or technical problems would be presented during the case. The researchers quietly graded the quality of the anesthesia checkout and found that the subjects, on average, checked 50% or fewer of 20 key items. Performance was noted to be poor regardless of the age or experience of the anesthesiologist.

As tempting as it may be to implicate the checklists in these failures, human factors and training issues are more likely to blame. In particular, a lack of cultural discipline in the routine, proper use of a PAC is seemingly the principal problem. As noted, pivotal work by Cooper and colleagues[8] demonstrated that in 22% of equipment-related mishaps, a failure to check or inspect was identified as an associated factor. Similarly, in a 1981 survey of anesthetic misadventures, human error was found to be more often responsible than equipment failure, and a failure to perform a machine checkout was the factor most likely associated with an equipment-related issue.[25] In 1992 Mayor and Eaton[26] found that almost 41% percent of anesthesia providers admitted to performing inadequate machine checks, and few followed published guidelines. In an Internet-based survey of anesthesiology providers and anesthesia technicians published in abstract form in 2005, 29% of respondents rated their competence in performing the 1993 FDA preuse checkout as poor.[27] Reasons cited in the same survey for *skipping* the checkout included unfamiliarity with the procedure, a belief that the machine self-check alone was sufficient, and that checkout took too long to perform. Finally, in a 2007 survey conducted in the United Kingdom, researchers found that most anesthetists admitted to only partially checking the anesthesia machine; only 12% performed a check between cases, and only 27% identified an alternate means for ventilation prior to anesthesia.[11]

It seems that no matter how well conceived and heavily promoted PAC recommendations have been, their adoption and routine use has not been consistent. Underlying this issue seems to be an inconsistent understanding of the anesthesia machine. What currently compounds the issue is the growing assortment of anesthesia machine designs and features that depart significantly from the more generic, older-generation gas machines and workstations. When these factors are combined with a misunderstanding of and overreliance on "automated" machine checkout functions, the potential for a suboptimal PAC is significant.

To improve PAC compliance and performance, it is recommended that individual anesthesia departments align the ASA's most recent 2008 Guideline for Designing Pre-Anesthesia Checkout Procedures with their respective manufacturer's suggested checkout procedures in order to develop their own effective, workstation-specific PAC checklists (Table 32-1).[28] In addition to developing effective PACs, it is also important that anesthesia providers remain knowledgeable about their equipment and embrace a "checklist culture." The 2008 guideline can be found at http://www.asahq.org for members within the "Standards, Guidelines, and Statements" tab (under Recommendations and Clinical Management Tools, ASA Committees: Anesthesia Machine Preoperative Checkout Procedures section) along with workstation-specific PACs from individual departments that can be used for PAC development.[28]

2008 Recommendations for Preanesthesia Checkout Procedures

The 2008 recommendations were developed with the knowledge that the existing PAC was not well understood, nor was it reliably used by anesthesia providers, and that anesthesia delivery systems have evolved to the point where one checkout procedure is no longer universally applicable.[28] Although anesthesia providers were encouraged to modify the 1993 PAC to meet their own equipment needs, it was essentially applicable to almost any machine when it was published. As stated, it was a nearly universal checklist. However, diligent users of the 1993 PAC came to realize that it became increasingly difficult to strictly apply as a newer generation of machines began to emerge. The newer generation machines differed in their functions and features and in their checkout procedures, and they have become increasingly diverse even among themselves. For precisely these reasons, the authors of the ASA's 2008 Recommendations for Pre-Anesthesia Checkout Procedures created a *template* to develop "checkout procedures that are appropriate for each individual anesthesia machine design and practice setting," instead of a detailed PAC.[28] Their goal was to provide guidelines applicable to all machines, so that individual departments could develop their own PAC, which could be performed consistently and expeditiously. In fact, the footer of the document reads "Guideline for Designing Pre-Anesthesia Checkout Procedures."

The 2008 recommendations warn against an overreliance on automated machine checkouts, alerting that anesthesiology providers may be unaware of what is actually assessed by these features and that they may omit important preuse checkout items if they place all their faith in an automated checkout. When developing a local PAC, a detailed understanding of what is actually checked by the machine is required. However, this is not always easy to ascertain by simply reviewing user manuals.

The 1993 version of the PAC placed all of the responsibility of the preuse checkout on the anesthesia provider. The authors of the 2008 guidelines recognized that using anesthesia technicians and/or biomedical technicians to perform some aspects of the checkout procedures may improve compliance with a department's PAC and could add redundancy to critical steps. Although the 2008 guidelines suggest which steps may be checked by "a qualified anesthesia technician, biomedical technician, or manufacturer-certified technician," this should indeed be an institutional decision, because skill levels, work flow

TABLE 32-1 **Summary Recommendations of the 2008 Preanesthesia Checkout Procedures**[28]

Item	Task	Responsible Parties
To Be Completed Daily		
1	Verify auxiliary oxygen cylinder and self-inflating manual ventilation device are available and functioning	Provider and technician
2	Verify patient suction is adequate to clear the airway	Provider and technician
3	Turn on anesthesia delivery system and confirm that AC power is available.	Provider or technician
4	Verify availability of required monitors, including alarms	Provider or technician
5	Verify that pressure is adequate on the spare oxygen cylinder mounted on the anesthesia machine	Provider and technician
6	Verify that the piped gas pressures are ≥50 psig	Provider and technician
7	Verify that vaporizers are adequately filled and, if applicable, that the filler ports are tightly closed	Provider only
8	Verify that there are no leaks in the gas supply lines between the flowmeters and the common gas outlet	Provider or technician
9	Test scavenging system function	Provider or technician
10	Calibrate, or verify calibration of, the oxygen monitor and check the low-oxygen alarm	Provider or technician
11	Verify carbon dioxide absorbent is not exhausted	Provider or technician
12	Perform breathing system pressure and leak testing	Provider and technician
13	Verify that gas flows properly through the breathing circuit during both inspiration and exhalation	Provider and technician
14	Document completion of checkout procedures	Provider and technician
15	Confirm ventilator settings and evaluate readiness to deliver anesthesia care (anesthesia time out)	Provider only
To Be Completed Before Each Procedure		
1	Verify patient suction is adequate to clear the airway	Provider and technician
2	Verify availability of required monitors, including alarms	Provider or technician
3	Verify that vaporizers are adequately filled and, if applicable, that the filler ports are tightly closed	Provider
4	Verify carbon dioxide absorbent is not exhausted	Provider or technician
5	Perform breathing system pressure and leak testing	Provider and technician
6	Verify that gas flows properly through the breathing circuit during both inspiration and exhalation	Provider and technician
7	Document completion of checkout procedures	Provider and technician
8	Confirm ventilator settings and evaluate readiness to deliver anesthesia care (anesthesia time out)	Provider

patterns, and training requirements vary greatly. The 2008 guidelines did not intend to make the use of technician checks mandatory. Regardless of who participates in the PAC, *the anesthesia care provider is ultimately responsible for the proper and safe functioning of the equipment.*

The items and rationale statements listed below, excerpted directly from the 2008 Recommendations for Pre-Anesthesia Checkout Procedures, are intended to describe a basic approach to developing sound institution-specific PAC procedures designed "for the equipment and resources available." They identify items that need to be checked as part of a complete PAC. The *method* used to check each item will be dependent upon the specific equipment. Also identified in the recommendations are the suggested frequency of the checks, and the suggested responsible parties either individually, alternatively ("or"), or redundantly ("and"). It is important to recognize that the guidelines are not all inclusive; they simply suggest the minimum machine-related items that should be assessed prior to use. A local PAC checklist should represent a workable merger between these guidelines and the manufacturer's checkout recommendations. As in the prior PAC guidelines, items that require checkout prior to each procedure are distinguished from those that need only to be checked daily.

Minimum PAC Checklist

Item 1: Verify auxiliary oxygen cylinder and self-inflating manual ventilation device are available and functioning

Frequency: Daily
Responsible Parties: Provider and technician

> *Failure to be able to ventilate is a major cause of morbidity and mortality related to anesthesia care. Because equipment failure with resulting inability to ventilate the patient can occur at any time, a self-inflating manual ventilation device (e.g., Ambu bag) should be present at every anesthetizing location for every case and should be checked for proper function. In addition, a source of oxygen separate from the anesthesia machine and pipeline supply, specifically an oxygen cylinder with regulator and a means to open the cylinder valve, should be immediately available and checked. After checking the cylinder pressure, it is recommended that the main*

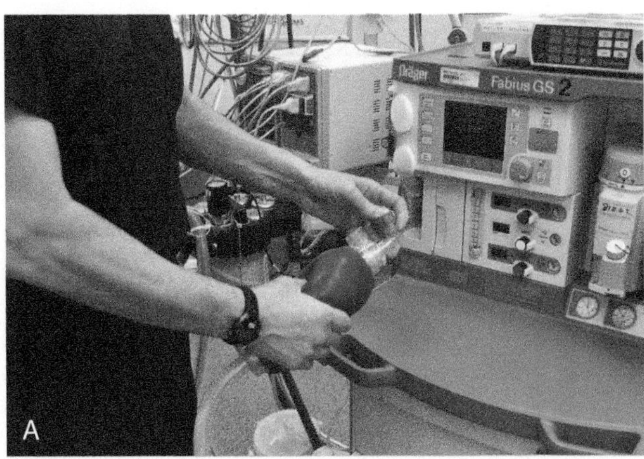

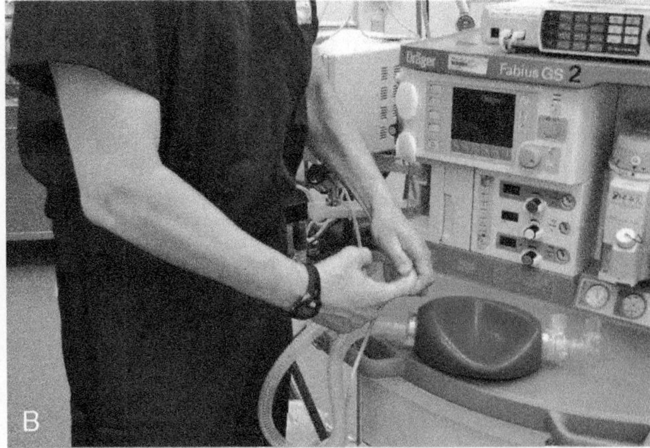

FIGURE 32-2 Inspection of a self-inflating resuscitation bag. Squeeze the bag and ensure that air flows out of the elbow connection. **A**, Next, occlude the elbow connection and squeeze the bag to check the inlet valve, bag, and other components for significant leaks. **B**, Occlude the reservoir tube inflow, then collapse the bag to assess the outlet check valve. The bag should remain collapsed if inflow is occluded.

cylinder valve be closed to avoid inadvertent emptying of the cylinder through a leaky or open regulator.[28]

This step was item 1 on the 1993 PAC and remains so in the 2008 recommendations. It is the *most important* item on the checklist. No matter what happens to the machine, you should always be prepared to keep the patient alive without it. The auxiliary ventilation device should be self-inflating, which would *exclude* the disposable Mapleson circuits often found in and out of the operating room (OR); these devices should be located at "every anesthetizing location," and the guideline further recommends that they be checked for proper function (Fig. 32-2). The recommendation also states that the auxiliary oxygen source should be separate from the machine and its pipeline supply, "specifically an oxygen cylinder." Ensuring that properly filled portable cylinders with attached flowmeters are available at specific locations requires an institutional logistic commitment and careful attention to detail by support staff. Incorporating technicians into this step would likely be very useful.

Item 2: Verify patient suction is adequate to clear the airway
Frequency: Prior to each use
Responsible Parties: Provider and technician

"Safe anesthetic care requires the immediate availability of suction to clear the airway if needed."[28]

This step moved up from the last position on the 1993 PAC recommendations. Suction is critically important to anesthesia care, because it is the only major piece of equipment used routinely by anesthesiologists whose function cannot be replaced in a life-threatening crisis by the anesthesiologist's own body. An anesthesiologist can monitor, ventilate, and even intubate if necessary without any equipment at all. An anesthesiologist cannot, however, adequately clear a pharynx full of secretions or vomitus without an adequately functioning suction; thus suction is a genuinely vital piece of anesthesia equipment. One simple way to check the suction is to determine whether there is enough negative pressure for the tubing to attach to the operator's finger and support its own weight while suspended in the air (Fig. 32-3).

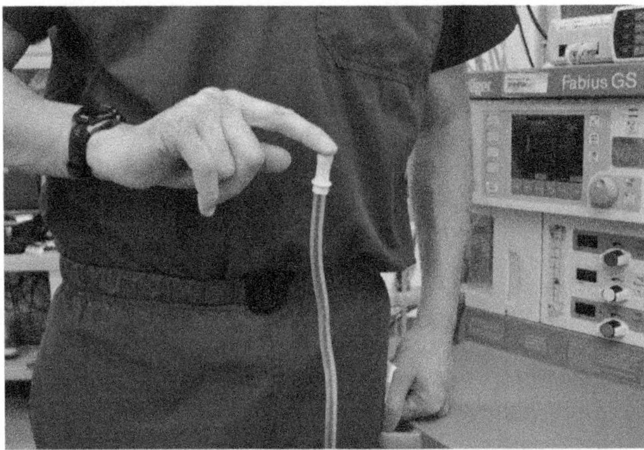

FIGURE 32-3 Checking the negative pressure of the suction. The force of the suction should be adequate if this maneuver can be performed.

Item 3: Turn on anesthesia delivery system and confirm that AC power is available
Frequency: Daily
Responsible Parties: Provider or technician

Anesthesia delivery systems typically function with back-up battery power if AC power fails. Unless the presence of AC power is confirmed, the first obvious sign of power failure can be a complete system shutdown when the batteries can no longer power the system. Many anesthesia delivery systems have visual indicators of the power source showing the presence of both AC and battery power. These indicators should be checked, and connection of the power cord to a functional AC power source should be confirmed. Desflurane vaporizers require electrical power and recommendations for checking power to these vaporizers should also be followed.[28]

Most anesthesia machines provide some indication that the machine is plugged into AC power, or that it is not and is on battery power (Fig. 32-4). Ensuring that the machine is plugged into AC power should be a checklist item. Some newer generation machines perform a battery check automatically and report problems to the operator during start-up checks, whereas some machines require a manual assessment of battery power, such as unplugging the machine from the outlet and pressing a battery test button. If not an automated function, checking the battery power is another example of how an anesthesia technician could unburden anesthesia providers.

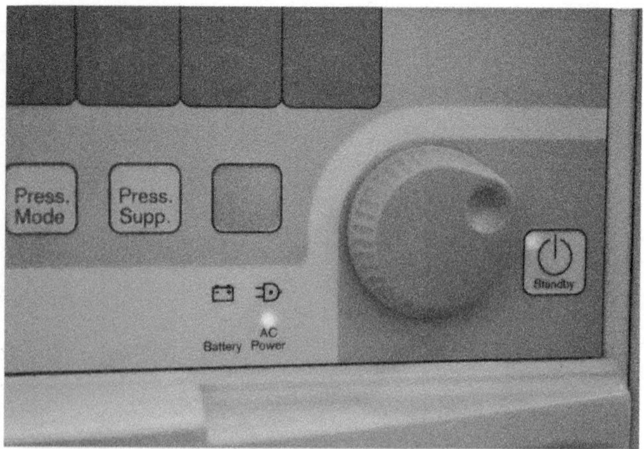

FIGURE 32-4 ■ Machine connection to alternating current (AC) power should be confirmed during preuse checkout procedures. Abrupt system failure could occur during battery-powered operations.

Item 4: Verify availability of required monitors and check alarms

Frequency: Prior to each use
Responsible Parties: Provider or technician

> *Standards for patient monitoring during anesthesia are clearly defined. The ability to conform to these standards should be confirmed for every anesthetic. The first step is to visually verify that the appropriate monitoring supplies (BP cuffs, oximetry probes, etc.) are available. All monitors should be turned on and proper completion of power-up self-tests confirmed. Given the importance of pulse oximetry and capnography to patient safety, verifying proper function of these devices before anesthetizing the patient is essential. Capnometer function can be verified by exhaling through the breathing circuit or gas sensor to generate a capnogram, or verifying that the patient's breathing efforts generate a capnogram before the patient is anesthetized. Visual and audible alarm signals should be generated when this is discontinued. Pulse oximeter function, including an audible alarm, can be verified by placing the sensor on a finger and observing for a proper recording. The pulse oximeter alarm can be tested by introducing motion artifact or removing the sensor. Audible alarms have also been reconfirmed as essential to patient safety by ASA, American Association of Nurse Anesthetists, Anesthesia Patient Safety Foundation, and the Joint Commission. Proper monitor functioning includes visual and audible alarm signals that function as designed.*[28]

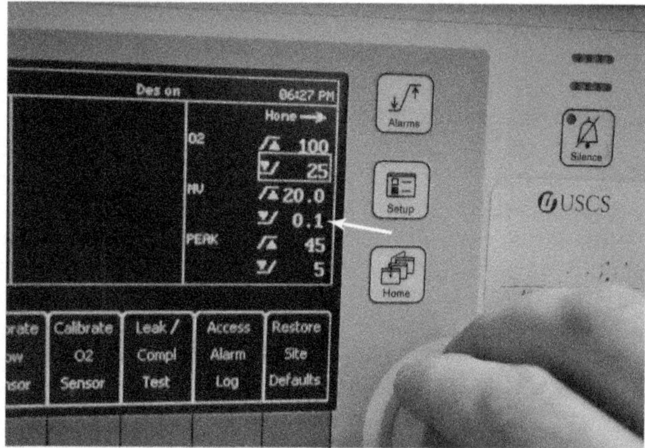

FIGURE 32-5 ■ Setting machine alarm limits. Alarm limit values are easy to adjust, although this task could be time consuming during routine preuse checkout. Safe default values can be established locally and set by trained technicians, which will help keep limits consistent. Note the inappropriately low minute ventilation threshold default on this machine (*arrow*).

Verifying the availability and proper functioning of standard and other required monitors is a relatively straightforward task. However, the process of checking alarm thresholds, and possibly resetting them, can be tedious. It is possible for alarm settings on monitors to vary within individual facilities, because of provider manipulation of alarms for case requirements, a lack of standard default settings, and a failure to routinely reset alarm limits. Departmental alarm default settings can be established and programmed into anesthesia workstation monitors. Alarm limit settings also include anesthesia machine alarms such as volume, pressure, and inspired oxygen concentration limits (Fig. 32-5). It is advisable to ensure that critical alarm limits are set to values that allow them to do what they were intended to do. Here, anesthesia technicians can improve the quality of the preuse checkout by checking the function of standard monitors and confirming that critical alarm thresholds are set to established default values.

Item 5: Verify that pressure is adequate on the spare oxygen cylinder mounted on the anesthesia machine

Frequency: Daily
Responsible Parties: Provider and technician

> *Anesthesia delivery systems rely on a supply of oxygen for various machine functions. At a minimum, the oxygen supply is used to provide oxygen to the patient. Pneumatically powered ventilators also rely on a gas supply. Oxygen cylinder(s) should be mounted on the anesthesia delivery system and determined to have an acceptable minimum pressure. The acceptable pressure depends on the intended use, the design of the anesthesia delivery system, and the availability of piped oxygen.*[28]

Verification of oxygen cylinder pressure is accomplished by opening the oxygen cylinder(s) on the back of

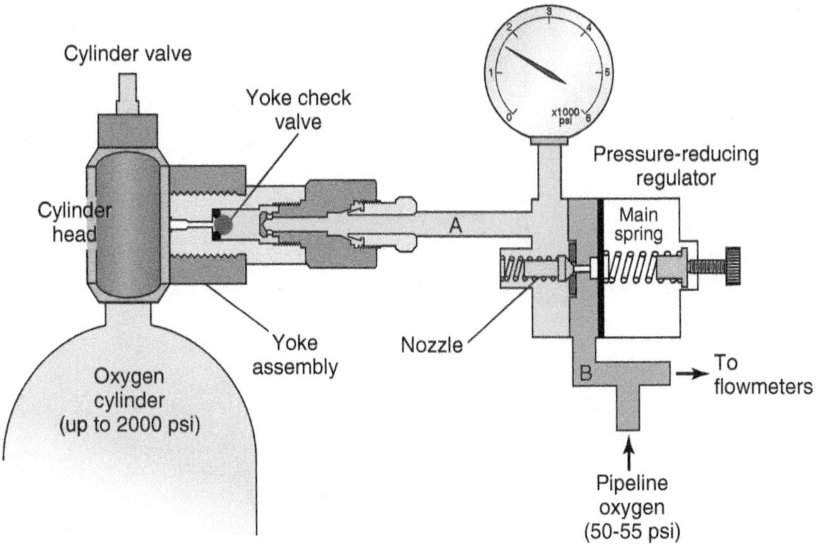

FIGURE 32-6 ■ High-pressure inlet segment of many anesthesia machines. When the cylinder valve is opened on the tank, gas flows through the yoke check valve from the tank into the high-pressure segment (*A*). If the pressure in the *pipeline* oxygen segment (*B*) is sufficient—that is, high enough to overcome the pressure-reducing regulator main spring pressure—it will hold the regulator nozzle closed, and cylinder gas and its corresponding pressure will be confined to segment A. (This is why it is important to disconnect the pipeline supply at the wall in the case of an oxygen pipeline contamination). Segment A will remain pressurized even if the tank is removed, or if the tank is open and bleeding down, because the yoke check valve will be held closed by segment A pressure. This can cause the cylinder gauge pressure reading to be erroneous because of its connection to segment A rather than the cylinder itself. (Modified from *Operating principles of Narkomed anesthesia systems,* ed 2. Telford, PA, 1998, Dräger Medical.)

the machine and evaluating the tank gauge pressure located on the front of the machine, although some newer machines may also have a tank gauge located on the back of the machine. The 1986 PAC guideline recommended to "replace any cylinder with less than 600 psig."[29] The 1993 PAC guideline recommends that the oxygen cylinder be "at least half full (about 1000 psig)" during checkout. The current recommendations do not provide a specific value, but some manufacturer's manuals still suggest the 1000 psig minimum.[30]

It is important to understand that it is theoretically possible for the tank gauge pressure to read higher than the actual pressure in the tank; this is because on many machines, the tank gauge pressure reflects the pressure *in the pipeline segment* between the yoke check valve and low-pressure side of the pressure-reducing regulator (Fig. 32-6). When the tank pressure falls below the pressure it contained when it was previously opened, the gauge will continue to reflect the higher pressure in the segment unless the *wall* supply pressure within the machine dips low enough for the pressure-reducing regulator to open to the tank supply route. A situation like this could occur, theoretically, if the provider were to leave the tank valve open during the PAC, and the tank were to drain down low or even empty through a leak at the yoke assembly. If a provider or technician then opened the tank valve, the gauge pressure would read the pressure remaining *in the piping segment,* not within the tank, because the segment pressure is higher than the pressure in the tank. This is due to the one-way nature of the yoke check valve. Unless tank pressure can overcome the upstream segment pressure, actual tank pressure will not be reflected on the gauge. In fact, even if the tank is *completely removed,* segment pressure will still be reflected on the gauge (Fig. 32-7).

This possible error can be overcome by bleeding the oxygen tank gauge down to zero prior to checking oxygen tank pressure. This can only be accomplished by disconnecting the wall oxygen source, closing the O_2 tank valve, and draining down all machine oxygen pressure using the oxygen flush button or the oxygen flow control valve. Disconnection of the oxygen pipeline supply was a recommended step in the 1986 FDA PAC but not in the 1993 version. Likewise, there is no mention in the 2008 guideline, although many machine users' manuals recommend this step in their respective daily checkout procedures.[30-35] During development of the 1993 PAC, it was noted that provider failure to reconnect the main oxygen supply line during the PAC was not a rare occurrence. There was also a concern that daily removal and reconnection of the oxygen supply line connector could contribute to wear or breakdown. Given these concerns, disconnection of the oxygen pipeline supply is not a specified recommendation within the 1993 and 2008 guidelines.[36] Some newer generation machines measure tank pressure prior to the outlet check valve, which eliminates this concern completely. Additional bulleted comments in this item of the 2008 guidelines include:

> *Typically, an oxygen cylinder will be used if the central oxygen supply fails.*[28]

Auxiliary oxygen cylinders will be used if the pipeline supply of oxygen fails *or becomes contaminated.* During a simulated gas pipeline crossover accident, researchers found that several participants used the machine's auxiliary oxygen flowmeter as a presumed external source of

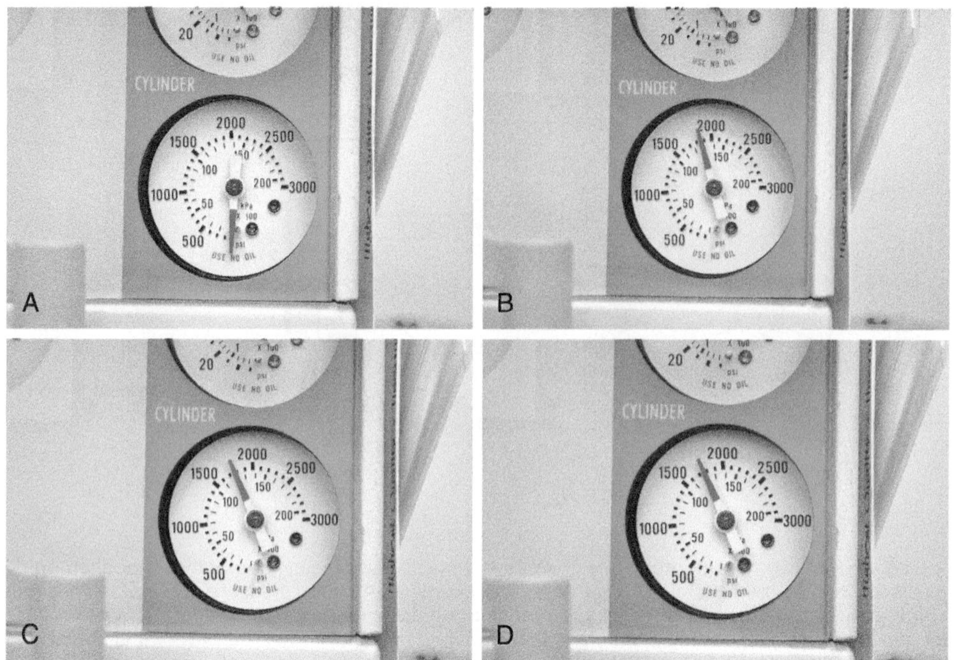

FIGURE 32-7 ■ Erroneous oxygen cylinder pressure caused by the presence of the yoke check valve. **A,** Closure of the oxygen cylinder valve, disconnection of the wall oxygen supply, and depression of the O_2 flush button results in zero gauge pressure. **B,** Connection of the O_2 supply line and opening of the O_2 cylinder valve demonstrates approximately 1850 psig cylinder pressure. **C,** *Removal* of the O_2 cylinder and depression of the O_2 flush results in minimal gauge deflection. **D,** Attaching an *empty* O_2 cylinder to the yoke assembly and opening the cylinder valve results in no change in gauge pressure.

oxygen, yet none properly disconnected the wall oxygen line while the inspired oxygen concentration declined in the face of sustained pipeline pressure.[3]

If the cylinder is intended to be the primary source of oxygen (e.g., remote-site anesthesia), then a cylinder supply sufficient to last for the entire anesthetic is required.[28]

The amount of oxygen required for a case begins with estimating the patient's anticipated needs and then determining the requirements of the mechanical ventilator if driven by gas (see below). It is always wise to estimate finite-source oxygen needs (e.g., a tank) by applying a wide margin on the side of safety.

If a pneumatically powered ventilator that uses oxygen as its driving gas will be used, a full 'E' oxygen cylinder may provide only 30 minutes of oxygen. In that case, the maximum duration of oxygen supply can be obtained from an oxygen cylinder if it is used only to provide fresh gas to the patient in conjunction with manual or spontaneous ventilation. Mechanical ventilators will consume the oxygen supply if pneumatically powered ventilators that require oxygen to power the ventilator are used. Electrically powered ventilators do not consume oxygen so that the duration of a cylinder supply will depend only on total fresh gas flow.[28]

Generally speaking, mechanical ventilators using a bellows are typically gas driven, with either oxygen or air, and piston driven ventilators are electrically driven. This underscores the importance of machine familiarity.

The oxygen cylinder valve should be closed after it has been verified that adequate pressure is present, unless the cylinder is to be the primary source of oxygen (i.e., piped oxygen is not available). If the valve remains open and the pipeline supply should fail, the oxygen cylinder can become depleted while the anesthesia provider is unaware of the oxygen supply problem.[28]

The interface between the oxygen tank and the yoke assembly is very vulnerable to leaking. As alluded to above, if the oxygen tank pressure were to steadily decrease during the day, the provider would possibly be unaware, because real-time tank pressure measurement could be blocked by the yoke check valve. If tank pressure on the machine was measured prior to the yoke check valve, which is currently the exception, actual tank pressure would be continuously displayed, and this problem would be immediately recognized.

Other gas supply cylinders (e.g. Heliox, CO_2, Air, N_2O) need to be checked only if that gas is required to provide anesthetic care.[28]

Item 6: Verify that piped gas pressures are 50 psig or greater

Frequency: Daily
Responsible Parties: Provider and technician

A minimum gas supply pressure is required for proper function of the anesthesia delivery system. Gas supplied from a central source can fail for a variety of reasons.

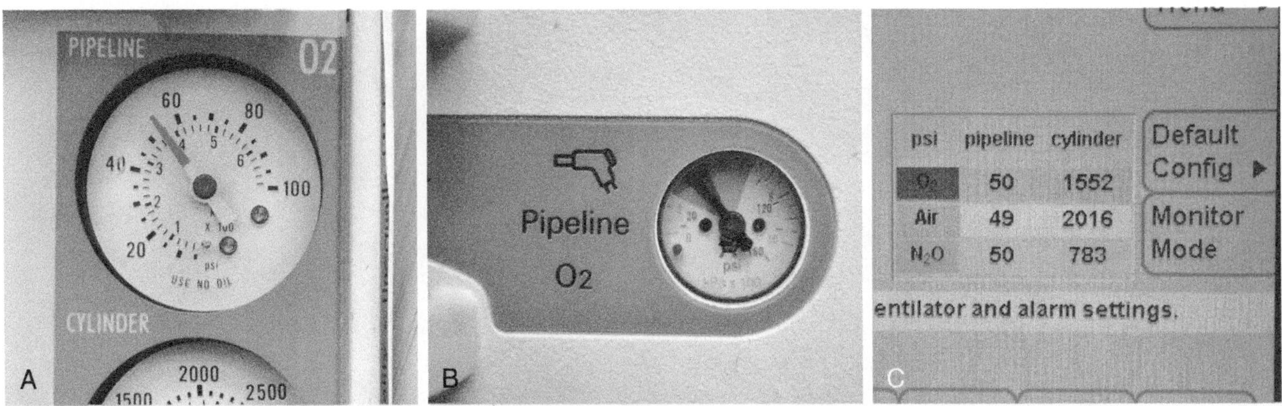

FIGURE 32-8 Pipeline pressure gauge examples. **A,** Standard analog gauge. **B,** Analog gauge with standard pressure ranges highlighted for psi (*dark green*) and kPa (*light green*). **C,** Digital pressure gauge.

Therefore the pressure in the piped gas supply should be checked at least once daily.[28]

Normal pipeline pressures in the United States for common gases (O_2, air, N_2O) are 50 to 55 psig (345 to 380 kPa).[37] Pipeline pressure gauges on anesthesia machines include standard numeric analog gauges, analog gauges that highlight acceptable ranges, and digital pressure gauges (Fig. 32-8). Although the guideline suggests verifying gauge pressures, an inspection of the supply hoses and connections is also recommended by some manufacturers. Checking that "hoses are connected" was a checklist item on the 1993 PAC. Despite gas-specific connectors, misconnections of gas hoses have been reported.[38-40] Likewise, medical gas supply lines behind the walls of the OR are not immune from misconnection or contamination.[41-45] A preuse check that includes a quick daily inspection of connections, supply hoses, gas pressures, and the presence of more than 90% oxygen in the inspiratory limb will greatly minimize risk.

An important safety item on all machines is an audible and visual alarm that warns the operator of diminishing oxygen supply pressure. The only way to evaluate this item is to disconnect the wall oxygen supply and shut off any oxygen supply tanks. Likewise, an evaluation of the machine's oxygen failure protection device or fail-safe feature would also require disconnection of the O_2 supply hose. These two checks were not included in the 1993 guideline or in the current version, presumably because they are too time consuming relative to their risk-preventative value. Also, and as alluded to above, daily removal of the oxygen supply hose may introduce a risk greater than that posed by the potential for failure of these features. An evaluation of these features is usually part of routine preventative maintenance.

Item 7: Verify that vaporizers are adequately filled and, if applicable, that the filler ports are tightly closed

Frequency: Daily
Responsible Parties: Provider and also the technician if redundancy is desired

If anesthetic vapor delivery is planned, an adequate supply is essential to reduce the risk of light anesthesia or recall. This is especially true if an anesthetic agent monitor with a low agent alarm is not being used. Partially open filler ports are a common cause of leaks that may not be detected if the vaporizer control dial is not open when a leak test is performed. This leak source can be minimized by tightly closing filler ports. Newer vaporizer designs have filling systems that automatically close the filler port when filling is completed. High and low anesthetic agent alarms are useful to help prevent over- or under-dosage of anesthetic vapor. Use of these alarms is encouraged, and they should be set to the appropriate limits and enabled.[28]

Although not part of the 2008 guideline, some manufacturers recommend a check of their machine's vaporizer interlock system, which if present prevents more than one vaporizer from being activated simultaneously. If this step is added to a local checklist, make sure that when one vaporizer handwheel is turned to a setting greater than zero that any other vaporizers remain locked in the zero position. Test the system for all mounted vaporizers, and then ensure all vaporizers are placed back to the zero position. This is also a good time to make certain that the vaporizers are firmly mounted.

Item 8: Verify that there are no leaks in the gas supply lines between the flowmeters and the common gas outlet

Frequency: Daily and whenever a vaporizer is changed
Responsible Parties: Provider or technician

The gas supply in this part of the anesthesia delivery system passes through the anesthetic vaporizer(s) on most anesthesia delivery systems. In order to perform a thorough leak test, each vaporizer must be turned on individually to check for leaks at the vaporizer mount(s) or inside the vaporizer. Furthermore, some machines have a check valve between the flowmeters and the common gas outlet, requiring a negative pressure test to adequately check for leaks. Automated checkout procedures typically include a leak test but

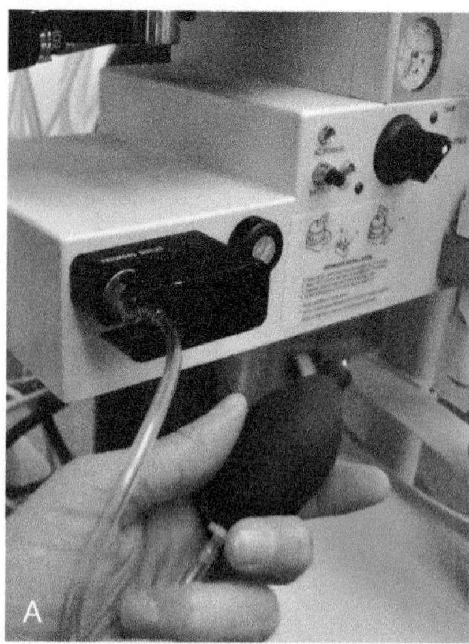

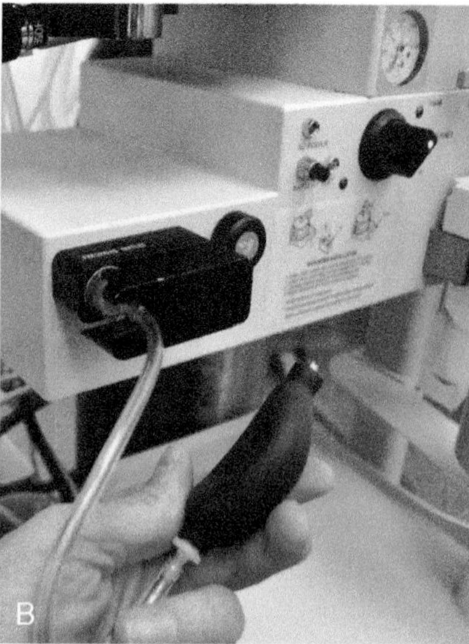

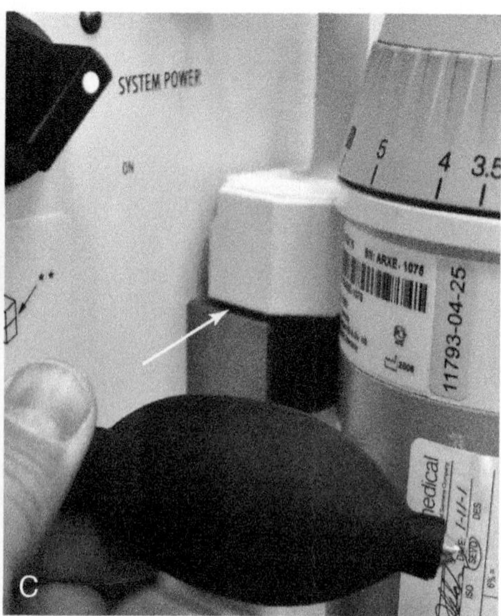

FIGURE 32-9 ■ The universal negative-pressure low-pressure system leak test. **A,** With the machine off and the flow control valves fully closed, a specially configured suction bulb is connected to the common (fresh) gas outlet. **B,** The bulb is pumped until it is fully collapsed; it is then observed to verify that it stays collapsed for more than 10 seconds, indicating that the low-pressure side of the machine is gas tight. Then, each vaporizer is opened in turn, and the maneuver is repeated to establish that no leak is associated with that vaporizer. **C,** The vaporizer was intentionally tilted on its mount in order to cause a low-pressure system leak resulting in immediate reexpansion of the suction bulb.

may not evaluate leaks at the vaporizer, especially if the vaporizer is not turned on during the leak test. When relying upon automated testing to evaluate the system for leaks, the automated leak test would need to be repeated for each vaporizer in place. This test should also be completed whenever a vaporizer is changed. The risk of a leak at the vaporizer depends upon the vaporizer design. Vaporizer designs where the filler port closes automatically after filling can reduce the risk of leaks. Technicians can provide useful assistance with this aspect of the machine checkout, since it can be time consuming.[28]

This step checks the integrity of the so-called low-pressure system (LPS) of the anesthesia machine, which is traditionally defined as the section downstream from the flow control valves to the common gas outlet. Leaks in this section of the machine are associated with hypoxemia or patient awareness under anesthesia.[46,47] Leaks here are commonly related to the anesthetic vaporizer, the vaporizer mounting, or the flowmeter tubes.

Because of significant machine design differences, several tests have been described to check for leaks within the LPS.[47] These tests use either positive pressure, assessing either leak flow or system pressure stability, or negative pressure to facilitate leak detection in this vulnerable part of the anesthesia machine (Figs. 32-9 and 32-10). Historically, selecting the proper test was confusing, because some machines have an outlet check between the common gas outlet and the vaporizers (many Ohmeda machines), but others do not. The check valve is meant to minimize the effects of intermittent backpressure on vaporizer output. For machines without an outlet check valve, positive-pressure tests of the LPS are generally sufficient. These include simple pressurization of the patient breathing circuit or more complex positive-pressure testing of the LPS using specialized bulbs, manometers, and/or flowmeters.[24,32,48]

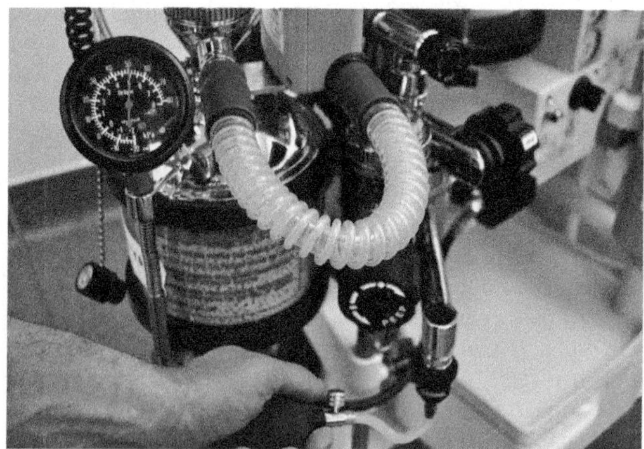

FIGURE 32-10 ■ Dräger (Telford, PA) positive-pressure breathing system leak test specified for the Narkomed 2, 3, 4, GS & M model anesthesia workstations. This particular procedure uses a sphygmomanometer bulb with bag-mount adapter and a length of tubing that short circuits inspiratory and expiratory ports. The test is negative if bulb-generated pressure decreases no more than 20 cm H_2O from 50 cm H_2O in 30 seconds.

Again, the presence of an outlet check valve precludes manual positive-pressure testing of the low-pressure system, because the valve is held closed by downstream positive pressure. To eliminate confusion with this, the 1993 PAC's "Leak Check of the Machine Low-Pressure System" prescribed the so-called universal leak test, a *negative-pressure test* that checks for leaks in the LPS regardless of whether an outlet check valve is present. When compared to several other LPS leak tests performed on machines with and without outlet check valves, the universal leak test was found to be the most sensitive.[49] This simple-to-perform

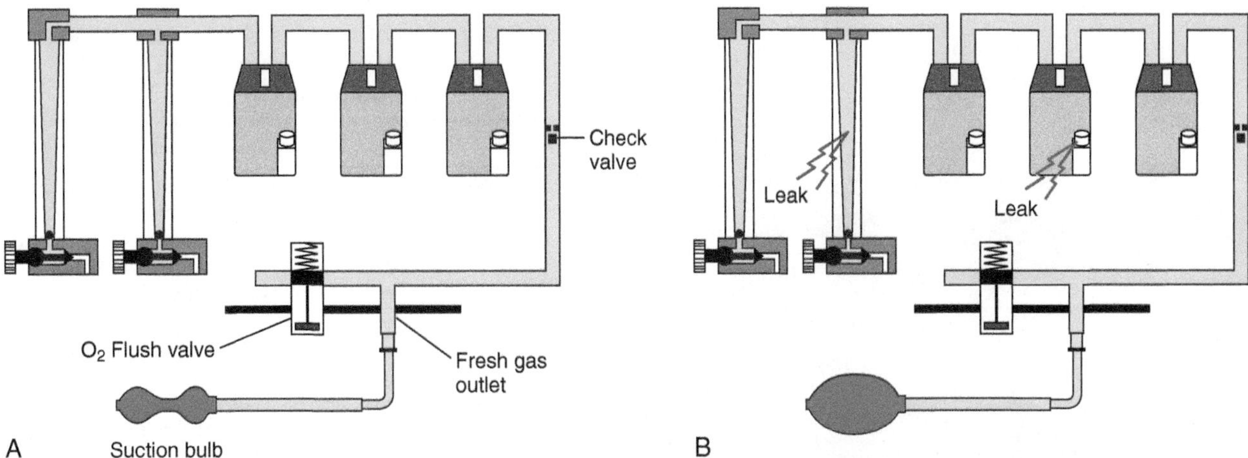

FIGURE 32-11 ■ The universal negative-pressure low-pressure system leak test. **A,** With the specially configured suction bulb connected to the common (fresh) gas outlet and collapsed, subatmospheric pressure is created in the low-pressure circuit, opening the outlet check valve (if present) and exposing the vaporizers, tubing, and associated piping and connections to the vacuum. **B,** Leaks in the system will draw in ambient air and reexpand the suction bulb. (Modified from *Operating principles of Narkomed anesthesia systems,* ed 2. Telford, PA, 1998, Dräger Medical.)

yet often neglected test requires that the machine be turned off and that the flow control valves be fully closed to prevent any flow of gas into the low-pressure system. A specially configured suction bulb, which can either be constructed or obtained from the manufacturer, is then attached to the common gas outlet via tubing and a 15 mm adapter (Figs. 32-11 and 32-12; see also Fig. 32-9). The bulb is then squeezed repeatedly until it is fully collapsed. If the bulb does not stay collapsed for a specified period of time, air is being sucked by the bulb into the machine via a leak that will allow gas to escape when the machine is pressurized. The same maneuver is carried out with each vaporizer opened in turn to check for associated leaks. The specified period of bulb collapse varies by reference from 10 seconds in popular texts to 30 seconds in some workstations' user manuals.[31,32,47,50,51] Although small leaks may require more than 10 seconds for bulb reinflation, it is likely that the collapsed bulb will be noted to be steadily expanding before that time.[49] The most important aspect about the universal negative-pressure leak test is that it eliminates any potential for error where an operator might mistakenly apply a positive-pressure leak test to a machine with an outlet check valve.

Many of the newer generation anesthesia machines do not have an accessible common gas outlet; therefore manual LPS testing cannot be performed. These machines presumably test the integrity of the LPS via an automated checkout. However, some machines of the current generation still require a manual LPS leak test (Table 32-2). For those that do, the universal leak test can be applied unless clearly instructed otherwise by the manufacturer. A locally developed PAC should indicate which steps are required on the specific machine to accomplish this important step.

Item 9: Test scavenging system function

Frequency: Daily
Responsible Parties: Provider or technician

A properly functioning scavenging system prevents room contamination by anesthetic gases. Proper function depends upon correct connections between the scavenging system and the anesthesia delivery system. These connections should be checked daily by a provider or technician. Depending upon the scavenging system design, proper function may also require that the vacuum level is adequate, which should also be confirmed daily. Some scavenging systems have mechanical positive and negative pressure relief valves. Positive and negative pressure relief is important to protect the patient circuit from pressure fluctuations related to the scavenging system. Proper checkout of the scavenging system should ensure that positive and negative pressure relief is functioning properly. Due to the complexity of checking for effective positive and negative pressure relief, and the variations in scavenging system design, a properly trained technician can facilitate this aspect of the checkout process.[28]

A test of the scavenging system begins by checking the proper assembly and integrity of each component and connection within the system, including the gas-transfer tubes leading from the adjustable pressure-limiting (APL) valve and the ventilator relief valve to the scavenging interface. In the case of many modern machines, a single transfer tube may lead from a compact breathing system to the scavenger interface. The integrity of the vacuum tubing leading from the wall outlet to the scavenger interface should also be checked.

There exist two types of scavenging interface systems, open and closed. *Closed scavenging systems* are isolated from the environment by pressure relief valves, so the relationship between waste-gas flow, vacuum flow, and the size of the system's reservoir bag determine the effectiveness of the gas elimination. Some closed systems may contain only a positive-pressure relief valve, which protects the breathing circuit from overpressurization (positive end-expiratory pressure [PEEP]) if obstruction occurs downstream from the scavenger interface. These systems rely on passive outflow of waste gas, not a central vacuum, and they do not require a reservoir bag (Fig. 32-13). They are designed to vent into nonrecirculating

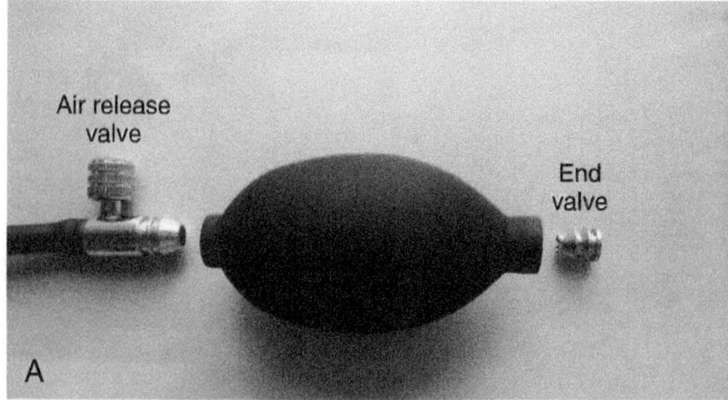

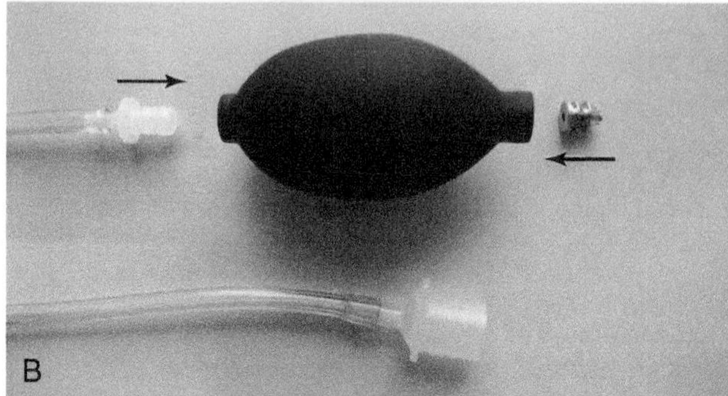

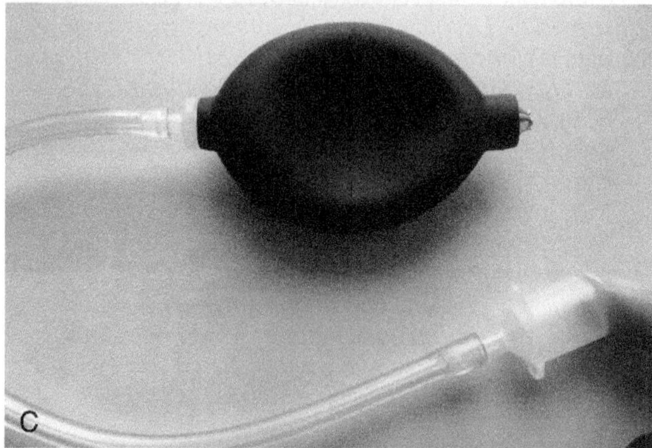

FIGURE 32-12 Constructing a negative-pressure system leak test suction bulb from a sphygmomanometer bulb. **A,** Remove the air release valve and discard. Remove the end valve. **B,** Reverse the end valve and reinsert. Find or purchase a tight-fitting connector, some extra tubing, and a suitable endotracheal tube adapter. Insert the connector into the bulb. **C,** Squeeze the bulb and occlude the adapter. The apparatus should remain collapsed for more than 60 seconds.[31]

heating, ventilation, and air conditioning (HVAC) systems or simply to the building's exterior. They are uncommon. A manufacturer's recommended test of this "passive" scavenger interface involves creating gas flow (pressure) within the breathing system by occluding the patient Y-piece, or short-circuiting the inspiratory and expiratory limbs of the breathing circuit with the breathing hose, occluding the exhaust hose outlet on the scavenging interface, and ensuring that the flow of gas exits the system through the positive-pressure safety relief valve, so excess pressure (>10 cm H_2O) does not build up in the breathing circuit.

Closed systems with positive- and negative-pressure relief valves, a reservoir bag, and active gas elimination via central vacuum are more common (Fig. 32-14).

TABLE 32-2 **Low-Pressure System Leak Tests for Various Anesthesia Workstations**

Machine	Test Method
Datex-Ohmeda Aestiva/5	Manual: negative pressure or positive pressure*‡
Datex-Ohmeda Aisys with ACGO	Manual: negative pressure or positive pressure*‡
Datex-Ohmeda Aisys without ACGO	Automatic
Datex-Ohmeda S/5 Aespire	Manual: negative pressure or positive pressure*‡
Datex-Ohmeda ADU	Automatic
Dräger Narkomed 2B	Manual: positive pressure†‡
Dräger Narkomed M	Manual: positive pressure†‡
Dräger Narkomed MRI	Manual: positive pressure†‡
Dräger Fabius MRI	Automatic†
Dräger Fabius Tiro	Automatic†
Dräger Narkomed Julian	Automatic†
Dräger Narkomed 6000 & 6400	Automatic†
Dräger Fabius GS	Automatic‡
Dräger Apollo	Automatic‡
Penlon Prima SP3	Manual: positive pressure‡
Mindray (Datascope) AS 3000	Automatic‡

Information from user's manuals from Dräger Medical (Telford, PA), Datex-Ohmeda (GE Healthcare, Waukesha, WI), Mindray DS USA Inc. (Mahwah, NJ), and Penlon Limited (Abingdon, UK).
*ISO 5358 or BSI standard positive low-pressure leak test.
†Must manually open vaporizers to check them.
‡Narkomed positive-pressure test using sphygmomanometer squeeze bulb, adapter, and inspiratory-expiratory port interconnection hose (universal negative-pressure leak test will work as well).
ACGO, auxiliary common gas outlet.

Negative-pressure relief valves within these systems prevent subatmospheric pressure from occurring within the patient breathing circuit as a result of the application of excessive suction. An adjustable needle valve regulates the waste-gas exhaust flow. A check of positive-pressure relief is conducted as described above. Some manufacturers recommend that the suction needle valve be turned off for this step. A check of negative-pressure relief is conducted by setting the scavenger interface suction to a routine setting, turning off all flow control valves on the anesthesia machine, and occluding inflow into the patient breathing circuit at the patient Y-piece, or short-circuiting the inspiratory and expiratory limbs of the breathing circuit with the breathing hose and at the breathing bag mount. At this point, the breathing pressure gauge should indicate a negligible negative pressure (e.g., no lower than -1.0 cm H_2O). Generally speaking, the scavenger suction on active systems should be adjusted so the reservoir bag is never overinflated or underinflated; rather, it should remain slightly inflated during routine use. Because the volume of gas being passed into the scavenging system varies, it may be necessary to adjust the needle valve. Given the diversity of breathing systems, this check serves as another instance in which users must consider manufacturer specified protocols when developing a local PAC.

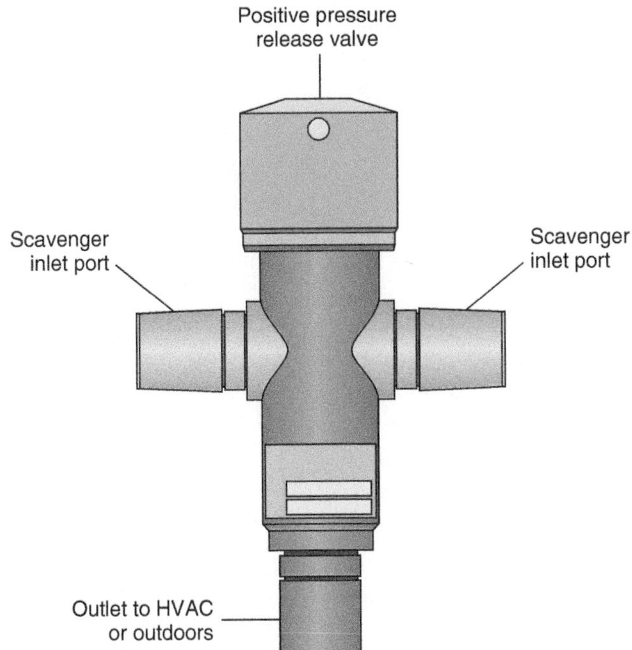

FIGURE 32-13 Passive "closed" scavenger assembly. Formal testing involves occluding the exhaust hose outlet on the scavenging interface, pressurizing the breathing circuit, and ensuring that gas exits the system through the positive-pressure safety relief valve, preventing pressure buildup in the breathing circuit. HVAC, heating, ventilation, and air conditioning unit. (Modified from *Operating principles of Narkomed anesthesia systems,* ed 2. Telford, PA, 1998, Dräger Medical.)

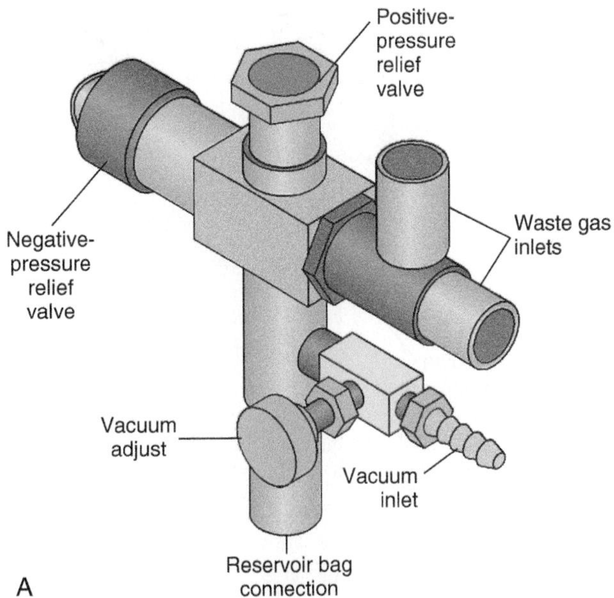

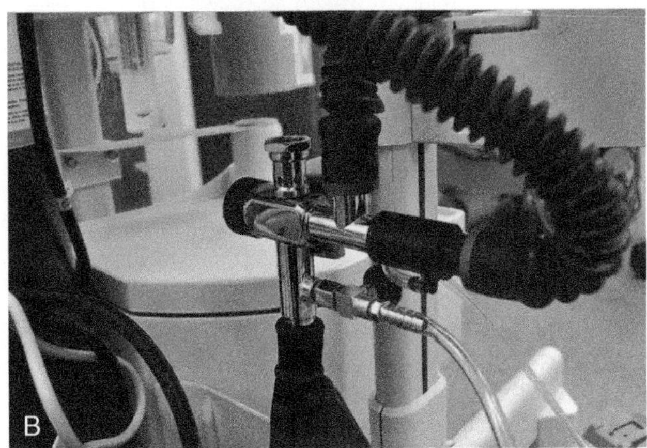

FIGURE 32-14 Active "closed" scavenger assembly. Positive-pressure relief testing can be conducted as described for passive systems. Negative-pressure relief testing involves occluding the patient Y-piece after turning off all flow control valves and ensuring that circuit breathing pressure indicates only a negligible negative pressure (e.g., more than −1.0 cm H_2O). Scavenger suction should be adjusted so the reservoir bag is neither overinflated or underinflated during routine use. (Modified from *Operators instruction and setup manual: Narkomed M anesthesia system,* Telford, PA, 2001, Dräger Medical.)

Open scavenger systems are simpler to understand and use, and they are easier to check out. Open systems contain no valves and are open to the environment (Fig. 32-15). The patient breathing circuit is much less likely to be subject to overpressure or negative pressure, assuming the conduits are patent, and adequate suction is present. As in the case of the active closed scavenger system, inadequate suction will result in waste anesthetic gases venting into the room. After ensuring that all gas-transfer tubes and suction lines are properly connected, the scavenger suction needle valve is adjusted to place the flowmeter bobbin between the indicator lines. A positive- and negative-pressure test is then conducted as described above.

The 1993 PAC prescribed a simple procedure for checking the scavenging system that eliminated several steps described in manufacturer's user's manuals. It can be applied to both closed and open scavenging systems. For every machine, the evaluation of the scavenging system is a manual evolution; there are no automated checks.

Item 10: Calibrate, or verify calibration of, the oxygen monitor and check the low oxygen alarm

Frequency: Daily
Responsible Parties: Provider or technician

> *Continuous monitoring of the inspired oxygen concentration is the last line of defense against delivering hypoxic gas concentrations to the patient. The oxygen monitor is essential for detecting adulteration of the oxygen supply. Most oxygen monitors require calibration once daily, although some are self-calibrating. For self-calibrating oxygen monitors, they should be verified to read 21% when sampling room air. This is a step that is easily completed by a trained technician. When more than one oxygen monitor is present, the primary sensor that will be relied upon for oxygen monitoring should be checked. The low oxygen concentration alarm should also be checked at this time by setting the alarm above the measured oxygen concentration and confirming that an audible alarm signal is generated.*[28]

The importance of the oxygen monitor cannot be overstated; therefore a proper evaluation of its function is imperative. It is the only monitor positioned to detect oxygen delivery problems downstream from the flow control valves.[47] All other oxygen-related safety devices

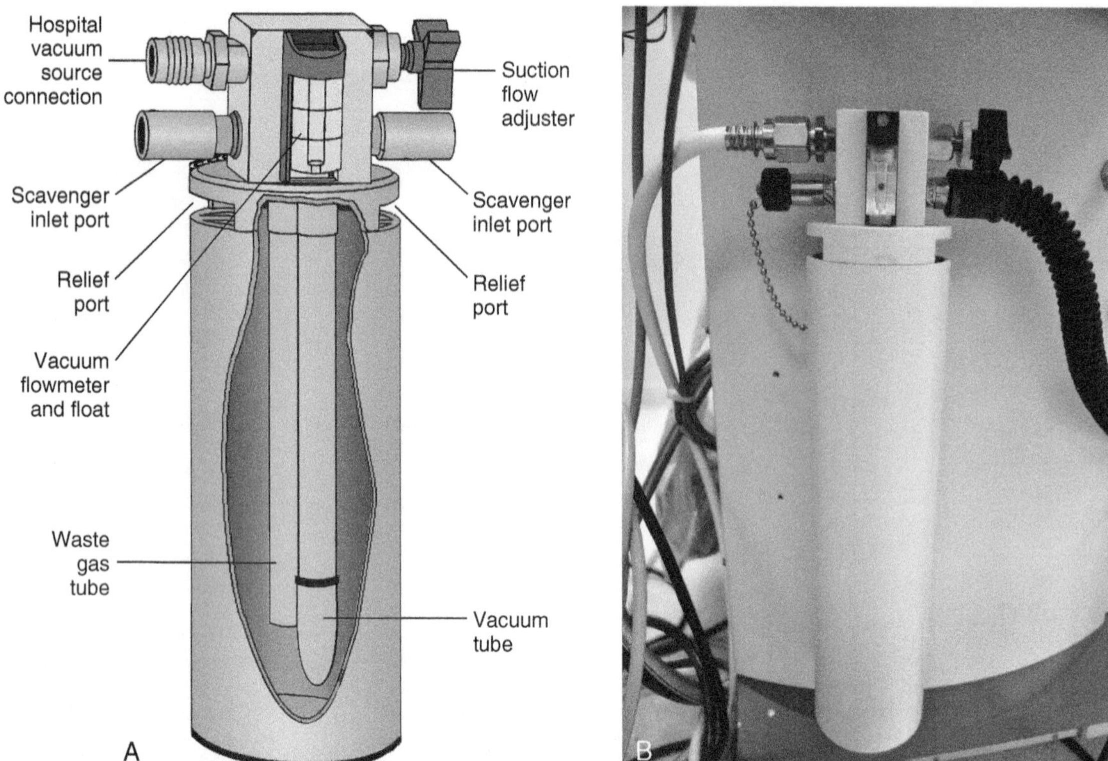

FIGURE 32-15 ■ "Open" scavenger assembly. The preuse check involves ensuring that gas flows freely from the patient breathing circuit into the scavenger and that the vacuum flow to the scavenger is adequate. (Modified with permission from *Operating principles of Narkomed anesthesia systems,* ed 2. Telford, PA, 1998, North American Dräger. Courtesy Dräger Medical.)

are located upstream from the flow control valves.[51] Traditionally, most machines have used a galvanic cell oxygen sensor located near the patient breathing circuit inspiratory valve. In most cases it is simple to access. In this position, the sensor is exposed to the gas as it flows toward the patient after the fresh gas flow is introduced. These electrochemical devices have a finite life span that is inversely proportional to the amount of oxygen exposure.[50] They are also vulnerable to drift; therefore daily verification of calibration is recommended, with recalibration as necessary.

The procedure to verify 21% fraction of inspired oxygen (F_IO_2) calibration varies among machines, but it often involves removing the sensor housing from the breathing circuit (Fig. 32-16, *A*). At this time, the low-oxygen alarm should also be tested. It should alarm if the low limit is set above 21% (see Fig. 32-16, *B*). A prudent default setting would be somewhere between 25% and 30%, unless oxygen concentrations below this value are used routinely. In any case, it should always be set to at least 21%. The steps involved in *recalibrating* the sensor to room air always involve removing the sensor from the breathing circuit. After calibration verification or recalibration, the breathing system is flushed with 100% oxygen. This should result in an oxygen concentration reading of more than 90% (see Fig. 32-16, *C*). Users and technicians should be aware that when a new oxygen sensor is placed into the sensor housing, it may take up to 90 minutes before it stabilizes and is ready for calibration.[52]

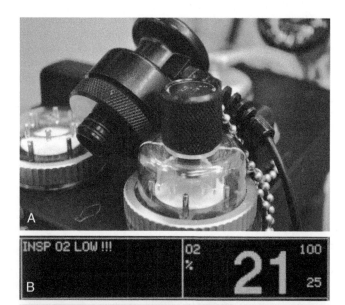

FIGURE 32-16 ■ Testing the low oxygen concentration alarm and calibrating the oxygen sensor. **A,** Removal of the oxygen-sensor housing exposes the sensor to ambient air. **B,** When the oxygen concentration decreases below the alarm threshold value, which in this case is set at 25%, the visual and auditory low inspired oxygen concentration alarms should activate. **C,** After replacing the oxygen sensor, the oxygen flush button should be used to bring the fraction of inspired oxygen to at least 90%.

Some newer generation anesthesia machines *do not* contain an in-circuit galvanic sensor. These machines rely on the sidestream-sampling gas analyzer to measure FiO_2. In this case, it is the FiO_2 sensor on the gas analyzer that requires some sort of daily check. Removal of the sample line can be done to check room air calibration. This serves as another example of growing machine diversity and the importance of machine familiarity as it pertains to daily use and local PAC development.

Item 11: Verify carbon dioxide absorbent is not exhausted
Frequency: Prior to each use
Responsible Parties: Provider or technician

> *Proper function of a circle anesthesia system relies on the absorbent to remove carbon dioxide from rebreathed gas. Exhausted absorbent as indicated by the characteristic color change should be replaced. It is possible for absorbent material to lose the ability to absorb CO_2, yet the characteristic color change may be absent or difficult to see. Some newer absorbents do change color when desiccated. Capnography should be used for every anesthetic and, when using a circle anesthesia system, rebreathing carbon dioxide as indicated by an inspired CO_2 concentration >0 can also indicate exhausted absorbent.*[28]

It is important for providers to know that absorbent color change is not as reliable as is the presence of *inspired* CO_2 on capnography in identifying exhausted absorbent. Absorbent “regeneration,” indicator deactivation, inner canister channeling, and coloration of the absorbent canister wall are examples of circumstances that can mislead the practitioner regarding the actual absorptive capacity.[50,53] Therefore a normal-appearing absorbent may be significantly degraded in its ability to remove CO_2. However, it is no longer advised for providers to manually exercise (i.e., breathe in and out of) the breathing circuit and absorbent to assess the absorbent during preuse checkout. Visual inspection must suffice.

In addition to the exhaustion of CO_2 absorptive capacity, absorber desiccation is another potential hazard. Exposure of volatile anesthetics to desiccated carbon dioxide absorbents that contain sodium, potassium, or barium hydroxide may result in severe exothermic reactions and/or the production of toxic byproducts such as carbon monoxide.[54] Whereas colorimetric indicators identify the exhaustion of most absorbents, currently only one absorbent provides a permanent colorimetric indicator of *both* desiccation and exhaustion (Amsorb Plus, Armstrong Medical, Lincolnshire, IL).[54,55] Currently no consistently reliable steps can be included in a PAC procedure to identify absorbent desiccation. However, certain scenarios increase the risk of absorbent desiccation, and if recognized these should prompt the provider performing the preuse check to ensure that the absorbent is replaced. Prolonged fresh gas flow during periods of nonuse is thought to be the main factor associated with absorber desiccation. Situations in which gas has been flowing for indeterminate periods—such as over a weekend, with an infrequently used remote-site machine, when gas flows are found during the daily preuse check—should therefore prompt concern. In 2005 the Anesthesia Patient Safety Foundation (APSF) convened a Carbon Dioxide Absorbent Desiccation Safety Conference and published a consensus statement aimed at reducing the risk of adverse reactions associated with carbon dioxide absorbents (Box 32-1). These recommendations should be referenced in developing a departmental risk-management strategy.

BOX 32-1 Anesthesia Patient Safety Foundation (APSF) Carbon Dioxide Absorbent Desiccation Safety Conference Consensus Statement and Recommendations[54]

The APSF recommends use of carbon dioxide absorbents whose composition is such that exposure to volatile anesthetics does not result in significant degradation of the volatile anesthetic. The APSF further recommends that there should be institutional, hospital, and/or departmental policies regarding steps to prevent desiccation of the carbon dioxide absorbent, should conventional carbon dioxide absorbents be chosen that may degrade volatile anesthetics when absorbent desiccation occurs. In such circumstances of using absorbents that may degrade volatile anesthetics, conference attendees generally agreed that users could take the following steps, consistent with ECRI Institute recommendations:

1. Turn off all gas flow when the machine is not in use.
2. Change the absorbent regularly, on Monday morning for instance.
3. Change absorbent whenever the color change indicates exhaustion.
4. Change all absorbents, not just one canister in a two-canister system.
5. Change absorbent when uncertain of the state of hydration, such as if the fresh gas flow has been left on for an extensive or indeterminate period.
6. If compact canisters are used, consider changing them more frequently.

Item 12: Breathing system pressure and leak testing
Frequency: Prior to each use
Responsible Parties: Provider and technician

> *The breathing system pressure and leak test should be performed with the circuit configuration to be used during anesthetic delivery. If any components of the circuit are changed after this test is completed, the test should be performed again. Although the anesthesia provider should perform this test before each use, anesthesia technicians who replace and assemble circuits can also perform this check and add redundancy to this important checkout procedure. Proper testing will demonstrate that pressure can be developed in the breathing system during both manual and mechanical ventilation and that pressure can be relieved during manual ventilation by opening the APL valve. Automated testing is often implemented in the newer anesthesia delivery systems to evaluate the system for leaks and also to determine the compliance of the breathing system. The compliance value determined during this testing will be used to automatically adjust the volume delivered by the ventilator to maintain a constant volume delivery to the patient. It is important that the circuit configuration that is to be used be in place during the test.*[28]

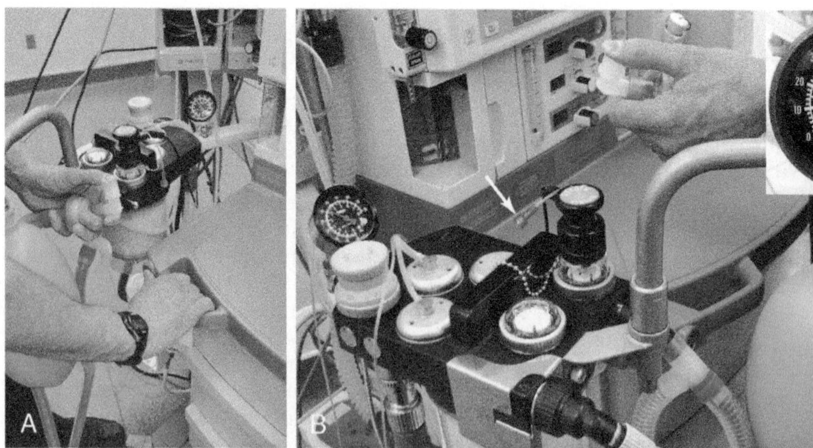

FIGURE 32-17 ■ Manual breathing system pressure and leak testing. The breathing system pressure and leak testing should be performed with the circuit configuration to be used during anesthetic delivery. **A,** The patient Y-piece or elbow is occluded, and the oxygen flush button is used to pressurize the breathing circuit to approximately 30 cm H_2O. **B,** The circuit should hold pressure at this level for at least 10 seconds. It is important to ensure that the gas flows are set to zero, or their minimal values, and that the gas sample line is removed (*arrow*) and its circuit port is occluded.

It is not rare for either the disposable breathing circuit components or the fixed anesthesia machine components to leak; therefore a leak check of the breathing system is of paramount importance. Traditionally, this test has been performed manually after an inspection of the breathing circuit, removal of the gas sampling line, and capping of the gas sampling line port. With the machine set in the "bag" or manual mode of ventilation, the gas flows are set to zero (or the minimal settings), the APL valve is closed, the patient Y-piece is occluded, and the breathing system is pressurized with the oxygen flush button to about 30 cm H_2O (Fig. 32-17). The circuit passes the leak test if it holds this pressure for at least 10 seconds. Some manufacturers may specify a low oxygen flow rate during the test.[32] PAC developers should refer to the user's manual in this regard. A decrease in pressure during the test should prompt a check of all plug-in, push-fit, and screw connectors and the seal of the absorber canister along with a careful inspection of the disposable tubing.

One of the most common locations of a circuit leak is at the absorber canister, and it is particularly important for the anesthesia provider to apply this check rigorously immediately after the absorbent has been changed, because obstructed disposable canisters (plastic wrapper still on) or incorrectly seated or poorly sealed reusable canisters (often an absorbent granule on the rubber gasket) probably constitute the most frequent anesthesia machine problem still occurring.

On many modern anesthesia machines, breathing circuit leak testing is an automated feature, although manual steps are still required for test preparation. Circuit compliance is often also automatically assessed during this phase to guide ventilator tidal volume delivery. It is therefore important that the test be performed with the circuit that will be used.

The APL valve can also be assessed at this time by opening it widely after the pressure test and ensuring that the breathing circuit pressure decreases rapidly to zero. A prompt pressure drop should occur regardless of APL valve design. Modern APL valves differ from the traditional variable-resistor valves in that they are designed to maintain a relatively stable circuit pressure through a range of fresh gas flows, living more up to the name "pressure limiting." Like any mechanical device, however, this feature has been reported to fail.[56] The ability of a modern APL valve to maintain stable circuit pressure can be easily assessed, if deemed necessary, by setting the APL valve to 30 cm H_2O, occluding the patient Y-piece in a manual mode of ventilation, increasing gas flow to approximately 5 L/min, and ensuring that the circuit pressure, once stable, remains within a range close to that set on the APL valve. This range may be specified in some user's manuals and altogether absent in others.[57]

Item 13: Verify that gas flows properly through the breathing circuit during both inspiration and exhalation

Frequency: Prior to each use
Responsible Parties: Provider and technician

> *Pressure and leak testing does not identify all obstructions in the breathing circuit or confirm proper function of the inspiratory and expiratory unidirectional valves. A test lung or second reservoir bag can be used to confirm that flow through the circuit is unimpeded. Complete testing includes both manual and mechanical ventilation. The presence of the unidirectional valves can be assessed visually during the PAC. Proper function of these valves cannot be visually assessed, since subtle valve incompetence may not be detected. Checkout procedures to identify valve incompetence that may not be visually obvious can be implemented but are typically too complex for daily testing. A trained technician can perform regular valve competence tests. Capnography should be used during every anesthetic, and the presence of carbon dioxide in the inspired gases can help to detect an incompetent valve.*[28]

The original 1986 FDA checklist recommended that the person checking the anesthesia machine inhale and exhale into the patient connector while observing the unidirectional valves for free gas flow in the correct direction and no flow in the opposite direction. Although it is controversial for the anesthesia provider to breathe in

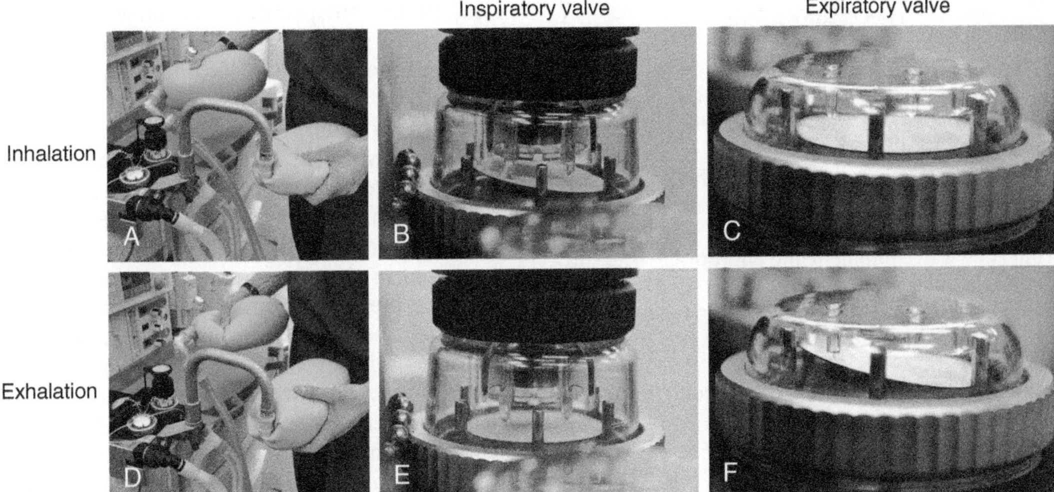

FIGURE 32-18 ■ Verification that gas flows properly through the breathing circuit during both inspiration and exhalation with the to-and-fro flow test. *Top,* A test lung or second reservoir bag can is placed on the patient elbow piece. A squeeze of the breathing bag should cause flow through inspiratory limb, open the inspiratory valve, fill the test lung, and hold the expiratory valve closed. *Bottom,* A reciprocal squeeze of the test lung should cause flow through expiratory limb, open the expiratory valve, fill the breathing bag, and hold the inspiratory valve closed. Circuit flow during the test should be smooth and unimpeded.

and out of the machine and through the next patient's breathing circuit, it is still important that the circuit be exercised to ensure that unidirectional flow is present and unimpeded. This test of circuit flow is easily accomplished by placing a "test lung" or an extra breathing bag at the patient elbow. In the "bag" or manual mode of ventilation, the operator ventilates the artificial "lung" with the breathing bag then actively "exhales" (squeezes) the test lung back to the breathing bag in a to-and-fro motion (Fig. 32-18). This is the so-called *flow test*. During inspiration, the inspiratory valve should open and the expiratory valve should close, and vice versa for exhalation. A major malfunction of a unidirectional valve can be visually assessed, although subtle valve leaks (reverse flow) may only be apparent via capnography during anesthesia or through formal machine evaluation. Obstruction to flow during the flow test manifests as a "tight" breathing bag on inspiration, whereas expiratory limb obstructions cause impeded exhalation. Some form of flow test should be conducted, because leak testing does not reliably identify circuit obstruction or unidirectional valve malfunction. Undetected circuit obstructions are particularly ominous and can manifest dramatically and sometimes immediately following induction.[58-60]

It cannot be stated definitively that all automated machine checks routinely assess for unimpeded circuit flow. Although most users' manuals for machines that perform automated aspects of the preuse checkout describe a leak test function, none were identified that specifically describe a flow test. In fact, some modern machines that incorporate automated checkout steps, including a leak test, recommend a manual assessment of the inspiratory and expiratory valves.[57]

Item 14: Document completion of checkout procedures

Responsible Parties: Provider and technician

Each individual responsible for checkout procedures should document completion of these procedures. Documentation gives credit for completing the job and can be helpful if an adverse event should occur. Some automated checkout systems maintain an audit trail of completed checkout procedures that are dated and timed.[28]

Documentation of completion of the anesthetic checkout procedure by *providers* should be contained within the anesthetic record. Currently, there is no guidance regarding where anesthesia or biomedical technician documentation of checkout procedures should occur. However, it would be prudent to maintain a detailed departmental log as a QA tool (see below).

Item 15: Confirm ventilator settings and evaluate readiness to deliver anesthesia care (anesthesia time out)

Frequency: Immediately prior to initiating the anesthetic
Responsible Parties: Provider

This step is intended to avoid errors due to production pressure or other sources of haste. The goal is to confirm that appropriate checks have been completed and that essential equipment is indeed available. The concept is analogous to the "time out" used to confirm patient identity and surgical site prior to incision. Improper ventilator settings can be harmful, especially if a small patient is following a much larger patient or vice versa. Pressure limit settings (when available) should be used to prevent excessive volume delivery from improper ventilator settings. Items to check: Monitors functional? Capnogram present? Oxygen saturation by pulse oximetry measured? Flowmeter and ventilator settings proper? Manual/ventilator switch set to manual? Vaporizer(s) adequately filled?[28]

This last step serves as a recommended final preinduction checklist of the machine and other important items, including the application of essential monitors. It is a "pre-takeoff" checklist for anesthesia providers. Some providers rely on final check mnemonic devices such as

BOX 32-2 MS MAIDS Mnemonic

Machine: The machine checkout is complete; the vaporizers are filled, closed, and set to "0"; all gas flow knobs are set to zero flow; the ventilator is set up for an upcoming patient.
Suction: Patient suction is adequate to clear the airway.
Monitors: All required monitors are present and ready to go.
Airway: Primary airway equipment and appropriate back-up equipment are ready to go.
IV: Lines, fluids, and associated equipment are ready to go.
Drugs: All necessary medications are available and are properly labeled.
Special Items: Any special or unique items required for the case are available and ready.

the "MS MAIDS" checklist (Box 32-2). Regardless of the configuration, a final checklist that verifies key safety items is just as important in anesthesia as it is in aviation.

Although the 2008 Guidelines for Designing Pre-Anesthesia Checkout Procedures are comprehensive, there are several steps that were part of the 1986 or 1993 recommendations that do not appear in the current guideline yet are sometimes found within machine users' manuals. The use of these steps should be based on local needs and/or requirements, because the 2008 recommendations are not restrictive or intended to be limiting. Some of these items have been mentioned above:

1. Disconnecting the central oxygen supply line to assess the low oxygen supply pressure alarm and to purge the tank pressure gauges to zero
2. Inspecting the gas supply hoses for cracks or wear
3. Testing the flowmeters for smooth operation
4. Testing the proportioning system by attempting to create a hypoxic O_2/N_2O mixture

Automated Anesthesia Machine Checkout Procedures

Important points to consider regarding automated PAC features or self-tests are that 1) they differ among manufacturers *and* models, 2) it is sometimes difficult to determine precisely which segments or components are actually being checked from reading the user's manual, and 3) *no* machine automatically checks all of the items on an effective PAC; at least some manual steps will be required. It has been suggested that many providers do not understand exactly what is being checked by automated checks, or they make false assumptions regarding their respective machine's automated checkout procedure. It is therefore easy to understand why the authors of the ASA's 2008 Recommendations for Pre-Anesthesia Checkout Procedures warned about an overreliance on the automated machine checkout. For example, one manufacturer's self-test screen reports a "leakage" amount, but the display or manual does not specify which segments and components are assessed. The operator must make an assumption that the LPS is also being tested for leaks, and the manual does not state that any vaporizer should be turned on during leak testing. Finally, it is not clear in this unspecified manual whether the circuit is assessed for proper unidirectional flow or obstruction.

When developing a local PAC procedure, providers should gain familiarity with their machine's automated checkout procedure via the user's manual and direct communication with the manufacturer if necessary. Once clear on the actual scope of the automated test, an effective departmental PAC checklist can be created. If an important item is not actually part of the described self-check or is not suggested in the user's manual, it should not be assumed that it is not important. Not requiring that conventional vaporizers be opened during a leak test of the LPS is an example of this problem. Further, if an important checklist item cannot be confirmed to be accomplished by the machine's self-test function, through either the user's manual or the manufacturer, it should be assumed that it *does not occur*, and this step should be accomplished manually if possible. An example of this would be a circuit "flow test."

Machine-Embedded Preanesthesia Checklists

Some anesthesia machines have embedded checklists that are displayed during machine checkout (Fig. 32-19). Like their paper counterparts, they help guide users through manual and self-test functions. If an embedded checklist provides a complete solution for a respective department, it can be used exclusively. However, it is possible that local requirements may exceed or depart to some degree from the workstation's embedded checklist. In these cases, the use of the embedded checklist, or a modification thereof, can become a line item within the local PAC.

Using Technicians to Perform Aspects of the Preanesthesia Checklist

The 2008 recommendations for Pre-Anesthesia Checkout Procedures identify aspects of the PAC that could be completed by a "qualified anesthesia and/or biomedical technician," although the ultimate responsibility for the preuse check remains with the provider. This represents a departure from the previous guidelines, which placed all of the tasks upon the anesthesia provider. The main benefit of using technicians to perform some aspects of the PAC is enhanced compliance by balancing tasks between anesthesia providers and technicians. Other potential benefits include redundant checks of critical items; possible identification of machine problems earlier in the day, so they can be addressed sooner; and enhanced technician familiarity with the anesthesia workstation. A training syllabus may be required for anesthesiology technicians, because a multistep anesthesia workstation precheckout is often not part of their responsibilities. If they are incorporated into daily and precase machine checks, their specific responsibilities can be outlined in the form of a separate technician checklist.

Preuse Checkout of the Anesthesia Machine in an Emergency Situation

During certain emergency circumstances, there may be no time to perform a proper PAC. These are usually

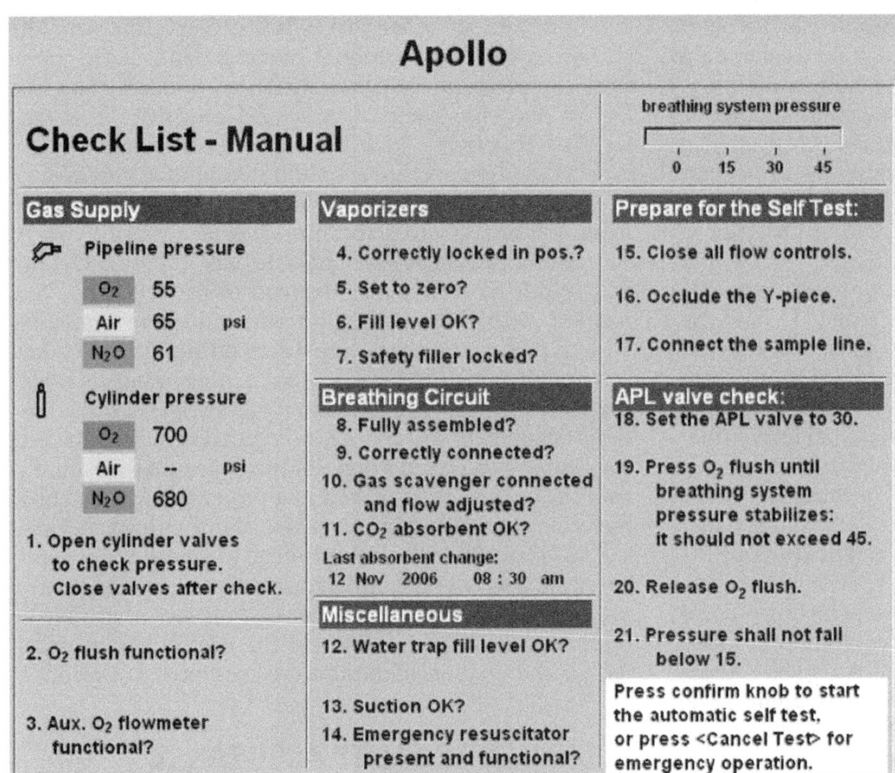

Apollo
Check List - Manual
breathing system pressure
0 15 30 45
Gas Supply
Pipeline pressure
O2 55
Air 65 psi
N2O 61
Cylinder pressure
O2 700
Air -- psi
N2O 680
1. Open cylinder valves to check pressure. Close valves after check.
2. O2 flush functional?
3. Aux. O2 flowmeter functional?
Vaporizers
4. Correctly locked in pos.?
5. Set to zero?
6. Fill level OK?
7. Safety filler locked?
Breathing Circuit
8. Fully assembled?
9. Correctly connected?
10. Gas scavenger connected and flow adjusted?
11. CO2 absorbent OK?
Last absorbent change:
12 Nov 2006 08 : 30 am
Miscellaneous
12. Water trap fill level OK?
13. Suction OK?
14. Emergency resuscitator present and functional?
Prepare for the Self Test:
15. Close all flow controls.
16. Occlude the Y-piece.
17. Connect the sample line.
APL valve check:
18. Set the APL valve to 30.
19. Press O2 flush until breathing system pressure stabilizes: it should not exceed 45.
20. Release O2 flush.
21. Pressure shall not fall below 15.
Press confirm knob to start the automatic self test, or press <Cancel Test> for emergency operation.

FIGURE 32-19 ▪ Dräger Apollo embedded preanesthesia checkout (PAC) checklist. Departments may consider including embedded machine checklists as a line item within a local PAC. (From *Apollo operating instructions*, ed 2. Telford, PA, 2008, Dräger Medical.)

circumstances in which the pace of events is impossible to control (e.g., a "crash" cesarean section, trauma surgery, or emergency cardiac surgery). Ideally, daily or morning checks at potential anesthetizing locations should ready machines for use. However, emergent situations often occur at odd hours and prior to daily PACs. Also, circuit changes, routine maintenance tasks such as an absorbent change, and other manipulations may occur during the day that are unbeknownst to the anesthesia providers. Such events could introduce serious faults, such as leaks or obstructions (see above), or other failures.[61-63] Under these conditions it is still important to know that the machine is, at least, potentially usable, and a minimal check should be performed (Table 32-3).

Anesthesia providers may encounter machines that are not turned on when needed in an emergency. Older generation anesthesia machines were usually ready for immediate use after powerup. However, some modern machines either automatically self-test or anticipate a user-initiated self-test after startup. For example, after turning on the Dräger Julian anesthesia workstation, about 40 seconds elapse for software loading, then an embedded checklist is presented.[64] Normally, after manual completion of the checklist items, the user confirms completion, which then initiates a 3- to 4-minute self-test. This would be obviously unsatisfactory during an emergency; in such as case, the patient can be manually ventilated immediately after turning on the machine. However, software loading still requires about 40 seconds, and the user still must initiate, and then cancel, the self-test. Although this entire process takes only about a minute, the user must be familiar with the steps involved in bypassing normal startup procedures. It may be useful then to include a small "Emergency PAC" within departmental PAC procedures, particularly when

TABLE 32-3 **Proposed Emergency Situation Preanesthesia Checkout**

Ambu bag	Present
Machine status	On
Self-test	Bypass if applicable
Breathing circuit	Circuit intact, absorbent canister closed
Pipeline pressure	50 to 55 psig
Circuit, manual leak test	Circuit holds pressure
Suction	Available
Monitors	Ready
Airway	Ready
IV	Ready
Drugs	Ready

Some modern machines may require an operator-selected bypass of the start-up or automated check-out procedure to ready the machine for routine use.

local machines require a nonintuitive emergency start-up process.

Developing a Local Preanesthesia Checkout Checklist

The goal of a PAC is to properly evaluate and configure the anesthesia workstation, so it is nearly ensured that it can perform its functions properly and safely. Similar to a pre-takeoff checkout of an aircraft, the PAC is a systematic task list consisting of numerous critical steps. It is therefore the perfect situation in which to use a *checklist*. The goals of the *checklist* are to guide the operator through an effective PAC and to promote compliance through ease of use. A checklist is a visual memory aid used to help overcome the limitations of short-term human memory, ensuring that a particular series of specified actions or procedures are accomplished.[65] A PAC checklist can also serve as a quality control tool by codifying important items onto an organized list used by all providers.[66] Although checklists have historically seen of little use in medicine, recent successes have highlighted their effectiveness.[67,68] As useful as they may be, however, a simple checklist like the PAC cannot stand alone. It must be combined with a general foundational knowledge of the anesthesia delivery system, knowledge about the respective workstation, and a positive attitude toward the use of the checklist. This concept is well understood in aviation. Pilots are very familiar with their aircraft, they use procedural checklists as memory aids in checking out their machinery, and they work within a safety culture that embraces the checklist. Based on the current available literature, anesthesia professionals seem to have less understanding of equipment used, have not been shown to be consistent when it comes to checking equipment prior to use, and tend to reject the use of checklists.[11,21,69,70] Anesthesia providers and their patients stand to benefit if we, too, commit to maintaining a sound knowledge of our workstations and advocate the use of checklists.

The essential items required for local PAC checklist development are the 2008 Recommendations for Pre-Anesthesia Checkout Procedures, the respective workstation user's manual, and an anesthesia machine reference text, such as this book. It should be understood that the ASA 2008 Recommendations do not relieve users of their responsibility to be aware of any special procedures or precautions outlined by the manufacturer of their specific machine. However, the PACs found in manufacturer's users' manuals tend to be several pages long, and they may contain items not specified in professional society recommendations, such as the ASA's guidelines. Local PAC developers will quickly recognize these competing objectives of completeness and brevity during the design process. An excessively long checklist will probably not be routinely completed properly, and an underinclusive PAC could miss key items. Alternatively, some manufacturers omit important steps in their PAC recommendations; not opening the vaporizers during leak testing is such an example.

Several basic premises are involved in effective checklist design. First, a checklist like the PAC is a series of read-and-do tasks, either action items ("Open the O_2 cylinder") or verification items ("Verify that the tank pressure reads >1000 psig"). In aviation it would be referred to as a "do-list," and like an aircraft checklist, it should avoid elaboration or explanation.[65,66] Next, the principle that form should follow function is operative when designing an effective PAC. The design of the checklist must support its function to the fullest extent possible, and the checkout procedure should be ergonomically ordered so as to minimize redundant movements and save time by placing procedures in a rational sequence. This is a well-recognized factor in the design of aviation checklists. A Federal Aviation Administration (FAA) monograph addressing human performance considerations in the use and design of aviation checklists states that "The [designer] should ensure that the checklist is configured in an order that is both compatible with the aircraft system's operational sequence and at the same time complement the crew's ability to perform tasks in a logical and consistent order."[71] An effective "flow pattern" will contribute to efficiency and compliance.

Finally, the checklist should be as short as possible yet be detailed enough so that critical items are not omitted. From a human factors and performance point of view, a shorter and less elaborate checklist will enhance use, but it may not be sufficiently detailed to provide those less familiar with the workstation with adequate guidance. Unlike pilots, anesthesia providers do not spend countless hours on equipment-focused training, which is where the aviation/anesthesia analogy weakens significantly. PAC developers will quickly recognize this dilemma and may choose to create a slightly more detailed version for trainees or new employees and another version for those more familiar with their respective workstations. Because a PAC should ideally be confined to one page, a laminated card with the detailed, instructional version on one side and the succinct, true checklist on the other may be optimal (Tables 32-4 and 32-5). Additional checklist design and use considerations are presented in Box 32-3.

EQUIPMENT QUALITY ASSURANCE

As opposed to the "acute" preanesthesia checkout, the "chronic" component of anesthesia equipment management is a comprehensive QA program that involves equipment evaluation, purchasing, installation, initial inspection, periodic safety inspections, preventive maintenance, repair, record keeping, and machine retirement. Coupled with specific attention to pieces of equipment can be a periodic safety inspection of the anesthetizing environment. A classic comprehensive review article[72] includes a 49-point safety inspection that is intended to be performed annually and covers anesthetizing areas (i.e., a suite of operating rooms), individual anesthetizing locations, and equipment. All facilities in which anesthesia is given should have this type of thorough safety inspection at least annually.

Prepurchase Evaluation

The QA or quality management program begins well before any anesthesia equipment is purchased. When new equipment is needed or contemplated, designated members of the anesthesia department must take responsibility for writing specifications for what is needed and then evaluating potential products. Anesthesiologists who will actually be using the equipment must be involved; these tasks should not be delegated to support personnel, purchasing agents, or a product evaluation committee of the facility as a whole. A proposed piece of equipment must meet applicable codes and standards. This usually will be the case when major manufacturers are involved. Thorough questioning of sales representatives and further investigation if there are any doubts should prevent the purchase of new equipment that does not meet current standards. Additional information can often be obtained from the ECRI Institute through its monthly publication *Health Devices*. The ECRI Institute

TABLE 32-4 Departmental Preanesthesia Checklist for the Dräger Fabius*

Check the emergency ventilation equipment

❑ Verify that a self-inflating ventilation bag ("Ambu" type) is available in the operating room.

Pre-Conditions

❑ Ensure that AC power is connected ("Mains Power" LED is illuminated) and that the machine is turned on (back of machine).
❑ Visually inspect the integrity of the breathing circuit.
❑ Check the vaporizer mounting, interlock, agent fill levels, & ensure caps are closed if applicable.
❑ Verify that the CO2 absorber color change is no > than 1/2 the canister.

> * Failure of the 02-tank gauge to deflect clockwise with valve opening suggests that tank pressure is lower than gauge value!

Check oxygen / gas supply sources

❑ Visually inspect the gas supply hoses and connections.
❑ Ensure 02 tank (s) secure → open valve with wrench, then close → ensure 02 tank gauge deflects clockwise & ≥ 1000 PSIG after valve opening*
❑ Verify that the gas pipeline pressure gauges are in dark green range (≈ 50-55 PSIG).

Perform the system test, calibrate the flow sensor, calibrate/check 02 sensor and low 02 alarm

❑ Remove the 02 sensor → plug the hole → set the Low FI02 alarm limit between 25-30% → in the STANDBY screen perform "Run System Test" → select "Calibrate Flow Sensor" (follow instructions) → select "Calibrate 02 Sensor" (follow instructions) →check the function of the "INSP 02 LOW" alarm as the FI02 drops → Reconnect the 02 sensor → flush 0_2 and ensure ≥ 90% FIO2 is eventually displayed.

Perform breathing circuit and low pressure system leak testing

❑ In the STANDBY screen perform the "Leak / Compl Test" with vaporizer that you plan to use set to 1 VOL %. Follow the instructions.
❑ **Be sure to turn the vaporizer off (to "0") when the test is complete.**

Check Adjustable Pressure Limiting Valve (APL) Function

❑ With Y-piece still plugged, go to "Man Spont" mode → set the APL to 30 cm & set 02 the flow to 5 LPM → use 02 flush to bring pressure to about 30 cm → release and ensure pressure levels settle @ 26-35 cm H20 → open the APL → ensure pressure rapidly drops to 0 cm H20.

Verify that gas flows through the patient breathing circuit without obstruction and that the inspiratory and expiratory valves function properly, check ventilator function

❑ Reconfigure the circuit, including the elbow, and place a spare breathing bag on the patient elbow → in the "Man Spont" mode hand ventilate the "test lung" in a to-and-fro manner; verify that gas flows without obstruction through the circuit and that the one-way valves function properly.
❑ Go to the "Volume Control" mode and ventilate the "test lung" with the ventilator → Verify "test lung" ventilation.

Check the 02 Flush Function

❑ Remove "test lung" from the patient elbow → press the 02 flush button: Gas should flow from patient elbow piece.

Check Anesthetic Gas Scavenging System

❑ Check the scavenge hose connections including the vacuum line.
❑ Verify that the vacuum float in the scavenge container is between the Min & Max marks.
❑ Occlude the patient elbow piece with your thumb → Place the APL valve set to SPONT (wide open) → Select "Man Spont" mode → Press and hold the 02 flush button → Verify that that the airway pressure remains < 10 cmH20 during 02 flush.

Check the oxygen flow control valve

❑ Turn the oxygen flow control valve through its full range and ensure that oxygen flows through the flow meter (the bobbin rises).

Check monitors

❑ Exhale into the gas sampling line to ensure that C02 is detected via the capnogram.
❑ Verify the availability of all ASA standard and other required monitors.

Evaluate your final readiness to deliver Anesthesia Care (the "MS MAIDS" Checklist)

❑ **Machine:** Machine checked; vaporizers filled, closed, and **set to "0"**; all gas flows knobs turned fully clockwise to **set to "0.0" flow**; ventilator set up for upcoming patient, APL valve fully open. Ensure that "Des Comp" is **off** if not using Desflurane.
❑ **Suction:** Verify that patient suction is adequate to clear the airway.
❑ **Monitors:** All required monitors present, alarms on and set
❑ **Airway:** All airway equipment and appropriate backup ready
❑ **IV:** IV lines, fluids, and equipment ready
❑ **Drugs:** Ensure all drugs are ready and are properly labeled
❑ **Special:** Any special or unique items required for the case are available and ready.

Anesthesia Apparatus Checkout Prior to Each Procedure

❑ Verify that the CO2 absorber color change is no > than 1/2 the canister.
❑ Perform a breathing system pressure leak test.
❑ Verify that gas flows through the breathing circuit without obstruction and that the inspiratory and expiratory valves function properly.
❑ Verify that the **vaporizers** are set to "0" , are adequately filled, and the ports are closed.
❑ Verify that the **flow meters** are all dialed clockwise to "0.0" flow.
❑ Perform the ***"MS MAIDS"*** checklist.

*Dräger Medical, Telford, PA.

conducts evaluations and gives ratings of the various brands and models of a specific type of product. The anesthesia literature occasionally may be of help, and when major purchases are contemplated, a computerized literature search for information may reveal relevant publications. Further, proprietary services will, for a contract fee, survey an anesthesia department's practice patterns, existing equipment, current needs, and projected future needs and then provide recommendations for purchases of specific capital equipment by brand and model.

When purchasing new equipment, such as an integrated monitoring system, it is prudent to consider several factors. The system must be user friendly and human engineered so that the anesthesia personnel can easily set up the parameters they need for a given case and be able to acquire the data from the monitor. The monitoring system should be easy to interface with current or future electronic record-keeping systems, and the system should be trialed using actual cases for a significant period of time. The system needs to be tested with all possible

TABLE 32-5 **Sample Departmental PAC Checklist for Dräger Fabius*—New User Version**

AMBU BAG	present in the room
AC POWER	connected ("Mains Power" illuminated)
MACHINE POWER	on
BREATHING CIRCUIT	intact
VAPORZERS	secured; filled; closed
C02 ABSORBENT COLOR	white more than half the canister
PIPELINE HOSES	properly connected
02 TANK PRESSURE	deflects to ≥ 1000 PSIG with valve opening
PIPELINE PRESSURES	dark green range (≈ 50-55 PSIG).
PERFORM "Run System Test"	pass
PERFORM "Calibrate Flow Sensor"	complete
PERFORM "Calibrate 02 Sensor"	complete
CHECK INSP LOW 02 ALARM	alarm sounds (low FI02 alarm limit should be set between 25-30%)
CHECK HIGH RANGE OF 02 SENSOR	> 90% FI02
PERFORM "Leak / Compl Test " WITH VAPORIZER @ 1%	pass
VAPORIZER STATUS AFTER TEST	**"0" Volume % (off)**
APL FUNCTION AT 30 CM	circuit pressure stays between 26-35 CM H20
APL FUNCTION WHEN OPEN WIDE	circuit pressure drops to 0 CM H20
HAND VENTILATE BREATHING CIRCUIT	unobstructed flow, good unidirectional valve function
MECHANICALLY VENTILATE THE BREATHING CIRCUIT	test lung ventilates
02 FLUSH	gas flows from elbow
SCAVENGER CONNECTIONS	connected
SCAVENGER VACUUM	bobbin between the Min & Max marks
SCAVENGER INTEGRITY	< 10 cmH20 circuit pressure with 02 flush button
FLOW CONTROL VALVE FUNTION	oxygen adjustable through full range and flow meter bobbin rises
CHECK FLOW CONTROL VALVE POSITIONS	**All set to "0.0" flow (off)**
TEST C02 SAMPLE LINE	exhaled C02 displayed
MS MAIDS Checklist	
MACHINE	check OK, vaporizers off, flows off, ventilator set, "Des Comp" set
SUCTION	functional
MONITORS	standard and required monitors present and functional
AIRWAY	primary and alternate equipment ready
IV	lines, fluids, equipment ready
DRUGS	ready and properly labeled
SPECIAL	special or unique items ready
Anesthesia Apparatus Checkout Prior to Each Procedure	
CHECK C02 ABSO RBENT COLOR	white more than half the canister
PERFORM "Leak / Compl Test" with vaporizer @ 1%	pass
HAND VENTILATE BREATHING CIRCUIT	unobstructed flow, good unidirectional valve function
VAPORIZER STATUS	vaporizers set to "0," filled, ports are closed
FLOWMETERS	dialed clockwise to "0.0" flow
MS MAIDS CHECKLIST	completed

*Drager Medical, Telford, PA.
AAPL, adjustable pressure-limiting

monitoring modes running simultaneously, because an integrated system may function properly when just the electrocardiogram (ECG), blood pressure, and pulse oximeter modules are in use but may fail when multiple invasive pressures, cardiac output, and electroencephalogram (EEG) are added. Finally, multiple people in the department must trial the system. This should include the most and the least technologically adept personnel, because all will have to eventually be comfortable using it.

A similar analysis must be performed when purchasing new anesthesia machines. This is especially important if the department is considering buying electronic anesthesia machines for the first time. As previously discussed, these machines will have a totally different checkout procedure than the traditional anesthesia machine. Even though they have self-test programs, it may actually take longer to properly check the electronic machine than it would to check a traditional machine. Other important

BOX 32-3 PAC Checklist Design and Use Tips[65,66,70,71]

Checklist Design

1. The PAC checklist should be designed in a read-and-do or read-and-confirm format (e.g., Self-inflating resuscitation bag…available and functioning")
2. The flow pattern of the checklist should lend itself to efficiency and compliance. Sequence the items in a logical order, minimizing redundant movements.
3. The checklist should be as short as possible yet include all key checks.
4. Where applicable, responses to checklist challenges should be provided so that the value or status of an item is verified rather than just a check of task completion (e.g., "verify O_2 tank pressure" is not good; "O_2 tank pressure >1000 psig" is good).
5. The challenges and responses on the checklist should be consistent with the labeling and text on the switches, screens, and controls of the machine.
6. Choose an easy-to-read font and character size.
7. Avoid the overuse of *italics*, **bold**, underline, and UPPERCASE words.
8. Use familiar, accessible, and unambiguous language.
9. Avoid excessive verbiage.
10. For long checklists, identify pauses between key steps, or divide the checklist into logical task groups as opposed to one long, continuous series of tasks.
11. Fit the checklist on one page; large type size is preferred for legibility, but small type size may be needed to keep the number of pages to a minimum.

Checklist Testing

1. Perform rigorous testing and validation of the checklist before implementation.
2. Apply a trial-and-error approach to checklist design by having multiple potential users test the checklist.

Checklist Use

1. Periodically evaluate and update the checklist based on user feedback, workstation modifications, manufacturer safety alerts, and compelling literature.
2. Checklist users should be made aware that the PAC procedure is vulnerable to production pressure. The checklist should not be relegated to a second level of importance.
3. The checklist should be kept in sight each time it is used. Its benefit will be defeated if it dangles from the side of the machine during the checkout.
4. Develop a "checklist culture" through sound checklist design, leadership, and the promotion of a positive departmental attitude regarding the procedure.

factors include emergency case usage, usability in a power failure, and functional changes from traditional machines; for example, to increase gas flow on many electronic machines, the flow control knob is turned clockwise; this is opposite to mechanical machines, in which increases in flow require the flow control knob to be turned counterclockwise. In addition, interfacing with electronic record keepers and the cost and availability of manufacturer-specific disposable parts, such as carbon dioxide absorbents, must be considered. Once again, the machine should be trialed by various anesthesia personnel, in different case scenarios, prior to purchase.

Incoming Inspection

When new equipment arrives, it must be inspected and checked for proper function before it is put into service. Any electrical device must be tested for leakage current and compliance with standards, usually in the facility's own maintenance shop or by an outside evaluator not associated with the manufacturer. Complex equipment such as anesthesia machines, ventilators, and physiologic monitoring systems should be assembled and then tested for correct function by a person from the equipment manufacturer or an associated manufacturer's agent. This leads to the manufacturer's certification that the equipment is safe and ready for use. (Note that these certification documents become the start of the unique file of records and information that will stay in the anesthesia department and track the piece of equipment throughout its life.) Allowing relatively untrained or inexperienced personnel to assemble and certify new equipment, even if they do it perfectly, can present serious adverse medicolegal implications. Any untoward development in the future involving the new equipment will prompt a review of the records and an automatic assumption of malfeasance, if the people initially handling the equipment were not fully qualified to do so.

Record Keeping

As noted, a unique record must be kept for each piece of capital equipment (anything with a serial number) that comes into the anesthesia workplace. This record can be a page or, more likely, a section in a master equipment logbook that should be maintained in every anesthesia department or environment. In addition to the certifying document, the exact make, model, serial number, and any in-house identification must be recorded. This not only allows immediate identification of any equipment involved in a recall or product alert but also serves as the permanent repository of the record of every instance of inspection, problem, problem resolution, maintenance, and servicing until that particular piece is discarded. For electrical equipment that will undergo periodic inspection and testing, it is convenient to create stickers with blanks for all the necessary information to be entered and to have these filled out by the technician performing the inspection. These stickers are then affixed in sequence in the master log over the life of that piece of equipment. This log should be kept up to date at all times. There have been rare but frightening examples of potentially lethal problems with anesthesia machines leading to product alert notices that require immediate identification of certain equipment, its location, and its service status.

Maintenance and Service

There is a distinction between equipment failure as a result of progressive deterioration of components over time from continued use and catastrophic, unexpected failure, which usually is not predictable. Preventive maintenance is intended to anticipate what is essentially predictable failure—such as worn O-rings, gaskets, and rubber bellows—and to replace the weakened component before it eventually does fail. Because of the potential liability implications of a catastrophic failure, manufacturers expend a great deal of effort constructing a preventive maintenance schedule for their capital equipment. Preventive maintenance should be performed often enough and thoroughly enough to prevent most predictable failures while still maintaining reasonable cost. Users sometimes believe manufacturers are too cautious and that they prescribe too much periodic maintenance in order to generate service business. These users are tempted to lengthen the maintenance cycles or to limit the extent of the service. Although this can save money in the short term, the liability implications in the event of a catastrophic anesthesia equipment failure that causes or contributes to patient harm are unacceptable. This functionally obligates users to attempt to adhere to the prescribed maintenance and service regimen that comes with the equipment from the manufacturer.

Safety inspections and functional testing are integral components of preventive maintenance. Clear protocols that use discrete, highly visible checklists for each type of equipment often come from the manufacturer and, if not, these should be developed by agents of the users. In facilities with a large number of each type of equipment, use of such protocols should simplify the repetitive tasks for service personnel and help to ensure that all the points are covered for each unit of that type. Of course, copies of the completed form should be stored permanently in the departmental master equipment log.

The question of who should maintain and service anesthesia equipment has been widely debated and is very important. Needs and resources differ. The fundamental options are 1) factory service representatives, who are directly employed by the manufacturer or the manufacturer's agent to work on the equipment made by that company; 2) independent service contractors, who usually work on all brands of equipment and who may or may not have some type of relationship with the various manufacturers but are not employed by them; and 3) personnel within the anesthesia group or department or the maintenance and engineering department of the health care facility; these can be either formal biomedical engineers or less formal technicians. The order of the three options approximately represents decreasing average cost and increasing liability implications for the practitioners using the equipment. These issues should not necessarily drive the decision as to which to choose, but they certainly can be taken into consideration. The fundamental issue is straightforward: the person performing preventive maintenance and service must be qualified to do so, and documentation of that qualification must be maintained.

Whether service personnel are qualified may be, at times, somewhat difficult to ascertain, but judicious investigation of references and direct questioning of the service personnel regarding their education, training, and experience is appropriate. Direct contact with the supervisor or manager responsible for the work of the service person is strongly advised. This indicates the importance that the practitioners attach to maintenance and service. Whether a technician who spent a week at a course at an equipment manufacturer's factory can perform the most complex repairs of computerized gas machines, for example, depends on a variety of factors.

Ultimately, the practitioner using the equipment must decide the competence level of the personnel who repair the equipment. Failure to be involved and to have some oversight in this process exposes the practitioner to increased liability in the event of an untoward outcome associated with improperly maintained or serviced equipment. Importantly, such situations are fortunately very rare. However, as with so many things in modern anesthesia practice, the continual background threat of liability implications is enough to prompt specific plans and actions in this regard.

Daily Support

In addition to periodic preventive maintenance and servicing, adequate day-to-day clinical maintenance of anesthesia equipment must be addressed. Because budgets of facilities with surgical suites are constantly under scrutiny, anesthesia technicians seem to be a popular target for cost cutters. It is dangerous false economy to decrease the number of technicians to below that genuinely needed to retrieve, clean, sort, disassemble, sterilize, reassemble, store, and distribute the equipment of daily anesthesia practice. Inadequate service in this area truly creates an accident waiting to happen. Although it is desirable that all anesthesia practitioners be able to change the carbon dioxide absorbent on their anesthesia machines, some might be sufficiently unfamiliar with the procedure as to create a hazard in the process. Many other sources of potential danger arise from a lack of adequate technical support personnel, intended to execute tasks such as this and thereby provide the correctly functioning wherewithal for anesthesia practice.

Retirement of Equipment

There appears to be a strong sentiment against using the word *obsolete* to refer to older anesthesia equipment. The concept has adverse medicolegal implications and dwells in the past, whereas a safety improvement effort involving new equipment looks to the future. It has been stated, however, that replacement of "obsolete" anesthesia machines and monitoring equipment is one key element of a risk-modification program.[73] Ten years has been frequently cited as an estimated useful life for an anesthesia machine, but this is simply an opinion and is probably at least in part related to depreciation tables used by hospital actuaries. Certainly, unmodified anesthesia machines that are significantly more than 10 years old may not meet the minimum specifications outlined by the ASTM F1850-00 (2005) Standard Specification for Particular Requirements for Anesthesia Workstations and Their Components. Furthermore, there is every indication that technology will continue to advance at an accelerating rate. Note that some anesthesia equipment manufacturers, anxious to minimize their own potential liability, have refused to support with parts and service some of their older pieces of equipment still in use, particularly gas machines. This fact should send a very strong message to practitioners that such equipment must be replaced as soon as possible.

The ASA published a guideline in 2004, developed by its Committee on Equipment and Facilities, entitled "Guideline for Determining Anesthesia Machine Obsolescence," which stated:

> *Anesthesia equipment can become obsolete if essential components wear out and cannot be replaced. It may also become obsolete as a result of changes in medical practices, changes in the training and experience of anesthesia providers, and/or development of new safety features. An anesthesia machine should not be considered obsolete solely because it has reached an arbitrary age. Furthermore, a machine should not be expected to meet all of the performance and safety requirements specified in United States or international equipment standards published after the machine was manufactured. It is the responsibility of the anesthesia provider to determine if a machine's failure to meet newer standards represents a sufficient threat to patient safety to render the machine obsolete.*

This type of statement emphasizes that the users of anesthesia equipment should be able to knowledgeably decide whether equipment is obsolete, again illustrating that anesthesia professionals need to know their equipment thoroughly and must ask many questions of the personnel who service and maintain it (see also Chapter 30 and Box 30-6).

The summary message is that a great many technologic advances have been made in anesthesia equipment, particularly in gas machines, that were specifically intended to increase the safety of the patients anesthetized with that equipment. Exactly how fast these improvements are incorporated into daily use will depend on the circumstances of a given anesthesia practice, published and de facto standards and guidelines, applicable regulations, and the relevant medicolegal climate.

Equipment Crisis Management

Finally, should equipment fail, it must be removed from service and replaced if that anesthetizing location will still be used. Groups or departments are obligated to have sufficient back-up equipment to cover any reasonable incidence of failure, predicted on the basis of past experience and manufacturer's guidelines. The equipment removed from service must be clearly marked with a sign to that effect, so that it is not put back into service by well-meaning support personnel or even other practitioners; the sign should include the date, time, person discovering the fault, and details of the problem. The responsible personnel must be notified so that they can remove the equipment, make an entry in the log, and initiate repair. A piece of equipment either directly or indirectly involved in possibly causing an anesthesia accident must be immediately sequestered and not touched by anybody, particularly not by any equipment service personnel. There may be strong pressure to return a major piece of equipment, such as a gas machine, to service if there is no spare available; this temptation must be resisted. If a severe accident occurred, it may be necessary for the equipment in question to be inspected at an appointed time by a group consisting of qualified representatives of the manufacturer, the service personnel, the plaintiff's attorney, the insurance companies involved, and the practitioner's defense attorney. Also, major equipment problems involving obvious or suspected hazards should be reported immediately to the electronic Medical Device Reporting system of the FDA and thus to the Manufacturer and User Facility Device Experience Database (http://www.fda.gov/MedicalDevices/Safety/ReportaProblem/default.htm). This system accepts voluntary reports from users and requires reports from manufacturers when there is knowledge that a medical device has been involved in a serious incident. This is a logical progression of an equipment QA process.

CONCLUSION

Implementation of the acute and chronic components of an anesthesia equipment QA program should help to minimize the likelihood of equipment-related untoward events during anesthesia care. Both the preanesthesia checklists and the equipment management programs outlined in this chapter are intended as models. Individual anesthesia practitioners, groups, and departments must adapt these principles to their own particular situations, taking into account the type of equipment, practice environments, and local characteristics. Incorporation of the spirit of the recommendations more than the letter is the key. It is important to recall that human error is implicated in the vast majority of adverse outcomes from anesthesia care; overt equipment failure or problems appear to be involved in only a small fraction of these cases. Nonetheless, this fraction is virtually reducible to zero with rigorous application of the principles of equipment checkout and QA.

REFERENCES

1. Lees DE: Anesthesia machine and equipment standards. In Eichhorn JH, editor: *Problems in anesthesia*, vol. 5, Philadelphia, 1991, Lippincott, pp 205–218.
2. Waldrop WB, Murray DJ, Boulet JR, et al: Management of anesthesia equipment failure: a simulation-based resident skill assessment, *Anesth Analg* 109:426–433, 2009.
3. Mudumbai SC, Fanning R, Howard SK, et al: Use of medical simulation to explore equipment failures and human-machine interactions in anesthesia machine pipeline supply crossover, *Anesth Analg* 110:1292–1296, 2010.
4. Petty C: *The anesthesia machine*, New York, 1987, Churchill Livingstone.
5. Rendell-Baker L: Problems with anesthetic gas machines and their solutions. *Problems with anesthetic and respiratory therapy equipment*, Boston, 1984, Little Brown, pp 1–82.
6. Spooner RB, Kirby RR: Equipment-related anesthetic incidents. In Pierce EC, Cooper JB, editors: *Analysis of anesthetic mishaps*, Boston, 1984, Little Brown, pp 133–147.
7. Caplan RA: Liability arising from gas delivery equipment, *ASA Newslett* 62:7–9, 1998.
8. Cooper JB, Newbower RS, Long CD, et al: Preventable anesthesia mishaps: a study of human factors, *Anesthesiology* 49:399–406, 1978.
9. Cooper JB, Newbower RS, Kitz RJ: An analysis of major errors and equipment failures in anesthesia management: considerations for prevention and detection, *Anesthesiology* 60:34–42, 1984.
10. Eichhorn JH: Prevention of intraoperative anesthesia accidents and related severe injury through safety monitoring, *Anesthesiology* 70:572–577, 1989.

11. Langford R, Gale T, Mayor A: Anaesthetic machine checking guidelines: have we improved our practice? *Eur J Anaesth* 24:1050–1056, 2007.
12. Arbous M, Anneke E, Jack W, et al: Impact of anesthesia management characteristics on severe morbidity and mortality, *Anesthesiology* 102(2):257–368, 2005.
13. Buffington CW, Ramanathan S, Turndorf H: Detection of anesthesia machine faults, *Anesth Analg* 63(1):79–82, 1984.
14. Carstensen P: FDA issues pre-use checkout, *APSF Newslett* 1(3):13–20, 1986.
15. March MG, Crowley JJ: An evaluation of anesthesiologists' present checkout methods and the validity of the FDA checklist, *Anesthesiology* 75(5):724–729, 1991.
16. Lees DE: FDA preanesthesia checklist being evaluated, revised, *APSF Newslett* 6(3):25–36, 1991.
17. Withiam-Wilson MJ: FDA pre-use equipment checklist spurred by accidents, studies, *APSF Newslett* 6(3):25–36, 1991.
18. FDA Publishes final version of revised apparatus checkout, *APSF Newslett* 9(3):26–27, 1994.
19. Anesthesia apparatus checkout recommendations. *Federal Register* 1994 July 11. Document number 94-16618. Accessed 2011 Mar 2 at http://www.federalregister.gov/articles/1994/07/11/94-16618/anesthesia-apparatus-checkout-recommendations-1993-availability.
20. Manley R, Cuddeford JD: An assessment of the effectiveness of the revised FDA checklist, *AANA J* 64(3):277–282, 1996.
21. Blike G, Biddle C: Preanesthesia detection of equipment faults by anesthesia providers at an academic hospital: comparison of standard practice and a new electronic checklist, *AANA J* 68(6):497–505, 2000.
22. Larson ER, Gregory AN, Brian DO, et al: A prospective study on anesthesia machine fault identification, *Anesth Analg* 104(1):154–156, 2007.
23. Olympio MA, Goldstein MM, Mathes DD: Instructional review improves performance of anesthesia apparatus checkout procedures, *Anesth Analg* 83(3):618–622, 1996.
24. Armstrong-Brown A, Devitt JH, Kurrek M, et al: Inadequate preanesthesia equipment checks in a simulator, *Can J Anaesth* 47(10):974–979, 2000.
25. Craig J, Wilson M: A survey of anaesthetic misadventures, *Anaesthesia* 36(10):933–936, 1981.
26. Mayor AH, Eaton JM: Anaesthetic machine checking practices: s survey, *Anaesthesia* 47(10):866–868, 1992.
27. Lampotang S, Moon S, Lizdas DE, et al: Anesthesia machine preuse check survey—preliminary results, *American Society of Anesthesiologists Annual Meeting*, Oct 24, 2005. abstract #A1195.
28. Sub-Committee of ASA Committee on Equipment and Facilities: Recommendations for pre-anesthesia checkout procedures, 2008. Accessed 2011 Mar 1 at http://www.asahq.org/clinical/fda.htm.
29. Eichhorn JH: Anesthesia equipment: checkout and quality assurance. In Ehrenwerth J, Eisenkraft JB, editors: *Anesthesia equipment*, ed 1, St Louis, 1993, Mosby, pp 473–491.
30. *Operators instruction manual: Narkomed 6400 anesthesia system*, Lübeck, Germany, 2002, Dräger Medical.
31. *Operation manual, part 1: Aestiva/5 7100.* Madison, WI, 2001, Datex-Ohmeda.
32. *User's reference manual-part 1: S/5 Aespire*. Madison, WI, 2002, Datex-Ohmeda.
33. *Service manual: Datascope AS3000 anesthesia delivery system*. Mahwah, NJ, 2008, Mindray North America.
34. *Operator's instruction and setup manual: Narkomed M anesthesia system*, Lübeck, Germany, 2001, Dräger Medical.
35. *Operator's instruction and setup manual: Narkomed 2B anesthesia system*, Lübeck, Germany, 1998, Dräger Medical.
36. J. Jeffrey Andrews, M.D., Professor and Chair, University of Texas Health Science Center San Antonio. Personal communication, February 9, 2011.
37. National Fire Protection Association: *NFPA 99: Standard for health care facilities*, 2005, NFPA. Accessed 2011 Feb 24 at http://www.nfpa.org/aboutthecodes/AboutTheCodes.asp?DocNum=99.
38. O'Connor CJ Jr, Hubin KF: Bypassing the diameter-indexed safety system, *Anesthesiology* 71(2):318–319, 1989.
39. Ellett AE, Justin CS, Ifune C, et al: A near miss: a nitrous oxide-carbon dioxide mix-up despite current safety standards, *Anesthesiology* 110(6):1429–1431, 2009.
40. Neubarth J: Another hazardous gas supply misconnection, *Anesth Analg* 80(1), 1995.
41. Krenis LJ, Berkowitz DA: Errors in installation of a new gas delivery system found after certification, *Anesthesiology* 62(5):677–678, 1985.
42. Jardine DS: An epidemic of hypoxemia in two intensive care units: cause and human response, *Anesthesiology* 77(5):1038–1043, 1992.
43. Sprague DH, Archer GW: Intraoperative hypoxia from an erroneously filled liquid oxygen reservoir, *Anesthesiology* 42(3):360–362, 1975.
44. Moss E: Medical gas contamination: an unrecognized patient danger, *J Clin Monit* 11(1):73–76, 1995.
45. Eichhorn JH: Medical gas delivery systems, *Int Anesthesiol Clin* 19(2):1–26, 1981.
46. McIntyre JW: Anesthesia equipment malfunction: origins and clinical recognition, *Can Med Assoc J* 120(8):931–934, 1979.
47. Riutort KT, Brockwell EC, Brull SJ, Andrews JJ: The anesthesia workstation and delivery systems. In Barash PG, Cullen BF, Stoelting RK, editors: *Clinical anesthesia*, ed 6, Philadelphia, 2009, Lippincott Williams & Wilkins, pp 644–694.
48. *Prima SP3 anaesthetic machine range user's manual.* Abingdon, UK, 2005, Penlon Limited.
49. Myers JA, Good ML, Andrews JJ: Comparison of tests for detecting leaks in the low-pressure system of anesthesia gas machines, *Anesth Analg* 84(1):179–184, 1997.
50. Dorsch JA, Dorsch SE: *Understanding anesthesia equipment*, ed 5, Philadelphia, 2008, Lippincott Williams & Wilkins.
51. Brockwell RC, Andrews JJ: Inhaled anesthesia delivery systems. In Miller R, Eriksson LI, Fleisher LA, editors: *Miller's anesthesia*, ed 7, Philadelphia, 2010, Churchill Livingstone, pp 667–718.
52. *Aisys user's reference manual.* Madison, WI, 2009, Datex-Ohmeda.
53. Andrews Johnston RV Jr, Bee DE, Arens JF: Photodeactivation of ethyl violet: a potential hazard of sodasorb, *Anesthesiology* 72(1):59–64, 1990.
54. Olympio M: Carbon dioxide absorbent desiccation safety conference convened by APSF, *APSF Newslett* 20(2):25–44, 2005.
55. Dr. Ciarán Magee: Technical Director, Armstrong Medical Limited, Coleraine, Ireland. Personal communication, January 20, 2011.
56. Souvatzis X, Askitopoulou H: Malfunction of an adjustable pressure limit valve, *Eur J Anaesthesiol* 24(11):978–980, 2007.
57. *Operator's instruction and setup manual: Fabius GS*, Lübeck, Germany, 2002, Dräger Medical.
58. Dean HN, Parsons DE, Raphaely RC: Case report: bilateral tension pneumothorax from mechanical failure of anesthesia machine due to misplaced expiratory valve, *Anesth Analg* 50(2):195–198, 1971.
59. Norman PH, Daley MD, Walker JR, et al: Obstruction due to retained carbon dioxide absorber canister wrapping, *Anesth Analg* 83(2):425–426, 1996.
60. Monteiro JN, Ravindran MN, D'Mello JB: Three cases of breathing system malfunction, *Eur J Anaesthesiol* 21(9):743–745, 2004.
61. Ianchulev SA, Comunale ME: To do or not to do a preinduction check-up of the anesthesia machine, *Anesth Analg* 101(3): 774, 2005.
62. Ezaru CS: Preinduction check-up of the anesthesia machine, *Anesth Analg* 102(5):1588–1589, 2006.
63. McLean JS, Houston P, Dumais R: Erroneous connection of the fresh gas flow to the anesthesia circuit, *Can J Anaesth* 50(1):93, 2003.
64. *Julian anesthesia workstation operating instructions*, Lübeck, Germany, 2000, Dräger Medical.
65. Federal Aviation Administration [FAA]: Flight Standards Information Management System. General technical administration, Chapter 32: Manuals, procedures, and checklists for 14 CFR parts 91K, 121, 125, and 135; Section 12, aircraft checklists for 14 CFR parts 121/135. Washington, DC, 2007, FAA. Accessed online 2011 Feb 24 at http://fsims.faa.gov/wdocs/8900.1/v03%20tech%20adm in/chapter%2032/03_032_012.pdf.
66. Degani A, Wiener EL: Cockpit checklists: concepts, design, and use, *Hum Factors* 35(2):345–359, 1993.
67. Pronovost P, Needham D, Berenholtz S, et al: An intervention to decrease catheter-related bloodstream infections in the ICU, *N Engl J Med* 355(26):2725–2732, 2006.
68. de Vries EN, Prins HA, Crolla RMPH, et al: Effect of a comprehensive surgical safety system on patient outcomes, *N Engl J Med* 363(20): 1928-1937, 2010.

69. Gawande A: *The checklist manifesto: how to get things right*, New York, 2009, Metropolitan Books.
70. Winters BD, Ayse PG, Lehmann H, et al: Clinical review: checklists—translating evidence into practice, *Crit Care* 13(6), 2009.
71. FAA Office of Integrated Safety Analysis, Human Factors Analysis Division: Human performance considerations in the use and design of aircraft checklists, January 1995. Accessed online 2011 Feb 24 at http://www.faa.gov/about/office_org/headquarters_offices/avs/offices/afs/afs200/branches/afs210/training_aids/media/checklist.doc.
72. Duberman SM, Wald A: An integrated quality control program for anesthesia equipment. In Chapman-Cliburn G, editor: *Risk management and quality assurance: issues and interactions*, Chicago, 1986, Joint Commission on Accreditation of Healthcare Organizations, pp 105–112. (A special publication of the *Quality Review Bulletin*).
73. Pierce EC: Risk modification in anesthesiology. In Chapman-Cliburn G, editor: *Risk management and quality assurance: issues and interactions*, Chicago, 1986, Joint Commission on Accreditation of Healthcare Organizations, pp 20–23. (A special publication of the *Quality Review Bulletin*).

CHAPTER 33

Risk Management and Medicolegal Aspects of Anesthesia Equipment

John T. Sullivan • Jeffrey B. Cooper

CHAPTER OUTLINE

OVERVIEW

To prevent harm resulting from anesthesia care and to continuously improve patient safety, active effort is needed to manage risk. The concept of *risk management* (RM) is widely applied in many domains, including health care, and especially in anesthesia. Successful RM is composed of several elements, beginning with the identification of problems that should be addressed to avoid poor outcomes and followed by the implementation of an overall strategy with appropriate tactics to minimize the opportunities for failures and their ensuing accidents. Because adverse outcomes will still occur despite the best intentions and efforts, a process is needed to appropriately respond so that the correct course is pursued for the patient, providers, organization, and even for the insurer. The general principles of RM are applicable to the spectrum of causes of poor outcomes. This chapter focuses on how these principles can be applied specifically to problems to which anesthesia equipment may contribute. Problems and circumstances that lead to adverse outcomes are discussed, and a set of processes that can constitute an RM strategy are provided. RM has elements that involve medicolegal processes and concerns.

ELEMENTS OF RISK MANAGEMENT IN ANESTHESIA

RM is an established discipline with professional organizations, such as the American Society for Healthcare; in addition, there are RM meetings, periodicals, and textbooks.[1-3] The terms frequently used in this discipline are summarized in Table 33-1. Traditionally and even currently, the emphasis has been on managing risk for the primary purpose of avoiding financial loss. More recently, it has been recognized that financial losses can best be prevented by avoiding problems before they result in accidents and potential financial loss and that RM is intimately tied to patient safety.[4] Formal processes have been developed in high-technology industries such as nuclear power, aviation, aerospace, and the chemical industry. Probability risk assessment (PRA),[5] failure mode effect analysis (FMEA),[6] and other quantitative and qualitative techniques are applied to estimate risk and plan for reaching "acceptable" risk levels. Such formal approaches have been less common in health care, but they are increasingly being adopted. Management of the risk associated with anesthesia equipment, especially for the clinician or administrator confronted with purchasing and process decisions, must often rely on more intuitive and

TABLE 33-1 **Frequently Used Risk Management Terminology**

Adverse event	An injury resulting from a medical intervention (i.e., not due to the underlying medical condition of the patient).
Error	Failure of a planned action to be completed as intended or the use of a wrong plan to achieve an aim; not all errors result in injury. In an effort to thoroughly consider all of the relevant issues related to medical errors, the Quality Interagency Coordination Task Force report expanded the Institute of Medicine's definition to read as follows: "An error is defined as the failure of a planned action to be completed as intended, or the use of a wrong plan to achieve an aim. Errors can include problems in practice, products, procedures, and systems."
Human factor	The study of relationships among human beings, the environments in which they live and work, and the tools they use.
Preventable adverse event	An adverse event that was attributable to a medical error. Negligent adverse events represent a subset of preventable adverse events that satisfy legal criteria used in determining negligence, whether the care provided failed to meet the standard of care reasonably expected of an average physician qualified to take care of the patient in question.
Safety	Freedom from accidental injury.
System	A set of interdependent elements working to achieve a common aim. The elements may be both human and nonhuman (e.g., equipment, technologies).
Types of failure	Errors of execution are those in which the correct action does not proceed as intended; errors of planning are those in which the original intended action is not correct.

qualitative assessments to judge the relative risks and benefits. Even in the absence of robust quantitative data, the general principles of RM are the same: defining potential problems, estimating the likelihood of occurrence, weighing the relative benefits of expenditure of available resources, applying the solutions, and monitoring how well the solutions have been applied. Perhaps the greatest problem with management of risk—especially for the rare, catastrophic events that are so devastating to all parties—is that it is virtually impossible to know whether the approach has been effective as a result of the absence of major problems, such as large or even many smaller malpractice claims. This is especially so for equipment, because such major events are relatively rarer than for other types of anesthesia-associated adverse outcomes.

Nature of Risk Associated with Anesthesia Equipment

The study of anesthesia mishaps provides insight into their causes and leads to interventions that should decrease their occurrences. Greater attention to improving patient safety and the introduction of new technology is believed to be associated with a declining trend in the overall incidence of anesthesia mishaps and probably also those associated with the use of anesthesia gas delivery equipment.[7,8] Nevertheless, adverse outcomes related to equipment failure and/or misuse persist, and the results are often severe. In fact, the inherent rarity of serious complications from anesthesia likely creates an additional hazard: most anesthesiologists are not well experienced in responding to them. Studies of anesthesia practice have yielded valuable data that quantify the frequent causes of errors and have provided insight into the complex environment in which they occur.

Anesthesia is delivered in a complex, dynamic environment that involves the interactions of a surgical insult with unpredictable physiology, numerous pharmacologic interventions, and the use of multiple electromechanical devices.[9] The system involves the interactions of numerous physicians, nurses, and ancillary personnel influenced by a "host of administrative, political, and cultural factors."[10] In this environment, deviations or "incidents" arise frequently, occurring spontaneously from the patient's disease (e.g., hypertension), from planned interventions, (e.g., disconnecting the breathing circuit to suction the tracheal tube), or as the result of human error or equipment failure. The majority of these incidents or "near misses" have little or no impact on patient outcome. Events that could or did lead to an undesirable outcome have been termed "critical incidents."[11] When an event does lead to an undesirable outcome, it is referred to as an "adverse event."[12]

The chain of events associated with accident evolution has been studied extensively in other domains in which RM is commonly practiced.[13] Many of the insights gained are equally applicable to prevention of anesthesia accidents. One more modern concept introduced into accident understanding and prevention in health care and anesthesia specifically is that errors and failures do not stand alone; rather they are elements embedded within a larger system, of which equipment forms one of several categories of latent risk factors for adverse events (Table 33-2).[14] It is now widely accepted that human error must be thought of in this context, that the operator is rarely the primary "fault." For that matter, neither is the technology ever the sole "fault" or cause of an adverse outcome. The science of patient safety has embraced these ideas, which are critical for establishing measures to avoid adverse outcomes associated with equipment.[4]

INCIDENCE AND CHARACTERISTICS OF ADVERSE EQUIPMENT EVENTS

Sources

Important sources from the English language literature that serve to define risk associated with the use of anesthetic equipment include the ASA Closed Claims Project

TABLE 33-2 **Latent Risk Factors**

Latent Risk Factor	Issues
Equipment, design, and maintenance	Availability, functioning, standardization design, and maintenance of machines
Staffing	Adequate staffing, skills
Communication	Work-directed communication, openness, interrelation, atmosphere
Training	Training for machines, procedures, team training
Teamwork and team training	Team performance
Procedures	Presence of protocols, adherence to protocols
Situational awareness	Awareness of present situation, own tasks, and future developments
Incompatible goals	Balance between goals and safety
Planning and organization	Process of care
Housekeeping	Hygiene

From van Beuzekom M, Boer F, Akerboom S, Hudson P: Patient safety: latent risk factors, *Br J Anaesth* 105(1):52–59, 2010.

(CCP); seven anonymous reporting systems in Australia (the Australian Incident Monitoring Study [AIMS]),[15] Britain (National Patient Safety Agency adverse events reporting),[16,17] and France (French Health Ministry's national registry of incidents)[18]; prospectively collected institutional quality data[19,20]; retrospective critical incident surveys[11,21]; and case reports.[22] Methodological challenges exist to prospectively investigate adverse anesthetic events related to equipment, foremost of which is the rarity of occurrence. Additional challenges in investigating this topic include heterogeneity in research aim and design, varied definitions used to characterize adverse events, and the subjective evaluation of these incidents. The sum of this body of literature forms a representative picture of adverse events related to anesthetic equipment and can help form strategies for their prevention.

The CCP is an evolving database on more than 9500 adverse anesthetic events[23] with data provided by numerous malpractice insurers in the United States to physicians for review and evaluation. The database contains 150 details about each claim, ranging from objective items, such as age of the patient and monitors used, to judgments about causes of anesthetic mishaps. The AIMS is a coordinated anonymous reporting system of critical incidents by anesthesiologists from 90 Australian and New Zealand hospitals and practices.[24] The first 2000 reports formed the basis of several studies that have reviewed subsets of adverse events in anesthesia practice, including anesthetic equipment failure.[15] No subsequent report has been published specifically analyzing anesthetic equipment from the AIMS database. The CCP and AIMS databases provide some of the largest and most published collections of significant anesthetic events from which to glean information about the occurrence of problems possibly associated with accidents. However, because the number of cases represented (i.e., the denominator) is unknown, neither study provides a measure of event incidence. Anonymous reporting systems related to anesthetic safety have been reproduced in many countries, and the data are readily available online.[25]

Incidence

The majority of adverse events in anesthetic practice are multifactorial and involve a combination of systems problems, human factors ("use error"), and actual technical failures.[14] Isolated anesthetic equipment failures are rare and contribute to the minority of adverse events. Nonetheless, it is valuable for the clinician to understand the incidence of such events and to what degree each is associated with patient injury. Attempts made to identify the incidence of these isolated failures and compare them are limited by varied methodology (e.g., extended timeframe of event collection, definitions used by investigators). In addition, many of the landmark studies in this field are now several decades old and may not accurately represent the current risk associated with anesthetic equipment. Other investigators[11] included in their analyses adverse events associated with intensive care unit (ICU) ventilators, infusion pumps, and anesthetic equipment not necessarily related to gas delivery equipment (e.g., tracheal tubes).[18] Also, the nature of reporting in this field of study is more subjective than in many other clinical investigations in anesthesiology. Nonetheless, in adverse event databases, anesthetic equipment failures account for 1% to 9% of cases.[7,15]

The most comprehensive reports on adverse events that specifically focused on anesthetic equipment include an analysis of the CCP database and the AIMS report. Although both of these were published in the 1990s, they still provide the most comprehensive analyses of patterns of adverse events involving anesthetic equipment. The comprehensive report on adverse events in the CCP database revealed that 2% (72 of 3791 total claims) were associated with gas delivery equipment.[26] There was a greater representation of anesthetic equipment-related adverse outcomes in the AIMS report; 9% of the first 2000 reported adverse anesthetic events were due to what was analyzed to be "pure" equipment failure.[15] An updated brief report of the CCP database in 2011 on the prevalence of equipment claims accounted for a smaller 1.2% (114 of 9214 total claims).[8] From a more practical standpoint, the incidence of equipment failure has been reported in single-institution, consecutive record audits at 0.04% to 2% or 1 in 50 to 1 in 2252 general anesthetics.[19,27,29]

It is not clear how generalizable these data are to individual anesthetic practices given the range of equipment used, audit reporting compliance, and definitions of "equipment problems." It is also possible that clinicians may be more likely to report on equipment-related events; hence those may be overrepresented in databases

TABLE 33-3 **American Society of Anesthesiologists Closed Claims Project Adverse Outcomes**

Equipment Group	Death	Brain Damage	Awareness	Recovery Delayed	Tracheostomy Scar	Pneumothorax
Breathing circuit (n = 28)	10	10	1	5	1	1
Vaporizer (n = 15)	7	3	5	0	0	0
Ventilator (n = 12)	7	5	0	0	0	0
Supply tanks or lines (n = 8)	6	2	0	0	0	0
Anesthesia machine	3	0	1	0	1	0
Supplemental O_2 tubing (n = 4)	1	1	0	0	0	2
Total (n = 72)	34 (47%)	21 (29%)	7 (10%)	5 (7%)	2 (3%)	3 (4%)

From Caplan RA, Vistica MF, Posner KL, Cheney FW: Adverse anesthetic outcomes arising from gas delivery equipment: a closed claims analysis. Anesthesiology *1997;87:741-748.*

that include noninjurious events. Fortunately, some of these equipment failures have led to practice improvement either through mandated removal from the market or design improvements.[18]

In contrast to isolated equipment failure, "use error," or what had been referred to in earlier publications as "human error," has been reported as being responsible for the majority of adverse events and thus represents a far more significant contributor to adverse outcomes.[15,26,30-33] Yet the user and technology are now understood to be intertwined. It may not be wise to label them in this way, but it still suffices for practical purposes. In addition, there is currently a deemphasis on personal blame in evaluating adverse events; rather, addressing systems problems has been deemed more fruitful in building a sustainable culture of safe health care delivery.[14]

Characteristics of Adverse Events

It is unclear whether adverse events in anesthesia involving equipment are associated with a great severity of injury. In publications from the 1990s, equipment-related claims were more likely to be associated with serious injury or death and larger financial settlements than other anesthetic adverse outcomes that did not implicate equipment directly (Table 33-3).[26] Certainly, the use of financial settlement size is an imperfect surrogate measure of outcome severity, and it is possible that some equipment-related claims were settled out of court by a manufacturer and were not represented in the CCP database.

The AIMS report identified that the leading sources of equipment problems included unidirectional valves, ventilators, anesthesia machines, breathing circuits, gas supplies, and electricity.[15] More recently, the CCP database added only 39 claims related to anesthesia gas delivery equipment from 1990 to 2011.[8] These include 10 problems related to breathing circuits, 13 with vaporizers, 7 with the anesthesia machine itself, 5 with ventilators, and 4 described as "supplemental oxygen line events." The management of many specific hazards and failures associated with anesthesia equipment are described in Chapter 30.

Anesthesia gas delivery is complex, with multiple connections and moving parts that would make it easy to suspect that equipment failure would play a prominent role in adverse events, but misuse of equipment appears to be more common than equipment failure per se, emphasizing the role of use error in equipment-related critical incidents and adverse outcomes (Table 33-4). Breathing circuits are an excellent example of this phenomenon; simple misconnection or disconnection of breathing circuits was the initiating event in a large proportion of cases.[15,19,20,26] More importantly, perhaps, this subset of adverse event type made the largest single contribution to injury when compiled over the entire course of the CCP (Table 33-5). It seems intuitive that the use of capnography, breathing circuit pressure, and pulse oximetry monitoring would have led to a reduction in patient injury related to those events over time, but there has not been convincing evidence to support that assertion.

Mitigating Factors

Although substantial changes have been made over the past few decades in some aspects of anesthetic equipment-related adverse events, little change has occurred in the mitigating factors reported to be associated with them. Failure to check equipment and lack of familiarity with it, inexperience, haste, inattention, distraction, fatigue, and lack of supervision are leading associated factors.[11,24,30,34] Little published evidence associates the relationship of equipment modification or lack of service to adverse events; maintenance inadequacy has only been reported to be related to medical gas line problems and not anesthesia machines or their components.[18] This suggests that either these factors play less of a role in adverse events than the others described above or that they may not have been as thoroughly investigated.

Trends

Because no detailed analysis of the CCP data has been published pertaining specifically to anesthesia gas delivery equipment since 1997, only the most general trends can be reported. The overall number of closed claims reported annually to the ASA database has declined from a peak in the mid-1990s (Fig. 33-1).[7] In addition, the number of severe claims related to death or permanent brain injury has also declined.[7] It is noteworthy that there have been no gas delivery system claims since 2003. Overall, however, it appears that gas delivery equipment problems are decreasing as a proportion of total claims.

TABLE 33-4 **American Society of Anesthesiologists Closed Claims Project Initiating Events**

Equipment Group	Initiating Event	No. of Claims	% (n = 72)
Breathing circuit (n = 28)	Misconnect	14	19
	Disconnect	11	15
	Leak	1	1
	Valve failure	1	1
	CO_2 canister defect	1	1
Vaporizer (n = 15)	Valve failure	5	7
	Leak	2	3
	Wrong dial/setting	2	3
	Tipped over	1	1
	Hooked up backwards	1	1
	Not turned on	1	1
	Knob turned inadvertently	1	1
	Uncertain	2	3
Ventilator (n = 12)	Not turned on	3	4
	Valve misinstalled	2	3
	Wrong ventilator chosen	1	1
	Valve failure	1	1
	Wrong setting	1	1
	Uncertain	4	6
Supply tanks or lines (n = 8)	Oxygen switch	7	10
	Uncertain	1	1
Anesthesia machine (n = 5)	Leak	3	4
	Wrong knob turned	1	1
	Uncertain	1	1
Supplemental oxygen tubing (n = 4)	Direct connection		
	Wall to patient	4	6

From Caplan RA, Vistica MF, Posner KL, Cheney FW: Adverse anesthetic outcomes arising from gas delivery equipment: a closed claims analysis. Anesthesiology *1997;87:741-748.*

Anesthesia gas delivery equipment claims represented 4% of all claims in the CCP database in the 1970s, 32% in the 1980s, 1% in the 1990s, and 1% from 2000 through 2008.[8] The outcomes in anesthesia gas delivery equipment claims from 1990 through 2010 also seem to be less severe than earlier claims. From 1990 through 2008, 38% of anesthesia gas delivery system claims resulted in severe injury or death compared with 80% from 1970 through 1989 ($P < .001$). Among the 39 claims from 1990 through 2010, 10 deaths, 5 cases of permanent brain damage, 6 pneumothoraces, and 9 awareness claims were reported. Payments reflect the lower severity of injury, with a median payment (in 2011 dollars) of $199,000 in the 1990 through 2003 claims period compared with $780,000 (adjusted to 2011 dollars) for earlier gas delivery equipment claims. Thirty-two (82%) of the 39 post-1990 claims resulted in payment.[8]

TABLE 33-5 **American Society of Anesthesiologists Closed Claims Project Claims Characterization**

Equipment Group	Misuse	Failure	Uncertain
Breathing circuit (n = 28)	26	2	0
Vaporizer (n = 15)	7	8	0
Ventilator (n = 12)	8	3	1
Supply tanks/lines (n = 8)	7	1	0
Anesthesia machine (n = 5)	2	3	0
Supplemental oxygen tubing (n = 4)	4	0	0
Total (n = 72)	54 (75%)	17 (24%)	1 (1%)

From Caplan RA, Vistica MF, Posner KL, Cheney FW: Adverse anesthetic outcomes arising from gas delivery equipment: a closed claims analysis. Anesthesiology *1997;87:741-748.*

PREVENTION

One of the principal components of RM is the development of preventive strategies for avoiding accidents.[34] With respect to anesthesia equipment, this strategy includes thoughtful equipment selection, preventive maintenance, personnel training, and supervision.

Equipment Selection

An RM strategy begins with the selection of appropriate equipment that meets current standards and is configured in a way that will minimize new types of errors. National standards for anesthetic equipment have been promulgated with the goal of reducing overt failures and errors associated with equipment misuse or unfamiliarity.[35] Voluntary consensus standards exist for anesthesia machines, ventilators, workstations, and essentially all of the commonly used anesthesia delivery technologies.[36,37] Although many features of anesthesia machines are now required as standard features—such as fail-safe devices, position of the oxygen flow control knob, and oxygen failure alarm—there is no design for a "universal anesthetic machine." Factors that have contributed to the variety of equipment available to anesthesiologists in the United States include the demand by consumers for different features and antitrust laws that require competition in the marketplace. No specific data are currently available from which to justify the costs of retooling the entire industry to impose more standardization.

Individual anesthesia departments should formulate plans for defining equipment obsolescence and replacing machines as necessary. No consensus exists on defining obsolescence in anesthesia equipment.[38] In 2004, the ASA promulgated its "Guidelines for Determining Anesthesia Machine Obsolescence" (see Chapter 30 for details). The introduction to these guidelines states:

This document has been developed by the ASA Committee on Equipment and Facilities, and has not been reviewed or

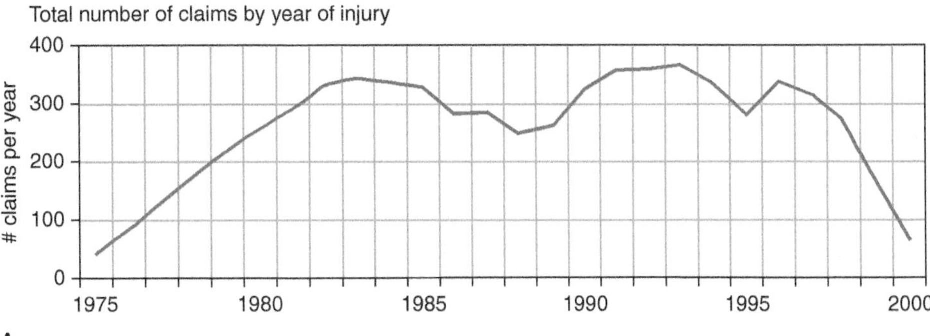

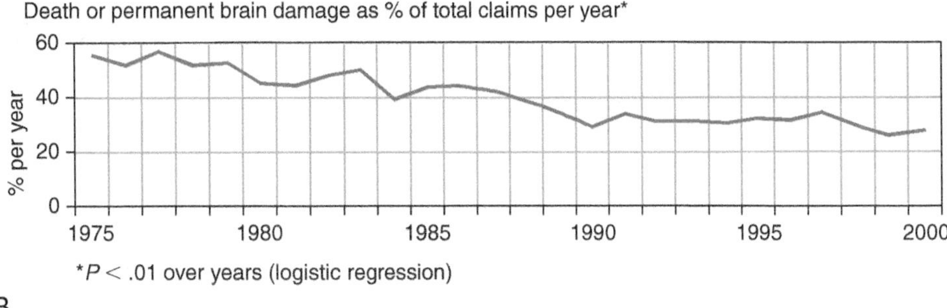

FIGURE 33-1 Overall number of closed claims reported annually. **A,** Total number of claims by year of injury. **B,** Death or permanent brain damage as a percentage of total claims per year. (From Cheney FW, Posner KL, Lee LA, et al: Trends in anesthesia-related death and brain damage: a closed claims analysis. *Anesthesiology* 2006;105:1081-1086.)

approved as a practice parameter or policy statement by the ASA House of Delegates. Variances from the recommendations contained in this document may be acceptable based on the judgment of the responsible anesthesiologist. The recommendations are designed to encourage quality patient care and safety in the workplace but cannot guarantee a specific outcome. They are subject to revision from time to time as warranted by the evolution of technology and practice.[39]

In essence, several issues should be addressed: compliance with ASTM International (formerly the American Society of Testing and Materials) standards, maintenance history, and policy regarding anesthetic machine uniformity (e.g., same manufacturer and model) in all anesthetizing locations for consistency.[38] Because unfamiliarity with equipment has been reported as a source of critical incidents, it would seem that standardizing equipment should reduce these errors.[30] Anesthetizing locations outside a main operating suite (e.g., the obstetric, radiology, gastroenterology, and cardiac units) are perhaps more likely to have atypical equipment, which may create a special risk. Other considerations for the replacement of existing anesthesia machines are manufacturer-defined life cycle, inability to obtain replacement parts, or development of new features not present on existing models. The medical equipment consumer organization, the ECRI Institute, publishes a monthly periodical, *Health Devices*, and maintains a large database on medical device problems, hazards, and recalls.[40] The database can help anesthesiologists keep abreast of recent developments in anesthesia equipment as well as alerting users to equipment safety concerns. Information available through the ECRI Institute's Problem Reporting Network and the Food and Drug Administration's (FDA) Medical Device Safety programs[41] may be timelier than information available in professional journals, which have inherently longer delays in publishing case reports or studies. Also, the Anesthesia Patient Safety Foundation (APSF) publishes a column in its quarterly newsletter in which current equipment-related hazards are discussed.[42]

Training

Active training programs geared to increased familiarity with new and existing anesthetic equipment and monitors should prevent many incidents. It is unlikely that even the most experienced, well-trained anesthesia provider will retain knowledge of the myriad ways in which equipment can fail. Although it is prudent to take specific actions to avoid problems that have been identified, it is equally important to define a generic strategy for prevention of equipment problems and injuries. This is certainly necessary to prevent the many ways in which equipment will fail, either from introduction of new designs and features or from circumstances that will cause failures that have not occurred previously with older designs.

Because appropriate response to critical events is important to stop an evolving accident, maintenance of skills and certification is prudent; this includes specialty board certification and relevant auxiliary skills, such as Advanced Cardiac Life Support. Documentation of all training activities is worthwhile, particularly from a medicolegal standpoint. Specific team-based performance skills are being taught to enhance skills in responding to crisis and critical events of all types. Anesthesia crisis resource management (ACRM) has been adapted from the aviation domain, stressing generic skills to optimize effectiveness in crisis response.[43] These skills include effective team communication; appropriate leadership and followership; enhanced dynamic decision making; and allocation and management of resources, such as delegation, prioritizing, and monitoring and validating information. The use of simulation has also become a popular method of training anesthesiologists in crisis management and is being evaluated in a wide array of health care fields for certification and licensing.[44,45] For anesthesiologists first licensed after 2008, the American Board of Anesthesiology requires participation in a simulation-based educational program for maintenance of certification in anesthesiology (MOCA).[46] Simulation is especially useful for training related to errors and critical events associated with equipment. Many specific training scenarios that involve the use of equipment can be effectively performed in realistic and computer-based simulators.[47,48]

Training and periodic review of basic environmental safety topics is also necessary and is mandated by The Joint Commission (TJC). Subjects relevant to equipment used by anesthesiologists and ancillary personnel include fire and electrical safety (see Chapter 31); hazards of toxic substances, such as inhalational anesthetics and carbon dioxide absorbent (see Chapter 30); and infectious disease control (see Chapter 20).

Supervision

Anesthetic practice frequently involves the additional risk of supervising residents, nurse anesthetists, and ancillary personnel. This can often become a complex and difficult task, requiring assessment of an individual's skills, judgment, and ability to function independently on a given task. One study that reviewed a form of significant adverse events involving residents in training pointed to several areas that require closer supervision; among these was incomplete knowledge about the construction, function, and hazards of breathing circuits and ventilators.[30] Noteworthy in the CCP study was the contribution of ancillary personnel—anesthesia technicians, engineers, nurses, and respiratory technicians—to the misuse of gas delivery equipment (16 of 54 claims).[26] Ancillary personnel figured most prominently in errors related to oxygen supply switches and misuse of supplemental oxygen tubing. This reinforces that the anesthesiologist is responsible not just for his or her own actions but for all of those assisting in the delivery of an anesthetic. The risk does not exist solely for the supervisor. As the supervisee, acknowledging limitations and knowing when to call for help may be two of the most important risk-reduction strategies.

Preventive Maintenance

Maintaining equipment according to manufacturer's guidelines at recommended intervals is implicit in delivering a safe anesthetic. Maintenance should be performed only by manufacturer-certified technicians, hospital biomedical technicians, or clinical engineers who have undergone training to maintain that particular device.

Preoperative Preparation

Preoperative preparation for anesthesia was the most commonly cited associated factor in critical incident studies.[30] This preparation includes thorough familiarization with the patient's history and the procedure and construction of a sound anesthetic plan and back-up plans. The patient should be adequately monitored and prepared medically prior to the induction of anesthesia. The anesthesiologist should be completely familiar with the anesthesia machine and any auxiliary equipment to be used, such as pacemakers and transport monitors. The anesthesia workspace should be arranged for maximal ergonomics with machine, drug cart, and back-up equipment all within close reach. Medications should be clearly labeled to avoid the various common administration errors. The anesthesiologist should also be familiar with the closest location of emergency equipment—including a defibrillator, an emergency airway cart, and a malignant hyperthermia cart—in every anesthetizing location.

The specifics of preparing the anesthesia machine prior to use have been the subject of extensive discussion with the goal of reducing critical incidents. In 1986, the FDA published a recommended preanesthetic equipment checklist, which was most recently revised in 2008 (see Chapter 32).[49] Production pressure is a familiar reality in many anesthesia practices and should not eclipse the need for adequate preoperative preparation.[9] The World Health Organization's campaign to improve surgical safety worldwide centers around the use of preprocedural checklists designed to address errors potentially vulnerable to poor communication and production pressure. The checklist requires pausing before the start of surgery to align team goals and review the details of the surgical plan, which include anesthetic equipment preparation.[50]

Use of Monitors

The appropriate use of redundant monitoring systems with their associated alarms can significantly improve an anesthesiologist's ability to detect and prevent errors in clinical practice. Several studies have reviewed the role of monitoring in the prevention of significant adverse events. In the CCP database, 56 of 72 gas delivery claims (78%) from the CCP were deemed preventable with the use, or better use, of monitors.[26] Most noteworthy were that nine claims (13%) occurred with a monitor alarm disabled or nonfunctional.

In a retrospective analysis of closed claims data, it was determined that a significant portion of the preventable mishaps would have been prevented with a combination of pulse oximetry and capnography.[51] This is particularly relevant, because nearly 40% of claims in the CCP involved breathing circuit misconnects or disconnects.[26] These technologies are now used almost universally, and despite the widely held belief that they have substantially reduced adverse anesthetic events, there is surprisingly limited evidence to support that thus far.

Data Validation and Situational Awareness

Any single observation in clinical anesthesia has an inherent level of error that reinforces the need for redundancy in monitoring and frequent validation of data. For example, the adequacy of ventilation relies primarily on capnography but should also be confirmed via alternative means, including direct clinical observation. In the complex environment of clinical anesthesia, frequent prioritizing of goals is paramount, particularly in a crisis situation. For example, when an arrhythmia develops, it is important to first quickly confirm adequate ventilation and oxygenation prior to treating rhythm disturbance.

Fixation error is a term used to describe a source of incident propagation in complex systems whereby a single incident distracts an operator from discovering a more dangerous one.[52] An example would be an anesthesiologist becoming focused on an infusion pump alarm while failing to identify a breathing circuit disconnection. An important quality for anesthesiologists to develop is a situational awareness, or a firm grasp of the "big picture" when responding to a variety of incidents.[52] This is a commonly addressed principle in crisis management training.

Compensation for Stressors

Numerous stressors and distracters exist in the practice of anesthesia, and they can contribute to errors.[52] These include fatigue, hunger, boredom, production pressure, interpersonal interactions, multitasking, noise, and so on. The first step to reduce their effects is to acknowledge their presence and effect on performance. An appropriate relief schedule should be maintained to avoid fatigue, and it should include a thorough debriefing of events and issues.[52] Effective procedures for handing off responsibilities between providers must be developed and used whenever responsibility for care changes.[53] Judgment must be used in short cases, or when continuity of care is critical and the risk of relieving an individual outweighs the benefit. A careful review of the status of anesthesia equipment is important and can detect ongoing problems that may have been missed or that may lead to additional preparation for an emergency.

RESPONSE

Recovery

Because the majority of adverse events in the practice of anesthesia are multifactorial, and many may never be completely eliminated, an important focus of RM is attempting to recover from simple incidents before they become more severe. Most accident models portray the escalation of small errors that compound into greater ones. In one landmark study, 93% of all critical incidents were "near misses" that did not evolve into serious accidents.[52] Perhaps the most essential feature of quality anesthesia care is breaking this "chain of accident evolution" with early and appropriate intervention.[9]

Elements required for successful recovery from anesthesia incidents and those associated with an unsuccessful recovery have been identified (Boxes 33-1 and 33-2).[9] These demand an existing knowledge base, adequate response training and planning, and an established system of preparedness that includes appropriate monitors and back-up equipment. Recovery also depends on less tangible elements such as operator vigilance, anticipation, and judgment. The first elements of successful recovery—detecting the incident, validating its existence, and acknowledging its threat to the patient—were discussed in the earlier section on prevention. The latter elements of successful incident recovery begin with implementing generic corrective strategies. An accurate diagnosis of the cause of a decreased pulse oximeter reading (SpO_2) should not delay an initial treatment by increasing the fraction of inspired oxygen (FiO_2). A decrease in blood pressure may be treated most appropriately by first administering fluids or decreasing inhaled anesthetic concentration.

The availability of back-up equipment also figures prominently in adequate recovery from critical incidents. Because the primary mechanism of most adverse anesthesia events is hypoxia, and many equipment failures involve the breathing circuit,[26] it is important to ensure availability and functionality of a self-inflating resuscitation bag, spare laryngoscope handles, and auxiliary oxygen cylinders. A back-up pulse oximeter, capnograph, and other critical equipment should also be available.

BOX 33-1 Requirements for Successful Recovery from Anesthesia Incidents

- Detect one or more manifestations of the incident in progress
- Verify the manifestations and reject false alarms
- Recognize that the manifestations represent an actual or potential threat
- Ensure continued maintenance of life-sustaining functions
- Implement "generic" diagnostic or corrective strategies to provide failure compensation and allow continuation of surgery if possible
- Achieve specific diagnosis and therapy of the underlying causes
- Provide follow-up of recovery to ensure adequate correction or compensation

From Gaba DM, Maxwell M, DeAnda A: Anesthetic mishaps: breaking the chain of accident evolution. *Anesthesiology* 1987;66:670-676.

BOX 33-2 Factors Associated with Unsuccessful Recovery from Anesthesia Incidents

- Lack of recognition of the most serious problem
- Failure to initiate life-sustaining therapies first
- Lack of adequate back-up or safety equipment
- Ignorance of appropriate recovery procedures
- Improper implementation of known recovery procedures
- Inadequate follow-up of recovery status
- Lack of patient response to properly applied appropriate recovery procedures

From Gaba DM, Maxwell M, DeAnda A: Anesthetic mishaps: breaking the chain of accident evolution. *Anesthesiology* 1987;66:670-676.

Administrative Response

The primary responsibility of an anesthesiologist involved with an anesthetic-related injury is to minimize harm to the patient. However, several other serious responsibilities exist that include patient follow-up, communicating with the family, activating appropriate administrative procedures, impounding equipment, and conducting an investigation. Because serious events in anesthesia are rare, it is important to attempt to systematically identify the cause of the accident to prevent future harm to patients. Critical pieces of information about anesthetic accidents have been lost in the past because of improper handling of evidence. These include hasty disposal of equipment or supplies; returning equipment to a service manager or the equipment manufacturer for testing and repair; and destructive testing, dismantling equipment, and loss of stored data by unplugging monitors with microprocessors. Failure to preserve evidence may give rise to additional legal claims, including spoliation of evidence.[54]

Several protocols exist to assist in responding to the administrative details of an anesthetic accident.[55,56] More recently, general procedures following an adverse event have been promulgated.[57] Currently, no body of evidence exists to support specific actions in response to an accident. Because accidents vary greatly, the recommendations serve primarily to organize the process of gathering information rather than serving as a strict protocol. Although the guidelines are intended primarily for responding to anesthetic deaths or serious injuries, the principles are equally useful for investigating "near misses."

An important component for minimizing patient injury is to mobilize the best medical resources as soon as is prudent. This includes appropriate specialist consultation, such as a neurologist in cases of hypoxic brain injury or a burn specialist for thermal injuries. It is prudent to provide frequent patient follow-up after the incident and to maintain close communication with the other physicians involved.

Administrative responsibility for accident investigation and follow-up should be shifted to other appropriate individuals soon after an incident occurs. This may include informing an appropriate administrator who can coordinate contacting others in the accident-response chain of command. The hospital risk manager should be contacted for specific advice on hospital policy for responding to accidents, communicating with families, and coordinating an investigation. Insurance carriers should be contacted for legal recommendations regarding the impounding of evidence and to ensure compliance with policy coverage requirements. Guidelines for impounding equipment that include specific actions for disposition, record keeping, communication with manufacturers, and legal implications are outlined by the ECRI Institute.[58] Under some circumstances, such as when accidents involve medical equipment and result in serious injury or death, the hospital may be required by law under the Safe Medical Devices Act of 1991 to report the event to the manufacturer and the FDA (see Chapters 32 and 34).

The primary anesthesiologist and others directly involved in the incident must document relevant information as soon as it is safe to do so. For the anesthesiologist, this involves completing the patient record, whether hand-kept or electronic, and filing an incident report. Attention should be paid to stating only the facts and avoiding judgments about causality or responsibility. If corrections must be made to the anesthetic record, they should be annotated in an appropriate fashion that includes date, time, and signature. Under no circumstances should information be erased, nor should any attempt be made to rewrite the entire record. Following these types of procedures in the aftermath of an equipment-related adverse outcome can be vital in determining cause and in preventing inappropriate financial loss.

MEDICOLEGAL ISSUES

Relationship Between Anesthesia Providers and Equipment Manufacturers

Both the anesthesia provider and the manufacturer share the responsibility for anesthesia equipment. Ideally, the two should function as partners with the common goal of safe patient care. However, the evolution of the medicolegal tort system in the United States in the past three decades has imposed additional constraints on this relationship.[59] The plaintiff in an anesthesia malpractice case may involve the equipment manufacturer as an additional defendant, even if it is only remotely connected to the incident. A motivation for this strategy is the perception that the manufacturer may have "deep pockets"; that is, it is more able to pay because of excess liability insurance and corporate assets. Consequently, cases believed to have little or no merit are pursued against manufacturers. Some states, such as California, limit the damages that may be awarded for noneconomic losses in medical malpractice cases. If, however, a case can be made for product liability, there may be no cap on the amounts that can be awarded. Companies often view these cases as having the potential for great liability, and they may offer to settle outside the courts for some nominal amount. If litigated, a successful strategy for these cases with multiple defendants—surgeon, anesthesiologist, hospital, and equipment manufacturer—is to maintain a unified defense and avoid finger-pointing among parties. It is believed that finger-pointing among defendants both increases the likelihood of a plaintiff's verdict and increases the dollar value of the plaintiff's case.

Product liability litigation has evolved from a focus on warranties to claims of product and design defects and a manufacturer's "post-sale duty to warn" users. Product warranties define a manufacturer's responsibilities, including circumstances in which a product is expected to function and specifies abuses of the product that will negate the responsibility of the manufacturer. Litigation against manufacturer defects on the basis that the seller failed to satisfy the buyer's belief of an implied warranty have become less prevalent because of the difficulty to prove negligence in the courts.[60]

Recent litigation strategies have included suits of alleged manufacturer negligence to warn a buyer of specific product safety hazards that are discovered after the date of sale (post-sale duty to warn). The legal responsibility for a manufacturer to warn or retrofit a product that is determined to be hazardous after sale varies from state to state. This has particular relevance when considering the controversies of defining obsolete equipment. From a manufacturer's standpoint, older anesthesia equipment is more difficult to defend in such cases, as is equipment that has not been actively serviced by the manufacturer. Other factors that may reduce the legal responsibility of the manufacturer are modification of equipment by the user and equipment used for purposes other than those intended or approved by the FDA.[60]

Despite continuing improvements in the safety of anesthesia care, errors and accidents related to use of equipment continue to occur, sometimes with devastating results. To further improve safety, a strategy for RM must be applied to anesthesia practices at the local level as well as throughout all processes of equipment acquisition and utilization. Individual events should be closely examined to identify causes and to develop interventions to prevent recurrence. In those cases in which poor outcomes have resulted, administrative actions should be implemented to properly manage follow-up in the best interests of all parties.

REFERENCES

1. American Society for Healthcare Risk Management (www.ashrm.org/ashrm/about/index/shtml/?page=index).
2. Carroll R: *Risk management handbook for health care organizations*, ed 5, San Francisco, 2009, Jossey-Bass.
3. Spath PL: *Error reduction in health care: a systems approach to improving patient safety*, ed 2, San Francisco, 2011, Jossey-Bass.
4. Wachter RM: *Understanding patient safety*, ed 2, Chicago, 2012, McGraw-Hill.
5. Pate-Cornell ME, Murphy DM, Latkis LM, et al: Patient risk in anesthesia: probabilistic risk analysis, management effects and improvements, *Ann Operations Res* 67:211–233, 1997.
6. Institute for Healthcare Improvement: *Failure Mode Effects Analysis*, 2004. Accessed online at http://app.ihi.org/Workspace/tools/fmea.
7. Cheney FW, Posner KL, Lee LA, Caplan RA, Domino KB: Trends in anesthesia-related death and brain damage: a closed claims analysis, *Anesthesiology* 105:1081–1086, 2006.
8. Eisenkraft JB: *ASA refresher course: hazards of the anesthesia workstation* 37(1):37–55, 2009.
9. Gaba DM, Maxwell M, DeAnda A: Anesthetic mishaps: breaking the chain of accident evolution, *Anesthesiology* 66:670–676, 1987.
10. Runciman WB, Webb RK, Lee R, Holland R: System failure: an analysis of 2000 incident reports, *Anaesth Intensive Care* 21:506–519, 1993.
11. Cooper JB, Newbower RS, Long CD, McPeek B: Preventable anesthesia mishaps, *Anesthesiology* 49:399–406, 1978.
12. Institute of Medicine: Definition of key terms. Accessed online at https://www.premierinc.com/safety/topics/patient_safety/index_1.jsp#IOM-1definitionsofkeyterms.
13. Reason JT: *Managing the risks of organizational accidents*, Farnham, UK, 1997, Ashgate.
14. van Beuzekom M, Boer F, Akerboom S, Hudson P: Patient safety: latent risk factors, *Br J Anaesth* 105(1):52–59, 2010.
15. Webb RK, Russell WJ, Klepper I, Runciman WB: Equipment failure: an analysis of 2000 incident reports, *Anaesth Intensive Care* 21:673–677, 1993.
16. Catchpole K, Bell MD, Johnson S: Safety in anaesthesia: a study of 12,606 reported incidents from the UK National Reporting and Learning System, *Anaesthesia* 63:340–346, 2008.
17. Cassidy CJ, Smith A, Arnot-Smith J: Critical incident reports concerning anaesthetic equipment: analysis of the UK National Reporting and Learning System (NRLS) data from 2006-2008, *Anaesthesia* 66:879–888, 2011.
18. Beydon L, Ledenmat PY, Soltner C, et al: Adverse events with medical devices in anesthesia and intensive care unit patients recorded in the French safety database in 2005-2006, *Anesthesiology* 112:364–372, 2010.
19. Fasting S, Gisvold SE: Equipment problems during anaesthesia—are they a quality problem? *Br J Anaesth* 89:825–831, 2002.
20. James RH: 1000 anaesthetic incidents: experience to date, *Anaesthesia* 58:856–863, 2003.
21. Kawashima Y, Takahashi S, Suzuki M, et al: Anesthesia-related mortality and morbidity over a 5-year period in 2,363,038 patients in Japan, *Acta Anaesthesiol Scand* 47:809–817, 2003.
22. Carter JA: Checking anaesthetic equipment and the Expert Group on Blocked Anaesthetic Tubing (EGBAT), *Anaesthesia* 59:105–107, 2004.
23. Caplan R, University of Washington, 2011, Personal communication.
24. Runciman WB, Webb RK, Lee R, Holland R: System failure: an analysis of 2000 incident reports, *Anaesth Intensive Care* 21:684–695, 1993.
25. Swiss Medical Association: Critical Incident in Anesthesiology. Accessed online at http://www.medana.unibas.ch/cirs.
26. Caplan RA, Vistica MF, Posner KL, Cheney FW: Adverse anesthetic outcomes arising from gas delivery equipment: a closed claims analysis, *Anesthesiology* 87:741–748, 1997.
27. Spittal MJ, Findlay GP, Spencer I: A prospective analysis of critical incidents attributable to anaesthesia, *J Int Soc Qual Health Care* 7:363–371, 1995.
28. Reference deleted in proofs.
29. Klanarong S, Chau-in W, Pulnitiporn A, Pengpol W: The Thai Anesthesia Incidents Study (THAI Study) of anesthetic equipment failure/malfunction: a qualitative analysis for risk factors, *J Med Assoc Thailand* 88(7):S134–S140, 2005.
30. Cooper JB, Newbower RS, Kitz RJ: An analysis of major errors and equipment failures in anesthesia management: considerations for prevention and detection, *Anesthesiology* 60:34–42, 1984.
31. Craig J, Wilson ME: A survey of anaesthetic misadventures, *Anaesthesia* 36:933–936, 1981.
32. Kumar V, Barcellos WA, Mehta MP, Carter JG: An analysis of critical incidents in a teaching department for quality assurance: a survey of mishaps during anaesthesia, *Anaesthesia* 43:879–883, 1988.
33. Chopra V, Bovill J, Spierdijk J, Koornneef F: Reported significant observations during anaesthesia: a prospective analysis over an 18-month period, *Br J Anaesth* 68:13–17, 1992.
34. Cooper JB, Longnecker D: Safety and quality: the guiding principles of patient-centered care. In Longnecker D, editor: *Anesthesiology*, New York, 2012, McGraw Hill Medical Publishing, pp 16–26.
35. American Society for Testing and Materials: *ASTM Standard F1208–89(2005), Standard Specification for Minimum Performance and Safety Requirements for Anesthesia Breathing Systems*, West Conshohocken, PA, 2005, ASTM International, DOI:10.1520/F1208/89R05, www.astm.org.
36. American Society for Testing and Materials: *ASTM Standard F1101–90(2003)e1, Standard Specification for Ventilators Intended for Use During Anesthesia*, West Conshohocken, PA, 2003, ASTM International, DOI:10.1520/F1101-90R03E01.
37. American Society for Testing and Materials: *ASTM Standard F1850–00(2005), Standard Specification for Particular Requirements for Anesthesia Workstations and Their Components*, West Conshohocken, PA, 2005, ASTM International, DOI:10.1520/F1850-00R05.
38. Petty WC: The aging anesthesia machine, *J Clin Monit* 13:129, 1997.
39. ASA Committee on Equipment and Facilities: *Guidelines for Determining Anesthesia Machine Obsolescence*, 2004. Accessed online at http://www.asahq.org/for-members/standards-guidelines-and-statements.aspx.
40. ECRI Institute, Plymouth Meeting, PA. Accessed online at http://www.ecri.org/pages/default.aspx.
41. U.S. Food and Drug Administration. Medical Device Safety. Accessed online at http://www.fda.gov/MedicalDevices/Safety/default.htm.
42. Anesthesia Patient Safety Foundation. Accessed online at http://www.apsf.org/resources.php.
43. Howard SK, Gaba DM, Fish KJ, et al: Anesthesia crisis resource management: teaching anesthesiologists to handle critical incidents, *Aviat Space Environ Med* 63:763–770, 1992.
44. Gaba DM, Howard SK, Fish KJ, et al: Simulation-based training in anesthesia crisis resource management (ACRM): a decade of experience, *Simulation Gaming* 32(2):175–193, 2001.
45. Holmboe EH, Rizzolo MA, Sachdeva AK, Rosenberg M, Ziv A: Simulation-based assessment and the regulation of healthcare professionals, *Sim Healthcare* 6:S58–S62, 2011.
46. American Board of Anesthesiology: Maintenance of certification anesthesiology (MOCA). Accessed online at http://www.theaba.org/Home/anesthesiology_maintenance.
47. Waldrop WB, Murray DJ, Boulet JR, Kras JF: Management of anesthesia equipment failure: a simulation-based resident skill assessment, *Anesth Analg* 109:426–433, 2009.
48. Mundumbai SC, Fanning R, Howard SK, Davies F, Gaba DM: Use of medical simulation to explore equipment failures and human-machine interactions in anesthesia machine pipeline supply crossover, *Anesth Analg* 110: 1292–1286, 2010.

49. ASA Subcommittee of ASA Committee on Equipment and Facilities: *Recommendations for Pre-Anesthesia Checkout Procedures*, 2008. Accessed online at http://www.asahq.org/for-members/clinical-information/2008-asa-recommendations-for-preanesthesia-checkout.aspx.
50. World Health Organization, Geneva Switzerland: Safe Surgery Initiative. Accessed online at http://www.who.int/patientsafety/safesurgery/en.
51. Tinker JH, Dull DL, Caplan RA, Ward RJ, Cheney FW: Role of monitoring devices in prevention of anesthetic mishaps: a closed claims analysis, *Anesthesiology* 71(4):541–546, 1989.
52. Cooper JB: Do short breaks increase or decrease anesthesia risk? *J Clin Anesth* 1:228–231, 1989.
53. Goldhaber-Feibert S, Cooper JB: Safety in anesthesia. In Dunn P, editor: *Clinical anesthesia procedures of the Massachusetts General Hospital*, ed 8, Philadelphia, 2010, Lippincott Williams & Wilkins, pp 127–134.
54. Casamassima AC: Spoliation of evidence and medical malpractice, *Pace L Rev* 14(1):235–299, 1994.
55. Cooper JB, Cullen DJ, Eichhorn JH, et al: Administrative guidelines for response to an adverse anesthesia event, *J Clin Anesth* 5:79–84, 1993.
56. Bacon AK: Major anaesthetic mishaps—handling the aftermath, *Curr Anaesth Crit Care* 1:253–257, 1990.
57. Conway J, Federico F, Stewart K, Campbell M: *Respectful management of serious clinical adverse events*, IHI Innovation Series white paper, ed 2, Cambridge, MA, 2011, Institute for Healthcare Improvement. Accessed online at www.IHI.org.
58. ECRI Institute: Reporting equipment-related incidents under new FDA regulations, *Health Devices* 14(1):3–8, 1984.
59. Studdard DM, Mello MM, Gawande AA, et al: Claims, errors and compensations payments in medical malpractice litigation, *N Engl J Med* 354:2024–2033, 2006.
60. Stolzer P: BOC Group, Murray Hill, NJ, 1997, Personal communication.

CHAPTER 34

STANDARDS AND REGULATORY CONSIDERATIONS

Michael B. Jaffe • David G. Osborn

CHAPTER OUTLINE

OVERVIEW

It was once possible to practice "safe" and "modern" anesthesia without any knowledge of the regulatory and voluntary standards governing anesthesia equipment and practice. This has changed, however, and individual practitioners are now subject to federal and state regulations regarding the use of these devices and are strongly influenced by international standards and agreements. The arena of medical device standards and regulations is complex and arcane, and there is much overlap of authority. This chapter reviews the history, present status, interested parties, relevant standards, standards processes, and pending developments that will affect the clinician in the future. The reader should be left with a good understanding of both the processes and the interested parties in the constantly evolving international setting of standards and regulations.

What Is a Standard?

A standard is a document, established by consensus and approved by a recognized body, that provides for common and repeated use, rules, guidelines, or characteristics for activities or their results, aimed at the achievement of the optimum degree of order in a given context.[1] Standards should be based on the consolidated results of science, technology, and experience, and they should be aimed at the promotion of optimum community benefits. In reality, a standard is an agreed restriction for a common good and a shared benefit.[1]

REGULATION OF MEDICAL DEVICES

The rules governing medical devices differ throughout the world.[2] Many different models exist, such as the U.S. Food and Drug Administration (FDA), European Union (EU) CE-marking system, and various registrations, listings, licenses, and approvals in other countries. Efforts have been under way since the early 1990s via organizations such as the Global Harmonization Task Force (GHTF) to better achieve uniformity among national medical device regulatory systems around the world. This is being done with two aims in mind: enhancing patient safety and increasing access to safe, effective, and clinically beneficial medical technologies.

Global Harmonization Task Force

A partnership between regulatory authorities and regulated industry, the GHTF consisted of five founding members: the European Union, United States, Canada, Australia, and Japan. The GHTF intended to foster international harmonization in the regulation of medical devices by the development of a regulatory model and supporting documents to underpin globally harmonized regulation of medical technologies. Regulatory and industry representatives from Europe, the Asia-Pacific region, and North America were encouraged to collaborate and actively participate in the development of guidance documents that describe regulatory practices to ensure the safety, effectiveness, and quality of medical devices. This task has been substantially completed, the GHTF has published many final documents on their Web site, and some countries have based their newly developed regulatory processes on these documents. Notwithstanding this success, little progress has been made by the founding members of the GHTF in the harmonization of their regulatory processes to this model. Many other countries, particularly some of the BRIC countries—Brazil, Russia, India, and China—unsuccessfully attempted to join the GHTF.

The FDA proposed, and the five founding members agreed, that the time had come to dissolve the GHTF and create a new, regulator-only forum with global reach that would consult with other interested groups—including industry, health care professionals, and consumers—in the advancement of regulatory harmonization. In October 2011, the regulatory authorities of Australia, Brazil, Canada, China, the European Union, Japan, and the United States and the World Health Organization (WHO) announced the establishment of the International Medical Device Regulators' Forum (IMDRF) to replace the GHTF. The IMDRF intends to provide guidance on strategies, policies, directions, and activities to accelerate international medical device regulatory harmonization. Unlike the GHTF, various stakeholder groups, such as industry, academia, health care professionals, and consumer and patient groups, are no longer invited to participate in the steering committee or management committee, although they can be invited to participate in ad hoc working groups.

Medical Device Regulation in the United States

Manufacturers of medical devices distributed in the United States must comply with certain basic regulatory requirements:

- Establishment registration
- Quality Systems (QS) regulation
- Labeling requirements
- Premarket Notification 510(k), unless exempt, or Premarket Approval (PMA)
- Medical device listing
- Medical Device Reporting (MDR)

Definition of Terms

Establishment Registration. A manufacturer must file its name and all places of business with the FDA. Any additional place of business must be registered immediately. Registration is performed electronically.

Quality System Regulation. The QS regulation requires the manufacturer to have a written quality system that is subject to periodic audit by the FDA. The QS regulation requires every medical device to be designed, manufactured, packed, stored, and installed in conformity with current Good Manufacturing Practices (GMP). The QS regulation requires use of design validation, investigation of complaints, and a corrective and preventive action plan to identify root causes of product nonconformance with standards and specifications and to implement effective actions to prevent recurrence.

Labeling Requirements. Medical devices must be labeled either on the medical device or on its immediate container. The label must identify the company name, trade name, or trade symbol of the manufacturer as well as the name and place of business of the manufacturer, packager, or distributor and the identity of and quantity of the contents of the package. In addition, the labeling of a medical device must provide adequate directions for use and adequate warnings against unsafe use for a layperson, unless the medical device is a prescription medical device, in which case the labeling may be written for health care professionals. The labeling of a prescription medical device may be made available electronically.

Premarket Notification 510(k). The 510(k) process is designed to ensure, through a quality review process, that marketed medical devices, subject to general and applicable special controls, provide a reasonable assurance of safety and effectiveness. It is also designed to foster innovation. This is achieved by comparing the (new) device to an existing (predicate) moderate-risk medical device and demonstrating that the new medical device is substantially equivalent to the predicate. The 510(k) process applies to moderate-risk medical devices (typically class II; Table 34-1).

Premarket Approval. The premarket approval (PMA) process is designed to ensure that a specific marketed medical device provides a reasonable assurance of safety and effectiveness through a scientific review process of safety and effectiveness data (clinical trials). The PMA process applies to novel medical devices or new high-risk medical devices (typically class III; see Table 34-1).

Medical Device Listings. A manufacturer must file a list identifying each medical device made or processed for commercial distribution in the United States and its

TABLE 34-1 **Comparison of FDA 510(k) Premarket Notification and Premarket Approval**

Factor	510(k) Premarket Notification	Premarket Approval
Classes of devices	Class I and II devices	Class III devices
Number annually	2428*	24*
Documentation (length)	Depends on type of submission (special, traditional) Typically 50 to 250 pages	Typically thousands of pages
Regulatory requirement	Reasonable assurance of safety and effectiveness	Reasonable assurance of safety and effectiveness
Evidence	"Substantial equivalence": comparison to an existing predicate medical device	Scientific review process of safety and effectiveness data
Clinical studies provided?	Varies depending on device type, overall about 10% with clinical studies	Required for both safety and effectiveness
Review period (goal/typical)	90/120 days† (traditionally 74% of submissions†) Average time for anesthesiology branch: 140 days†	180/410 days‡
Source of required information	21 CFR 807.87	Section 515(c)(1) of the federal Food, Drug, and Cosmetic Act
Outside review?	No	FDA Advisory Panel meeting
User fees	$4717§	$220,050§
		Additional changes made via PMA supplements

*2011 actual.
†An analysis of FDA 510(k) data from 2006 to 2010, Emergo Group (January 9, 2012).
‡Three-year average, fiscal years 2006 to 2008.
§2012 actual.
CFR, Code of Federal Regulations; FDA, Food and Drug Administration; PMA, Premarket Approval.

labels and labeling. Additionally, the manufacturer must provide a notice of discontinuance once a medical device is no longer made. Listing is performed electronically.

Medical Device Reporting. Manufacturers of moderate- and high-risk medical devices (class II or class III) must report to the FDA when they learn of information that reasonably suggests that a medical device has or may have caused or contributed to the death or serious illness of or serious injury to a patient, or when they learn of an event that might contribute to the death or serious illness of or serious injury to a patient should it reoccur.

Medical Device Regulation in the European Union

In the EU, medical devices are regulated by one of three directives: the Medical Devices Directive (MDD), the Active Implantable Medical Devices Directive (AIMDD), or the In Vitro Diagnostic Directive (IVDD). Directives are an instrument from the European Parliament directing each member state to enact a law that embodies the content of the directive. The directives establish the regulatory scheme based on a risk-based classification system and, for higher risk devices, a certified quality system. The directives establish broad safety and performance criteria called the *Essential Requirements* (ERs). All medical devices are required to demonstrate compliance with the ERs.

Medical Device Regulation in Japan

The Pharmaceutical Affairs Law (PAL) applies to all medical devices in Japan. PAL is controlled by the Ministry of Health, Labor, and Welfare (MHLW). All medical devices are classified with a Japanese classification rule that was basically an adopted GHTF rule. Based on the classification, a medical device can require *notification*, *certification*, or *approval* (respectively, from lower to higher risk and from lower to higher effort). Additionally, certain measuring devices require a separate metrological (pattern) approval.

Medical Device Regulation in China

The State Food and Drug Administration (SFDA) is the central government agency in charge of drug and medical device administration with functions similar to those of the FDA in the United States. All medical devices must be registered with the SFDA before they are exported to or sold in China. The SFDA process requires in-country testing of medical devices for the Chinese market. Additionally, certain measuring devices require a separate metrological approval.

The General Administration of Quality Supervision, Inspection, and Quarantine (AQSIQ) is tasked with oversight, inspection, and quarantine as well as with establishing the technical standards for imported and exported goods. AQSIQ maintains responsibility for certifying electrical safety for a wide variety of products with the so-called China Compulsory Certificate (CCC). The CCC safety license process requires manufacturers to obtain the CCC mark before exporting or selling products listed in the CCC catalog into the Chinese market. The CCC mark is administered by the Certification and Accreditation Administration (CNCA). The China Quality Certification Centre (CQC) is designated by the CNCA to process CCC mark applications. Electrical medical devices require CCC certification prior to SFDA registration.

ROLE OF STANDARDS IN MEDICAL DEVICE REGULATION

In almost all jurisdictions, *standards* are used for the detailed requirements used to regulate medical devices, and *regulations* are used to set the high-level principles. The exception is China, where the standards are written into the law and become part of the regulation.

The U.S. FDA reviews standards and, when found appropriate, recognizes them as suitable by publishing them in the *Federal Register* (FR). Manufacturers may then use those standards to simplify regulatory submissions. The EU harmonizes standards that they find acceptable by publishing them in the *Official Journal* (OJ). A harmonized standard has a special status. Medical devices that comply with the relevant harmonized standards are presumed to demonstrate compliance with the relevant essential requirements, and this presumption cannot be easily challenged.

Early Efforts in the United States

The passage of the Federal Food, Drug, and Cosmetic Act (FD&C Act) of 1938 was hastened by a tragedy the previous year in which nearly a hundred people died after ingesting "Elixir Sulfanilamide."[3] This act included new provisions to:

- Extend control to cosmetics and therapeutic medical devices
- Start a new system of drug regulation that requires new drugs to be shown to be safe
- Loosen misbranding requirements by eliminating the need to prove intent to defraud
- Ensure that safe limits be created for unavoidable poisonous substances
- Authorize food standards created for identity, quality, and container filling
- Authorize medical device factory inspections
- Add the remedy of court injunctions against violative manufacturers

Increasing public concern over the safety and effectiveness of medical devices in the late 1960s and early 1970s led to the formation of a study group within the Department of Health, Education, and Welfare, the predecessor of the present Department of Health and Human Services (DHHS). This study group, chaired by Dr. Theodore Cooper of the National Heart, Lung, and Blood Institute, estimated, as did other studies at the time, that over the previous decade more than 10,000 injuries and hundreds of deaths were linked to medical devices still on the market.[4]

Recommendations from this study group formed the basis of the Medical Device Amendments of 1976. The members of the group felt that performance standards would be more effective than a PMA in ensuring the safety and effectiveness of most new medical devices. Since 1976, the FDA and medical device regulation has evolved. A timeline showing significant events since 1976 is shown in Figure 34-1.

Food and Drug Administration

History

The Food and Drug Administration is a scientific, regulatory, public health agency whose mission is to protect and promote public health. One of its purposes is to establish a reasonable assurance of the safety and effectiveness of medical devices marketed in the United States. Regulation of medical devices in the United States by the FDA has been undergoing an evolution since the passage of the Medical Device Amendments in 1976. This evolution (see Fig. 34-1) has included the passage of several pieces of legislation and the establishment of important reporting and disclosure tools, such as MedWatch (www.fda.gov/Safety/MedWatch/ucm170520.htm) and ClinicalTrials.gov.

The meaning of the terms *safety* and *effectiveness* is dependent on the risk profile of the medical device. For low-risk medical devices (class I), general postmarketing controls are considered sufficient to provide reasonable assurances of safety and effectiveness. For moderate-risk devices (class II) for which there is sufficient information, so-called *special controls*—typically a combination of standards and guidance documents—are considered sufficient to provide reasonable assurances of safety and effectiveness. For high-risk devices (class III) or for those medical devices on which there is not sufficient information, scientific evidence from well-controlled clinical trials is required to provide reasonable assurances of safety and effectiveness.

Medical Device Amendments of 1976. In 1976, the Medical Device Amendments (21 U.S.C. Secs. 513 through 521)

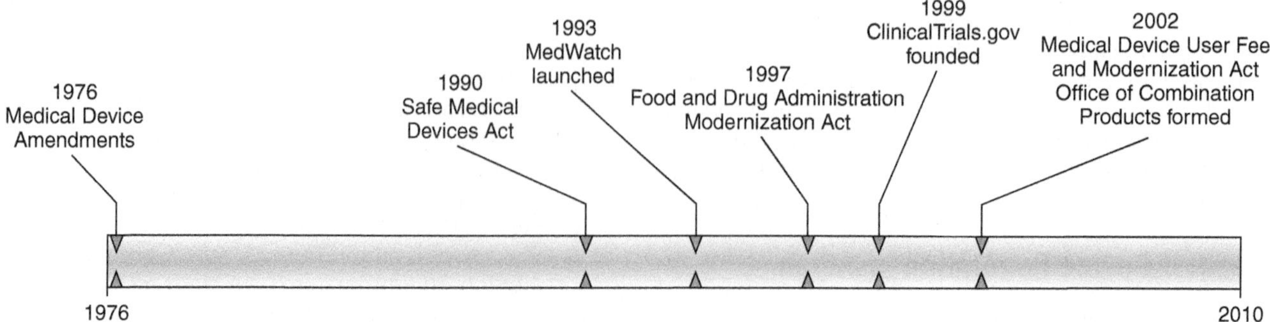

FIGURE 34-1 Timeline of Food and Drug Administration–related medical device legislation since 1976.

supplemented the original Federal FD&C Act, which required a "reasonable assurance of safety and effectiveness" before a medical device can be marketed. Section 201(h) of the FD&C Act defined a medical device as:

> *An instrument, apparatus, implement, machine, contrivance, implant, in vitro reagent, or other similar or related article including any component, part or accessory which is (1) recognized in the official National Formulary, or the United States Pharmacopoeia, or any supplement to them, (2) intended for use in the diagnosis of disease or other conditions, or in the cure, mitigation, treatment, or prevention of disease, in man or other animals, or (3) intended to affect the structure of the body in man or other animals and which does not achieve any of its principal intended purposes through chemical action within or on the body of man or other animal and which is not dependent upon being metabolized for the achievement of any of its principal intended purposes.*

These amendments provided the FDA with the authority to regulate medical devices by establishing a three-tiered system of regulation. Manufacturers were required, at the very least, to register with the FDA any new low-risk device. High-risk devices, on the other hand, required PMA, and moderate-risk devices required PMN and FDA clearance prior to being marketed. In all cases, however, the FDA was required to conduct postmarket surveillance of devices after introduction into clinical use, and manufacturers were required to report significant incidents to the FDA.

After the 1976 amendments, problems with an anesthesia machine that led to the death of four patients exposed problems with the regulatory framework in place at that time. This led to congressional hearings and helped lead to the MDR regulations, issued shortly thereafter, which required all manufacturers and distributors of medical devices to report deaths and serious injuries from medical devices to the FDA.[5] During those hearings, the FDA agreed to work to minimize the dangerous use of medical devices, and real efforts for extending the FDA's Good Manufacturing Practices to cover the design of medical devices began.

A series of legislative changes have been made by Congress to the FD&C Act. They include:

- Safe Medical Devices Act (SMDA) of 1990
- Medical Device Amendments of 1992
- FDA Modernization Act (FDAMA) of 1997
- Medical Device User Fee and Modernization Act (MDUFMA) of 2002

Safe Medical Devices Act. The Safe Medical Devices Act (SMDA) was signed into law on November 28, 1990 (Public Law 101-629).[6] Elements of the new law included user reporting of probable device-related issues, distributor/manufacturer reporting of device incidents, changes to the 510(k) clearance and PMA processes, changes to the classification of devices, and changes to the FDA's internal performance standards process, recall authority, postmarket surveillance, and greater enforcement powers. One of the most important features of this law is that it imposed mandatory requirements on facilities that use medical devices. The user shared the onus, which previously only had fallen to the manufacturer. Thus the FDA has gained some regulatory access and control in the local hospital. With this new law, the emphasis was supposed to have been moved from premarket review to postmarket surveillance. Consistent with this change in philosophy, the processes by which devices are classified and approved were to have been relaxed. There is little evidence that this has happened. All institutions—from major medical centers to small, freestanding ambulatory surgical centers—are now expected to report any information on the death or injury of a patient that may have been caused by a medical device. Both the FDA and the manufacturer must be notified within a specified period of time and in a prescribed manner. In addition, institutions are required to produce biannual reports summarizing all individual reports filed over the past 180 days.

The SMDA made important changes in the law compared with the 1976 Medical Device Amendments, including certain changes in the requirements for all classes of medical devices. The Medical Device Amendments of 1992 were intended to clarify both the Medical Device Amendments of 1976 and the SMDA.

It is interesting to note that within the medical industry, medical devices are now subject to more stringent regulation than is the pharmaceutical industry. This is the case despite the fact that most of the recent congressional investigations and public scandals have been associated with pharmaceuticals.

MedWatch. The act causes the FDA to consolidate several adverse reaction reporting systems under the name MedWatch. The program is designed to provide a single portal for health professionals for the voluntary reporting of problems associated with medical devices. In this program, the FDA partners with a wide variety of organizations, which are encouraged to play an active role in postmarketing surveillance.

Food and Drug Administration Modernization Act (FDAMA) of 1997. The FDAMA included provisions that require the FDA to accelerate review of devices. In response the FDA completed dozens of guidance documents, most of which added requirements for manufacturers. FDAMA included a mandate that the Center for Devices and Radiological Health (CDRH) create a standards program, which has been very successful. FDAMA included provisions for regulation of advertising of unapproved uses of drugs and devices as well as regulation of health claims for foods.

Medical Device User Fee and Modernization Act (MDUFMA) of 2002. The MDUFMA included provisions that permit the FDA to assess fees from sponsors of medical device applications for evaluation. In return the FDA agrees to improve performance to certain goals. MDUFMA included provisions for device establishment inspections by accredited third parties, and new requirements emerged for reprocessed single-use devices. MDUFMA also included provisions that led to the formation of the Office of Combination Products within the

Office of the Commissioner to oversee review of products that fall into multiple jurisdictions within the FDA. An excellent review of the regulatory history of the FDA may be found in Section 2 of the recent Institute of Medicine (IOM) report.[7] In late 2012, the MDUFMA was reauthorized for an additional 5 years. This reauthorization includes numerous incremental improvements to the device approval process.

Organization of the Food and Drug Administration

The FDA is an agency within the DHHS. It consists of the following centers and offices:

- Office of the Commissioner
- National Center for Toxicological Research
- Office of Operations
- Center for Veterinary Medicine
- Office of Medical Products and Tobacco
- Center for Devices and Radiological Health (CDRH)
- Center for Biologics Evaluation and Research (CBER)
- Center for Drug Evaluation and Research (CDER)
- Center for Food Safety and Applied Nutrition
- Center for Tobacco Products
- Office of Regulatory Affairs

The parts of the FDA of most interest to anesthesiologists include the CDRH (devices), CDER (drugs), and CBER (biologics/vaccines, gene therapies). The discussion will focus on the CDRH and its activities.

Center for Devices and Radiological Health. In 1982, the FDA established the CDRH, which was formed from elements of the old Bureau of Medical Devices and the Bureau of Radiological Health. The CDRH has evolved over the past 30 years and now has seven divisions, or offices, that report to the Director's Office: 1) Compliance, 2) Management Operations, 3) in Vitro Diagnostic Device Evaluation and Safety; 4) Surveillance and Biometrics, 5) Communication, Education, and Radiation Programs, 6) Science and Engineering Laboratories, and 7) Device Evaluation.

The Office of Device Evaluation (ODE) is responsible for the program areas through which medical devices are evaluated or cleared for clinical trials and marketing. These programs include PMA, product development protocol, humanitarian device exemption, investigational device exemption, and premarket notification programs. The ODE is presently divided into five scientific divisions:

1. Anesthesiology, General Hospital, Infection Control, and Dental Devices
2. Cardiovascular Devices
3. Reproductive, Gastro-Renal, and Urological Devices
4. Ophthalmic, Neurological, and ENT Devices
5. Surgical, Orthopedic, and Restorative Devices

Each division is further subdivided. The Anesthesiology, General Hospital, Infection Control, and Dental Devices division is divided into four branches, each with a separate branch chief.

Medical Devices Advisory Committee. The 1976 amendments also established the Medical Devices Advisory Committee, which currently consists of 18 medical device advisory panels that range from immunology to radiology for the purpose of advising the FDA on issues related to the safety and effectiveness of medical devices. These advisory panels include the Anesthesiology and Respiratory Therapy Devices Panel. Each panel has nine members in addition to an FDA employee, who serves as the executive secretary. Seven of the panelists are voting members, and the consumer and industry representatives are nonvoting members. A panel can request consultants when necessary.

In 2010, the FDA changed the procedures of the medical device advisory panels. The panels are no longer being asked to vote on whether to recommend a medical device's approval or conditions of approval. Instead, they are being asked to vote on the device's safety and effectiveness and how the device's benefits compare with its risks. Typically, each of these attributes is voted separately with questions phrased along the lines of:

1. Do the data included in the product submission provide substantial evidence of safety for the requested indication?
2. Do the data included in the product submission provide substantial evidence of effectiveness for the requested indication?
3. Do the available data indicate that the benefits outweigh the risks of the device when used for the requested indication?

This change permits the panel members to focus on the scientific issues, which are more likely related to their expertise, instead of the regulatory issues with which they might not be familiar.

Classification of Devices

Different parts of the world use different classification approaches as illustrated in Table 34-2.

Europe

Europe's classification system of medical devices is defined in EU directives on medical devices.[8] These top-down classification rules are based on criteria such as the duration of contact with the patient (less than 60 minutes, not more than 30 days, and more than 30 days), the degree of invasiveness, and the part of the body affected by the use of the device.

United States

In the United States, the FDA was required to classify all medical devices into one of three categories per the 1976 amendments, based on the intended use of the device. *Intended use* refers to objective intent of the persons legally responsible for the labeling of a medical device. The FDA expects the intended use to address:

- The intended medical indication
- The intended patient population
- The intended part of the body or type of tissue applied to or interacted with
- The intended user
- The conditions of use
- The operating principle

TABLE 34-2 **Summary of Classification Systems and Approval and Clearance Processes of Medical Devices in Selected Countries and Regions**

Country	Primary Agency	Classification (Legal Basis/Classes)	Premarket Placing on Market*
Canada	Health Canada (www.hc-sc.gc.ca)	Food and Drugs Act (RSC, 1985, c. F-27) Invasive vs. noninvasive vs. active devices Classes I to IV	Establishment license Device license
China	State Food and Drug Administration (former. sfda.gov.cn). The General Administration of Quality Supervision, Inspection, and Quarantine is responsible for electrical safety	Regulations for the Supervision and Administration of Medical Devices (Decree 276 of State Council, 2000) Class I: routine administration Class II: further control Class III: strict control Includes devices implanted into the human body, those used for life support or sustenance, and those that pose potential risk to the human body	Product registration certificate Licensing of manufacturers and distributors
European Union	European Union (ec. europa.eu/)	Active Implantable Medical Device Directive 90/383/EEC Medical Device Directive 93/42/EEC In Vitro Diagnostic Medical Device Directive 98/79/EC Risk-based classification	Compliance label (CE marking) Responsible person registration
Japan	Ministry of Health Labor and Welfare (MHLW) (www.mhlw.go.jp/english/)	Pharmaceutical Affairs Law Class I: general Class II: certification Class II: approval Class III: approval Class IV: approval	PMDA Notification Third-party certification MHLW approval
United States	Food and Drug Administration (www.fda.gov)	Title 21 United States Code Class I: general controls	Establishment registration
		Class II: performance standards/special controls Class III	Classification and finding of substantial equivalence (510[k]) or PMA

*Premarket (product control/tools for acknowledging product cleared for the market); placing on market (medical device/establishment control).

EC, European Commission; EEC, European Economic Community; PMA, premarket approval; PMDA, premarket drug approval.

The class I to class III designations are used by the FDA to denote increasing scrutiny and controls. The classification of devices was originally determined by panels of experts, who advised the FDA following the adoption of the 1976 amendments. Of the initial 1750 generic types of devices classified, 40% were class I, 50% were class II, and 10% were class III. Device types were grouped into 16 medical specialties referred to as *panels*. The panels assigned each device type to one of the three regulatory classes based on their assessment of the "level of control necessary to assure the safety and effectiveness of the device." The classification is risk based, that is, the risk the device poses to the patient and/or the user is a major factor in the class to which it was assigned. Class I includes devices with the lowest risk, and class III includes those with the greatest risk. The class to which a device is assigned determines, among other things, the type of premarketing submission/application required for FDA clearance to market. If a device is classified as class I or II, and if it is not exempt, a 510(k) notification is required for marketing. All medical devices classified as exempt are not subject to premarket review, but the manufacturer is required to register the device with the FDA. For class III devices, a PMA is required unless the device is a preamendment device (on the market prior to the passage of the Medical Device Amendments in 1976, or substantially equivalent to such a device), in which case a 510(k) is required. The FDA has nearly completed the task of either downgrading all preamendment class III devices into class II or calling for a PMA. Once this task has been completed, there will no longer be any class III preamendment devices on the market via the 510(k) process. In essence, the FDA classification system is bottom-up and based on the state of knowledge and medical devices in the late 1970s with some subsequent modification.

All classes of medical devices are subject to General Controls, which are the baseline requirements of the FD&C Act that apply to all medical devices, class I, II, and III.

Despite the congressional mandate to write performance standards for all class II medical devices, this task overwhelmed the CDRH, which had inadequate resources. In response the FDA gave tacit approval to existing national or international standards for this purpose. In doing so, the FDA was not relieved of the responsibility to formulate mandatory performance standards; however, they had indicated informally that their limited resources would not be used where voluntary standards were in effect. The process by which the FDA was to develop a mandatory performance standard was quite complex and involved an FDA-appointed Standards Advisory Committee. To date, only the apnea monitor standard has been developed by this process.[9] As such, voluntary standards were sought and have become widely used, because they represent an excellent starting point. The use of externally developed voluntary consensus standards was helped by the Pentagon and its allies, who persuaded the Office of Management and Budget to issue Circular A-119 in 1982, urging "federal participation in the development and use of voluntary consensus standards."[10] Circular A-119 was revised and strengthened in 1993.

At present, it is noted that the "CDRH believes that conformance with recognized consensus standards can support a reasonable assurance of safety and/or effectiveness for many applicable aspects of medical devices."[11]

The current list of recognized standards maintained on the FDA's Web site (www.accessdata.fda.gov/scripts/cdrh/cfdocs/cfStandards/search.cfm) and the standards program are managed by the CDRH Standards Management Staff (SMS). The SMS had been part of the Office of Science and Engineering Laboratories (OSEL) but was elevated to the Office of the Center Director in 2011. SMS is responsible for facilitating the recognition of national and international medical device consensus standards within the CDRH and FDA. The CDRH standards program was created to address the Congressional mandate contained in the FDA Modernization Act (FDAMA) of 1997. SMS ensures appropriate medical device standards are published in the *Federal Register* at least twice annually. Manufacturers are permitted to use recognized standards to simplify their premarket applications to the FDA. Although CDRH had been involved in the development of medical device standards for decades, FDAMA formalized the process.

Class I: General Controls. Class I medical devices were subject only to general controls to ensure safety and effectiveness. These controlling regulations 1) required that devices be registered; 2) prohibited adulteration or mislabeling of items; 3) provided for notification of risks, repair, replacement, or refund; 4) restricted the sale and distribution of certain devices; and 5) required GMPs as defined by the FDA.

Class II: Performance Standards and Special Controls. Medical devices in class II had to meet performance standards, because general controls were not considered sufficient to guarantee their safety and effectiveness. These devices had to fulfill all requirements of class I in addition to FDA performance standards.

Class III: Substantial Equivalence. A new class III medical device that was available commercially after the enactment date could attempt to claim substantial equivalence to an existing preamendment class III device and thus "ride on the coattails" of similar, older devices. This was provided for under section 510(k) of the FD&C Act. If a manufacturer chose the 510(k) route, the FDA needed PMN. Should the FDA have decided that substantial equivalence did not apply to the particular device, it had to be classified as a class III device. As such, it required PMA and review by the Anesthesiology and Respiratory Devices Review Panel before it could be marketed. The manufacturer's only other option was to re-petition for reclassification of their device to class I or class II. The FDA generally ruled that a device was not substantially equivalent if 1) its intended use was different, 2) it raised new questions about safety or effectiveness, or 3) it did not perform as well as devices already on the market.

Classifying a Device in the United States

To find the classification of a device, the classification regulation for the device of interest needs to be found either using the FDA's on-line classification database (Web site) or using the device panel. Part 868, entitled *Anesthesiology Devices*, includes subparts for diagnostic, monitoring, therapeutic, and miscellaneous devices. Each classified device within each part has a seven-digit number associated with it, referring to the specific code in Title 21 of the Federal Regulations, where it is defined. An anesthesia machine is listed under 21 CFR §868.5160 as a gas machine for anesthesia or analgesia and is defined as:

> *(a) Gas machine for anesthesia—*
> *(1) Identification. A gas machine for anesthesia is a device used to administer to a patient, continuously or intermittently, a general inhalation anesthetic and to maintain a patient's ventilation. The device may include a gas flowmeter, vaporizer, ventilator, breathing circuit with bag, and emergency air supply.*
> *(2) Classification. Class II (performance standards).*
> *(b) Gas machine for analgesia—*
> *(1) Identification. A gas machine for analgesia is a device used to administer to a patient an analgesic agent, such as a nitrous oxide–oxygen mixture (maximum concentration of 70 percent nitrous oxide).*
> *(2) Classification. Class II (performance standards).*

Premarket and Placing-on-Market Processes

The processes and tools used to evaluate a product before permitting its introduction to market vary considerably among countries (see Table 34-2). In the United States, the approval process (PMA) and marketing clearance (510[k]) of the FDA (see Table 34-1) are most often used to place products on the market in the United States. The EU requires compliance with its directives prior to applying CE-marking and the placement of a product in commerce. For medical devices, a manufacturer must demonstrate that the medical device meets the essential requirements of the Medical Device Directive[8] by creating a technical file with the appropriate evidence and creating a Declaration of Conformity signed by a representative of the company prior to introduction. For manufacturers outside the EU, this material must be accessible to a designated Authorized Representative within the EU. The CE-marking approach is intended to ensure free movement of goods and services within the European common market.

Canada requires obtaining a license with the process similar to that of the 510(k) in the United States, from a paperwork perspective. In Asia a wide variety of listings, registrations, and approvals for medical devices exist that range from a simple addition of the medical device to a list to very involved approval processes that require in-country clinical evaluations.

Pending Regulatory Changes in the United States

What is happening in the United States with respect to changes in to the 510(k) and other processes? Following a 1-year internal assessment in August 2010, CDRH's 510(k) Working Group published a preliminary report[12] consisting of more than 60 recommendations grouped under six findings aimed at improving the Center's effectiveness in implementing its various missions. The preliminary report focused on three major areas: the need for 1) a rational, well-defined, and consistently interpreted review standard; 2) well-informed decision making; and 3) continuous quality assurance. The report found:

1. There is insufficient clarity with respect to the definition of "substantial equivalence."
2. CDRH's current practice allows for the use of some types of predicates that may not be appropriate.
3. The de novo pathway is important and has not been optimally used across the Center.
4. It is challenging for reviewers to obtain the information they need to make well-supported clearance decisions.
5. The CDRH's knowledge management infrastructure is limited.
6. Variations in the expertise, experience, and training of reviewers and managers, including third-party reviewers, may contribute to inconsistency or uncertainty in 510(k) decision making.

The report committed the FDA to create a large number of new or revised guidance documents aimed at improving the 510(k) program.

The FDA also commissioned the IOM to evaluate the current 510(k) process to see whether it protects patients and promotes innovation, and if not, to evaluate what legislative, regulatory, or administrative changes are recommended to best achieve the goals of the 510(k) process. The IOM report includes an excellent summary of the history of the reform of the 510(k) process. It was issued in July of 2011 and found that the current 510(k) process:

- Does not determine safety or efficacy of a medical device
- Lacks the legal basis to screen a medical device for safety and efficacy
- Was never intended to do either of the above

The IOM report indicated that "rather than continuing to modify the 35-year-old 510(k) process, the IOM concludes that the FDA's finite resources would be better invested in developing an integrated premarket and postmarket regulatory framework."[7] The day the IOM report was published, the FDA immediately rejected its conclusion and announced "the 510(k) process should not be eliminated, but the FDA is open to additional proposals and approaches for continued improvement of our device review program."[13]

The FDA has continued to follow through on its commitments from the 510(k) preliminary report with the following objectives:

- Create new or update existing guidances for clarity
- Integrate systems and databases to make information more accessible
- Issue regulations to cover previously neglected items and transfer of ownership of a 510(k).[13]

MEDICAL DEVICE VOLUNTARY STANDARDS

Overview

Work on standardizing medical equipment began because of incompatibilities that became obvious during World War II.[10] Voluntary consensus standards for medical devices have been in use for the past few decades, and commercial standards have existed for well over 100 years. These standards often codify commonly used and long-standing practices. Commercial standards may be developed solely within a company, by a trade group, or by a technical society. Generally, in the United States the writing of standards is essentially a bottom-up process that formalizes existing and accepted commercial or industrial processes and experience.

On the international level, standards are dichotomized much as they are nationally. Older multinational standards organizations, such as the International Organization for Standardization (ISO) and the International Electrotechnical Commission (IEC), work on the basis of voluntary consensus. ISO members are the National Standardization Institutes of 163 countries and its staff at the Central Secretariat in Geneva, Switzerland, coordinating and supporting the creation and marketing of ISO standards. ISO member bodies (www.iso.org/iso/about/iso_members.htm) may directly develop standards (e.g., Germany's DIN and the United Kingdom's BSI) or may delegate another body to do so (e.g., ANSI in the United States; Table 34-3). Other newer, multinational organizations with official regulatory authority are now emerging.

The arena of voluntary consensus standards for medical equipment may not appear as orderly and regimented as that of government regulation. In fact, it can be a source of considerable confusion to the practicing anesthesiologist. This is especially true when an anesthesiologist wants to determine the current voluntary consensus standard for a particular piece of equipment. Several different sets of voluntary standards from a number of different organizations often apply to a single medical device (Table 34-4). Even the "alphabet soup" used to describe the different organizations—AAMI, ANSI, NFPA, IEEE, IEC, ISO, and ASTM—can be confusing.

Development of standards by the voluntary consensus method is faster and more responsive to the marketplace than methods used by either state or federal agencies. Organizations that propose voluntary standards are not subject to the cumbersome bureaucratic and legal intricacies that govern both federal and state governments. This is not to say, however, that voluntary consensus organizations

TABLE 34-3 **Selected Standard Development Organizations of Interest to Anesthesia**

Scope	Organizations	Committee of Interest	Committee Focus/Comment
United States (domestic)	ASTM	F29	Anesthesia
	AAMI	U.S. TAG for IEC/SC 62D	Safety
	ANSI		
	IEEE	EMB/11073	Communications
	NEMA	MITA	
	NCCLS		Radiology, in vitro diagnostics
	CGA		
United States (foreign)	BSI, DIN, JISC, SAC, ABNT	TC 121	Anesthesia
Regional	CEN (EU)	TC 215	ISO TC 121 mirror
	CENELEC (EU)	TC 62	IEC TC 62 mirror
International	ISO	TC 121; TC 210	Anesthesia; quality systems and risk management
	IEC	SC 62A, 62D	Electrical aspects

AAMI, Association for the Advancement of Medical Instrumentation; ABNT, Associação Brasileira de Normas Técnicas (Brazilian Association of Technical Standards); ANSI, American National Standards Institute; ASTM, American Society for Testing and Materials; BSI, British Standards Institute; CEN, Comité Européen de Normalisation (European Committee for Standardization); CENELEC, Comité Européen de Normalisation Électrotechnique (European Committee for Electrotechnical Standardization); CGA, Compressed Gas Association; DIN, Deutsches Institut für Normung (German Standards Institute); IEC, International Electrotechnical Commission; IEEE; Institute of Electrical and Electronic Engineers; ISO, International Organization for Standardization; JISC, Japanese Industrial Standards Committee; MITA, Medical Imaging and Technology Alliance; NCCLS, National Clinical and Laboratory Standards Institute; NEMA, National Electrical Manufacturers Association; SAC, Standardization Administration of China; SC, Scientific Committee; TAG, Technical Advisory Group; TC, Technical Committee.

TABLE 34-4 **Selected Recognized, Harmonized, and Particular Standards in Relation to Technology**

		FDA		MDD	
Equipment	**Latest International Particular Standard (ISO, IEC, ASTM)**	**Product Code(s)***	**"Recognized Consensus" Standard†**	**"Harmonized" Standard‡**	**Related Clinical Guidelines**
Anesthesia workstation	IEC 60601-2-13: 2011	BSZ	IEC 60601-2-13 Ed 3.1: 2009	EN 60601-2-13: 2006	Machine checklist, obsolescence, gas disposal (ASA, FDA, institutional, government)
Anesthetic agents monitor	IEC 80601-2-55: 2011	CBQ, CBS, CBR	ISO 21647: 2004	EN ISO 21647: 2009	Regulatory bodies with respect to gases
Carbon dioxide monitor	IEC 80601-2-55: 2011	CCK	ISO 21647: 2004	EN ISO 21647: 2009	AARC (CPG, 2011) Numerous anesthesia guidelines for different settings (e.g., ASA)
Pulse oximetry	IEC 80601-2-61: 2011	DQA	ISO 9919: 2005 IEC 80601-2-61 Ed 1.0: 2011	EN ISO 9919: 2009	CLSI (POCT11-A2) AARC (CPG-1992) ASA
Oxygen monitor	IEC 80601-2-55: 2011	CCL	ISO 21647: 2004	EN ISO 21647: 2009	AARC (various CPGs)

*Per http://www.accessdata.fda.gov/scripts/cdrh/cfdocs/cfpcd/classification.cfm.
†As of March 1, 2012, per http://www.accessdata.fda.gov/scripts/cdrh/cfdocs/cfStandards/search.cfm.
‡As of March 1, 2012, per http://ec.europa.eu/enterprise/policies/european-standards/harmonised-standards/medical-devices.
AARC, American Association for Respiratory Care; ASA, American Society of Anesthesiologists; CLSI, Clinical Laboratory and Standards Institute; CPG, clinical practice guideline; EN, European Committee standard designator; FDA, Food and Drug Administration; IEC, International Electrotechnical Commission; ISO, International Organization for Standardization; MDD, Medical Device Directive; POCT, point-of-care testing.

can be cavalier or ignorant with regard to legal requirements. In the interest of fairness and to prevent legal ramifications, all interested parties are allowed to participate in the process of creating standards in accordance with the individual organization's bylaws.

Compliance with voluntary standards is not mandatory, because the parent organization has no legal jurisdiction. Voluntary consensus standards, however, often have an influence even before they are finalized. Responsible manufacturers find both legal protection and sales advantages in claiming that their equipment meets various voluntary standards, such as those of AAMI, ANSI, IEC, ISO or ASTM. New voluntary standards cannot require that a manufacturer remove from the marketplace earlier equipment that does not conform to the new standard. Only a municipal, state, or federal authority having jurisdiction can demand compliance or remove an item from the market. Often, voluntary consensus standards, such as those of the National Fire Protection Association (NFPA), are adopted by local agencies that have the authority to turn the standards into law. Voluntary equipment standards can also be adopted by a government agency as part of their procurement or purchasing policies. On occasion, however, a governmental regulation may be adopted before the voluntary standard has been finalized.

Stages in the Development of International Standards

An international standard is the result of an agreement among the member bodies of an organization. It may be used as such, or it may be implemented through incorporation in national standards of different countries. International standards are developed by technical committees and subcommittees. Many such committees follow a six-step process. The six-step process followed by ISO affiliated committees is shown in Figure 34-2 with the activity, documents, and elapsed time for each stage noted.[14] ISO standards are reviewed at the least 3 years after publication and every 5 years thereafter by all the ISO member bodies. A majority of the participating members of the technical committee (TC) or scientific committee (SC) decides whether an international standard should be confirmed, revised, or withdrawn.

Within organizations such as ISO, standardization is an open, voluntary process built around consensus, and it is stakeholder driven. Within the ISO, the committee of relevance to anesthesia is TC 121, Anaesthetic and Respiratory Equipment. The stakeholders in TC 121 include equipment manufacturers, clinicians, regulatory agencies, test houses, and others. Created in 1966, TC 121 has a scope defined as "standardization of anaesthetic and respiratory equipment and supplies, related devices, and supply systems." It is responsible for 85 standards among its subcommittees (see Table 34-3) and includes 25 participating and 24 observing countries. Also of importance is the IEC, which has a committee responsible for developing international standards for electrical equipment used in medical practice (IEC TC 62), whose subcommittee D is responsible for electromedical equipment (e.g., the nonradiology particular medical electrical device standards of the 60601-2 series).

Given the wide variety of equipment on the market, it is often not clear which organization should be responsible. So that the expertise of both organizations may be made available in the development of standards, joint working groups (JWGs) between ISO and IEC are often formed. In these cases, either ISO or IEC may take the lead. For each JWG, one of national standards bodies, which for ISO is a member body and for IEC is a national committee, accepts responsibility for administering the JWG, and that organization holds the secretariat and appoints one or two individuals to handle the technical and administrative work. A convenor (chairman) runs the meetings and works to reach consensus. Frequently a JWG has a secretary who manages the documents and works closely with the convenor.

Within each committee, and as part of the standards development processes, are important roles to play, both nationally and internationally. Clinician involvement is crucial to the development and revision of medical device standards. Participation can be as an expert in a working group, a member of a national delegation, and even as a head of a national delegation. Experts attend meetings in their own capacity as experts, but they must be aware of the position of the national body of the country they represent. Influence may be wielded

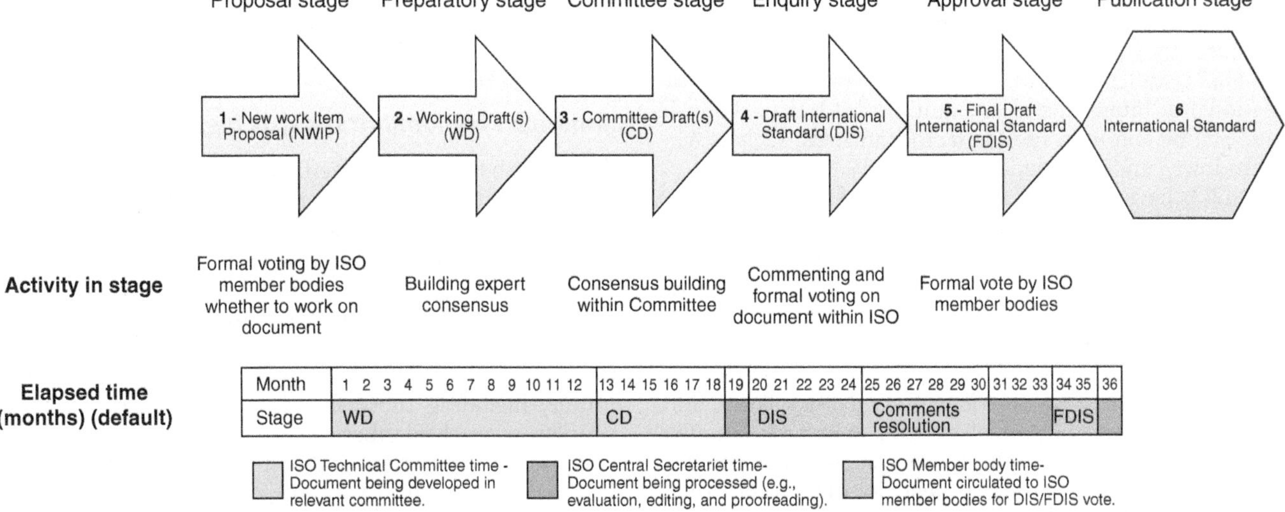

FIGURE 34-2 ■ The consensus-building stages of standards. Note: Committee draft, draft International Standard, and final draft International Standard documents are approved only if a two-thirds majority of the participating member bodies of the technical and scientific committees are in favor, and not more than one quarter of the total number of votes cast are negative.

through formal approaches—written comments, discussions, drafting of resolutions, and voting—and by informal means, such as lobbying members of other delegations and through personal relationships.

Organization of Standards Development Organizations

The scope of standards that the standards development organization (SDO) develops varies considerably. It may represent a technical area (e.g., electrical, pneumatic), or it may be application oriented (e.g., clinical). Sometimes the scope may not be clear. In the case of ISO and IEC, the technical divisions are often not clear, and JWGs exist to allow members of both bodies to participate. Agreements have been signed between different regional and international SDOs to help clarify the roles and responsibilities to reduce duplicative activities and promote cooperation. The Committee for European Standardization (CEN) and Committee for European Electrotechnical Standardization (CENELEC) have agreements with their international counterparts, ISO and IEC, defining the rules governing cooperation. The Vienna (1991) and Dresden (1996) Agreements signed between CEN and ISO and CENELEC and IEC, respectively, helped to create the framework for cooperation between European and international standards activity with the explicit recognition of the "primacy of international standards" and goal of simultaneous recognition at the international and European level.

For in vitro diagnostics, the Clinical and Laboratory Standards Institute (CLSI), formerly the National Committee for Clinical Laboratory Standards (NCCLS), develops the preponderance of relevant standards. The CLSI also is the international secretariat of ISO TC 212, Clinical Laboratory Testing and In Vitro Diagnostic Test Systems, which gives CLSI a pathway to have its standards become European standards via the Vienna Agreement with CEN.

Other standards or guidelines may be developed primarily by medical societies, which include societies such as the American Thoracic Society, American Society of Anesthesiologists (ASA), and American Association for Respiratory Care.

Standards come into existence in three ways: 1) by national or international recognition (ISO, IEC, ASTM, etc.); 2) by common use (de facto standards, such as MS Windows), and 3) by industry consortia.

SDOs have certain defining characteristics. First, they follow a very formal standards development process. Second, they have broadly inclusive participation structures composed of representatives from all members of a given class, because an international SDO must include a representative from each nation. Third, open discussion and debate occurs on all issues, and due process gives members the opportunity to lodge formal complaints and appeals to the establishment of given standards. Finally, democratic voting procedures are available that emphasize consensus as opposed to majority or plurality rule. Because of these characteristics, standards issued by SDOs have a high degree of legitimacy, derived from the process that created them.

SDO standards do offer stability and support. On the other hand, these same characteristics generate criticism of SDOs, which are often too slow with respect to market time frames. Redundant and parallel structures exist, especially within the country representatives to international SDOs. Therefore SDOs are inefficient; they are too focused on consensus and hence are often reduced to choosing the least common denominator, which often is not an ideal solution to many users. Voting structures are out of sync with the economic investment of participating members, and participation of nonstakeholder members drags out the process. SDOs cost too much (e.g., AAMI), and their processes are out of date. While technically apt, committee members lack experience and writing skills to produce draft standards quickly, and SDOs do not effectively prioritize drafts that need to be considered first. Unlike European and Pacific Rim countries, the United States is not represented at international standards organizations by any official governmental representative, and the United States does not have a single body that speaks for all standards activities within the country.

At present ANSI serves as the coordinator and formal representative for the United States before the ISO and the IEC. However, ANSI delegates the responsibility for actually doing the work to other SDOs within the United States (e.g., AAMI, ASTM, CLSI). The General Agreement on Tariffs and Trade (GATT), to which the United States has been a signatory since the late 1940s, was replaced by the World Trade Organization (WTO) in 1994. Under these international trade agreements, there exists a Standards Code that provides ground rules for preparing, ratifying, and implementing international technical standards to be used to prevent technical barriers to trade. ANSI has assumed the role of representative for the United States, but in contrast to many of its counterparts in Europe, it has no official governmental sanction.

Several non-U.S. SDOs of interest include both regional (e.g., CEN and CENELEC) and national SDOs (e.g., DIN, BSI), which also may serve as the ISO or IEC member body.

U.S. Standards Development Organizations of Interest

American National Standards Institute (ANSI)

The anesthesia community has a long history of involvement with ANSI, a private, nonprofit organization founded more than 70 years ago to coordinate and facilitate the development of standards. In 1956 the ASA assumed the secretariat of ANSI Committee Z-79 for Anesthesia and Respiratory Therapy Equipment, and they maintained this position until 1983. During this time, many standards were produced by the Z-79 Committee, including those for humidifiers, reservoir bags, ventilators, tracheal tubes, and anesthesia machines. Probably the most important and best-known standard created by the Z-79 Committee was the Z-79.9 1979 standard for anesthesia machines.[15] This was the first attempt by the manufacturers and users of anesthesia equipment to ensure compatibility and performance among the various types of anesthesia machines. Although this standard contained flaws, it was the best standard that could be developed at the time through voluntary consensus efforts. However, the standard was deficient in some major areas. For example, it permitted the use of in-circuit vaporizers and required neither oxygen analyzers nor a method to prevent the administration of a hypoxic mixture. It did, however, serve the anesthesia community well, both manufacturer and user, during the 10 years it functioned as the ruling anesthesia machine standard. National standards activity in this area was transferred by committee vote in 1983 from ANSI to ASTM.

ASTM International

Formerly the American Society for Testing and Materials, ASTM International currently handles most of the activities concerning voluntary standards that affect anesthesia durable equipment. Committee F-29 on Anesthetic and Respiratory Therapy Equipment has 10 subcommittees that focus on safety and performance standards rather than on design or specific engineering standards. Design and engineering decisions are best left to the individual manufacturer. ASTM views standards-writing activities as a method to achieve an orderly approach to a specific activity or problem. All committee members are volunteers; the formal ASTM staff provides only administrative support. ASTM does not fund any participants, nor does it have its own laboratory facilities; individual members must have their own funding. At present, the ASA funds the travel of its liaison to Committee F-29.

Under ASTM bylaws, the members of any committee should reflect a balance of users, producers, ultimate consumers, technical representatives, insurers, educators, and those with an interest in the area. The last category can include members of the FDA or of nonprofit health care organizations that deal with medical devices directly or indirectly.

Almost anyone can initiate the creation of a standard within ASTM. The proponent must first submit a written request detailing the various companies, individuals, and organizations participating. The executive staff of ASTM then decides whether the proposal has merit. If accepted, the proposal is then referred to a particular committee.

Association for the Advancement of Medical Instrumentation (AAMI)

AAMI is a nonprofit organization founded in 1967. It is a unique alliance of more than 6000 members from around the world united by one mission: to provide global multidisciplinary leadership and programs that enhance the goals and capabilities of the professions, health care institutions, government, industry, and other organizations that relate to the delivery, development, management, use, and other aspects of safe and effective medical instrumentation and related technologies. The AAMI standards program consists of over 100 technical committees and working groups that produce Standards, Recommended Practices, and Technical Information Reports for medical devices. Standards and Recommended Practices represent a national consensus, and many have been approved by ANSI as American national standards. AAMI also administers a number of international health care technical committees of ISO and IEC in addition to U.S. Technical Advisory Groups (TAGs).

National Fire Protection Association (NFPA)

The anesthesia community has been involved with voluntary standards for almost 40 years. Initially, the ASA participated in the development of standards by the NFPA, which writes standards for many aspects of fire prevention, detection, and suppression. The NFPA also addresses standards for different types of facilities, such as multiple dwellings, factories, and hospitals. Initially, when cyclopropane and ether were used in operating rooms (ORs), the input of anesthesiologists was important in developing standards for anesthetizing locations. Their input was again needed with the advent of centralized medical-gas distribution systems, such as for oxygen and nitrous oxide. What initially developed as fire safety regulations for all occupants of a facility eventually evolved into patient safety standards. An example of this is the present NFPA standard for nonflammable medical-gas piping systems.

Anesthesiology input has remained vital to the NFPA throughout the years, both to provide user input and to ensure that proposals by fire professionals for changes or modifications do not adversely affect the hospital's clinical practice. For instance, a firefighter cannot elect to turn off the hospital's entire oxygen supply because of a fire in one wing of the facility. Obviously, the drafting of such a standard requires compromise on the part of both clinicians and fire professionals.

All standards published by the NFPA that affect hospitals are now published in one document: the NFPA 99 Health Care Facilities Code.[16] This document is generally updated every 3 years and was most recently updated in 2012. It contains standards governing anesthetizing locations, emergency power supplies, high-frequency electricity, medical-gas pipeline systems, and hyperbaric oxygen facilities.

In the newest edition, NFPA-99 has changed from a standard to a code. It has been rewritten to be a risk-based, rather than an occupancy-based, document. That means the requirements are based on whether a system failure would cause a high, moderate, or low risk to a patient. Therefore wherever general anesthesia is being administered to patients, appropriate back-up systems must be in place for things such as oxygen and electrical power: it no longer matters if the facility is a 50 OR medical center or a two-room freestanding outpatient facility.

Other changes to NFPA-99 include a provision that all new or remodeled ORs will default to being a wet location. That means that special electrical protection in the form of isolated power or ground fault circuit interrupters (GFCIs) will have to be installed, unless the facility does a risk assessment to prove that certain ORs are not wet locations. Other relevant changes include a requirement for all electrical/gas booms to be inspected on a regular basis and for a minimum of 18 electrical outlets to be installed in a critical care area and 36 in an OR.

Although ether and cyclopropane are no longer used in modern ORs, the threat of fire has in no way been eliminated. Each year the amount of electrical equipment in the OR increases. Many of these devices, such as electrosurgical units (ESUs) and lasers, can ignite drapes, sponges, and other disposable items in an OR. In the presence of oxygen or nitrous oxide, a spark can become a conflagration (see also Chapter 31). A number of organizations have become interested in the prevention of OR fires. In 2008 the ASA issued a Practice Advisory on OR fire prevention.[17] Also, in 2010 the Anesthesia Patient Safety Foundation (APSF; www.apsf.org) produced a video with new recommendations on the prevention of OR fires, *Prevention and Management of Operating Room Fires*. Other organizations that have made efforts to prevent OR fires include the ECRI Institute[18] and the Association of Operating Room Nurses (AORN).

Institute of Electrical and Electronics Engineers (IEEE)

The IEEE has traditionally written standards that directly concern only engineers. One project within IEEE of particular interest to the anesthesia community concerns the work of IEEE Committee P-1073, which has been developing medical communications standards since 1987; the idea originated during the early 1980s, after the AAMI sponsored a roundtable discussion in 1982 on developing standards for data management in monitoring. Many of those attending the session thought that a standardized method for data communication among monitoring equipment was needed in the OR. A proposal was subsequently made by the AAMI Standards Board that a technical committee be formed to develop standards for monitoring system data management. However, no further action was taken by AAMI.

In 1987, this subject was taken up by Committee P-1073 of the IEEE Engineering in Medicine and Biology Society (EMBS), which consisted of device manufacturers, computer experts, clinicians, and biomedical engineers. The Committee undertook to produce standards for local area networks (LANs) to enable communication among freestanding monitors, infusion and life-support devices, and a host computer system. This was not to serve laboratory or pharmacy functions but rather was intended solely to support the clinician in an acute patient-care setting, such as the intensive care unit (ICU) or OR.

These standards specifically make provisions for anesthesia machines and ventilators with the purpose of developing an automated anesthesia record using "local intelligence," which can be uploaded to a large host computer system. The goal is to eliminate the need for individual institutions to write software or design connectors for devices. The standards therefore are vendor independent.

It has taken more than two decades, but Committee P-1073 has written a series of standards for point-of-care medical device communication, the IEEE 11073 series, many of which have also been adopted by ISO TC 215, Health Informatics.

Medical Device Standards

ISO and IEC standards follow the same basic structure:

- *Scope* defines without ambiguity the subject of the standard and the aspects covered, thereby indicating the limits of applicability of the standard.
- *Normative references* give a list of the referenced documents cited in the standard in such a way as to make them indispensable for the application of the standard.
- *Terms and definitions* give the definitions necessary for the understanding of certain terms used in the standard.
- *Requirements* contain clauses that have all of the dictates, statements, and recommendations or references to them necessary to claim compliance to the standard.
- *Annexes*, both normative and informative, give provisions additional to those in the body of the document. Annex AA, which is found in many ISO and IEC health care standards, contains particular guidance and rationale that includes useful explanations to the reader and user of the standard. This allows an interpretation more aligned to what was intended by the developer of the standard. Another annex commonly found is an Annex reference to the essential principles (of ISO 16142).

The General Standard (60601-1)

The IEC 60601-1, developed by IEC TC 62, is a family of technical standards for the basic safety and essential performance of medical electrical equipment, comprising the general standard, a series of 11 collateral standards, and over 70 particular standards. At present, three editions have been published: the first in 1977, the second in 1988, and the third in 2005. The general standard is formally known as IEC 60601-1, Medical Electrical Equipment, Part 1: General requirements for basic safety and essential performance.[19] IEC 60601-1 contains the general requirements for medical electrical equipment. Compliance with IEC 60601-1 has become a de facto requirement for the commercialization of electrical medical equipment in many countries. It is harmonized with the MDD, needed for CE-marking, and is recognized by the FDA.

Although this is an international standard, each country does have the right to recognize the standard in whole or with deviations, changes to specific clauses, for country-specific requirements. The deviations may be minor or significant. The U.S. deviations are published as a "cover" to the international standard and are known as AAMI ES 60601-1.

The latest edition of this standard, the third edition, was published in 2005. It resulted from an understanding of the recognized deficiencies of the second edition and in particular the need to address the safety performance of medical electrical equipment. It is the work of 11 working groups involving over 200 people over a period of 10 years.

Key changes in the third edition include the overall structure and the numbering scheme of the clauses. The application and visibility of risk management was increased by adding requirements for the establishment of a risk management process per ISO 14971, the establishment of acceptable levels of risk, and demonstration that the residual risks are acceptable (according to the manufacturer's policy for determining acceptable risk).[20] The concept of essential performance (EP) or safety-related performance was introduced and defined as the "performance of a clinical function, other than that related to basic safety, where loss or degradation beyond the limits specified by the manufacturer results in an unacceptable risk."[19] EP is most easily understood by considering whether its absence or degradation would result in an unacceptable risk. The process of creating third edition–compliant versions of all of the related published standards is ongoing, and manufacturers and users of the standards will have to deal with both the second and third edition versions of the particular standards until the transition periods in all countries are completed.

For many specific product types, a standard has been developed using the general standard as a template with additions, deletions, and changes made to specific clauses, thereby creating what is known as a *particular standard*, numbered as IEC 60601-2-xx, where *xx* references the particular device. Where the particular standard is the product of an ISO/IEC joint working group, the standard can be numbered 80601-2-xx, with either an ISO or IEC prefix, determined by which organization had the lead for the work. This is shown graphically for a couple of devices in Figure 34-3.

Collateral standards (Table 34-5) have been created over the years to add requirements for a subgroup of equipment, such as for certain safety and performance aspects specific to environments of use (e.g., home care), or related to a specific characteristic of all equipment not fully addressed in IEC 60601-1 (e.g., alarm systems or electromagnetic capability [EMC]). For an FDA perspective on the role of standards in medical devices EMC, see Silberberg.[21]

Standards of Particular Interest

Particular standards take precedence over the general standard and collateral standards. Standards of particular relevance to anesthesia are numerous. A number of these standards that are the domain of TC 121 (Table 34-6) are shown in Table 34-7. In addition, the breadth of coverage of these standards is shown graphically in Figure 34-4. This section highlights the key aspects and history of three standards of particular interest to anesthesiologists: 1) anesthetic workstations, 2) respiratory gas monitors, and 3) pulse oximeters. These medical device standards and other standards can be given much of the credit for the reduction in mortality and morbidity from anesthesia over the past 30 years. These standards have included important safety innovations, such as the introduction of the *diameter index safety system* for connections for medical-gas hoses; the *pin index safety system* for medical-gas cylinders with post-type valves and cylinder mounting yokes; color coding of gas cylinders and equipment; and the incorporation of various fail-safes and protective features, such as the keyed filling system for vaporizers, vaporizer interlocks (which permit the use of only one vaporizer at a time), and hypoxia prevention systems. Additionally, many aspects of the anesthesia machine that have been made standard often directly relate to solving known problems or helping to reduce "use errors." Over time

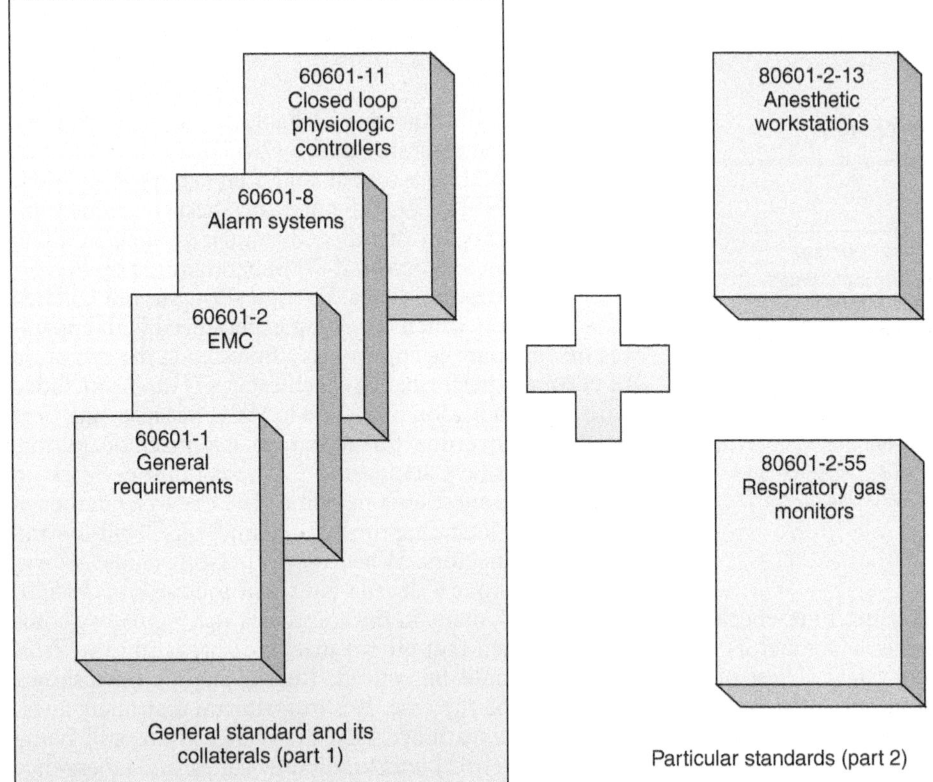

FIGURE 34-3 ■ Organization of International Electrotechnical Commission 60601, its collaterals, and particular standards. Note that the particular standard is dominant and amends the general standard and its collaterals.

TABLE 34-5 **Collateral Standards**

Collateral Standard: Year of Latest Edition	Title	Comments*
60601-1-1	Medical Electrical Systems	Discontinued as a stand-alone document; incorporated into the third edition.
60601-1-2: 2007	Electromagnetic Compatibility (EMC)	Compliance means that the equipment will neither generate excessive unwanted electromagnetic radiation nor be unduly affected by it.
60601-1-3: 2008	Radiation Protection for Diagnostic X-ray Systems	Ensures that radiation is kept as low as reasonably achievable for the safety of patient and operator.
60601-1-4	Programmable Electrical Medical Systems (PEMS)	This is a collateral standard for software. It has been discontinued as a stand-alone document and is now incorporated into the third edition.
60601-1-6: 2007	Usability	Increases emphasis on ergonomics; manufacturers must take the requirements into account during the design phase. Many adverse incidents in the past have been traced to "use error"; intended to control risks caused by usability problems.
60601-1-8:2007+A1: 2012	Medical Alarm Systems	Gives guidance and requirements in the prioritizing and management of alarm functions in medical equipment. Alarm systems can be chaotic if the user does not know what is going off and whether the alarm condition is trivial or serious.
60601-1-9: 2008	Environmentally Conscious Design	Design process requiring the manufacturer to consider contamination of the air, water, and biosphere; the use of raw materials; and transport and packaging in the design of new products.
60601-1-10: 2008	Physiologic Closed Loop Controllers	Design process to be considered when designing medical devices used to control the parameters they are measuring. Such systems have to be stable, reliable, and fault tolerant. Software must be designed methodically and validated comprehensively.
60601-1-11: 2010	Home Health Care Equipment	Puts considerable emphasis on the use of home health care equipment by non-specialist users. Electrical safety is also a factor here and the equipment must be tolerant of poor wiring in the building and wide environmental limits.
60601-1-12 Ed 1 (under development)	Equipment for Use in Emergency Medical Services Environment	Puts considerable emphasis on the use of emergency medical equipment by users in crisis situations. Electrical safety is also a factor, and the equipment must be tolerant of the extremely wide environmental limits that can be found at the scene of an emergency.

*Modified from http://www.mddionline.com/article/collateral-standards-iec-60601-1.

TABLE 34-6 **Subcommittees of TC 121**

Subcommittee/ Working Group	Title
CAG	Chairman Advisory Group
SC 1	Breathing Attachments and Anaesthetic Machines
SC 2	Airways and Related Equipment
SC 3	Lung Ventilators and Related Equipment
SC 4	Terminology and Semantics
SC 6	Medical Gas Systems
SC 8	Suction Devices for Hospital and Emergency Care Use

the addition of monitors, anesthesia machine checkout procedures, and the use of anesthesia simulators for teaching have helped increase patient safety. These monitors include airway pressure monitors, tidal volume monitors, oxygen analyzers positioned to sample inspiratory gases, carbon dioxide analyzers placed to monitor exhaled gases from the patient, and pulse oximeters.

Anesthetic Workstations. Table 34-8 highlights the changes in anesthesia machine/workstation standards, both U.S. and international, and their sequence since the advent of ANSI Z-79.8, the first anesthesia machine standard.[15] Activity on the Z-79.8 standard began in about 1970, as members on the Z-79 Subcommittee on Performance of Anesthesia Gas Machines sought and collated "the problems which are being experienced with apparatus throughout the country, as a first step in the evolution of pertinent performance specifications"[22] and concluded with the publication of Z-79.8 in 1979, because "the time (was) long overdue for action on gas machine performance and safety standards."[23] The committee work on Z-79 for the anesthesia machine gave rise to a number of standards,[24] including those for humidifiers[25] and 15- and 22-mm connectors. When the F1161-88 standard[26] was published about a decade later and followed by F1850-00[27] in 2000, many in the anesthesia and regulatory community hoped that all gas machines predating the Z-79 standard would be retired. Recent studies have shown this not to be the case. It is unfortunate that many anesthesia machines more than 30 years old are still being used in obstetrical units, radiology suites, and emergency rooms, even though they do not reflect the current state

TABLE 34-7 **Selected Published Standards under the Responsibility of ISO TC 121 SC/1 and SC/6**

Title	Standard
Anaesthetic and respiratory equipment, Conical connectors. Part 1: Cones and sockets	ISO 5356-1:2004
Anaesthetic and respiratory equipment, Conical connectors. Part 2: Screw-threaded weight-bearing connectors	ISO 5356-2:2006
Anaesthetic machines for use with humans	ISO 5358:1992
Low-pressure hose assemblies for use with medical gases	ISO 5359:2008, Amd 1:2011
Anaesthetic vaporizers: Agent-specific filling systems	ISO 5360:2012
Inhalational anaesthesia systems. Part 7: Anaesthetic systems for use in areas with limited logistical supplies of electricity and anaesthetic gases	ISO 8835-7:2011
Gas mixers for medical use: Stand-alone gas mixers	ISO 11195:1995
Inhalational anaesthesia systems: Draw-over vaporizers and associated equipment	ISO/TS 18835:2004
Medical electrical equipment. Part 2-13: Particular requirements for basic safety and essential performance of an anaesthetic workstation	ISO 80601-2-13:2011*
Medical electrical equipment. Part 2-55: Particular requirements for the basic safety and essential performance of respiratory gas monitors	ISO 80601-2-55:2011†
Medical supply units	ISO 11197:2004
Medical gas pipeline systems	
Part 1: Pipeline systems for compressed medical gases and vacuum	ISO 7396-1:2007
Part 2: Anaesthetic gas scavenging disposal systems	ISO 7396-2:2007
Terminal units for medical gas pipeline systems	
Part 1: Terminal units for use with compressed medical gases and vacuum	ISO 9170-1:2008
Part 2: Terminal units for anaesthetic gas scavenging systems	ISO 9170-2:2008
Pressure regulators for use with medical gases	
Part 1: Pressure regulators and pressure regulators with flow-metering devices	ISO 10524-1:2006
Part 2: Manifold and line pressure regulators	ISO 10524-2:2005
Part 3: Pressure regulators integrated with cylinder valves	ISO 10524-3:2005
Part 4: Low-pressure regulators	ISO 10524-4:2008
Anaesthetic and respiratory equipment: Compatibility with oxygen	ISO 15001:2010
Flow-metering devices for connection to terminal units of medical gas pipeline systems	ISO 15002:2008
Oxygen concentrator supply systems for use with medical gas pipeline systems	ISO 10083:2006
High-pressure flexible connections for use with medical gas systems	ISO 21969:2009
Rail systems for supporting medical equipment	ISO 19054:2005
Medical gas systems: Systems for evacuation of plume generated by medical devices	ISO/WD 16571

From http://www.iso.org/iso/iso_catalogue/catalogue_tc/catalogue_tc_browse.htm?commid=51986&published=on
Replaces IEC 60601-2-13:2003+A1:2006.
†Replaces ISO 21647.
Amd, amendment; TS, technical specification.

of technology. Although obsolescence is difficult to define, a gas machine that has been in operation for more than two decades should be retired, because it will be missing many important safeguards. Failure to retire an outdated machine can significantly jeopardize the safety of the patient, and it can create liability issues for the anesthesia provider and the institution. Unfortunately, no legal mechanism exists to ensure that such equipment is not used.

In 1990 CEN began working on a standards project entitled "Anesthetic Workstations and Their Modules: Essential Requirements." The Anesthetic and Respiratory Devices Committee of ISO was actively involved in the development of this European standard, which established the important safety and performance requirements for anesthetic workstations, or *anesthetizing locations*, as they are known in the United States. The standard, EN 740:1999, outlined the complete requirements for individual modules that together constitute a complete anesthetic workstation (i.e., anesthesia ventilator, breathing system, scavenging system, vaporizers, monitors, and alarm systems). Here, the goal was not to specify a universal world anesthesia machine but rather to ensure that each component used clinically meets minimum, specific, identifiable requirements. Subsequently, a version of this standard became ISO 60601-2-13:2003, which became ISO/IEC 80601-2-13:2011, rewritten under the third edition of the general standard.[28]

Each of these standards applies the same requirements to both the workstation as a whole and the individual modules. These standards cover environmental conditions, electrical shock hazards, mechanical hazards, excessive or unwanted radiation, and excessive temperature; they also set requirements for construction as well as for minimum accuracy. Although these standards recognize the practice standards both in the United States and in other countries, they do expect minimum monitoring configurations. Additionally, they require that certain performance standards be met for those elements that are present.

Hazards inherent in the intended physiologic function of an anesthetic workstation and its individual components

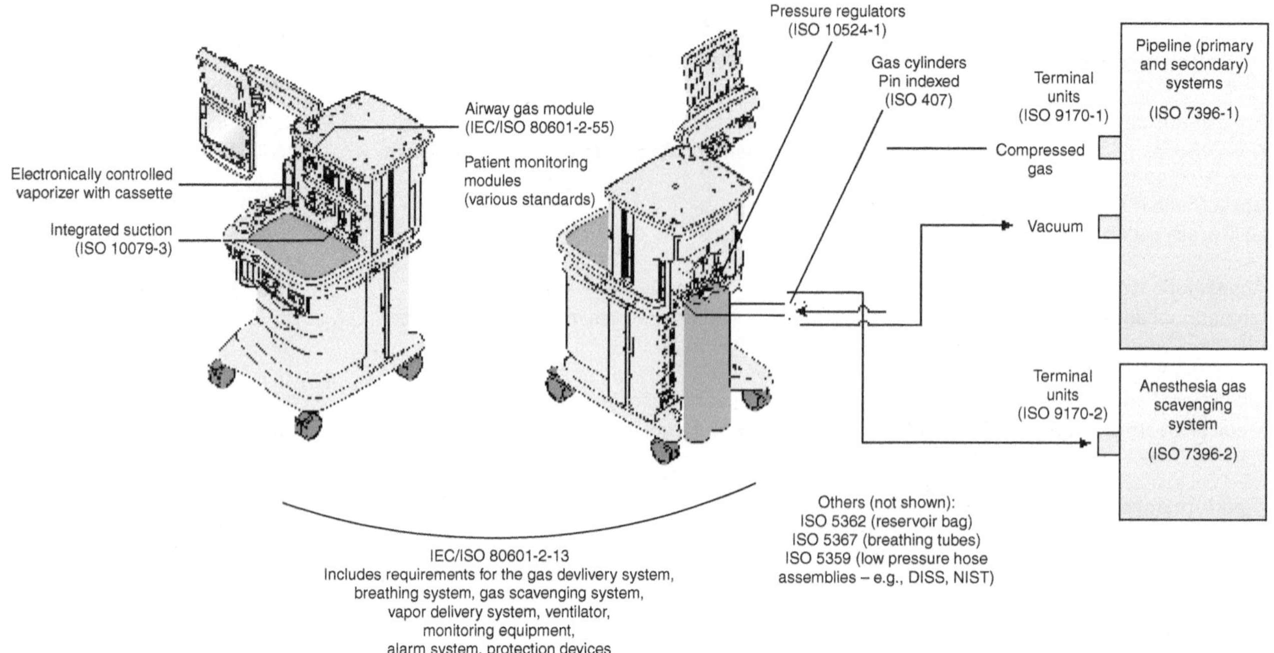

FIGURE 34-4 Selected "standardized portions" of the anesthesia workstation and its connections. DISS, diameter index safety system; IEC, International Electrotechnical Commission; ISO, International Organization for Standardization; NIST, National Organization for Standards and Technology. (Courtesy GE Healthcare, Waukesha, WI.)

within the scope of ISO/IEC 80601-2-13:2011 are not covered by specific requirements therein, and it is not applicable to any anesthetic workstation intended for use with flammable anesthetic agents.

Respiratory Gas Monitors. The latest international standard for respiratory gas monitors is ISO 80601-2-55:2011, prepared by ISO/IEC Joint Working Group 6 of TC 121 SC/1, and it specifies the "particular requirements for the basic safety and essential performance of a respiratory gas monitor (RGM) intended for continuous operation for use with a patient."[29] It is not applicable to an RGM intended for use with flammable anesthetic agents. It cancels and replaces previous international standard ISO 21647, which had combined the previous standards for anesthetic gas monitors (ISO 11196:1995), carbon dioxide monitors (ISO 7767:1997), and oxygen monitors (ISO 9918:1993) into a single standard. ISO 80601-2-55:2011 was the first RGM standard to be harmonized with the third edition of the general standard. Additional reporting requirements have been added to the standard that impact test requirements. Separate requirements as applicable are specified for diverting and nondiverting respiratory gas monitors. These include disclosure of the minimum sampling flow rate for a diverting gas monitor. Minimum accuracy using the test procedure described in the standard is specified in the standard and is shown in Table 34-9.

Note that previous standards may have used different units of measure (e.g., partial pressure for carbon dioxide) to express accuracy, and it was the intent of the RGM standard to use consistent units for all of the gases. The accuracy of each gas is expressed as an offset error at zero with a slope error specified in the table. For example, at 5% carbon dioxide (38 mm Hg at sea level pressure of 760 mm Hg), the measurement accuracy requirement in the form of a line described by "mx + b" (where m is the slope and b is the intercept) would be calculated as ([0.43 ÷ 100] + [8 ÷ 100] × [0.05]), or ±0.0083 vol% or ±6.3 mm Hg (0.0083 × 760).

Additionally, there are test requirements for drift, total system response and rise time, and gas interferences with the appropriate gas mixtures listed for each type of gas monitor. The standard attempts not to be design restrictive. However, for the sake of safety, connector requirements exist for the exhaust and input and restrictions on flow direction as well as for alarm condition priority requirements.

In addition to this international standard, the requirements and guidelines from numerous clinical American and other societies—Association of Anaesthetists of Great Britain and Ireland (AAGBI), ASA, American College of Emergency Physicians (ACEP), American Association for Respiratory Care (AARC), American Heart Association (AHA), American Society for Gatrointestinal Endoscopy (ASGE), European Resuscitation Council (ERC), and Society of Critical Care Medicine (SCCM)—and government bodies (e.g., New York, New Jersey, North Carolina, and Ohio) with respect to the use of carbon dioxide monitors grows every year. This often includes specific requirements for continuous carbon dioxide monitoring.

Pulse Oximeters. The latest international standard for pulse oximeters is ISO 80601-2-61:2011, prepared by a joint working group of TC 121 SC 3, and it cancels and replaces ISO 9919:2005 and has been harmonized with the third edition of the general standard.[30] It specifies the basic safety and essential performance of pulse oximeter equipment intended for use on humans, including the pulse oximeter monitor, pulse oximeter probe, and any

TABLE 34-8 **Key Differences Between Selected U.S. Anesthesia Machine/Workstations: Standards from 1979 to the Present**

	ANSI Z-79.8* (1979)[15]	ASTM F1850-00† (2005)[27]
Key changes	First standard for anesthesia machines, structured as a requirements list for machine components (59 pages)	F1850 (anesthesia workstation; 32 pages) structured as a particular standard of IEC 60601-1 second edition; includes data interface requirements for workstation, interfaced infusion pump, and automated anesthesia record keeper (AARK)
Cancels or replaces	NA	F1850 replaced F1161 (1988, reapproved 1994),[26] which replaced ANSI Z-79.8
Selected requirements		**Selected additions or changes from Z-79.8**
Anesthetic gas delivery system, breathing system, and ventilator	5.1.3 Pin-indexing system on gas cylinder yokes 5.1.5 Elimination of cross filling between cylinders 6.1.1 Pipeline pressure and cylinder pressure gauges 7.1.2 Pressure regulators to preferentially seek oxygen from central as opposed to cylinder supplies 10.1.1 Manually operated single-purpose oxygen flush valves 11.1.1 Single flowmeter knobs for each gas‡ 11.1.4 Oxygen enters the common manifold downstream of other gases 14.1.1 Common gas outlet with standard 15 mm female port to accept connector with coaxial 22-mm male connector designed to prevent accidental disconnection and misconnection 15.1.3 Pipeline inlet fitting shall be diameter-indexed safety system–threaded body fittings	64.3 Each flow control is next to a flow indicator. 64.5 Profile of oxygen flow control knob is physically distinguishable.§ 65.4 Oxygen flow indicator is to the right most extremity of a bank of flow indicators. 76 An auxiliary oxygen flowmeter is strongly recommended. 51.9.3.3 Maximum limited pressure is protected during intended use and single-fault conditions. Various connection requirements were added for patient connection port, exhaust port, reservoir and other ports, Y-piece, and exhaust valve.
Anesthesia vapor delivery system	12.1.8 Vaporizer "lockout" for multiple vaporizers 13.1 Concentration-calibrated vaporizers 12.1.7 Liquid level indicated, designed to prevent overfilling 12.1.8 "Should" use keyed-filling devices	68.8 No discharge of liquid anesthetic occurs from the vaporizer even at maximum fresh gas flow.
Patient monitoring equipment	16.1.2 Oxygen analyzer for "inadequate oxygen percentage"	Greater emphasis on patient monitoring includes: 51.9.4 Exhaled volume 51.10.5 Carbon dioxide 51.11 FiO_2 51.12 Oxygen supply pressure 51.13 Hypoxic guard 51.14 Inhaled agents concentration 51.8.2 Volume, gas concentration, and pressure monitors must be enabled by machine automatically (no separate power switches). 51.15 SaO_2, BP, and ECG (to reflect ASA minimum monitoring guidelines)
Scavenging system	4.1.13 A means to convey surplus gas to a system for its disposal should be provided	Separate standard (integrated with ISO 80601-2-13)
Alarm system	16. 1.1 and 16.1.2 Alarms (auditory/visual; O_2 supply pressure or inadequate oxygen percentage)	51.7 Hierarchical alarm prioritization: high, medium, low 51.8.2.1 Automatic enabling of monitors and alarms
Protection module(s)	Various protection measures (e.g., loss of O_2 pressure)	51.9.3.2 and 51.9.3.3 Maximum pressure limits on ventilator and anesthesia breathing system 51.13.1 Hypoxia prevention system (O_2 >21%)
Other		72 Preoperational checklist must be provided (it may be electronic, or performed manually by the user; developed in conjunction with FDA). 78 Data interface 80 Record keeper

*Z79.8 developed by Writing Group on Gas Machine Safety and Performance, chaired by Leslie Rendell-Baker, MD.

†ISO 80601-2-13 (2011)[28] in the international version, which is harmonized with the third edition of IEC 60601-1; note separate requirements for integrated scavenging systems. Clause numbers from each standard are shown.

‡Parallax error is possible; a rotameter could be read against wrong scale.

§When working in the dark, such as in the x-ray room, the anesthesiologist would often use the sense of touch to determine which knob is the oxgyen control knob.

ANSI, American National Standards Institute; ASA, American Society of Anesthesiologists; ASTM, American Society for Testing and Materials; BP, blood pressure; ECG, electrocardiogram; FDA, Food and Drug Administration; IEC, International Electrotechnical Commission; ISO, International Organization for Standardization.

TABLE 34-9 **Measurement Accuracy of Respiratory Gas Monitors***

	Measurement Accuracy (Volume Fraction)	
Gas	Slope Error (%)	Offset Error (%)
Halogenated agent	15	0.2
Carbon dioxide	8	0.43
Nitrous oxide	8	2.0
Oxygen	2.5	2.5

*Modified from ISO 80601-2-55:2011.

probe cable extender. This standard is not applicable to pulse oximeter equipment intended for use in laboratory research applications or to oximeters that require a blood sample from the patient. The intended use of pulse oximeter equipment includes, but is not limited to, the estimation of arterial oxygen hemoglobin saturation and pulse rate of patients in professional health care institutions and in the home health care environment.

This standard specifies temperature limits at the tissue interface and includes reporting requirements for pulse oximetry (SpO_2) over 70% to 100% with A_{rms}, root-mean-squared difference, and reported and accuracy requirements of functional oxygen saturation as A_{rms} of less than or equal to 4% SpO_2 over the range of 70% to 100%. The accuracy claims are required to be supported by controlled desaturation studies over the full range with appropriate testing during motion and/or low perfusion.[31] An additional requirement for response time and alarm condition delay particular to a rapid desaturation is included. Of interest is a lengthy discussion of the differences between patient simulators of SpO_2, none of which are available; calibrators to test accuracy of the device; and functional testers that provide a simulated input using an artificial finger with light sources modulated to simulate the plethysmographic signals.

Other Standards and Changes

Interoperability

The term *interoperability* as applied to health care often means different things to different people. Various medical device interoperability initiatives are in process.[32] Lesh and colleagues[33] discuss the challenges of interoperability:

> *The concept of interoperability for an increasingly instrumented and computerized healthcare environment is intuitively appealing, but what does this enticing goal entail? From a user's point of view this can be the ability of medical devices and people to interact at multiple levels with seemingly little effort. Underlying this goal is an enormous amount of complexity, because interoperability creates dynamic relationships that must be manageable over time. There are technical, business, regulatory, legal, and administrative relationships that cumulatively create a grand challenge.*[33]

There are more than 101,000 devices that fall into one of 5267 generic device product categories described in 21 C.F.R. Subchapter H, Medical Devices (e.g., an anesthesia machine is described in section 868.5160). The continuum of interoperability based on complexity varies from *physical interoperability*, defined as the ability for one device to connect to or be used with another device and perform individual functions without alteration of the individual device, to data/information exchange with understanding.[30] This understanding requires both a common syntax (messaging standard) and common semantics (terminology). At present, most medical devices are not interoperable for reasons that may include:

- Lack of incentives or regulatory requirements to interoperate with other manufacturers' devices
- Scarcity of accepted medical device interoperability standards
- Slow response of health care sector with respect to computerization and networking
- Liability and regulatory issues[33]

The potential benefits of medical devices that are interoperable include improved quality of care and patient safety, improved clinical decision support, and closed-loop control of therapies such as medication, delivery of fluids, and mechanical ventilation.

For example, Arney and colleagues[34] demonstrate in a use case how automatic synchronization of the x-ray exposure with ventilation eliminates the need to turn off the ventilator to obtain a radiograph and thereby improves patient safety by helping to alleviate those circumstances when an anesthesiologist would turn off the anesthesia ventilator for a radiograph and forget to turn it back on. Cortes and colleagues[35] propose a design on an interoperable, integrated clinical environment (ICE)–compliant system (see below) for patient-controlled analgesia (PCA) infusion pumps using integrated decision support and closed-loop control to detect overmedication using a capnograph and pulse oximeter and to respond to resultant respiratory depression.

Several consortia working on medical device interoperability include the Medical Device Plug-and-Play Program (MD PnP; www.mdpnp.org/home.php), the Continua Health Alliance (www.continuaalliance.org/index.html), and Integrating the Healthcare Enterprise (IHE; www.ihe.net).

The MD PnP is described as a "multidisciplinary, multi-institutional program committed to simplifying and standardizing medical device connectivity in support of improving patient safety and healthcare efficiency."[33] Some of their projects include:

- Medical Device Clock Errors: A study to address this issue (e.g., standards) is important given the general lack of automatic clock setting and time synchronization in medical devices used in the clinical environment and the potential negative impact on the electronic medical record (EMR) and analysis of adverse events.
- ICE Standard: This set of standards allows comprehensive data acquisition for the EMR and the integration of devices to enable real-time decision support, safety interlocks, and closed-loop control through the functions described in a new series of

standards for the "patient-centric integrated clinical environment" (ASTM F2761-2009).

- MD Fire: This project is intended "to promote the awareness and knowledge of medical device interoperability throughout the medical and healthcare community."[36]
- Prototype Health Care Intranet for Improved Health Outcomes: This project was funded by a $10M National Institutes of Health (NIH) Phase II Quantum Grant (2010).
- Medical Device Interface Data Sheets (MDIDS): This project is working to create a reference compendium of medical device interface capabilities and data elements to serve as a reference for SDOs, manufacturers, researchers, and clinical organizations.

Small-Bore Connectors

As explained in the introduction and rationale of ISO 80369-1:2010, in the 1990s, concern grew regarding the proliferation of medical devices fitted with Luer connectors and the reports of patient death or injury arising from misconnections that resulted in the inappropriate delivery of enteral solutions, intrathecal medication, or compressed gases. Advances in modern medicine have led to a significant rise in the number of medical devices connected to patients, including monitoring, diagnostic, and therapeutic devices. Unfortunately, the tubing of many of these medical devices is equipped with the same 6% Luer tapered connector as specified in ISO 594-1:1996 and ISO 594-2:1998. These medical devices perform a variety of similar, but not interchangeable, functions and are connected to a variety of different sites on a patient.

Using compatible connectors in combination with the proximity of several different connections around a single patient makes accidental tubing misconnections inevitable. The consequences of such misconnections vary. Serious and usually fatal misconnections include intravenous (IV) injection of air, IV injection of enteral feeds, and intrathecal injection of vincristine.[37] To solve this problem, new connectors are needed for each functional application that cannot be interconnected with each other or with the traditional Luer connector. A JWG of ISO TC 210 and IEC 62D was formed in 2008 to create and validate new tubing connectors for breathing system ancillary connections; driving gases; enteral, urinary, and cuff-limb inflation; and neuraxial applications, reserving the traditional Luer connector for vascular access and hypodermic syringe applications.

ISO 80369, which pertains to small-bore connectors for liquids and gases in health care applications,[38] is being developed in seven parts; part 1 defines the general requirements for small-bore connectors, and it is all that has been published at this writing. The remaining six parts reflect the division of small-bore connectors by application areas. They include breathing systems and driving-gas applications (part 2), enteral applications (part 3), urethral and urinary applications (part 4), limb cuff inflation applications (part 5), neuraxial applications (part 6), and intravascular or hypodermic applications (part 7, the new Luer standard).

These standards will have a profound impact on the delivery of health care, because many practices and processes will have to change as medical devices begin to incorporate new tubing connectors. Parts 2, 5, and 6 will directly impact the delivery of anesthesia.

Alarm Systems

The ISO TC 121 began the development of standardization is this area with the publication of the ISO 9703 series of standards beginning in 1992. These early standards specified the requirements for alarm signals from anesthetic and respiratory equipment, the beeping sounds and flashing lights found on many medical devices today. The next step in alarm system standardization occurred when a JWG of ISO TC 121/SC3 and IEC 62A created the collateral standard, IEC 60601-1-8:2003, in the IEC 60601-1 family for the alarm systems of all medical electrical equipment.

Despite 20 years of published standards for medical device alarm systems, many problems and challenges remain with alarm systems used on medical devices today. In October of 2011, AAMI co-convened with the FDA, The Joint Commission, ECRI Institute, and American College of Clinical Engineering a summit to explore the issues associated with medical alarm system safety. The summit brought together 300 multidisciplinary stakeholders, and they developed the following seven clarion themes and priority issues:

1. Deepen all stakeholders' understanding of use environments
2. Improve alarm system management
3. Innovate to improve alarm system integration
4. Reconcile challenges and differences in use environments
5. Strengthen medical electrical equipment standards and contracting language to promote success in all intended use environments
6. Clarify regulatory requirements
7. Share illuminating practices and lessons learned with all stakeholders[39]

Acknowledgment

The authors acknowledge Gregory Welyczko of GE Healthcare (retired), Stand Weitzner, MD, and Mark Graber of GE Healthcare for their contributions to the anesthesia equipment standards in Table 34-8.

REFERENCES

1. ISO/IEC Guide 2:2004, Standardization and related activities. General vocabulary. Available at www.iso.org.
2. *Medical device regulations: global overview and guiding principles*, Geneva, Switzerland, 2003, World Health Organization.
3. Elixir Sulfanilmide-Massengill: Report of the United States Secretary of Agriculture, *Cal West Med* 48(1):68–70, 1938.
4. Department of Health and Human Services: *Everything you always wanted to know about the medical device amendments… and weren't afraid to ask*, Publication FDA 84-4173, ed 2, 1984, US DHHS, Public Health Service, FDA Center for Devices and Radiological Health.
5. Anesthesia machine failures: hearing before the Subcommittee on Oversight and Investigations of the Committee on Energy and Commerce, House of Representatives, Ninety-eighth Congress, second session, September 26, 1984.
6. Safe Medical Devices Act of 1990. 21 CFR Part 821, *Federal Register* 57(60), 1992.

7. *Medical devices and the public's health: The FDA 510(k) clearance process at 35 years, Committee on the Public Health Effectiveness of the FDA 510(k) Clearance Process*. 2011, Institute of Medicine.
8. Council of the European Union: Council Directive 93/42/EEC of 14 June 1993 concerning medical devices (OJ No L 169/1 of 1993-07-12).
9. Class II Special Controls Guidance Document: Apnea Monitors; Guidance for Industry and FDA. Issued July 17, 2002, Food and Drug Administration Center for Devices and Radiological Health.
10. Hedley-Whyte J, Milamed DR: Equipment standards: history, litigation, and advice, *Ann Surg* 230(1):120–127, 1999.
11. Guidance for Industry and FDA Staff: Recognition and Use of Consensus Standards. Issued on September 17, 2007, Food and Drug Administration Center for Devices and Radiological Health.
12. CDRH Preliminary Internal Evaluations, Vol I, 510(k) Working Group -Preliminary Report and Recommendations. August 2010, Food and Drug Administration Center for Devices and Radiological Health.
13. Henza C, Hutchin G: Reforming the 510(k) process: where we are, how we got here, and what's to come, *MDDI*, 2012 Jan 5.
14. ISO/IEC Directives. *Part 1: Procedures for the technical work*, ed 8, Geneva, 2011.
15. *Minimum Performance and Safety Requirements for Components and Systems of Continuous-Flow Anesthesia Machines for Human Use, ANSI Z-79.8*, New York, 1979, American National Standards Institute.
16. *NFPA 99: Health Care Facilities Code, 2012 Edition*, Quincy, MA, 2012, National Fire Protection Association.
17. Caplan RA, Barker SJ, Connis RT, et al: Practice advisory for the prevention and management of operating room fires, *Anesthesiology* 108:786–801, 2008.
18. Surgical Fire Prevention Guide, *Health Devices* 38(10):314–332, 2009.
19. IEC 60601-1: 2005. Medical electrical equipment. Part 1: General requirements for basic safety and essential performance, 2005 + Amendment 1, Piscataway, NJ, 2012, IEEE.
20. ISO 14971: 2007. Medical devices. Application of risk management to medical devices, Geneva, 2007.
21. Silberberg JL: Achieving medical device EMC: the role of regulations, standards, guidelines and publications. 2001 IEEE International Symposium on Electromagnetic Compatability. Volume 2, 2001, pp 1298–1303.
22. Meyer JA, Rendell-Baker L: Safety and performance of anesthesia and ventilatory equipment, *Anesthesiology* 32(5):473–474, 1970. (correspondence).
23. Rendell-Baker L: Some gas machine hazards and their elimination, *Anesth Analg* 55(1):26–33, 1976.
24. Richard Imbruce, personal communication, 2005.
25. ANSI: Standard tor humidifiers and nebulizers for medical use, ANSI Z-79.9. 1979, American National Standards Institute.
26. ASTM: *Standard specifications for minimum performance and safety requirements for components and systems of anesthesia gas machines*, ASTM F-1161–88, Philadelphia, 1989, American Society for Testing and Materials.
27. ASTM: *Standard Specification for Particular Requirements for Anesthesia Workstations and Their Components, F1850–00*, Philadelphia, 2005, ASTM.
28. ISO 80601-2-13:2011 Medical electrical equipment. Part 2-13: Particular requirements for basic safety and essential performance of an anaesthetic workstation, ed 1, Geneva, 2011.
29. ISO 80601-2-55:2011 Medical electrical equipment. Part 2-55: Particular requirements for the basic safety and essential performance of respiratory gas monitors, ed 1, Geneva, 2011.
30. ISO 80601-2-61:2011 Medical electrical equipment. Part 2-61: Particular requirements for basic safety and essential performance of pulse oximeter equipment, ed 1, Geneva, 2011.
31. Severinghaus JW, Naifeh KH: Accuracy of response of six pulse oximeters to profound hypoxia, *Anesthesiology* 67:551–558, 1987.
32. Moorman B: Medical device interoperability: overview of key initiatives, *Biomed Instrum Technol* 44(2):132–138, 2010.
33. Lesh K, Weininger S, Goldman JM, Wilson B, Himes G: Medical Device Interoperability-Assessing the Environment High Confidence Medical Devices, Software, and Systems and Medical Device Plug-and-Play Interoperability, *Joint Workshop on Publication Year: 2007*, 3–12, 2007.
34. Arney D, Goldman JM, Insup Lee Llukacej E, Whitehead S: *Use Case Demonstration: X-Ray/Ventilator*, Joint Workshop on High-Confidence Medical Devices, Software, and Systems and Medical Device Plug-and-Play Interoperability. 160, 2007.
35. Cortes PA, Krishnan SM: Insup Lee Goldman JM: Improving the Safety of Patient-Controlled Analgesia Infusions with Safety Interlocks and Closed-Loop Control High Confidence Medical Devices, Software, and Systems and Medical Device Plug-and-Play Interoperability, *Joint Workshop on Publication Year:2007*, 149–150, 2007.
36. MD FIRE Contracting Language: Medical Device Free Interoperability Requirements for the Enterprise, August 2012. Available at www.mdpnp.org/uploads/MD_FIRE?August_2012_v2.0.pdf.
37. Joint Commission on Accreditation of Healthcare Organizations: Sentinel event alert: tubing misconnections—a persistent and potentially deadly occurrence. 2006 Apr 3;36. Accessed online at http://www.jointcommission.org/SentinelEvents/SentinelEventAlert.
38. ISO 80369-1. Small-bore connectors for liquids and gases in healthcare applications, Geneva, 2010.
39. AAMI: *A Siren Call to Action: Priority Issues from the Medical Device Alarms Summit*, 2011, AAMI. Accessed online at http://www.aami.org/publications/summits/2011_Alarms_Summit_publication.pdf.

INDEX

A

Page numbers followed by *f* refer to figures, *t* refer to tables, and *b* refer to boxes.

C

D

F

G

H

I

J

M

N

O

P

Q

R

S

T

W

X

Y

Z